BRADY

PARAMEDIC EMERGENCY CARE

THIRD EDITION

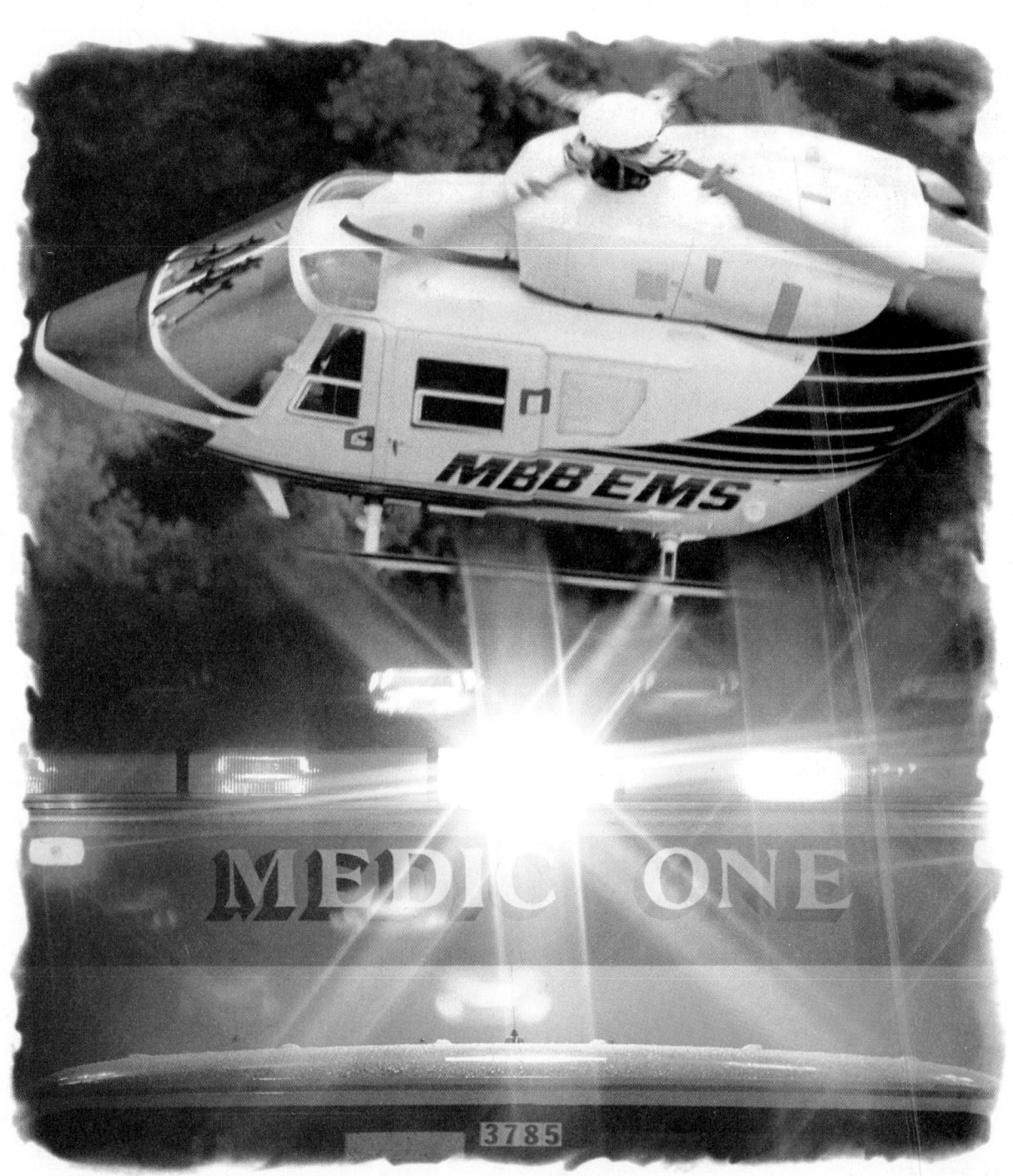

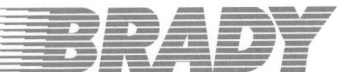

PARAMEDIC EMERGENCY CARE

THIRD EDITION

Bryan E. Bledsoe, D.O., EMT-P

Medical Director, Emergency Department
Baylor Medical Center—Ellis County
Waxahachie, Texas
and
Clinical Associate Professor of Emergency Medicine
University of North Texas Health Sciences Center
Fort Worth, Texas

Robert S. Porter, M.A., NREMT-P

Flight Paramedic
Air One, Onondaga County Sheriff's Department
Syracuse, New York

Bruce R. Shade, EMT-P

Commissioner, Cleveland Emergency Medical Services
Cleveland, Ohio

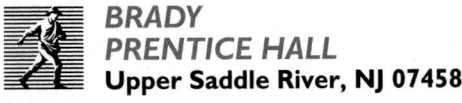

BRADY
PRENTICE HALL
Upper Saddle River, NJ 07458

Library of Congress Cataloging-in-Publication Data
Bledsoe, Bryan E., *(date)*
    Paramedic emergency care / Bryan E. Bledsoe, Robert S. Porter, Bruce R.
Shade; with contributions from Richard A. Cherry . . . [et al.]. — 3rd ed.
        p. cm.
    Rev. ed. of: Brady paramedic emergency care. 2nd ed. c1994.
    Includes bibliographical references and index.
    ISBN 0-8359-4987-7 (case)
        1. Medical emergencies. 2. Emergency medical personnel.
I. Porter, Robert S.   II. Shade, Bruce R.   III. Bledsoe, Bryan E. Brady
paramedic emergency care. IV. Title.
        [DNLM: 1. Emergency Medical Services—methods. 2. Emergency
Medical Technicians.   WX 215 B46p 1997]
RC86.7.B596   1997
616.02′5—dc20
DNLM/DLC   96–19776
for Library of Congress   CIP

Publisher: Susan Katz
Marketing manager: Judy Streger
Managing development editor: Lois Berlowitz
Development editors: Deborah Parks, Sandra Breuer
Managing production editor: Patrick Walsh
Editorial/production supervision: Julie Boddorf
Interior design: Linda J. Den Heyer Rosa/Laura Ierardi
Cover design: Bruce Kenselaar
Cover photography: Helicopter: ©George Hall/Check Six;
    Ambulance: ©Walter Hodges/Westlight
Managing photography editor: Michal Heron
Assistant photography editor: Baylen Leonard
Interior photographers: George Dodson, Michal Heron,
    Richard Logan
Page makeup: Laura Ierardi
Formatters: Julie Boddorf, Dean Fiorino, Freddy Flake,
    Suzanne Graziano, Stephen Hartner, Adele Kupchik,
    Mark LaSalle, Ken Liao, Lorraine Patsco, Gary J. Sella
Senior production manager: Ilene Sanford

© 1997, 1994, 1991 by Prentice-Hall Inc.
A Simon & Schuster Company
Upper Saddle River, New Jersey 07458

Printed in the United States of America

10 9 8 7 6 5 4 3 2

ISBN 0-8359-4987-7

Prentice Hall International (UK) Limited, *London*
Prentice Hall of Australia Pty. Limited, *Sydney*
Prentice Hall Canada Inc., *Toronto*
Prentice Hall Hispanoamericana, S.A., *Mexico*
Prentice Hall of India Private Limited, *New Delhi*
Prentice Hall of Japan, Inc., *Tokyo*
Simon & Schuster Asia Pte. Ltd., *Singapore*
Editora Prentice Hall do Brasil, Ltda., *Rio de Janeiro*

Art Acknowledgments:

Network Graphics, Hauppauge, New York

Rolin Graphics, Plymouth, Minnesota

Appendix illustrations redrafted with permission of Ciba-Geigy.

Photo Acknowledgments:

The following individuals and institutions graciously provided
photographs for use in **Paramedic Emergency Care**:

Center for Emergency Medicine, Pittsburgh, Pennsylvania:
    Figures 1-5, 5-8, 5-11, 5-12, 10-19, 14-1, 14-17, opening
    photos for Chapters 5, 9, 19, 23, 25, 26.
Thomas W. McCarthy, Chicago Fire Department: Figures 1-6,
    14-2, opening photos for Chapters 7, 8.
District of Columbia Fire Department EMS: Opening photos
    for Chapters 13, 16, 21.
Jack Jordan, Phoenix Fire Department: Figures 6-4, 6-5, 6-6,
    6-7, opening photos for Chapters 2, 10, 14, 15.
Doug Key, MedStar: Figures 2-14, 3-1, 14-18, 27-2, opening
    photo for Chapter 27.
Bob Porter: Figures 5-13, 14-8, 14-9, 14-14, 14-16, 19-6, 19-7,
    27-3, opening photo for Chapter 28.
Bryan Bledsoe, D.O.: Figures 5-1, 5-4, 5-6, 17-5, 17-6, 20-17,
    opening photos for Chapters 12, 17, 20.
MIEMSS: Figure 2-11, opening photo for Chapter 3.
Charles C. Freeman, Pinellas County EMS: Opening photo for
    Chapter 4.
Rod Dennison: Figures 5-5, 5-7, 5-9.
Bruce Turney, Milwaukie, Oregon: Figure 5-10.
Ohmeda: Figure 11-11.
Nelcor, Inc.: Figures 11-12, 11-13, 11-39.
Pace Tech, Inc.: Figure 11-14.
Watson P. Roye, M.D.: Figure 11-38.
Ron Stewart, M.D.: Figure 11-47.
Matrx: Figure 11-76.
Scott and White Memorial Hospital: Figures 14-28, 18-2, 18-3,
    18-4, 18-5, 18-8, 18-9, 18-10, 18-11, 18-15, 18-17, 18-18, 18-19,
    18-20, 26-3, 26-4, 30-10, 30-11, 30-12, opening photo for
    Chapter 10.
Ken Phillips, D.O.: Figures 18-21, 18-22.
David Zehr, M.D.: Figure 18-23.
Baptist Hospital, San Antonio, Texas: Opening photo for
    Chapter 24.
Fred Koenig, Bell Helicopter: Opening photo for Chapter 31.
Harriette Hartigan, ARTEMIS, 14 Short Trail, Hartford, CT 06903:
    Figures 32-10, 32-17, 32-21, opening photo for Chapter 32.
Pool/Gamma Liaison: Opening photo for Chapter 6, Figure 6-1e
Allan Tannenbaum/Sygma: Figure 6-1a.
Lisa Quinones/Black Star: Figure 6-1b.
Porter Gifford/Gamma Liaison: Figure 6-1c.
Sygma: Figure 6-1d.
William Philpot/Sygma: Figure 6-1f.
Robert J. Bennett: Figures 10-2, 10-3.
Nite-Light Photo/Glen Jackson: Figure 10-10.
Mark C. Ide: Opening photo for Chapter 11.

SPECIAL NOTES

To my wife Emma, my son Bryan, and my daughter Andrea. They remain my biggest supporters. They help me weave this life of medicine, writing, and family into a package which has somehow worked for over 17 years. They are indeed the inspiration and love of my life.

B.E.B

To my students, who have taught me much more about prehospital emergency care and education than I have ever taught them.

R.S.P.

This book is dedicated to all the EMS providers, educators, and administrators working to make the delivery of prehospital care a true profession.

B.R.S.

PARAMEDIC EMERGENCY CARE
THIRD EDITION

A complete package for Paramedic students and instructors

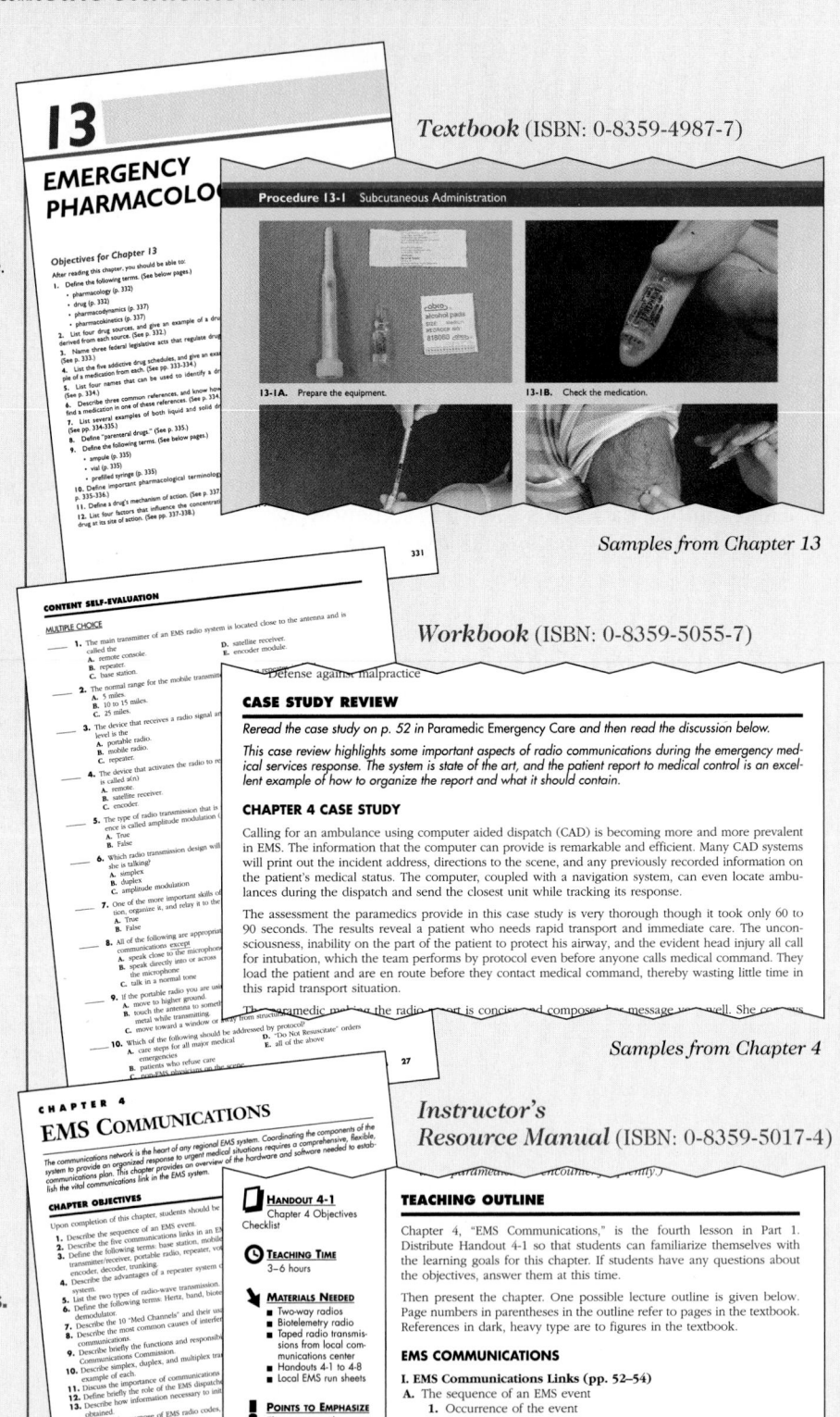

Textbook (ISBN: 0-8359-4987-7)

Samples from Chapter 13

Workbook (ISBN: 0-8359-5055-7)

Samples from Chapter 4

Instructor's Resource Manual (ISBN: 0-8359-5017-4)

Samples from Chapter 4

Contents

I. PREHOSPITAL ENVIRONMENT.

1. Roles and Responsibilities of the Paramedic.
2. Emergency Medical Service Systems.
3. Medical-Legal Considerations of Emergency Care.
4. EMS Communications.
5. Rescue Operations.
6. Major Incident Response.
7. Stress Management in Emergency Services.

II. PREPARATORY INFORMATION.

8. Medical Terminology.
9. Anatomy and Physiology.
10. Comprehensive Patient Assessment.
11. Airway Management and Ventilation.
12. Pathophysiology of Shock.
13. Emergency Pharmacology.

III. TRAUMA EMERGENCIES.

14. The Kinetics of Trauma.
15. Head, Neck, and Spine Trauma.
16. Body Cavity Trauma.
17. Musculoskeletal Injuries.
18. Soft-Tissue Trauma and Burns.
19. Shock Trauma Resuscitation.

IV. MEDICAL EMERGENCIES.

20. Respiratory Emergencies.
21. Cardiovascular Emergencies.
22. Endocrine and Metabolic Emergencies.
23. Nervous System Emergencies.
24. Gastrointestinal, Genitourinary, and Reproductive System Emergencies.
25. Anaphylaxis.
26. Toxicology and Substance Abuse.
27. Infectious Diseases.
28. Environmental Emergencies.
29. Emergencies in the Elderly Patient.
30. Pediatric Emergencies.

V. OBSTETRICAL AND GYNECOLOGICAL EMERGENCIES.

31. Gynecological Emergencies.
32. Obstetrical Emergencies.
33. Emergency Management of the Neonate.

VI. PSYCHIATRIC EMERGENCIES.

34. Behavioral and Psychiatric Emergencies.

Appendix: 12 Lead ECG Monitoring and Interpretation.
Glossary.
Index.

Textbook

(©1997, 1136 pp., case cover, ISBN: 0-8359-4987-7)

The Third Edition retains your favorite features from the previous editions, including...

- Margin glossary and key concepts
- A case study at the beginning of each chapter
- Glossary at the end of the book
- Objectives listed at the start of each chapter with page references where content is covered.

New to this edition...

- Revised and expanded chapters, including...

  Major Incident Response includes information on METTAG as well as the START system

  Advanced Patient Assessment features *Pop Out* study aids, use of mnemonics such as AMPLE questions and OPQRST questions, body substance isolation, more on mechanisms of injury assessment, new segment on ongoing assessment, new management segment with primary assessment section

  Advanced Airway presents additional information on trauma intubation

  Shock offers a new feature called *Understanding Chemical Notation* and revised information on Fluids, Electrolytes, Acid-Base Balance with new pH scale table

  Pharmacology completely updated and expanded—new information on side effects, pediatric dosages, and an alphabetical index to drugs

  Anaphylaxis entirely rewritten and updated.

- New cardiovascular appendix includes information on 12 Lead ECG
- New photo summaries (scan sheets) of key procedures
- Expanded Index.

Workbook (ISBN: 0-8359-5055-7)

The workbook includes test-taking tips. Each chapter features...

- Review of Chapter Objectives
- Multiple-choice, matching, labeling, and sequencing questions
- Case Study Reviews that discuss case studies in the text
- Worksheets and crossword puzzles
- Division Reviews at the end of each division are built around scenarios with multiple-choice questions
- National Registry Skill Sheets
- Answer key with page references where answers can be found or supported
- Emergency Drug Cards
- Patient Care Scenario Cards displaying signs and symptoms on one side and assessment and treatment on the other.

CONTENTS OVERVIEW

PART 1

Prehospital Environment

1 ROLES AND RESPONSIBILITIES OF THE PARAMEDIC
Richard A. Cherry   2
2 EMERGENCY MEDICAL SERVICE SYSTEMS
Richard A. Cherry   16
3 MEDICAL-LEGAL CONSIDERATIONS OF EMERGENCY
CARE   Bryan E. Bledsoe, D.O.   38
4 EMS COMMUNICATIONS   Bryan E. Bledsoe, D.O.   50
5 RESCUE OPERATIONS   Rod Dennison   68
6 MAJOR INCIDENT RESPONSE   Gary P. Morris and Paul
Maniscalco   86
7 STRESS MANAGEMENT IN EMERGENCY SERVICES
Bryan E. Bledsoe, D.O.   110

PART 2

Preparatory Information

8 MEDICAL TERMINOLOGY   Bryan E. Bledsoe, D.O.   122
9 ANATOMY AND PHYSIOLOGY
Bryan E. Bledsoe, D.O.   140
10 COMPREHENSIVE PATIENT ASSESSMENT
Robert S. Porter   164
11 AIRWAY MANAGEMENT AND VENTILATION   Bryan E.
Bledsoe, D.O. and
Bruce R. Shade   204
12 PATHOPHYSIOLOGY OF SHOCK   Bruce R. Shade and
Bryan E. Bledsoe, D.O.   284
13 EMERGENCY PHARMACOLOGY
Bryan E. Bledsoe, D.O.   330

PART 3

Trauma Emergencies

14 THE KINETICS OF TRAUMA   Robert S. Porter   400
15 HEAD, NECK, AND SPINE INJURY   Robert S. Porter   432
16 BODY CAVITY TRAUMA   Robert S. Porter   468
17 MUSCULOSKELETAL INJURIES   Robert S. Porter   498
18 SOFT-TISSUE TRAUMA AND BURNS   Robert S. Porter   520
19 SHOCK TRAUMA RESUSCITATION   Robert S. Porter   552

PART 4

Medical Emergencies

20 RESPIRATORY EMERGENCIES
Bryan E. Bledsoe, D.O.   570
21 CARDIOVASCULAR EMERGENCIES
Bryan E. Bledsoe, D.O.   600
22 ENDOCRINE AND METABOLIC EMERGENCIES
Bryan E. Bledsoe, D.O.   724
23 NERVOUS SYSTEM EMERGENCIES
Bryan E. Bledsoe, D.O.   738
24 GASTROINTESTINAL, GENITOURINARY, AND
REPRODUCTIVE SYSTEM EMERGENCIES
Bryan E. Bledsoe, D.O.   768
25 ANAPHYLAXIS   Bryan E. Bledsoe, D.O.   792
26 TOXICOLOGY AND SUBSTANCE ABUSE
Bryan E. Bledsoe, D.O. and Dexter W. Hunt   804
27 INFECTIOUS DISEASES   Bryan E. Bledsoe, D.O.   838
28 ENVIRONMENTAL EMERGENCIES
Bryan E. Bledsoe, D.O.   862
29 EMERGENCIES IN THE ELDERLY PATIENT
Bryan E. Bledsoe, D.O.   892
30 PEDIATRIC EMERGENCIES   Bryan E. Bledsoe, D.O.   910

PART 5

Obstetrical and Gynecological Emergencies

31 GYNECOLOGICAL EMERGENCIES
Bryan E. Bledsoe, D.O.   952
32 OBSTETRICAL EMERGENCIES
Bryan E. Bledsoe, D.O.   964
33 EMERGENCY MANAGEMENT OF THE NEONATE
Bryan E. Bledsoe, D.O.   994

PART 6

Psychiatric Emergencies

34 BEHAVIORAL AND PSYCHIATRIC EMERGENCIES
Bryan E. Bledsoe, D.O.   1012

APPENDIX

12 Lead ECG Monitoring and Interpretation   1031

CONTENTS

PREFACE *xxi*

ACKNOWLEDGMENTS *xxiii*

ABOUT THE AUTHORS *xxvii*

NOTICES *xxix*

PRECAUTIONS ON BLOODBORNE PATHOGENS AND INFECTIOUS DISEASES *xxx*

PART I

Prehospital Environment

1 ROLES AND RESPONSIBILITIES OF THE PARAMEDIC *Richard A. Cherry 2*

Objectives   3
Case Study   4
Introduction   4
Changes in the Field   5
Professional Ethics   6
Professionalism   9
Role of the Paramedic   10
Post-Graduate Responsibilities   12
   Continuing Education   13
   Professional Organizations   13
   National Registry   14
   Professional Journals   14
Summary   14
Further Reading   15

2 EMERGENCY MEDICAL SERVICES SYSTEMS *Richard A. Cherry 16*

Objectives   17
Case Study   18
Introduction   18
The History of the EMS System Development   20
The Systems Approach   21
   System Administration   21
   Medical Control   22
   Public Information and Education   24

   EMS Communications   25
   Emergency Medical Dispatching   26
   Education and Certification   28
   Patient Transportation   29
   Quality Assurance and Quality Improvement   32
   Research   34
   Receiving Facilities   34
   Mutual Aid/Mass-Casualty Preparation   36
   System Financing   36
Summary   36
Further Reading   37

3 MEDICAL-LEGAL CONSIDERATIONS OF EMERGENCY CARE *Bryan E. Bledsoe, D.O. 38*

Objectives   39
Case Study   40
Introduction   40
Legal Principles   41
Laws Affecting EMS   41
   Medical Practice Acts and State EMS Legislation   41
   Right to Die   42
Standard of Care   44
   Negligence and Medical Liability   44
   Areas of Potential Medical Liability   45
   Problem Patients   47
Medical Liability Protection   47
Summary   48
Further Reading   49

4 EMS COMMUNICATIONS *Bryan E. Bledsoe, D.O. 50*

Objectives   51
Case Study   52
Introduction   52
EMS Communication Links   52
Communications Systems: Technical Aspects   54
   Base Station   54
   Mobile Two-Way Radios   55
   Portable Radios   55
   Repeater Systems   55
   Remote Consoles   56
   Satellite Receivers   56
   Encoders and Decoders   56
   Mobile Telephones   57

Radio Communications 58
  Frequencies 58
  Biotelemetry 59
  Transmission Types 60
Equipment Maintenance 61
Rules and Operating Procedures 61
  Dispatch Procedures 61
  Radio Codes 63
  Radio Communications Techniques 63
Communication of Medical Information 64
  General Concepts 65
  Communication of Patient Information by the Paramedic 65
  Biotelemetry 66
  Written Communications 66
Summary 66
Further Reading 67

5 RESCUE OPERATIONS Rod Dennison **68**
Objectives 69
Case Study 70
Introduction 70
Safety 70
  Personal Safety 70
  Patient Safety 72
  Safety Procedures 73
The Rescue Operation 74
  Assessment 74
  Gaining Access 76
  On-Scene Emergency Care 78
  Disentanglement and Removal 80
  Transportation 82
Rescue Resources 82
Summary 84
Further Reading 85

6 MAJOR INCIDENT RESPONSE
Gary P. Morris and Paul Maniscalco **86**
Objectives 87
Case Study 88
Introduction 88
The Prehospital Emergency Response 88
Benefits of the Incident Command System 90
  Organization of Command 91
  Organization of Sectors 91
Operation of the Incident Command System 93
  The Incident Commander 93
  Transfer of Command 96
  Extrication Sector 97
  Treatment Sector 98
  Transportation Sector 99
  Staging Sector 101
  Supply Sector 102
  Triage Sector 102
  Communications 105
Plans, Procedures, and Equipment 107
Inter-Community and Inter-Agency Planning 107
Incident Duties 107
Essential Items 108
Summary 109
Further Reading 109

**7 STRESS MANAGEMENT IN EMERGENCY
SERVICES** Bryan E. Bledsoe, D.O. **110**
Objectives 111
Case Study 112
Introduction 112
Stress 112
  Physiology of Stress 113
  The Body's Response to Stress 113
  Types of Stress Reactions 113
Anxiety 116
  Normal Anxiety Levels 116
  Detrimental Anxiety Levels 116
Paramedic Job Stress 117
  Managing EMS Job Stress 118
  Dealing With Critical Incident Stress 119
  Critical Incident Stress Debriefings 120
Death and Dying 120
  Grief Process 120
  Management of the Dead or Dying Patient 121
Summary 121
Further Reading 121

PART 2

Preparatory Information

8 MEDICAL TERMINOLOGY
Bryan E. Bledsoe, D.O. **122**
Objectives 123
Case Study 124
Introduction 124
Medical Dictionary 125
Medical Terminology 125
  Root Words 125
  Prefixes and Suffixes 130
Abbreviations 134
Summary 139
Further Reading 139

9 ANATOMY AND PHYSIOLOGY
Bryan E. Bledsoe, D.O. **140**
Objectives 141
Case Study 142
Introduction 142
Structure 143
  The Cell 143
  Tissues 144
  Organs 144
  Organ Systems 145
  Organism 146
Topographical Anatomy 159
  Anatomic Terms 159
  Topographical Anatomy of the Chest 160
  Topographical Anatomy of the Abdomen 161
Body Cavities 162
Summary 163
Further Reading 163

10 COMPREHENSIVE PATIENT ASSESSMENT
Robert S. Porter 164

Objectives 165
Case Study 166
Introduction 166
Phases of Prehospital Assessment 166
Scene Size-up 167
   Review Dispatch Information 167
   Survey the Scene 167
   Identify Potential Hazards 168
   Body Substance Isolation 168
   Secure the Scene 168
   Determine the Mechanism of Injury or the
      Nature of the Illness 168
   Locate Patients 169
Primary Assessment 170
   Airway and Breathing 170
   Circulation 172
   Disability 173
   Expose 173
   Critical Management Priorities 174
Secondary Assessment 175
   Examining the Trauma Patient 176
   Examining the Medical Patient 176
   Techniques for Conducting the Physical Exam 177
Head-to-Toe Evaluation 178
   Head 178
   Facial Region 182
   Neck 184
   Chest 185
   Abdomen 187
   Genitalia 188
   Lower Extremities 188
   Upper Extremities 189
   Posterior Body 189
   Analysis of the Head-to-Toe Evaluation 189
   Neurological Assessment 189
Vital Signs 191
   Blood Pressure 191
   Pulse 192
   Respiration 192
   Body Temperature 192
   Other Assessment Techniques 194
Patient History 196
   Questioning Techniques 196
   The Chief Complaint 196
   Circumstances of the Present Illness or Injury 197
   Past Medical History 198
Ongoing Assessment 200
Communication and Documentation 200
   Radio/Phone Communication 200
   Emergency Department Arrival 201
   Documentation 201
Summary 202
Further Reading 203

**11 AIRWAY MANAGEMENT
AND VENTILIATION** *Bryan E. Bledsoe, D.O.
and Bruce R. Shade 204*

Objectives 205
Case Study 206
Introduction 206

Anatomy of the Respiratory System 206
   Anatomy of the Upper Airway 207
   Anatomy of the Lower Airway 210
Physiology of the Respiratory System 212
   Respiration and Ventilation 212
   Respiratory Cycle 212
   Pulmonary Circulation 212
   Gas Exchange in the Lungs 213
   Regulation of Respiration 215
   Modified Forms of Respiration 216
   Measures of Respiratory Function 217
Respiratory Problems 217
   Airway Obstruction 218
   Inadequate Ventilation 220
Assessment of the Respiratory System 220
   Primary Assessment 220
   Secondary Assessment 221
Basic Airway Management 225
   Manual Airway Manuevers 226
   Basic Mechanical Airways 228
Advanced Airway Management 232
   Esophageal Obturator Airways 232
   Esophageal Gastric Tube Airway 236
   Endotracheal Intubation 236
   Pharyneo-Tracheal Lumen Airway 265
   Esophageal Tracheal Combitube (ETC) Airway 267
   Surgical Airways 269
Suctioning 275
   Equipment for Suctioning 275
   Techniques for Suctioning 276
Oxygenation 276
   Oxygen Administration 277
   Oxygen Devices 277
Ventilation 279
   Mouth-to-Mouth/Mouth-to-Nose 279
   Pocket Mask 279
   Bag-Valve Devices 280
   Demand Valve 280
   Automatic Ventilators 281
Summary 282
Further Reading 283

12 PATHOPHYSIOLOGY OF SHOCK
Bruce R. Shade and Bryan E. Bledsoe, D.O. 284

Objectives 285
Case Study 286
Introduction 286
Fluid and Electrolytes 287
   Water 287
   Hydration 288
   Electrolytes 289
   Osmosis and Diffusion 292
   Intravenous Therapy 294
Acid-Base Balance 299
   The pH Scale 299
   Bodily Regulation of Acid-Base Balance 299
   Acid-Base Derangements 302
Physiological Background to Shock 303
   Physiology of Perfusion 304
   Oxygen Transport 307
   Tissue Perfusion 307

Physiological Responses to Shock   308
  Systemic Response to Shock   308
  Shock at the Cellular Level   308
  Stages of Shock   309
Types of Shock   310
  Hypovolemic Shock   310
  Cardiogenic Shock   311
  Neurogenic Shock   311
Evaluation of the Shock Victim   311
  Primary Assessment   312
  Secondary Assessment   314
General Management of Shock   315
  Maintaining a Patent Airway   315
  Maintaining Adequate Respiratory Function   316
  Oxygenation of the Patient   317
  Control of Major Bleeding   317
  Managing Hypotension   317
  Maintaining Body Temperature   328
  Use of Medications in the Treatment of Shock   328
Rapid Packaging and Transport   329
Summary   329
Further Reading   329

13 EMERGENCY PHARMACOLOGY
Bryan E. Bledsoe, D.O.   330

Objectives   331
Case Study   332
Introduction   332
Basic Pharmacological Background   332
  Drug Sources   332
  Drug Laws   333
  Drug Names   334
  Drug References   334
  Drug Forms   334
  Pharmacological Terminology   335
  Studying Medications   336
Actions of Drugs   337
  Pharmacokinetics   337
  Pharmacodynamics   339
The Autonomic Nervous System   340
  Basic Anatomy and Physiology   340
  The Sympathetic Nervous System   341
  Adrenergic Receptors   344
  The Parasympathetic Nervous System   345
Administration of Drugs   348
  Weights and Measures   348
  Medication Administration Routes   352
Drugs Used in Prehospital Care   360
  Drugs Used in Cardiovascular Emergencies   361
  Drugs Used in the Treatment of Respiratory
    Emergencies   384
  Drugs Used in the Treatment of Endocrine and
    Metabolic Emergencies   389
  Drugs Used in the Treatment of Neurological
    Emergencies   391
  Drugs Used in the Treatment of Obstetrical and
    Gynecological Emergencies   393
  Drugs Used in the Management of Toxicological
    Emergencies   394
  Drugs Used in the Management of Behavioral
    Emergencies   398
  Other Medications   398

Summary   399
Further Reading   399

PART 3

Trauma Emergencies

14 THE KINETICS OF TRAUMA
Robert S. Porter   400

Objectives   401
Case Study   402
Introduction   402
Trauma Triage Protocols   403
  Mechanism of Injury   403
  Index of Suspicion   404
  The Golden Hour   404
  Decision to Transport   404
Kinetics of Trauma   406
  Inertia   406
  Conservation of Energy   406
  Kinetic Energy   406
  Force   407
Kinds of Trauma   407
Blunt Trauma   408
  Automobile Accidents   408
  Motorcycle Accidents   419
  Pedestrian Accidents   420
  Recreational Vehicle Accidents   421
  Other Blunt Trauma   422
Penetrating Trauma   425
  Ballistics   426
  Pathologies of Penetrating Trauma   429
Summary   431
Further Reading   431

15 HEAD, NECK, AND SPINE INJURY
Robert S. Porter   432

Objectives   433
Case Study   434
Introduction   434
Anatomy and Physiology   435
  Central Nervous System Protection   435
  The Central Nervous System   439
  Special Sense Organs   442
  The Neck   443
Head, Neck, and Spinal Trauma   444
  Superficial Injury   444
  Internal CNS Injury   447
  Sense Organ Injury   452
  Neck Injury   453
Assessment   453
  Primary Assessment   454
  Secondary Assessment   456
Management   460
  Immediate Spinal Immobilization   460
  Oxygen and Hyperventilation   460
  Endotracheal Intubation   461
  Hemorrhage Control/Shock Care   462
  Spinal Immobilization   462

    Wound Care   464
    Drug Therapy   466
Summary   467
Further Reading   467

16 BODY CAVITY TRAUMA   Robert S. Porter   468

Objectives   469
Case Study   470
Introduction   470
Anatomy and Physiology   471
    The Thorax   471
    The Abdomen   474
    The Pelvic Cavity   475
Body Cavity Injuries   475
    Chest Injuries   476
    Abdominal Injury   481
    Genitalia Injury   482
Assessment   482
    Mechanism of Injury   482
    Primary Assessment   483
    Secondary Assessment   485
Management   489
    Thoracic Trauma Care   490
    Abdominal Trauma Care   495
Summary   496
Further Reading   497

17 MUSCULOSKELETAL INJURIES
Robert S. Porter   498

Objectives   499
Case Study   500
Introduction   500
Anatomy and Physiology   501
    The Skeleton   501
    The Muscular System   505
Pathophysiology   506
    Muscular Injury   506
    Joint Injury   507
    Fractures   508
    General Musculoskeletal Considerations   510
    Specific Musculoskeletal Considerations   510
Assessment   513
    Primary Assessment   513
    Secondary Assessment   513
Management   515
    Immediate Transport   515
    On-Scene Care   516
Summary   519
Further Reading   519

18 SOFT-TISSUE TRAUMA AND BURNS
Robert S. Porter   520

Objectives   521
Case Study   522
Introduction   522
Overview of Soft-Tissue Injuries   523
Anatomy and Physiology of the Skin   523
    Layers of Skin   523
    Blood Vessels   524
    Functions of the Skin   525

Pathophysiology of Soft-Tissue Injury   525
    Wounds   525
    Hemorrhage   528
    Burns   528
Assessment of Soft-Tissue Injury   538
    Wounds   538
    Thermal Burns   539
    Chemical Injuries   542
    Electrical Injuries   543
    Radiation Exposure   543
Management of Soft-Tissue Injury   543
    Wounds   544
    Burns   548
Summary   551
Further Reading   551

19 SHOCK TRAUMA RESUSCITATION
Robert S. Porter   552

Objectives   553
Case Study   554
Introduction   554
Trauma Management   554
Anatomy and Physiology of the Cardiovascular
    System   556
Pathophysiology   557
    Compensated Shock   557
    Decompenstated Shock   558
    Irreversible Shock   559
Assessment   559
    Review of Dispatch Information   560
    Survey of the Scene   560
    Primary Assessment   560
    Decision to Transport   563
    Trauma Score   564
Shock/Trauma Resuscitation   564
    Correction of Critical Life Threats   564
    Application of the PASG   565
    Fluid Therapy   566
Air Medical Transport   567
Summary   569
Further Reading   569

PART 4

Medical Emergencies

20 RESPIRATORY EMERGENCIES
Bryan E. Bledsoe, D.O.   570

Objectives   571
Case Study   572
Introduction   572
Review of Respiratory Anatomy and
    Physiology   572
Assessment of the Respiratory System   575
    History   575
    Physical Examination   575
    Pulse Oximetry   580

Pathophysiology and Management of Respiratory
    Disorders   581
  Management Principles of Respiratory Emergencies   581
  Upper-Airway Obstruction   581
  Obstructive Lung Disease   583
  Asthma   586
  Pneumonia   594
  Toxic Inhalation   595
  Carbon Monoxide Inhalation   596
  Pulmonary Embolism   597
  Hyperventilation Syndrome   597
  Central Nervous System Dysfunction   598
  Dysfunction of the Spinal Cord, Nerves, or
      Respiratory Muscles   598
Summary   599
Further Reading   599

21   CARDIOVASCULAR EMERGENCIES
Bryan E. Bledsoe, D.O.   600

Objectives   601
Case Study   602
Introduction   602
Anatomy and Physiology   602
  Anatomy of the Heart   603
  Anatomy of Peripheral Circulation   607
  Physiology of Circulation   609
  Nervous Control of the Heart   610
  Role of Electrolytes   612
  Electrophysiology   612
Recognition of Dysrhythmias   616
  Introduction to ECG Monitoring   616
  Interpretation of Rhythm Strips   625
  Introduction to Dysrhythmias   627
Dysrhythmias Originating in the SA Node   630
  Sinus Bradycardia   631
  Sinus Tachycardia   633
  Sinus Dysrhythmia   635
  Sinus Arrest   637
Dysrhythmias Originating in the Atria   638
  Wandering Pacemaker   639
  Premature Atrial Contractions   641
  Paroxysmal Supraventricular Tachycardia   643
  Atrial Flutter   647
  Atrial Fibrillation   649
Dysrhythmias Originating in the AV Junction   652
  Premature Junctional Contractions   653
  Junctional Rhythm   655
  Accelerated Junctional Rhythm   657
  Paroxysmal Junctional Tachycardia   658
Dysrhythmias Originating in the Ventricles   660
  Ventricular Escape Complexes and Rhythms   661
  Premature Ventricular Contractions   662
  Ventricular Tachycardia   665
  Ventricular Fibrillation   669
  Asystole   671
  Artificial Pacemaker Rhythm   672
Dysrhythmias That Are Disorders of Conduction
    674
  AV Blocks   675
  First-Degree AV Block   675
  Second-Degree AV Block (Mobitz I) Wenckebach   677

  Second-Degree AV Block (Mobitz II)   679
  Third-Degree AV Block   681
  Disturbances of Ventricular Conduction   682
  Pre-excitation Syndromes   682
Assessment of the Cardiac Patient   683
  Common Chief Complaints and Symptoms   683
  Significant Past Medical History   685
  Physical Examination   685
Pathophysiology of Cardiovascular Disease   688
  Atherosclerosis   688
  Left Ventricular Failure With Pulmonary Edema   694
  Right Ventricular Failure   697
  Cardiogenic Shock   699
  Cardiac Arrest/Suddent Death   701
  Peripheral Vascular and Other Cardiovascular
      Emergencies   704
  Hypertensive Emergency   709
Management of Cardiovascular Emergencies   709
  Drugs Used in Cardiovascular Emergencies   710
  Management Techniques   712
Summary   721
Further Reading   723

22   ENDOCRINE AND METABOLIC
EMERGENCIES   *Bryan E. Bledsoe, D.O.*   724

Objectives   725
Case Study   726
Introduction   726
Anatomy and Physiology   726
  Pituitary   726
  Thyroid Gland   728
  Parathyroid Gland   728
  Pancreas   729
  Adrenal Glands   729
  Gonads   730
Endocrine Emergencies   730
  Diabetes Mellitus   730
  Diabetic Ketoacidosis (Diabetic Coma)   732
  Hypoglycemia (Insulin Shock)   733
Summary   736
Further Reading   737

23   NERVOUS SYSTEM EMERGENCIES
Bryan E. Bledsoe, D.O.   738

Objectives   739
Case Study   740
Introduction   740
Anatomy and Physiology   740
  Anatomy and Physiology of the Central Nervous
      System   741
  Anatomy and Physiology of the Peripheral Nervous
      System   747
Assessment of the Neurological System   749
  Primary Assessment   749
  Secondary Assessment   749
Nervous System Emergencies   754
  Altered Mental Status   754
  Seizures   760

Status Epilepticus 763
Stroke (Cerebrovascular Accident) 763
Summary 767
Further Reading 767

24 GASTROINTESTINAL, GENITOURINARY, AND REPRODUCTIVE SYSTEM EMERGENCIES
Bryan E. Bledsoe, D.O. 768

Objectives 769
Case Study 770
Introduction 770
Anatomy and Physiology of the Abdomen 771
The Gastrointestinal System 772
The Circulatory System 773
The Genitourinary System 774
The Reproductive System 774
Abdominal Pathophysiology 776
Gastrointestinal System Emergencies 776
Genitourinary System Emergencies 779
Reproductive System Emergencies 781
Assessment of the Acute Abdomen 783
Primary Assessment 783
Secondary Assessment 783
History 786
Management of the Acute Abdomen 786
Special Patients: Dialysis 787
Types of Dialysis 787
Complications of Dialysis 788
Complications Related to Vascular Access 790
Management of the Dialysis Patient 790
Summary 790
Further Reading 791

25 ANAPHYLAXIS *Bryan E. Bledsoe, D.O.* 792

Objectives 793
Case Study 794
Introduction 794
The Immune System 794
Allergies 796
Delayed Hypersensitivity 796
Immediate Hypersensitivity 796
Anaphylaxis 797
Clinical Features of Anaphylaxis 798
Assessment 798
Primary Assessment 798
Secondary Assessment 799
Management 799
Fluid and Pharmacological Therapy 799
Summary 803
Further Reading 803

26 TOXICOLOGY AND SUBSTANCE ABUSE
Bryan E. Bledsoe, D.O. and Dexter W. Hunt 804

Objectives 805
Case Study 806
Introduction 806
Poisoning—An Overview 807
Routes of Toxic Exposure 807
Poison Information Centers 809

General Principles of Toxicologic Management 809
Scene Survey 809
Primary and Secondary Survey 809
Decontamination 810
Ingested Poisons 810
General Principles of Assessment 810
General Principles of Management 812
Specific Ingested Toxins 814
Inhaled Poisons 817
Presentation of Toxic Inhalations 817
General Management of Toxic Inhalations 818
Specific Inhaled Toxins 818
Injected Poisons 821
General Principles of Management 821
Insect and Arthropod Bites and Stings 821
Snake Bites 825
Marine Animal Injection 828
Surface Absorbed Poisons 829
General Principles of Management 829
Organophosphates 829
Drug Overdose and Substance Abuse 830
Alcohol Abuse 830
Physiological Effects 833
General Alcoholic Profile 834
Consequences of Chronic Alcoholism 835
Withdrawal Syndrome 835
In-Field Treatment of Alcohol Abuse 836
Summary 836
Further Reading 837

27 INFECTIOUS DISEASES
Bryan E. Bledsoe, D.O. 838

Objectives 839
Case Study 840
Introduction 840
Pathogenesis of Infectious Disease 841
Bacteria 841
Viruses 841
Fungi 842
Parasites 842
Immunity 842
Immune Response 842
The Lymphatic System 843
Transmission of Infectious Disease 843
Routes of Disease Transmission 843
Increased Risk of Disease Transmission 843
Post-Exposure Considerations 844
Infection Control in Prehospital Care 845
Preparation for Response in Emergency Incidents 845
Response to Emergency Incidents 846
Actions at Emergency Incidents 846
Recovery From Emergency Incidents 848
Infectious Diseases and Emergency Care 850
Infections of the Nervous System 850
Infections of the Respiratory System 851
Skin Infections 853
Childhood Diseases 854
Infections of the Gastrointestinal System 855
Sexually Transmitted Diseases 857
HIV Infection 858

Summary 861
Further Reading 861

28 ENVIRONMENTAL EMERGENCIES
Bryan E. Bledsoe, D.O. 862

Objectives 863
Case Study 864
Introduction 864
Thermoregulation 864
  Generation and Loss of Heat 864
  Heat-Controlling Mechanisms 865
Thermal Disorders 867
  Hyperthermia 867
  Fever (Pyrexia) 871
  Hyperpyrexia 871
  Hypothermia 871
  Frostbite 876
Near-Drowning and Drowning 877
  Pathophysiology 877
  Factors Affecting Survival 879
  Prehospital Management 879
Nuclear Radiation 880
  Basic Nuclear Physics 880
  Effects of Radiation on the Body 881
  Principles of Safety 881
  Prehospital Management 883
Diving Emergencies 884
  Physical Principles of Pressure 884
  Common Diving Injuries 885
  General Assessment of Diving Emergencies 886
  Pressure Disorders 887
Summary 890
Further Reading 891

29 EMERGENCIES IN THE ELDERLY PATIENT
Bryan E. Bledsoe, D.O. 892

Objectives 893
Case Study 894
Introduction 894
Anatomy and Physiology of Aging 895
  General Age-Related Changes 895
  Systemic Age-Related Changes 895
Assessment of the Geriatric Patient 897
  Complicating Factors 897
  History 898
  Physical Examination 899
Pathophysiology and Management 899
  Trauma in the Elderly Patient 899
  Respiratory Emergencies in the Elderly Patient 900
  Cardiovascular Disease in the Elderly Patient 902
  Neurological Emergencies in the Elderly Patient 903
  Psychiatric Disorders in the Elderly Patient 905
  Gastrointestinal Emergencies Among Elderly Patients 906
  Environmental Emergencies Among Elderly Patients 907
Pharmacology in Geriatrics 908
  Complicating Factors 908
Geriatric Abuse/Neglect 909

Summary 909
Further Reading 909

30 PEDIATRIC EMERGENCIES
Bryan E. Bledsoe, D.O. 910

Objectives 911
Case Study 912
Introduction 912
General Approach to Pediatric Emergencies 912
  The Child's Response to Emergencies 912
  Development Stages—A Key to Assessment 913
  The Parents' Response to Emergencies 917
General Approach to Pediatric Assessment 917
  History 917
  Physical Examination 918
  Pediatric Vital Signs 919
  Non-Invasive Monitoring 920
Pediatric Trauma Emergencies 921
  Head, Face, and Neck Injuries 922
  Chest and Abdomen Injuries 922
  Extremity Injuries 923
  Burns 923
  Child Abuse and Neglect 923
Pediatric Medical Emergencies 927
  Neurological Emergencies 927
  Respiratory Emergencies 930
  Gastrointestinal Emergencies 935
  Cardiovascular Emergencies 936
  Other Pediatric Emergencies 940
Pediatric Advanced Life Support (PALS) 941
  Anticipating Cardiopulmonary Arrest 941
  Rapid Cardiopulmonary Assessment 941
  Management of the Critically Ill Infant of Child 945
Summary 951
Further Reading 951

PART 5

Obstetrical and Gynecological Emergencies

31 GYNECOLOGICAL EMERGENCIES
Bryan E. Bledsoe, D.O. 952

Objectives 953
Case Study 954
Introduction 954
Anatomy and Physiology 954
  Female Reproductive Organs 954
  Menstrual Cycles 957
Assessment of the Gynecological Patient 957
  History 958
  Physical Examination 958
Gynecological Emergencies 959

Medical Gynecological Emergencies 959
Traumatic Gynecological Emergencies 960
Summary 962
Further Reading 963

32 OBSTETRICAL EMERGENCIES
Bryan E. Bledsoe, D.O. 964

Objectives 965
Case Study 966
Introduction 966
The Prenatal Period 966
  Anatomy and Physiology of the Obstetric Patient 966
  Obstetric Terminology 969
  Assessment of the Obstetrical Patient 970
  Complications of Pregnancy 971
The Puerperium 981
  Deliveries 981
  Management of a Patient in Labor 982
  Unscheduled Field Delivery 983
  Complications of Delivery 987
  Maternal Complications of Labor and Delivery 991
Summary 993
Further Reading 993

33 EMERGENCY MANAGEMENT OF THE NEONATE *Bryan E. Bledsoe, D.O.* 994

Objectives 995
Case Study 996
Introduction 996
Anatomic and Physiologic Changes at Birth 997
Routine Care of the Newborn 998
  Establishment of the Airway 998
  Prevention of Heat Loss in the Neonate 998
  Cutting the Umbilical Cord 999
  Assessment of the Neonate 999
  The APGAR Score 999
The Premature Neonate 1000
The Distressed Neonate 1001
  Airway and Ventilation 1001
  Resuscitation of the Distressed Neonate 1001
Neonatal Transport 1009
Summary 1011
Further Reading 1011

PART 6

Psychiatric Emergencies

34 BEHAVIORAL AND PSYCHIATRIC EMERGENCIES *Bryan E. Bledsoe, D.O.* 1012

Objectives 1013
Case Study 1014

Introduction 1014
Understanding Behavioral Emergencies 1014
  Intrapsychic Causes 1014
  Interpersonal/Environmental Causes 1015
  Organic Causes 1015
Assessment of Behavioral Emergencies 1016
  Scene Survey 1016
  Assessment 1016
  Interviewing Techniques 1017
General Management and Intervention Techniques 1018
Specific Psychiatric Disorders 1019
  Depression 1019
  Suicide 1019
  Anxiety Disorders 1021
  Manic Disorders 1021
  Schizophrenia 1022
Age-Specific Behavioral Emergencies 1023
  Behavioral Emergencies in the Aged 1023
  Crisis in the Pediatric Patient 1023
Controlling the Violent Situation 1024
  Methods of Restraint 1025
  Positioning and Restraining Patient for Transport 1027
  Methods of Avoiding Injury to the Paramedic 1029
Domestic Violence 1029
Summary 1030
Further Reading 1030

APPENDIX
12 Lead ECG Monitoring and Interpretation 1031

Introduction 1031
The Cardiac Conductive System 1031
ECG Recording 1032
ECG Leads 1033
  Bipolar Limb Leads 1034
  Unipolar or Augmented Limb Leads 1035
  Precordial Leads 1038
Mean QRS Axis Determination 1039
Axis Deviation 1039
The Normal 12 Lead ECG 1042
Disease Findings 1044
  Evolution of Acute Myocardial Infarction 1045
  Localizationof Acute Myocardial Infarction 1048
Conduction Abnormalities 1051
  AV Blocks 1051
  Bundle Branch Blocks 1055
  Prehospital ECG Monitoring 1059
Summary 1066
Further Reading 1066

GLOSSARY 1067

INDEX 1085

PREFACE TO THE THIRD EDITION

Congratulations on your decision to further your EMS career by undertaking the course of training required for certification as an Emergency Medical Technician-Paramedic! The world of paramedic emergency care is one that you will find both challenging and rewarding. Whether you will be working as a volunteer or paid paramedic, you will find the field of advanced prehospital care very interesting.

This textbook will serve as your guide to advanced prehospital care. It is based upon the 1985 United States Department of Transportation National Paramedic Training Curriculum and extensively updated with current information and procedures. The text is divided into 34 chapters, separated into 6 divisions. The first division is entitled *Prehospital Environment* and presents the basics of advanced prehospital care. The second division, *Preparatory Information,* reviews the basics of emergency medical care. It also addresses the fundamentals of paramedic practice, including patient assessment, advanced airway management, shock, and emergency pharmacology. *Trauma Emergencies,* the third division of the text, discusses advanced prehospital care of injuries. The trauma presentation is based upon the management principles taught in Prehospital Trauma Life Support and Basic Trauma Life Support courses. The fourth division of the book, *Medical Emergencies,* is the longest and addresses paramedic level care of medical problems. Particular emphasis is placed upon cardiovascular emergencies, including interpretation of the electrocardiogram. The last two divisions address advanced prehospital care of *Obstetrical and Gynecological Emergencies* and *Psychiatric Emergencies.* An Appendix addressing 12 Lead ECG Monitoring and Interpretation has been added to the Third Edition for those EMS systems venturing into Rapid Acute Myocardial Infarction Identification and Treatment.

SKILLS

Advanced prehospital skills are best learned in the classroom, laboratory, and clinical setting. The common advanced prehospital skills are presented in both the text and in the Procedure Sheets. Review these before practicing the skill.

It is important to point out that this text cannot teach skills. These are only learned under the watchful eye of a paramedic instructor.

HOW TO USE THIS TEXTBOOK

Paramedic Emergency Care is designed to accompany a paramedic education program that follows the 1985 United States Department of Transportation *Emergency Medical Technician-Paramedic: National Standard Curriculum.*

The education program should include ample classroom, practical laboratory, inhospital clinical, and prehospital field experience. These educational experiences must be guided by instructors and preceptors with special training and experience in their areas of participation in your program.

It is intended that your program coordinator will assign reading from *Paramedic Emergency Care* in preparation for each classroom lecture and discussion section. The knowledge gained from reading this text will form the foundation of the information you will need in order to function effectively as a paramedic in your EMS system. Your instructors will build upon this information to strengthen your knowledge and understanding of advanced prehospital care so that you may apply it in your work. The inhospital clinical and prehospital field experiences will further refine your knowledge and skills under the watchful eyes of your preceptors.

In preparing for each classroom session, read the assigned chapter carefully. First, review the chapter objectives. They will identify what the authors feel are important concepts to be learned from the reading. Read the case study to get a feeling of why a chapter is important and how the knowledge it contains can be applied in the field. Read the content carefully, while keeping the chapter objectives in mind. Last, re-read the chapter objectives and be sure that you are able to answer each one completely. If you aren't, re-read the section of the chapter to which the objective relates. If you still do not understand the objective or any portion of what you have read, ask your instructor to explain it at your next class session.

Ideally, you should read this entire text at least three times. The chapter should be read in preparation for the class session, the entire division should be read before the division test, and the entire text should be re-read before the course final exam. While this might seem like a lot of reading, it will improve your classroom performance and your knowledge of emergency care.

The workbook that accompanies this text can also assist in improving classroom performance. It contains information, sample test questions, and exercises designed to assist learning. Its use can be very helpful in identifying the important elements of paramedic education, in exercising the knowledge of prehospital care, and in helping you self-test your knowledge.

Paramedic Emergency Care attempts to present the knowledge of emergency care in as accurate, standardized, and clear a manner as is possible. However, each EMS system is uniquely different, and it is beyond the scope of this text to address all differences. You must count heavily on your instructors, the program coordinator, and ultimately the program medical director to identify how specific emergency care procedures are applied in your system.

Bryan E. Bledsoe, D.O.
Robert S. Porter
Bruce R. Shade

**Visit Brady's Web Site
www.bradybooks.com**

ACKNOWLEDGMENTS

PRODUCTION

The task of writing, editing, reviewing, and producing a textbook the size of *Paramedic Emergency Care* is complex. Many talented people have been involved in the revision of this book.

First, the authors would like to acknowledge the support of Susan Katz and Lois Berlowitz. Their belief in us, and support of EMS, has allowed us to assure that *Paramedic Emergency Care* is in the forefront of paramedic education. Special thanks also go to Sandra Breuer, who served as Development Editor for the third edition. Sandra first learned about the special world of EMS and then, with new insight, tackled incredibly complex stacks of manuscript pages. Her efforts and attention to detail have made the text much cleaner, easier to read, and better organized.

The challenges of production were assigned to Pat Walsh and Julie Boddorf. Together they took material from the earlier editions of the work and intergrated the material new to the third edition. The result is a cohesive text that covers the essential elements of advanced prehospital care.

The art and photographs came from many sources. Most of the staged photographs were by Michal Heron of New York City and Richard Logan of Tampa, Florida. The new art was drafted by Rolin Graphics of Plymouth, Minnesota. Thanks to these professionals for their commitment to excellence.

Finally, the job of selling and marketing the text is handled by the Prentice Hall Marketing Department and the Brady Telesales Department. As a result of their close customer contacts, these professionals are able to provide essential feedback from readers and instructors throughout the world. They are the primary reason behind the success of *Paramedic Emergency Care*.

CONTRIBUTORS

The people listed on the following page contributed chapter material to the third and previous editions of *Paramedic Emergency Care*. They have been an important part of the development and revision process. Our appreciation goes to:

Richard A Cherry, M.Ed., NREMT-P
Director of Paramedic Training/Clinical Instructor
Department of Emergency Medicine
State University of New York Health Science Center
Syracuse, New York

Rodney L. Dennison, B.S., EMT-P
Emergency Medical Services Program Manager
Texas Department of Health
Public Health Region 7
Temple, Texas

Dexter W. Hunt, M.Ed., EMT-P
Senior Field Paramedic Preceptor
Ada County Emergency Medical Services
Boise, Idaho

Paul M. Maniscalco, B.S., NREMT-P
Deputy Chief / New York City EMS
Commanding Officer
Special Operations Division
New York, New York

Gary P. Morris, EMT-P
Deputy Fire Chief / Phoenix Fire Department
Phoenix, Arizona

REVIEWERS

The reviewers of *Paramedic Emergency Care* have provided many excellent suggestions and ideas for improving the text. The quality of the reviews has been outstanding, and the reviews have been a major aid in the preparation and revision of the manuscript. The assistance provided by these EMS experts is deeply appreciated.

The following people reviewed chapters new to the Third Edition of *Paramedic Emergency Care*

Brenda J. Beasley, B.S., R.N., EMT-P
EMS Program Director, Southern Union College
Opelika, Alabama

Richard W.O. Beebe, M.Ed., R.N., REMT-P
Hudson Valley Community College
Institute of Prehospital Emergency Medicine
Troy, New York

Chip Boehm, R.N., EMT-P
Portland Fire Dept., Medical Devision
Portland, Maine

Harold C. Cohen, M.S., EMT-P
Battalion Chief
Baltimore County Fire Department
Catonsville, Maryland

Judy G. Dyke, R.N., NREMT-P
Paramedic Technology Program Coordinator
Rogers State College
Claremore, Oklahoma

Steven English, R.N., C.C.R.N., C.E.N., EMT
University of Kentucky / Aeromedical Services
Lexington, Kentucky

Lisa Evenbly, R.N., B.S.N., M.I.C.N., C.E.N., EMT-P
Director of Clinical Education
Tacoma County College
Tacoma, Washington

Carol Gallager, M.P.A., B.S.N.
Director of Education and Training
Daniel Freeman Hospitals, Inc.
Inglewood, California

William E. Gandy, J.D., EMT-P
Director, Department of Emergency Medical Technology
Tyler Junior College
Tyler, Texas

Jeffrey L. Hayes, B.S., NREMT-P
Dept. Head, Emergency Medical Services Technology
Austin Community College
Austin, Texas

Linda Honeycutt
Education Coordinator / Maine EMS
Augusta, Maine

Jeffrey L. Jarvis, M.S., EMT-P
State Training Coordinator / Texas Dept. of Health
Austin, Texas

David M. LaCombe, EMT-P
Paramedic Instructor
University of Miami School of Medicine
Miami, Florida

Joseph F. Peters, Jr., EMT-P
Assistant Professor/Field Coordinator
UTHSCSA - Dept. of EMT
San Antonio, Texas

Lorna Ramsey, R.N., M.S.N., NREMT-P
Program Director, Emergency Medical Technology
Tidewater Community College
Virginia Beach, Virginia

Virginia K. Reidy, R.N., NREMT-P
Program Diector
Northwest Ohio Paramedic Program
Medical College Hospitals
Toledo, Ohio

Andrew W. Stern, M.P.A, M.A, EMT-P
Senior Paramedic
Town of Colonie Emergency Medical Services
Colonie, New York

Beth S. Toups, R.N., C.C.R.N., NREMT-P
Program Director, Emergency Health Science
Our Lady of the Lake College
Baton Rouge, Louisiana

We wish to thank the ESM professionals listed below who reviewed earler editions of *Paramedic Emergency Care.* They have contributed to the success of this program.

Jane W. Ball, R.N., Dr.P.H.
Richard S. Bennett, R.N., NREMT-P
Marvin Birnbaum, M.D., Ph.D.
Scott Bolleter, EMT-P
Chief Kevin S. Brame
Dena Brownstein, M.D.
Debra Cason, R.N., M.S., EMT-P
Richard A. Cherry, M.Ed., NREMT-P
Dwayne E. Clayden, EMT-P
Daniel J. Cobaugh, Pharm.D.
Captain Harold C. Cohen, M.S., EMT-P
Neil Coker, EMT-P
Judith A. Cremeens, R.N., M.Ed., CEN, NREMT-P
Howard Cummings, RN, Ed.D.
Ken D'Alessandro, NREMT-P
John Davanzo, EMT-P
Bonnie S. Dean, R.N., B.S.N., D.A.B.A.T.
C. Scott Dembowski, A.A.S., NREMT-P
Pamela B. doCarmo, Ph.D., NREMT-P
Martin R. Eichelberger, M.D.
David Fair, C.C., C.T.C., EMT
Phil Fontanarosa, M.D.

Rusty R. Fowler, B.S., NREMT-P
Captain Steven K. Frye, EMT-P
Herbert G. Garrison, M.D., M.P.H.
Greg Gibson, EMT-P
Carol Goodykoontz, EMT-P
Owen M. Grossman, M.D., F.A.A.F.P.
Greg L. Kennedy, A.S., B.B.A., NREMT-P
Laura Kitzmiller
Ken Koch, EMT-P
Alexander E. Kuehl, M.D., M.P.H.
Mark Lockhart, NREMT-P
Paul Maniscalco, B.S., EMT-P
Gregg S. Margolis, B.S., EMT-P
Bill Metcalf, EMT-P
Linda D. Metcalf, EMT-P
Charly D. Miller, NREMT-P
Chief Gary P. Morris, EMT-P
Jim Moshinskie, Ph.D., EMT-P
Kevin Parrish, R.N., EMT-P
Dwight A. Polk, B.A., NREMT-P
David Potashnick, EMT-P
Laura Randall, R.N.
Ham Robbins, R.N., EMT-P
Ronald Roth, M.D., F.A.C.E.P.
Nels Sanddal, EMT-P
Ray Shelton, Ph.D., EMT-CC
Ellen Shopes, R.N., M.S.N., C.C.R.N.
Andrew Stern, NREMT-P
Douglas Stevenson, EMT-P
Mike Taigman, EMT-P
Patricia L. Tritt, R.N., B.S.
Michael Wainscott, M.D.
Katherine West, R.N., M.S.Ed.
Chief Richard Wiederhold, B.A., EMT-P
Jean B. Will, R.N., M.S.N., C.E.N., EMT-P
Douglas R. Williams
Mark Winstead, EMT-P
Frank M. Yeiser, M.D., F.A.C.E.P.

ORGANIZATIONS AND INDIVIDUALS

The authors would like to gratefully acknowledge the assistance and support of the following organizations and persons who contributed significantly to the development of this textbook.

Georgetown Hospital
Kenneth Potete, Administrator
Georgetown, Texas

Williamson County EMS
George Stephenson, Director
John Sneed, Training Coordinator
Georgetown, Texas

East Texas Medical Center Emergency Medical Services
Keith Bundick, Regional Operations Manager
Waxahachie, Texas

City of Annapolis Fire Department EMS
Annapolis, Maryland
Anne Arundel Medical Center Emergency Department
Annapolis, Maryland

Scott and White Memorial Hospital
Department of Plastic and Reconstructive Surgery
    Charles N. Verheyden, M.D., Ph.D., F.A.C.S.
    Raleigh R. White, IV, M.D., F.A.C.S.
    Dennis J. Lynch, M.D., F.A.C.S.
    Peter Grothaus, M.B., Ch.B., F.R.C.S.(C)
Texas A & M University College of Medicine
Temple, Texas

Scott and White Memorial Hospital
Department of Medical Photography
David Hansen
Texas A & M University College of Medicine
Temple, Texas

Maryland Institute for Emergency Medical Services Systems
Baltimore, Maryland

Center for Emergency Medicine of Western
Pennsylvania
Pittsburgh, Pennsylvania

Acadian Ambulance Service, Inc.
W. Keith Simon
Lafayette, Louisiana

City of Phoenix Fire Department
Chief Alan Brunacini
Deputy Chief Gary Morris
Phoenix, Arizona

Presbyterian University Hospital
Rich Boland, EMS Coordinator
Trauma Services
Pittsburgh, Pennsylvania

Publications Committee
National Council of State EMS Training Coordinators

We wish to express our appreciation to the following people at the LifeFleet Ambulance Service, A MedTrans Company, Tampa, Florida for their extraordinary efforts on the photography program, including the valuable contribution of equipment and models.

Conrad T. Kearns, M.B.A, Paramedic
Director of Government Affairs

Walt Eisemann, Managing Director
Fort Lauderdale, Florida

Nestor Berrios-Torres, Supervisor
Hillsborough Office

Herman Cortez, Operations Manager

Tom Maiolo, Area Service Manager

Ted Rodgers, NREMT-P, Field Training Officer

Carol Hawthorne, NREMT, Operations Supervisor

The following persons gave freely of their time to act as models or to provide technical support for many of the photographs used in this book:

Ronnie Hahn, LVN, EMT-P, Baylor Medical Center
Shannon Hargrove, EMT-P, East Texas EMS
Tommy Camp, EMT-P, East Texas EMS
Robin Potete, EMT-P, East Texas EMS
Vernon Wickliffe, EMT-P, East Texas EMS
Scott Gibson, EMT-P, Williamson County EMS
Dave Reimer, EMT-P, Williamson County EMS

Bobby Slaughter, EMT-P, Williamson County EMS
John Sneed, EMT-P, Williamson County EMS
Paul Ward, EMT, Round Rock Fire Department
Janice Ward, LVN, EMT, Georgetown Hospital
Reta Reimer, LVN, Austin MediCenter
Cyndi Gibson, Georgetown Hospital
Jana Slaughter, Georgetown Hospital

In addition, the following children served as models for various photographs in the book: Andrea Bledsoe, Bryan Bledsoe, II, Jennifer Dean, Nicholas Hargrove, Brian Slaughter, Melanie Slaughter, Erin Ward, and Julie Ward.

Special thanks go to Ronnie Taylor, EMT-P, with the City of Austin EMS, who provided excellent moulage injuries for the photography sessions.

ABOUT THE AUTHORS

BRYAN E. BLEDSOE, D.O., EMT-P

Dr. Bledsoe is an emergency medicine physician with special interest in prehospital care. He received a B.S. degree from the University of Texas at Arlington in Arlington, Texas and received his medical degree from the University of North Texas/Texas College of Osteopathic Medicine. His internship was at Texas Tech University and residency training at Scott and White Memorial Hospital/Texas A & M College of Medicine. Prior to attending medical school, Dr. Bledsoe, a Texas native, worked as an EMT, Paramedic, and Paramedic Instructor. He completed EMT training in 1974 and paramedic training in 1976 and worked for 6 years as a field paramedic in Fort Worth. In 1979, he joined the faculty of Texas College of Osteopathic Medicine and served as coordinator of EMT and Paramedic programs at the college. He is active in emergency medicine and a member of numerous professional organizations. He is medical director for many EMS services and fire departments in the Dallas area

Dr. Bledsoe has authored several other EMS books published by Brady Communications including *Manual of Emergency Drugs*, *Prehospital Emergency Pharmacology*, *Paramedic Pocket Reference*, and *Atlas of Paramedic Skills*. He is married to Emma Bledsoe. They have two children, Bryan and Andrea, and live in Arlington, Texas.

ROBERT S. PORTER, M.A., NREMT-P

Mr. Porter has served as Director of the Central New York Emergency Medical Services Program, which serves an eleven-county region with a population of 1.4 million people. Mr. Porter is a Wisconsin native and received his bachelor's degree in education from the University of Wisconsin. He completed his master's degree in Health Education from Central Michigan University. Mr. Porter was certified as a Basic EMT and EMT Instructor in 1973 and was nationally registered as a paramedic in 1978. Mr. Porter has been an EMS educator since 1973 and has taught Basic EMT and paramedic programs in Wisconsin, Michigan, Louisiana, and Pennsylvania. Mr. Porter is past chairman of the National Society of EMT Instructors/Coordinators and is a site evaluator for accreditation of paramedic programs. He has published numerous articles in EMS periodicals and is the author of the workbook that accompanies this text.

BRUCE R. SHADE, NREMT-P

Mr. Shade is currently Commissioner for the Cleveland Emergency Medical Service in Cleveland, Ohio. Cleveland EMS is a third city service operation that responds to over 70,000 EMS call per year. Mr. Shade has attended Cuyahoga Community College and Lakeland Community College in Cleveland, Ohio. Mr. Shade, an Ohio native, was certified as an EMT in 1972 and as a paramedic in 1976. He was educational supervisor and paramedic instructor for the city of Cleveland from 1980-1986. Mr. Shade is currently Chairperson, Society of EMT Instructor/Coordinators with the NAEMT and a member of many other professional organizations. He is co-author of *Advanced Cardiac Life Support: Certification, Preparation, and Review,* published by Brady Communications. In addition, he is a frequent contributor to EMS periodicals. He is married to Cheri Shade. They have two children, Katie and Christopher. He and his family live in Willoughby, Ohio.

NOTICES

It is the intent of the authors and publisher that this textbook be used as part of a formal paramedic education program taught by a qualified instructor and supervised by a licensed physician. The care procedures presented here represent accepted practices in the United States. They are not offered as a standard of care. Paramedic-level emergency care is to be performed only under the authority and guidance of a licensed physician. It is the reader's responsibility to know and follow local care protocols as provided by medical advisors directing the system to which he or she belongs. Also, it is the reader's responsibility to stay informed of emergency care procedure changes.

Notice on Drugs and Drug Dosages

Every effort has been made to ensure that the drug dosages presented in this textbook are in accordance with nationally accepted standards. When applicable, the dosages and routes are taken from the American Heart Association's Advanced Cardiac Life Support Guidelines. The American Medical Association's publication *Drug Evaluations,* and the material published in the *Physician's Desk Reference,* are followed with regard to drug dosages not covered by the American Heart Association's guidelines. It is the responsibility of the reader to be familiar with the drugs used in his or her system, as well as the dosages specified by the medical director. The drugs presented in this book should only be administered by direct order, either verbally or through accepted standing orders, of a licensed physician.

Notice on Gender Usage

The English language has historically given preference to the male gender. Among many words, the pronouns "he" and "his" are commonly used to describe both genders. Society evolves faster than language and the male pronouns still predominate in our speech. The authors have made great effort to treat the two genders equally, recognizing that a significant percentage of paramedics are female. However, in some instances, male pronouns may be used to describe both male and female paramedics solely for the purpose of brevity. This is not intended to offend any readers of the female gender.

Notice on Photographs

Please note that many of the photographs contained in this book are taken of actual emergency situations. As such, it is possible that they may not accurately depict current, appropriate, or advisable practices of emergency medical care. They have been included for the sole purpose of giving general insight into real-life emergency settings.

PRECAUTIONS ON BLOODBORNE PATHOGENS AND INFECTIOUS DISEASES

Prehospital emergency personnel, like all health care workers, are at risk for exposure to bloodborne pathogens and infectious diseases. In emergency situations it is often difficult to take or enforce proper infection control measures. However, as a paramedic, you must recognize your high-risk status. Study the following information on infection control before turning to the main portion of this book.

Infection control is designed to protect emergency personnel, their families, and their patients from unnecessary exposure to communicable diseases.

Laws, regulations, and standards regarding infection control include:

- *Centers for Disease Control (CDC) Guidelines.* The CDC has published extensive guidelines regarding infection control. Proper equipment and techniques that should be used by emergency response personnel to prevent or minimize risk of exposure are defined.

- *The Ryan White Act.* The Ryan White Act of 1990 and allows emergency personnel to find out if they were exposed to an infectious disease while rendering patient care. Employers are required to name a "designated officer" to coordinate communications with the treating hospital.

- *Americans with Disabilities Act.* This act prohibits discrimination against individuals with disabilities including those with contagious diseases. It guarantees equal employment opportunities and job protection if the infected individual can perform essential job functions and does not pose a threat to the safety and health of patients and coworkers.

- *Occupational Safety and Health Administration (OSHA) Regulations.* OSHA recently enacted a regulation entitled Occupational Exposure to Bloodborne Pathogens that classifies emergency response personnel as being at the greatest risk of occupational exposure to communicable diseases. This regulation requires employers to provide hepatitis B (HBV) vaccinations free of charge, maintain a written exposure control plan, and provide personal protective equipment (PPE). These requirements primarily apply to private employers. Applicability to local and state governmental employees varies by locality. Many states have developed their own OSHA plans.

- *National Fire Protection Association (NFPA) Guidelines.* This is a national organization that has established specific guidelines and requirements regarding infection control for emergency response agencies, particularly fire departments and EMS services.

Body Substance Isolation Precautions and Personal Protective Equipment

Emergency response personnel should practice *Body Substance Isolation (BSI),* a strategy that considers ALL body substances potentially infectious. To achieve this, all emergency personnel should utilize *personal protective equipment (PPE).* Appropriate PPE should be available on every emergency vehicle. The minimum recommended PPE includes the following.

- *Gloves.* Disposable gloves should be donned by all emergency response personnel BEFORE initiating any emergency care. When an emergency incident involves more than one patient, you should attempt to change gloves between patients. When gloves have been contaminated, they should be removed as soon as possible. To properly remove contaminated gloves, grasp one glove approximately one inch from the wrist. Without touching the inside of the glove, pull the glove half-way off and stop. With that half gloved hand, pull the glove on the opposite hand completely off. Place the removed glove in the palm of the other glove, with the inside of the removed glove exposed. Pull the second glove completely off with the ungloved hand, only touching the inside of the glove. Always wash hands after gloves are removed, even when the gloves appear intact.

- *Masks and Protective Eyewear.* Masks and protective equipment should be present on all emergency vehicles and used in accordance with the level of exposure encountered. Masks and protective eyewear should be worn together whenever blood spatter is likely to occur, such as arterial bleeding, childbirth, endotracheal intubation, invasive procedures, oral suctioning, and clean-up of equipment that requires heavy scrubbing or brushing. Both you and the patient should wear masks whenever the potential for airborne transmission of disease exists.

- *HEPA Respirators.* Due to the resurgence of tuberculosis (TB), prehospital personnel should protect themselves from TB infection through use of a high-efficiency particulate air (HEPA) respirator, a design approved by the National Institute of Occupational Safety and Health (NIOSH). It should fit snugly and be capable of filtering out the tuberculosis bacillus. The HEPA respirator should be worn when caring for patients with confirmed or suspected TB. This is especially true when performing "high hazard" procedures such as administration of nebulized medications, endotracheal intubation, or suctioning on such a patient.

- *Gowns.* Gowns protect clothing from blood splashes. If large splashes of blood are expected, such as with childbirth, wear impervious gowns.

- *Resuscitation Equipment.* Disposable resuscitation equipment should be the primary means of artificial ventilation in emergency care. Such items should be used once, then disposed of.

Remember, the proper use of personal protective equipment ensures effective infection control and minimizes risk. Use ALL protective equipment recommended for any particular situation to ensure maximum protection.

Consider ALL body substances potentially infectious and ALWAYS practice body substance isolation. See Chapter 27 for additional information on bloodborne pathogens and infectious diseases.

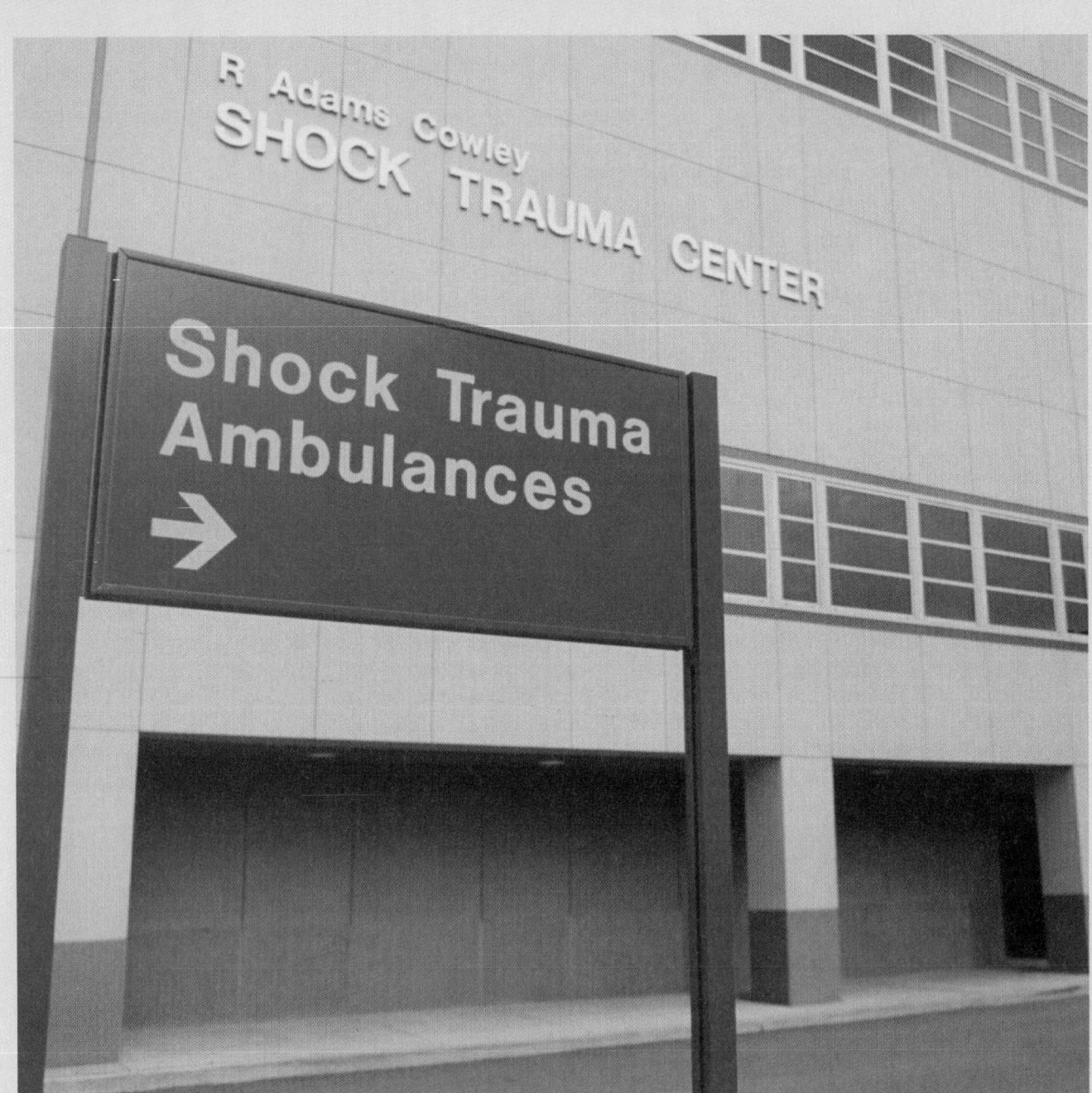

1

ROLES
AND RESPONSIBILITIES
OF THE PARAMEDIC

Objectives for Chapter 1

After reading this chapter, you should be able to:

1. Define the role of the EMT-Paramedic. (See pp. 4–6, 10–12.)

2. Define and give examples of professional ethics. (See pp. 6–9.)

3. Define and give examples of behavior that characterizes the health care professional. (See p. 9.)

4. List the duties of the EMT-Paramedic in preparation for handling emergency medical responses. (See p. 10.)

5. List the duties of the EMT-Paramedic during an emergency response. (See pp. 10–11.)

6. List the duties of the EMT-Paramedic after an emergency response. (See pp. 11–12.)

7. List the post-graduation responsibilities of the EMT-Paramedic. (See pp. 12–14.)

8. Recognize differences among certification, licensure, and reciprocity. (See pp. 12–13.)

9. State the benefits and responsibilities of continuing education for the EMT-Paramedic. (See p. 13.)

10. State the major purposes of a national organization. (See p. 13.)

11. List some national organizations for EMS providers. (See p. 13.)

12. State the major purposes of the National Registry of Emergency Medical Technicians. (See p. 14.)

13. Describe the major benefits of subscribing to professional journals. (See p. 14.)

Imagine it's a warm summer evening in July, 1958. That night, two speeding cars collide at an urban intersection. Bystanders immediately recognize the seriousness of the accident and notify the police. The police dispatcher relays the call to patrolling officers by way of two-way radios. Three ambulance services in the vicinity hear about a "10-50 major" on their police monitors. After noting the address, the ambulance drivers race to their vehicles.

The first ambulance to hit the street is owned by Nathan-Crigler Funeral Home. The ambulance is truly a work of art. It is a dark blue Mercury station wagon, with a chrome mechanical siren and a fire-ball beacon on the roof. Most impressive, however, is what's inside. The vehicle contains a high-performance Ford engine, four-speed transmission, four-barrel carburetor, and racing suspension.

As the ambulance turns onto the highway, the driver floors the accelerator. The ambulance quickly reaches a cruising speed of more than 100 miles per hour. Down the road, the driver sees the flashing beacons of the police cars and decelerates, down-shifting and pulling right up to the most damaged automobile. Immediately, the driver and the attendant jump out and start looking for the most injured patient. Near the corner, they find an unconscious female with multiple facial lacerations. The attendant runs to the ambulance, grabs the stretcher, and quickly returns to the patient. The driver and the attendant grab the patient—one under her armpits, the other under her knees—and quickly lift her onto the stretcher. During the lift, the patient's head falls back and she moans lightly. She moans again as her head hits the top of the stretcher. After putting the patient in the ambulance, both the driver and the attendant return to the front seat. The driver states: "She looks bad.... Let's haul!" With a jolt, the ambulance sets out for the hospital. With the road straight, the driver soon hits 110 miles per hour. The crew rushes to St.

INTRODUCTION

So you want to become a paramedic! Before you begin this long but rewarding journey, it is important to understand what a paramedic is, what your future role will be, and what society will expect from you. In addition, you must understand how to maintain a professional attitude in a field that has evolved from primitive roots to the sophisticated industry known as **Emergency Medical Services** (EMS) in less than 30 years.

It's not all flashing lights and sirens. The paramedic is expected to provide not only competent emergency medical care, but also emotional support for the patient and family members. Often, you will be providing these services for people who are unaware of your extensive training and neither understand nor appreciate what you did. But if self-satisfaction and pride in a job well done are reward enough for you, and if you have a genuine desire to help people in need, being a paramedic can be a very fulfilling career.

As the highest-trained prehospital emergency care provider in the EMS system, the paramedic accepts the awesome responsibility for patient care. While others manage a variety of factors during an emergency medical incident, the paramedic concentrates on the care and well-being of the patient. Your willingness to accept this role during a medical emergency and an interest in learning how to devise effective treatment plans are the first steps toward becoming a paramedic.

■ **emergency medical services** a complex health care system that provides immediate, on-scene patient care to those suffering sudden illness or injury.

✳ The paramedic's primary responsibility in any emergency is patient care.

Mary's hospital and delivers the patient to a waiting stretcher. Without changing the sheets, they return the stretcher to the ambulance and race back to the accident scene. After 22 weeks, the patient finally leaves the hospital. The doctors have determined that nothing else can be done for her neck-down paralysis, so they send the woman to a home for the crippled.

Now imagine that a similar accident takes place *today* at the same intersection. As before, bystanders immediately know that it is serious. A passerby grabs his cellular telephone and dials 9-1-1. The EMS dispatcher takes the essential information and activates the EMS system.

The first members of the EMS system to arrive on the scene are EMT-trained firefighters. The lieutenant in charge quickly assesses the scene and requests additional equipment and personnel. Within a minute, the first ambulance arrives. The senior paramedic quickly surveys the scene and notes that five people have been injured, two seemingly seriously. He declares a Multiple-Casualty Incident and implements the Incident Command System. The patients are triaged. Each responding ambulance now has its assignment. The most critical patient is an unconscious female lying near the curb. An EMT manually stabilizes the patient's cervical spine, while the paramedic performs the primary assessment. Next, the paramedic completes the secondary assessment. The patient's Glasgow Coma Scale is 10, but her vital signs are stable.

The paramedics quickly, but gently, completely immobilize the patient from head to toe. They administer oxygen and establish an IV. They now transport the patient to a Level I trauma center, where a neurosurgeon assumes her care upon arrival. The patient responds well. She will have to spend five weeks in cervical traction and faces a long rehabilitation. However, she exhibits no paralysis and the doctors expect her to recover.

CHANGES IN THE FIELD

What will the public expect from you? Prior to the late 1960s, emergency medical services differed greatly from those available today. Most local fire departments had primitive rescue squads whose members had little training in emergency procedures and little or no knowledge of spinal immobilization or airway management techniques. Funeral homes operated ambulance services that offered little more than fast, horizontal transport in vehicles ill-suited for patient care. The public did not expect much from prehospital emergency medical care—and did not receive much.

In 1966, a major research project conducted by the National Academy of Sciences, National Research Council led to the publication of a landmark paper titled "Accidental Death and Disability: The Neglected Disease of Modern Society." This historic document, commonly called "The White Paper," described the inadequacies of emergency medical care in this country. It criticized both hospital emergency rooms and prehospital emergency care. It made recommendations for establishing emergency medical services systems, starting emergency medical technician training programs, and upgrading ambulances. Through the efforts of the U.S. Department of Transportation Curriculum Committee, the Emergency Medical Technician (EMT), a professionally trained and certified basic life-support provider, evolved. The EMT would be trained to administer oxygen and cardiopulmonary resuscitation,

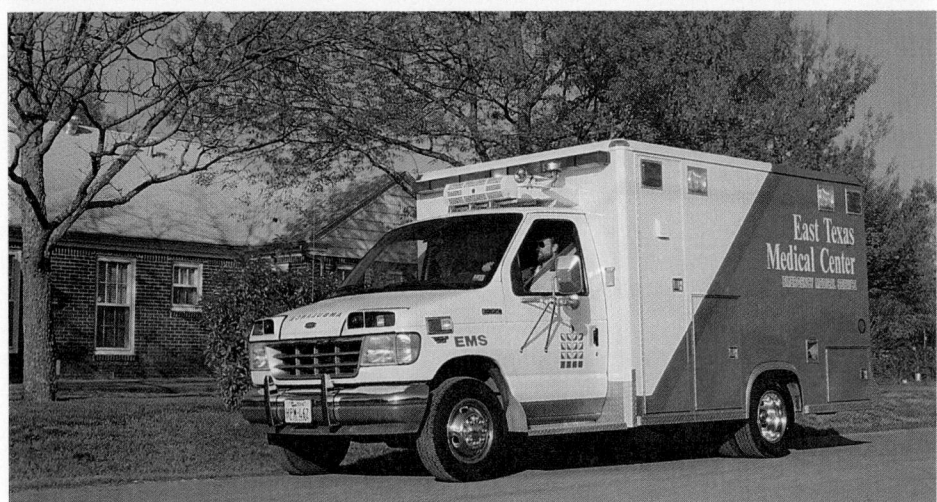

FIGURE 1-1 EMS has evolved into a comprehensive health care system providing state of the art emergency care at the scene and en route to the hospital. The modern ambulance is truly a mobile emergency department.

perform basic splinting and bandaging, and immobilize patients who had spinal cord injuries. Thus, the EMT became the first certified prehospital emergency care provider.

The innovative work of Dr. J. Frank Pantridge, a physician at the Royal Victoria Hospital in Belfast, Northern Ireland, introduced the concept of bringing advanced cardiac life support to the patient in the field. Shortly thereafter, the United States enacted legislation allowing specially trained EMTs to provide services that previously required a physician. Dr. Eugene Nagel, with the University of Miami School of Medicine, trained the first U.S. paramedics in Miami. Formal paramedic programs were soon organized in Los Angeles, Seattle, and Columbus, Ohio. These important developments began as bold initiatives by a few dedicated physicians who believed that prehospital emergency care would reduce preventable deaths. Today, there are more than 400 paramedic education programs in the United States.

The greatest cultural impact, however, came in 1971. The television series *Emergency*, which popularized two young firefighter paramedics in weekly episodes, set the first standard for the professional paramedic. The two clean-cut paramedics responded promptly to emergencies, had a solution for everything, and remained calm in the most stressful situations. The young people who watched that show in the 1970s are today's taxpayers. They expect the same skillful, compassionate, top-quality care portrayed on *Emergency*. Achieving such a high level of patient care and customer service is a major challenge for the paramedic of the 1990s.

Much of this chapter will deal with conceptual and highly specialized information. However, the ability to accept these concepts and apply them to one's professional conduct ultimately separates the outstanding paramedic from an average one.

PROFESSIONAL ETHICS

■ **ethics** the rules, standards, and morals governing the activities of a group or profession.

Ethics are the rules or standards that govern the conduct of members of a particular group. Physicians have long subscribed to a body of ethical standards that were developed primarily for the benefit of the patient. These standards have subsequently been extended to the allied health professions. Ethics are not laws, but standards for honorable behavior designed by the group;

The Oath of Geneva

I solemnly pledge myself to consecrate my life to the service of humanity; I will give to my teachers the respect and gratitude which is their due; I will practice my profession with conscience and dignity; the health of my patient will be my first consideration; I will respect the secrets which are confided in me; I will maintain by all the means in my power the honor and noble traditions of the medical profession; my colleagues will be my brothers; I will not permit considerations of religion, nationality, race, party, politics, or social standing to intervene between my duty and my patient; I will maintain the utmost respect for human life from the time of conception; even under threat, I will not make use of my medical knowledge contrary to the laws of humanity. I make these promises solemnly, freely and upon my honor.

FIGURE 1-2

conformity by all members is expected. As members of an **allied health** profession, paramedics must recognize a responsibility not only to their patients, but also to society, to other health professionals, and to themselves. In 1948, the World Medical Association adopted the "Oath of Geneva." (See Figure 1-2.) In 1978, the National Association of Emergency Medical Technicians adopted the EMT Oath (see Figure 1-3) and a Code of Ethics (see Figure 1-4). These documents detail the guiding principles for professional EMT service.

■ **allied health** term used to describe ancillary health care professionals, apart from physicians and nurses, such as paramedics, respiratory therapists, and physical therapists.

The EMT Oath

Be it pledged as an Emergency Medical Technician, I will honor the physical and judicial laws of God and man. I will follow that regimen which, according to my ability and judgment, I consider for the benefit of patients and abstain from whatever is deleterious and mischievous, nor shall I suggest any such counsel. Into whatever homes I enter, I will go into them for the benefit of only the sick and injured, never revealing what I see or hear in the lives of men unless required by law.

I shall also share my medical knowledge with those who may benefit from what I have learned. I will serve unselfishly and continuously in order to help make a better world for mankind.

While I continue to keep this oath unviolated, may it be granted to me to enjoy life and the practice of the art, respected by all men, in all times. Should I trespass or violate this oath, may the reverse be my lot. So help me God.

Adopted by The National Association of Emergency Medical Technicians, 1978

FIGURE 1-3

The EMT Code of Ethics

Professional status as an Emergency Medical Technician-Paramedic is maintained and enriched by the willingness of the individual practitioner to accept and fulfill obligations to society, other medical professionals, and the profession of Emergency Medical Technician. As an Emergency Medical Technician at the basic level or an Emergency Medical Technician-Paramedic, I solemnly pledge myself to the following code of professional ethics:

A fundamental responsibility to the Emergency Medical Technician is to conserve life, to alleviate suffering, to promote health, to do no harm, and to encourage the quality and equal availability of emergency medical care.

The Emergency Medical Technician provides services based on human need, with respect for human dignity, unrestricted by consideration of nationality, race creed, color, or status.

The Emergency Medical Technician does not use professional knowledge and skills in any enterprise detrimental to the public well being.

The Emergency Medical Technician respects and holds in confidence all information of a confidential nature obtained in the course of professional work unless required by law to divulge such information.

The Emergency Medical Technician, as a citizen, understands and upholds the law and performs the duties of citizenship; as a professional, the Emergency Medical Technician has the never-ending responsibility to work with concerned citizens and other health care professionals in promoting a high standard of emergency medical care to all people.

The Emergency Medical Technician shall maintain professional competence and demonstrate concern for the competence of other members of the Emergency Medical Services health care team.

An Emergency Medical Technician assumes responsibility in defining and upholding standards of professional practice and education.

The Emergency Medical Technician assumes responsibility for individual professional actions and judgement, both in dependent and independent emergency functions, and knows and upholds the laws which affect the practice of the Emergency Medical Technician.

The Emergency Medical Technician has the responsibility to be aware of and participate in matters of legislation affecting the Emergency Medical Technician and the Emergency Medical Services System.

The Emergency Medical Technician adheres to standards of personal ethics which reflect credit upon the profession.

Emergency Medical Technicians, or groups of Emergency Medical Technicians, who advertise professional services, do so in conformity with the dignity of the profession.

The Emergency Medical Technician has an obligation to protect the public by not delegating to a person less qualified, any service which requires the professional competence of an Emergency Medical Technician.

The Emergency Medical Technician will work harmoniously with and sustain confidence in Emergency Medical Technician associates, the nurse, the physician, and other members of the Emergency Medical Services health care team.

The Emergency Medical Technician refuses to participate in unethical procedures, and assumes the responsibility to expose incompetence or unethical conduct of others to the appropriate authority in a proper and professional manner.

The National Association of Emergency Medical Technicians.

FIGURE 1-4

■ **moral dilemma** issue involving the principles of right and wrong as governed by individual conscience.

While legal guidelines obligate the paramedic to certain actions, ethical standards suggest that certain behaviors are right or wrong. The paramedic will encounter many situations that present a **moral dilemma**. For example, the paramedic must decide between a patient's rights and family members' wishes when called upon to resuscitate a terminally ill patient in cardiac arrest. Another example is that of the intoxicated, belligerent patient who has sustained a head injury, but refuses transport. The paramedic must choose between the risk of abandonment and a possible charge of false imprisonment when deciding how best to manage the patient. How paramedics act in such cases will depend mostly on their personal values and ethical convictions. Legally, a paramedic must provide for the physical well-being of the patient. Ethically, the paramedic also must care for the emotional welfare of the patient and others at the scene.

The science of EMS involves advanced technology, research, and the delivery of sophisticated prehospital emergency medical care. The art of EMS means carrying out the duties with sincerity, compassion, grace, and a respect for human dignity. The best paramedics are excellent technicians who never forget that their patients are human beings with rights and feelings. If you always place the patient's welfare above everything but your own safety, you will probably never commit an unethical act. Treating all patients as you would members of your own family is all that can be expected from you as a paramedic. The best paramedics are aware of not only their legal obligations, but also the ethical and moral responsibilities of the job.

PROFESSIONALISM

Professionalism describes the conduct or qualities that characterize a practitioner in a particular field or occupation. Health care professionals promote quality patient care and take pride in their profession; they set high goals. They earn the respect and confidence of team members by performing their duties to the best of their abilities and by exhibiting a high level of respect for their profession. Attaining professionalism is not easy. It requires an understanding of what distinguishes the professional from the non-professional. To develop this skill, keep the following points in mind.

Professionals place the patient first; non-professionals place their egos first. Professionals practice their skills to the point of mastery, then keep practicing them to improve and stay sharp. Non-professionals do not believe their skills will fade and see no reason to constantly strive for improvement. Professionals understand the importance of response times; non-professionals get to an accident when it's convenient. Professionals take refresher courses seriously, because they know they have forgotten a lot and because they are eager for new information. Non-professionals believe they don't need training sessions and dislike being required to attend them. Professionals set high standards for themselves, their crew, their agency, and their system. Non-professionals aim for the minimum standard and can be counted on to take the path of least resistance. Professionals critically review their performance, always seeking a way to improve. Non-professionals look to protect themselves, to hide their inadequacies, and to place blame on others. Professionals check out all equipment prior to the emergency response. Non-professionals *hope* that everything will work, supplies will be in place, batteries will be charged, and oxygen levels will be adequate.

Maintaining professionalism requires effort. But, the result of that effort—the admiration and respect of one's peers—is the highest compliment a person can receive. True professionals establish excellence as their goal and never allow themselves to become satisfied with their performance. Professionalism is an attitude, not a matter of pay. It cannot be bought, rented, or faked. Although a young industry, EMS has achieved recognition as a bona fide allied health care profession. Gaining professional stature is the result of many hard-working, caring individuals who refused to compromise their standards. The paramedic must always strive to maintain that level of performance and commitment known as professionalism.

■ **professional** a person who exhibits the conduct or qualities that characterize a practitioner in a particular field or occupation.

✱ The paramedic is a health care professional.

ROLE OF THE PARAMEDIC

The role of the paramedic is diverse. It includes not only patient care, but a variety of responsibilities before, during, and after an emergency response. Prior to responding to a medical incident, preparation is the key. The paramedic must be prepared mentally, physically, and emotionally. At the very least, the paramedic is expected to maintain a high level of medical knowledge, expert recall of local treatment protocols, and a mastery of practical skills. Because the public has the right to quality patient care, these items are non-negotiable.

The physical demands of the job require ongoing training: aerobics for cardiovascular fitness, exercises for muscular strength and endurance, stretching for increased flexibility, and an understanding of the biomechanics of lifting (to prevent early retirement caused by lower-back injuries). Psychological stability is also essential to withstand the emotional strain of the job. Recognizing the effects of stress, and practicing ways to alleviate it, are the keys to long-term survival. The paramedic must also become familiar with the following:

❑ Policies and procedures of the local EMS system.
❑ The communications system, both hardware (radios) and software (frequency utilization and communication protocols).
❑ Local geography, including populations during peak loads and alternative routes during rush hours.
❑ Support agencies—what is available from neighboring departments and how to coordinate efforts and resources.

✳ The paramedic is the prehospital team leader.

Leadership is an important, but often forgotten, aspect of paramedic training. Paramedics are the prehospital team leaders. They must develop a leadership style that both suits their personalities and gets the job done. Although there are many successful styles of leadership, certain characteristics are common to all great leaders. These include:

❑ Self-confidence
❑ Established credibility
❑ Inner strength
❑ The ability to remain in control
❑ The ability to communicate
❑ The willingness to make a decision
❑ The willingness to accept responsibility for the consequences of the team's actions

The successful team leader knows the members of the crew, including their capabilities and limitations. Ask crew members to do something beyond their capabilities, and they will question your ability to lead, not their ability to perform. (See Figure 1-5.)

During an emergency response, the paramedic has the responsibility to:

✳ The paramedic is responsible for ensuring that the scene is safe, thus protecting the safety and well-being of both the patient and rescuers.

1. Size up and assure scene security.
2. Determine the needs of the incident and communicate that information to the emergency medical dispatcher.
3. Conduct the patient assessment.
4. Assign priorities of care and develop a treatment plan.
5. Communicate the plan to crew members.

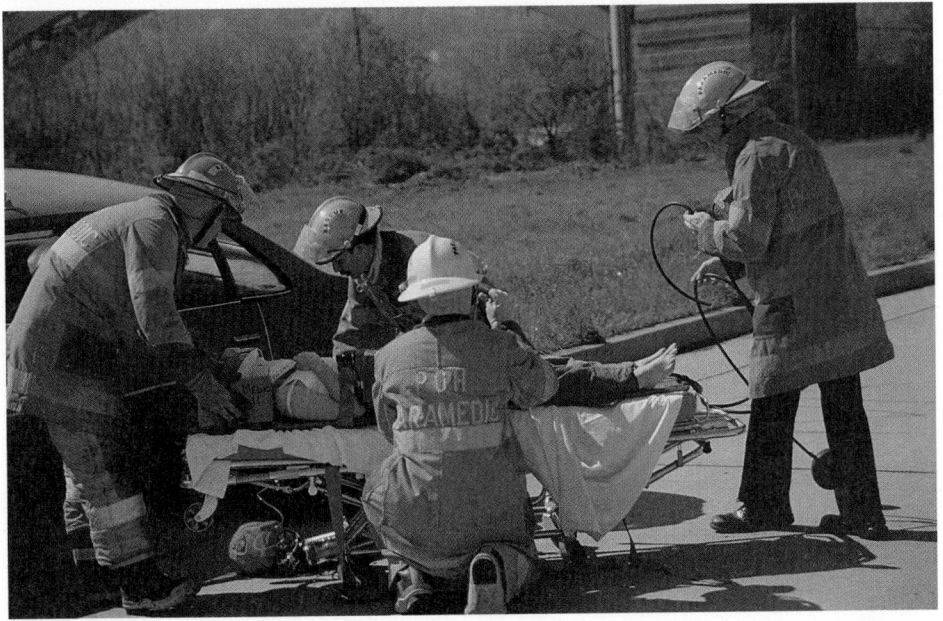

FIGURE 1-5 The paramedic is the leader of the emergency medical services team and must interact with patients, bystanders, and other rescue personnel in a professional and efficient manner.

6. Initiate basic and advanced life-support procedures, according to established standing orders. (See Figure 1-6.)
7. Assess the effects of treatment.
8. Establish contact with the medical control physician to discuss further treatment.
9. Direct and coordinate transport of the patient to the appropriate medical facility.
10. Maintain rapport with the patient, with support agencies, and with hospital personnel.

After the response, the paramedic must restock the ambulance in preparation for the next call. The paramedic must also gather or write all documentation concerning the incident. The importance of accurate and complete

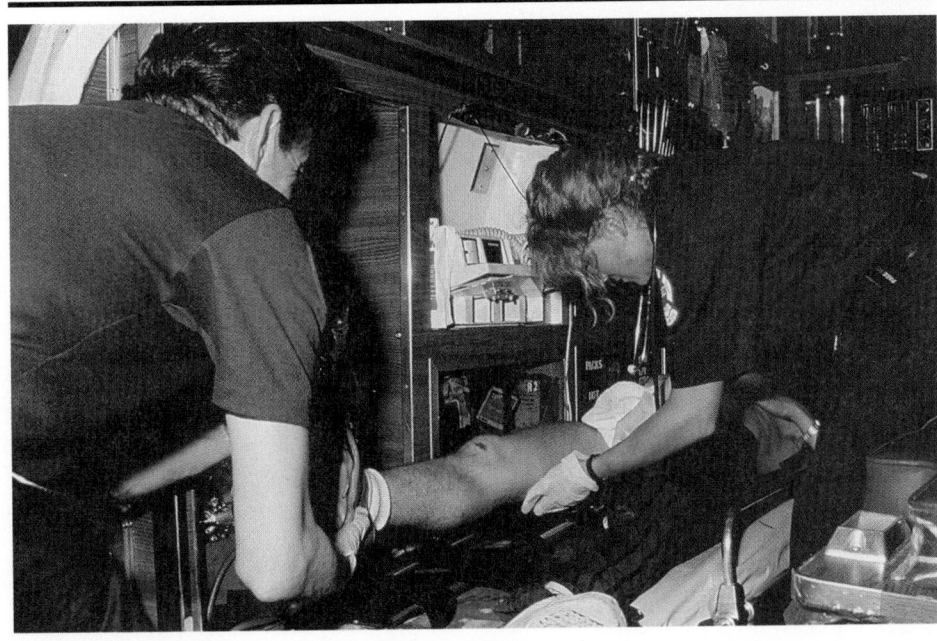

FIGURE 1-6 The paramedic's primary responsibility in any emergency situation is patient care.

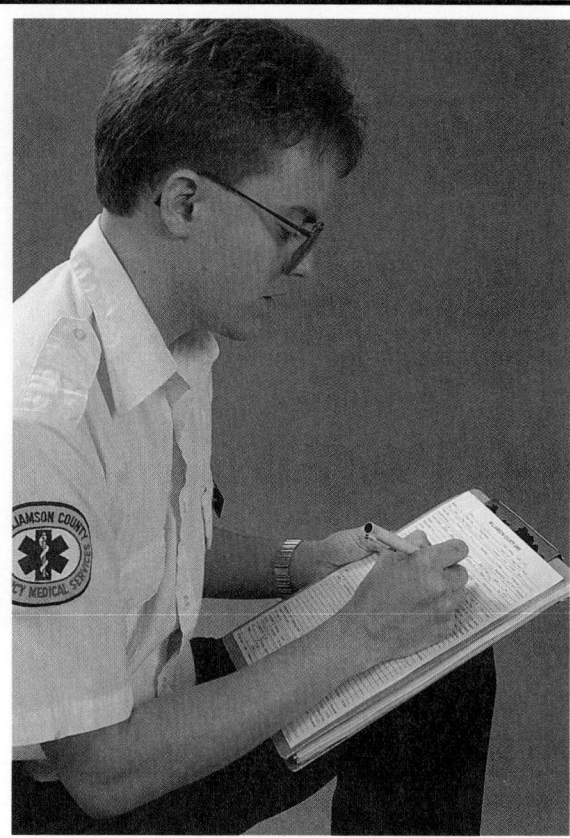

FIGURE 1-7 The responsibility of the paramedic does not end with delivery of the patient to the emergency department. Post-call documentation, restocking, and run critique are as important as the call itself.

documentation cannot be overemphasized. Proper record-keeping helps to ensure continuity of patient care from the prehospital to the hospital setting. To avoid potential legal problems and embarrassing court situations, the paramedic should record observations only on the runsheet (the patient had an odor of alcohol on his breath), not opinions (the patient was drunk). The former cannot be disputed and the latter cannot be proved. (See Figure 1-7.) Reviewing the call with crew members will improve future team performance. Finally, the paramedic team leader should check the crew members for signs of **critical-incident stress**, and assist anyone who needs help.

The role of the paramedic also includes duties not associated with emergency responses: CPR training, EMS demonstrations, seminars, teaching first-aid classes, accident prevention programs, and more. In addition, paramedics must also educate the public about how to recognize a medical emergency, how to initiate basic life support procedures, and how to promptly access the EMS system.

POST-GRADUATE RESPONSIBILITIES

Upon successful completion of a course following the **National Standard Curriculum for EMT-P**, the paramedic usually will become certified. **Certification** is the process by which an agency or association grants recognition to an individual who has met its qualifications. Many states certify emergency medical technicians and paramedics. After attaining state certification, paramedics are permitted to work within an established emergency medical services system under the direct supervision of a physician medical director.

■ **critical-incident stress** reaction commonly experienced by emergency personnel after a large or particularly stressful emergency response.

■ **National Standard Curriculum** paramedic training curriculum published by the United States Department of Transportation; widely used as the standard guidelines for paramedic education.

■ **certification** the process by which an agency or association grants recognition to an individual who has met its qualifications.

Licensure is the process by which a governmental agency grants permission to engage in a given occupation to an applicant who has attained the degree of competency required to ensure the public's protection. For example, a state grants licenses to physicians, teachers, and barbers to perform the duties associated with those professions. Some states choose to license paramedics instead of certifying them.

Reciprocity is the process by which an agency grants automatic certification or licensure to an individual who has comparable certification or licensure from another agency. For example, some states grant reciprocity to paramedics who are certified in another state.

Maintaining certification is the responsibility of the paramedic. Each state, region, and local system may have its own policies, regulations, and procedures for certification. Paramedics cannot function without satisfying those requirements.

Continuing Education

Certification or licensure marks the beginning, not the end of the paramedic's education. Paramedics have an important responsibility to continue their education. Everyone is subject to the decay of knowledge and skills. Skills and knowledge, both basic and advanced, suffer from infrequent use. As a rule of thumb, remember that as the volume of calls decreases, training should correspondingly increase.

Field paramedics have many choices in continuing education for keeping up their interest and staying informed. A few alternatives include: case reviews, videotapes, cassette lectures, in-hospital rotations in patient care areas, field drills, mobile classrooms that bring educational presentations to outlying squads, self-study exercises, and periodic "teaching days," in which a variety of topics are covered in lectures and presentations. When designing continuing education programs, administrators are limited only by their imagination and ingenuity.

Since EMS is a relatively young industry, new technology and data emerge rapidly, and the paramedic must make a conscious effort to keep up. A variety of journals, seminars, computer bulletin boards, and learning experiences are available to help. Only through continuing education and recertification requirements can the public be assured that quality patient care is being delivered. Refresher requirements vary from state to state, but the goal of this training is the same—to review previously learned materials and to receive new information.

✷ The paramedic must continually strive to stay abreast of changes in EMS.

Professional Organizations

Belonging to a professional organization is a good way to keep abreast of the latest technology. Communicating with members from other parts of the country provides an excellent opportunity to share ideas with people of similar backgrounds. Some national EMS organizations include:

❑ National Association of Emergency Medical Technicians (NAEMT)
❑ National Association of Search and Rescue (NASAR)
❑ National Association of State EMS Directors (NASEMSD)
❑ National Association of EMS Physicians (NAEMSP)
❑ National Flight Paramedics Association (NFPA)
❑ National Council of State EMS Training Coordinators (NCSEMSTC)

These are just some examples of organizations through which paramedics, emergency physicians, and nurses can enrich themselves and pursue their particular interests.

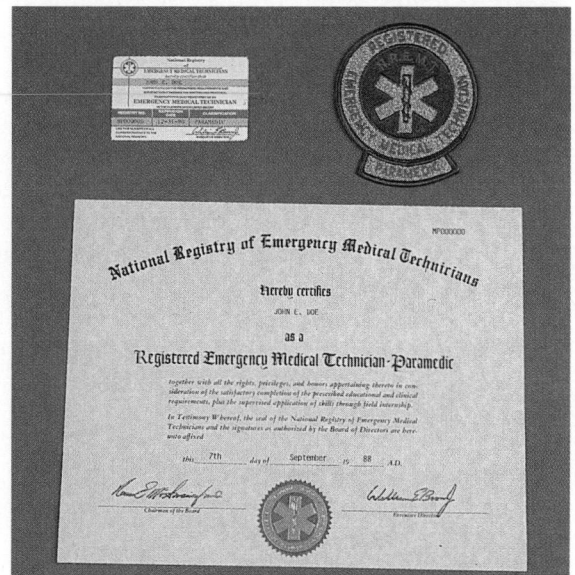

FIGURE 1-8 The National Registry of Emergency Medical Technicians develops and administers standardized testing for all levels of EMT from EMT-Basic to EMT-Paramedic. Completion of the National Registry testing may follow completion of an approved paramedic training program.

National Registry

The National Registry of EMTs is an agency that prepares and administers standardized testing materials for First Responder, EMT-Basic, EMT-Intermediate, and EMT-Paramedic. (See Figure 1-8.) This agency assists in developing and evaluating EMT training programs. It establishes the qualifications for registration and biennial re-registration. The registry is currently the only vehicle for establishing a national minimum standard of competency. As such, it serves as a major tool for reciprocity. The exam provides verification at the national level of paramedic training and sets a medical-legal standard for evaluating the competence of paramedics to deliver quality ALS patient care.

Professional Journals

A variety of journals are available to keep the paramedic aware of the latest changes in an ever-changing industry. These journals also provide an abundant source of continuing education material, as well as an excellent opportunity for EMS professionals to write and publish articles.

SUMMARY

To become a paramedic, you must be willing to accept the responsibility of being a leader in the prehospital phase of emergency medical care. The responsibilities include on-call emergency duties and off-duty preparation. When the emergency call comes in, you must already be prepared to respond. If you are not, it is too late.

It is important to begin your paramedic training with the understanding that you will not be spending the majority of your time in emergency medical situations. Instead, you will spend most of your time preparing yourself to do the job properly. If you can accept this reality and if you are willing to undertake the responsibility of preparing for this dynamic occupation, then you are ready to begin your paramedic education. Remember: The best paramedics are those who make a commitment to excellence.

FURTHER READING

Ampolsk, A.G. "Paramedics, EMTs push for licensing." *Emergency.* 22(4) 48, 1990.

Dick, T. and L. Federoff. "Why Do Paramedics Intimidate Their Leaders." *JEMS* 17(2) 63, 1992

Gregory, A. "Playing Prophet." *Emergency.* 24(12) 28-35, 1992.

Iserson, K.V., *et al. Ethics in Emergency Medicine.* Baltimore: Waverly Press, 1986.

National Academy of Sciences, National Research Council. *Accidental Death and Disability: The Neglected Disease of Modern Society.* Washington, DC: U.S. Department of Health, Education, and Welfare, 1966.

Page, James O. *The Paramedics.* Morristown, NJ: Backdraft Publications, 1979.

_____ *The Magic of 3 AM.* Solana Beach, CA: JEMS Publishing, 1986.

Pantridge, J.F., and J.S. Geddes. "A Mobile Intensive Care Unit in the Management of Myocardial Infarction." *Lancet,* 2 (1967) 271–273.

U.S. Department of Transportation. *National Standard Curriculum: Emergency Medical Technician–Paramedic.* Washington, DC, 1985.

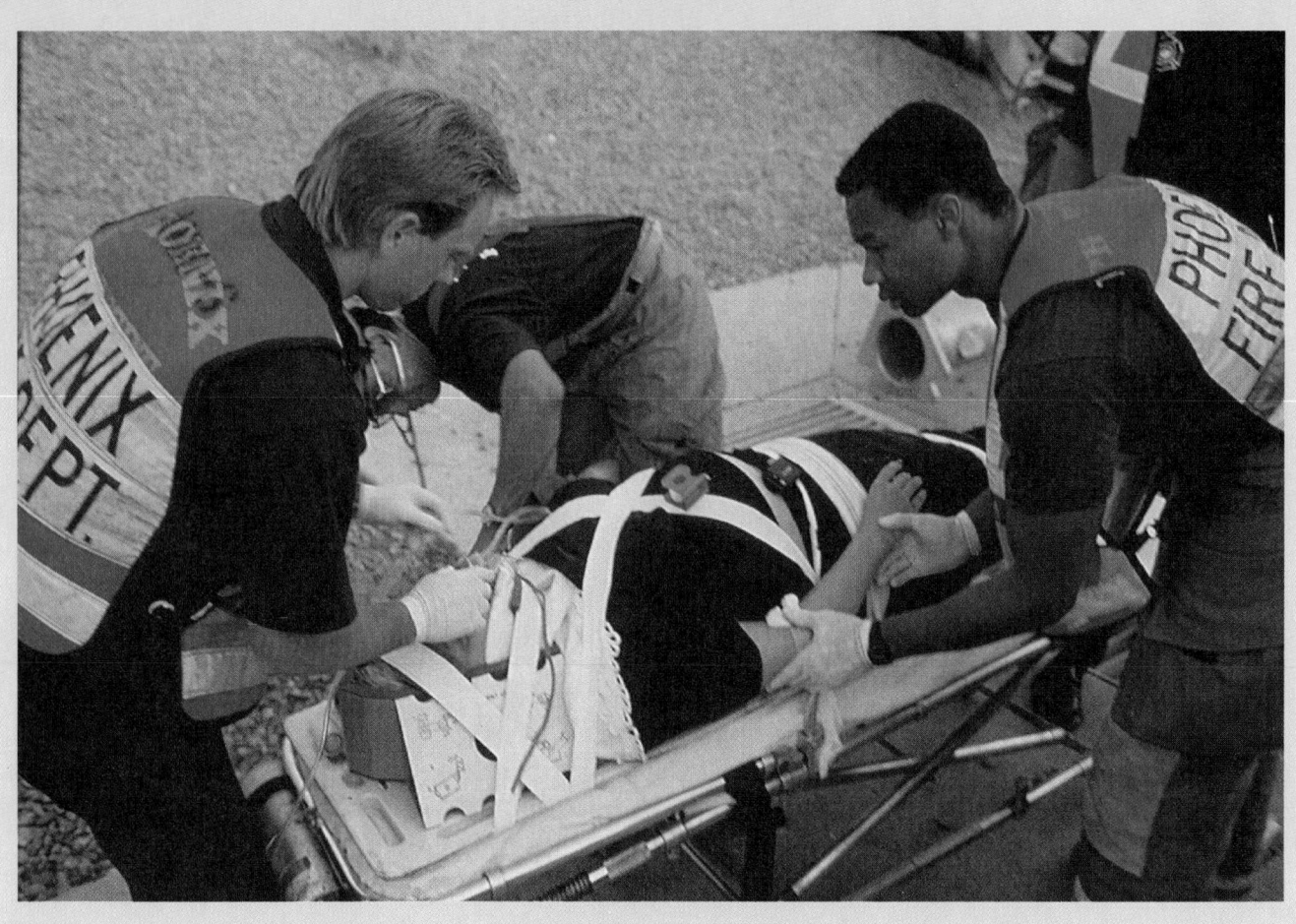

2

EMERGENCY MEDICAL SERVICES SYSTEMS

Objectives for Chapter 2

After reading this chapter, you should be able to:

1. Describe the development of the EMS system in the United States. (See pp. 20–21.)

2. List and define the components of an EMS system. (See pp. 20–21.)

3. Explain the oversight duties of an EMS administrative agency. (See pp. 21–22.)

4. Discuss the responsibilities of the physician medical director regarding direct-line and indirect-line medical control. (See pp. 22–24.)

5. Describe public involvement in an EMS system, with regard to system access, recognition of an emergency, and initiation of basic life support. (See pp. 24–25.)

6. Describe the components of an effective medical and operational communications system. (See pp. 25–26.)

7. Describe the components of emergency medical dispatching: system status management, interrogation guidelines, response protocols, pre-arrival instructions, and dispatcher training. (See pp. 26–28.)

8. Describe the use of patient transfer protocols for ground and air transport services. (See pp. 31–32.)

9. Describe the importance of quality evaluation in EMS, and discuss the similarities and differences between Quality Assurance and Quality Improvement programs. (See pp. 32–33.)

10. Discuss the value of research in EMS. (See p. 34.)

11. Describe the categorization of receiving facilities, and explain how the coordination of resources is attained. (See pp. 34–35.)

12. List the components of mutual aid and mass-casualty planning. (See p. 36.)

13. Outline the various designs and financing methods for an EMS system. (See p. 36.)

On Saturday morning, Mr. Chlopek gets up as usual at 7:30 to mow the yard. He hasn't been feeling right the last few days and dreads the yard work. Nonetheless, he starts the mower and begins to mow. After making the first pass, he develops a terrible pressure in his chest. He feels as if he's been kicked in the chest. He leaves the mower running and sits down on the gasoline can. By now, he is pale and is sweating profusely. Shortly, his vision goes black, and he falls to the ground.

Across the street, Mr. Webber is retrieving his morning paper and sees Mr. Chlopek collapse. Mr. Webber, a high school football coach, runs across the street. He quickly sees that his friend is in cardiac arrest. He calls for help and starts CPR. Another neighbor arrives to help. Mr. Webber instructs him to call EMS. When he calls 9–1–1, the badly shaken neighbor blurts out to the dispatcher: "Hurry! Bill collapsed and John is doing CPR." In his excited state, he could not recall his neighbor's address and hangs up to go help.

The dispatcher is able to determine the address through the enhanced 911 system. He then dispatches the appropriate EMS response. Within two minutes, the First Responders, who are members of the volunteer fire department, arrive. They assume care of the patient and begin two-person CPR. Within another two minutes, the EMT-Intermediate (EMT-I) crew arrives by rescue unit. The EMTs quickly apply an automatic defibrillator, and a countershock is delivered within five minutes of the patient's collapse. Two minutes later, the paramedics arrive and assume care from the EMTs. The patient now has a pulse and is being effectively ventilated with supplemental oxygen. The paramedics place an IV and administer 100 milligrams of lidocaine and start a lidocaine drip. They package the patient and transport him to Central Hospital.

In the emergency department, the physician quickly evaluates the patient. An ECG confirms the presence of an anterior wall myocardial infarction. Tissue Plasminogen Activator (TPA) is administered and the patient is transferred to the coronary care unit. Here a cardiologist assumes his care. The patient does well. Two weeks after his heart attack, he undergoes a coronary artery bypass graft (bypass surgery). He is discharged 10 days later.

INTRODUCTION

■ **EMS System** a comprehensive approach to providing emergency medical services.

The **Emergency Medical Services (EMS) system** is a complex health care system made up of personnel, equipment, and resources. The EMS system has several components. The prehospital component includes:

- ❏ Lay persons trained in CPR
- ❏ The First Responder
- ❏ The Emergency Medical Technician
- ❏ The paramedic

The hospital component includes:

- ❏ The emergency department nurse
- ❏ The emergency physician
- ❏ Specialty physicians (e.g., trauma surgeons, cardiologists)

Support personnel also help the EMS system operate smoothly. In the prehospital phase, they include EMS dispatchers, law-enforcement personnel, firefighters, and other public-safety workers. In the hospital, respiratory therapists, radiologic technicians, and other specialists provide important support services. All components of the system must work together to assure quality patient care.

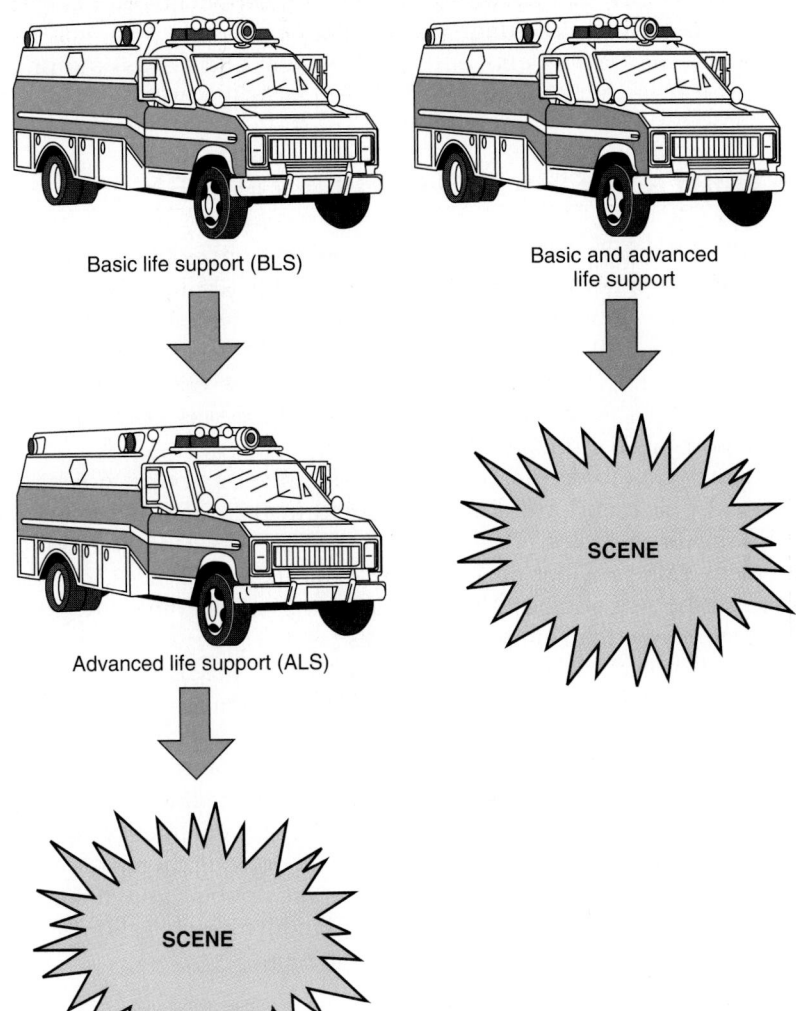

Basic life support (BLS)

Basic and advanced
life support

Advanced life support (ALS)

SCENE

SCENE

FIGURE 2-1 Some systems utilize a tiered response. BLS responders arrive first. ALS care, if required, arrives later. Other systems simply dispatch an ALS vehicle on each call.

Usually, the first EMS person to respond to a medical emergency is the First Responder. The First Responder may be a police officer, firefighter, or lay person who has received basic emergency medical training in an approved First Responder program. The First Responder's role is to stabilize the patient until the EMT or paramedic arrives. First Responders are trained in CPR, basic airway management, and other basic skills.

The next component is the EMT. The EMT may respond in a fire department vehicle or in an ambulance. He or she should either continue the stabilization started by the First Responder or initiate life support measures. The next component, the paramedic, should provide advanced life support care, if indicated. Several EMS systems are **"tiered"** in this order of incident response. (See Figure 2-1.) Care is handled by EMTs unless advanced life support is indicated. In many other EMS systems, however, paramedic personnel respond to every incident in case advanced life support care is needed.

Upon arrival at the hospital emergency department, patients are usually assigned priorities for care by a nurse or physician. Then the emergency department nurse and physician take over. If needed, a surgeon or other specialist will be summoned to the emergency department.

■ **tiered response** a type of EMS system where BLS-level vehicles are initially dispatched to all calls unless ALS-level care is needed.

The system depends on the strength of all its components. A weakness in any one of them weakens the entire system, and patient care suffers. This chapter will address the components of the EMS system and discuss the problems that may arise in such a system.

THE HISTORY OF EMS SYSTEM DEVELOPMENT

Emergency Medical Services (EMS) is a health care system requiring the integration of several components. It is designed to provide appropriate care for all emergency patients. Until the late 1960s, few areas provided adequate prehospital emergency medical care. The prevailing thought was that care began in the hospital emergency room. Rescue techniques were crude, ambulance attendants poorly trained, and equipment minimal. There was no radio communication and no physician involvement.

Eventually, as costs forced many mortician-operated ambulance services to withdraw, local police and fire departments had to provide this service. In many areas, volunteer groups were formed. The result was a proliferation of local, independent EMS provider agencies that could barely, if at all, communicate with each other. In addition, it was impossible to coordinate response activities on a scale larger than simple, local calls.

The publication in 1966 of "Accidental Death and Disability: The Neglected Disease of Modern Society," by the National Academy of Sciences, National Research Council, focused national attention on the problem. "The White Paper," as the report came to be called, spelled out the deficiencies in prehospital emergency medical care. It also suggested guidelines for the development of EMS systems, the training of prehospital emergency medical providers, and the upgrading of ambulances and their equipment. Although many improvements have been made since the report's publication, a surprising number of inadequate services still exist. This landmark publication set off a series of federal and private initiatives. They included:

1966—Congress passed the National Highway Safety Act, which forced the states to develop effective EMS systems or risk losing federal highway construction funds.

1971—The White House funded nearly $9 million toward EMS demonstration projects. These projects were designed to be models for subsequent system development.

1972—The Robert Wood Johnson Foundation provided grants for establishing regional EMS projects and communications systems.

1973—Congress passed the Emergency Medical Services Systems Act, which provided funding in a series of projects awarded to develop regional systems. In order to be eligible for this funding, an EMS system had to include the following 15 components specified by the act:

1. Manpower
2. Training
3. Communications
4. Transportation
5. Emergency facilities
6. Critical care units
7. Public safety agencies
8. Consumer participation
9. Access to care

10. Patient transfer
11. Standardized record–keeping
12. Public information and education
13. System review and evaluation
14. Disaster management
15. Mutual aid

Unfortunately, the designers of this legislation left out two major components: system financing and medical control. When federal funding was significantly reduced in the early 1980s, many systems faced economic disaster and lacked a solid plan for financial recovery. Even worse, many systems were operating without physician direction. The legislative oversights have meant a long, uphill battle for medical directors attempting to re-establish authority and accountability for medicine practiced by EMTs and paramedics in the streets. In many ways, the EMS Systems Act paved the way for system development. But in some respects, it sent EMS in the wrong direction. This act was amended in 1976 and again in 1979. A total of $215,000,000 was appropriated over a seven-year period toward the establishment of regional EMS systems.

In 1981, the passage of the Consolidated Omnibus Budget Reconciliation Act (COBRA) wiped out all federal funding for EMS, except block grant programs administered by the Department of Transportation and the Health and Human Services Administration. Only a small portion of this money, however, is available for EMS activities. These funds are given to the states, which in turn disburse the money to formally established regional systems. Since 1972, some areas have been able to manage their grant monies effectively. These areas have developed strong, efficient systems of prehospital emergency medical care. But many other areas have not. Today, in this technologically advanced country, there are still startling regional differences in the quality of prehospital care.

THE SYSTEMS APPROACH

The efficient delivery of emergency medical care requires a team effort and a systematic approach to get the best use of existing resources. There is no "best" method for providing prehospital emergency medical care in a given area. However, certain essential elements are considered "standard" for ensuring the best possible patient care in any region. Each system must develop operational policies for its components. Included among these policies are the items described in the rest of this chapter.

System Administration

An administrative agency should first be established. This agency will be responsible for managing the local system's resources and for developing operational guidelines and standards for each component. A budget is created to operate the system and to select a qualified administrative staff. The agency should incorporate a planning board—composed of providers, representatives of the medical community, emergency physicians, and consumers—that will advise and assist the agency in setting policy.

Once established, the agency will designate who may function within the system. It will develop policies consistent with existing state requirements. The EMS agency must develop a quality assurance or quality improvement program to evaluate the system's effectiveness and to ensure that the best interest of the patient is always top priority. In short, the needs of the patient are determined first; then the system is designed to meet those needs. The coordination of system components to meet the patient's needs is the responsibility of the EMS agency.

In addition to regional and municipal EMS agencies, EMS agencies also exist on the state level. The state EMS agencies are typically responsible for allocating funds to local systems, enacting legislation concerning the prehospital practice of medicine, licensing and certifying field providers, enforcing all state EMS regulations, and appointing regional advisory councils. In essence, EMS is a series of systems within a system. The integration of these systems and the cooperation of all participants result in a better quality of emergency medical care.

Medical Control

■ **medical director** a physician, who by experience or training, handles the clinical and patient care aspects of the EMS system.

The EMS system will retain a **medical director**, who will be actively involved in, and ultimately responsible for, all clinical and patient care. All prehospital medical care provided by non-physicians is considered an extension of the medical director's license. Every prehospital ambulance or rescue service must have a medical director who is responsible for that service. Prehospital care providers are designated agents of the medical director, regardless of whose employees they may be. For this reason, the medical director determines which providers may care for patients within the system. The medical director is the ultimate authority in all direct-line and indirect-line medical control issues. (See Figure 2-2.)

■ **direct medical control** communications between field personnel and a medical control physician during an emergency run; also known as on-line control.

Direct Medical Control **Direct medical control** exists when prehospital providers communicate directly with a physician at a medical control or resource hospital. The physician's direction is usually based on established protocols for managing specific problems. This physician assumes responsibility and gives treatment orders for patients. Direct medical control physicians should be experienced in emergency medicine. They should have completed a training program that emphasizes system particulars, treatment protocols, and communications policies and procedures. Once they've become proficient in these areas, they should go through a formal certification process. They

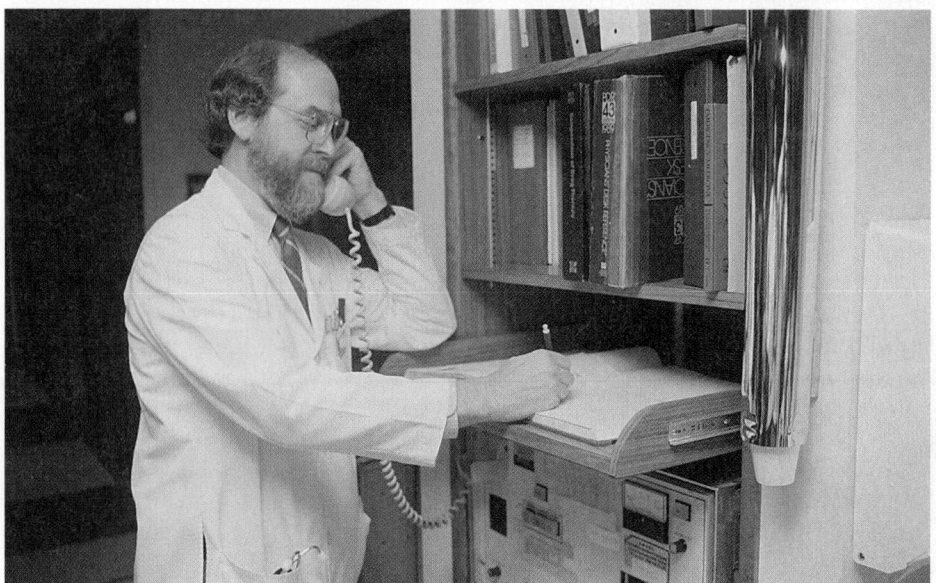

FIGURE 2-2 Medical control is an essential component of EMS. There are two aspects of medical control—direct and indirect. On-line medical control, as depicted here, provides immediate direction for on-scene care.

should also be required to ride with crews to get a feel for the realities of pre-hospital field medicine. Medical control communications are sometimes delegated to a mobile intensive care nurse (MICN), physician assistant (PA), or paramedic. In all circumstances, however, ultimate on-line responsibility rests with the medical control physician.

Control of a medical emergency scene should go to the individual with the most knowledge and best training in prehospital emergency stabilization and transport. When an advanced life support unit, under medical direction, is requested and dispatched to the emergency scene, a physician/patient relationship is established by the physician providing medical control. The paramedic is responsible for the subsequent management of the patient and acts as the medical control physician's agent, unless the patient's physician is present (as in a doctor's office). If a private physician is present and assumes responsibility for the patient's care, the paramedic should defer to the physician's orders.

The ALS unit's responsibility reverts to the direct medical control physician whenever the private physician is not in attendance (in the back of the ambulance, for example). If an **intervener physician** is present and on-line medical control does not exist, the paramedic should relinquish responsibility to the physician. But first, the physician must identify himself or herself and demonstrate a willingness to accept responsibility and to document the intervention as required by the local EMS system. If the treatment differs from established protocol, however, the physician should accompany the patient to the hospital. If an intervener physician is present and direct medical control does exist, the on-line physician is ultimately responsible. In case of disagreement between the intervener physician and the on-line physician, the paramedic must take orders from the on-line physician and put him or her in contact with the intervening physician.

Indirect Medical Control   **Indirect medical control** includes training and education, protocol development, audit, chart review, and quality assurance. To be effective, medical control must have official and clearly defined authority, with the power to discipline, or limit the activities of, those who deviate from the established standard of care. (See Figure 2-3.)

✳ All advanced life support activities may only be carried out under the direction of the medical control physician.

■ **intervener physician** a licensed physician, professionally unrelated to patients on the scene, who attempts to assist paramedic field crews.

■ **indirect medical control** the establishment of system policies and procedures, such as treatment protocols and case reviews; also known as off-line medical control.

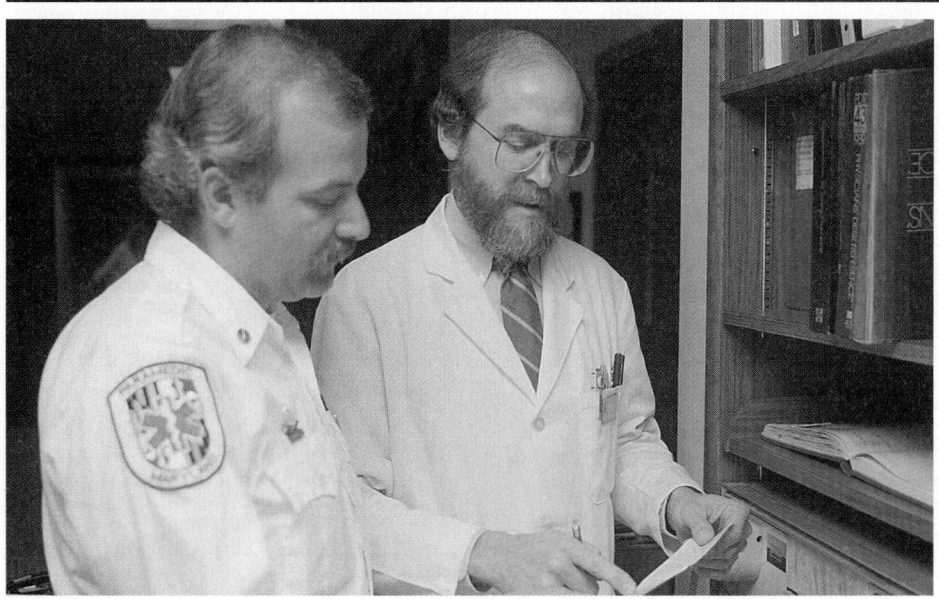

FIGURE 2-3   Indirect medical control includes training, chart review, protocol development, audit, and quality assurance.

Protocols are designed by the off-line medical control system to provide a standardized approach to common patient problems and a consistent level of medical care. When treatment is based on such protocols, the on-line physician assists prehospital personnel in interpreting the patient's complaint, understanding the findings of their evaluation, and applying the appropriate treatment protocol. Protocols will be designed around the four T's of emergency medical care. They include:

❏ Triage
❏ Treatment
❏ Transport
❏ Transfer

Triage guidelines help the physician make decisions involving patient flow through an EMS system. This simply means allocating the system's resources to the needs of victims. The EMS dispatcher will determine the type, level, and priority of response to the victim. The victim will then be directed to the appropriate receiving facility, which can provide definitive care or stabilize the victim until he or she is transferred to a definitive care facility.

Treatment often includes emergency interventions by field personnel. Some procedures will be done upon a direct order from the medical control physician. Others will be **standing orders**. Treatment protocols should be kept current with new research.

Transport involves decisions about mode (air vs. ground) and the level of care during transport (ALS vs. BLS, paramedic vs. nurse, nurse vs. physician, etc.). Most plans call for taking the patient to the closest appropriate facility, as designated by the system. Transport plans are based on three factors:

1. Nature of the injury or illness
2. Condition of the patient
3. Estimated transport time

Transfer protocols cover the management of inter-hospital patient transfer. They allow for region-wide continuity of care when patients are transferred. Agreements between receiving facilities within the system ensure that the patient is admitted to the definitive care facility.

Protocols will also be established for special circumstances, such as the proper handling of "Do Not Resuscitate" orders, patients who refuse treatment, sexual abuse, abuse of children or elderly persons, initiation and termination of CPR, and intervener physicians. (See Chapter 3.) Although protocols standardize field procedures, they should allow the paramedic flexibility to improvise and adapt to special circumstances. Protocols establish a basis for medical care and a standard for accountability in an EMS system.

Public Information and Education

The public is an essential, yet often overlooked, component of an EMS system. An EMS system should have a plan to educate the public about recognizing an emergency, accessing the system, and initiating basic life support.

The American Heart Association (AHA) estimates that 350,000 cardiac arrests per year occur before the patient reaches the hospital. Most happen within two hours of the onset of cardiac symptoms, because many patients deny that something is wrong and delay calling for help. If the patient, a family member, friend, or bystander can recognize the emergency and intervene in time, many cases of sudden death can be prevented. Families of patients with coronary artery disease should be targeted for instruction in recognizing emergency symptoms.

The second aspect of public education is system access. Systems with 9-1-1 telephone service make emergency access easy. The phone number should be well-publicized, and citizens should be taught how to give information to the emergency medical dispatcher. For regions with a single, seven-digit access number, the process is similar. For areas with multiple access numbers, however, the problem may be overwhelming. In any case, the public must learn how to access the system efficiently in an emergency, thereby avoiding life-threatening delays.

After recognizing that a medical emergency exists, the bystander must initiate basic life support (BLS) procedures such as cardiopulmonary resuscitation (CPR). This could also include initial patient care after major trauma and hemorrhage control. Abundant research in the last 10 years indicates a relationship between response times and the patient's ultimate recovery. Communities that have many citizens trained in BLS, plus a rapid paramedic response, have proven that a large number of patients can be successfully resuscitated. On the other hand, communities weak in prompt bystander CPR have shown a much lower rate of recovery. The role of the bystander in emergency medical care is critical to successful resuscitation of a cardiac arrest victim. The AHA estimates that 100,000–200,000 lives could be saved each year in the United States with implementation of community CPR programs and fast paramedic response.

Future public involvement may include bystander defibrillation. Research shows increasing numbers of successful first-responder defibrillation programs. With the advent of automatic external defibrillators, the technology may someday allow affordable, portable automatic defibrillators in public places—such as theaters, churches, and malls—or in the homes of cardiac patients. The public component must not be overlooked when designing or improving an EMS system.

EMS Communications

The communications network is the heart of any regional EMS system. Coordinating the components into an organized response to urgent medical situations requires a comprehensive, flexible, communications plan. The basic components of a communications system include the following six elements:

1. Citizen access
2. Single control center
3. Operational communications capabilities
4. Medical communications capabilities
5. Hardware
6. Software

Any citizen with an urgent medical need should have a simple and reliable mechanism for accessing the EMS system. A well-publicized universal number, such as 9-1-1, provides direct citizen access to the communications center. Multiple community telephone numbers add life-threatening minutes to any emergency response system. The basic emergency telephone number, 9-1-1, available from American Telephone and Telegraph (AT&T) since 1967, is a toll-free telephone service that enables the caller to dial three digits to reach a single public safety answering point. Enhanced 9-1-1 (E-911) gives automatic location of the caller, instant routing of the call to the appropriate public emergency service (fire, EMS, police), and instant callback capabilities should the caller hang up too soon.

A single communications center that can communicate with and direct all emergency medical units in the system is best. (See Figure 2-4.) Systems with multiple control points cannot ensure the best use of resources or the best emergency response. The EMS dispatcher should be in charge of all emergency vehicle movements in the area to maintain system readiness. Ideally, all public service agencies should be dispatched from the same communications center. The communications center should be able to reach emergency vehicles throughout a large geographical area. In some regions, repeaters and relays may be needed.

Operational communications allow efficient and effective use of the system's resources. After the caller has successfully accessed the system, the EMS dispatcher must be able to communicate with emergency units to provide the best response and to facilitate operations on the scene. Emergency units must also be able to communicate with each other and with other agencies during mutual aid and disaster operations. Hospitals must be able to communicate with other hospitals in the region to assess specialty capabilities. The organizational plan enables the EMS dispatcher to manage effectively all aspects of system response and to assess the system's readiness for the next response.

Medical communications allow the paramedic to communicate with the receiving facility and, in many areas, to transmit ECG telemetry signals to the on-line physician. Hospitals must also be able to communicate with each other (usually by a land-line or microwave network) to facilitate patient transfer.

Communications hardware includes radios, consoles, pagers, transmission towers, repeaters, telephone land lines, and any other telecommunications equipment required to operate the system. Communications hardware is discussed in more detail in Chapter 4.

Software includes the radio frequencies used for various functions and the communications protocols used by the system. Radio procedures, policies consistent with FCC standards and local protocols, and backup communications plans for disaster operations are essential.

An EMS system must have an effective, practical communications network. No one system design will meet the needs of all communities. Each regional system should design a communications network that is simple, flexible, and practical.

Emergency Medical Dispatching

Emergency medical dispatching is the nerve center of an EMS program. The activities of medical dispatchers are crucial to the efficient operation of the system. Dispatch is the means of assigning and directing appropriate medical care to the victim. An emergency medical dispatching plan should include pre-established interrogation protocols, pre-assigned response configurations, system status management, and pre-arrival telephone instructions. Medical direction for the emergency medical dispatcher should be given by the EMS medical director. Quality assurance of the EMS dispatch program is an EMS agency responsibility.

Any effective emergency medical dispatching system has certain key components. EMS dispatchers do more than send ambulances; they make sure the system's resources are in a constant readiness to respond. System status management relies on projected call volumes and locations, not geographical or political tradition, to strategically place ambulances and crews. The system is used to reduce response times.

* The EMS communications system must be tailored to the individual needs of the local EMS system.

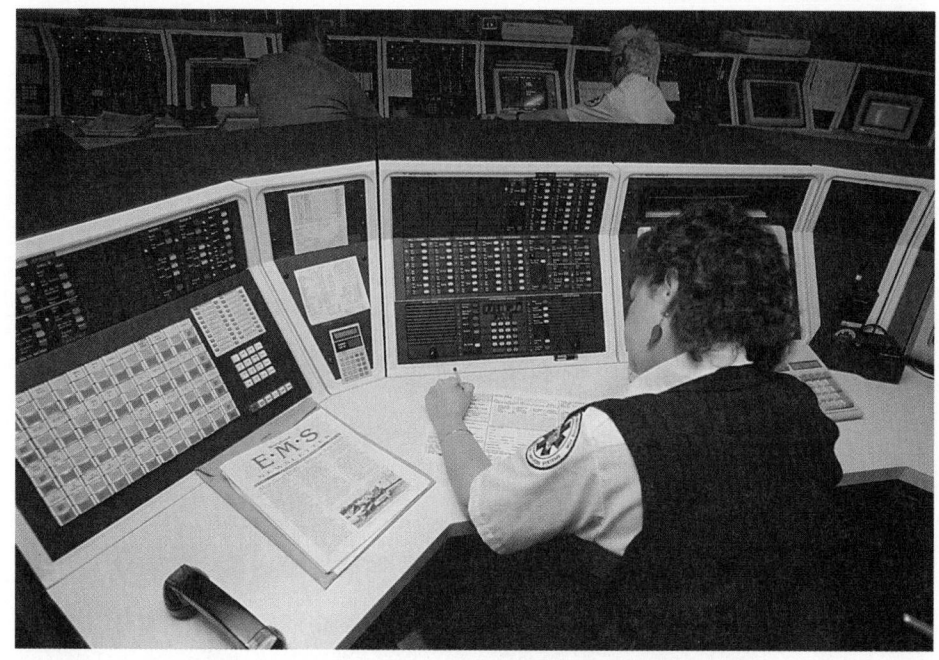

Another dispatch system is priority dispatching. In this system, first used by the Salt Lake City Fire Department, medical dispatchers are trained to medically interrogate a distressed caller, prioritize symptoms, select the appropriate response, and give lifesaving pre-arrival instructions. A set of medically approved protocols is used by all dispatchers. These priorities must reflect the level of appropriate response, including types of personnel, number of vehicles, and mode of response. During the interrogation, the dispatcher asks a set of standard questions to determine the level of response.

In 1974, the Phoenix Fire Department introduced a pre-arrival instruction program developed by medically trained dispatchers. While emergency units are responding, the caller may initiate lifesaving first-aid techniques with the dispatcher's help. In 1985, the Seattle EMS system initiated a successful program of instructing callers in CPR. Critics of this service point out the increased liability of priority dispatching and of treatment instruction by dispatchers. Even so, the increased liability of not providing the service may far outweigh the risk of providing it.

Medical dispatchers must be both medically and technically trained. Emergency Medical Dispatch (EMD) training should cover basic telecommunication skills, medical interrogation, the giving of pre-arrival instructions, and dispatch prioritization. The course should be standardized and should include certification by a governmental agency. (See Figure 2-5.)

✱ EMS Dispatchers must be both medically and technically trained.

An effective EMS dispatching system will place first responding units on the scene within four minutes following the onset of the emergency. The AHA reports that brain resuscitation will be unsuccessful if response times exceed four minutes, unless there was proper BLS intervention (CPR). While systems must be prepared for the worst-case scenario (sudden death), their design must provide for a rapid BLS response.

Many studies have suggested that definitive care (defibrillation) in sudden death victims within eight minutes can produce 43 percent successful outcomes with patients in ventricular fibrillation. Many systems are now using EMTs or First Responders for this definitive care. Early defibrillation programs have been extremely successful across the country in reversing sudden death

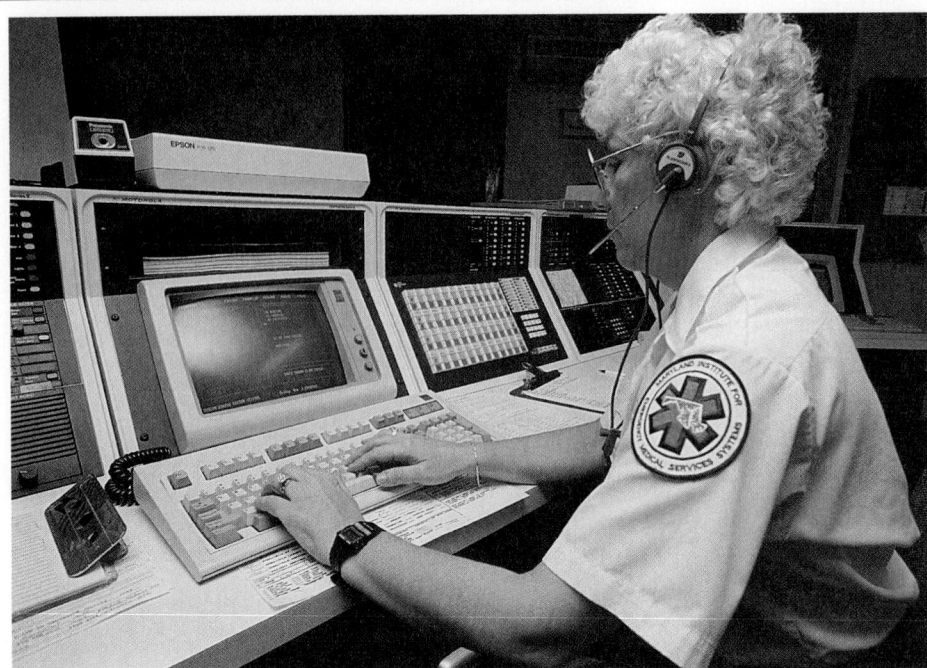

FIGURE 2-5 The EMS dispatcher of today is a skilled professional. Ideally, all EMS dispatchers should complete an approved Emergency Medical Dispatch training program. Concurrent EMT or paramedic certification is desirable.

mortality. The goal of emergency response is: BLS care in less than four minutes, and ALS care in less than eight minutes following the event. High-performance systems meet this standard more than 90 percent of the time.

An effective emergency medical dispatching program should include pre-established caller interrogation protocols, pre-determined response configurations, system status management, and pre-arrival caller instructions. It should be under full control of the physician medical director and the EMS agency.

Education and Certification

The two kinds of education programs for EMS personnel are original education and continuing education. Original education programs are the initial training courses for prehospital providers. They involve the completion of a standardized course that meets or exceeds the United States Department of Transportation (USDOT) national curriculum for that level (EMT-Basic, EMT-I, EMT-P). Continuing education programs include refresher courses for recertification and periodic in-service training sessions. All education programs should have a medical director who is involved in the EMS system. The EMS agency is responsible for assuring funding for these programs.

There is a variety of prehospital certification levels for communities to choose from. In 1983, because of variations in state and regional EMS terminology, there were as many as 30 levels of prehospital care providers. Since then, the National Registry of EMTs has recognized, and the Department of Transportation has developed curricula for, three levels. These include:

- ❏ *EMT-Basic*. The EMT-basic should be competent at CPR, airway management, hemorrhage control, stabilization of fractures, emergency childbirth, basic extrication, communications, and use of the pneumatic anti-shock garment. In some cases, the EMT may undergo additional training in defibrillation.
- ❏ *EMT-Intermediate*. The EMT-Intermediate (EMT-I) should possess all the EMT-Basic skills. In addition, he or she should be competent at

■ **EMT-Basic** a person, currently certified, who has successfully completed the U.S. Department of Transportation (USDOT) National Standard Curriculum for EMT-Basic.

■ **EMT-Intermediate** a person, currently certified, who has successfully completed the USDOT National Standard Curriculum for EMT-I.

advanced airway management, intravenous fluid therapy, and certain other advanced skills. (See Figure 2-6.)

❑ *EMT-Paramedic.* The EMT-Paramedic should possess all the skills required of an EMT-Basic and EMT-I. In addition, he or she should be trained in advanced patient assessment, trauma management, pharmacology, cardiology, and other medical emergencies. Paramedics should successfully complete Advanced Cardiac Life Support (ACLS) and Pediatric Advanced Life Support (PALS) courses as offered by the American Heart Association. Basic Trauma Life Support (BTLS) or Prehospital Trauma Life Support (PHTLS) course completion is also desirable. (See Figure 2-7.)

The curricula for these primary education programs include classroom lectures, practical skills lab work, hospital clinical experience, and, at the advanced levels, a supervised field internship.

The training of prehospital personnel is a critical phase of EMS system design. Attitudes and values that are learned in the classroom carry over into the streets. EMS instructors should remember that the process of training is as important as the training itself. The goal is for personnel to graduate from the program with a high regard for human dignity and a passion for excellence. In addition, graduates realize that certification marks the beginning—not the end—of their education. Instructors who inspire excellence and set an example for being punctual and reliable will graduate students who value those virtues.

Patient Transportation

Patients who are transported under the direction of an emergency medical services system should be taken whenever possible to the closest appropriate medical facility. The medical control physician should be the authority to designate that facility, based on the needs of the patient and the availability of services. In some cases, the patient's need for special services—trauma, burn, pediatric, etc.—means designating a facility that is not nearby. At other times, the closest facility will be designated for stabilization of the patient while transfer is arranged. The ultimate authority for this decision, however, remains with the on-line medical control physician.

All transport vehicles, ground and air, should be licensed and locally approved. Equipment lists should be consistent with system-wide standards. In 1983, the American College of Surgeons' Committee on Trauma recommended a standard set of equipment to be carried by providers of basic life-support services. In 1988, the American College of Emergency Physicians (ACEP) published a recommended list of advanced life-support supplies and equipment to be carried on ALS units. Both sets of recommendations serve as excellent guidelines for any prehospital EMS system. Regional standardization of all equipment and supplies would best facilitate interagency efforts during disaster operations.

In 1974, in response to a request from the Department of Transportation, the General Services Administration developed the KKK-A-1822 Federal Specifications for Ambulances. This was the first attempt at standardizing an ambulance design to permit intensive life support for patients en route to a definitive care facility. The act defined the following three basic types of ambulances:

❑ *Type I.* Conventional cab and chassis on which a modular ambulance body is mounted, with no passageway between driver's and patient's compartments. (See Figure 2-8.)

■ **EMT-Paramedic** a person, currently certified, who has successfully completed the USDOT National Standard Curriculum for EMT-P.

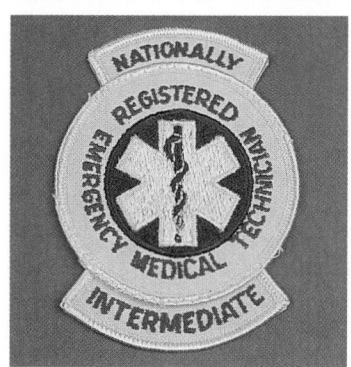

FIGURE 2-6 The EMT-Intermediate provides limited, advanced life support care typically including IV therapy and advanced airway management.

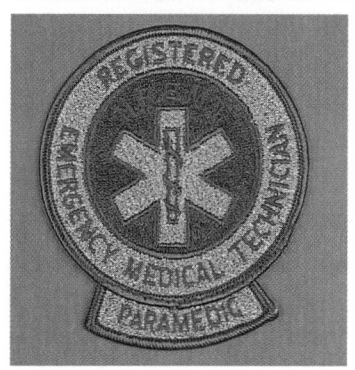

FIGURE 2-7 The EMT-Paramedic is the highest level of training for prehospital providers. He or she should be trained in all aspects of advanced prehospital care.

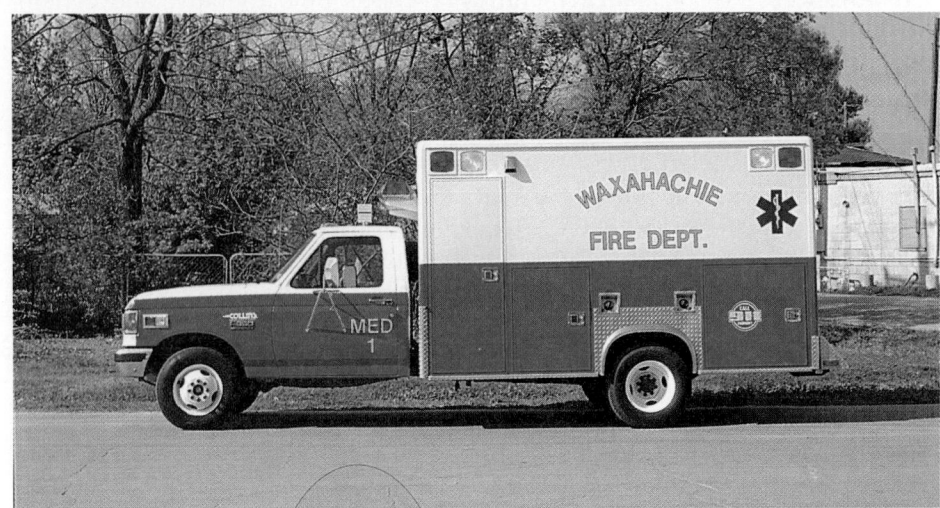

FIGURE 2-8   Type I ambulance.

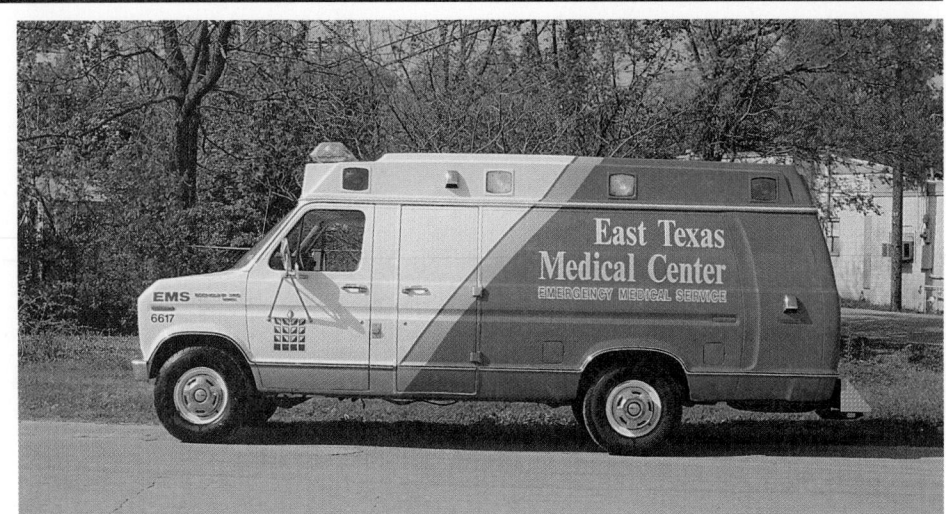

FIGURE 2-9   Type II ambulance.

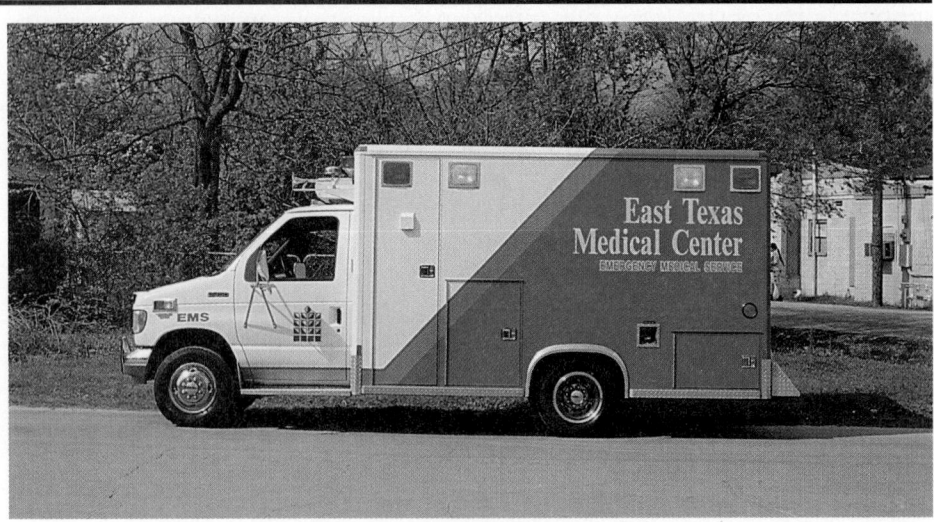

FIGURE 2-10   Type III ambulance.

- ❑ *Type II.* Standard van, body, and cab form an integral unit; most have a raised roof. (See Figure 2-9.)
- ❑ *Type III.* Specialty van with forward cab and integral body, with passageway from driver's compartment to patient's compartment. (See Figure 2-10.)

Only these certified ambulances may display the registered "Star of Life" symbol as defined by the USDOT's National Highway Traffic Safety Administration (NHTSA). The word "AMBULANCE" should appear in mirror image on the front of the vehicle so that other drivers can identify the ambulance in their rear view mirrors.

In 1980, revision KKK-A-1822A aimed at improving ambulance electrical systems by designing a low-amp lighting system to replace antiquated light bars and beacons. This standard helped to reduce electrical system overloads. In 1985, revision KKK-A-1822B specified changes based on National Institute for Occupational Safety and Health (NIOSH) standards. These include reduced internal siren noise, high engine temperatures, and exhaust emissions; safer cot-retention systems; wider axles; hand-held spotlights; battery conditioners for longer life; and venting systems for oxygen compartments. The KKK specifications are intended to improve the safety, reliability, and function of ambulances. All ambulances purchased with federal funds during the 1970s were required to comply with these criteria. Since then, however, some states have adopted their own stricter criteria.

Aeromedical Transportation   Patients can be transported by ground or air. The use of helicopters for medical transport was introduced during the Korean War and expanded in Vietnam. The success of these military evacuation procedures led to their use in civilian ambulance systems. In 1970, the Military Assistance to Safety and Traffic (MAST) program was established. This demonstration project set up 35 programs nationwide to test the feasibility of using military helicopters and paramedical personnel in civilian medical emergencies. Today, trauma care systems use military, law enforcement, municipal, hospital-based, and private helicopter transport services to transfer patients. (See Figures 2-11 and 2-12.) Fixed-wing aircraft are also used when patients must be transported long distances, usually more than 120 miles.

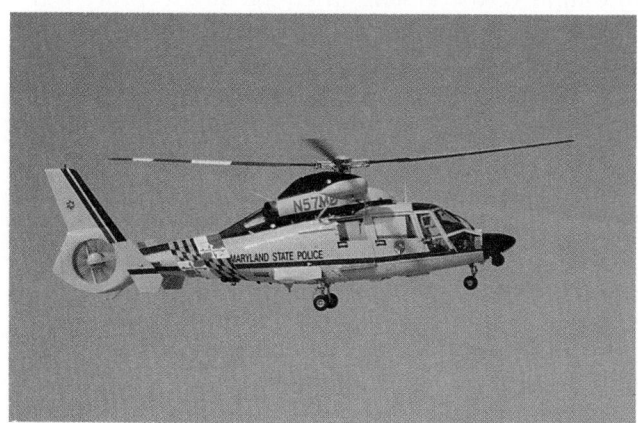

FIGURE 2-11 The helicopter has become an integral and important aspect of prehospital care. The helicopter offers smooth and rapid transport as well as a mechanism for providing specialized emergency care, once limited to the hospital, at the scene of the medical emergency.

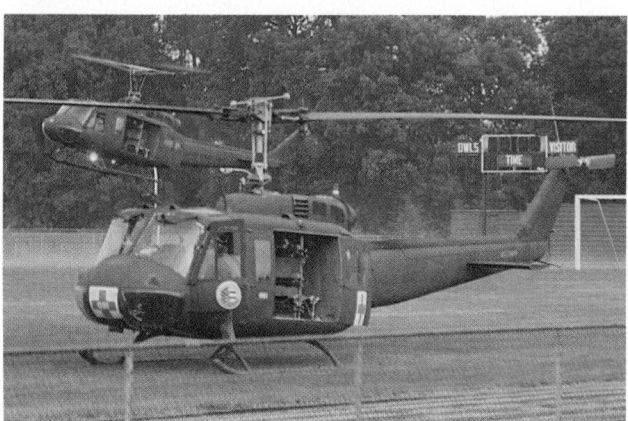

FIGURE 2-12 The military helicopter proved its value in reducing morbidity and mortality in the Vietnam war. Military helicopters are frequently made available to assist civilian EMS systems.

Getting the right patient to the right facility requires a transport system that includes specific patient transfer protocols coordinated by a single agency. These protocols should be based on severity of injury, length of travel, and availability of resources at the facility. Since the early 1970s, trauma care systems, such as the Maryland Institute for Emergency Medical Services Systems (MIEMSS), have designated various levels of receiving facilities around the state. MIEMSS employs a single system communications center (SYSCOM) to coordinate the aeromedical transport of critical trauma patients to the appropriate facility. The state is divided into five regions, in which ground and air transport resources are strategically placed for the maximum benefit of all Maryland residents. The Maryland system works well because it is a coordinated, well-organized operation.

Quality Assurance and Quality Improvement

An EMS system must be designed to meet the needs of the patient. In EMS, patients are the users of the system and hence the "customer." The quality of an EMS system is reflected in the daily medical practices of its prehospital care providers. *In EMS, the only acceptable quality is excellence.* Because of this, the EMS system of today must have a program to evaluate the quality of service provided. For a quality evaluation program to be effective, it must be comprehensive and continuously ongoing. In addition, the EMS system must be willing to react to the quality evaluation program and to adjust its practices and procedures accordingly.

Many EMS systems have ongoing quality assurance programs, while others have gone a step further and initiated quality improvement programs. A **Quality Assurance (QA)** program is primarily designed to maintain continuous monitoring and measurement of the quality of clinical care delivered. QA programs emphasize evaluation of objective clinical data such as response times, adherence to protocols, patient survival, and other key indicators of system performance. QA programs document the effectiveness of the care provided. They also help identify problems and select areas that need improvement. A common complaint of QA programs is that they tend only to identify problems and focus on punitive corrective action. Thus, prehospital personnel often view QA programs negatively.

As a result, many EMS systems have taken QA a step further and now utilize **Quality Improvement (QI)** for evaluating system performance. A QI program focuses on customer perceptions of the service provided. It is an ongoing effort to refine and improve the system in an attempt to provide the highest level of service possible. In addition to clinical issues, a QI program evaluates other aspects of the EMS system such as billing, maintenance, supply, and so on. Ultimately, all components of an EMS system, whether they be clinical or non-clinical, affect patient care. In a QI program, the emphasis is on service with customer satisfaction being the ultimate indicator of quality. In contrast to QA programs, QI programs focus on recognizing, rewarding, and reinforcing good performance instead of simply pointing out problems.

"Take-It-for-Granted" Quality   EMS quality can be divided into two broad categories. The first is something we can call "take-it-for-granted" quality. These aspects of our system are traditionally clinical and something that our customers take for granted. People take it for granted that when they call 9-1-1 we will respond quickly and that the ambulance will not break down. Most of our patients are not medical professionals and must assume that we are always acting in their best interest. Thus, they take it for granted that the care they receive from us is safe, appropriate, and the best that is available. Quality improvement in this area is best accomplished through ongoing education of personnel and continuous evaluation of the system.

* In EMS, the only acceptable quality is excellence

■ **Quality Assurance (QA)** quality evaluation program that is designed to objectively identify problems within the system. A QA program deals primarily with clinical issues.

■ **Quality Improvement (QI)** quality evaluation program that emphasizes service and uses customer satisfaction as the ultimate indicator of system performance.

Clinical evaluation and improvement should be subject to rigorous examination prior to implementation and periodically thereafter. When we want to add a new medication, process, or procedure to the system, we should follow set rules. These rules, often called the "Rules of Evidence," were developed by Joseph P. Ornato, M.D., Ph.D. They include the following guidelines.

1. *There must be a theoretical basis for the change.* That is, the change must make sense based on relevant anatomy, physiology, biochemistry, and other basic medical sciences. For example, automatic defibrillators and intravenous fluid therapy have a solid theoretical basis for their use.

2. *There must be ample scientific human research to support the idea.* Any device or drug used in patient care must have adequate scientific human research to justify its use. The pneumatic anti-shock trouser (PASG) is a device that has been frequently used in EMS. However, there is an inadequate amount of scientific human research to support its use. Therefore, the evaluation process should stop here for the PASG. It would have never been put into wide-spread use if EMS systems had ongoing programs for evaluating quality.

3. *It must be clinically important.* The device, medication, or procedure must make a significant clinical difference to the patient. For example, a device such as an automated external defibrillator may mean the difference between living and dying for some patients, while color-coordinated stretcher linen has little clinical significance.

4. *It must be practical, affordable, and teachable.* Some medical devices remain too expensive and too impractical for use in routine prehospital emergency care. Prehospital placement of intra-aortic balloon pumps may save a few lives. However, the equipment is both expensive and impractical for field use. It would also be difficult to train prehospital personnel to place the balloon properly.

If a clinical innovation or improvement meets all these guidelines, then the change should probably be made. Only devices, drugs, and procedures that pass these rigorous tests should be implemented.

Paramedics can improve their aspect of "take-it-for-granted" quality by reading, taking classes, reviewing each other's patient charts, soliciting feedback on clinical performance from nurses and physicians at receiving hospitals, and following up on patients. We expect excellence from the system, and we should accept no less than excellence from ourselves.

Service Quality   The second type of quality can be categorized as "service quality" or "relationship quality." In the business world, this type of quality is called "customer satisfaction." This is the kind of quality that individual customers get excited about, feel good about, and tell stories about. These are the little extras that exceed customer's expectations and elicit thank you letters. Prime examples of customer satisfaction include such patient statements as: "You fed my cat before we left." "You remembered my name and introduced me to the nurse." "You held my hand." "You seemed like a friend when I needed one."

Customer satisfaction can be either created or destroyed in a brief moment with a simple word or deed. A significant part of the way we communicate with one another is through the subconscious use of body language or through tone of voice. Paramedics who genuinely care about their patients communicate this in many subtle ways. From the patient's perspective, this is much more important than IVs, backboards, and EKGs. It is essential to remember the ultimate reason for our existence: To serve the patient and to provide the highest quality service and patient care available.

Research

In order to provide a scientific basis for prehospital EMS, a formal ongoing **research** program is an essential component of the system. Existing and future procedures, techniques, and equipment must be evaluated scientifically. For moral, educational, medical, financial, and practical reasons, an EMS system design must include research. Unfortunately, many protocols and procedures that paramedics use today have evolved without clinical evidence of their usefulness, safety, or benefit to the patient.

Future EMS research projects must address the following issues:

1. Which prehospital field interventions actually reduce morbidity and mortality?
2. Are the benefits of certain paramedic field procedures worth the potential risks?
3. What is the cost/benefit ratio of sophisticated prehospital EMS systems?
4. Is field stabilization possible, or should paramedics begin immediate transport in every case?

As a paramedic, you should be familiar with the components of a research project. First, you identify a problem and explain the reason for the study. Next, you state a hypothesis, or the precise question to be asked. Third, you research the literature to identify the body of published knowledge. Then you select the best design for study, with all logistics clearly outlined and all patient-consent issues examined and approved. When you have completed these steps, the study can begin. The raw data are then collected, analyzed, and correlated in a statistical application. The results are assessed and evaluated against the original hypothesis. The final step is writing a cohesive, comprehensive paper for publication in a medical journal.

Paramedics are encouraged to participate in research projects. Current EMS practice must be justified by hard clinical data derived from an objective, valid program of ongoing research.

Receiving Facilities

Not all hospitals are equal in emergency and support service capabilities. Hospital categorization identifies the readiness and capability of a hospital and its staff to receive and effectively treat emergency patients. Categorization originated from the realization that patients have varying degrees of illness and injury and that receiving facilities have varying capabilities to provide initial or definitive care. A facility categorization system lets the EMS system's coordinators know in advance of specialty areas within the EMS delivery system. This knowledge expedites the transportation of emergency patients to hospitals that will provide definitive treatment, or lifesaving stabilization, until transfer can be arranged.

Once categorization has been established, regionalizing available services helps give all patients reasonable access to the appropriate level of facility. Burn, trauma, pediatric, psychiatric, perinatal, cardiac, spinal, and poison control centers are examples of specialty-service facilities that offer high-level care for specific groups of patients. Large EMS systems should designate a resource hospital that will coordinate the system's specialty resources and ensure appropriate patient distribution.

Ideally, receiving facilities should have the following capabilities: an emergency department with an emergency physician on duty at all times; surgical facilities; a lab and a blood bank; and X-ray capabilities available around

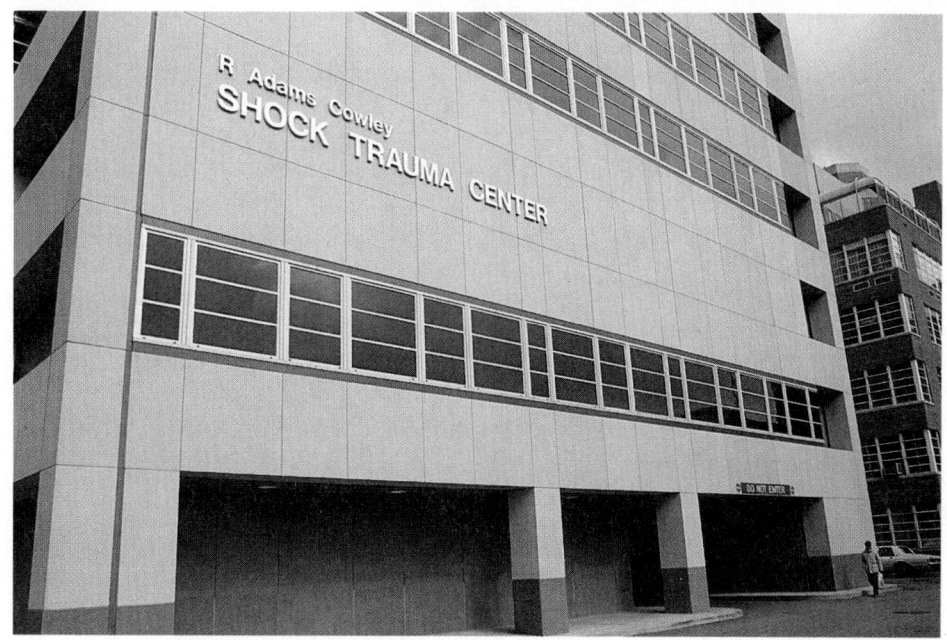

FIGURE 2-13 Hospital emergency departments have evolved along with EMS. A prime example is the R. Adams Cowley "Shock Trauma Center" in Baltimore, Maryland.

the clock. In addition, receiving facilities should have critical intensive care units, a documented commitment to participate in the EMS system, and a willingness to receive all emergency patients in transport, regardless of their ability to pay. They should also have the ability to provide medical audit procedures to ensure quality assurance and medical accountability. Finally, receiving facilities should exhibit a desire to participate in mass-casualty preparedness plans. (See Figure 2-13.)

A hospital categorization inventory is designed to match the clinical needs of emergency patients with the emergency facility best prepared to treat them. This should result in a system of regional hospitals that provides highly specialized emergency care. (See Figure 2-14.)

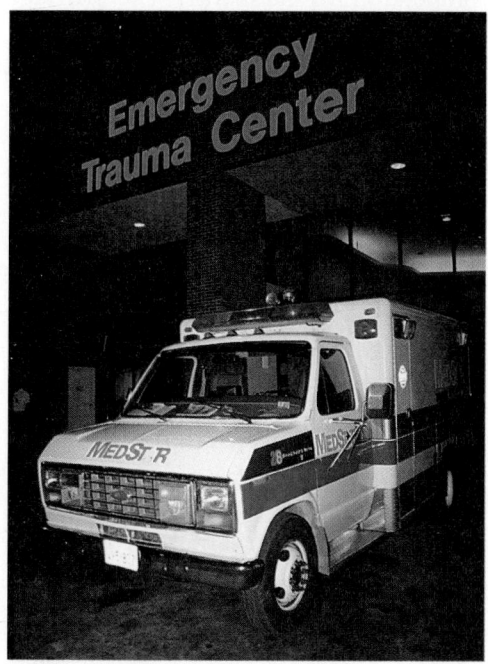

FIGURE 2-14 Hospital emergency departments should be categorized based on their ability to provide care. This categorization should be based upon staffing, physical plant, equipment, and availability of specialty care.

Mutual Aid/Mass-Casualty Preparation

No system is an island, and the resources of any region will sometimes be overwhelmed. A formalized mutual-aid agreement policy will ensure that help is available when needed. Mutual-aid agreements can be between neighboring departments, municipalities, systems, and even states. Cooperation among all EMS agencies must supersede geographical, political, and historical boundaries.

Each system should put in place a mass-casualty plan for unexpected catastrophes that may overwhelm available resources and normal operations. There should be a coordinated central management agency that identifies commanders within the framework of the incident command system and the existing mutual aid plan. The plan should integrate all EMS system components and have a flexible communications system. Frequent drills should test the plan's effectiveness and practicality. The communications, dispatch, and control systems should be capable of coordinating a system-wide response to a major medical incident without a major change in personnel, equipment, or operating protocol. Standardized apparatus, equipment, supplies, and radio hardware and software will facilitate shifting from everyday operations to disaster mode. Specific components of a mass-casualty plan will be discussed in Chapter 6.

System Financing

At present in the United States, there is a wide variety of EMS system design. EMS services can be hospital-based, fire department- or police department-based, municipal third service, private commercial business, volunteer, or some combination thereof. Major differences exist in the philosophy of EMS system finance, from fully tax-subsidized municipal systems to all-volunteer squads supported solely by contributions. EMS funding can come from the following sources: tax subsidies, contributions, corporate sponsorship, subscription plans, Medicare, Medicaid, private medical and auto insurance, fund-raising activities, prepaid health care programs (HMO), and user fees.

Two new approaches to system financing include the Public Utility Model and the Failsafe Franchise. In these systems, a municipality establishes the design and standards for the contract bid, then periodically—usually every three or four years—holds wholesale competition for the market. The provider firm that wins the contract must manage services properly and efficiently throughout the contract term or face severe penalties.

SUMMARY

An EMS system comprises a number of components, all of them crucial to providing emergency medical care for sick and injured people. The system is a continuum of care: from the EMT who conducts public education classes; to the mechanic who keeps the ambulance fleet running; to the emergency medical dispatcher who calms a distressed caller and provides lifesaving instructions over the phone; to the paramedic who provides field intervention; to the emergency department physician, surgeon, and physical therapist who will see the patient through definitive care and rehabilitation. No one component, no one person, is more important than another. EMS is a total team effort.

EMS systems are designed with the patient as the highest priority. They begin with a strong administrative agency, which structures the system around the patients' needs and grants the medical director ultimate authority in all issues of patient care. The medical director is an emergency physician who remains actively involved in all components of the system.

An EMS system aims to get help to patients as quickly as possible. Most EMS systems use a single-number access (911). They also rely on a centralized communications center that handles all medical emergencies in the area and coordinates all levels of communication—operational and medical—within the region. EMS dispatchers, who are trained and certified, control the movement of all emergency medical units within the area. They have pre-designed interrogation protocols, pre-established priority response modes, and system status management procedures. They also give pre-arrival instructions. On at least 90 percent of all emergency calls, the system places BLS units on the scene in four minutes, ALS units in eight minutes. Coordination of ground and air transport service follows established protocols at the communications center.

Mutual-aid agreements ensure a continuum of care during peak-load periods and personnel shortages. Disaster plans are formalized, rehearsed regularly, and revised when necessary. Hospitals are categorized according to their readiness to provide essential and specialty services within the region. Personnel are trained according to the USDOT national standard curricula. An ongoing continuing education program encourages each system provider to achieve excellence. A quality improvement program documents the system's performance daily. An ongoing research program attempts to validate the actions of prehospital providers through scientific, clinical evaluation. Finally, the system flourishes because of a strong, stable financial plan that ensures consistent patient care of the highest quality.

FURTHER READING

American College of Emergency Physicians, Emergency Medical Services Committee. "Control of Advanced Life Support at the Scene of Medical Emergencies." *Ann Emerg Med*, 23: 1994, pp. 1145–46.

American College of Emergency Physicians. "Prehospital Advanced Life Support Skills, Medications, and Equipment." *Ann Emerg Med*, 17: 1988, pp. 1109–1111.

American Heart Association: Committee on Cardiac Care. "Guidelines for Cardiopulmonary and Emergency Cardiac Care." *JAMA*, 268: 16, October 21, 1992, pp. 21, 2171–2299.

American Medical Association, Joint Review Committee on Educational Programs for EMT–Paramedic. "Essentials and Guidelines of an Accredited Educational Program for the Emergency Medical Technician–Paramedic," revised 1989.

Clawson, J. J., and K.B. Dernocoeur. *Principles of Emergency Medical Dispatch*. Englewood Cliffs, NJ: Prentice Hall, 1986.

Cowley, R. A., *et al.* "An Economical and Proved Helicopter Program for Transporting the Emergency and Critically Injured Patient in Maryland." *J. Trauma*, 13: 1973, pp. 1029–1038.

Eisenberg, M., *et al.* "Paramedic Programs and Out–of–Hospital Cardiac Arrest: Factors Associated with Successful Resuscitation." *American Journal of Public Health*, 69: 1979, pp. 30–38.

Eisenberg, M. S., *et al.* "Emergency CPR Instruction via Telephone." *American Journal of Public Health*, 75: 1985, pp. 47–50.

"Essential Equipment for Ambulances." *Am Coll Surg Bull*, 68: 1983, pp. 36–38.

Hacker, L. P. "Time and Its Effects on Casualties in World War II and Vietnam." *Arch Surg*, 98: 1969, pp. 39–40.

Hunt, R. C., *et al.* "Influence of Emergency Medical Services Systems and Prehospital Defibrillation on Survival of Sudden Cardiac Death Victims." *American Journal of Emergency Medicine*, 7: 1989, pp. 68–82.

Kuhl, A., "National Association of EMS Physicians," *EMS Directors' Handbook*. St. Louis, MO: CV Mosby, 1989.

National Academy of Sciences, National Research Council. "Accidental Death and Disability: The Neglected Disease of Modern Society." Washington, DC, U.S. Department of Health, Education, and Welfare, 1966.

National Association of EMS Physicians: Consensus Document on Emergency Medical Dispatching.

Page, J.O., *et al.* "Twenty Years Later." *JEMS*, 11: 1988, pp. 30–43.

Powers, Robert J., and Mike Taigman, "Debating Quality Assurance vs. Quality Improvement." *JEMS*, January 1992, pp. 65–70.

Stout, J.L. "Measuring Your System." *JEMS*, January 1983, pp. 84–91.

_____. "System Status Management." *JEMS*, 1983, pp. 22–30.

_____. "Ambulance System Designs." *JEMS*, January 1986, pp. 85–99.

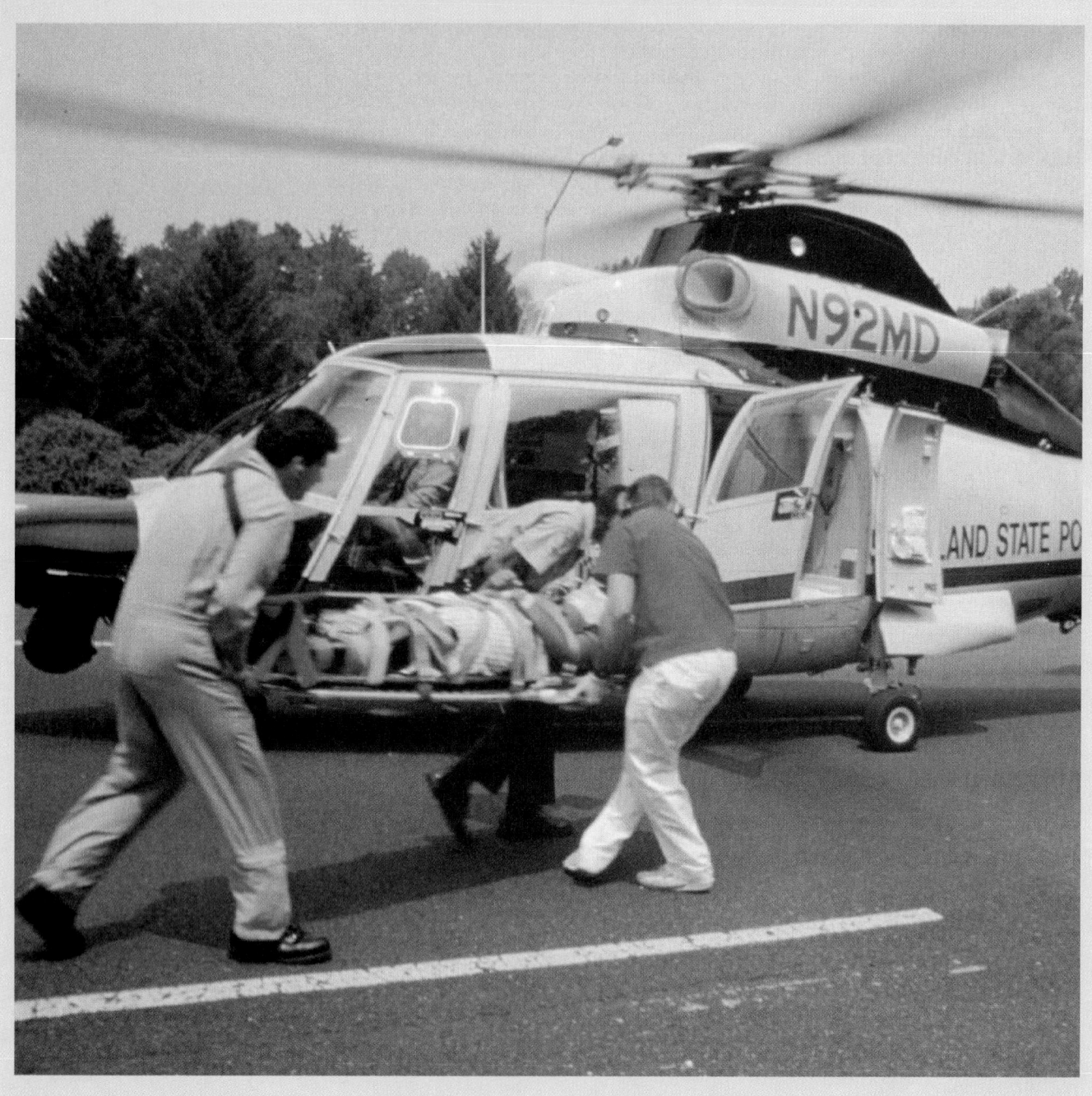

3

MEDICAL-LEGAL CONSIDERATIONS OF EMERGENCY CARE

Objectives for Chapter 3

After reading this chapter, you should be able to:

1. Describe the two general categories of law in the United States. (See pp. 41.)

2. Define the following terms. (See below pages.)
- tort (p. 41.)
- negligence (p. 44.)
- duty to act (p. 44.)
- abandonment (p. 46.)
- false imprisonment (p. 46.)
- slander (p. 47.)
- libel (p. 47.)

3. Describe the medical practice act and its implications in prehospital care. (See pp. 41.)

4. Explain what is meant by the term "delegation of authority." (See pp. 41.)

5. Describe the purpose and limitations of Good Samaritan Laws. (See pp. 41.)

6. Explain the need to know state motor vehicle laws that apply to emergency vehicles. (See pp. 41.)

7. Define a "Living Will" and a "Durable Power of Attorney for Health Care." (See pp. 42.)

8. Discuss the concept of "standard of care" as it applies to prehospital care. (See pp. 44.)

9. List and define the four components required to prove negligence in a malpractice proceeding. (See pp. 44.)

10. Discuss the concept of *res ipsa loquitur*. (See pp. 44–45.)

11. Discuss the following types of consent. (See below pages.)
- expressed consent (p. 45.)
- implied consent (p. 45.)
- involuntary consent (p. 45.)

12. Define the term "informed consent," and relate it to the practice of prehospital emergency care. (See pp. 45.)

13. Define assault and battery, and give examples of each. (See pp. 46.)

14. Discuss the importance of the medical record. (See pp. 47–48.)

15. List several methods of protecting yourself from malpractice liability. (See pp. 47–48.)

EMS Unit 706 receives a call to assist a person with altered mental status. A bystander has given the dispatcher only limited information. She reports that the police are en route to the scene, which is reported to be near the intersection of highways 38 and 317.

Although traveling from different directions, the ambulance and police officers arrive simultaneously. The paramedics immediately notice a middle-aged male staggering near the shoulder of the road. A truck is parked nearby. The paramedics deem the scene safe and approach the patient behind the police officers. The lead police officer asks the patient if anything is wrong. The patient immediately turns and lunges at the officer. The officer subdues the patient, who thrashes around briefly before losing consciousness.

The paramedics rush in to do their job. They quickly assess airway, breathing, and circulation. They detect no other problems during this primary assessment. Upon beginning the secondary assessment, however, they note a Medic-Alert bracelet that says "Diabetic." They now suspect hypo-glycemia. While one paramedic completes the secondary survey, the other performs a rapid glucose determination with a Glucometer and notes the blood sugar to be 26 mg/dL. Per approved standing orders, an IV is established and 50 mL of 50 percent dextrose is administered.

The patient immediately arouses. He becomes fully oriented and politely thanks the paramedics. He then notes some recent problems with dosing his insulin and reports two other episodes of hypo-glycemia in the past two weeks.

The paramedics urge the patient to go to the hospital for additional evaluation. The patient declines, stating that he already has scheduled a physician's appointment and that he is late for a business meeting. The paramedics assure themselves that the patient is fully conscious and that he is oriented and capable of refusing consent. They then aseptically discontinue the IV, have the patient sign a "refusal of transport" form, and have it witnessed by a police officer. They return their equipment to the ambulance and notify the dispatcher that they are back in service.

INTRODUCTION

Legal issues are an important concern of the paramedic. As a paramedic, you will interact with the legal system frequently, and you must be familiar with all its components. In addition, you must be familiar with all laws affecting pre-hospital care. This chapter will address the medical-legal aspect of emergency care, with emphasis on prehospital care. (See Figure 3-1.)

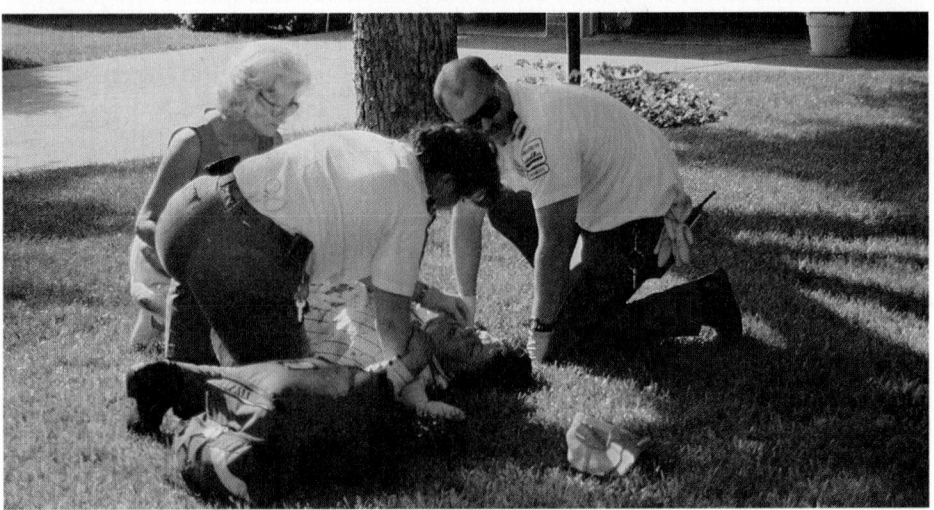

FIGURE 3-1 Each EMS response has the potential of involving EMS personnel in the legal system.

LEGAL PRINCIPLES

The United States has two general categories of law—civil law and criminal law. Both are subject to principles set forth in the U.S. Constitution. **Criminal law** deals with crime and punishment. Criminal **litigation** involves legal action by a state against an offending individual. Homicide and rape are examples of criminal wrongs. **Civil law**, on the other hand, deals with non-criminal issues, such as contracts and domestic relations. Civil litigation involves conflicts between two or more parties. Examples of civil litigation include disputes over divorce, contracts, and child custody. **Tort law**, a branch of civil law, deals with civil wrongs committed by one individual against another (rather than against society). A malpractice suit is an example of a tort.

As an EMT or paramedic, you may become involved in any aspect of the legal system. You may be called as a witness in a criminal offense. You may be asked to testify in a civil matter, such as a divorce or a contract dispute. And you could be named in malpractice litigation.

■ **criminal law** the division of the legal system that deals with wrongs against society or its members.

■ **litigation** the act or process of carrying on a lawsuit.

■ **civil law** the division of the legal system that deals with non-criminal issues and conflicts between two parties.

■ **tort law** a branch of civil law concerning civil wrongs between two parties.

LAWS AFFECTING EMS

Most laws that affect emergency medical services and paramedics are state laws. Although these laws often vary from state to state, they have several principles in common. This section will address common legal principles, laws, and legislation that affect the paramedic.

Medical Practice Acts and State EMS Legislation

A *medical practice act* is state legislation that defines the scope and role of the paramedic and all prehospital workers. Often, a state will have a general medical practice act that governs all health care professionals.

Paramedics are not licensed to practice independently. Paramedics may only function under the direct supervision of a licensed physician, through a **delegation of authority**. This term means that, as a paramedic, you are practicing under the auspices and license of the physician. Supervision may be direct—by telephonic or radio communications—or by accepted, approved standing orders. Failure to adhere to this requirement could make you criminally liable for practicing medicine without a license.

Most states have EMS laws that govern paramedics and set forth the requirements for certification, or licensure, and recertification, or relicensure. In addition, most states have laws and regulations that define the skills and procedures a paramedic may perform. It is your responsibility to understand fully the EMS laws and regulations of your state.

■ **delegation of authority** the granting of privileges by a physician to a non-physician to perform well-delineated skills and procedures.

✷ The paramedic may only function under the direct supervision of a licensed physician.

Good Samaritan Laws   Virtually every state has **Good Samaritan Laws**, which protect from liability people who assist at the scene of a medical emergency. Many states have expanded these laws to cover prehospital personnel. Generally, a person is immune from liability for assisting at the scene of a medical emergency if he or she acts in good faith, is not negligent, acts within the scope of his or her training, and does not accept payment for his or her services. The Good Samaritan Laws of many states now protect prehospital personnel, even though they may be paid.

■ **Good Samaritan Laws** laws designed to protect from liability persons who assist at the scene of a medical emergency.

Motor Vehicle Laws   As with EMS laws, motor vehicle laws vary from state to state. It's important that you know the laws of your state. Generally, there are special motor vehicle laws governing the operation of emergency vehicles. These laws may apply to such considerations as speed and use of the siren and emergency lights. In addition, many municipalities have local rules and regulations for emergency vehicles. You should keep up to date on state and municipal laws where you work.

Other Laws   Many states have enacted laws to protect the public. The paramedic must abide by these laws. Most states have laws requiring a health care worker who suspects child abuse or abuse of the elderly to report the incident. Violent crimes, such as rape and shootings, should also be reported to law enforcement officials. Emergencies that threaten public health, such as animal bites, must be reported to the appropriate authority.

As a paramedic, you should be familiar with local laws and regulations governing the use of physical restraints for violent or confused patients. You should also be familiar with the regulations governing entry into restricted areas, such as military installations, nuclear power plants, and sites with hazardous materials.

Right to Die

Advances in medical technology have saved thousands of lives. However, in some instances, the use of sophisticated medical technology may only be prolonging inevitable death instead of sustaining life. When a person is seriously injured or gravely ill, family members must make very difficult decisions regarding the intensity of medical care to be rendered, including the use or withdrawal of life-support systems. To improve communications between patients, their family members, and physicians regarding these important issues, the federal government enacted the Patient Self-Determination Act of 1990. This act requires hospitals and physicians to provide patients and their families with sufficient information to make informed decisions about medical treatment and use of life-support measures, including cardiopulmonary resuscitation (CPR).

■ **living will** a written request to withhold heroic life support measures from a patient with a terminal condition. A living will is usually executed before the person becomes ill or injured and is used to express that person's wishes.

Living Wills   Many patients choose to make their personal decisions regarding medical treatment and artificial life-support known ahead of time through the use of a living will. A **living will** is a legal document that allows the patient to specify the kinds of medical treatment he or she wishes to receive should the need arise. (See Figure 3-2.) Many states will allow patients to specify in a living will their desires on a number of sensitive issues: Whether to die in a hospital or at home, whether to receive CPR in the event of a cardiac arrest, whether to donate organs and other body parts, or whether to specify a particular person to speak on their behalf. Living wills, once signed and witnessed, are effective until they are revoked by the patient.

Patients with prolonged illnesses sometimes invoke the right to choose a person to make health care decisions for them in the event that their mental functions become impaired. They might formalize this decision either through a special notation in a living will or through execution of what is known as a

■ **Durable Power of Attorney for Health Care** a legal document whereby a patient designates another person to make health care decisions for them.

Durable Power of Attorney for Health Care. Paramedics should respect patient requests expressed through valid living wills and properly executed Durable Powers of Attorney for Health Care. If a question arises concerning these issues, the medical control physician should be contacted for further direction.

Do Not Resuscitate Orders   "Do Not Resuscitate" (DNR) orders are a particular problem. Paramedics will often be called to nursing homes or residences where they may find a patient in cardiac arrest and in need of resusci-

TEXAS

LIVING WILL
DIRECTIVE TO PHYSICIANS

Directive made this_____day of _____(month/year).

I, _____, being of sound mind, willfully and voluntarily make known my desire that my life shall not be artificially prolonged under the circumstances set forth below, and do hereby declare:

　　If at any time I should have an incurable or irreversible condition caused by injury, disease, or illness certified to be a terminal condition by two physicians, and where the application of life-sustaining procedures would serve only to artificially prolong the moment of my death and where my attending physician determines that my death is imminent whether or not life-sustaining procedures are utilized, or will result within in a relatively short time without application of such procedures, I direct that such procedures be withheld or withdrawn, and that I be permitted to die naturally.

　　In the absence of my ability to give directions regarding the use of such life-sustaining procedures, it is my intention that this directive shall be honored by my family and physicians as the final expression of my legal right to refuse medical or surgical treatment and accept the consequences from such refusal.

　　If I have been diagnosed as pregnant and that diagnosis is known to my physician, this directive shall have no force or effect during the course of my pregnancy.

　　Other directions: *(You may use this space to make other requests of your caregivers.)*

　　This directive shall be in effect until it is revoked.

　　I understand the full impact of this directive and I am emotionally and mentally competent to make this directive.

　　I understand that I may revoke this directive at any time.

　　A duplicate copy of this directive shall have the same force and effect as the original.

Signed_____

City, County and State of Residence_____

　　I am not related to the declarant by blood or marriage; nor would I be entitled to any portion of the declarant's estate on his/her decease; nor am I the attending physician of the declarant or an employee of the attending physician; nor am I a patient in the health care facility in which declarant is a patient, or any person who has a claim against any portion of the estate of the declarant upon his/her decease. Furthermore, if I am an employee of a health care facility in which the declarant is a patient, I am not involved in providing direct patient care to the declarant, nor am I directly involved in the financial affairs of the health care facility.

Witness_____　Witness_____

This directive complies with the Natural Death Act, section 672.001
et seq. of the Texas Health and Safety Code (eff. Sept. 1, 1989).

FIGURE 3-2　Example of a living will.

tation. As a rule, the paramedic is legally obligated to resuscitate a patient. If a physician has written a specific order to avoid resuscitation, the EMS system should not have been summoned. However, legal living wills and bonafide "Do Not Resuscitate" orders should be honored. If there is any doubt, however, resuscitation should be initiated.

Occasionally, you may be requested to treat a patient as a "slow code" or "chemical code only." This is nonsense. Cardiac resuscitation is an "all-or-none" proposition. There is no such thing as treating a cardiac arrest with medications only, abandoning airway management and defibrillation. To do so amounts to negligence and must be avoided.

STANDARD OF CARE

* The paramedic is expected to practice the same level of care as any other competent paramedic in the community with equivalent training.

A paramedic is expected to practice the same level of care as any other competent paramedic in the community who has equivalent training. As a rule, you are expected to perform as any other "prudent person" would in a similar situation. Any deviation from this standard might open you to allegations of negligence.

Negligence and Medical Liability

■ **negligence** a deviation from an accepted standard of care. It is synonymous with malpractice in the context of medical care.

Negligence is defined as deviation from accepted standards of care recognized by law for the protection of others against unreasonable risks of harm. In medical care, negligence is synonymous with malpractice.

Grounds for Negligence In a malpractice proceeding, the complaining party must establish and prove four particular elements in order to win a lawsuit for negligence. First, the complainant must establish that the paramedic had a *duty to act*. This duty may be established by a contract, such as that between a private ambulance company and a city or county. In this case, the paramedic has a legal obligation to care for the patient. Often, however, the act of voluntarily assuming care of a patient implies that there was a duty to act.

Second, the complainant must prove there was a breach of duty by the paramedic. This simply means that the paramedic's conduct was not that expected of a reasonable, competent paramedic, given the same or similar circumstances. This breach can be failing to act, acting inappropriately, or acting beyond the level of certification or training.

Third, the complainant must prove there were damages—in other words, that he or she was harmed by the actions of the paramedic. This is an essential component. A lawsuit cannot be won if the defendant's actions caused no ill effects.

■ **proximate cause** a legal concept describing a person, who, through his or her actions, does something that produces an effect. In current usage, it usually means that a person was the immediate causative factor in a civil or criminal wrong.

Finally, the complaining party must prove that the paramedic's actions were the **proximate cause** of the damages. Proximate cause means that the actions of someone or something immediately caused the problem. For example, a patient who is injured in an ambulance accident could prove that his or her injuries resulted from the accident, and the accident was the "proximate cause" of the injuries. On the other hand, a patient who suffered a heart attack while in the ambulance would have difficulty proving that the ambulance ride was the "proximate cause" of his or her illness.

■ **res ipsa loquitur** a Latin phrase meaning "the thing speaks for itself," used in negligence proceedings.

Doctrine of *Res Ipsa Loquitur* Unlike criminal cases, which require proof "beyond a reasonable doubt," civil causes require only a proof of guilty by "preponderance of the evidence." As a result, a complainant may sometimes invoke the doctrine of ***res ipsa loquitur***, Latin for "the thing speaks for itself." The doctrine is used in cases in which it would be difficult for the complainant to prove all four elements of negligence. To support *res ipsa loquitur*, the complainant must prove that the damages would not have occurred in the absence of somebody's negligence, that the instruments causing the damages were under the defendant's control at all times, and that the patient did nothing to contribute to his or her own injury. When the doctrine of *res ipsa loquitur* is invoked in court, the burden of proof shifts from the plaintiff to the defendant.

An example of a case in which *res ipsa loquitur* might be used in the prehospital setting is the defibrillation of a conscious patient who does not have cardiac disease or dysrhythmia. To prove negligence, the plaintiff's attorney would have to show that the damage would not have occurred without the defibrillation, that the defibrillator was under the paramedic's control, and that the patient did not contribute to the injury. Many cases in which *res ipsa loquitur* would be successful are settled out of court.

Areas of Potential Medical Liability

There are several areas of potential liability that you should recognize and take into account when you care for patients.

Consent   **Consent** is the granting of permission to treat. More accurately, it is the granting of permission to touch. Consent is based on the concept that every human being of adult years and sound mind has the right to determine what shall be done with his or her own body. Touching a patient without appropriate consent may subject you to charges of assault and battery.

■ **consent** the granting of permission to treat by a patient to a health care provider.

For consent to be legally valid, it must be informed. That is, a patient must be made to understand the nature and risks of the procedures to be performed. The benefits and risks of planned treatments must be explained to the patient in a manner in which he or she understands. **Informed consent** must be obtained from every conscious, mentally competent adult person before treatment is started. In most states, a patient must be eighteen years of age or older in order to give or refuse consent. Persons under eighteen years of age who are married, in the armed services, or legally emancipated are considered adults. As such, they too may legally give consent or refuse treatment.

■ **informed consent** consent obtained only after the patient has had the risks and benefits of treatment explained in a manner which the patient understands.

✳ Patient care should always be preceded by valid patient consent.

Patients who do not meet the above criteria are considered minors. In the case of a minor, consent should be obtained from a parent, blood relative, or legal guardian. If one of these people cannot be located, and if the child is suffering an apparent life-threatening injury or illness, treatment may be rendered under the doctrine of implied consent, explained in the paragraphs that follow.

There are three general forms of consent. **Expressed consent** is the most common form of consent and occurs when a person, either verbally, non-verbally, or in writing, grants permission to treat. Often, the act of the patient requesting an ambulance is considered an expression of a desire to be treated. Unconscious patients cannot express consent. When treating the unconscious patient, consent for treatment is considered to be implied. With **implied consent**, it is assumed that the patient would want life-saving treatment if he or she were able to provide express consent. Children with life-threatening injuries or illnesses, who do not have a responsible adult immediately available, can also be treated under the doctrine of implied consent, even if the child is conscious.

■ **expressed consent** verbal, non-verbal, or written communication by a patient that he or she wishes to receive medical care.

■ **implied consent** situation involving an unconscious patient where care is initiated under the premise that the patient would desire such care if he or she were conscious and able to make the decision.

Occasionally, courts will order a patient to undergo treatment, even though they may not want it. This is considered **involuntary consent** and is most commonly encountered with regard to patients who are mentally ill. It is used on occasion to force patients to undergo treatment for a disease that

■ **involuntary consent** consent to treat based upon a court order or magistrate's order that is against the desires expressed by the patient.

threatens the community at large such as tuberculosis and other types of infectious illnesses. Often law-enforcement personnel will accompany patients who are undergoing court-ordered treatment.

Withdrawal of Consent A mentally competent adult may withdraw consent for treatment at any time. However, such refusal must also be informed. That is, the patient must understand the risks of not continuing treatment or transport to the hospital. A common example of this problem is the unconscious hypoglycemic patient. When the patient regains consciousness after being given dextrose, he or she may refuse transport to the hospital. The patient should be encouraged—*but cannot be forced*—to go to the emergency department. He or she has regained consciousness and is now capable of making consent decisions. In these cases, advanced life support measures, such as IV fluids, should be discontinued, and the patient should complete a release-from-liability form (see paragraph below).

Refusal of Service Many EMS runs do not result in transport of a patient to the hospital. Emergency care should always be offered a patient, no matter how minor the injury or illness appears to be. Often, the patient will refuse emergency care or transport. In such cases, the patient should be asked to sign a "release from liability" or "refusal of transport" form. If possible, the signing should be witnessed by an individual who is not part of the EMS system, such as a police officer or family member. A patient's refusal to sign the form should be documented and witnessed, if possible, by a non-EMS individual. The refusal must be informed. That is, the patient must be informed of all possible risks of refusing care.

✴ Refusal of care by a patient must be informed and properly documented.

Abandonment **Abandonment** is the termination of the paramedic-patient relationship without assuring a mechanism for continuation of the care. Thus, you should not initiate patient care, then arbitrarily discontinue it. In addition, you should not turn over care of a patient to personnel with less training than you have. For example, a paramedic who has initiated advanced life support care should not turn the patient over to an EMT crew for transport. Physically leaving a patient unattended may be grounds for a charge of abandonment. An example would be an elderly patient on an ambulance stretcher, who, while briefly left unattended by the paramedic, fell off the stretcher and fractured a hip. A plaintiff's attorney could charge abandonment as the breach-of-duty component in a negligence proceeding.

■ **abandonment** the termination of a health care provider-patient relationship, without assurance that an equal or greater level of care will continue.

Assault and Battery Failing to obtain appropriate consent could open the paramedic to allegations of assault and battery. **Assault** is defined as unlawfully placing a person in apprehension of immediate bodily harm without his or her consent. **Battery** is the unlawful touching of another individual without his or her consent. Assault and battery can be either a criminal offense, or civil offense, or both.

■ **assault** an action that places a person in immediate fear of bodily harm.

■ **battery** the unlawful touching of a person without his or her consent.

False Imprisonment Like assault and battery, false imprisonment is a tort that can be prevented by obtaining appropriate consent. False imprisonment is defined as intentional and unjustifiable detention. It is a particular problem with psychiatric patients. In most cases, you can avoid allegations of false imprisonment by having a law enforcement officer apprehend the patient and accompany you to the hospital. If no officer is available, you must carefully judge the risks of false imprisonment against the benefits of detaining the patient. You should determine whether medical treatment is immediately necessary, whether the patient poses a threat to himself or herself or to the public, and whether the physical facilities and equipment are available for the patient.

Libel and Slander **Libel** is the act of injuring a person's character, name, or reputation by false or malicious writings. **Slander** is the act of injuring a person's character, name, or reputation by false or malicious spoken words. Allegations of libel can be avoided by respecting the patient's confidentiality. The medical record should be accurate and confidential. Slang and labels should be avoided. Since many states consider ambulance run reports part of the public record, you should never write anything on the run report that could be labeled as libel.

Slander can be avoided by limiting oral reporting of a patient's condition to the appropriate personnel. Many EMS systems record ambulance-hospital radio transmissions. In addition, scanners, which give the public access to EMS transmissions, are common in the United States. Information transmitted over the radio should be limited to essential matters of patient care. In most cases, the patient's name and the status of his or her insurance should not be broadcast.

Problem Patients

As a paramedic you will occasionally encounter a "problem patient." The problem patient will often present a medical-legal dilemma for the paramedic. Examples of problem patients include victims of drug overdoses, intoxicated adults, intoxicated minors, and minors in accidents without an available adult to provide consent.

A common example of a problem patient is a person who has taken a possible overdose of medication. Concerned family members call EMS. However, the patient is alert and oriented and refuses consent for treatment or transport. In a case such as this, one of the paramedics should develop a rapport with the patient. If the paramedic can gain the patient's trust, then he or she may agree to treatment and transport. If the patient refuses, and still remains alert and oriented, then he or she cannot be forced to accept treatment. Paramedics should explain the situation to family members. A refusal-of-transport form should be completed and witnessed by a police officer. If the patient will not sign the refusal, have a police officer or family member sign it, indicating that the patient verbally refused care. If the situation truly becomes dangerous, police officers or family members should consider legal measures to force the patient to receive treatment.

A similar problem patient is the intoxicated person who refuses treatment or transport. Every effort should be made to encourage the patient to accept care and transport to the hospital. If the patient refuses, explain to him or her in a calm and timely manner the implications of refusal. Then have the patient sign a release from liability form. The conversation and the refusal of transport should be witnessed.

Regardless of the type of problem patient, always document the encounter in detail. The record should include a description of the patient, the results of any physical examination carried out (or the lack thereof), important statements made by the patient and other persons at the scene, and the names and addresses of any witnesses. Ideally, a police officer should respond to the scene of all problem patients.

✱ Involve law enforcement personnel in a problem patient encounter and document in detail all factors pertaining to the encounter.

MEDICAL LIABILITY PROTECTION

The best protection from potential liability is practicing good prehospital care. In addition, all actions, procedures, and medications should be adequately documented on the run report. A complete, well-written run report is your

✱ The best protection from potential liability is practicing good prehospital care.

best protection in a malpractice proceeding. To the court, observations and treatments not documented on the run report were not performed. Documentation has become so important that some EMS systems have started requiring paramedics to dictate their reports. These dictations are later transcribed and placed on the permanent record. (See Figure 3-3.)

The medical record should never be altered. An intentional alteration amounts to an admission of guilt by the paramedic. If a medical run report is inaccurate, a written amendment should be attached to the report. The date and time the amendment *was written*—not the date of the original report—should be noted on the paper.

Another important step to take is the purchase of personal malpractice insurance. (See Figure 3-4.) Malpractice insurance is one of the best investments you can make. Although many employers provide malpractice insurance, it is still a good idea to get your own coverage. Some corporate policies are inadequate. Many are written to protect the policyholder—city, county, private company owner—not the paramedic. These policies will not cover you off duty. Also, some cities claim governmental immunity from liability, even though such claims are controversial. The courts are increasingly striking down governmental immunity statutes. The claim of governmental immunity is not good protection. Alternative coverage should be obtained.

SUMMARY

Paramedics cannot avoid becoming involved in the legal system. The nature of the job requires interaction with law enforcement authorities. It also requires paramedics to be at scenes where they may be material witnesses to a crime or domestic dispute. The paramedic is not immune from allegations of malpractice. However, malpractice charges may be avoided by adhering to the following guidelines:

❑ Always obtain informed consent before initiating treatment.
❑ Practice only those skills and procedures that a reasonable and prudent paramedic would, given the same or similar circumstances.

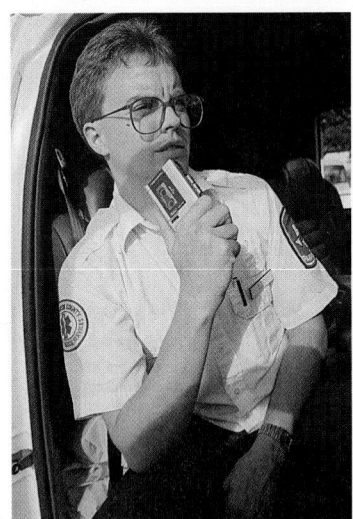

FIGURE 3-3 Some EMS systems now require their paramedics to dictate the patient report. The dictation is transcribed later and placed on the patient's record. This saves time and allows for a more legible document.

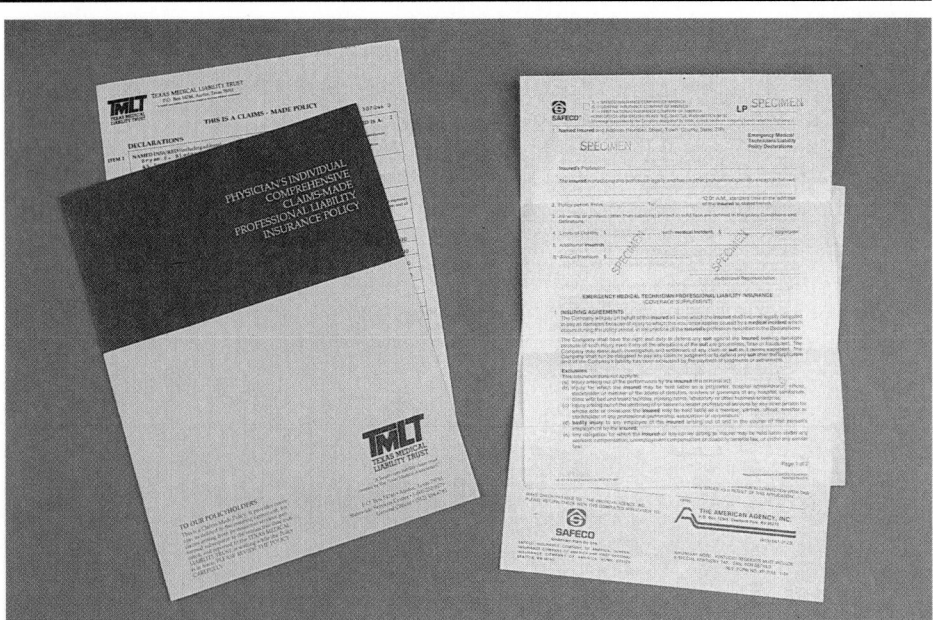

FIGURE 3-4 All prehospital personnel should consider the purchase of professional malpractice insurance. This is especially important in cases where the employer's policy may be inadequate.

- ❏ Practice only those procedures authorized directly by the base station physician or by approved local standing orders.
- ❏ Prepare accurate and legible medical records that thoroughly document the entire EMS incident—from scene response to hospital emergency department.
- ❏ Discuss patient information with only those who need to know. Limit writings and oral reports to information essential to patient care.
- ❏ Purchase and maintain malpractice insurance, and see that your employer does the same.

High-quality patient care is always your best protection.

FURTHER READING

Brody, Howard. *Ethical Decisions in Medicine.* 2nd ed. Boston: Little Brown, 1981.

George, James E. *Law and Emergency Care.* St. Louis: C.V. Mosby, 1980.

Page, James O. "Anatomy of a Lawsuit." *JEMS,* 14(4):36, 1989.

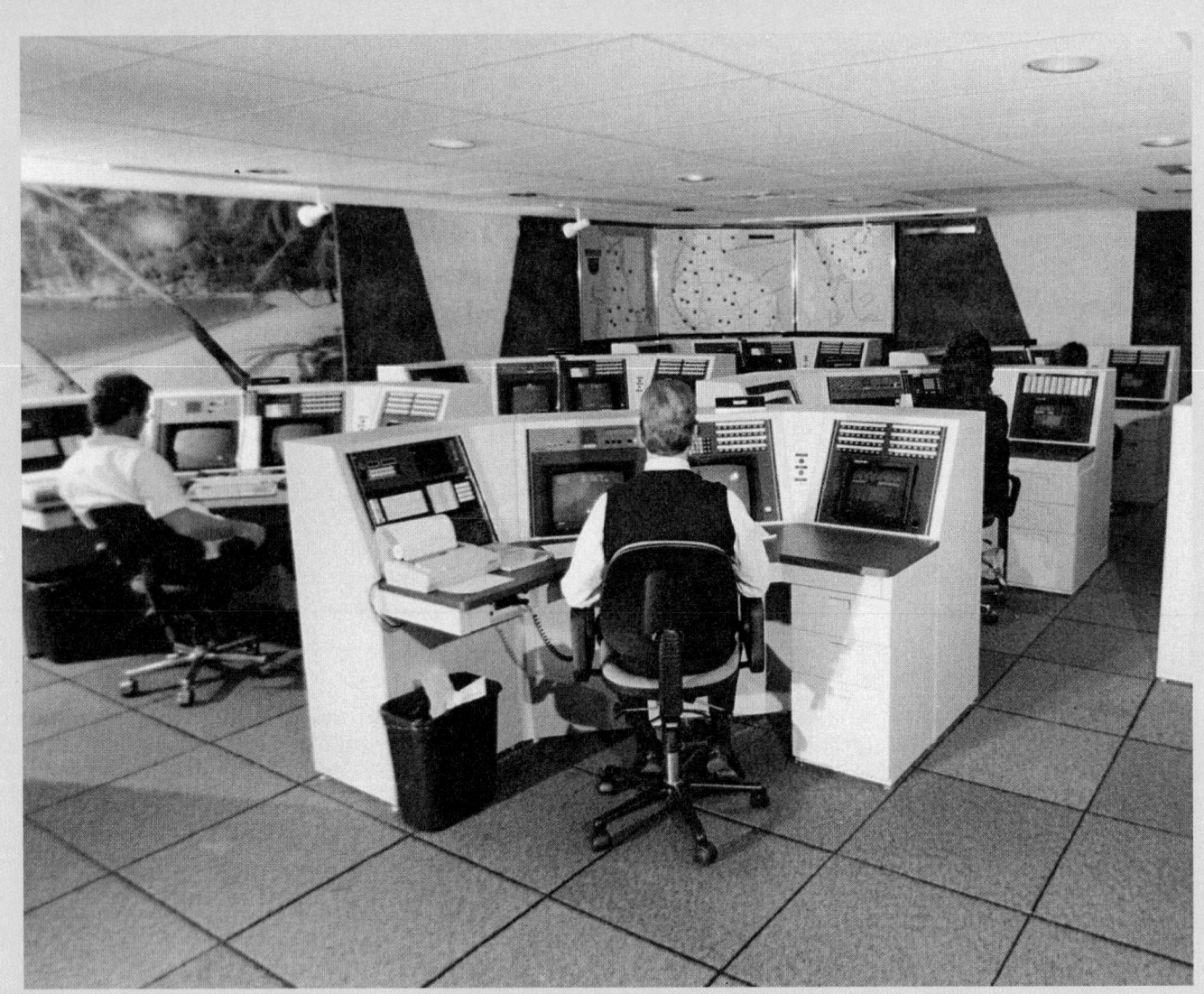

4

EMS COMMUNICATIONS

Objectives for Chapter 4

After reading this chapter, you should be able to:

1. Describe the sequence of an EMS event. (See pp. 52–53.)

2. Describe the five communication links in an EMS event. (See pp. 53–54.)

3. Define the following terms. (See below pages.)
- base station (p. 54.)
- mobile two-way radio transmitter/receiver (p. 55.)
- portable radio (p. 55.)
- repeater (p. 55.)
- voting (p. 55.)
- remote console (p. 56.)
- encoder (p. 56.)
- decoder (p. 57.)
- trunking (p. 58.)

4. Describe the advantages of a repeater system over a nonrepeater system. (See pp. 55–56.)

5. List the two types of radio-wave transmission. (See p. 56.)

6. Define the following terms. (See below pages.)
- Hertz (p. 58.)
- band (p. 58.)
- biotelemetry (p. 59.)
- modulator (p. 59.)
- demodulator (p. 59.)

7. Describe the 10 "Med Channels" and their usage. (See p. 59.)

8. Describe the most common causes of interference in biotelemetry communications. (See pp. 60.)

9. Describe briefly the functions and responsibilities of the Federal Communications Commission. (See p. 61.)

10. Describe simplex, duplex, and multiplex transmissions, and give an example of each. (See pp. 60–61.)

11. Discuss the importance of communications equipment maintenance. (See p. 61.)

12. Define briefly the role of the EMS dispatcher. (See pp. 61–62.)

13. Describe how information necessary to initiate an EMS response is obtained. (See pp. 62–63.)

14. Describe the purpose of EMS radio codes, and give examples of local radio codes. (See p. 63.)

15. List radio techniques that improve efficiency. (See pp. 63–64.)

16. List the important components of the patient medical report. (See pp. 64–66.)

17. Describe the importance of written medical protocols. (See p. 66.)

18. Name five uses of the written EMS form. (See p. 66.)

On a dry, warm Sunday afternoon, a 31-year-old male loses control of his motorcycle and strikes a highway sign. Several people witness the incident. The first bystander to reach the patient rushes to his automobile to dial 9-1-1 on his cellular telephone. The dispatcher takes the necessary information and dispatches an ALS ambulance and an engine company. After the units depart, the dispatcher instructs the caller in basic emergency care. The EMS unit and engine company get the call via a computer print-out of all essential information. They quickly arrive at the scene and initiate the appropriate care. Because the patient has a severe head injury, the paramedics perform only a limited assessment and immediately transport him.

As the ambulance departs, the paramedic relays the following:

Paramedic: Medic 801 to EMS receiving.

Medical Control: Go ahead, Medic 801.

Paramedic: We are leaving the scene of a one-person motorcycle accident on Interstate 35. We have one victim, a male who appears to be in his 30s. He was apparently the rider of a motorcycle that went off the roadway and struck a sign. He is unconscious, with obvious facial and chest trauma. Medical history is unknown. Vital signs are: Blood pressure 110/60, pulse 110, respirations 10. Glasgow coma scale is 3. An endotracheal tube has been placed. There is a large laceration above the right eye with an exposed skull fracture.

There is also blood draining from the right ear. Pupils are dilated and minimally reactive, yet equal. Palpation of the cervical spine does not reveal any obvious deformity. A rigid C-collar is in place and the spine has been stabilized. There is no tracheal deviation. Breath sounds are symmetrical, yet diminished. There is subcutaneous emphysema on the right as well as several palpable rib fractures. The abdomen is soft, and the pelvis appears stable. There may be some lower-extremity fractures. Respirations are being assisted with a demand valve using 100 percent oxygen. We will attempt an IV en route. Our ETA is 10 minutes.

Medical Control: We copy, Medic 801. Attempt an IV en route, but transport immediately. Hyperventilate the patient and notify us of any further problems.

Paramedic: We copy, EMS receiving: Attempt an IV en route and hyperventilate the patient.

Medical Control: The patient will be going into Trauma 1. The trauma team will be in the ED awaiting your arrival.

Upon arrival, the patient is met by the trauma team and a neurosurgeon. Despite comprehensive care, the patient dies as a result of his head injury. However, at the family's request, the patient's organs are harvested. They are sent to cities more than 1,500 miles away and used in two transplant operations.

INTRODUCTION

Knowledge of communications plays an important role in your training as a paramedic. All aspects of prehospital care require constant, efficient communications. In addition to using routine radio communications, you must organize and present patient information through spoken communication or in written reports.

EMS COMMUNICATION LINKS

The sequence of an EMS event illustrates the importance of communications in prehospital care. The order of events usually includes:

- ❑ Occurrence
- ❑ Detection
- ❑ Notification and response
- ❑ Treatment and preparation for transport
- ❑ Transport and delivery
- ❑ Preparation for the next event

As the above list shows, a typical EMS response begins with the occurrence of an accident or illness. Next, someone must detect the emergency and summon EMS. Upon receipt of essential information, the dispatcher sends the appropriate EMS unit to the scene of the emergency. At the scene, treatment will be initiated and the patient prepared for transport to the appropriate medical facility. The patient will then be transported to the hospital, where care of the patient is transferred to the hospital staff. Following delivery of the patient, the medical record must be completed. Then all equipment must be prepared for the next response.

Communications play a significant role throughout each stage of an EMS event. The first link in EMS communications is notification of the EMS system. (See Figure 4-1.) Notification occurs between a party requesting help and the EMS dispatcher. In much of the country, notification is made through the public telephone system, by dialing 9-1-1 or another well-publicized emergency number. EMS can also be summoned by other means, such as radio communications from another emergency agency. The EMS dispatcher will quickly determine the nature of the emergency, the address, the cross street, and a call-back telephone number. The appropriate EMS unit is then dispatched. After the EMS unit is dispatched, many systems have a paramedic or other health care worker give the caller simple first aid instructions until the vehicle reaches the scene.

The second link in the communications sequence is notification of the appropriate EMS personnel. (See Figure 4-2.) It may occur through direct telephone link, a radio dispatch system, pagers, or computer-generated dispatch instructions. Personnel are then directed to the scene and progress is monitored throughout the response. The EMS dispatcher may also alert the hospital personnel who will receive the patient.

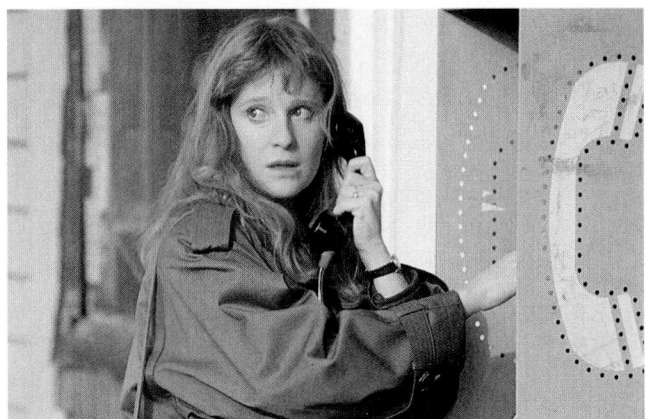

FIGURE 4-1 The first link in EMS communications is notification of the emergency. Citizen access to EMS is most efficient by having a standard emergency number for the entire system such as 9-1-1.

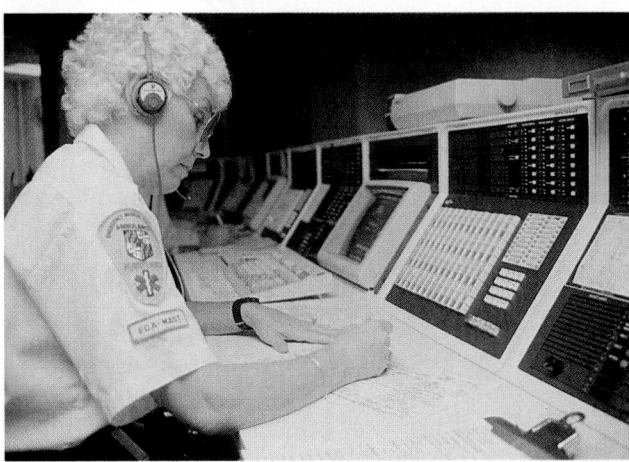

FIGURE 4-2 The second link in EMS communications is notification and dispatch of appropriate EMS personnel.

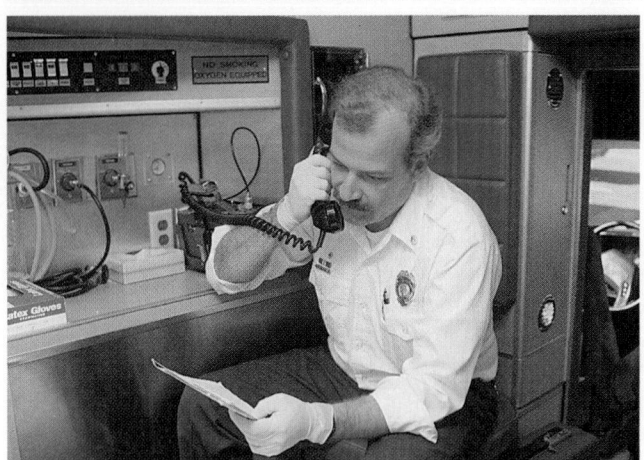

FIGURE 4-3 The third link in EMS communications is communications between the paramedic and the hospital.

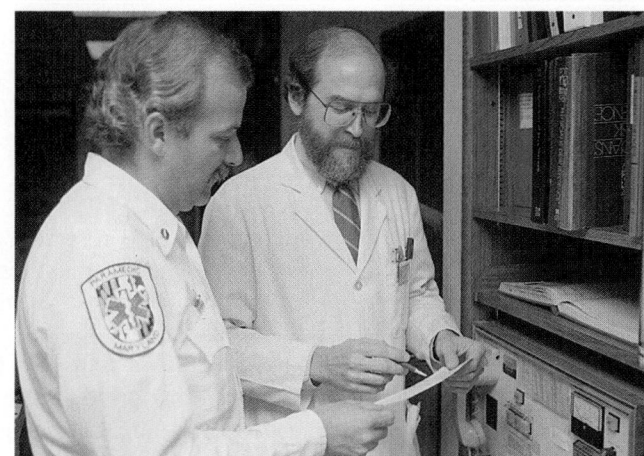

FIGURE 4-4 The fourth link in EMS communications is direct communications with the emergency department staff upon arrival.

■ **ECG** electrocardiogram (ECG); a graphic recording of the electrical activities of the heart.

The third link in the system is communications between the paramedic and medical control. (See Figure 4-3.) Following their initial assessment, the paramedics contact the hospital and relay a report of the patient's condition. The paramedic may have to communicate directly with the emergency physician. Telemetry of the patient's **ECG** may be necessary.

The fourth link is direct communication with hospital personnel after arrival in the emergency department. (See Figure 4-4.) This frequently includes making a detailed verbal patient report, which may address the patient's response to ordered drugs and therapies. A detailed written patient report should also be completed. In many systems, this report becomes a part of the patient's permanent medical record.

The fifth, and final, link is notification of EMS dispatch that the EMS unit is back in service and available for response. The EMS unit should be restocked, cleaned, and refueled before being declared in-service. This chapter will address the fundamentals of the EMS communications system necessary for rapid efficient patient care.

COMMUNICATIONS SYSTEMS: TECHNICAL ASPECTS

Communications systems vary in complexity and cost. A simple communications system may include a self-contained desktop transmitter/receiver, a speaker, a microphone, an antenna, and a one-piece, vehicle-mounted **radio**. A complex system, on the other hand, may include remote consoles, high-power transmitters, repeater stations, satellite receivers, multiple-frequency radios, and encoders. The communications system is usually custom-designed for each EMS system.

■ **radio** an electronic device that transmits sound waves and telemetry over distances using electromagnetic waves.

Base Station

The base station is the principal transmitter and receiver of an EMS communications system. It is usually the most powerful radio in the system and may be controlled by remote console. The power output is typically 45 to 275 **watts**. The maximum allowable base station power is set by the Federal Communications Commission (FCC) and is stated on the base station license.

■ **watt** a fundamental unit of electrical power.

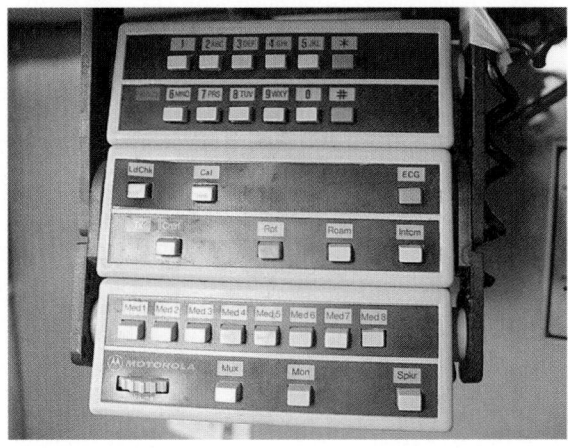

FIGURE 4-5 Control head of ambulance mounted two-way radio.

When determining maximum allowable wattage, the FCC considers the size of the service area, as well as the surrounding geography. Some base stations are multiple-channel systems, but most can only communicate on one channel at a time.

Mobile Two-Way Radios

The mobile two-way transmitter/receiver is usually a vehicular-mounted device that operates at much lower power than a base station—typically, 20–50 watts. Normal range, without a repeater system, is 10–15 miles over average terrain. Transmissions over flatlands or water will increase the range, while transmissions over mountains, through dense foliage, or in urban areas with large buildings, will decrease the range. The mobile radio may be single- or multiple-channel and may have telemetry capability. (See Figure 4-5.)

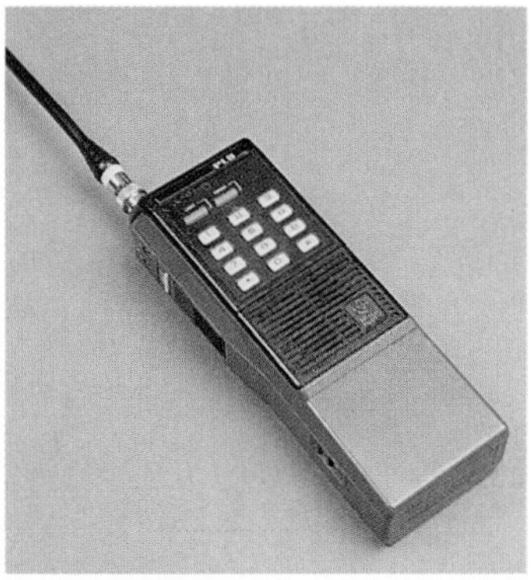

Portable Radios

Portable radios are handheld devices, with a low-power output, typically 1–5 watts, that limits their range. Considerably smaller than mobile radios, they allow radio communications away from the vehicle. Portable radios may be single- or multiple-channel. Often, they must be used with a repeater system. (See. Figure 4-6.)

FIGURE 4-6 Portable radio like the ones commonly used in EMS communications.

Repeater Systems

A **repeater** is a device that receives a transmission from a low-power portable or mobile radio on one frequency, and re-transmits it at a higher power on another frequency. Repeaters are important in large geographical areas because portable and mobile radios may not have enough range either to communicate with each other or with medical or dispatch facilities. Repeaters often have tower-mounted antennas to facilitate the reception of low-power transmissions. Use of a repeater allows two users of low-power radios to hear each other, thus preventing simultaneous transmitting.

Many larger EMS systems have more than one repeater. Often, when a mobile unit transmits, more than one repeater will pick up the transmission. The system is designed so that the repeater receiving the strongest signal will transmit the message. This process is called "**voting**." Some systems use repeaters mounted in the vehicle. These repeaters receive the transmission

■ **repeater** a radio base station modified to retransmit a radio broadcast so the range of the broadcast can increase.

■ **voting** a process by which the repeater station receiving the strongest incoming signal is chosen to rebroadcast that signal.

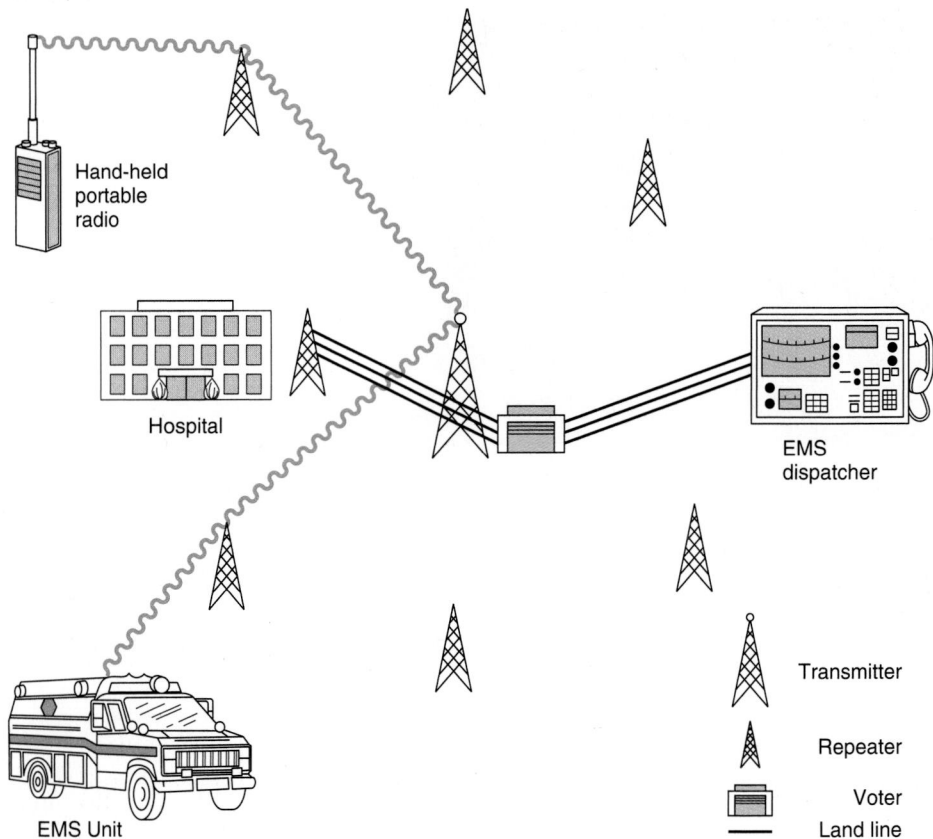

FIGURE 4-7 Example of typical EMS communications system showing the relationship of repeaters, portable radios, voter, and remote consoles.

Hand-held portable radio

Hospital

EMS dispatcher

EMS Unit

Transmitter

Repeater

Voter

Land line

from the low-power portable radio and boost the signal for transmission to the base station. This method is used especially for transmitting remote telemetry. (See Figure 4-7.)

Remote Consoles

Generally, the base station should be placed where it will provide the widest range. It is not always possible, or desirable, to have the dispatch center at the base station. Thus, the base station can be controlled by a remote console. The remote console allows complete operation of the base station from any location. (See Figure 4-8.) This is achieved by using dedicated telephone lines or microwave transmitter links. It many cases, more than one remote may be attached to a base station.

Satellite Receivers

Satellite transmissions may be used to cover large areas. Often, repeaters are placed strategically to receive low-power portable transmissions. The repeater then relays the information to a satellite, which in turn relays it to the remote base station. (See Figure 4-9.)

Encoders and Decoders

There may be a number of base stations on one frequency. This is common for channels used to transmit patient information to the hospital. Several hospitals receive and transmit on the same frequency. Thus, these hospital receivers can be activated by an **encoder**. An encoder is a device that resem-

■ **encoder** a device for generating unique codes or tones that are recognized by another radio's decoder.

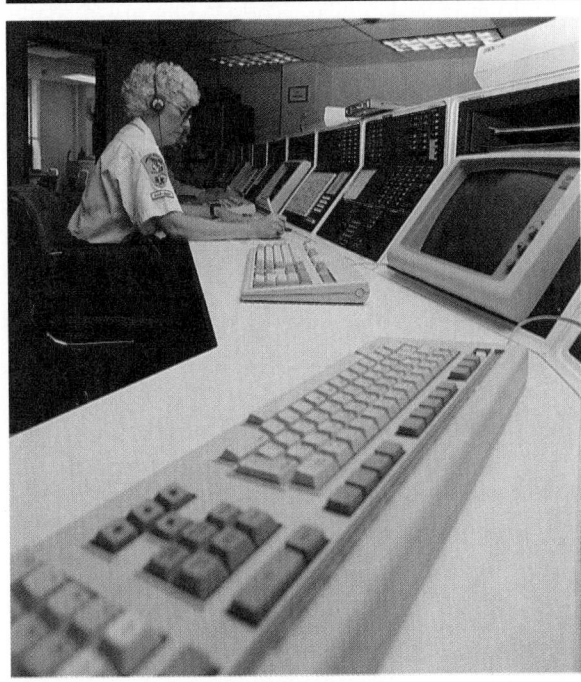

FIGURE 4-8 EMS remote console. Often it is not practical to locate the dispatch console at the transmitter site. Instead, it can be located anywhere and connected by way of telephone lines, microwave, or satellite links.

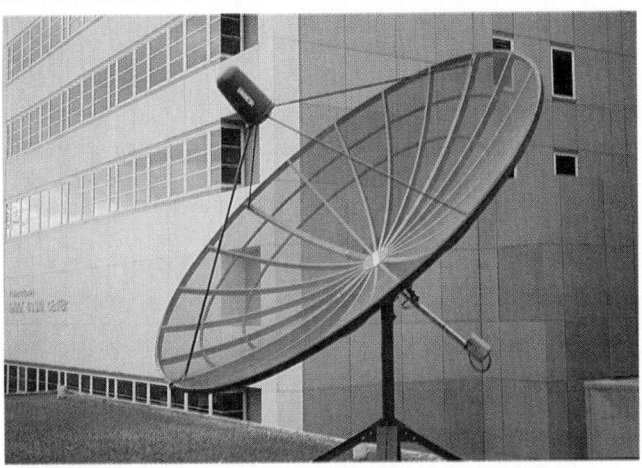

FIGURE 4-9 Satellite communications allow a tremendously increased range and versatility.

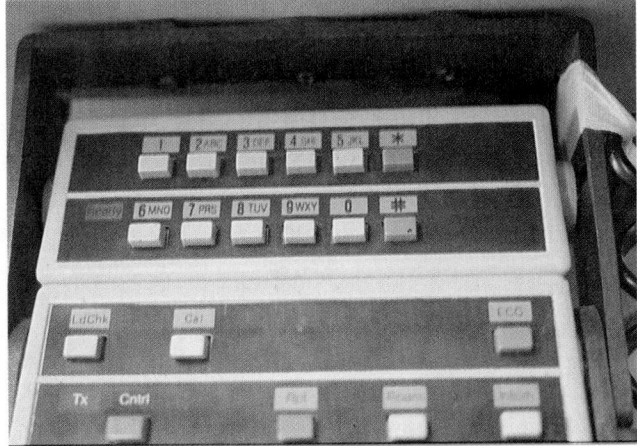

FIGURE 4-10 Typical ambulance mounted encoder. This device will allow paramedics to access hospital radios by way of electronically generated tones.

bles a telephone keypad. When activated by pressing the buttons, it sends specific tones over the air. (See Figure 4-10.) Each receiver has a **decoder**, which recognizes the tones and activates the remote base station. Only the sequence of tones specific for the base station will activate it. Most pagers work on the same principle.

■ **decoder** a device that receives and recognizes unique codes or tones sent over the air.

Mobile Telephones

Many EMS systems have found that mobile telephones are a cost-effective way to transmit essential patient information to medical control. The advantages of mobile telephones became apparent with the advent of "cellular telephones," now in operation throughout most of the United States. A cellular telephone

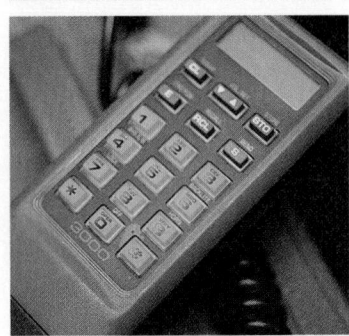

FIGURE 4-11 Cellular telephone technology has opened a whole new era in EMS communications. Now, high-quality transmission of telefacsimile (FAX), computer data, and 12-lead ECGs from the ambulance to the base station is possible.

service is divided into various regions called "cells." These cells are actually radio base stations, with which the mobile telephone communicates. When the transmission becomes out of range for one cell, it is immediately picked up by another cell without interruption. (See Figure 4-11.)

Hospitals may have a telephone line dedicated for use by paramedics to talk with the medical control physician. Since the cellular system provides so many frequencies, accessing a line is rarely a problem. Telemetry can be performed on the same frequency by use of a demodulator. Cellular technology has opened a new era in EMS communications. Now, an ambulance can transmit 12-lead ECGs, telefacsimiles (FAX), and computer data to the dispatcher or hospital.

RADIO COMMUNICATIONS

Radios function by the transmission of sound waves over designated radio frequencies. There are two types of radio wave transmissions: amplitude modulation (AM), and frequency modulation (FM). AM transmissions have greater range because they follow the curvature of the earth. But they are more subject to interference and are generally not acceptable for EMS use. FM transmissions are strictly "line of sight"; that is, they do not follow the curvature of the earth, but travel in a straight line. However, FM transmissions are much cleaner than AM transmissions and are less subject to interference. The majority of EMS units communicate via FM.

Frequencies

■ **Hertz** a measurement of radio frequency, one cycle per second.

The radio frequency is designated by its number of cycles per second. One cycle per second is referred to as a **Hertz (Hz)**. Prefixes are commonly added to simplify frequency description. These include:

- ❏ Kilohertz (KHz) = 1,000 cycles per second
- ❏ Megahertz (MHz) = 1,000,000 cycles per second
- ❏ Gigahertz (GHz) = 1,000,000,000 cycles per second

■ **band** a group of radio frequencies close together on the electromagnetic spectrum.

Radio communications are typically in the 100 KHz to 3,000 GHz range.

A group of radio frequencies fairly close together is called a **"band."** Such frequencies are usually assigned a special use by the Federal Communications Commission (FCC). Bands designated for EMS usage include:

- ❏ Very High Frequency (VHF) Low Band = 30 MHz–50 MHz
- ❏ Very High Frequency (VHF) High Band = 150 MHz–170 MHz
- ❏ Ultra High Frequency (UHF) = 450 MHz–470 MHz

■ **trunking** a system to expedite radio transmissions by automatically routing, usually by computer, the transmissions to the next available frequency in the order they are received.

Many EMS systems have expanded their communications system and now use frequencies in the 800 MHz range. This band offers even clearer communications with minimal interference. Many communications systems operating in the 800 MHz range utilize **trunking** to expedite communications. In a trunked system, all frequencies are pooled together. When a radio transmission comes in, it is routed, usually by computer, to the first available frequency. The next transmission is routed to the next available frequency, and so on. When the transmission terminates, the frequency is freed up and goes back into the pool of available frequencies. In this way trunking eliminates the need to search through different frequencies in an attempt to find one which is not being utilized.

TABLE 4-1	Designated EMS Channels		
Channel	**Transmit Frequency**	**Receive Frequency**	**Usage**
MED 1	463.000 MHz	468.000 MHz	EMT/MD
MED 2	463.025 MHz	468.025 MHz	EMT/MD
MED 3	463.050 MHz	468.050 MHz	EMT/MD
MED 4	463.075 MHz	468.075 MHz	EMT/MD
MED 5	463.100 MHz	468.100 MHz	EMT/MD
MED 6	463.125 MHz	468.125 MHz	EMT/MD
MED 7	463.150 MHz	468.150 MHz	EMT/MD
MED 8	463.175 MHz	468.175 MHz	EMT/MD
MED 9	462.950 MHz	467.950 MHz	Dispatch
MED 10	462.975 MHz	467.975 MHz	Dispatch

The FCC controls all licensing and frequency allocations. It has designated 10 EMS channels for use nationwide. Eight are for paramedic/physician communications, two are reserved for EMS dispatch. (See Table 4-1.)

Biotelemetry

Vital patient information, such as ECGs, can be transmitted over the radio by a process called **biotelemetry**. (See Figure 4-12.) In the ambulance, ECG voltage is converted from an electrical impulse to audio tones via a **modulator**. The audio tones are then transmitted to the hospital over the radio. At the hospital, they are converted back to electrical impulses by a demodulator and displayed on an oscilloscope, on ECG paper, or both. Most new EMS radios have a built-in modulator and most base stations have a built-in demodulator.

■ **biotelemetry** the process of transmitting physiological data, such as an electrocardiogram, over distance, usually by radio.

■ **modulator** a device that transforms electrical energy into sound waves.

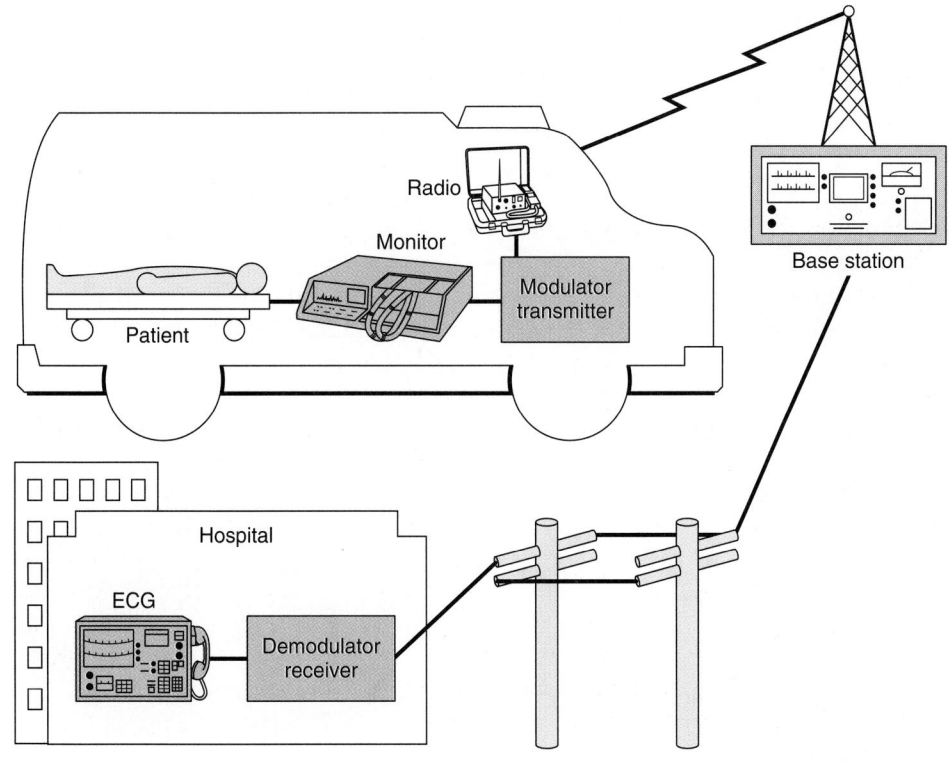

FIGURE 4-12 Biotelemetry allows the transmission of patient data, such as the ECG, from the scene to the hospital. This technology opened the door for the development of prehospital advanced life support.

Telemetry is subject to interference by such things as muscle tremor, loose electrodes, 60 Hz interference (from other electrical sources), fluctuations in transmitter power, and by the transmission of voice communications while telemetry is in progress.

Transmission Types

Several types of radio transmission are possible. Usage may vary from system to system. The most simple communications systems use **simplex transmissions** (see Figure 4-13), in which both transmission and reception occur on the same frequency. In a simplex system, transmission and reception cannot occur at the same time. A person must transmit a message, release the transmit button, and wait for a response. Most dispatch systems use simplex transmissions.

Duplex transmissions allow simultaneous two-way communications by using two frequencies. (See Figure 4-14.) This method works like telephone communications. Use of a repeater to boost signal strength is another form of duplex transmission. It allows the receipt of a transmission on one frequency

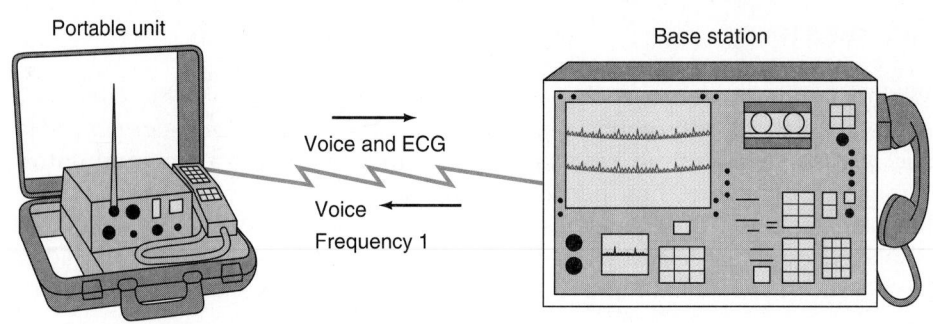

FIGURE 4-13 Simplex communications.

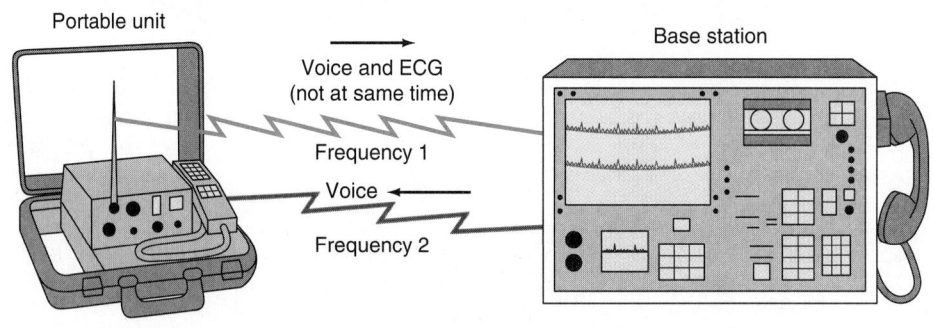

FIGURE 4-14 Duplex communications.

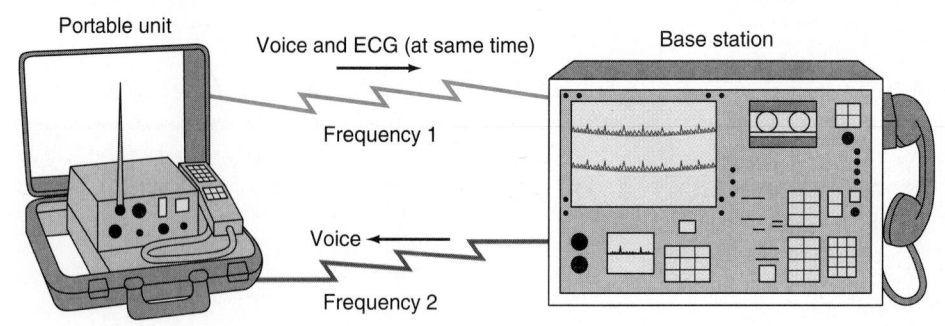

FIGURE 4-15 Multiplex communications.

and rebroadcast of the same transmission on another. It functions as a simplex system, however, because the user must release the transmit button to hear the response. Because it transmits and receives the same message at the same time, it is classified as a duplex system.

Some systems have the capability of **multiplex communications**. Such systems make it possible to carry on a conversation with the medical control physician while transmitting telemetry at the same time. (See Figure 4-15.)

EQUIPMENT MAINTENANCE

Communications equipment is expensive and fragile. It must be protected from harsh environments and dusty or wet conditions. Dropping a radio is a common cause of equipment damage that can usually be avoided by careful handling.

Regular cleaning of radio equipment will improve the radio's physical appearance and life expectancy. Clean exterior surfaces with a slightly damp rag and very mild detergent. Do not use cleaning solvents.

Malfunctioning radio equipment should be repaired by a qualified technician. Preventive maintenance will reduce breakdowns and increase the radio's service life.

Most portable radios and ambulance-based defibrillator/monitors are powered by rechargeable batteries. These batteries are very expensive and must be carefully maintained. Fresh, recharged batteries should be placed daily in the radio and defibrillator/monitor. Spare batteries should always be available. The manufacturer's recommendations for charging, cycling, and replacing batteries should be closely followed.

RULES AND OPERATING PROCEDURES

The Federal Communications Commission (FCC) is the governmental agency responsible for controlling and regulating all radios and radio communications in the United States. Primary functions of the FCC include:

❑ Licensing and allocating radio frequencies.
❑ Establishing technical standards for radio equipment.
❑ Licensing and regulating the technical personnel who repair and operate radio equipment.
❑ Monitoring frequencies to assure appropriate usage.
❑ Spot-checking base stations and dispatch centers for appropriate licenses and records.

The FCC requires all EMS communications systems to adhere to appropriate governmental regulations and laws.

Dispatch Procedures

The **emergency medical dispatcher** is a central component of the EMS system. (See Figure 4-16.) Comprehensive EMS dispatch training is based upon the EMS Dispatcher National Standard Curriculum, produced by the U. S. Department of Transportation. Major responsibilities of the EMS dispatcher include:

❑ Obtaining necessary information about the emergency, as quickly as possible.

■ **multiplex transmissions**
method of radio transmission in which voice and other data can be transmitted simultaneously by use of multiple frequencies.

■ **emergency medical dispatcher**
person responsible for assignment of emergency medical resources to a medical emergency.

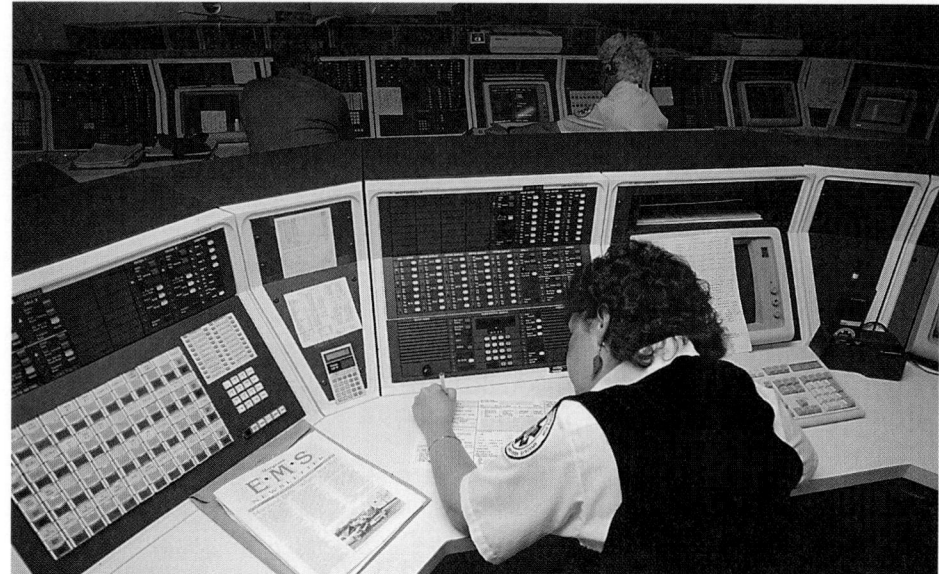

FIGURE 4-16 The EMS dispatcher has evolved into a highly trained and important member of the EMS team. In addition to technical expertise, EMS dispatchers must have knowledge of medical emergencies, local geography, and available resources.

❑ Directing the appropriate emergency vehicle to the right address.
❑ Monitoring and coordinating communications among providers in the system.
❑ Instructing the caller in basic first aid measures that can be undertaken until emergency assistance arrives.
❑ Maintaining written records.

Dispatchers may be dedicated solely to EMS events. Or, they may handle dispatching for an entire public safety system, including fire and law-enforcement agencies.

The dispatcher must decide which vehicles to dispatch. In the larger systems, this may be handled by **computer-aided dispatch (CAD)**. To use EMS resources most efficiently, the dispatcher must know the location of all vehicles and their capabilities (ALS or BLS). The dispatcher must also determine whether rescue or other support services are required.

The skilled dispatcher must know what information to get from a caller before dispatching an EMS vehicle. Necessary information includes:

❑ The location and nature of the emergency. (The vehicle may be dispatched as soon as these facts are known.)
❑ An appropriate "call back" number in case of accidental telephone disconnect.

The following example shows the sequence of events in a properly executed EMS dispatch.

❑ THE EMS DISPATCHER ANSWERS A CALL.
❑ What is the caller's name and call-back number?
❑ What is the address of the event and the closest cross-street?
❑ What is the nature of the event?
❑ DISPATCH FIRST AMBULANCE.
❑ Is the patient unconscious, not breathing, or bleeding severely?

■ **computer-aided dispatch**
enhanced dispatch system in which computerized data is used to assist dispatchers in selection and routing of emergency equipment and resources.

❑ Is the patient trapped? Is there a fire or other hazard?

❑ UPDATE AMBULANCE CREW AND DISPATCH SUPPORT HELP.

❑ Are there emergency care measures the caller can perform until the ambulance arrives?

Radio Codes

Some EMS systems use radio codes, either alone or in a combination with English. Radio codes can shorten radio air time and provide clear and concise information. They can also allow transmission of information in a format not understood by the patient, family members, or bystanders. There are, however, some disadvantages. First, the codes are useless unless everyone in the system understands them. Second, medical information is often too complex for codes. Third, several codes are infrequently used, so valuable time may be wasted looking up a code's meaning.

Some systems still use the **ten-code system**. Published by the Associated Public Safety Communications Officers (APCO), it is used occasionally in EMS dispatch. Many EMS systems, however, have abandoned all codes in favor of standard English.

■ **ten-code system** radio code system published by the Association of Public Safety Communications Officers that uses the number "10" followed by another code number.

Radio Communications Techniques

Proper use of the radio results in efficient and professional communications. All transmissions must be clear and crisp, with concise and professional content. Below are some guidelines for efficient radio usage. (See Figures 4-17 and 4-18.)

1. Listen to the channel before transmitting to assure that it is not in use.

2. Press the transmit button for one second before speaking.

3. Speak at close range, approximately 2–3 inches, directly into, or across the face of, the microphone.

4. Speak slowly and clearly. Pronounce each word distinctly, avoiding words that are difficult to understand.

5. Speak in a normal pitch, keeping your voice free of emotion.

6. Be brief. Know what you are going to say before you press the transmit button.

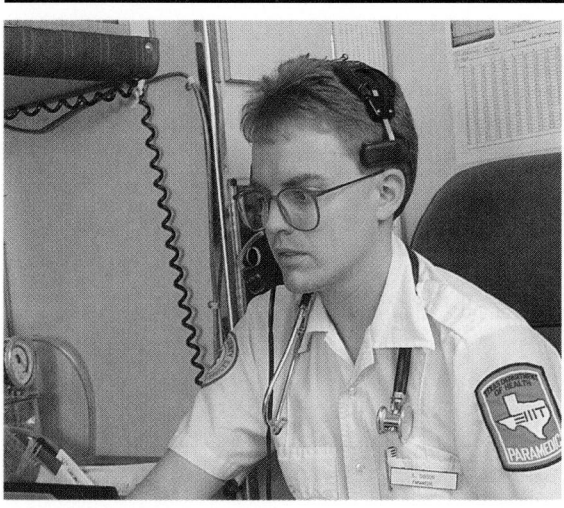

FIGURE 4-17 The patient report should be accurate, clear, and concise. Microphone systems, such as that pictured, allow hand-free operation so that patient care activities can continue.

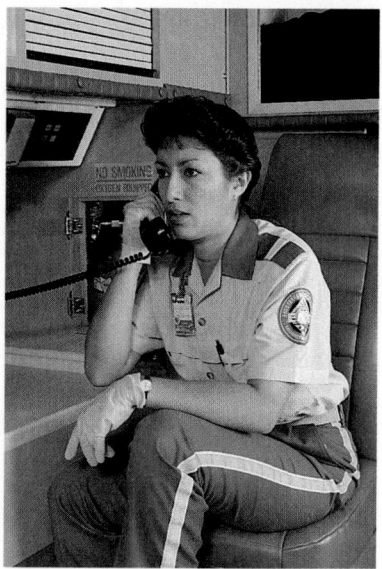

FIGURE 4-18 A clear, concise patient report will enable the emergency department staff to prepare for the needs of the patient.

7. Avoid codes unless they are part of your EMS system.
8. Do not waste air time with unnecessary information.
9. When transmitting information:
   - ❏ Protect the privacy of the patient. When appropriate:
     - • Use telephone rather than radio.
     - • Turn off external speaker or radio.
     - • Don't use the patient's name.
   - ❏ Use proper unit or hospital numbers, and correct names or titles.
   - ❏ Do not use slang or profanity.
   - ❏ Use standard formats for transmission.
10. Use the "echo" procedure when receiving directions from the dispatcher or orders from the physician. Immediate repetition of the statement confirms accurate reception and understanding.
11. Always write down addresses, important dispatch communications, and physician orders.
12. When completing a transmission, obtain confirmation that your message was received and understood.

Occasionally, communications equipment will not function properly. If you are far from the base station, particularly if you have a portable radio, try to get to higher terrain to broadcast. Also, structures that contain steel and concrete can interfere with radio transmission. Simply moving outside the building or near a window will improve communications. If communications still aren't working, try to telephone.

COMMUNICATION OF MEDICAL INFORMATION

Medical information must be effectively relayed to the receiving hospital staff. Initially, this may occur over the radio or by using cellular telephones. Later, when the patient is delivered to the emergency department, additional information should be communicated in-person to the appropriate receiving hospital personnel.

General Concepts

One of the most important skills of the paramedic is to gather essential patient information, organize it, and relay it to the medical control physician. The medical control physician will then issue appropriate orders for patient care. In many instances, written protocols are available. Written protocols are predetermined guidelines for patient care developed by the medical control board of the EMS system. Protocols may vary from system to system. Specific written protocols should be available for all major types of medical emergencies. In addition, there should be protocols to deal with problem situations such as the obviously ill patient who refuses transportation, a non-EMS physician who interferes at the scene, questions relating to "Do Not Resuscitate" (DNR) directives, and so on.

Communication of Patient Information by the Paramedic

The communication of patient information to the hospital or to the medical control physician is a fundamental component of the EMS system. Verbal communications, which may occur via radio or land line, provide the hospital with enough information on the patient's condition to prepare for care. In addition, these communications should initiate required medical orders for patient treatment in the field.

A standard format for transmission of patient assessment information serves several key functions. First, it enables efficient use of the medical communications system. Second, it permits the physician to assimilate information about the patient's condition quickly. Third, a standard format assures that medical information is complete. Although the format should be concise, it should include the following data.

✴ The patient report should be accurate, clear, and concise.

1. Unit call name and name or number of the paramedic
2. Description of the scene
3. Patient's age, sex, and weight
4. Patient's chief complaint
5. Patient's primary problem
6. Associated symptoms
7. Brief history of the present illness
8. Pertinent past medical history, including surgeries, medications, and medication allergies
9. Physical exam findings, including:
   ❑ Level of consciousness (AVPU system)
   ❑ Vital signs
   ❑ Neuro exam
   ❑ General appearance and degree of distress
   ❑ ECG (if applicable)
   ❑ Trauma Index and Glasgow Coma Scale (if applicable)
   ❑ Other pertinent observations, including significant positive and negative findings
10. Treatment given thus far
11. Estimated time of arrival (ETA) at the hospital
12. Name of private physician

After transmitting further information, await further questions and orders from the medical control physician. When communicating from the field with the physician, remember to do the following.

- Be accurate and complete.
- Provide whatever information is requested.
- "Echo" back the physician's orders.
- Question unclear or inappropriate orders.
- Report back when orders have been carried out, describing the patient's response.
- Keep the physician informed of any changes in the patient's condition.
- Protect patient privacy.
- Consult with the physician when transport of the patient is deemed unnecessary.
- Contact the medical control physician for advice on what course to take.

Upon arrival, verbally report essential patient information to the provider assuming care. This report should include a brief history, pertinent physical findings, treatment, and responses to that treatment.

Biotelemetry

Some systems use telemetry for every patient; others never use it. Use of telemetry alone, without field interpretation, is not appropriate. You should always verify your interpretation with medical control, either over the radio or after arrival at the hospital. A 15- to 20-second telemetry strip is usually sufficient. Continuous telemetry is rarely required, since it uses excessive airtime and depletes batteries.

Written Communications

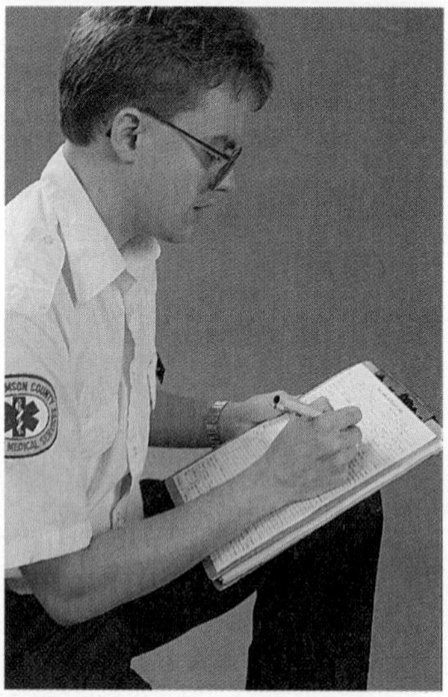

The written patient report is as important as any verbal communication. From a legal standpoint, it may be more important. Most EMS systems use a standard set of forms to document prehospital care. The forms have several purposes.

- The written record of the patient's initial condition and care remains at the hospital after the EMS unit has left.
- The patient report becomes a legal record of the patient's prehospital care and usually becomes a part of the patient's permanent medical record.
- The written record can document a patient's refusal of care or refusal of transport.

FIGURE 4-19 Post-call documentation is as important as the run itself. It should be completed promptly, accurately, and legibly.

The patient report is essential for medical audits, quality control, data collection, and billing. In addition, a complete and accurate patient report form is your best defense against malpractice. (See Figure 4-19.) EMS forms should be as complete as possible. They should show response times, vehicle numbers, personnel, weather, and patient information. Other material, such as medication flow sheets and ECG strips, should be attached. All information must be legible. Also, you should sign all forms.

SUMMARY

As one of the most fundamental aspects of prehospital care, accurate communications help ensure efficient operation of an EMS system. Communications begin with the citizen accessing the EMS system and end with the completion of the patient report and subsequent run critique. Communications must be concise, legible, and complete. They must conform to national and local protocols. The more sophisticated and advanced an EMS system becomes, the more sophisticated and advanced the communications must also become.

FURTHER READING

Bledsoe, Bryan E. *Atlas of Paramedic Skills, 2nd ed.* Englewood Cliffs, NJ: Prentice Hall, 1994.

Clawson, Jeff, and Kate Dernocoeur. *Principles of Emergency Medical Dispatch.* Englewood Cliffs, NJ: Prentice Hall, 1988.

Johnson, Mark, and Robert Tredwell. "Rural EMS Communications." *Emergency Medical Services.* 20, no. 8 (August 1991).

Macneil, Cross, and Paul Maniscalco. "Cellular Technology: An EMS Overview." *Emergency Medical Services* 18, no. 7 (August 1989).

Stanford, Todd M. *EMS Report Writing: A Pocket Reference.* Englewood Cliffs, NJ: Prentice Hall, 1992.

Steele, Susi B. *Emergency Dispatching: A Medical Communicator's Guide.* Englewood Cliffs, NJ: Prentice Hall, 1993.

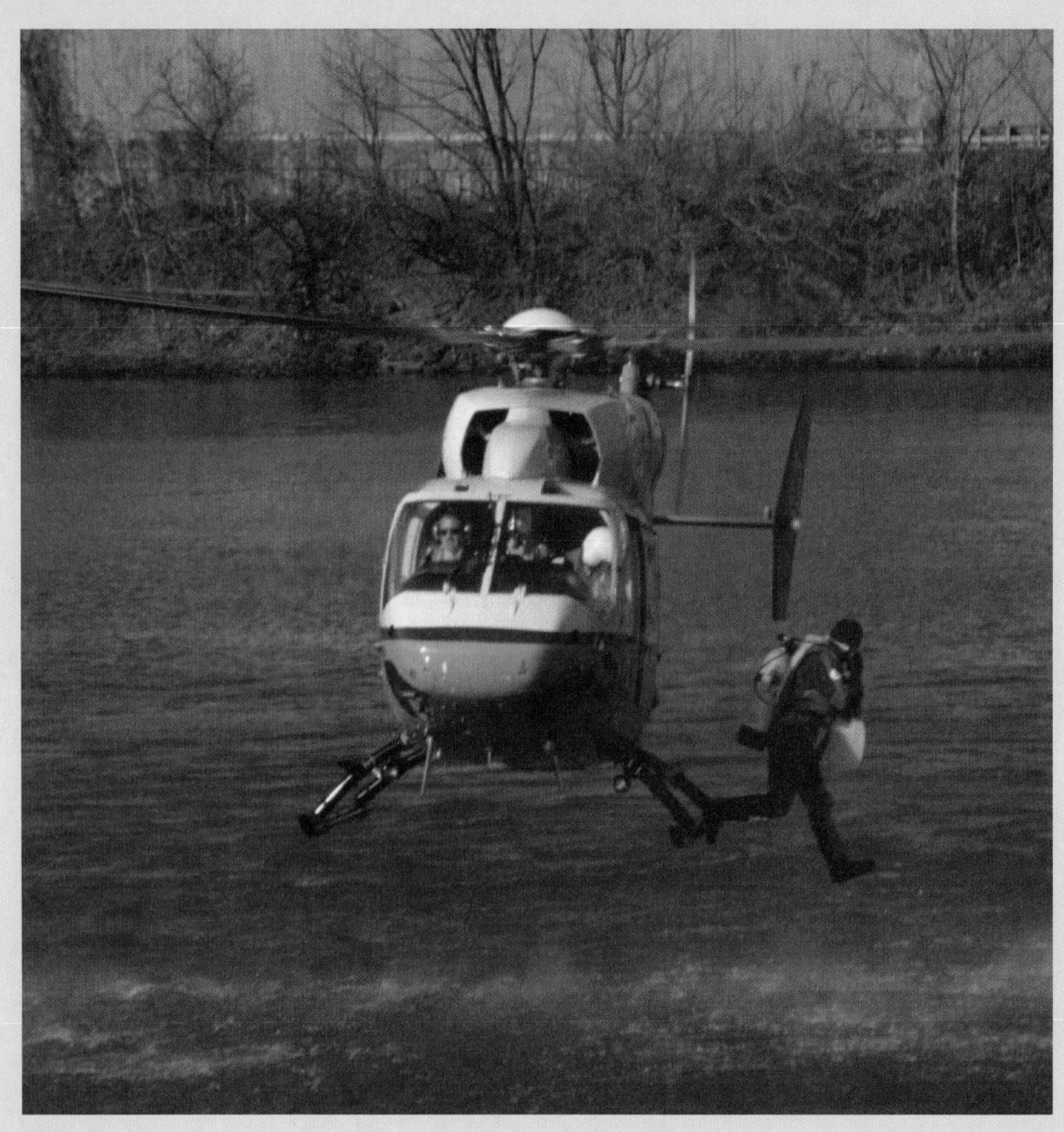

5

RESCUE OPERATIONS

Objectives for Chapter 5

After reading this chapter, you should be able to:

1. List the items required for personal and patient safety during a rescue. (See pp. 70–73.)

2. Discuss the purpose of written safety procedures. (See p. 73.)

3. Describe the role of the Safety Officer. (See p. 73.)

4. Describe how preplanning contributes to the safety and efficiency of a rescue operation. (See pp. 73–74.)

5. Describe the six phases of a rescue operation, and discuss the key elements of each rescue phase. (See pp. 74–82.)

6. List the types of hazards that might be encountered at a rescue scene. (See pp. 75–76.)

7. List types of information, in addition to hazards, that a paramedic should gather during scene assessment. (See pp. 75–76.)

8. List three special rescue operations that require special skills or equipment. (See pp. 77–78.)

9. Describe reasons a paramedic's technical capability must be guaranteed before he or she attempts to reach an entrapped patient. (See p. 78.)

10. Name the three major responsibilities of a paramedic in providing on-scene medical care during a rescue. (See p. 78.)

11. List the two key goals of patient assessment in a rescue. (See pp. 78–79.)

12. List five situations in which patients may have to be moved prior to complete stabilization. (See p. 79.)

13. Discuss how prolonged time in reaching—or in disentangling, removing, and transporting—a patient will necessitate modification of management protocols. (See pp. 80–82.)

14. List three responsibilities of the paramedic during patient disentanglement. (See pp. 80–81.)

15. Identify elements of a thorough patient survey upon removal. (See p. 81.)

16. Explain how the method of patient transport is determined. (See p. 82.)

17. Identify some of the scenarios that an EMS unit should consider in compiling a rescue resource list. (See p. 82.)

A dispatcher sends Fire Unit 1204, a volunteer-operated paramedic ambulance, to assist an injured person in a rural state park, approximately 15 miles from the station. Because of winding roads, the response takes nearly 20 minutes. A park ranger meets the paramedics upon arrival. The ranger informs them that an amateur rock climber has fallen off a vertical cliff popular with local climbers. The ranger then takes one of the paramedics by four-wheel-drive vehicle to a trail that leads to the victim. Because the portable radio will not reach dispatch from the park, the other paramedic stays with the ambulance.

From a vantage point along the trail, the paramedic spots the patient through binoculars. He is laying on a rock ledge, about 55 feet below the trail. The cliff is a straight face, and ropes will be required for the rescue. The on-scene paramedic relays the patient information to the paramedic at the ambulance. He, in turn, calls dispatch and requests the vertical-rescue team and the medical

evacuation helicopter. Dispatch quickly arranges for two members of the rescue team to be flown in with the medical evacuation helicopter. Upon arrival, the vertical-rescue team is taken to the site of the emergency. After assuring scene and personal safety, the rescuers prepare their equipment for descent and access to the patient.

One of the first rescuers down is a paramedic. She performs a primary and secondary assessment. Assessment reveals that the patient is unresponsive with multiple fractures. Nonetheless, blood pressure and pulse are stable. The paramedic immobilizes the patient and establishes an IV of lactated Ringer's. Because required rigging of the ropes will prolong removal time, she starts a second IV, cleans and dresses all wounds, and splints all fractures. It takes approximately 25 minutes for the entire vertical-rescue team to rig the rescue and remove the patient. They finally lift the climber to the trail and transport the patient to the waiting helicopter.

INTRODUCTION

■ **rescue** to free from confinement or danger.

Rescue can be defined as the freeing of a subject from entrapment or threat of danger. Because there are so many potential rescue situations, you cannot be trained to meet them all. (See Figure 5-1.) In fact, proficiency in more than a few rescue specialties is rare. Nonetheless, all EMS responders will eventually be called to a situation requiring rescue. Therefore, you must prepare yourself for such situations *before* they arise. Each paramedic—you and the other members of your crew—will have to make preparations that match specific training or ability with the planned responsibilities of the EMS system.

Because the field of "rescue" entails so many specialties, this chapter will not present step-by-step rescue procedures or extensive lists of specialty equipment. Instead, it will offer an overview of considerations that apply to most rescue scenarios.

SAFETY

✱ Personal safety is your first concern in any rescue situation.

Personal and patient safety must be the paramount issue in any rescue situation. Therefore, the first step in preparing for rescue response is to develop an individual protective equipment cache. This equipment is generalized because it has application in many rescue situations.

Personal Safety

You will jeopardize your own safety and the safety of the patient without the appropriate protective gear. As a minimum, you should have at least the following equipment immediately available. (See Figure 5-2.)

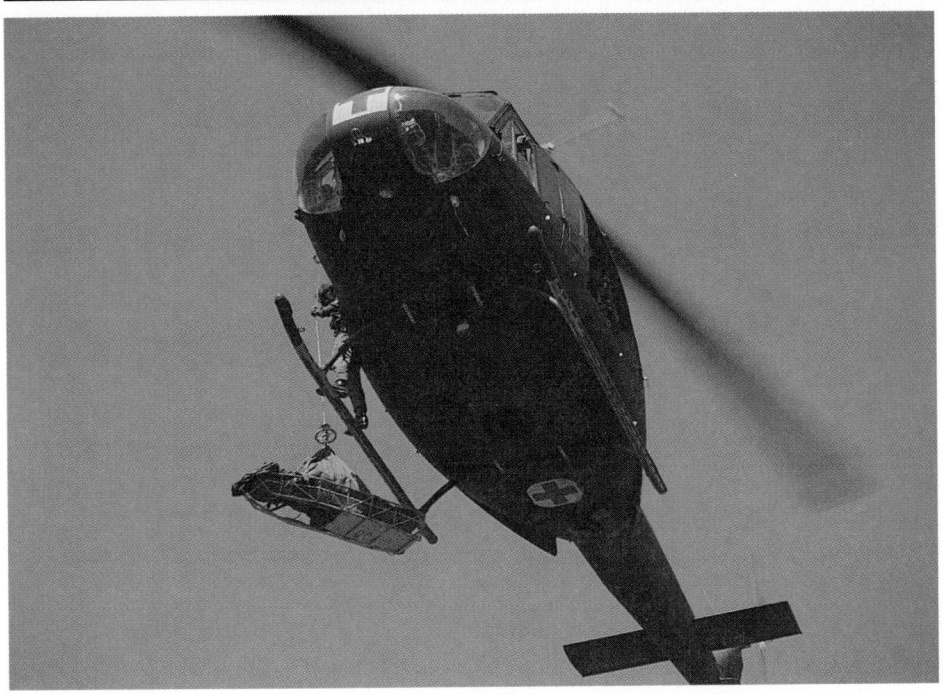

FIGURE 5-1 Rescue is a dangerous activity and safety is the number one priority. It is impossible for an individual paramedic to be highly trained in all types of rescue. Instead, specialized rescue teams should be utilized.

❏ *Helmets.* The best helmets have a 4-point, non-elastic suspension system, in contrast to the 2-point system found in construction hard hats. Most of the 4-point suspension helmets are designed to withstand more severe impacts than hard hats. Avoid helmets with non-removable "duck bills" in the back because a helmet should be compact enough to wear in tight spaces.

❏ *Eye Protection.* Two essential pieces of eye gear include goggles, vented to prevent fogging, and industrial safety glasses, held by an elastic band.

❏ *Hearing Protection.* From a purely technical standpoint, high-quality earmuff styles provide the best hearing protection. However, you must take into account more than technical considerations. Practicality, convenience, and availability will also play a role in your choice of hearing protectors. The multi-baffled rubber earplugs used by the military and the sponge-like disposable earplugs are good choices. They should be used by crews or patients whenever the protection of hearing is necessary, especially if superior hearing protectors are either unavailable or impractical.

❏ *Respiratory Protection.* Surgical masks or commercial dust masks are adequate for most occasions. These should be routine equipment on all EMS units.

❏ *Gloves.* Leather work gloves are usually best. They allow free movement of the fingers, as well as good protection. Heavy, gauntlet-style gloves are too awkward for most rescue work.

❏ *Boots.* High-top, steel-toed boots with a coarse lug sole are preferred. For rescue operations, lace-up boots will provide greater stability and better ankle support. They also don't pull off as easily as pull-on boots in deep mud. However, these benefits must be weighed against the call-to-call advantages of pull-on boots.

❏ *Coveralls.* Coveralls add some arm and leg protection and can be put on quickly. They also protect uniform pants and shirt. They can be designed

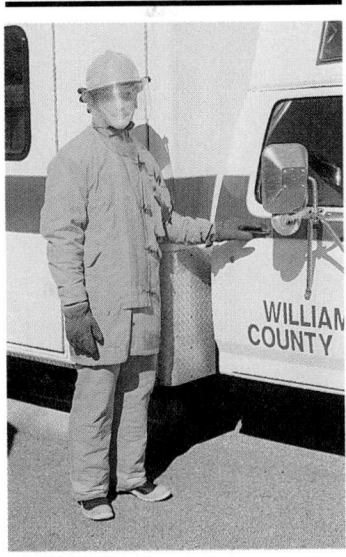

FIGURE 5-2 Each EMS unit should contain basic safety equipment to protect both the paramedics and the patient.

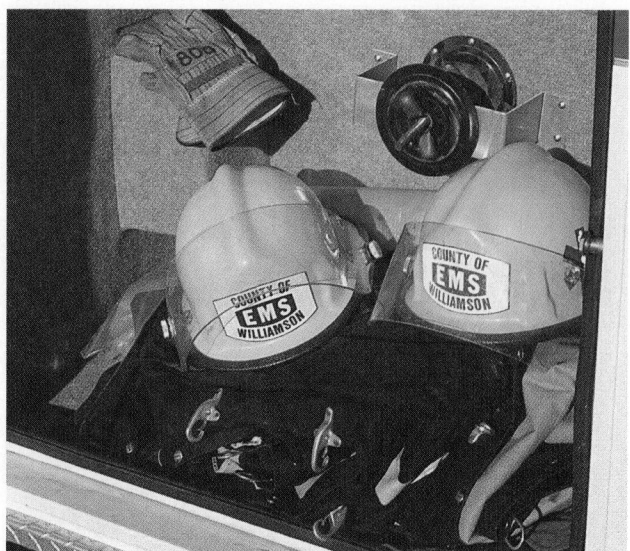

FIGURE 5-3 The quantity of safety and rescue equipment that can be carried on a standard ambulance is limited.

with bright colors or reflective symbols for high visibility. The insulated style is very helpful in cold weather.

❑ *Turnout Coat/Pants.* Turnout gear provides the best protection against the sharp, jagged metal or glass that you might find when extricating someone from vehicle wreckage or structural collapse. This equipment should be available to all paramedics.

❑ *Specialty Equipment.* Hazardous-materials suits or SCBA (self-contained breathing apparatus) should only be made available to personnel who are thoroughly trained in the applications of this equipment. These items are often supplied on specialty support vehicles, such as hazardous material (Haz-Mat) response units. (See Figure 5-3.)

Patient Safety

After you ensure that responding personnel have adequate safety equipment, you should consider patient safety. Although many of the considerations for rescuer safety also apply to patients, there are several significant differences. A patient safety equipment cache should include at least the following items.

❑ *Helmets.* There is usually no need for patient helmets to be as heavy duty as those of rescuers. So you will probably use patient helmets as protection against minor hazards. The less expensive, construction-type hard hats are adequate. If you anticipate severe hazards, outfit patients with the same high-grade helmets that rescuers use.

❑ *Eye Protection.* Vented goggles, held in place by elastic bands, are ideal. They are not as easily dislodged as safety glasses. Workshop face shields also may be used.

❑ *Hearing and Respiratory Protection.* The same considerations for protecting the rescuer's hearing should apply to protecting the patient's hearing. Earplugs are usually adequate.

❑ *Protective Blankets.* A variety of protective blankets should be available to shield patients from debris, fire, or weather. Inexpensive vinyl tarps do a good job of protecting patients from water, weather, and most debris. Aluminized rescue blankets should be available for protection from fire or heat. Commercially available wool blankets, or the less expensive variety at surplus stores, provide excellent insulation from the cold. Plastic sheeting (the kind used by landscapers) is inexpensive, durable (usually 3–4.5 millimeters thick), and comes in large rolls. Trash bags of many sizes and thicknesses are very useful. The 30- to 40-gallon trash/leaf bags are the most versatile. However, one 55-gallon-drum liner is large enough to cover a single patient. It also can be used as a disposable blanket, poncho, or vapor barrier.

❏ *Protective Shielding.* Circumstances may call for protective equipment more substantial than blankets or plastic sheets. All rescue teams should be trained to use backboards and other commonly found equipment as shields to protect patients from fire, weather, falling rock or debris, glass, or other sharp-edged objects. Shields specifically designed for litters and baskets should be available. These shields can be either purchased or homemade.

Keep in mind that a device that shields a patient from debris or the elements may also limit rescuers' access to the patient. The more securely that you package a patient, the more difficult it will be for you to monitor him or her. As a result, patient care becomes more complicated and changing patient conditions may be overlooked.

Safety Procedures

All teams should have written safety procedures that are familiar to every team member. Contents should include sections on all types of anticipated rescue. Procedures should specify required safety equipment, particular actions required or prohibited, and any rescue-specific modifications in assignments.

Manuals should include a statement requiring a **Safety Officer**. The Safety Officer should be someone with the knowledge and authority to intervene in unsafe situations. This person makes the "go/no go" decision for the operation.

In addition to written procedures and selection of a safety officer, an EMS unit must anticipate crew assignments and special needs *before* the rescue operation. These tasks can be done through personnel screening and careful preplanning.

Screening   Search and rescue planners often use personnel screening to determine the participants in the rescue process. Programs are available that identify physical capabilities of crew members. Findings of these programs could have significant impact on personnel assignments. In addition, psychological testing is recommended. It may even be desirable to screen for specific traits, such as phobias. For example, a rescuer's inordinate fear of heights or small spaces should be considered in assigning rescue duties.

Preplanning   A rescue plan contributes greatly to personnel safety and operational success. Preplanning starts with the identification of potential rescue locations, structures, or activities. Effective preplanning then evaluates the specific training and equipment needed to manage each of these incidents. The preplan also generates ideas on efficient use of existing personnel and equipment and anticipates the need for additional equipment, rescuers, and/or expertise. (See Figure 5-4.)

Because of the intensity and length of many rescue operations, provisions must be made for the maintenance and rotation of rescue personnel.

■ **safety officer** a person with the knowledge and authority to intervene in unsafe rescue situations. This person makes the "go/no go" decision for the rescue operation.

✱ Only personnel trained in the type of rescue needed should participate in dangerous rescue techniques.

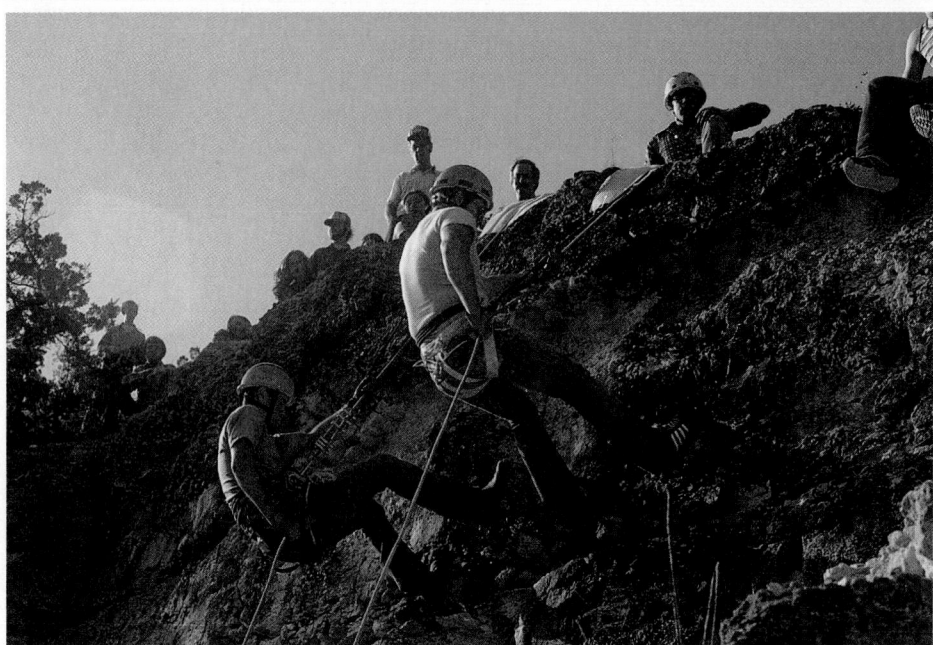

FIGURE 5-4 Dangerous rescue techniques, such as vertical rescue, should be frequently practiced to assure the utmost safety.

Plans should be made for "stand-by" or staging sites that offer protection from the weather. Sites should be away from the immediate operations area and secure from bystanders and the media. Personnel should be rotated at controlled intervals. The crew should follow predetermined policies regarding food and hydration. To maintain maximum personnel performance, rescuers should eat frequently, but in small amounts. The diet should be high in complex carbohydrates and low in sugars and fats. Fluid replacement should consist of plain water or relatively dilute electrolyte solutions. The classic coffee and donuts regimen should be avoided altogether.

THE RESCUE OPERATION

Rescue operations consist of six general phases. The phases include:

- ❑ Assessment
- ❑ Gaining access
- ❑ Emergency care
- ❑ Disentanglement
- ❑ Removal
- ❑ Transport

Assessment

Assessment begins with the dispatcher's call and subsequent arrival at the scene. (See Figure 5-5.) Although the dispatch message may indicate a rescue situation, the responding crew must determine the need for technical, rescue intervention upon arrival. The decision requires careful evaluation of information gathered at the scene. The following topics can serve as guidelines in

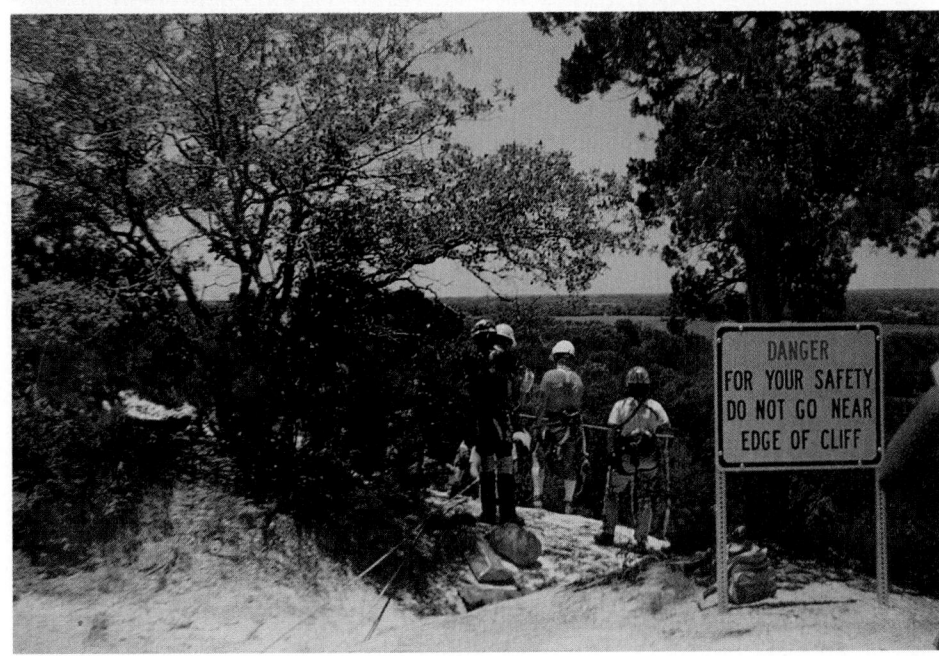

FIGURE 5-5 The first step of the rescue operation is assessment of the scene to determine what resources and equipment will be required.

assessing the need to request backup. As a tip in making this decision, remember that your primary function is medical.

Nature of the Situation   Once at the scene, quickly identify the type of emergency or rescue operation. For example, you may come upon a structural collapse, vehicle extrication, high-rise rescue, or climbing accident. Each of these situations can necessitate specialized crews, additional medical supplies, or sophisticated equipment. Because such backup requires additional time, this phase can be critical. A prompt call to medical control can save additional minutes in a life-threatening situation.

Scene Hazards   On-scene hazards need to be identified with equal speed and clarity. Often you must deal with these hazards *before* even attempting to reach the patient. To do otherwise will place you and other personnel at risk. Some situations involve hazardous materials—chemical spills, radiation, or gas leaks. Others pose the potential for fire or explosion. Only a spark is needed to set off a gas leak or oil spill. Electric wires hold out a double threat for fire and electric shock. The very environment in which you stand can be risk-filled. Look around to determine the possibility for lightning, avalanche, rock slides, cave-ins, and so on. Other potential hazards include the following conditions. As you skim through the list, keep in mind that these are only a sampling of conditions you may encounter.

❑ Poisonous or caustic substances.
❑ Biological agents or germ-infested materials.
❑ Water hazards such as swift-moving currents, floating debris, or toxic contamination.
❑ Confined spaces such as vessels, trenches, mines, or caves.
❑ Extreme heights, particularly in mountainous situations.

❑ Possible psychological instability such as those experienced in hostage crises, urban violence, mass hysteria, or individual emotional trauma on either the part of the victim or the crew (hence the need for pre-assessment of the crew).

The first on-scene EMS personnel can sometimes overestimate their capability to handle a rescue situation. Individual acts of courage may be called for. But rescue operations involve safety first, not heroics. If in doubt, err on the side of precaution. Remember, it is easier to send back a rescue crew than rectify a personal tragedy.

Specific Patient Location   On rare occasions you will come across rescue situations that "hide" patients. Such conditions involve entrapment in vessels, cave-ins, avalanches, and structural mishaps. If possible, ask dispatch to send an on-scene specialist to meet the crew. Search dogs, electronic detection devices, or experienced search managers may be required.

Number of Victims   First responding EMS units must notify dispatch if the magnitude of the incident exceeds the capability of either the EMS unit or routine backup. Initiation of mass-casualty response procedures, implementation of mutual-aid agreements, and contact of off-duty personnel can be an unfamiliar—and hence slow—process. Also, as the principal on-scene medical personnel, you will need to estimate the severity of injuries, the need for advanced life support (ALS), and patient transport needs.

Gaining Access

Following assessment, the next step is to gain access to the patient or patients. (See Figure 5-6.) Initially, a rescue plan should be formulated. Then, the plan should be instituted, the patient accessed, and emergency care provided.

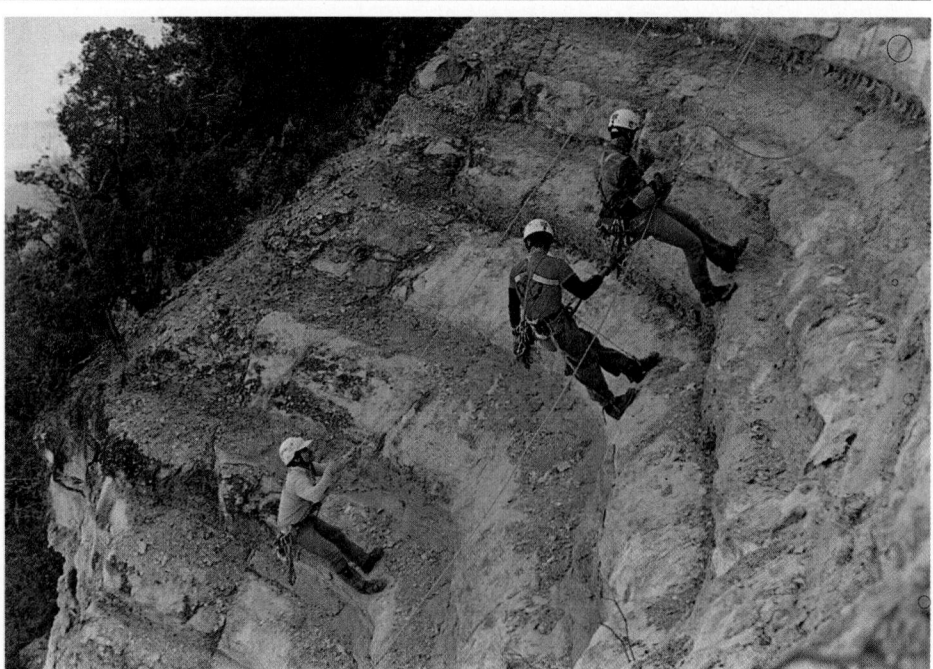

FIGURE 5-6   The second step of the rescue operation is gaining access. In specialized rescues, such as vertical rescue, this can be a long process.

The Rescue Plan   Access triggers the technical beginning of the rescue. Disentanglement and removal come later. While gaining access, you must use appropriate safety equipment and procedures. This is the point when you and your supervisory personnel should honestly evaluate the training and ability needed to access the patient. Undertrained, poorly equipped, or inexperienced rescue personnel must not put their safety at risk through foolhardy, heroic rescue attempts.

During the access phase, key medical, technical, and supervisory personnel must agree on the methods they will use to accomplish the rescue. To assure that everyone understands and supports the rescue plan, a formal briefing should be held for rescue personnel before the operation begins. Even with well-trained personnel and adequate equipment, rescue efforts are often poorly executed because team members do not understand the "big picture" or do not know what they, or their fellow rescuers, are supposed to do.

Special Rescue Operations   There are several types of rescue operations that include technically difficult procedures, very specialized equipment, or both. They should only be attempted by personnel with special training and experience in these areas. Special rescue operations include vertical operations, swift-water rescue, and rescue from confined spaces.

Vertical Rescue. Vertical rescues must constantly contend with the non-discriminatory effects of gravity. Any organization that could be assigned a vertical technical rescue must have extensive initial training, additional advanced training, frequent supervised practice, and top-of-the-line equipment. Members of a vertical rescue team should have individual competency in such techniques as rappelling, ascending, and self-rescue. Even so, most vertical rescues should be carried out using team techniques. There are several capabilities a vertical-rescue team must have. They include:

❏ Adequate equipment such as ropes, helmets, gloves, harnesses, descenders, ascenders, carabiners, and proper boots.
❏ Knowledge of equipment application.
❏ Knot tying, anchoring, and rigging skills.
❏ Competency in the operation of common technical systems, including hauls, lowers, and belays.
❏ Capability of packaging a patient for technical transport.

Swift-Water Rescues. Swift-water rescues require personnel to contend with another powerful and relentless force. Competency to cope with swift-water rescue situations comes only through extensive experience. Trained swift-water rescuers should have a background in the technical operations required in vertical-rope rescue. In addition, they must also be able to adapt these techniques to the specific demands of swift water. In addition to preparation for technical-rope rescues, swift-water rescuers must have the following items or skills.

❏ Adequate equipment, including a personal flotation device, exposure suit, helmet, knife, whistle, goggles or face mask.
❏ Competency in individual water skills such as crossing, defensive swimming, negotiating strainers, and use of throw bags and boogy boards.
❏ Proficiency in shore-based swimming and boat-based rescue techniques.

❑ Ability to manage water-specific emergencies.

❑ Capability to package the victims of water-related injuries and illnesses for transport.

Confined-Space Rescues. Confined-space rescues present a number of threats, any one of which can prove fatal. Most confined spaces appear to be relatively safe. As a result, rescue procedures may appear far less difficult, time consuming, or dangerous than they actually are. Consequently, as a rescue category, confined-space rescues have the highest fatality rate among potential rescuers.

Examples of confined spaces include storage or transport tanks, silos, hoppers, and underground vaults. While "confined space" can have a variety of general meanings, the particular definition for rescue purposes has certain key components. Confined spaces are areas or structures not designed or intended for human occupancy. They are large enough for entry (e.g., for maintenance or repair), but the means of entry and exit are limited. Confined spaces present threats to occupants—hazardous atmospheres (low oxygen, flammables, toxins), potential for engulfment (e.g., grain), or some other physical hazard (inward slopes, entrapping walls/floor, machinery, electrical wires), and so on.

Fortunately, most industries are required to develop a confined-space rescue program. This means that employers must provide a training program for their employees who work in and around confined spaces. These employees may be called upon to perform on-site rescues. Most industries have strict requirements such as continuous atmospheric monitoring, posted warnings, and work-site permits with detailed data on hazard management.

Rescuers should never be allowed to enter a confined space to perform a rescue unless they have training, equipment, and experience specific to this environment.

On-Scene Emergency Care

After the rescue plan is set, medical personnel can begin to make patient contact. But remember: No personnel should enter an area to provide patient care unless they are protected from hazards and have the technical skills to reach, manage, and remove patients safely. The interests of both rescuer and patient may be best served by a first responder with expertise in the type of rescue under way—e.g., a Haz-Mat, vertical, or swift-water expert. A paramedic who doesn't have such skills may end up having to be rescued.

In a rescue, you have three major responsibilities. These include:

1. Initiation of patient assessment and care as soon as possible.

2. Maintenance of patient care procedures during disentanglement.

3. Accompaniment of the patient during removal and transport.

Patient Assessment   To the extent possible, you should quickly assess each patient with regard to the standard primary survey (ABCDE and c-spine status). (See Figure 5-7.) The next critical steps include rapid, secondary assessment and medically oriented recommendations to evacuation teams.

Because a long time may pass before patients are ready for transport, their condition can change significantly during disentanglement and removal. As a result, you should perform patient assessment with two goals in mind:

1. First, identify and care for existing patient problems.

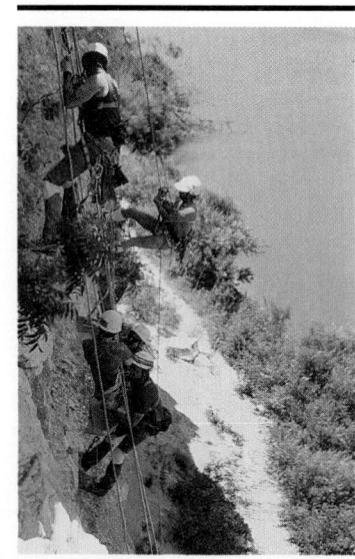

FIGURE 5-7   The third step in the rescue operation is patient assessment and emergency care. This must be modified based on the environment of the rescue.

2. Second, anticipate changing patient conditions and determine the assistance and equipment needed to cope with those changes.

Management   Continually evaluate risks to rescuers and patient. In many situations, the best overall patient care requires rapid basic stabilization and immediate removal. Final positive patient outcome may depend upon initial sacrifice of definitive patient care so the patient and rescuers can be removed from imminent danger. Example of such situations include:

❑ Injured, stranded window cleaners; workers on water, radio, or TV towers; high-rise construction workers.
❑ Victims of trench cave-ins.
❑ Persons stranded in swift-running, rising water.
❑ Victims of vehicular entrapment with associated fire.
❑ Persons overcome by life-threatening atmospheres.

In all these cases, rapid transport of a non-stabilized patient to a safer location is justified by the risk of injury to the rescuers and the possibility of worsening patient injuries by applying "definitive" patient care at the scene. This rapid movement might be required even though the transport itself will aggravate the patient's injuries.

Generally, care for the entrapped patient has the same foundation as all emergency care. Steps include:

1. Assessment, monitoring, and maintenance of the ABC's of the primary survey.
2. Control of life-threatening hemorrhage.
3. Immobilization of the spine.
4. Splinting of major fractures.
5. Packaging with consideration to patient injuries, extrication requirements, and environmental conditions.

■ **packaging** the completion of emergency care procedures needed for transferring a patient from the scene to an ambulance.

Prolonged Patient Care   Specifics of patient management during a rescue are often the same as protocols and procedures used "on the street." However, some specifics may be—or should be—significantly different. Differences are based mainly on the effects of lengthy time periods required to access, disentangle, or evacuate the patient. EMS personnel are trained in rapid stabilization and transport, particularly with trauma patients. However, during a rescue mission, the desire to achieve speedy transport, as well as to obey the cherished "Golden Hour" rule, may be irrelevant. You must be able to "shift gears" mentally when circumstances prevent application of familiar Basic Trauma Life Support (BTLS) or Prehospital Trauma Life Support (PHTLS) protocols.

Special Training.   For rescue operations, at least some personnel should have formal training in managing patients whose injuries have been aggravated by prolonged lack of treatment. Procedures adopted from wilderness medical research will prove useful in managing a patient who has had no care for hours or who cannot be evacuated promptly. The position papers of the Wilderness Medical Society or the Wilderness EMT course, sponsored by the National Association for Search and Rescue, can serve as guidelines for protocols that anticipate these situations. Regardless of their source, many protocols vary substantially from standard EMS procedures. A system's protocols for extended patient care must be negotiated through, and approved by, medical control. These protocols should address at least eight considerations. They include:

- ❑ Long-term hydration management.
- ❑ Repositioning of dislocations.
- ❑ Cleansing and care of wounds.
- ❑ Removal of impaled objects.
- ❑ Pain management.
- ❑ Assessment and care of head and spinal injuries.
- ❑ Hypothermia management.
- ❑ Termination of CPR.

Psychological Support. You should also be prepared to provide more in-depth psychological support for rescue patients than might otherwise be required. Establish a solid rapport with the patient, striking up a constant reassuring conversation. In quieting the fears of rescue patients, try to use the following tips.

- ❑ Learn and use the patient's name.
- ❑ Be sure the patient knows your name and knows that you will not abandon him or her.
- ❑ Be sure that other team members know and use the patient's correct name. The term "it" should never be substituted for the patient's name in any prehospital setting.
- ❑ Avoid negative comments regarding the operation or the patient's condition within earshot of the patient.
- ❑ Explain all delays to the patient, and reassure him or her if problems arise.
- ❑ Ask special rescue teams to explain technical aspects of the operation that could directly impact the patient's condition. Translate these operations into clear, simple terms for the patient.

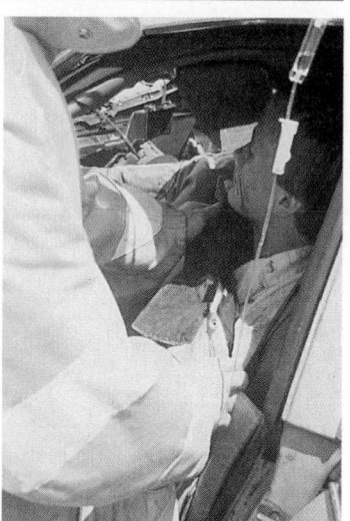

FIGURE 5-8 The fourth step in the rescue operation is disentanglement. It can be prolonged, as in the case of entrapment in autos.

■ **disentanglement** the processes of freeing a patient from wreckage, to allow for proper care, removal, and transfer.

Disentanglement and Removal

After determining preliminary on-scene medical care, the next phases of the rescue operation begin. Depending upon the situation, you could be involved in two processes—disentanglement and removal. Both may be required to ready the patient for transport.

Disentanglement   **Disentanglement** from such situations as wrecked vehicles, structural collapse, or cave-ins may be the most technical and time-consuming part of the rescue. (See Figure 5-8.) If you are assigned to patient care during this part of the rescue, you will have three responsibilities. They include:

- ❑ Personal and professional confidence in the technical expertise and gear needed to function effectively in the active rescue zone.
- ❑ Readiness to provide prolonged patient care.
- ❑ Ability to call for and/or use specialty rescue resources.

If you or another member of the rescue team cannot fulfill these requirements, reassess available rescue personnel and call for backup.

Removal   Removal of the patient may be one of the most difficult tasks to accomplish. (See Figure 5-9.) Activities involved in the removal of a patient will require the coordinated effort of all personnel.

Paramedic Responsibilities. As a paramedic, your responsibilities will include varied tasks, some of which may be performed under the supervision of rescue experts. During removal, you might expect to carry out some of the following activities.

❑ *Select Personnel.* In critical situations, you may be required to assist crews assigned to rigging, evacuation, or **extrication**. If you are the lead paramedic, select people with technical or equipment experience. Also, pick the strongest EMS members to handle lifting and litter-carrying. In such cases, however, constantly monitor team members for fatigue or injury.

❑ *Select Equipment.* Try to get the "right tool for the right job." Unless absolutely necessary, makeshift tools will increase the potential for further injury or risk. For example, you should never substitute a chicken wire Stokes basket for a SKED in a confined-space rescue.

❑ *Assess Terrain.* Evaluate evacuation routes for hazards and physical and/or technical difficulty. Make sure gear matches the terrain.

❑ *Ensure Patient Safety.* In technical operations, you must act as a patient advocate. It is your job to review recommendations that affect patient care. For example, in a cliff rescue, you will not decide which haul system to use. However, you will recommend that the litter be lifted either vertically or horizontally to avoid aggravation of such conditions as head trauma, lower extremity fractures, breathing difficulty, shock, or spinal injury.

❑ *Review Techniques.* Because of the medical implications of removal techniques, you will need frequently to discuss methods with all rescue personnel involved in the operation. With both rescuer and patient safety in mind, the team should balance good medical care against proper technical constraints.

> ■ **extrication** the use of force to free a patient from entrapment.

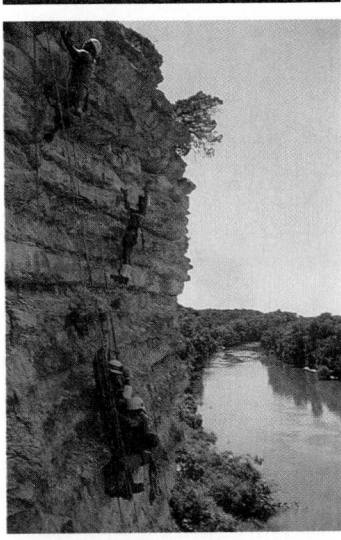

FIGURE 5-9   The fifth step in the rescue operation is removal of the patient.

Reassessment. During removal, you or another paramedic must remain with the patient at all times. You cannot completely evaluate or manage a patient in disentanglement or extrication. But you can check vital signs and patient responsiveness. Once the patient is free of debris or in a safe location, survey or perform as many of the following activities as feasible.

❑ Secure airway.
❑ Check oxygen delivery systems.
❑ Control hemorrhage.
❑ Assess spinal immobilization.
❑ Administer IV solutions, or implement other shock procedures.
❑ Administer drugs, as necessary.
❑ Monitor the ECG.
❑ Dress wounds.
❑ Splint fractures.

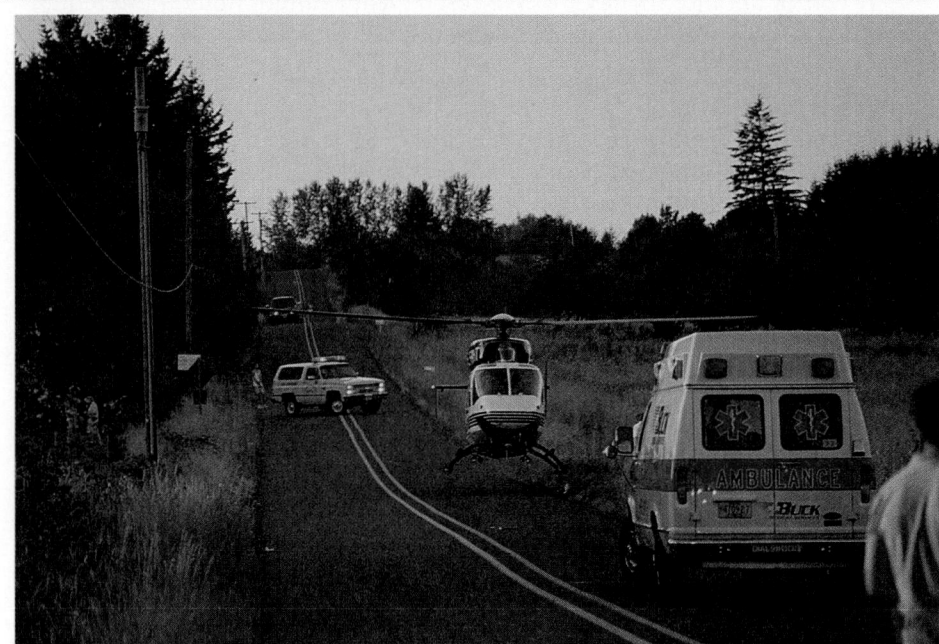

FIGURE 5-10 The sixth, and final step, in the rescue operation is transport of the patient. This can be either by helicopter or ground ambulance, depending upon the rescue situation.

Transportation

■ **transportation** the act of moving a patient from the scene into the ambulance or from the ambulance into the emergency department.

Transportation to a medical facility should be thought out well in advance, especially if you anticipate delays. Decisions regarding patient transport, whether by ground vehicle, by aircraft, or by physical carry-out, should be coordinated with advice from medical control. (See Figure 5-10.) En route to the hospital, update the patient's condition and administer additional therapy as ordered.

RESCUE RESOURCES

Although paramedics are not responsible for developing a rescue resource list, you should have ready access to such a list. No list can cover all scenarios or all kinds of assistance. However, a resource list should include expertise and equipment resources for at least the following types of rescues.

❑ Transportation accidents
❑ Hazardous materials release (See Figure 5-11.)
❑ Confined-space accidents
❑ High-angle accidents (See Figure 5-12.)
❑ Water accidents (See Figure 5-13.)

To develop your resource list, you might want to contact the following organizations.

International Fire Service Training Association
Oklahoma State University
Stillwater, OK 74078

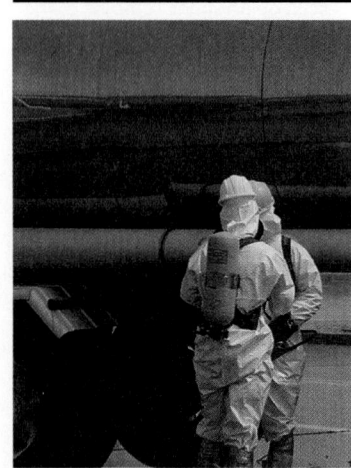

FIGURE 5-11 Hazardous materials require special training and special equipment. Most fire departments will have a Haz-Mat team.

National Institute of Occupational Safety and Health (NIOSH)
Washington, D.C.

The American Red Cross
National Headquarters
431 18th Street NW
Washington, D.C. 20006

Occupational Safety and Health Administration (OSHA)
Washington, D.C.

Department of Transportation (DOT)
Washington, D.C.

Ohio Department of Natural Resources
Division of Watercraft
Columbus, OH 43224

National Fire Academy
Emmitsburg, MD

Rescue 3
P.O. Box 4686
Sonora, CA 95370

Environmental Protection Agency (EPA)
Washington, D.C.

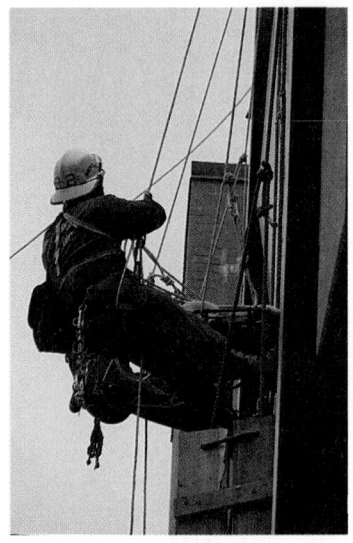

FIGURE 5-12 High-angle rescue is dangerous and difficult. It should be deferred to persons trained and experienced in high-angle rescue techniques.

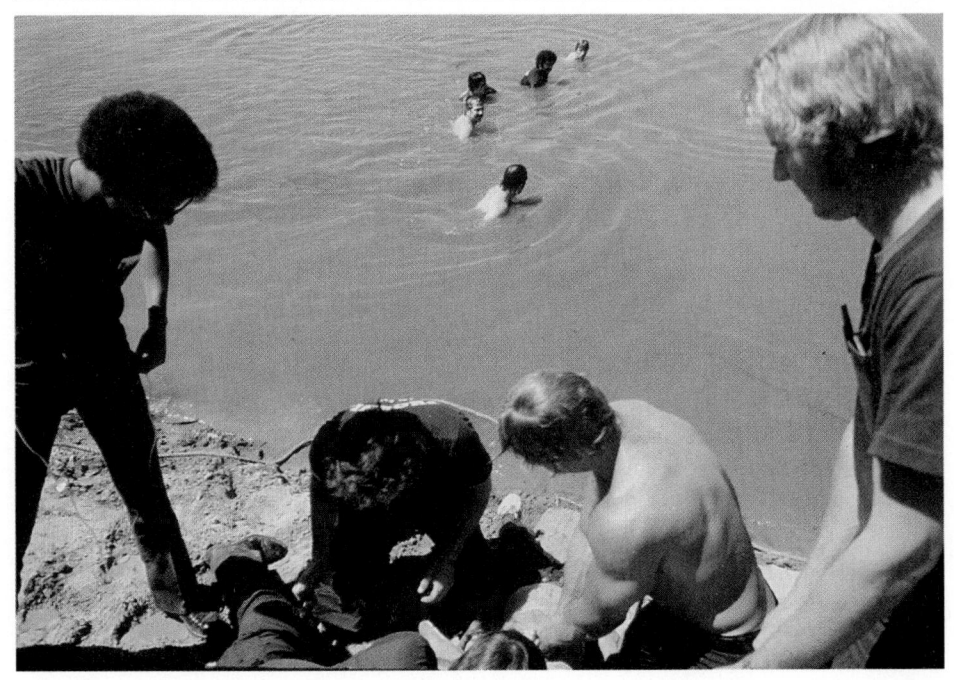

FIGURE 5-13 Water rescue can be deceptively dangerous. Paramedics should not enter the water unless they have been properly trained and have the appropriate equipment.

National Fire Protection Association
Batterymarch Park
Quincy, MA 02269

Air Force Rescue Coordination Center
Scott Air Force Base, IL

Federal Emergency Management Agency (FEMA)
Washington, D.C.

National Cave Rescue Commission (NCRC)
Cave Avenue
Huntsville, AL 35810

Mountain Rescue Association
P.O. Box 2513
Yakima, WA 98902-2513

National Association for Research and Rescue (NASAR)
P.O. Box 3709
Fairfax, VA 22038

The Ocean Corporation
10840 Rockley Rd.
Houston, TX 77099

Wilderness Medical Society
P.O. Box 3907
Point Reyes Station, CA 94956

National Association of Underwater Instructors
P.O. Box 14650
Montclair, CA 91763-1150

SUMMARY

All rescue operations can be divided into at least six functional phases: assessment, gaining access, emergency care, disentanglement, removal, and transport. Whenever you function in any one of these phases you must be properly outfitted with protective equipment. In addition, it is imperative that you have training specific to your assigned rescue.

In a rescue, you must access the scene quickly so assessment and management may begin. At times, situational threats to the rescuer or patient may dictate non-standard, expeditious patient removal. However, patients should be assessed and cared for as thoroughly as conditions permit. They should be continually reassessed and repackaged as removal progresses.

During the operational phases of the rescue, you must provide direct patient care and work with technical teams to assure optimal patient management. Any paramedic assigned to rescue duties should have training in the care of patients who require prolonged management. Such training results from the increased time to locate, access, remove, or transport a rescue patient.

Either you or a paramedic on your team must accompany the patient throughout the removal phase. This person should constantly monitor any changes in condition, while coordinating patient transport to an appropriate medical facility.

FURTHER READING

Auf der Heide E. *Disaster Response: Principles of Preparation and Coordination*. St. Louis, MO: C.V. Mosby, 1989.

Hafen, B. and K. Karren. *Prehospital Emergency Care and Crisis Intervention, Fourth Edition*. Englewood Cliffs, NJ: Prentice-Hall, 1992.

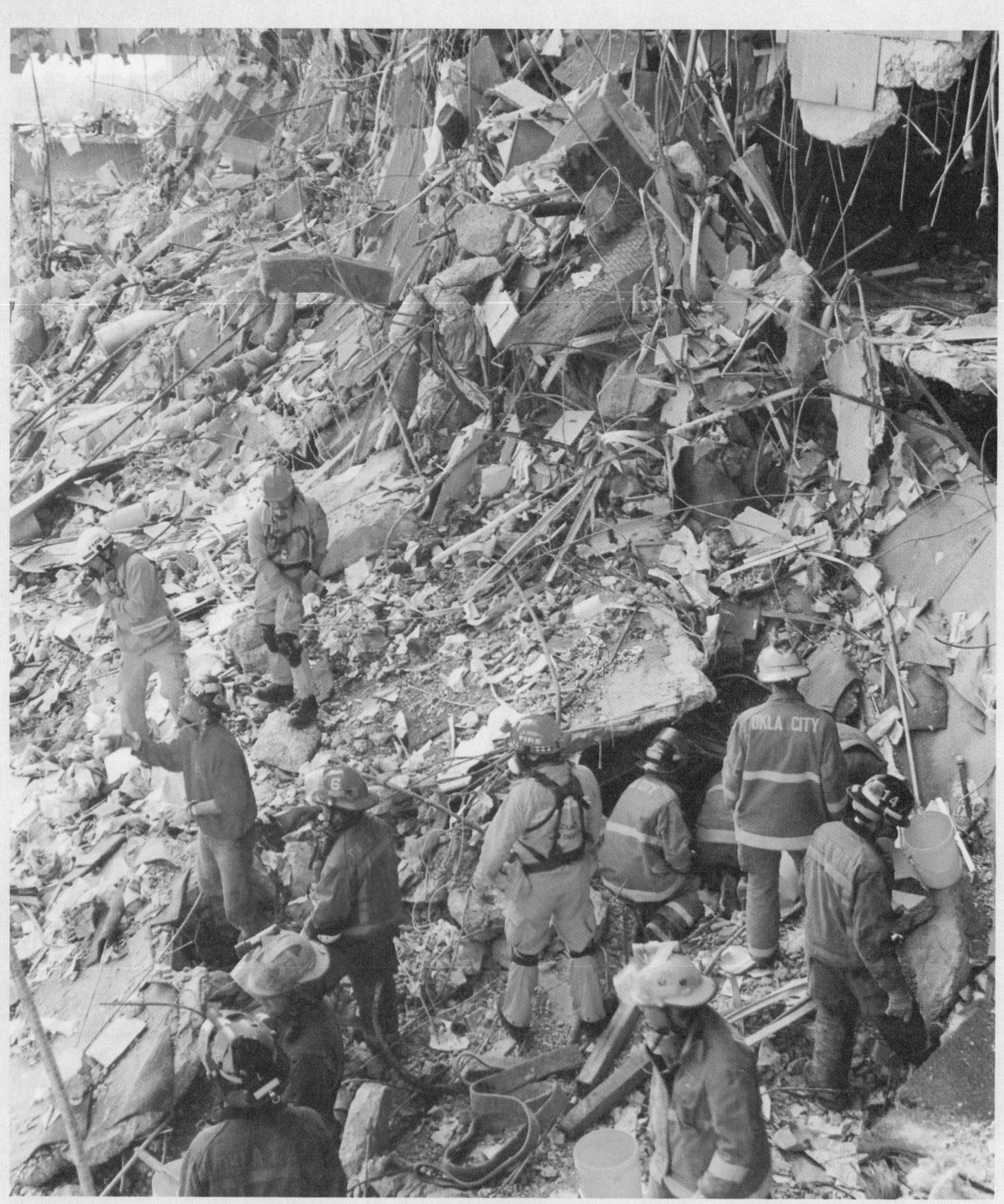

6

MAJOR INCIDENT RESPONSE

Objectives for Chapter 6

After reading this chapter, you should be able to:

1. Name the three categories of EMS response to a mass-casualty incident. (See pp. 88, 90.)

2. Describe the need for controlling and organizing responding rescuers at a mass-casualty incident. (See p. 91.)

3. Identify the Incident Commander, and explain how to contact him or her. (See p. 91–92, 93–94.)

4. Explain the responsibilities of an Incident Commander. (See p. 94.)

5. Describe the transfer-of-command process for the Incident Commander and sector officers. (See p. 96.)

6. Describe the sectors that are used at mass-casualty incidents, and explain the responsibilities of each sector. (See pp. 97–103.)

7. Explain the need for triage and tagging at mass-casualty incidents. (See pp. 91, 97, 102–105.)

8. Explain the START and METTAG methods of triaging patients. (See pp. 103–105.)

9. Explain the communication system requirements at a mass-casualty incident, and describe how to use the system to direct rescuers and process information for decision making. (See pp. 105–106.)

10. Explain the importance of plans and procedures in responding to mass-casualty incidents. (See p. 107.)

11. Cite some of the major duties of paramedics involved in a mass-casualty incident. (See pp. 107–108)

12. List essential items that help a commander and sector officers perform more effectively. (See pp. 108–109.)

A school bus transporting 50 students swerves off the roadway and overturns. Shortly thereafter, 9-1-1 receives multiple calls for the bus accident and, based upon initial information, dispatches several EMS, police, and fire department units to the scene.

Upon arrival of the first unit, the senior paramedic transmits a preliminary report to the dispatch center confirming the incident: "30X-Ray to Central, we're on the scene of an overturned school bus at Foster and 83rd Streets. Some occupants are out of the bus and the initial reports from them indicate multiple injuries. We are assuming the radio designation of Foster Command. Progress report to follow."

The senior paramedic leaves his vehicle and walks around the scene, performing a quick size-up/scene assessment to determine what additional resources will be required. He relays: "Foster Command to Central, I have a school bus on its side, fuel leaking. I have an estimated 40 patients; 10 or 12 appear critical. I am requesting the activation of the Multiple Casualty Incident plan with 10 ambulances in the first response wave. All units are to stage at Foster Avenue and 82nd Street. Instruct all units to change their radios to the tactical channel for assignment upon arrival at the staging sector. Advise the Police Department of this incident and request sufficient officers for traffic control."

Fortunately, the EMS system has a prepared Multiple Casualty Incident (MCI) plan and immediately implements it. In accordance with this plan, a pre-designated response matrix is activated that allows for a structured and effective response of resources. Later, the on-duty supervisor arrives and assumes command of the incident. Various sectors are set up—such as triage, extrication, treatment, and transportation sectors—to manage the victims quickly and efficiently. Incoming EMS personnel arrive at the staging sector and, from there, are directed to any sectors requiring additional staffing. Throughout the response, control of the incident remains in the hands of the Incident Commander and sector officers. Although the incident severely taxes emergency resources, the crews triage, extricate, treat, and transport all patients to an appropriate hospital in a rapid and coordinated fashion.

INTRODUCTION

mass-casualty incident (MCI) an incident involving a large number of patients.

✳ Organization and control of rescuers is essential in any mass-casualty event.

During your career as a paramedic, you can expect to respond to many multiple-patient incidents. These events will generally involve fewer than ten patients with varying levels of injury from stable to extremely critical. A large-scale, **mass-casualty incident (MCI)** involving 50, 100, or more patients is rare. Even so, these major events do occur. Understanding your role in mass-casualty-incident management and knowing how to organize rescuers who will respond to such an incident is important to the overall success of these responses. (See Figure 6-1, A-F.) This chapter will discuss the EMS response to multiple-casualty incidents with particular emphasis on prehospital medical care.

THE PREHOSPITAL EMERGENCY RESPONSE

low-impact incident a multiple-casualty incident that can be managed by local EMS personnel and resources without mutual aid from outside organizations.

high-impact incident a multiple-casualty incident that severely taxes local EMS personnel and resources and usually necessitates mutual aid from several outside agencies.

Multiple-casualty incidents can be divided into three categories that dictate the necessary level of response (resources, personnel, equipment). These categories are:

❑ **Low-impact incident.** A low-impact incident is a localized multiple-casualty incident that can be managed by local EMS personnel and resources without mutual aid from outside organizations. It will typically involve only one jurisdictional authority and follows the normal agency chain of command.

❑ **High-impact incident.** A high-impact incident is a multiple-casualty incident that severely taxes local EMS personnel and resources. A high-

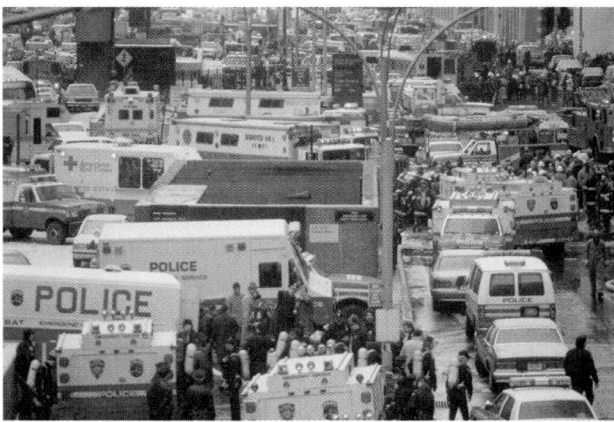

A. The scene of the World Trade Center bombing, February 26, 1993.

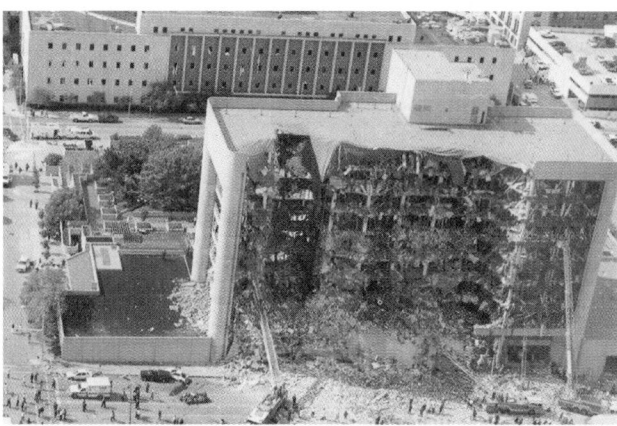

D. The scene of the Oklahoma City federal building bombing, April 19, 1995.

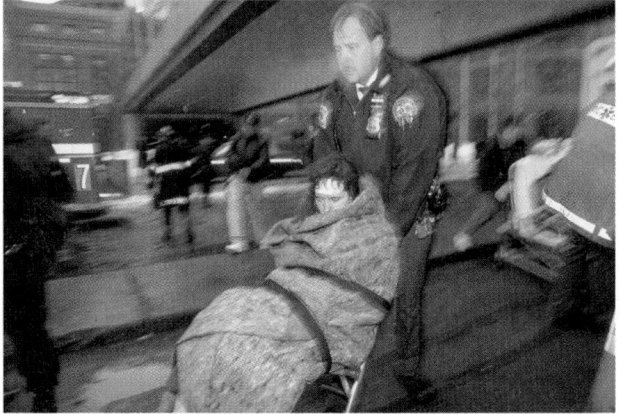

B. Triage, treatment, and transport at the World Trade Center bombing scene.

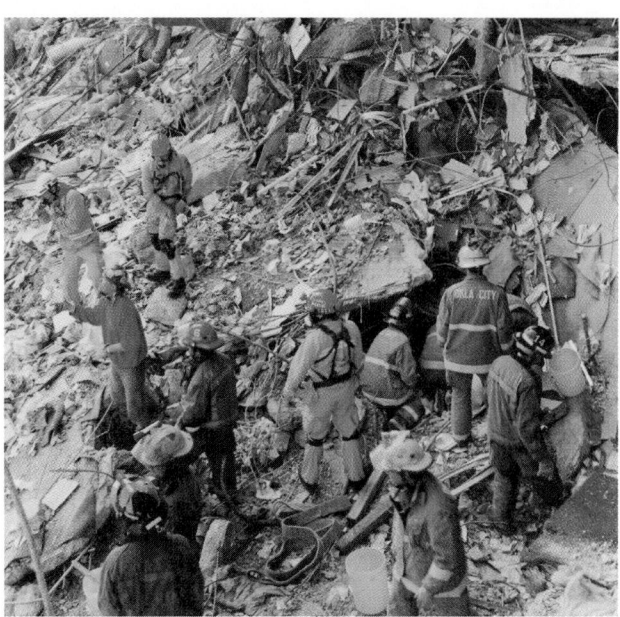

E. Extrication at the bombed federal building, Oklahoma City.

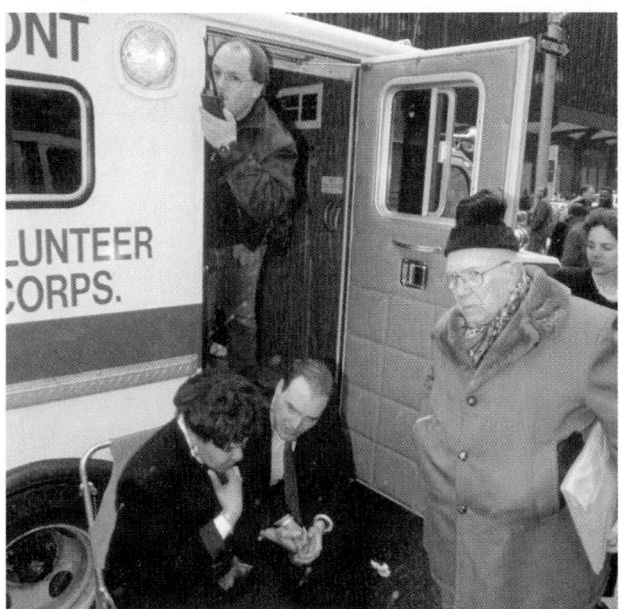

C. Communications at the World Trade Center scene.

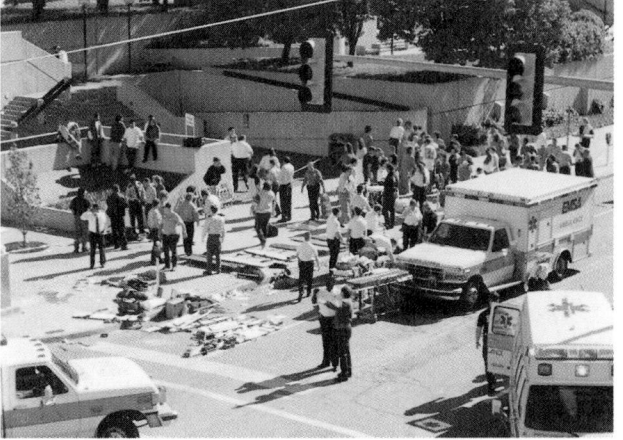

F. Staging of ambulances and supplies at the Oklahoma City bombing scene.

FIGURE 6-1 Two extremely serious mass-casualty incidents, well managed as a result of prior planning and training by public agencies and emergency service organizations: Left (Figures A, B, C)—the World Trade Center bombing, February 26, 1993; Right (Figures D, E, F)—the Oklahoma City bombing, April 19, 1995.

impact incident typically involves a large number of patients and may involve more than one incident site. Often, there may be overlapping of jurisdictional boundaries, thus requiring some inter-agency coordination. A high-impact-incident response usually necessitates mutual aid from several outside agencies.

❏ **Disaster/catastrophic incident.** A disaster/catastrophic incident is a mass-casualty emergency that overwhelms both local and regional EMS and rescue resources. In a disaster/catastrophic incident, there may be multiple patients spread over multiple or widespread incident sites. Typically, there will be overlapping of jurisdictional boundaries, thus requiring significant inter-agency coordination. A disaster/catastrophic incident will often necessitate establishment of an Emergency Operations Center (EOC) and implementation of secondary levels of management.

■ **disaster/catastrophic incident** a mass-casualty emergency that overwhelms both local and regional EMS and rescue resources, typically overlapping jurisdictional boundaries and requiring significant inter-agency coordination. A disaster/catastrophic incident will often necessitate establishment of an Emergency Operations Center (EOC) and implementation of secondary levels of management.

The first EMTs arriving at a multiple-patient or major mass-casualty incident will quickly be overwhelmed. There will be far more patients than treatment personnel can handle—a situation that will persist well into the event. In addition, there will be confusion and a great deal of chaos.

The initial actions of the first EMS members on the scene to organize the incoming wave of responders will directly affect the outcome of the incident. Correct actions will bring organization, efficiency, and calmness to a stressful event. On the other hand, improper or delayed actions will create more confusion and chaos.

As a paramedic, you must place your priority upon organization of rescuers in addition to patient care. If you are unable to organize rescuers, patient care can be delayed or even missed. In addition, duplication of efforts may occur thus delaying or misdirecting patient transportation.

BENEFITS OF THE INCIDENT COMMAND SYSTEM

■ **Incident Command System (ICS)** a management program designed for managing emergency response resources in situations such as fires, hazardous materials, and mass-casualty incidents, as well as other rescue operations. Major components of the system include the Incident Commander and a subdivided subordinate management team in charge of various sectors.

A proven program, called the **Incident Command System (ICS)**, has been developed over the past two decades to assist emergency services in managing a large-scale event. Originally designed to manage the huge numbers of firefighters who were combating California's major brush fires, it was found to be extremely effective in structural fire attack management as well. More recently, the program has been applied to mass-casualty management.

There are a number of different Incident Command Systems used in this country. Some are more complex than others. Each may have been modified to fit local circumstances. All, however, have common organizational elements, which will be discussed in this chapter.

There are also several nationally recognized standards that apply to Incident Command Systems and mass-casualty-incident management. This chapter will present a commonly used and uncomplicated application of the Incident Command System for MCI management—one that meets national standards. This chapter will also discuss plans and standard operating procedures that relate to MCI management, focusing on the positive effects that ICS, as a dynamic operational management tool, lends to your management of MCIs. Finally, it will discuss your role as a paramedic in the management of mass-casualties.

The following benefits are realized when the Incident Command System is utilized as the operational management tool for MCIs.

❏ It provides an organizational plan designed to manage incident needs effectively.

- ❏ It provides a blueprint for the command, control, and coordination of— and communications between—the substantial resources that are likely to respond to a major incident.
- ❏ It provides a framework within which similar functions are grouped.
- ❏ It identifies and defines responsibilities and lines of authority.
- ❏ It provides an orderly means to communicate and process information for decision making.
- ❏ It provides a common terminology.
- ❏ It identifies a transfer-of-command process.
- ❏ It offers performance evaluation criteria.

All these benefits will be explained further in the chapter.

Organization of Command

The cornerstone of the Incident Command System is the requirement that overall incident command responsibilities be assigned to one person. The system further requires that a strong, direct, and visible command mode be established as early as possible during an operation. An effective command organization must then be developed, including an orderly means of **transfer of command** to higher-ranking officers or supervisors who subsequently arrive on the scene.

The significance of having an immediate, single **Incident Commander** cannot be overemphasized. If incident command is not established immediately, rescuers will take independent actions, often in conflict with one another. These independent actions, also referred to as "freelancing," are dangerous and create an environment in which accountability and organization become difficult to establish. Within minutes, chaos may become irreversible. Similar chaos will occur if two or more people attempt to command the incident.

Organization of Sectors

Once command is established, the Incident Commander will begin to organize his or her forces by subdividing the incident into three to six (and sometimes more) components. (See Figures 6-2,3.) These components are often called **sectors**. Each sector will be assigned an officer in charge of all its activities. Portable radios will be used to maintain communication between the Incident Commander and the sector officers. The typical sectors established are extrication, treatment, transportation, staging, and supply. There may or may not also be a triage sector. (**Triage**—which will be described in detail later in this chapter—is the sorting of patients based on the severity of their injuries or condition. Triage is an ongoing process at an MCI, whether or not there is a separate triage sector.)

Each of these sectors becomes a component of the Incident Command organization. Each sector serves a group of similar functions, so there is no conflict in management objectives (e.g., more than one sector trying to manage patient extrication, or a single sector trying to manage extrication and a large patient treatment area at the same time).

The subdivision of an incident into sectors is necessary for two major reasons:

- ❏ The Incident Commander cannot be expected personally to direct the activities of all rescuers at a scene. To do so would require the Commander to run from one area of the scene to another giving orders. This is commonly referred to as the "chicken with its head cut off" syndrome. The inefficiency is obvious: An out-of-control leader is no leader at all.

■ **transfer of command** a process of transferring command responsibilities from one individual to another. Commonly, a formal procedure of face-to-face communication is followed by a briefing on the situation, and then a radio announcement to a dispatch center, that a certain individual has now assumed command of the incident. This process also applies to transfer of sector responsibilities.

■ **Incident Commander** the individual in charge of and responsible for all activities at an incident when the Incident Command System is in effect. All sector officers report to and are directed by the Incident Commander.

■ **sector** a component of the Incident Command System consisting of a group of rescuers performing similar functions under the supervision of a sector officer. Separate sectors are commonly formed to perform extrication, treatment, triage, transportation, staging, and supply. Fewer or more sectors may be formed according to local plans and the demands of the incident.

■ **triage** a process of sorting patients, based on severity of injury, for treatment and transportation. Critical patients are typically treated and transported before stable patients.

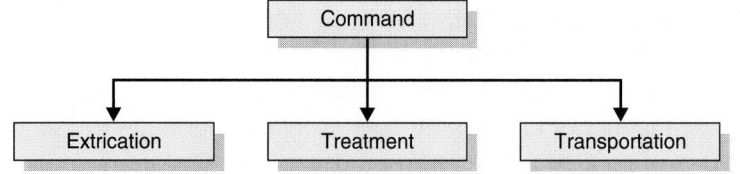

FIGURE 6-2 Organization of the Incident Command System for a small MCI.

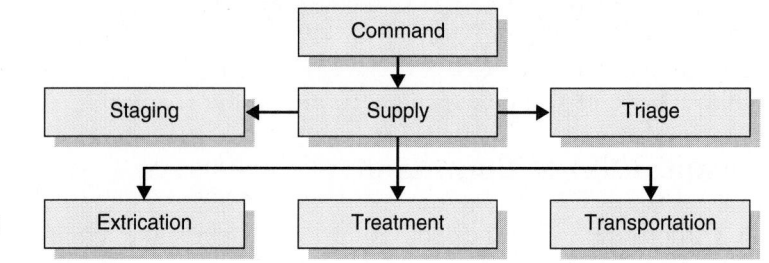

FIGURE 6-3 Organization of the Incident Command System for a large MCI.

■ **sector officer** the person supervising a group of rescuers who are performing a similar function such as extrication, treatment, or transportation.

❑ Management studies have shown that a group leader (e.g., a **sector officer**) provides the close leadership and direction necessary for efficient management of rescuers with common objectives.

Each sector generally assumes a radio designation consistent with its function. Therefore, the incident command component responsible for extricating patients would be called the "extrication sector," the component responsible for treating patients would be called the "treatment sector," and so on. Such common terminology is necessary when large numbers of rescuers are involved, particularly if multiple agencies respond. Some communities, however, may alter their sector titles to fit local circumstances. For example, the extrication sector may be called the "rescue sector," and the treatment sector may be called the "triage sector." In addition, some communities may call the various components divisions (e.g., "rescue division") rather than sectors. Even though the titles may be modified, task objectives remain basically the same. In special circumstances, it may be necessary to create sectors that meet the needs of a specific incident or event. For example, tracking of patients and their on-site care and transportation destinations may become necessary. In this case, a "tracking sector" may need to be established.

These titles will be used in radio communications throughout an incident. The Incident Commander will assume the radio designation of "Command" or some modification such as "Main Street Command," "IC," or other. A good rule of thumb is to adopt a command radio designation that is unique to the event being managed. This will diminish the possibility of confusion if your system is confronted with simultaneous, but unrelated, MCIs. When communicating with a transportation sector, the Incident Commander would use the radio call "Command to Transportation Sector."

The use of function/task titles for Command and the sectors makes it easy for rescuers to remember various responsibilities during a stressful event. In addition, it avoids the problem of trying to remember apparatus or unit identity numbers, which change as higher-ranking officers arrive and assume overall command or sector responsibilities. The titles "Command" and "Transportation," for instance, remain the same throughout all transfers of command and sector responsibilities.

OPERATION OF THE INCIDENT COMMAND SYSTEM

Many communities use the Incident Command System on a routine basis for smaller scale emergency incidents. For example, an EMS service, irrespective of delivery model (fire service, third service, private ambulance) may automatically implement the system any time three or more units are committed to an emergency. This routine use of the system has proven to be highly successful, and this kind of application is recommended. While this routine use might appear at first glance to be "overkill," such use of the system does provide better on-scene control of rescuers. As an additional benefit, routine use provides frequent and repeated training. When a major event does occur, rescuers will have been exposed to the system on numerous past occasions and will be very familiar with it. Remember the old adage: "They'll play as they've trained." This familiarity will provide a comfort level with the Incident Command System which will result in its effective and fluid implementation.

The Incident Commander

As noted earlier, the cornerstone of effective incident management is a single Incident Commander and the establishment of command by units first on the scene. The first on-scene unit must assume control of the incident and direct all initial rescue efforts. (See Figure 6-4.) As the incident develops and more resources arrive, command will be transferred to higher-ranking officers, as required. Some situations may not warrant the relinquishment of command to a higher ranking officer. In these cases, the senior officer may take the designation "Senior Advisor" and act in that capacity to help the subordinate officer become more confident in the utilization of ICS while ensuring that operations proceed safely and effectively. Experience is a great teacher, and these opportunities to boost subordinates' confidence in their use of ICS should not be passed up.

✳ The cornerstone of effective incident management is a single Incident Commander.

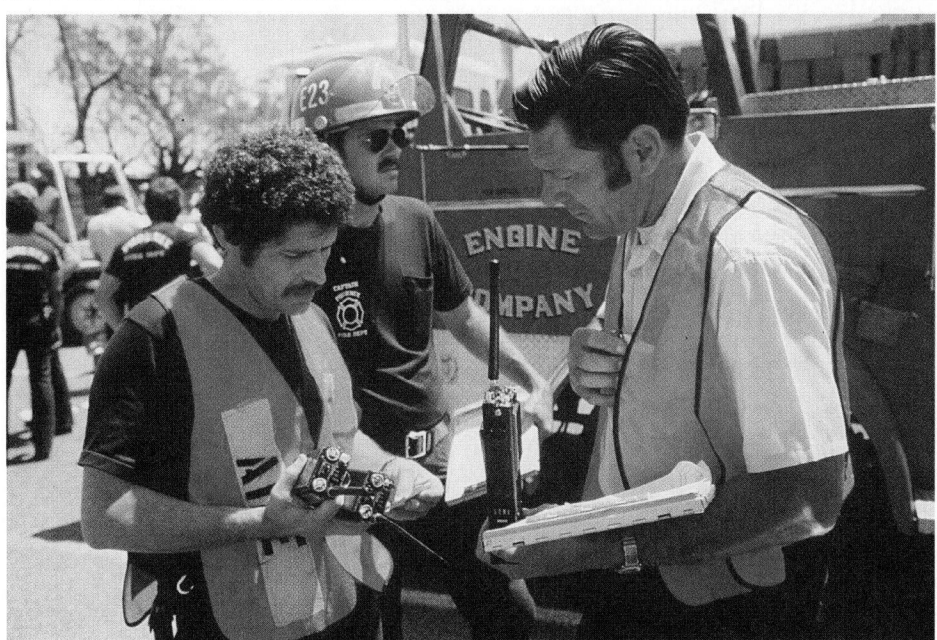

FIGURE 6-4 The first on-scene unit must assume command and direct all initial rescue efforts at an MCI.

TABLE 6-1	Command Officer Responsibilities

1. Assume an effective command mode and position.
2. Transmit a brief preliminary report to the communication center.
3. Rapidly evaluate the situation.
4. Request additional resources, and provide assignments as necessary.
5. Develop an effective and safe management strategy or plan.
6. Delegate authority and responsibility to subordinates in order to accomplish incident needs and objectives.
7. Assign units as required, consistent with the needs of the incident and standard operating procedures or disaster plans; then provide specific operating objectives for these units.
8. Provide continuing effective command until relieved by a higher-ranking official.
9. Review and evaluate the effectiveness of site operations through frequent progress reporting from sector officers, modifying the operation/command organization as required.
10. As an incident winds down, return units to 9-1-1 service and secure the incident when appropriate.

Basic Responsibilities Assuming command means accepting the responsibilities of command, namely providing the control and necessary direction and using the radio designation "Command." (See Table 6-1.) Normally, this is done via the radio on an assigned incident frequency, allowing other responding units to recognize that command has been established and who the party responsible for command is. From this point on, all additional responding units will announce their arrival on the scene at staging and await instructions from the Incident Commander or through the Staging Officer. As soon as the Incident Commander determines the appropriate use for arriving units, he or she will order them to the scene and commit them to areas of need, primarily to work within a sector.

After the first unit on-scene assumes control of the situation, the Incident Commander will transmit a brief radio report to dispatch. This report accomplishes a number of objectives.

❏ First, dispatch and other units know that a unit is on the scene and in command.
❏ Second, dispatch and other responding units know the nature and seriousness of the incident. If it's reported to be a major incident, responding crews can begin to mentally prepare and plan their activities upon arrival.
❏ Third, dispatch can automatically implement some behind-the-scenes support activities (e.g., to notify hospitals, helicopter services, etc.).

Sizing Up the Scene To explain how the Incident Command System works at a major incident, let's refer to the accident scenario described in the case study. As you recall, a school bus carrying 50 passengers swerved off the road and overturned. The dispatch center sent out a number of EMS units. When the first unit arrived at the scene, the paramedic reported:

> 30X-Ray to central, we're on the scene of an overturned school bus at Foster and 83rd Streets. Some occupants are out of the bus and the initial reports

from them indicate multiple injuries. We are assuming the radio designation of Foster Command. Progress report to follow.

The term "Command" remains the title of the Incident Commander throughout the incident—no matter how many times command responsibility is transferred to higher-ranking officers.

After making such an initial report, the Incident Commander will make a rapid evaluation to determine the exact situation and the number of patients involved. This evaluation, or size-up, of the overall scene is different from triage, which is an evaluation of individual patients. In a size-up, you quickly walk around the scene and quickly count the patients. Often the basic information will be obvious upon arrival, and a preliminary report can then be given.

A second size-up can be more accurate, allowing you to give a more detailed report to dispatch. The initial Incident Commander will request additional resources as necessary to meet the demands of the incident. Experience suggests that it is generally better to request more units than you think you need. Making piecemeal requests for individual units is not good practice; in fact, it may interfere with the communications center's ability to relocate units to balance the routine 9-1-1 demands for service. When requesting additional resources for a major incident, the Incident Commander will establish and identify a staging area. (See the information on the staging sector later in the chapter.)

In fire departments, additional resources are often grouped as "alarms." Each additional alarm brings a pre-determined number of fire units to the scene. Irrespective of delivery model (fire service, ambulance, or other), EMS systems should develop predefined response matrixes that can be activated for any MCI. These matrixes establish a disciplined and structured response to an MCI that assists in its overall effective management.

Developing a Plan of Action   The Command Officer then puts together a plan of action, or management strategy. This plan will help personnel to stabilize the situation and to begin extrication, triage, treatment, and, ultimately, transportation of patients.

Once an organizational structure is developed (i.e., all sectors are in place), the Incident Commander will be able to assign arriving resources to the various sectors based upon progress reports, incident needs, and other priorities in accordance with his or her strategic plan. The Incident Commander will continue to control, direct, organize, and coordinate all incident activities until the incident is secured. Each sector officer will implement tactical directions and manage all activities within his or her sector.

Monitoring Progress   An important part of the Incident Command System is the need for a continuous monitoring and reassessment of incident needs and progress. Every incident is a dynamic event, with constantly changing conditions and problems. The Incident Commander will stay abreast of conditions by continually seeking progress reports and other information from sector officers.

Experience has proven that it is best for the Incident Commander to remain at a fixed location, or command post. Typically, the Commander operates from his or her vehicle. (Some communities may have a special command vehicle that responds to major events, giving the Incident Commander a base from which to operate.) A Commander who is running about a scene has created a difficulty for subordinate officers who need to find the Incident Commander to conduct face-to-face communications. If it is absolutely necessary for the Commander to move about, he or she must carry a portable radio in order to maintain access with the sector officers and the command post.

The command post should be close to rescue operations, at a position where the Incident Commander can view as much of the operation as possible yet still be out of the way. The proximity of the command post to the event is necessary to enable the Commander to visualize events as they occur. Additionally, it is important to ensure a safe environment for command post operations. The command post must be located upwind and uphill to prevent any problems associated with hazardous materials.

Finally, as the incident winds down, the Incident Commander will coordinate the release of units and redeployment back into 9-1-1 service. At the proper time, hospitals and related agencies will be notified that the scene has been secured.

Transfer of Command

As additional higher-ranking officials arrive on the scene, transfer of command will usually take place. The mere fact that a higher-ranking official has arrived on the scene does not mean that he or she has assumed command. Even though the officer might have been monitoring radio transmissions en route, the official will have missed a lot of face-to-face communications. The transfer of command is a quick and simple, yet important, process. The arriving official will report to the officer in command for a briefing, after which command will be transferred. In most Incident Command Systems, a radio announcement is made to dispatch, alerting dispatch to the fact that command has been transferred. A typical radio report might state: "Command to Dispatch, Unit 6 has assumed command."

It is important to point out that the same transfer-of-command process takes place at the sector level. No officer should assume command of an incident or sector before he or she knows what has already taken place.

In the case of the bus accident scenario, the first on-scene unit would establish command. If additional crew members are aboard this unit, they would begin the triage process. It is important that rescuers rapidly assess all patients for injury priorities and stop only long enough to correct life-threatening medical problems. Shortly after the first unit arrives, additional rescuers will begin to appear on the scene. At this time, the Incident Commander will assign sector officer responsibilities.

TABLE 6-2 Extrication Officer Responsibilities

1. Determine whether triage and primary treatment are to be conducted on site or at the treatment sector.
2. Determine resources needed to extricate trapped patients, and deliver them to the treatment sector.
3. Provide for site safety for members and patients (very important!).
4. Determine resources needed for triage and primary treatment of patients.
5. Communicate resource requirements to command.
6. Allocate assigned resources.
7. Assign, direct, and supervise members and resources.
8. Collect, assemble, and assess patients with obvious minor injuries, and isolate them from the treatment and extrication sector operations.
9. Report progress to Command.
10. Report to the Incident Commander when all patients have been extricated and delivered to the treatment sector.

Extrication Sector

The Incident Commander normally establishes the **extrication sector** first. An Extrication Officer is assigned from the next arriving rescue crew. (See Table 6-2.) (Additional sectors follow as more rescuers arrive on the scene.) Normally, the extrication sector operates within the **hazard zone** (e.g., within the crashed aircraft or at a collapsed area. In the bus accident scenario, extrication activities would take place in and near the bus.) Typically, personnel will begin **primary triage and treatment** here (such as for airway problems and severe bleeding) and subsequently move patients to the treatment sector. (See Figure 6-5.)

Once the extrication sector has been established, and additional rescuers arrive, the Triage Officer will determine whether patients should be triaged and tagged where they're found or wait until they arrive in the treatment sector. The criteria involved in this decision will vary from community to community.

Normally, patients would be triaged where they're found and then moved to the treatment area based on life-threatening injury priorities. Critical patients would be extricated and tagged, delivered to the treatment sector, and transported before patients with more stable injuries. In order to do this, patients need to be triaged and tagged where they are found. However, if a life-threatening hazard exists, such as an uncontrolled fuel leak or a fire patients will need to be moved on a first-come, first-served basis. Triage and tagging can take place upon arrival in the treatment sector.

In the bus accident scenario, most patients would be triaged on-site prior to removal from the bus. Because of the confined space within the bus, however, it may be difficult to reach some patients until wreckage, or other patients around them, can be removed. Interior conditions may also mean that less-critical patients should be removed and delivered to the treatment sector first, allowing rescue crews to reach entrapped patients whose condition may be critical.

The extrication sector often operates in a significant hazard area, and the sector officer must take appropriate action to provide safety for patients and rescuers. In the bus scenario, a firefighter may have to stand by with a pressurized fire hose or apply foam to the vehicle's fuel leak for fire protection.

■ **extrication sector** the component of the Incident Command System that is responsible for freeing victims from wreckage and managing them at an accident site.

■ **hazard zone** an area of rescue operation that poses a significant physical threat to rescuers as well as to victims.

■ **primary triage and treatment** identification and treatment that targets life-threatening problems in three categories: airway, breathing, and circulation—including hemorrhage and inadequate pulse or perfusion. (Cardiac arrest patients are usually categorized as unsalvageable unless the Incident Commander or Treatment Officer makes the decision that enough personnel are available and orders on-site resuscitation efforts.)

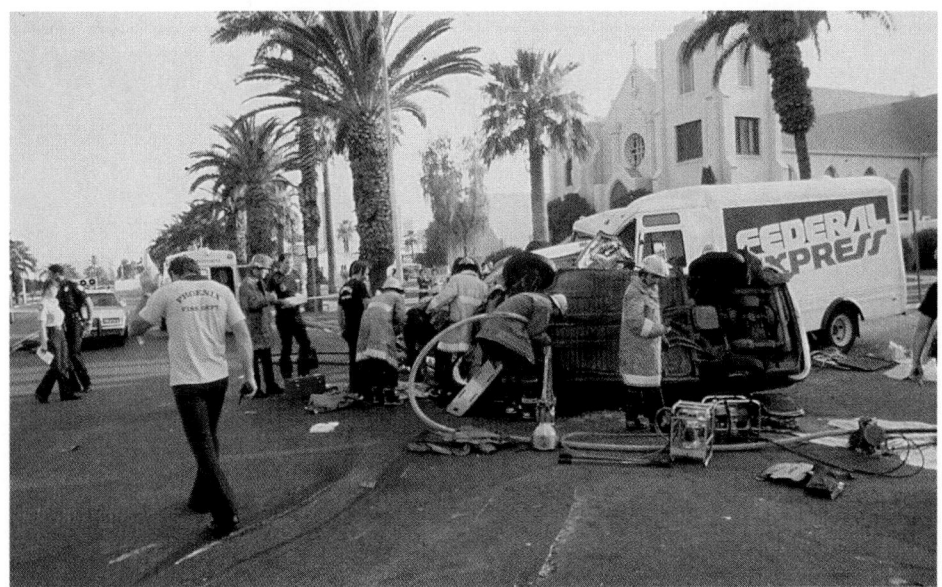

FIGURE 6-5 An MCI training session in Phoenix. Patients are triaged and freed from wreckage in the extrication sector.

■ **Site Safety Officer** a person assigned by the Incident Commander to handle incident safety responsibilities, especially when there are significant hazards at the site.

The bus may have to be blocked up or otherwise secured to prevent further slippage. Rescuers may have to wear protective clothing. As more resources arrive, the Incident Commander must appoint a **Site Safety Officer** to handle incident safety responsibilities.

The Extrication Officer will evaluate what personnel, backboards, extrication equipment, and other medical supplies will be required to extricate and move patients to the treatment sector. In some cases, paramedics will be needed to start IV lines on patients who are expected to remain entrapped a prolonged period of time. Typically, only a few paramedics will be needed in the extrication sector. The majority will be assigned to the treatment sector.

The Extrication Officer will report all resource requirements to the Incident Commander. The Commander, in turn, will provide resources based on availability and priority needs of the entire incident (and all sectors). As more and more personnel assigned to the extrication sector arrive, the sector officer will meet and direct them to appropriate patients and extrication duties. The Extrication Officer will supervise all personnel assigned to his or her sector and manage all activities within that sector.

Throughout the extrication operation, the Extrication Officer will update the Command Officer on progress. (The most significant notification comes when the Extrication Officer reports that the last survivor has been extricated.) The Extrication Officer will also coordinate activities with the Triage and/or Treatment Officer and other agencies and sectors involved in the extrication process.

Treatment Sector

■ **treatment sector** the component of the Incident Command System that is responsible for collecting and treating patients in a centralized treatment area.

Shortly after the extrication sector is established, a **treatment sector** must be created. (See Figure 6-6.) The Treatment Officer will establish an area where patients can be collected and treated. (See Table 6-3.) Central treatment areas permit maximum patient care in incidents that involve large numbers of patients.

The Treatment Officer will determine how many treatment personnel will be needed to handle all patients, as well as the necessary medical supplies. Various rules of thumb have been proposed, but the bottom line is that a minimum of one treatment person per serious patient (1:1) will be required. Multiple minor patients can be managed with a lesser (1:3) rescuer-to-patient

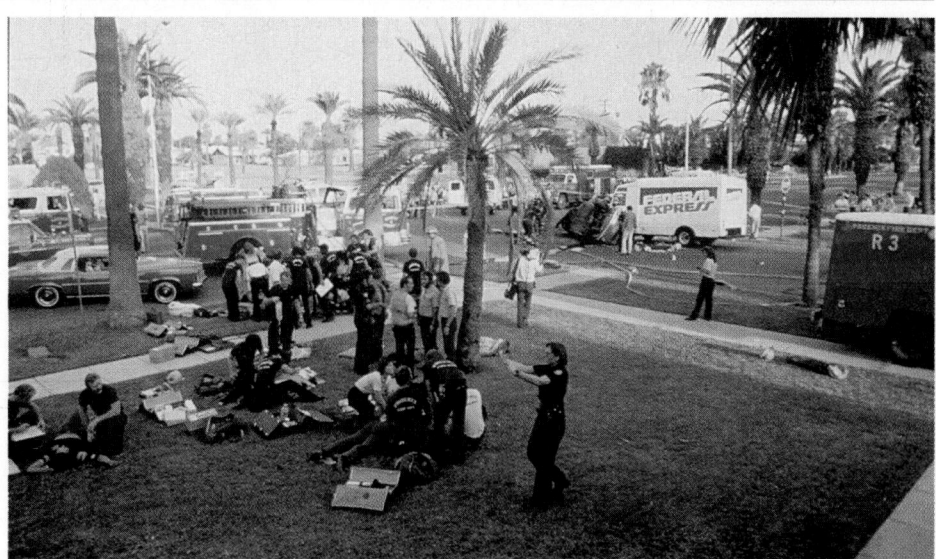

FIGURE 6-6 Patients are further triaged, treated, and packaged for transport in the treatment sector. In this scene, the extrication sector is operating in the background, the treatment sector in the foreground.

TABLE 6-3 Treatment Officer Responsibilities

1. Locate a suitable treatment sector area and report that location to the Extrication Officer and Command.
2. Evaluate resources required for patient treatment, and report those needs to Command.
3. Provide suitable "immediate" and "delayed" treatment areas.
4. Allocate resources.
5. Assign, direct, supervise, and coordinate personnel within the sector.
6. Report progress to Command.

ratio. This resource requirement will be reported to Command. The Command Officer will notify the Staging Officer that appropriate resources should be sent to the treatment sector. In some cases, such progress reports will lead the Incident Commander to call additional resources to the scene.

Paramedics should attend first to critical patients and then to patients triaged as less serious. With regard to paramedic use, the majority of these ALS-trained personnel will be assigned to treatment sector operations. Only a few paramedics, if any, will be needed in the extrication sector, and they will primarily treat entrapped patients who face a long extrication. Many systems give patient treatment needs such high priority that they avoid or minimize assigning sector officer responsibilities to paramedics.

The treatment area will be divided into two sections. One will be used to treat all critical patients, while the other will treat those who have been less seriously injured. As patients arrive, the Treatment Officer will determine to which area the patient should be routed. If triage tagging has not been done prior to the patients' arrival in the treatment sector, that will take place at this time. The Treatment Officer will ensure that all patients are placed in the proper treatment area and are attended to in a timely manner. All treatment personnel will be closely supervised. The Treatment Officer will provide the Incident Commander with progress reports, noting when the first patients arrive and when the last patient is transported. Other progress reports will be given to the Incident Commander as essential information or situations become known. The Treatment Officer's close coordination with both the Extrication and Triage Officers and the Transportation Officer will be maintained throughout the rescue effort.

Transportation Sector

As patients are treated and "packaged" for moving, the **transportation sector** becomes involved. This sector's officer has a real challenge: He or she will determine and obtain all transportation for the patients. (See Table 6-4.) The sector officer will also notify hospitals and coordinate patient allocation to those facilities. (Separate radios should be used to communicate with hospitals and with the dispatch center if possible.) Hospitals must be alerted early, and their capacity for receiving and treating patients must be determined. Communication will flow continuously between the Transportation Officer and medical facilities in regard to the number of patients, their injuries and conditions, hospital patient allocation, arrival times, and so on.

The transportation sector will set up operations near the exit of the treatment sector area and close to the ambulance/patient-loading site. The Transportation Officer will work closely with the Treatment Officer in determining which patients are to be transported, in what order, and to which medical facilities. (See Figure 6-7.) It is the Transportation Officer who deter-

■ **transportation sector** the component of the Incident Command System that is responsible for obtaining and coordinating all patient transportation.

TABLE 6-4 Transportation Officer Responsibilities
1. Establish ambulance staging (if Command has not done so) and patient loading areas.
2. Establish and operate a helicopter landing site.
3. Work with the communication center and hospitals to obtain medical facility status and treatment capabilities.
4. Coordinate patient allocation and transportation with the treatment sector, the communication center, and hospitals.
5. Report resource requirements to Command.
6. Supervise assigned personnel.
7. Coordinate with other sectors.
8. Report progress to Command.

mines to which hospital the patient will be sent, based on the hospital availability reports and patient conditions, then arranges appropriate transportation (e.g., ambulance, helicopters). The Transportation Officer normally communicates directly with the Staging Officer, so that ambulances can be sent to the treatment area as needed (generally one or two units at a time). As patients are loaded, the Transportation Officer or aide will tear off the triage tag stub (if used), enter that information on a tally sheet, and alert receiving hospitals about how many patients are en route, patient priorities, the nature of their injuries (in brief and general terms), and their estimated times of arrival.

The Transportation Officer may also be responsible for establishing a helicopter landing zone if helicopters are used. This usually requires an aide with a radio (communicating on the command channel). The aide may also need an additional radio for air-to-ground radio communications in order to provide landing instructions and coordination. Some agencies establish a separate Landing Zone Officer for air transportation operations.

The Transportation Officer typically employs several aides—one assigned to hospital radio communications, one to the landing zone (if helicopters are used), and one to the patient-loading area. Additional personnel may be required at larger disasters.

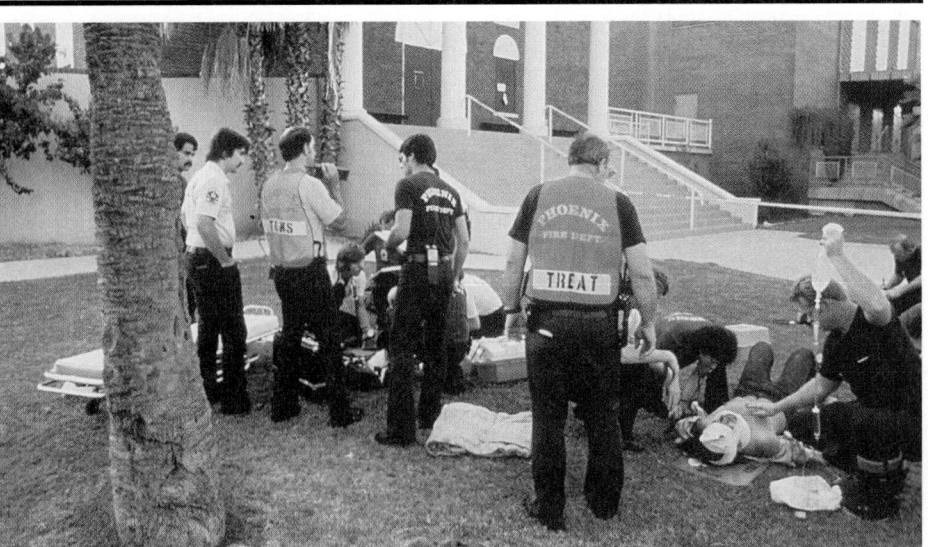

FIGURE 6-7 In this scene, the Transportation Officer (holding two-way radio) coordinates patient transportation with the Treatment Officer and hospital facilities.

The transportation sector will provide frequent progress reports to Command and, in many cases, to various hospitals. Command will be advised when the sector is in operation and when the first patients are transported. It is especially important that the Transportation Officer advise Command and hospitals when the last patient is transported.

Staging Sector

As soon as the Incident Commander sizes up a major operation, he or she will establish a **staging sector** and assign a sector officer (see Table 6-5). All additional apparatus—fire, police, EMS, or other vehicles and agencies—will report to the staging sector. Exceptions are made in the case of apparatus carrying specialized equipment requested by the Incident Commander. Such resources will be sent directly to the scene.

The staging sector will be established reasonably close to the incident, yet far enough away to minimize site congestion. In the case of the bus scenario described earlier, it would be important that the area immediately around the vehicle remain uncongested so that ambulances will have unobstructed access to the scene. The staging area will also be organized to avoid internal congestion and to allow apparatus the mobility to move up to or around the incident site.

As various sectors report their resource requirements to the Incident Commander, he or she will determine which units are available. In some cases, the Incident Commander will request more resources from Dispatch. The Command Officer then communicates these needs to the Staging Officer, who selects the appropriate units and sends them directly to the sectors in need. Within the staging sector, assignments are communicated face-to-face. The Staging Officer then advises the Incident Commander as to which units were detailed.

To further minimize congestion at the incident site, personnel assigned to sectors will, when possible, leave the staging sector on foot and hand-carry any additional medical equipment needed to function at the incident site. In some cases, a single pick-up truck, ambulance, or other vehicle can be used to shuttle large numbers of personnel and equipment from staging to the incident site.

■ **staging sector** the component of the Incident Command System that is responsible for assembling fire, police, EMS, and other vehicles and apparatus to be ready for deployment in an area close to the incident site.

TABLE 6-5 Staging Officer Responsibilities

1. Coordinate with the police department to block streets, intersections, and other access routes required for staging operations.
2. Ensure that all apparatus and vehicles are parked in an appropriate and orderly manner within staging, so that they may be easily moved to the incident site.
3. Maintain a log of units available in the staging area, as well as an inventory of all specialized equipment and medical supplies that might be required at the scene.
4. Confer with Command about essential resources in the staging area, and coordinate requests for these resources with the communications center.
5. Assume a position that is visible and accessible to incoming and staged units. This can best be accomplished by one unit leaving its emergency lights on, while all others turn their lights off upon entering the staging area. The staging officer will be located at the vehicle with its lights on. He or she should wear a sector vest.
6. Report progress to Command.

TABLE 6-6 Supply Officer Responsibilities
1. Establish a suitable location for supply sector operations, normally near the treatment sector.
2. Determine the medical supply and equipment needs of other sectors.
3. With the transportation sector, coordinate procurement of medical supplies from hospitals.
4. Coordinate the procurement of additional supplies that are not available from hospitals.
5. Report additional resource requirements to Command.
6. Allocate supplies and equipment as needed.
7. Report progress to Command.

Supply Sector

■ **supply sector** the component of the Incident Command System that is responsible for obtaining and distributing supplies at a major incident.

If an incident is so large that it exhausts routine stocks of medical supplies and equipment carried on apparatus, the Command Officer will establish a **supply sector** (otherwise known as "support" or "resource"). A Supply Officer should be designated to assure that the sector is operating well and that supplies are readily available. (See Table 6-6.) Radio designation for this sector could be "supply sector" or "resource sector." This sector is responsible for procuring and assembling the equipment and medical supplies necessary to meet the anticipated demands of the incident.

The location of the supply sector would typically be near the treatment sector, which generally has the greatest demand for the supply sector's services. All requests for the supply sector's services normally go through Command first. However, the Incident Commander may find it more practical to have the extrication, treatment, and transportation sectors communicate directly with the supply sector when requesting supplies. As always, face-to-face communications are preferred.

Triage Sector

The command organization presented thus far assumes that triage is a continuous process, initiated by the first arriving crews and closely monitored and reevaluated throughout the extrication, treatment, and transportation process.

TABLE 6-7 Triage Officer Responsibilities
1. Establish the triage sector in close proximity to the incident in a secure and safe area, upwind and uphill from the scene if possible.
2. Ensure the proper utilization of the START system or other local triage protocol.
3. Ensure that triage tags, if used, are being properly completed and secured to the patients.
4. Provide for site safety for members and patients (very important!).
5. Communicate resource requirements to Command.
6. Assign, direct and supervise members and resources.
7. Provide progress reports, as requested or appropriate, to the Incident Commander.

This is because patient conditions change, often rapidly. Therefore, all personnel, especially the people operating in the extrication and treatment sectors, must have the necessary medical training (EMT-Basic level or higher) to make triage decisions. For this reason, it may not be necessary to assign any individual solely to triage.

The local Incident Command System, however, may recommend that the Incident Commander designate a **triage sector** in addition to the extrication, treatment, and transportation sectors. This sector and its Triage Officer (see Table 6-7) would be responsible for triage and tagging of all patients, which could take place within the extrication sector or at the entrance to the treatment sector. (In Figure 6-6, note that the sidewalk divides the treatment sector into "critical" and "delayed" treatment areas.) In either case, close coordination with the Extrication and Treatment Officers will be important.

> ■ **triage sector** the component of the Incident Command System that is responsible for sorting all patients according to the severity of their injuries.

The START Method   **START** is an acronym for Simple Triage and Rapid Treatment, a method of triaging and treating patients that was developed in Newport Beach, California, in the early 1980s. The START method has proven to be an effective and rapid approach for triaging large numbers of patients. One of its advantages is that only limited medical training is required to use the method effectively. (See Figure 6-8.)

> ■ **START** the acronym for Simple Triage and Rapid Treatment. The START program describes a rapid method of triaging large numbers of patients in an emergency incident.

Under the START concept, the first on-scene rescuers clear the site of any walking wounded by telling them to walk to a designated location. These patients are then moved out of the wreckage area and told to remain in a predetermined area. Rescuers who arrive later will further assess these patients and treat any injuries. These survivors must always be thoroughly assessed when time and resources become available, as they may have hidden serious injuries.

> ✱ Prolonged and detailed triage techniques are not appropriate for a mass-casualty incident. Instead, a rapid triage system, such as the START system, should be used.

Once the walking wounded are out of the way, rescuers should continue their rapid triage. Patients will be triage-tagged at the completion of each assessment. Each patient's triage assessment should be completed in less than 60 seconds. The three clinical objectives of the START system are assessment of the following:

1. Respiratory status
2. Hemodynamic status
3. Mental status

The first assessment evaluates respirations. If they are adequate, the rescuer goes to the next item. If respirations are inadequate or absent, basic attempts to clear the airway, such as debris removal or repositioning the head, will be taken. Depending upon the results of these corrective actions, the patient is classified according to one of the following triage categories:

❏ No respiratory effort: **Dead/non-salvageable**.
❏ Respirations above 30 or patient requires assistance maintaining airway: **Critical/immediate**.
❏ Respirations below 30: Go to next assessment.

> ■ **dead/nonsalvageable** a triage term for patients who are obviously dead or who have mortal wounds.

> ■ **critical/immediate** a triage term for patients who are critically injured and require immediate transportation.

The next assessment evaluates hemodynamic status (pulse and/or perfusion). The rescuer checks the patient's radial pulse. If it is detected, the patient most likely has a systolic blood pressure of at least 80 mmHg (a lower blood pressure probably cannot be felt at distal pulse points). Note that only the presence of a radial pulse is checked at this point. Pulse rates are not considered.

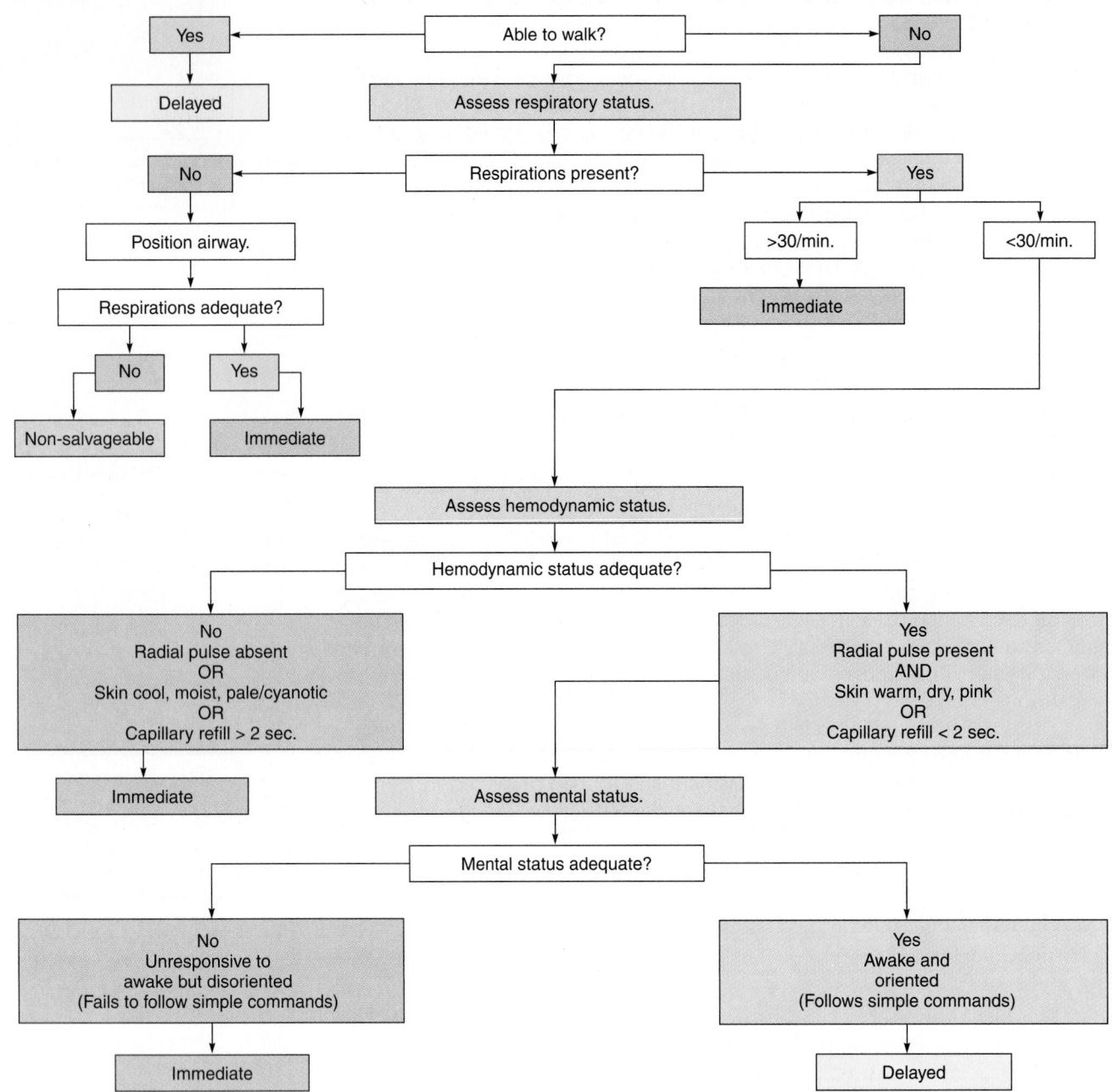

FIGURE 6-8 The START method is an effective and rapid approach for triaging large numbers of patients.

To evaluate perfusion, the rescuer can quickly check skin temperature, condition, and color. Cool, moist, and pale or cyanotic skin indicates poor perfusion, while warm, dry, pink skin indicates adequate perfusion. (Check color at the conjunctiva of the eyes, lips, or nail beds—especially in a dark-skinned patient.) Capillary refill time can also be checked. The rescuer presses the fleshy part of an arm or leg or a nail bed, holds it briefly, then releases the pressure. If the color returns to normal in 2 seconds or less, perfusion is normal. (Capillary refill time is a more reliable indicator of perfusion status in infants or young children than in adults.)

On the basis of the hemodynamic check, the patient falls into one of these categories:

❑ Absence of radial pulse OR skin cool, moist, and pale or cyanotic OR capillary refill greater than 2 seconds: **Critical/immediate**
❑ Palpable radial pulse AND skin warm, dry, and pink OR capillary refill less than 2 seconds: Go to next assessment.

The third assessment evaluates the mental status of the patient. Based upon this assessment, the patient is placed in one of the following four categories on the AVPU scale (see Chapter 10 for a detailed explanation of the AVPU evaluation of mental status):

❑ Unresponsive: **Critical/immediate**
❑ Responsive only to painful or verbal stimuli: **Critical/immediate**
❑ Alert but disoriented (not oriented to time, place or person/self): **Critical/immediate**
❑ Alert and oriented to time, place, and person/self: **Delayed**

■ **delayed** a triage term for patients who do not have immediately life-threatening injuries and who can wait a period of time for transportation and definitive treatment.

It should be pointed out that the first of these assessments that falls into a "critical/immediate" category will stop all further triage assessment. The patient is tagged "critical/immediate" at that time. Only correction of life-threatening problems, such as airway obstruction or severe hemorrhage, would be undertaken before moving to the next patient.

The START process permits a few rescuers to triage a large number of patients very rapidly. Little specialized medical training is required to make these initial triage decisions. After patients are moved to the treatment area, more detailed assessments can be conducted by paramedics.

The METTAG System   Some jurisdictions use the **METTAG** four-color system to categorize and tag patients during triage. (See Figure 6-9.) The colors have the following meanings:

❑ Red—Critical injuries; rapid transportation.
❑ Yellow—Less serious injuries; delayed transportation.
❑ Green—No or mild injuries; transportation unnecessary.
❑ Black—Dead or unsalvageable.

■ **METTAG** a four-color system of tagging patients during triage in which red denotes critical injuries requiring rapid transportation, yellow denotes less serious injuries and delayed transportation, green denotes no or mild injuries for which transportation is optional or unnecessary, and black denotes a dead or unsalvageable patient.

Remember to consult your local Medical Director and/or State Health Department for any specific limitations or mandates they may have relative to triage process and protocol for your local jurisdictions.

Communications

We have only superficially discussed communications as part of incident command organization. Radio communication is absolutely essential. All rescuers and agencies assigned to the various sectors must be able to communicate with the Incident Commander. Therefore, all sector officers will be equipped with a radio tuned to the same frequency as the Incident Commander's. Other channels can be used for support activities (e.g., alerting and briefing hospitals).

However, a great number of rescuers working on the same radio channel can create problems, especially when some are broadcasting non-essential information. Simply put, too much communication—or multiple rescuers operating on separate radio channels—can "gridlock" or even cripple the rescue effort.

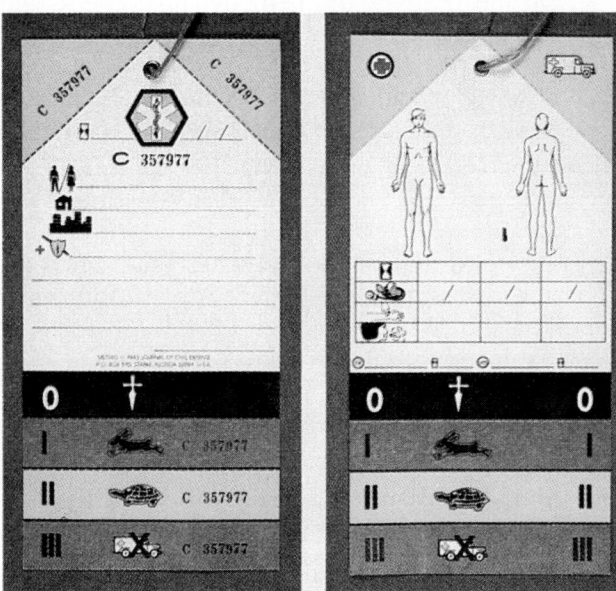

FIGURE 6-9 The METTAG system triages patients using a four-color tagging code.

The Incident Command System controls chaos to a great extent. Go back to the bus accident scenario. Such an incident could easily attract 30 rescue units (fire and ambulance). Without the Incident Command System and the organizational structure described in this chapter, the officer in charge would then have to communicate throughout the incident with 30 people via radio. And those 30 could also be communicating among themselves. It is easy to see how this situation would create a communications overload.

Under the Incident Command System, however, all personnel assigned to each sector work for and communicate only with their sector officer. In the vast majority of cases, because the sector officer is in the work area, this communication is face-to-face. Only occasionally would a member of a sector need to communicate by radio with his or her sector officer. In any case, only the sector officers should communicate with the Incident Commander. As a result, the Incident Command System minimizes radio overload while allowing the Incident Commander to control and maximize the use of available resources.

Progress reporting is also essential to the Incident Command System. Incident command is all about decision-making. Decisions cannot be made without accurate information. Thus, sector officers should frequently update their Incident Commander on what is happening in each sector. If a sector has a problem meeting its objectives, needs more resources, or faces other problems, the sector officer must advise and seek help from the Incident Commander. Otherwise the situation will worsen. If things are going well, the Incident Commander must also know this. Progress reports, however, should contain only essential information. If the sector officer does not have any significant information to give the Incident Commander, he or she should stay off the radio.

Radio codes (e.g., "10-83") pose tremendous problems and should be avoided. These codes can create misunderstandings and confusion, as resources from outside the jurisdiction (and even from within it) may not know what a particular code really means. The use of plain English for all communications is absolutely essential. The use of "clear speak" will ensure that "say what you mean and mean what you say" is adhered to when communicating directions or progress reports.

PLANS, PROCEDURES, AND EQUIPMENT

Inter-Community and Inter-Agency Planning

It is essential to have joint community and agency planning for disaster management. All parties likely to respond to a major incident must have compatible plans and procedures. The elimination of any "turf battles" is a must. Close coordination and cooperation will bring more efficient response to disasters and help in day-to-day operations.

The question of which emergency service should ultimately assume command of overall operations needs to be determined locally. In many cases, local ordinances and other laws make this determination. In most cases the assignment of command authority will fall upon the agency that has the greatest involvement because of the nature of the incident (e.g., civil disorder = police; multiple-alarm fire = fire/rescue service).

It's important that command responsibilities and procedures be worked out by all emergency agencies prior to any disaster. Protocols should describe how all agencies will respond, how they will function on the scene, and what their lines of authority and responsibility will be. Protocols should tell each rescuer what performance is expected.

All emergency agencies should integrate the Incident Command System into their daily operations. As a paramedic, you should consult your employer to determine whether an Incident Command System has been established and is in use. Also find out what, if any, systems are used by other local agencies responsible for incident management. Appropriate plans and procedures, as well as training in the Incident Command System, should be available to new employees. A progressive emergency service organization will already be using the system. For those systems that do not have a system on-line, it is imperative to research which system is best for your jurisdiction and proceed with implementation ASAP.

Organizations such as the National Fire Academy (NFA) in Emmitsburg, Maryland conduct training programs that will acquaint you with a system that is tailored to the needs of EMS. The NFA Incident Command System for Emergency Medical Services was developed by Senior EMS and Fire Chief officers from New York, Phoenix, Los Angeles, and Orange County, California. It provides the students with a solid background in ICS and prepares them to take that information home in order to design and implement the local ICS approach. Additionally, organizations such as the National Fire Service Incident Management System Consortium have published guidelines that are great resources on the design and implementation of ICS for EMS operations.

Incident Duties

A paramedic who reported to the scene in the bus accident scenario would either work in one of the sectors or be assigned as a sector officer. Occasionally, a paramedic will serve as Incident Commander.

Sector Duties Under the Incident Command System, after being assigned to work in a particular sector, the paramedic should report first to the sector officer for a specific assignment. He or she should then continue to report only to that sector officer. No "freelancing" of activities is permitted. Face-to-face communication with the sector officer is essential. Radio communication should be avoided. All problems, progress, and resource needs should be addressed to the sector officer. That officer will, in turn, provide progress reports and request additional resources from the Incident Commander.

Sector Officer Duties   The paramedic assigned as a sector officer must remember that he or she is a manager of rescuers and the rescue effort. Such an officer is not a treatment person. The sector officer might only get involved in hands-on activity very early in the operation when few rescuers are on the scene. Once additional resources begin to arrive, the sector officer must assume the management role. A sector officer who allows himself or herself to be pulled into a hands-on activity loses overall awareness and control of a sector's needs and responsibilities.

The sector officer must obtain a radio (preferably portable) that has a channel to communicate directly with Command. He or she must receive an initial briefing from the Incident Commander regarding the incident's current status and the Commander's plan and objectives. If a paramedic is assuming control of a sector from another paramedic, the transfer of command (for the sector) process must take place.

The objective of the sector officer is to assess quickly the situation as it relates to the responsibilities of his or her sector. The officer then obtains the resources necessary to fulfill those responsibilities. As rescuers arrive in a sector, the officer in charge must meet them and give them their tasks. The sector officer must closely supervise the rescuers to ensure that the sector's objectives are accomplished. Close coordination between adjacent sectors and with Command will be necessary.

The sector officer must be an aggressive manager. He or she cannot assume that another person is taking care of something or that something will naturally take care of itself. Close supervision of personnel assigned to a sector is a must. Patients must be quickly and safely extricated, treated, and transported. If you are a sector officer, it is your job to make things happen!

Essential Items

During mass-casualty incidents, there are items (command adjuncts) that can help an Incident Commander and sector officers perform more effectively. The first is a clipboard with pencils and paper. No one, under the stress of a major incident, can be expected to track everything from memory. The Incident Commander must continually be aware of, and have the ability to track, what units are assigned to various sectors, what remains in staging, and many other details. This sort of information must be written down and tracked. The same information-tracking efforts are required of sector officers. Each will need to know which units are assigned to that sector. The transportation sector, in particular, will need to document how many patients each hospital can take, which ambulances are transporting, and so on. The need for documentation and tracking is obvious. Some communities develop pads or worksheets that organize important information and provide reminders of what needs to be done.

Sector vests are also excellent tools in a rescue operation. These brightly colored garments identify sector officers (and aides) in a crowd of rescuers. Some vests have sector titles printed on them, which makes it easier for rescuers to locate sector officers quickly. Typically, these vests are carried in the supervisors' or other specialized vehicles. Some agencies include a vest in all vehicles. Vests should be issued as early as possible during an incident.

With regard to the use of ambulances and their personnel, past experience in mass-casualty events has provided some important lessons. There will always be fewer ambulances available than patients until well into an event. For the most part, rapid transportation of patients is of highest priority (especially during trauma-related events), so rescue personnel should quickly treat and package all patients. Multiple trips must be made to and from hospitals in order to clear a scene of all patients. The speed of patient transportation will depend on the number of ambulances available and how rapidly they can return to the scene.

It's important that ambulances and the personnel staffing them be used solely for transportation, whenever possible. Other paramedics, who are not assigned to a transport ambulance, should treat patients on the scene and assume sector officer responsibilities. Such organization will depend on local resources, personnel training levels, and mass-casualty plans, but ambulance transportation needs must be given the highest priority.

SUMMARY

During your career as a paramedic, you will almost inevitably be involved in some form of multiple-casualty-incident response. While most of these events will involve no more than two or three vehicles—and fewer than five or six patients—the Incident Command System should be employed. If a major incident develops, procedures used on a day-to-day basis, such as START or MET-TAG and the Incident Command System, can be immediately implemented, with all members of the response aware of their roles in the rescue, ensuring proper span of control along with an effective and safe organization.

FURTHER READING

Auf der Heide, E. *Disaster Response: Principles of Preparation and Coordination.* Saint Louis, MO: C.V. Mosby, 1989.

Brunacini, A.V. *Fire Command.* Quincy, MA: National Fire Protection Association, 1985.

Hafen, B., K. Karren, and J. Mistovich. *Prehospital Emergency Care,* 5th ed. Upper Saddle River, NJ: Prentice Hall, 1996, 794–807.

Leonard, R.B. *Approach to Mass Gatherings and Terrorism.* Dallas, TX: American College of Emergency Physicians, 1992.

Lilja, G.P., M.A. Madsen, and J. Overton. "Multiple Casualty Incidents," in A. Kuehl, *Prehospital Systems and Medical Oversight,* 2nd ed. Saint Louis, MO: Mosby-Yearbook, 1994, 441–446.

Maniscalco, Paul M. "Terrorism Hits Home—Terror at the Towers." *Emergency Medical Service: The Journal of Emergency Care and Transportation,* Vol. 22, No. 5 (May 1993).

Mauck, Robert A. "The Crash of American Eagle Flight 4184." *Street Skills—Rescue—EMS,* Vol. 13, No. 5 (September/October 1995).

START: A Triage Method. Newport Beach, CA: Hoag Memorial Hospital Presbyterian, 1989.

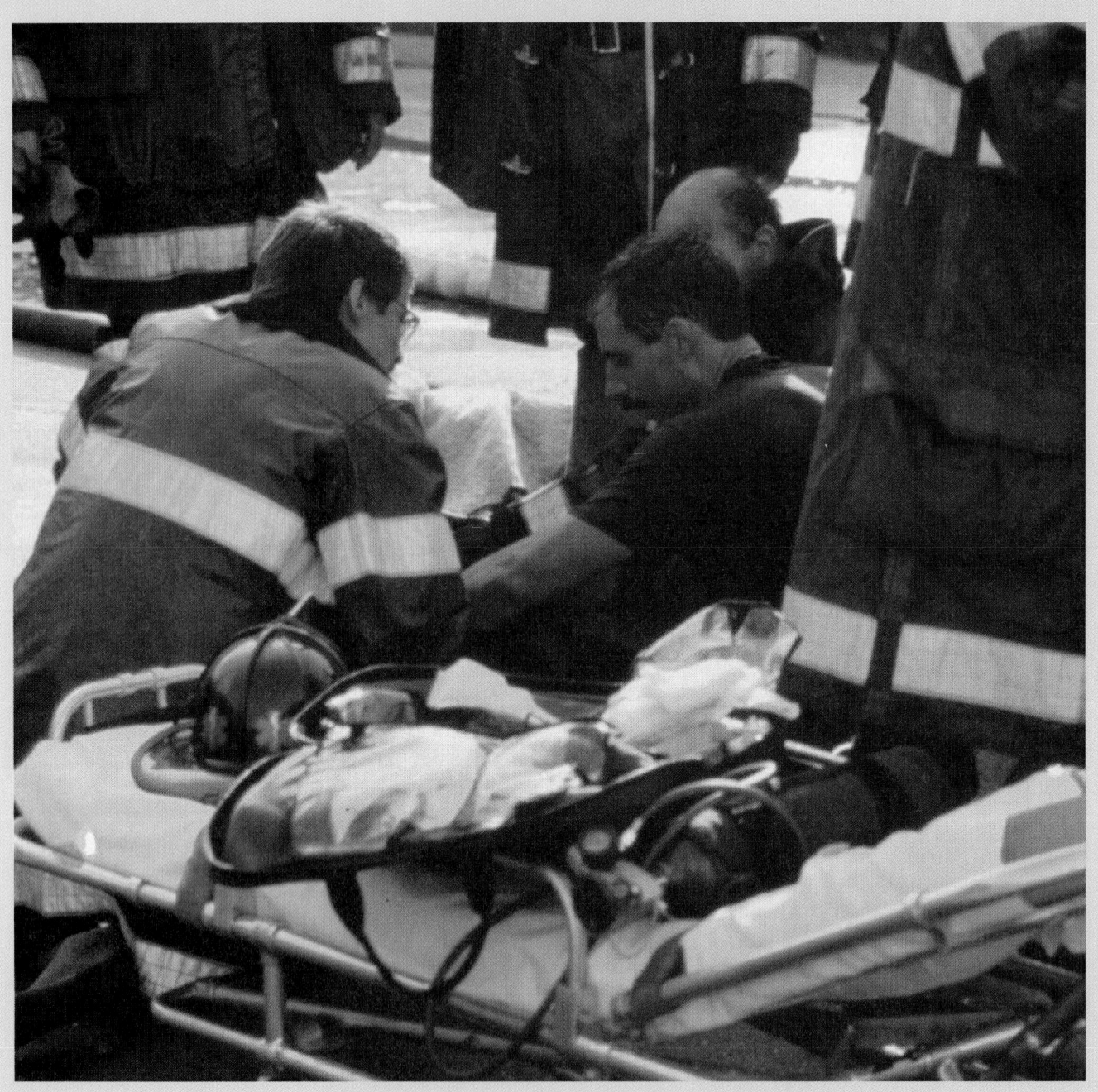

7

STRESS MANAGEMENT IN EMERGENCY SERVICES

Objectives for Chapter 7

After reading this chapter, you should be able to:

1. Define the term "stress." (See p. 112.)

2. Describe the stress reaction, including the various psychological and physiological components. (See pp. 113–116.)

3. Describe the three stages of the body's response to stress. (See p. 113.)

4. Define the term critical incident, and describe critical incident stress. (See pp. 113–114.)

5. Describe the three types of stress reactions. (See pp. 113–116.)

6. Describe anxiety, and discuss its role in helping us to cope with various stressors. (See pp. 116–117.)

7. Name common causes of job stress for the paramedic. (See pp. 117–118.)

8. List techniques the paramedic can use to deal with stress. (See pp. 118–120.)

9. Describe the purpose of Critical Incident Stress Debriefing. (See p. 120.)

10. Describe the stages of the grief process. (See pp. 120–121.)

11. Describe the needs of the dying patient, the family of the dying patient, and the EMT-P. (See p. 121.)

On November 22, a dispatcher sent Medic 16 to a local laundromat on an "unknown medical emergency." The dispatcher reported that the call had come through the police department, but she had no other information. Police officers, however, were en route. On that date, Medic 16 had a crew of three. The driver, and senior paramedic, was Bill Wyncek, who had three years of EMS experience. The other paramedic, Cathy Downley, had less than one year of experience, but she performed like a seasoned veteran. The third crew member was a paramedic student, serving his field internship.

Arriving at the scene, the paramedics found police officers crouched behind their cars with guns drawn. The paramedics could learn only that there was a shooting and that the suspect was still inside the laundromat. The stand-off lasted more than an hour. Police negotiators tried to reason with the suspect. They eventually learned that the suspect had recently separated from his wife, lost his job, and hurt his back in a fall. The suspect became more hostile as the ordeal continued. Finally, in anger, he sprayed the police cars with automatic weapon fire. The police returned the fire. Then, there was quiet. After about five minutes, the suspect appeared in the door with the pistol barrel in his mouth. He made an obscene gesture at the police and squeezed the trigger. Police officers then carefully advanced into the laundromat. They declared the scene safe and summoned the paramedics.

Nothing could have prepared the crew of Medic 16 for the scene inside. Bullet holes and blood covered the walls of the laundromat. Three victims were on the floor. A woman, probably the gunman's wife, was obviously dead, shot 20–30 times. Also dead were two young children, one an infant. Like the woman, bullet holes riddled their bodies.

With nothing to be done for any of the victims—including the gunman—the paramedics returned to the ambulance, slowly and in silence. Calmly, Bill picked up the EMS microphone: "Medic 16 clear, no transport." They returned to the station. Although Bill showed no outward signs of emotion, his internal emotions were in turmoil. He had never witnessed a person die violently. Beyond that, he and his wife had a baby girl, about the age of one of the children killed at the scene.

Fortunately, Cathy talked with supervisors about the incident. They soon called a Critical Incident Stress Debriefing. Supervisors took care to include the paramedic student. It took Bill a long time to open up and describe his feelings. He felt rage toward the gunman in particular and toward society in general. The meeting, and two later ones, helped Cathy, Bill, and the student deal with their emotions and feelings. All three still work in EMS.

INTRODUCTION

Stress is an inherent aspect of emergency medical services. Only in recent years has stress been recognized as a bona fide hazard of emergency work. Prehospital personnel must learn to manage stress, as well as the conditions that cause it. Dealing with stress in a positive manner promotes emotional and physical health and prevents **burnout**. This chapter will discuss EMS stress and how to cope with its effects.

■ **burnout** burnout occurs when coping mechanisms no longer buffer the job stressors. It can compromise personal health and well-being.

STRESS

The word **stress** literally means a hardship, force, or strain. From a psychological standpoint, stress can be defined as a state of physical and psychological arousal. It exists to some degree in everyone.

A **stressor** is any agent or situation that causes stress. Often stress results from a perceived imbalance between the demands of the job and our ability to meet those demands. In addition, stress may be increased by the demands imposed by people and events around us.

■ **stress** a state of physical or psychological arousal.

■ **stressor** any agent or situation that causes stress.

Physiology of Stress

The body's response to stress is termed a **stress reaction**. The stress reaction is complex and involves many body systems. After detection of the stressor, information received from the various senses is processed and interpreted in the cerebral cortex. The cerebral cortex is the part of the brain that controls higher mental functions and intellect. The limbic system, located in the mid-brain, is subsequently activated and an emotional reaction (fear, anger, rage, hostility, etc.) occurs. The response then proceeds to lower brain centers, including the hypothalamus.

The hypothalamus controls many bodily functions, including temperature and sleep. It also regulates the endocrine system. Once stimulated by the hypothalamus, the endocrine system releases hormones such as epinephrine (adrenalin) and norepinephrine (noradrenalin) in response to the stress. The release of epinephrine further stimulates the brain. The body quickly enters a hyperalert state commonly called the "fight-or-flight" response or "alarm reaction." The fight-or-flight response is characterized by an increase in heart rate and blood pressure, pupillary dilation, excessive perspiration, increased muscle tension, increased blood glucose levels, and a sense of anxiety. This response prepares the body to deal with any threats, real or perceived.

■ **stress reaction** complex response of the body to stress that prepares the body to deal with any perceived threats.

The Body's Response to Stress

The body is under various levels of stress at all times. However, after repeated exposure to the same stressor, the body will adapt by suppressing the typical emotional and physical responses. The body's response to stress generally goes through the following stages.

❑ *Stage I: Alarm.* An alarm reaction occurs at the first exposure to the stressor. The signs include increased pulse rate, pupillary dilation, and other responses of the sympathetic nervous system. If resistance to stress is diminished, the physiological and emotional response can be overwhelming.

❑ *Stage II: Resistance.* This stage starts when the individual begins to adapt to the stress. Resistance is often brought about by use of various coping mechanisms. Physiological parameters, such as pulse and blood pressure, may return to normal. As adaptation develops, resistance increases above the normal level.

❑ *Stage III: Exhaustion.* Prolonged exposure to the same stressors leads to the exhaustion of an individual's adaptation energy. The signs of the alarm reaction reappear, but they are now much more difficult to reverse.

■ **acute stress reaction** reaction that occurs soon after a catastrophic event that has a powerful emotional impact on the rescuer.

Types of Stress Reactions

A stress reaction has both physical and psychological components. There are three types of stress reactions that can occur: acute, delayed, and cumulative stress.

■ **critical incidents** an event that has a powerful emotional impact on a rescuer that causes an acute stress reaction.

Acute Stress Reaction   The **acute stress reaction** usually occurs after a catastrophic event. The reaction has a powerful emotional impact on the rescuer. Catastrophic events capable of evoking such a response have been labeled **critical incidents**. The acute stress reaction that follows is called **critical incident stress**.

■ **critical incident stress** reaction that occurs soon after a catastrophic event that has a powerful emotional impact on the rescuer. It is synonymous with acute stress reaction.

TABLE 7-1	Distress Signals Requiring Immediate Corrective Action	
Physical	**Cognitive**
Chest pain*	Decreased alertness to surroundings
Difficulty breathing*	Difficulty making decisions
Elevated blood pressure*	Hyperalertness
Collapse from exhaustion*	Generalized mental confusion
Cardiac arrhythmias*	Disorientation to person, place, time
Blood in stool*	Serious disruption in thinking
Dehydration*	Seriously slowed thinking
Dizziness*	Problems in naming familiar items
Vomiting*	Problems recognizing familiar people
Emotional	**Behavioral**
Panic reactions	Significant change in speech patterns
Shock-like state	Excessively angry outbursts
Phobic reaction	Crying spells
General loss of control	Antisocial acts (e.g. violence)
Inappropriate reactions	Extreme hyperactivity

* Indicates a need for medical evaluation

From Jeff Mitchell/Grady Bray, *Emergency Services Stress*, ©1990, pp. 42-43. Reprinted by permission of Prentice-Hall, Englewood Cliffs, New Jersey.

The acute stress reaction may begin at the scene or shortly after the event. Several warning signs or symptoms characterize its onset. (See Tables 7-1 and 7-2.) Some signs and symptoms require immediate intervention, while others do not. Early intervention will help minimize the long-term effects of the stress. **Critical Incident Stress Debriefing (CISD)** helps to effectively deal with stress and prevent post-traumatic stress disorder. If indicated, the CISD team may refer the rescuer for professional counseling. (For more information on CISD, see page 120.)

Delayed Stress Reactions   **Delayed stress reaction**, also called "post-traumatic stress disorder," occurs days, weeks, months, or even years after a critical incident. Not all personnel who experience a critical incident will suffer a delayed stress reaction—but some will. The following signs or symptoms characterize post-traumatic stress disorder.

❑ *Reexperiencing of the traumatic event.*
   • Recurrent and intrusive recollections of the event.
   • Recurrent dreams and nightmares related to the event.
   • Flashbacks, or sudden feelings that the event is recurring, usually after exposure to some triggering stimulus.
❑ *Diminished responsiveness to the external world.*
   • Decreased interest in life.
   • Feeling detached or estranged from others.
   • Suppression of normal emotional responses such as love, anger, or fear.
❑ *Physical and cognitive symptoms.*
   • Hyperalertness.
   • Difficulty sleeping.

■ **Critical Incident Stress Debriefing (CISD)** form of group support, developed by Jeff Mitchell, Ph.D., to assist rescuers in coping with highly stressful events.

■ **delayed stress reactions** a stress reaction that occurs days, weeks, or months after a critical incident, also called post-traumatic stress disorder.

TABLE 7-2 Common Signs and Symptoms of Distress Not Requiring
Immediate Action

Physical	Cognitive
Nausea	Confusion
Upset stomach	Lowered attention span
Tremors (lips, hands)	Calculation difficulties
Feeling uncoordinated	Memory problems
Profuse sweating	Poor concentration
Chills	Seeing an event over and over
Diarrhea	Distressing dreams
Rapid heart rate	Disruption in logical thinking
Muscle aches	Blaming someone
Sleep disturbance	
Dry mouth	
Shakes	
Vision problems	
Fatigue	

Emotional	Behavioral
Anticipatory anxiety	Change in activity
Denial	Withdrawal
Fear	Suspiciousness
Survivor guilt	Change in communications
Uncertainty of feelings	Change in interactions with others
Depression	Increased or decreased food intake
Grief	Increased smoking
Feeling hopeless	Increased alcohol intake
Feeling overwhelmed	Overly vigilant to environment
Feeling abandoned	Excessive humor
Feeling lost	Excessive silence
Worried	Unusual behavior
Wishing to hide	
Wishing to die	
Anger	
Feeling numb	
Identifying with victim	

From Jeff Mitchell/Grady Bray, *Emergency Services Stress*, ©1990, pp. 42-43. Reprinted by permission of
Prentice-Hall, Englewood Cliffs, New Jersey.

- Survivor guilt.
- Memory impairment and difficulty concentrating.
- Avoidance of any activities that may cause recall of the event.
- Avoidance of thoughts or feelings associated with the incident.
- Problems with interpersonal relationships.

Post-traumatic stress disorder can interfere with your life. It can provoke
marital problems, alcohol and drug abuse, personality changes, and even suicide. Because of this, persons suffering from a post-traumatic stress disorder
should seek expert professional help soon.

Cumulative Stress Reaction

Cumulative Stress Reaction The third type of stress reaction is called a **cumulative stress reaction**, or "burnout." Cumulative stress, unlike the types of stress discussed earlier, does not result from a single critical incident. Instead, it stems from recurring minor stressors, both work and non-work related.

A cumulative stress reaction typically takes years to develop. Initially, the person will experience depression, boredom, apathy, and emotional fatigue. As the reaction progresses, the person will experience sleep disturbances, increasing loss of emotional control, frequent physical complaints, physical and emotional fatigue, irritability, and worsening depression. Ultimately, the person will develop extreme fatigue, severe depression, feelings of paranoia, crying spells, loss of sexual drive, inability to perform a job, significant problems managing his or her personal life, and occasionally suicidal or homicidal thinking.

Failure to intervene in the early stages of cumulative stress will result in severe disability for the person involved. Often he or she will suffer destruction of close family relationships, divorce, and inability to work in his or her chosen profession. The best treatment for the cumulative stress reaction is prevention. EMS systems should have programs that routinely screen their personnel for signs and symptoms of cumulative stress. Such programs will allow for early intervention, thus avoiding the condition's devastating consequences. Also, stressful assignments, such as busy stations or those with a higher incidence of critical patients, should be shared among personnel.

ANXIETY

Anxiety is an emotional state caused by stress. It is a major cause for the development of **defense mechanisms**. Anxiety alerts a person to impending or perceived danger. Facilitated through the sympathetic nervous system, anxiety maintains all potential resources, emotional and physical, in readiness for emergencies. Anxiety is related to each individual's perception of the environment around him or her. It is based upon a person's psychological processes and personal history. The factors that lead to anxiety can be divided into two general categories: normal and detrimental.

Normal Anxiety Levels

A "normal" level of anxiety varies from individual to individual. It acts as a warning system to put us on guard, so we won't be overwhelmed by a sudden stimulation or immobilized in a critical situation. "Normal" anxiety may be considered adaptive, because it has evolved to help us cope with stressors by focusing our attention. It helps us increase our tolerance for stress by developing coping and/or defense mechanisms.

This process is evident in emergency medical services. The first emergency response that an EMT or paramedic makes is a very stressful event. The person experiences a high pulse rate, dilated pupils, poorly organized thought processes, and a feeling of tension. However, over time, the body adapts to stress. Each response becomes more and more routine. However, as long as the EMT or paramedic is "on call" for emergency response, his or her level of anxiety never returns to a non-work state. Keeping anxiety at an "on-alert" level is a coping mechanism. Because it is impossible to predict and prepare for the next problem, anxiety helps the paramedic maintain a level of readiness.

Detrimental Anxiety Levels

Although many reactions to anxiety and stress are positive, there are also detrimental ones. Detrimental reactions include the failure of anxiety to stimulate the appropriate coping mechanisms. Conversely, an increase in anxiety that is disproportionate to the actual danger would also be detrimental. These reactions may interfere with a rational thought process, disrupt performance, or cause physical problems. Symptoms of anxiety include:

- ❑ Heart palpitations
- ❑ Difficult or rapid breathing
- ❑ Dry mouth
- ❑ Chest tightness or pain
- ❑ Anorexia, nausea, vomiting, abdominal cramps, flatulence, or the classic "butterflies in the stomach"
- ❑ Flushing, diaphoresis, or fluctuation in body temperature
- ❑ Urgency or frequency of urination
- ❑ Dysmenorrhea, or decreased sexual drive or performance
- ❑ Aching muscles or joints
- ❑ Backache or headache

Effects that are not felt include:

- ❑ Increased blood pressure and heart rate
- ❑ Blood shunting to muscles
- ❑ Increased blood glucose levels
- ❑ Increased catecholamine production by the adrenal glands
- ❑ Reduced peristalsis in the digestive tract
- ❑ Pupillary dilation

People react differently to stress. The patient and family may react with anger, guilt, or indecisiveness. A a paramedic, you may react with impatience, fear, or anger. It is important to remember that the patient and family are not as adept at dealing with stress as you the professional. Because of indecisiveness, the patient and family members should not be given too many alternatives. Despite your emotions, you must maintain a professional attitude and remain non-judgmental.

PARAMEDIC JOB STRESS

EMS work involves a lot of stress. (See Figure 7-1.) Some of the occupational stressors include:

- ❑ *Multiple Role Responsibilities.* The paramedic is often a "jack of all trades." The various responsibilities may become overwhelming. This is particularly true of systems in which paramedics also function as firefighters, police officers, or safety officers.
- ❑ *Unfinished Tasks.* The requirements of the job often leave personal and work tasks incomplete. For example, once a patient is delivered to the hospital, you often lose track of the person with whom you spent a great deal of time and energy treating. On a continuous basis, this can result in stress.
- ❑ *Angry or Confused Citizens.* Paramedics do not see society at its best. The very people who require our help can be a source of stress, as a result of either their physical condition or their emotional response to stress.

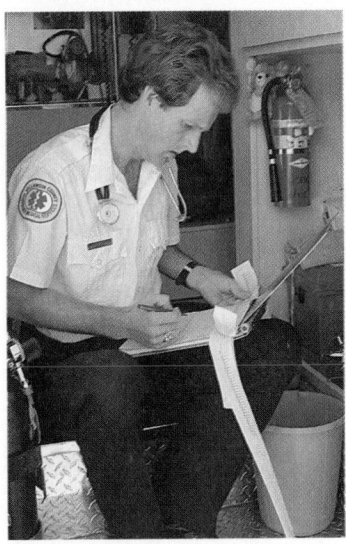

Figure 7-1 EMS is stressful. Paramedics must learn to deal with stress in order to avoid frustration and burnout.

- *Meeting Continuous Time Constraints.* Emergency medical services, like many other occupations, place time constraints on personnel. Eventually, these constraints can result in stress, especially if they are unreasonable.

- *Absence of Challenge.* It is hard to believe that emergency medical services can be unchallenging. But, routine runs (transfers) can get old. Also, in some systems, interesting and challenging runs are rare.

- *Overdemand on Time, Energy, Ability, or Emotions.* Emergency work often demands a great deal of time. Long hours are emotionally and physically demanding. In addition, overwork tends to stress our physical and emotional health.

- *Necessary Restrictions on Practice.* Restrictions limit the scope of the paramedic's practice. The limits can often be frustrating, especially for personnel with previous medical experience. For example, medical personnel in the military work more independently than paramedics. When such people enter EMS, they often feel frustrated when they are not allowed to conduct procedures that they performed routinely in the military.

- *Unpredictable Changes in the Workplace.* No one can deny that emergency medical services work varies day to day. However, lack of stability can become stressful.

- *Lack of Recognition.* Paramedics are often "silent heroes" who routinely do what many people feel is worthy of recognition. Continued lack of recognition can be stressful.

- *Limited Career Mobility.* Many EMS organizations do not provide much opportunity to move up. This deficiency can cause frustration and stress. The limited opportunities for advancement should be considered before entering the profession.

- *Abusive Patients and Dangerous Situations.* Emergency medical service is dangerous. Verbal and physical abuse by patients complicates the matter. You should never become complacent, but you should also be careful not to overreact to abuse from patients or inherent dangers at the scene.

- *Critically Ill or Dying Patients.* No matter how well-adapted you become, caring for critically ill and dying patients produces stress. Treating these patients is frustrating, since, all too frequently, medical intervention is too late or death is unpreventable.

Managing EMS Job Stress

* The paramedic must learn to manage stress in order to survive in EMS.

You must learn to manage stress in order to survive in emergency medical services. You must recognize the early warning signs of anxiety. Remember that some stress is valuable—it protects an individual and improves performance. Therefore, you need to discover your own optimal stress level and attempt to maintain it.

To monitor your own perception of a stressful event, ask yourself these questions.

- Do you see what is really happening?
- Are you blaming yourself unjustly?
- Are your expectations realistic?

Next, try to sort events into categories of importance, urgency, and degree of actual threat.

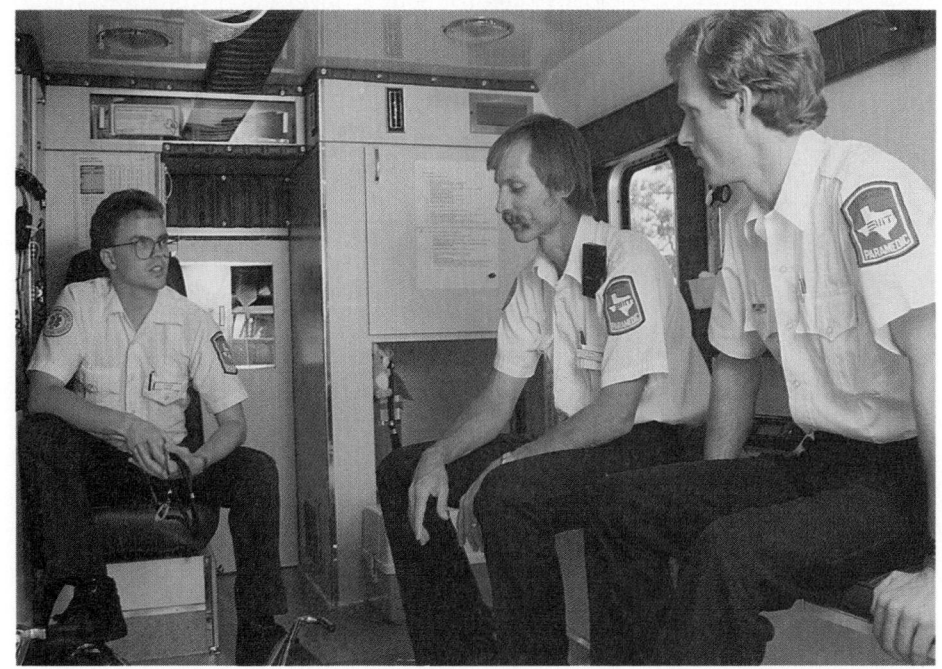

Figure 7-2 Informal discussions with colleagues concerning your feelings and frustrations are helpful and should be encouraged. Following particularly stressful incidents a Critical Incident Stress Debriefing may be warranted.

Another method of coping with stress is to seek and use situational support. Talking about the situation with someone, as soon as possible, is a simple and effective way of coping. (See Figure 7-2.) Particularly stressful situations, involving multiple personnel, may benefit from group discussion. A good example is Critical Incident Stress Debriefing, available in many systems.

Other tips for daily living also help manage stress. These include: adequate sleep and rest, "leaving the job at work," and balancing work and recreation. Physical activity or exercise provides a good release for stress. To balance your personal and professional lives, try to have friends who are both in and out of the EMS field. Remember, you're more than a paramedic. In addition to your job responsibilities, you have the same personal responsibilities as anyone else. Never neglect one aspect of your life and concentrate solely on the other. Learn to accept that certain things are beyond your control and cannot be changed. Above all, use appropriate coping mechanisms. Determine which defense mechanisms are effective for you and adopt those most likely to reduce stress.

Dealing With Critical Incident Stress

Some assignments may be more stressful than others. Although you may experience pain following a particularly stressful event, remember that it is a normal part of the healing process. Do not label yourself as "crazy." Instead, try to minimize the harmful effects of stress. There are several things you can do to help cope with particularly severe stress. These include:

❏ Within the first 24–48 hours, alternate strenuous physical exercise with relaxation. This will help alleviate some of the physical reactions.
❏ Structure your time to stay busy. This will help keep your mind off the stressful event.
❏ Keep your life as normal as possible. Don't make any major life changes during this time.

- Spend time with people and talk to them. Conversation will allow you to express your feelings and is therapeutic.
- Do not overuse drugs or alcohol to "numb" the pain. This only prolongs the stress.
- Help your co-workers as much as possible by sharing feelings and conversation. Realize that they too are under stress.
- Do things that feel good to you.
- Eat balanced meals on a regular basis.
- Get an adequate amount of sleep. Avoid the use of hypnotic drugs; they decrease the amount of quality sleep time. They also can cause rebound insomnia the following night.
- Keep a journal. Write down your thoughts. This too is therapeutic and makes time pass more quickly.
- Reach out. People do care.

Never be afraid to seek additional help. If necessary, request a Critical Incident Stress Debriefing session. Often, an informal session with a trained peer on the scene may be all that is required.

Critical Incident Stress Debriefings

Critical Incident Stress Debriefings are structured group meetings that allow emergency and rescue personnel to discuss their feelings and other reactions after a critical incident. They are not psychotherapy or psychological treatment. They are, however, designed to reduce the impact of a critical event and to accelerate the normal recovery of normal people. Remember that it is normal to suffer painful reactions to an abnormal event. Abnormal reactions occur when such feelings are not shared. Therefore, every system should offer Critical Incident Stress Debriefings or similar programs to personnel who encounter a critical incident.

DEATH AND DYING

Death and dying are a part of emergency medical services. It is important to develop an appropriate personal attitude about death and the dying patient, as well as about the patient's family.

Grief Process

The family of a dying patient, as well as the patient, goes through a grief process initially described by Dr. Elizabeth Kubler-Ross. The grief process has several identifiable stages.

- *Denial and Isolation.* This stage is used by most dying patients. It is healthy and acts as a mental buffer between the shock of dying and dealing with it. It happens throughout the illness. It is a temporary stage, often giving way to acceptance.
- *Anger.* In the anger phase, the patient and the family ask, "Why me?" People are angered at the loss and may project their anger to anything and anyone. It is important to remember that this anger has little to do with the people or things present; they are often simply "targets." The anger can be difficult for you to deal with. Try not to take the patient's or the family's anger personally. Be tolerant, and don't be afraid of anger. Don't become defensive. Listen to the patient and the family.

- *Bargaining.* Bargaining is a defense mechanism used by the dying patient to formulate some sort of "agreement," which, in the patient's mind, postpones the inevitable.
- *Depression.* Depression is common and expected. It is a normal response to the greatest loss. In "reactive depression," the dying patient reacts to the needs of a life situation. For example, who will care for the children or take care of funeral arrangements? There is also "preparatory depression." In this state, the patient is often silent and reassurance is not meaningful.
- *Acceptance.* Acceptance may not be a happy stage. At this point, the patient is without fear and despair. He or she is devoid of feelings. The patient becomes less involved with people as he or she prepares to face death alone. At this stage, the family needs help, understanding, and support more than the patient.

It is important to recognize the needs of individuals when dealing with the dead or dying. The dying patient needs dignity and respect, sharing, communication, hope, privacy, and control. The family has needs, too. They often go through a grief process similar to the patient's. They may need to express their feelings of rage, anger, and despair. In addition, they need to reduce their feelings of guilt. You may also go through some grief stages. This coping requires a lot of energy to cover feelings. It should be followed by adequate time for reflection and discussion.

Management of the Dead or Dying Patient

How you react to death and the dying patient reflects your own thoughts and beliefs. It is natural to feel uncomfortable. Don't bring up the subject of death. Let the patient do so. Don't falsely reassure the patient or the family. Do not be afraid to tell the patient that he or she is dying, if asked. Use non-verbal communications, such as a gentle tone of voice, appropriate facial expression, and a reassuring touch.

If the patient is already dead, the family becomes "the patient." Comfort the family with kind deeds, such as calling neighbors, family members, or a minister. The family needs to hear the word "dead." Avoid euphemisms like "expired," "passed away," or "moved on." Always refer to the deceased patient by their name. Recognize that the family will cope with death in much the same manner as they deal with everyday stresses.

SUMMARY

Stress is a part of emergency medical services. You should recognize that a certain level of stress is important. You should also recognize that increasing stress can seriously affect personal health and job performance. As a paramedic you must learn to adapt to stress and to deal with it positively. You must also learn to deal with stress in other people.

FURTHER READING

Asken, Michael J. *PsycheResponse: Psychological Skills for Optimal Performance by Emergency Responders.* Englewood Cliffs, NJ: Prentice-Hall, 1993.

Mitchell, Jeff, and Bray Grady. *Emergency Services Stress: Guidelines for Preserving the Health and Careers of Emergency Services Personnel.* Englewood Cliffs, NJ: Prentice Hall, 1990.

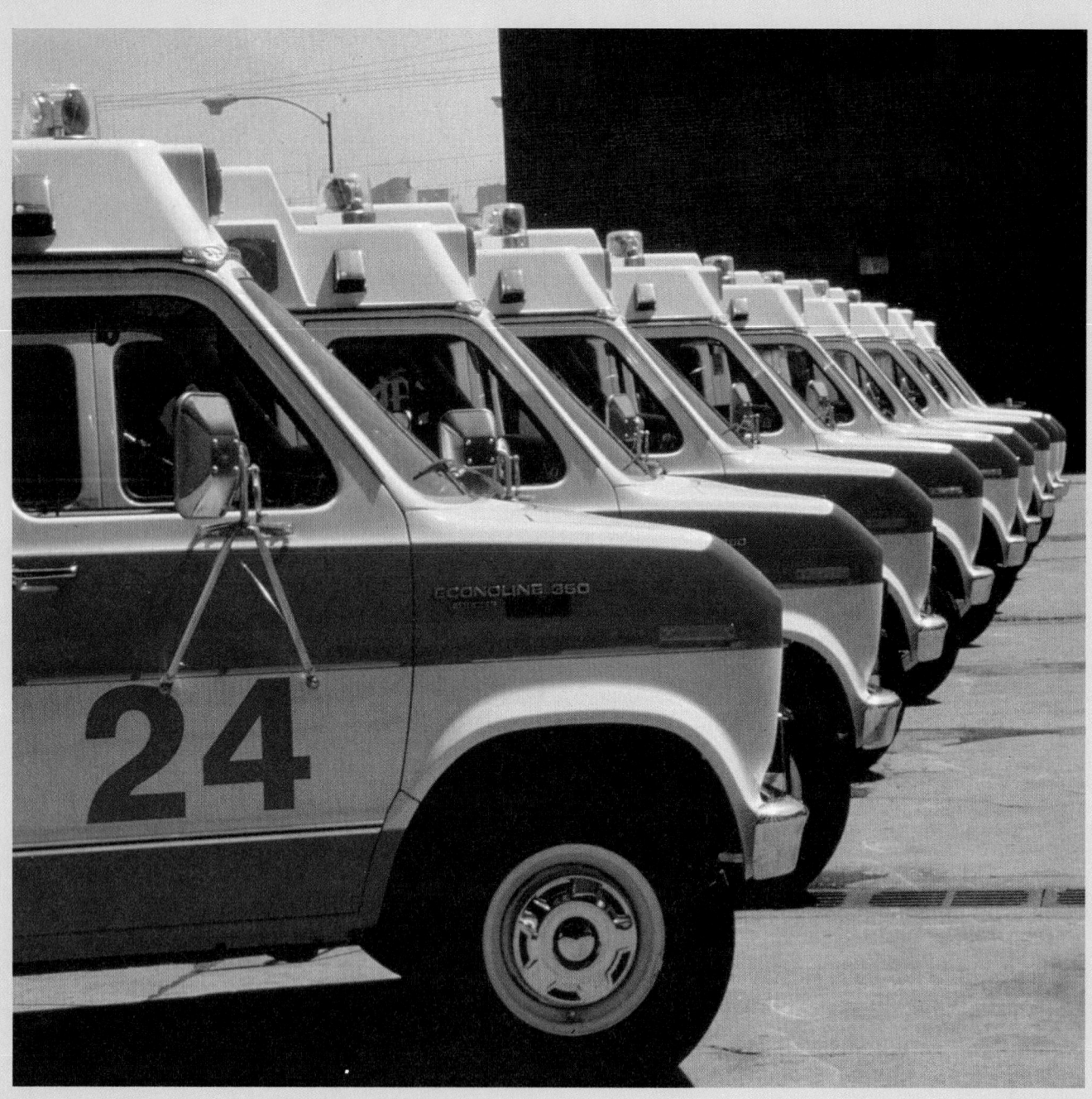

8

MEDICAL TERMINOLOGY

Objectives for Chapter 8

After reading this chapter, you should be able to:

1. Locate at least ten medical terms in a medical dictionary. (See p. 125.)

2. Identify common root words and define their meaning. (See pp. 125–129.)

3. Identify and define common suffixes and prefixes. (See pp. 130–133.)

4. Identify and determine the meaning of common medical terms. (See pp. 125–133.)

5. Identify common medical abbreviations. (See pp. 134–139.)

Air 1, an emergency medical helicopter unit, is dispatched to a rural community hospital to transfer a critically-ill patient to a large urban hospital for definitive care. The flight personnel are alerted and go immediately to the helipad. While the pilot is performing the pre-flight check and warm-up, the flight paramedic receives the initial patient report from the dispatcher. The crew learns that the patient is a 50-year-old male who suffered an acute anterior wall myocardial infarction. While in the emergency department, he suffered an episode of ventricular fibrillation and was successfully resuscitated. Additional information will be relayed when it becomes available.

The helicopter ascends from the helipad and heads south toward the community hospital. The dispatcher relays additional patient information to the flight crew. The patient's vital signs are stable, and he weighs approximately 90 kilograms. He received thrombolytic therapy and is currently receiving a heparin and lidocaine infusion. He has received morphine sulfate for his pain. There have been no reperfusion dysrhythmias noted.

After a short 15-minute flight, the helicopter descends and lands on the helipad at the community hospital. The flight personnel transfer needed medical equipment to a waiting stretcher and proceed to the emergency department. Upon arrival in the emergency department, one crew member begins patient assessment while the other obtains a medical report from the emergency department nurse. The nurse states: "The patient is a 50-year-

old male who suffered an acute onset of retrosternal chest pain approximately 30 minutes prior to arrival. The chest pain radiated to the left arm and jaw. It was accompanied by dyspnea, orthopnea, and diaphoresis. The EKG revealed an anterior wall myocardial infarction with lateral extension of the infarct. The patient has a long history of poorly-controlled hypertension and non-insulin dependent diabetes mellitus. He had a CABG three years ago and coronary angioplasty one year ago. He has also had a cholecystectomy and endoscopic polypectomy—both more than two years ago. Current medications include metoprolol, glyburide, and aspirin. He is allergic to penicillin."

She further states: "He received 1.5 million units of streptokinase as a thrombolytic. His pain has improved, although he is not completely pain-free. The streptokinase infusion was recently completed, and there have been no reperfusion dysrhythmias noted. He is being transferred for emergency coronary angiography because of the continued pain."

The flight crew complete their assessment, prepare the patient for transport, and move him to the waiting helicopter. The transfer proceeds without incident. Upon arrival at the receiving hospital, the patient is taken immediately to the coronary angiography suite. The angiogram reveals a 95 percent blockage of one of his coronary bypass grafts. Angioplasty is carried out and deemed successful. The patient soon becomes pain-free. He is discharged from the hospital eight days later.

INTRODUCTION

■ **medical terminology** the language and terms of medicine, based mostly on Latin and Greek.

Medical terminology is the language of medicine. Like other fields, medicine uses specialized terms and abbreviations. To communicate effectively, those who work in medicine must speak and understand the same language. A knowledge of medical terminology will help you to comprehend reading material and get more benefit from classes and lectures. Knowledge of medical terminology will also facilitate communication with physicians, nurses, and other health care personnel.

Initially, medical terminology may look like a foreign language—and in some ways it is so. The Greeks helped found modern medicine, and many of their terms still remain in use. When the seat of medicine passed to ancient Rome, Latin became the universal language of medicine. In the centuries that followed, Greek and Latin terms slipped into common usage. Even today, many new medical terms are derived from Greek or Latin.

MEDICAL DICTIONARY

A medical dictionary is a valuable tool, both in the classroom and on the job. Medical dictionaries not only define and spell terms, they also provide medical information. Some of the main features of a medical dictionary include: correct spelling, phonetic pronunciation (in parentheses), definitions, meanings, subtopics, etymologies, and medical synonyms. Subtopics in the dictionary offer related words; etymologies give the derivatives of words and their Greek or Latin meanings. After definition of the word will come a list of associated words or synonyms. Most medical dictionaries also provide sections on first aid, diseases, drugs, and anatomy.

MEDICAL TERMINOLOGY

The three parts of a medical term are the **prefix, root word**, and the **suffix**. Not all medical terms have both a prefix and suffix, but most have one or the other. To identify the meaning of a medical term involves identifying each of its parts. For example:

> Tonsil   +   itis   = Tonsillitis (inflammation of the tonsils)
> (root word) (inflammation)

Root Words

A root word is defined as the part of a word that conveys its essential meaning. It is distinguished from other word parts that modify this meaning. Roots may be attached to other roots to form words, or prefixes and suffixes may be attached to roots to form words. The following examples show how a root word may be modified by the addition of another root word or by a prefix or suffix. (Also, see Table 8-1.)

> algia (pain) }
> caus (burn) }   causalgia (burning pain)
>
> partus (labor)   postpartum (after birth)
> tropho (nourish)   hypertrophy (overnourishment)

■ **prefix** one or more syllables affixed to the beginning of a word to modify its meaning.

■ **root word** a word to which a suffix, prefix, or both is affixed.

■ **suffix** one or more syllables affixed to the end of a word to modify its meaning.

TABLE 8-1 Common Root Words	
Root Words	**Meaning**
abdomino-	belly or abdominal wall
acou-	to hear
acq-	water
acro-	extreme ends of a part
aden-	a gland
adip-	soft fat of animals
alb-	white
alg-	pain
all-	other, different
anc-, ang-, ank-	bend or hollow
andr-	male
angi-	blood vessel

TABLE 8-1   Common Root Words (Continued)

Root Words	Meaning
aort-	large artery exiting from the left ventricle
arter-	artery
arth-	joint
artic-	joint
asphyxia	unconsciousness due to suffocation
asth-	short drawn breath, panting
asthenia	weakness
aud-, aur-, aus-	to hear
bio-	life
brachy-	short
branchi-	arm
bronch-	one of the major divisions of the trachea
bucc-	cheek
burs-	pouch or sac
caes-, cis-	cut
call-	hard, thick skin
calx, calca-	heel
can-	malignant tumor
caput, capitis	head
carc-	cancer
card-, cardia-	heart
carotid	great arteries of the neck
carpus	wrist
caus-, caut-	to burn
celi-	hollow or cavity, specifically the abdomen
cent-	center/centimeter/centigrade
-centesis	puncture of a cavity
ceph-	head
cerv-	neck
chol-	bile
chond-	cartilage
chrom-	color
cil-	hairlike process
cleid-	collarbone (clavicle)
cochlea	part of the inner ear
coll-	gelatin, neck
cond-	knuckle
core	pupil
cori-	skin
corp-	the body
cry-	cold
cubitus	elbow
-cuss	shake violently
cyan-	blue
cyc-	circle
cyst	bladder, cyst
dent-	tooth
derm-	skin

TABLE 8-1 Common Root Words (Continued)

Root Words	Meaning
digit	finger
duct	to lead or guide
edem-	swelling
embryo	fetus
enter-	intestines
eryth-	red
-esth-	sensation
eti-	cause
facil-	easy
febr-	fever
flex	to bend
foramen	opening
fract-	to break into pieces
gangl-	tumor under the skin, junction of nerve cells
gangr-	gnawing sore
gast-	stomach, belly
gen-, gon-	become, produce
gest-	carry, produce
glomerulus	plexus of capillaries
gnosis	knowledge
-gram	something written
-graph	to write
gyn-	female
hem-, -em	blood
hepat-	liver
heter-	other, different
homo-	the same
humerus	upper arm
hydr-	water
hyster-	the womb
idi-	personal, one's own
idio-	distinct
ingui-	front of body between hips and groin
lact-	milk
lev-	left side
ligament	band of fibrous tissue connecting two bones
ling-	tongue
-lith-	stone
mal-	bad
meatus	external opening
med-	middle
mega-	large
melan-, melen-	black
men-, mena-	monthly
menin-	membrane covering brain and spinal cord
morb-	disease
myel-	marrow or spinal cord
myo-	muscle

TABLE 8-1 Common Root Words (Continued)

Root Words	Meaning
nephr-	kidney
noct-	night
nomen-, nomin-	name
oa-, oss-, ost-	bone
ocul-	eye
odon-	tooth
oo-, ov-	egg
ophthalm-	eye
orch-	testis
ot-	ear
palpate	to touch
pari-, part-	to bear
pariet-	wall
path-	disease
pea-, ped-	foot
ped-	child
percuss	to strike
phag-	to eat
photo-	light
placenta	organ supplying nutrients to the fetus during gestation
pleur-	membrane surrounding lung and lining the thoracic cavity
pneum-	breathing
pod-	foot
pseud-	false
psych-	mind
ptosis	falling down
pty-	spit out
pur-, pus-, py-	pus
pyel-	pelvis (including pelvis of kidney)
pyr-	fever
quad-, quar-, quat-	four
radius	rod
ren-	kidney
reticulum	network
retina	inner nerve-containing layer of the eye
rhin-	nose
rub-	red
salpinx	tube

TABLE 8-1 Common Root Words (Continued)

Root Words	Meaning
sang-	blood
scler-	hard
sebum	hard fat of animals
sect-, seg-	to cut
sepsis	containing growing bacteria
sept-	wall
serum	fluid formed when blood clots
sinus	cavity or hollow
somat-	body
sphincter	muscle that closes an opening when it contracts
spir-	coil
stasis	standing
stature	height
status	condition
stern-	chest
stoma	opening or mouth
sulc-	groove on surface of brain
tachy-	rapid
tact-	to touch
talus	heel
tarsus	bones of the forefoot
tel-	distance
temp-	time, or temple of the head
tendon	fibrous tissue connecting muscle to bone
tetr-	four
tom-	to cut
toxic	poisonous
trachea	windpipe
trich-	hair
ur-, urin-	urine
vagina	female genital canal
varic-	dilated vein
vertebra	bone supporting the spinal column
vertex	top of the skull
vertigo	dizziness
viscera	internal organs
viscous	sticky
xen-	foreign
xer-	dry

Prefixes and Suffixes

A root word's meaning may be modified by the placement of additional phrases either before or after the word. Phrases placed before a root word are called *prefixes,* while phrases placed after the word are called *suffixes.*

Prefixes   Prefixes are placed at the beginning of root words to modify a word's meaning. They are never used alone. If the root word starts with a vowel, and the prefix ends with one, then the final vowel of the prefix is dropped.

"Dys" is a prefix meaning disordered, painful, or difficult. Dysrhythmia would imply a disorder of a heart rhythm. Some other examples of prefixes include:

a (without or lack of)	apnea (without breath)
tachy (fast)	tachycardia (fast heart rate)
derma (skin)	dermatitis (inflammation of the skin)
erythro (red)	erythrocyte (red cell)

TABLE 8-2   Common Prefixes

Prefix	Meaning	Example
a, an-	without, lack of	apnea (without breath)
		anemia (lack of blood)
ab-	away from	abnormal (away from the normal)
acr-	pertaining to extremity	acromegaly (enlargement of the bones of the distal parts)
ad-	to, toward	adhesion (something stuck to)
aden-	pertaining to gland	adenitis (inflammation of a gland)
ana-	up, back, again	anastomosis (joining of two parts)
angio-	blood vessel, vessel	angiokinetic (pertaining to changes of blood vessels)
ante-	before, forward	antenatal (occurring or formed before birth)
anti-	against, opposed to	antipyretic (against fever)
arthro-	joint	arthrodynia (pain in a joint)
auto-	self	auto-intoxication (poisoning by a toxin generated within the body)
bi-	two	bilateral (two-sided)
blast-	germ or cell	blastoma (a true tumor of cells)
bleph-	pertaining to eye	bleparotomy (surgical cutting of eyelid)
brady-	slow	bradycardia (slow heart rate)
cardio-	pertaining to heart	cardiography (recording of the actions of the heart)
cephal-	pertaining to head	cephalopathy (any disease of the head or brain)
cerebro-	brain	cerebrospinal (referring to the brain and spinal cord)
chole-	pertaining to bile	cholelithiasis (stones in the biliary system)

TABLE 8-2 Common Prefixes (Continued)

Prefix	Meaning	Example
circum-	around, about	circumflex (winding around)
contra-	against, opposite	contralateral (on the opposite side)
cost-	pertaining to rib	costal margin (margin of the ribs)
cyst-	pertaining to bladder	cystitis (inflammation of the bladder or any fluid-containing sac)
derma-	skin	dermatitis (inflammation of the skin)
di-	twice, double	diplopia (double vision)
dia-	through, completely	diagnosis (knowing completely)
dys-	with pain or difficulty	dyspnea (difficulty breathing)
e-, ex-	from, out of	excise (to cut out or remove completely or surgically)
ecto-	out from	ectopic (out of place)
em-	in	empyema (pus in the chest)
endo-	within	endometrium (within the uterus)
enter-	pertaining to the intestines	enteritis (inflammation of the intestines)
epi-	upon, on	epidermis (the skin)
erythro-	red	erythrocyte (red blood cell)
eu-	healthy	eupnea (normal breathing)
exo-	outside	exogenous (produced outside the body)
extra-	outside, in addition	extrasystole (premature contraction of the heart)
gastr-	pertaining to the stomach	gastritis (inflammation of the stomach)
gynec-	pertaining to women	gynecology (study of women's diseases)
hem-, hemato-	pertaining to blood	hemoglobin (pigment of red blood cells)
hemi-	half	hemiplegia (paralysis of one side of the body)
hydro-	water	hydropenia (deficiency in body water)
hyper-	over, excessive in	hyperplasia (excessive formation)
hypo-	under, deficient in	hypotension (low blood pressure)
hyster-	pertaining to uterus	hysterectomy (removal of the uterus)
in-	not	inferior (beneath or lower)
infra-	below, after	infrascapular (below the scapula)
inter-	between	intercostal (between the ribs)
intra-	within	intralobar (within the lobe)
iso-	equal	isotonic (having equal tension)
laterad-, lateral-	side	laterodeviation (displace to one side)
leuk-	pertaining to anything white	leukocyte (white blood cells)
macro-	large	macroblast (abnormally large cell)
micro-	small; "one millionth part of"	microplasia (dwarfism)
myo-, mye-	pertaining to muscle	myoma (muscle tumor)
neo-	new	neoplasm (new growth)
nephr-	pertaining to kidney	nephrectomy (surgical excision of the kidney)
neuro-	nerve	neurocanal (central canal of the spinal cord)

TABLE 8-2 Common Prefixes (Continued)

Prefix	Meaning	Example
olig-	little	oliguria (little production of urine)
oophor-	pertaining to ovary	oophorectomy (surgical excision of an ovary)
ophthal-	pertaining to eye	exophthalmos (protruding eyeballs)
ot-	pertaining to ear	otitis media (inflammation of the middle ear)
para-	by the side of	parathyroids (along side of the thyroid)
patho-	disease	pathology (study of the nature and cause of disease)
per-	through	perforation (a breaking through)
peri-	around	pericardium (fibroserous sac enclosing the heart)
phago-	to eat	phagocyte (cells that eat debris)
pneumo-	air; lung	pneumothorax (abnormal presence of air in the thorax)
poly-	many	polycystic (containing many cysts)
post-	after, behind	postpartum (after childbirth)
pro-	before, in front of	prognosis (forecast as to the outcome of disease)
proct-	pertaining to rectum	proctoscopy (inspection of the rectum)
pseudo-	false	pseudoanemia (false anemia)
psych-	pertaining to the mind	psychiatry (treatment of mental diseases)
pulmo-	lung	pulmonary (involving the lungs)
py-	pertaining to pus	pyorrhea (discharge of pus)
pyel-	pertaining to renal pelvis	pyelitis (inflammation of the renal pelvis)
retro-	backward	retroflexion (bending backward)
rhin-	pertaining to nose	rhinitis (inflammation of nose)
salping-	pertaining to a tube	salpingectomy (excision of the oviduct)
semi-	half	semiflexion (partially flexed)
sub-	under, moderately	subacute (moderately sharp)
supra-	above	supraclavicular (above the clavicle)
sym-	with, together	symphysis (grow together)
tachy-	fast	tachycardia (fast heart rate)
trans-	across	transfusion (pour across)
tri-	three	tricuspid (having three cusps)
uni-	one	unilateral (one-sided)
vaso-	vessel	vasopressor (agent that increases vascular resistance)

Suffixes   Suffixes are placed at the end of the root word or prefix to alter the meaning of a word. Pronunciation sometimes requires changing the last letter or letters of the root word when the suffix is added. Also, it may be necessary to change the last vowel. An example is the word cardiology, derived from "cardia." The word neuritis, derived from "neuro," is an example of dropping the final vowel in the root word to add a suffix that begins with a vowel. Other examples of suffixes include:

'pnea (breathing)	dyspnea (difficulty breathing)
'ology (science of)	cardiology (science of the heart)
'cyte (cell)	leukocyte (white cell)
'rrhagia (bursting forth)	hemorrhage (burst forth of blood)

TABLE 8-3   Common Suffixes

Suffix	Meaning	Example
-algia	pertains to pain	neuralgia (pain along a nerve)
-blast	germ of immature cell	myeloblast (bone marrow cell)
-cele	tumor, hernia	enterocele (hernia of intestine)
-centesis	puncturing	thoracentesis (a procedure involving puncture and drainage of the pleural space)
-cyte	cell	leukocyte (white cell)
-ectomy	a cutting out	tonsillectomy
-emia	blood	anemia
-itis	inflammation	tonsillitis
-ostomy	creation of an opening	gastrostomy (artificial opening into the stomach)
-lysis	destruction or loosening	lysis (destruction or loosening of adhesions)
-oma	tumor, swelling	neuroma (tumor of a nerve)
-osis	condition of	psychosis (a mental disorder characterized by disordered thinking)
-pathy	disease	neuropathy (disease of the nervous system)
-phagia	eating	polyphagia (excessive eating)
-phasia	speech	aphasia (loss of speech)
-phobia	fear	hydrophobia (fear of water)
-plasty	repair of; or tying of	nephroplasty (suturing of a kidney)
-ptosis	falling	enteroptosis (falling of the intestine)
-rhythmia	rhythm	tachydysrhythmia (faster than a normal rhythm)
-rrhagia	bursting forth	hemorrhage (flowing of blood)
-rrhaphy	suture of; or repair of	herniorrhaphy (repair of a hernia)
-rrhea	flowing	pyorrhea (discharge of pus)
-scope	instrument for examination	bronchoscope (instrument for looking into the bronchi)
-scopy	examination with an instrument	bronchoscopy (examination of the bronchi)
-taxia	order, arrangement of	ataxia (failure of muscle coordination)
-trophia	nourishment	atrophy (a wasting away of something)
-uria	to do with urine	polyuria (excessive production of urine)

ABBREVIATIONS

Medical documentation tends to be lengthy and time-consuming. As a result, abbreviations become routine. The abbreviations in the following table pertain to prehospital care.

TABLE 8-4	Common Abbreviations
Abbreviation	**Meaning**
a	before
aa	of each
AED	automated external defibrillator
AO × 4	alert and oriented to person, place, time, and self
abd.	abdomen
Ab	abortion
a.c.	before meals
ACLS	advanced cardiac life support
adm.	administration
AF	atrial fibrillation
AIDS	Acquired Immune Deficiency Syndrome
aq.	water
ARDS	Adult Respiratory Distress Syndrome
ASA	aspirin
ASHD	atherosclerotic heart disease
AMA	against medical advice
ant.	anterior
AP	front-to-back (anteroposterior)
A & P	anatomy and physiology
APC	Aspirin, Phenacetin, and Caffeine
art.	artery
AT	atrial tachycardia
AV	atrioventricular
BBB	bundle branch block
b.i.d.	twice a day
BM	bowel movement
BP	blood pressure
BS	blood sugar, breath sounds
BSA	body surface area
BVM	bag-valve-mask
C°	centigrade
c̄	with
Ca	carcinoma, cancer
CABG	coronary artery bypass graft
CAD	coronary artery disease, computer-assisted dispatch
Caps.	capsule
CBC	complete blood count
cc	cubic centimeter
CC or C/C	chief complaint
CCU or MICU	coronary care unit or medical intensive care unit

TABLE 8-4 Common Abbreviations (Continued)

Abbreviation	Meaning
CHF	congestive heart failure
Cl⁻	chloride
cm	centimeter
CNS	central nervous system
c/o	complains of
CO	carbon monoxide
CO_2	carbon dioxide
COPD	chronic obstructive pulmonary disease
CP	chest pain
CPR	cardiopulmonary resuscitation
CSF	cerebrospinal fluid
CSM	carotid sinus massage
CVA	cerebrovascular accident
CVP	central venous pressure
CXR	chest x-ray
D/C	discontinue
D & C	dilatation and curettage
DM	diabetes mellitus
DOA	dead on arrival
DOE	dyspnea on exertion
DPT	diphtheria, pertussis, and tetanus vaccine
DT's	delirium tremens
D5W	dextrose 5 percent in water
DVT	deep venous thrombosis
Dx	diagnosis
ECG, EKG	electrocardiogram
EDC	estimated date of confinement
EEG	electroencephalogram
e.g.	for example
ENT	ear, nose, and throat
EOMI	extraocular muscles intact
ER/ED	emergency department
ETA	estimated time of arrival
ETOH	alcohol (ethanol)
F°	Fahrenheit
FHx	family history
fl	fluid
fx	fracture
GB	gall bladder
GI	gastrointestinal
→	going to or leading to
Gm., g	gram
gr.	grain
GSW	gunshot wound
gtt.	drop
GU	genitourinary
GYN	gynecologic
h, hr.	hour

TABLE 8-4 Common Abbreviations (Continued)

Abbreviation	Meaning
H/A	headache
H, (H)	hypodermic
Hb., Hgb.	hemoglobin
Hct.	hematocrit
H & H	hemoglobin & hematocrit
Hg	mercury
H & P	history and physical
hs	at bedtime
Hx	history
IC	intracardiac
ICP	intracranial pressure
ICU	intensive care unit
IM	intramuscular
inf.	inferior
IO	interosseous
IPPB	intermittent positive pressure breathing
IV	intravenous
JVD	jugular venous distention
K^+	potassium
kg	kilogram
KVO	keep vein open
L	left
L	liter
LAC	laceration
lb.	pound
LBBB	left bundle branch block
LBP	low back pain
liq.	liquid
LLL	left lower lobe of the lung
LLQ	left lower quadrant of abdomen
LOC	level of consciousness
LPM	liters per minute
LR	lactated Ringer's
LUL	left upper lobe of the lung
LUQ	left upper quadrant of abdomen
m	meter
MAEW	moves all extremities well
MAP	mean arterial pressure
mcg.	microgram
MCL	midclavicular line
MCL	modified chest lead
mEq.	milliequivalent
μg.	microgram
mg., mgm.	milligram
MI	myocardial infarction
MICU	mobile intensive care unit, medical intensive care unit
mL	milliliter
mm	millimeter

TABLE 8-4 Common Abbreviations (Continued)

Abbreviation	Meaning
MS	morphine sulphate, multiple sclerosis
MVA	motor vehicle accident
Na^+	sodium
NaCl	sodium chloride
NAD	no apparent distress
$NaHCO_3$	sodium bicarbonate
NC	nasal cannula
NG tube	nasogastric tube
NPO	nothing by mouth
NKA	no known allergies
NS	normal saline
NSR	normal sinus rhythm
NTG	nitroglycerine
N/V	nausea/vomiting
O_2	oxygen
OB	obstetrics
OBS	organic brain syndrome
OD	overdose
O.D.	right eye
OR	operating room
O.S.	left eye
oz.	ounce
$\bar{p}$	after
PAT	paroxysmal atrial tachycardia
p.c.	after meals
pCO_2	carbon dioxide pressure
P.E.	physical exam, pulmonary embolism
PEA	pulseless electrical activity
PERL	pupils equal and reactive to light
pH	hydrogen ion concentration
PID	pelvic inflammatory disease
PND	paroxysmal nocturnal dyspnea
p.o.	by mouth
PO	postoperative or "post op"
pO_2	oxygen pressure or tension
post.	posterior
1°	primary, first degree
PRN	as needed
psi	pounds per square inch
PSVT	paroxysmal supraventricular tachycardia
pt.	patient
PT	physical therapy
PTA	prior to admission
PVC	premature ventricular contraction
q	every
q.h.	every hour
q.i.d.	four times a day
RBBB	right bundle branch block

TABLE 8-4	Common Abbreviations (Continued)
Abbreviation	**Meaning**
RBC	red blood cell
RHD	rheumatic heart disease
RL	ringer's lactate
RLL	right lower lobe of the lung
RML	right middle lobe of the lung
R/O	rule out
ROM	range of motion
RUL	right upper lobe of the lung
RUQ	right upper quadrant of abdomen
Rx	take; treatment
$\overline{s}$	without
2°	secondary, second degree
SA	sino-atrial
S/S	signs/symptoms
SC, SQ	subcutaneous
SICU	surgical intensive care unit
SIDS	Sudden Infant Death Syndrome
SL	sublingual
S.O.B.	shortness of breath
ss	half
stat.	immediately
Sub. Q.	subcutaneous
SVT	supraventricular tachycardia
sym. or Sx	symptoms
tab.	tablet
tbsp.	tablespoon
TIA	transient ischemic attack
t.i.d.	three times a day
TKO	to keep open
TPR	temperature, pulse, respiration
tsp.	teaspoon
u	unit
URI	upper respiratory infection
USP	United States Pharmacopeia
VD	venereal disease
VO	verbal order
vol.	volume
V.S.	vital signs
WBC	white blood cell
WNL	within normal limits
wt.	weight
y.o.	year old
↑	increased, elevated
↓	decreased, depressed
Ø	none
®	right
Ⓛ	left
μ	micro

TABLE 8-4	Common Abbreviations (Continued)
Abbreviation	**Meaning**
α	alpha
β	beta
$\approx$	approximate
o	normal
X2	times two
··	two
···	three
/	per
$\neq$	not equal
>	greater than
<	less than
?	questionable, possible
♂	male
♀	female
+	positive
−	negative
Δ	change

SUMMARY

By learning the lists of root words, prefixes, and suffixes in this chapter, and by consulting the medical dictionary regularly, you will gain a command of medical terminology. Knowing medical terminology is essential for preparing medical records, learning new material, and communicating with other health care personnel.

This chapter has been a brief introduction to medical terminology. Paramedic personnel are encouraged to complete a course in medical terminology. Several self-programmed texts are available.

FURTHER READING

Dorland's Illustrated Medical Dictionary. 26th ed. Philadelphia: W.B. Saunders, 1981.

Yvorra, James. *Mosby's Dictionary: Quick Reference for Emergency Responders*. Saint Louis: C.V. Mosby, 1989.

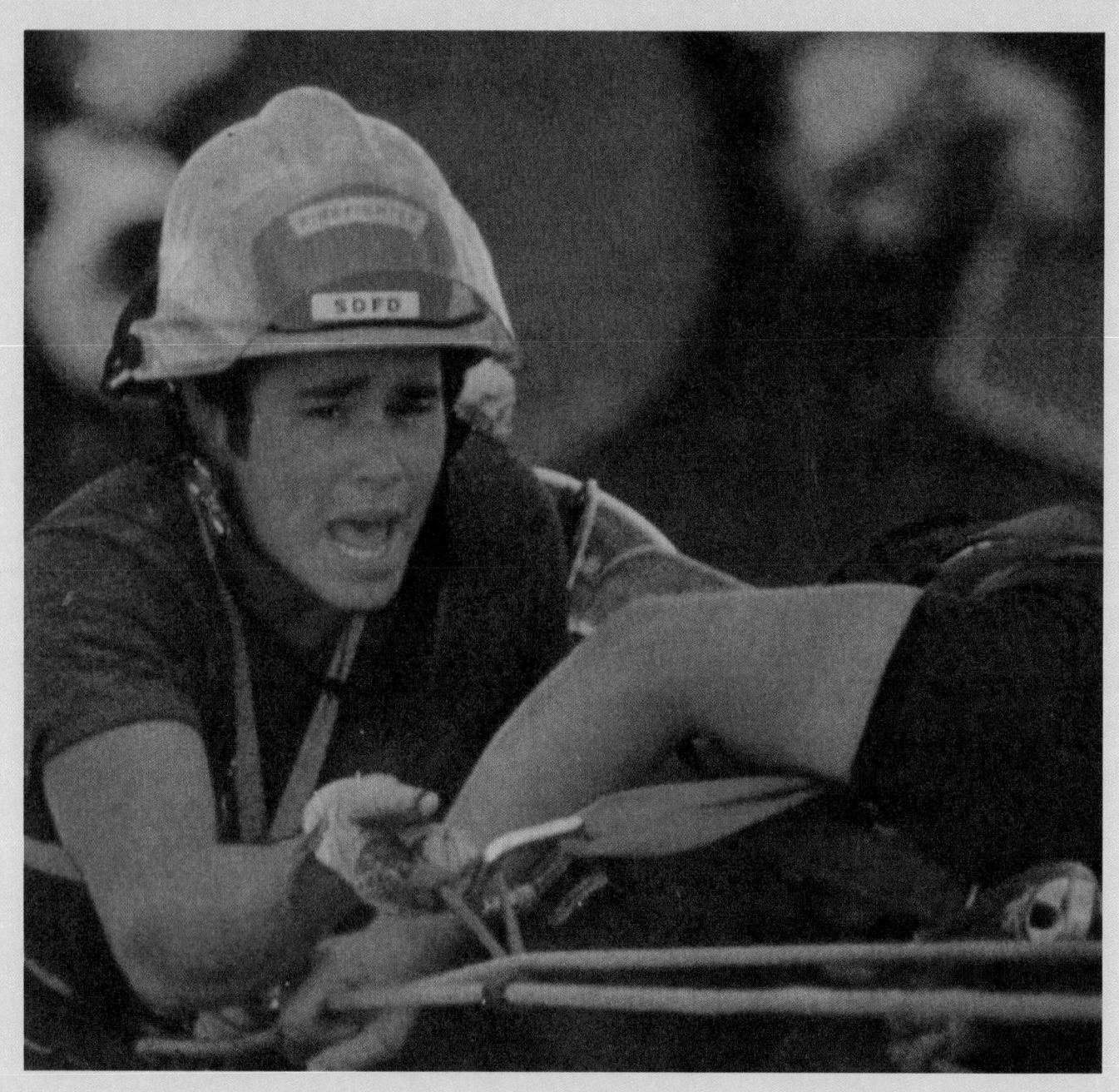

9

ANATOMY AND PHYSIOLOGY

Objectives for Chapter 9

After Reading this chapter, you should be able to:

1. Define the following terms. (See below pages.)
   - anatomy (p. 142.)
   - physiology (p. 142.)
   - biochemistry (p. 142.)
   - biophysics (p. 142.)
2. Describe the hierarchy of the human body. (See p. 143.)
3. Define the following terms. (See below pages.)
   - cell (p. 143.)
   - tissue (p. 144.)
   - organ (pp. 144–145.)
   - organ system (p. 145.)
   - organism (p. 146.)
4. List the four types of tissue. (See p. 144.)
5. List the major body organ systems, and describe their functions. (See pp. 145–146.)

6. Define homeostasis, and give an example of a homeostatic response. (See p. 146.)

7. List the topographical anatomy terms frequently used in emergency medical services, and give an example of each. (See p. 159.)

8. Describe, in topographical terms, the location of various lines on the chest. (See p. 160.)

9. Describe in anatomical terms, a mark on the chest and abdomen in a way that tells the medical control physician the precise location of the lesion. (See p. 160.)

10. Describe the four anatomical divisions of the abdomen, and list the organs within each. (See pp. 161–162.)

11. List the major body cavities and the important organs in each. (See pp. 162–163.)

Saturday night begins like many other Saturdays for the crew of Medic-4. The sun has been down only 15–20 minutes when the computer printout alerts the crew to a shooting at the Zodiac Bar and Grill on the south side of town. Fortunately, the bar is only two minutes from the station. Upon arrival, a police officer informs paramedics that this is a drug-related shooting. The officer also says that the alleged assailant and his assault rifle are in custody.

The paramedics see a male victim lying in the doorway. They now approach the patient. Noting several bloodstains on the shirt, the paramedics remove the garment.

The patient is alert, yet weak. Primary survey reveals no compromise of the airway, breathing, or circulation. There are three apparent entrance wounds in the anterior chest. While Paul is obtaining vital signs, Steve, the senior paramedic, contacts medical control. He reports: "We have a 22-year-old male, with multiple gunshot wounds to the chest. There are three entrance wounds and two apparent exit wounds. The first wound enters the chest in a mid-clavicular line on the right, at the level of the third rib. The second enters in an anterior axillary line, at the level of the tenth rib on the right side. The third wound appears to be a shallow wound in the right mid-axillary line, at the sixth intercostal space; it apparently doesn't penetrate the thorax. Blood pressure is 90 by palpation. The pulse is 110 and respirations are 20. We have placed the PASG, but have not inflated it. We are administering supplemental oxygen by nonrebreathing mask. We are preparing to transport the patient and will attempt an IV and secondary assessment en route. Our ETA is four minutes."

Dr. Johnson, the on-line medical control physician, alerts the surgical crew. Based on the paramedics' description of the wounds, the surgeons expect to find a penetrating wound to the liver and a probable pneumothorax. Within minutes, the surgical crew is opening instruments for both a thoracotomy and exploratory laparotomy. When the victim arrives at the hospital, two IVs are in place. The patient is quickly examined by Dr. Johnson and taken immediately to the operating room. The patient is in the operating room 18 minutes after the paramedics arrived at the emergency scene.

INTRODUCTION

This textbook presents a "systems approach" to medical emergencies and trauma. That is, each type of emergency is presented in the chapter corresponding to the body system most involved. For example: acute myocardial infarction is presented in the cardiovascular emergencies chapter; emphysema is presented in the respiratory emergencies chapter; and so on. Each chapter begins with the anatomy and physiology that pertain to the body system under discussion. This chapter will present the fundamentals of human anatomy and physiology, leaving detailed discussions of various body systems to later chapters.

Anatomy is the study of body structure, whereas **physiology** is the study of body functions. Two related disciplines are **biochemistry** and **biophysics**. Biochemistry is the study of chemical events occurring within a living organism. Biophysics is the application of the principles of physics to body mechanics. As a paramedic, you will be expected to understand relevant anatomy, physiology, and biochemistry. During EMT training, you learned a great deal of anatomy and physiology. As a paramedic, you will be expected to expand this knowledge in areas appropriate to advanced prehospital care.

■ **anatomy** the study of body structure.

■ **physiology** the study of body function.

■ **biochemistry** the study of chemical events occurring within a living organism.

■ **biophysics** the application of the principles of physics to body mechanics.

STRUCTURE

The human body consists of a hierarchical system, ranging from the smallest structural element—the cell—to the entire organism. This section will address human anatomy as it applies to emergency medical care.

The Cell

The fundamental component of the human body is the **cell**. (See Figure 9-1.) The cell is the basic unit of life. It contains all necessary components to turn essential nutrients into energy, remove waste products, reproduce, and carry on other essential life functions. Within the cell are several specialized structures, called **organelles**. Each organelle has a specific function. Examples of organelles and other cellular structures include the following items.

■ **cell** the basic unit of life and the fundamental element of which an organism, such as the human body, is composed.

■ **organelles** specialized structures within the cell that provide for cellular needs.

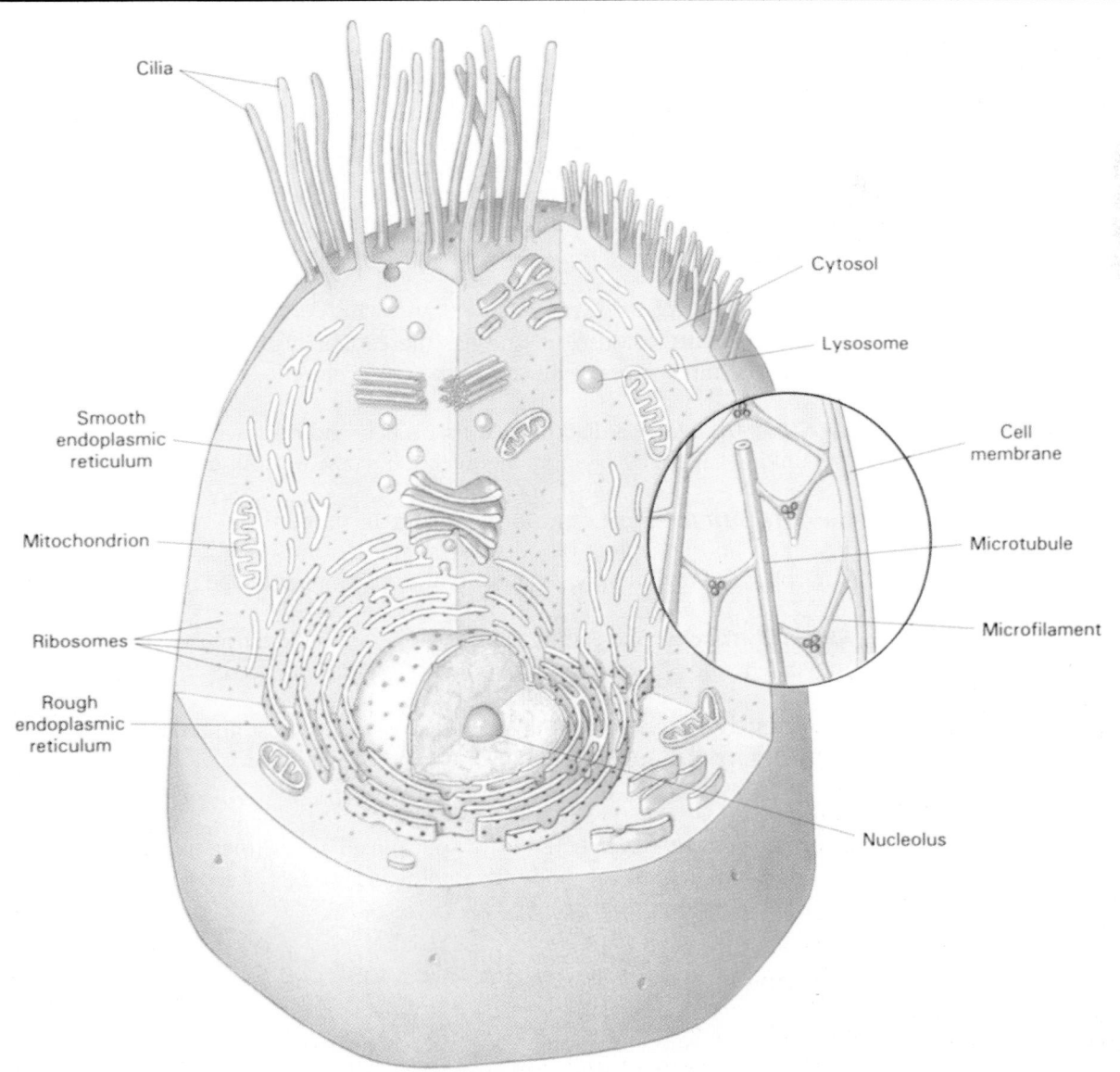

FIGURE 9-1 The cell.

nucleus cellular organelle which contains the genetic material (DNA).

Nucleus

The nucleus contains the genetic material, DNA, and the enzymes necessary for replication of DNA. DNA must be constantly copied and transferred to the new cells.

mitochondria organelle responsible for provision of cellular energy.

Mitochondria

The mitochondria are the energy factories of the cells. They convert essential nutrients into energy sources, often in the form of adenosine triphosphate (ATP).

cell membrane structure which surrounds the cell. It plays a major role in maintaining the internal environment of the cell.

Cell Membrane

The cell membrane is a very important structure that encircles the cell and protects it from the outer environment. Vital functions of the cell membrane—which will be discussed in a later chapter—include electrolyte and fluid balance and the transfer of enzymes, hormones, and nutrients into and out of the cell.

cytoplasm material within the cell that provides for structure, support, and certain biochemical functions.

Cytoplasm

As the substance that fills and gives shape to the cell, cytoplasm provides many biochemical functions.

Tissues

tissue a group of cells, which, together, have a common function or purpose.

The types of cells in the body depend on their location and function. **Tissue** refers to a group of cells that perform a similar function. The following are the four basic types of tissue.

Epithelial Tissue

Epithelial tissue lines body surfaces and protects the body. In addition, certain types of epithelial tissue perform specialized functions such as secretion, absorption, diffusion, and filtration. Examples of epithelial tissue are skin, mucous membranes, and the lining of the intestinal tract.

Muscle Tissue

Muscle tissue has the capability of contraction when stimulated. The three types of muscle tissue (see Figure 9-2) include the following:

Cardiac Muscle. Cardiac muscle tissue is found only within the heart. It has the unique capability of spontaneous contraction without external stimulation.

Smooth Muscle. The smooth muscle is that muscle found within the intestines and encircling blood vessels. Smooth muscle is generally under the control of the involuntary, or autonomic, component of the nervous system.

Skeletal Muscle. Skeletal muscle is the most abundant muscle type. It allows movement and is mostly under voluntary control.

Connective Tissue

Connective tissue is the most abundant tissue in the body. It provides support, connection, and insulation. Examples of connective tissue include bones, cartilage, fat, and blood.

Nerve Tissue

Nerve tissue is specialized tissue that transmits electrical impulses throughout the body. Examples of nervous tissue include the brain, spinal cord, and peripheral nerves.

Organs

organ a group of tissues with a common function.

A group of tissues functioning together is an **organ**. For example, the pancreas consists of epithelial tissue, connective tissue, and nervous tissue.

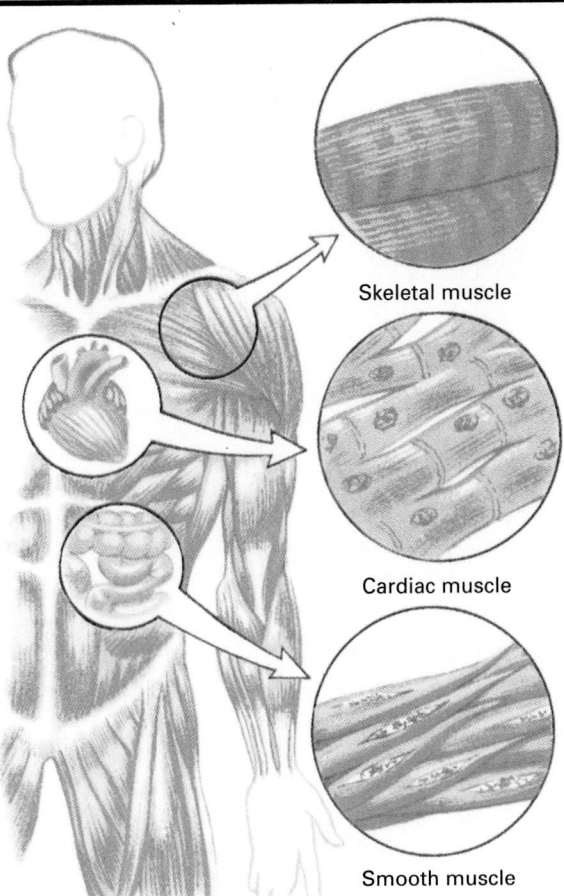

Skeletal muscle

Cardiac muscle

Smooth muscle

FIGURE 9-2 There are three types of muscle. Skeletal muscle, also called voluntary muscle, is found throughout the body. Cardiac muscle is limited to the heart. Smooth muscle, occasionally called involuntary muscle, is found in the intestines, arterioles, and bronchioles.

Together, these tissues perform the essential functions of the pancreas. These functions include production of certain digestive enzymes and regulation of glucose metabolism.

Organ Systems

A group of organs that work together is referred to as an organ system. (See Figures 9-3 to 9-14.) The following are examples of important organ systems.

Cardiovascular System   The cardiovascular system consists of the heart, blood vessels, and blood. It transports nutrients and other essential elements to all parts of the body.

Respiratory System   The respiratory system consists of the lungs and associated structures. It provides oxygen to the body, while removing carbon dioxide and other waste products.

Gastrointestinal System   The gastrointestinal system consists of the mouth, esophagus, stomach, intestines, liver, pancreas, gall bladder, and rectum. It takes in complex nutrients and breaks them down into a form that can be readily used by the body. It also aids in the elimination of excess wastes.

Genitourinary System   The genitourinary system consists of the kidneys, ureters, bladder, and urethra. It is important in the elimination of various waste products. It also plays a major role in the regulation of water, electrolytes, blood pressure, and other essential body functions.

Reproductive System   The reproductive system allows for reproduction of the organism. In the female, it consists of the ovaries, fallopian tubes, uterus, vagina, and breasts. In the male, it consists of the testes, prostate, seminal vesicles, vas deferens, urethra, and penis.

Nervous System   The nervous system consists of the brain, spinal cord, and all peripheral nerves. It controls virtually all bodily functions and is the seat of intellect and being.

Lymphatic System   The lymphatic system is often considered a part of the cardiovascular system. It consists of the spleen, lymph nodes, lymphatic channels, and the lymph itself. It is important in fighting disease, in filtration, and in removing waste products of cellular metabolism.

Endocrine System   The endocrine system is another control system closely associated with the nervous system. It consists of the pituitary gland, pineal gland, pancreas, testes (male), ovaries (female), adrenal glands, thyroid gland, and parathyroid glands. There is well-documented evidence that other organs—such as the heart, kidney, and intestines—have endocrine functions. The endocrine system exerts its effects through the release of chemical messengers called hormones.

Muscular System   The muscular system is responsible for movement, posture, and heat production. It consists, primarily, of the skeletal muscles.

Skeletal System   The skeletal system consists of the bones, cartilage, and associated connective tissue. It provides for support, protection, and movement. The bone marrow is the site for production of various blood cells, including the red blood cells and certain types of white blood cells.

Organism

■ **organism** a group of organ systems; the functional unit of life.

■ **homeostasis** the natural tendency of the body to maintain the internal environment relatively constant.

The sum of all cells, tissues, organs, and organ systems is the **organism**. As this book will make clear, the failure of any component, from the cellular level to the organ-system level, can cause the development of a serious medical emergency.

Homeostasis refers to the body's natural tendency to keep all physiological activities fairly constant. That is, whenever a change occurs in the body, the body immediately attempts to correct the change. At the cellular level, the body will strive to maintain a very constant environment, because cells do not tolerate extreme environmental changes. As an organism, the body uses each organ system to maintain its internal environment. For example, an accumulation of carbon dioxide and lactic acid occurs after exercise. The body immediately attempts to return itself to the resting state by eliminating the excess carbon dioxide and by removing the accumulated lactic acid.

The Eye and Ear

THE EYE

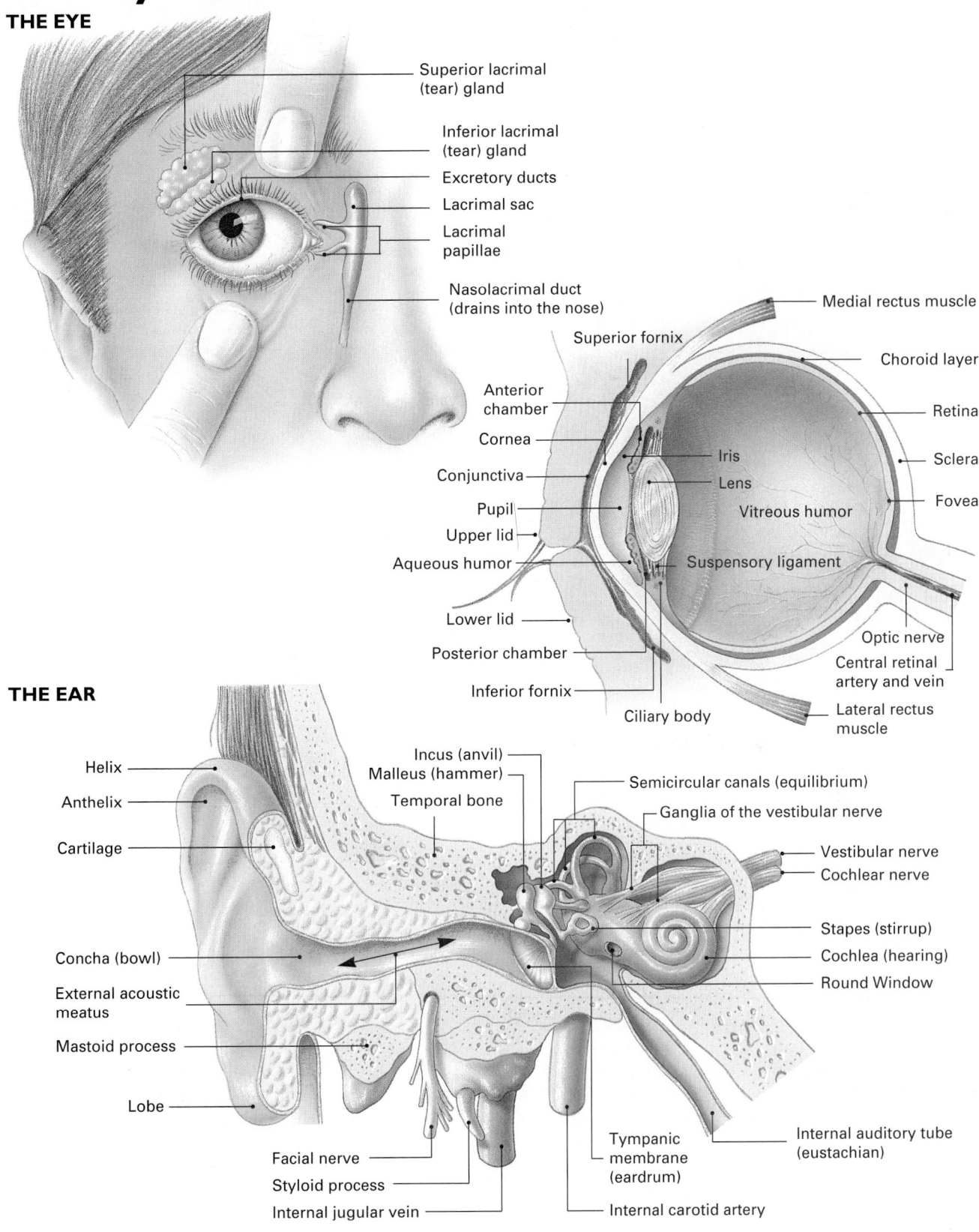

Superior lacrimal (tear) gland

Inferior lacrimal (tear) gland

Excretory ducts

Lacrimal sac

Lacrimal papillae

Nasolacrimal duct (drains into the nose)

Medial rectus muscle

Choroid layer

Retina

Sclera

Fovea

Superior fornix

Anterior chamber

Cornea

Conjunctiva

Pupil

Upper lid

Aqueous humor

Iris

Lens

Vitreous humor

Suspensory ligament

Lower lid

Posterior chamber

Inferior fornix

Ciliary body

Optic nerve

Central retinal artery and vein

Lateral rectus muscle

THE EAR

Helix

Anthelix

Cartilage

Concha (bowl)

External acoustic meatus

Mastoid process

Lobe

Incus (anvil)

Malleus (hammer)

Temporal bone

Semicircular canals (equilibrium)

Ganglia of the vestibular nerve

Vestibular nerve

Cochlear nerve

Stapes (stirrup)

Cochlea (hearing)

Round Window

Facial nerve

Styloid process

Internal jugular vein

Tympanic membrane (eardrum)

Internal carotid artery

Internal auditory tube (eustachian)

FIGURE 9-3 Special senses—the eye and ear.

Membranes

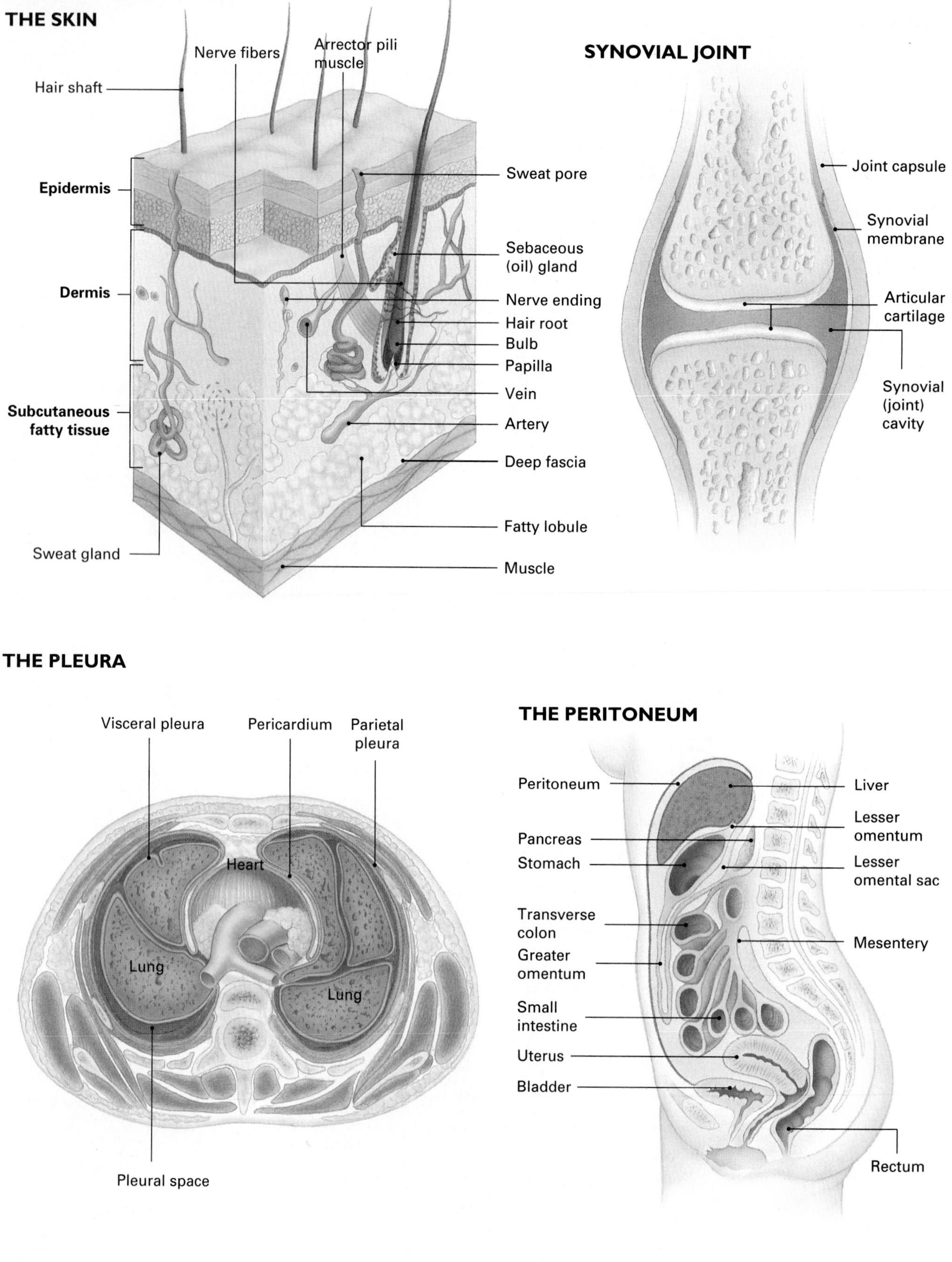

THE SKIN

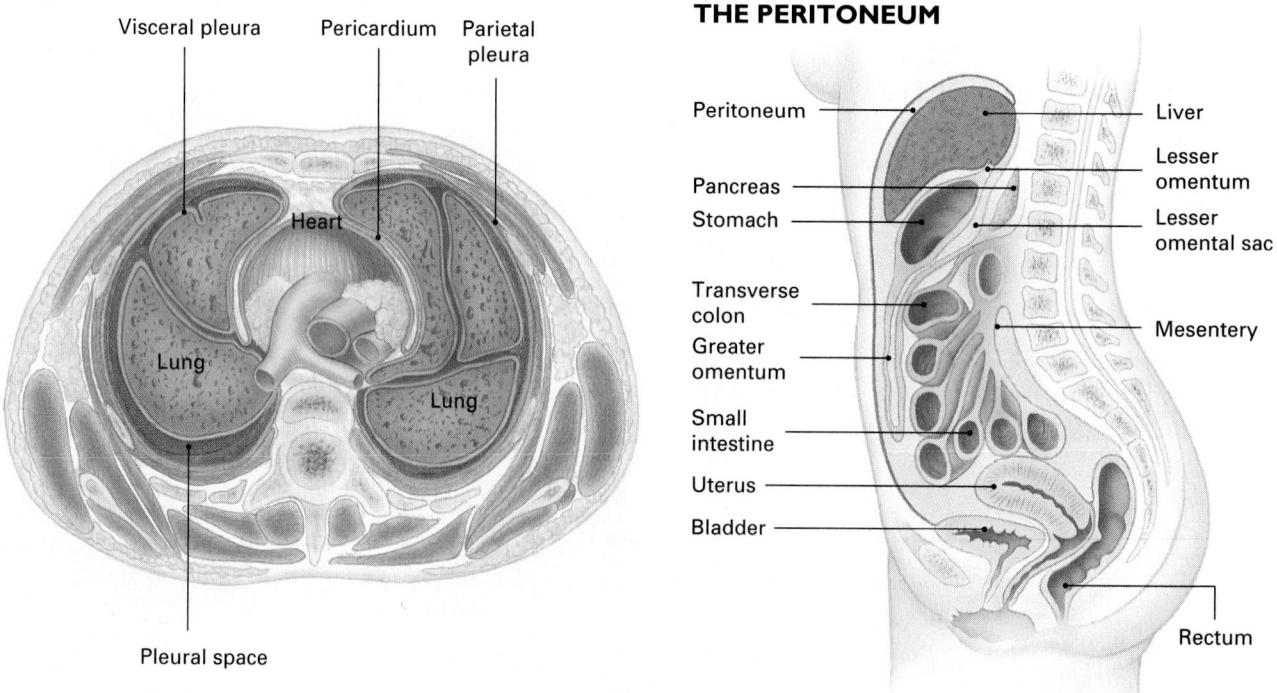

Hair shaft
Nerve fibers
Arrector pili muscle
Epidermis
Dermis
Subcutaneous fatty tissue
Sweat gland

Sweat pore
Sebaceous (oil) gland
Nerve ending
Hair root
Bulb
Papilla
Vein
Artery
Deep fascia
Fatty lobule
Muscle

SYNOVIAL JOINT

Joint capsule
Synovial membrane
Articular cartilage
Synovial (joint) cavity

THE PLEURA

Visceral pleura
Pericardium
Parietal pleura
Heart
Lung
Lung
Pleural space

THE PERITONEUM

Peritoneum
Pancreas
Stomach
Transverse colon
Greater omentum
Small intestine
Uterus
Bladder

Liver
Lesser omentum
Lesser omental sac
Mesentery
Rectum

FIGURE 9-4   Membranes.

The Skeletal System

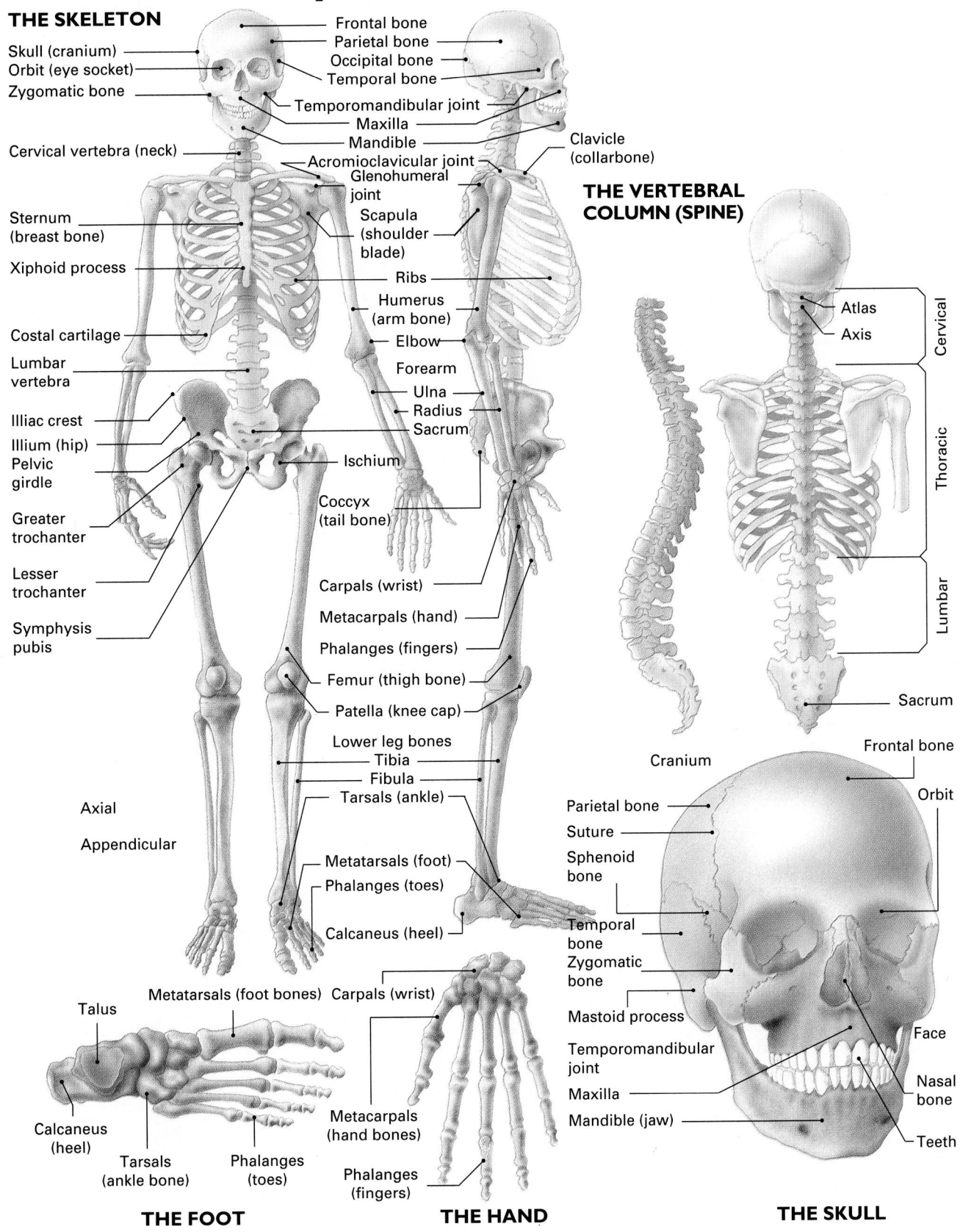

THE SKELETON

Skull (cranium)
Orbit (eye socket)
Zygomatic bone

Frontal bone
Parietal bone
Occipital bone
Temporal bone
Temporomandibular joint
Maxilla
Mandible

Cervical vertebra (neck)

Acromioclavicular joint
Glenohumeral joint
Scapula (shoulder blade)

Clavicle (collarbone)

Sternum (breast bone)

Xiphoid process

Ribs
Humerus (arm bone)
Elbow
Forearm
Ulna
Radius
Sacrum

Costal cartilage

Lumbar vertebra

Illiac crest
Illium (hip)
Pelvic girdle

Ischium

Coccyx (tail bone)

Greater trochanter

Lesser trochanter

Symphysis pubis

Carpals (wrist)
Metacarpals (hand)
Phalanges (fingers)
Femur (thigh bone)
Patella (knee cap)

Lower leg bones
Tibia
Fibula
Tarsals (ankle)

Axial

Appendicular

Metatarsals (foot)
Phalanges (toes)

Calcaneus (heel)

THE VERTEBRAL COLUMN (SPINE)

Atlas
Axis

Cervical

Thoracic

Lumbar

Sacrum

Cranium

Parietal bone
Suture
Sphenoid bone
Temporal bone
Zygomatic bone
Mastoid process
Temporomandibular joint
Maxilla
Mandible (jaw)

Frontal bone
Orbit
Face
Nasal bone
Teeth

Talus

Metatarsals (foot bones)
Carpals (wrist)

Calcaneus (heel)

Tarsals (ankle bone)
Phalanges (toes)

Metacarpals (hand bones)

Phalanges (fingers)

THE FOOT

THE HAND

THE SKULL

FIGURE 9-5   The skeletal system.

The Muscular System

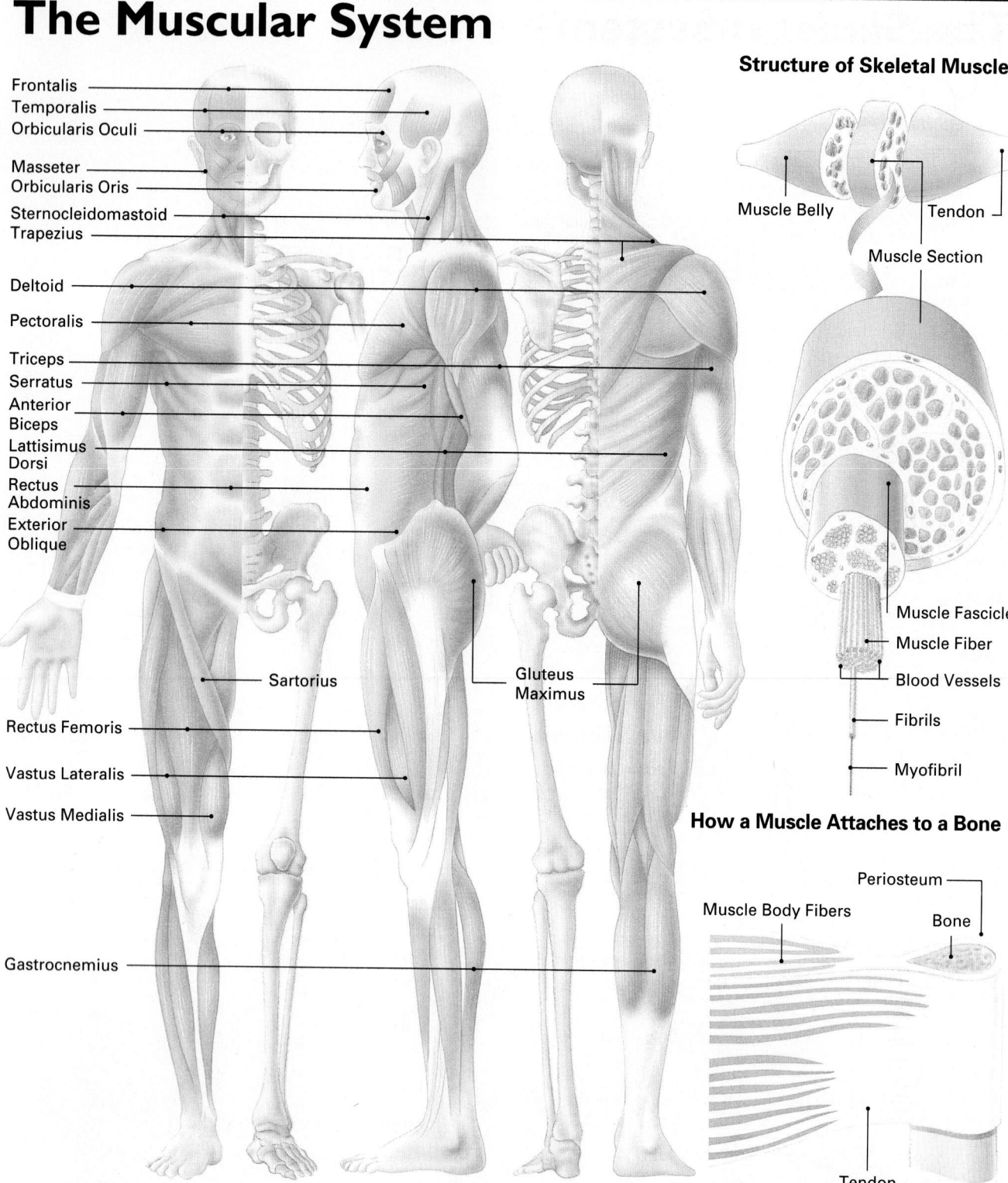

Structure of Skeletal Muscle

Frontalis
Temporalis
Orbicularis Oculi

Masseter
Orbicularis Oris
Sternocleidomastoid
Trapezius

Deltoid

Pectoralis

Triceps
Serratus
Anterior
Biceps
Lattisimus
Dorsi
Rectus
Abdominis
Exterior
Oblique

Sartorius

Rectus Femoris

Vastus Lateralis

Vastus Medialis

Gastrocnemius

Gluteus
Maximus

Muscle Belly
Tendon
Muscle Section

Muscle Fascicle
Muscle Fiber
Blood Vessels
Fibrils
Myofibril

How a Muscle Attaches to a Bone

Periosteum
Bone
Muscle Body Fibers
Tendon

FIGURE 9-6   The muscular system.

The Cardiovascular System

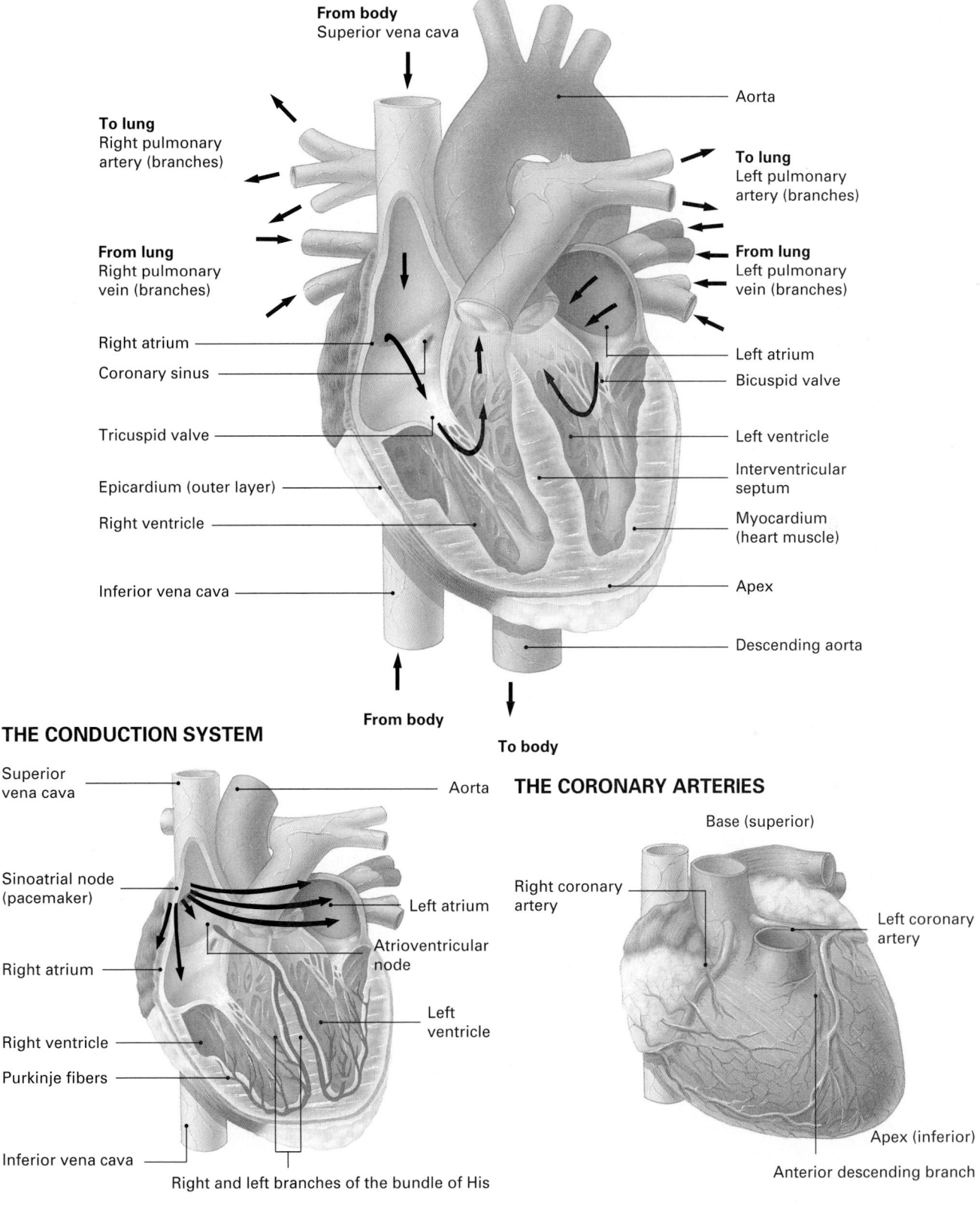

From body
Superior vena cava

To lung
Right pulmonary
artery (branches)

From lung
Right pulmonary
vein (branches)

Right atrium

Coronary sinus

Tricuspid valve

Epicardium (outer layer)

Right ventricle

Inferior vena cava

Aorta

To lung
Left pulmonary
artery (branches)

From lung
Left pulmonary
vein (branches)

Left atrium

Bicuspid valve

Left ventricle

Interventricular
septum

Myocardium
(heart muscle)

Apex

Descending aorta

From body

To body

THE CONDUCTION SYSTEM

Superior
vena cava

Sinoatrial node
(pacemaker)

Right atrium

Right ventricle

Purkinje fibers

Inferior vena cava

Aorta

Left atrium

Atrioventricular
node

Left
ventricle

Right and left branches of the bundle of His

THE CORONARY ARTERIES

Base (superior)

Right coronary
artery

Left coronary
artery

Apex (inferior)

Anterior descending branch

FIGURE 9-7   The cardiovascular system.

The Circulatory System

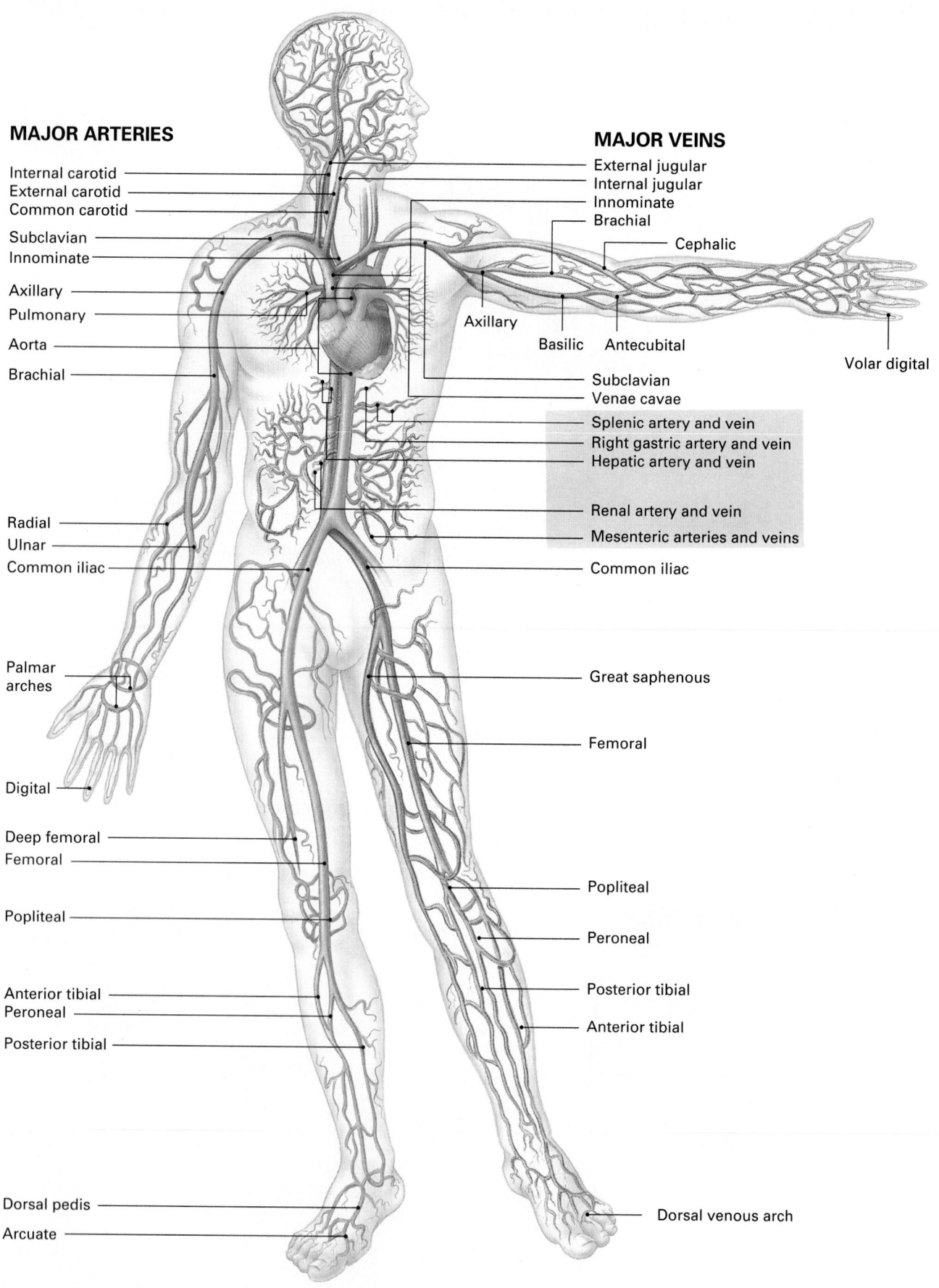

MAJOR ARTERIES

Internal carotid
External carotid
Common carotid
Subclavian
Innominate
Axillary
Pulmonary
Aorta
Brachial
Radial
Ulnar
Common iliac
Palmar arches
Digital
Deep femoral
Femoral
Popliteal
Anterior tibial
Peroneal
Posterior tibial
Dorsal pedis
Arcuate

MAJOR VEINS

External jugular
Internal jugular
Innominate
Brachial
Cephalic
Axillary
Basilic
Antecubital
Volar digital
Subclavian
Venae cavae
Splenic artery and vein
Right gastric artery and vein
Hepatic artery and vein
Renal artery and vein
Mesenteric arteries and veins
Common iliac
Great saphenous
Femoral
Popliteal
Peroneal
Posterior tibial
Anterior tibial
Dorsal venous arch

FIGURE 9-8   The circulatory system.

The Nervous System

THE BRAIN

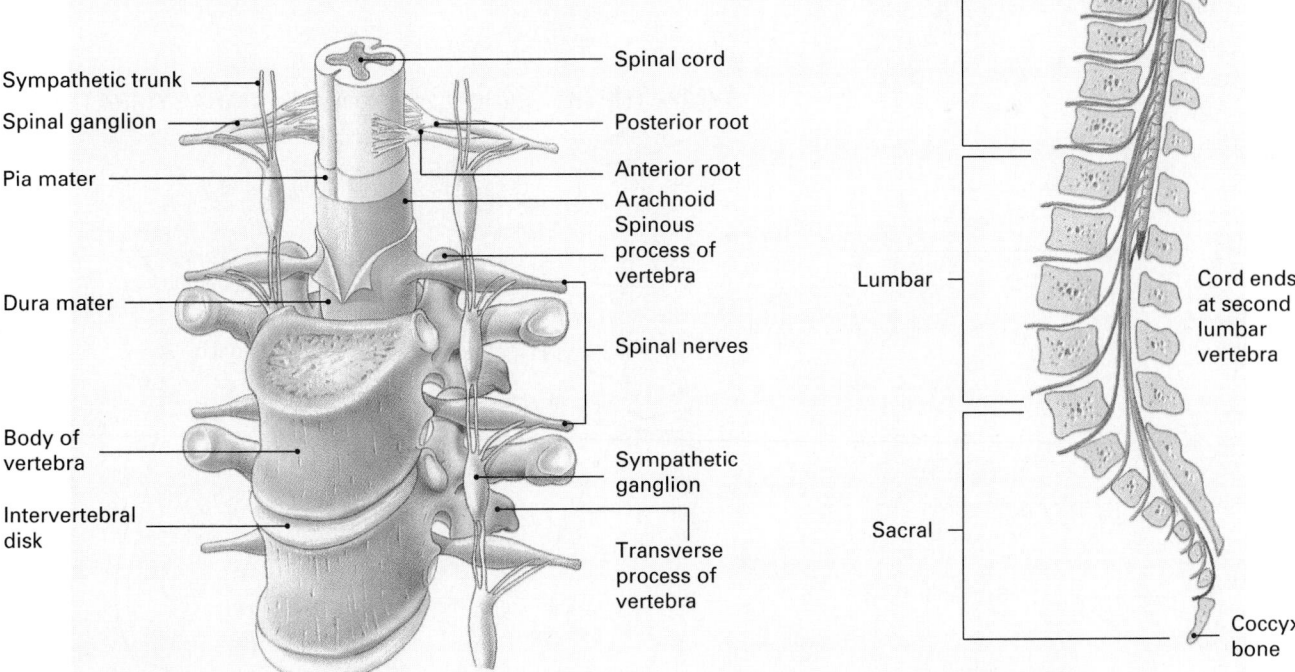

Frontal lobe

Frontal bone

Cerebrum

Frontal sinus

Pituitary gland

Sphenoid sinus

Parietal lobe

Fornix
Corpus callosum
Thalamus
Isthmus
Occipital lobe
Pons
Cerebellum

Medulla Oblongata

DIVISIONS OF THE SPINAL CORD

Cervical

Thoracic

Lumbar

Sacral

Cord ends at second lumbar vertebra

Coccyx bone

THE SPINAL CORD

Sympathetic trunk

Spinal ganglion

Pia mater

Dura mater

Body of vertebra

Intervertebral disk

Spinal cord

Posterior root

Anterior root
Arachnoid
Spinous process of vertebra

Spinal nerves

Sympathetic ganglion

Transverse process of vertebra

FIGURE 9-9   The nervous system.

Nervous System (continued)

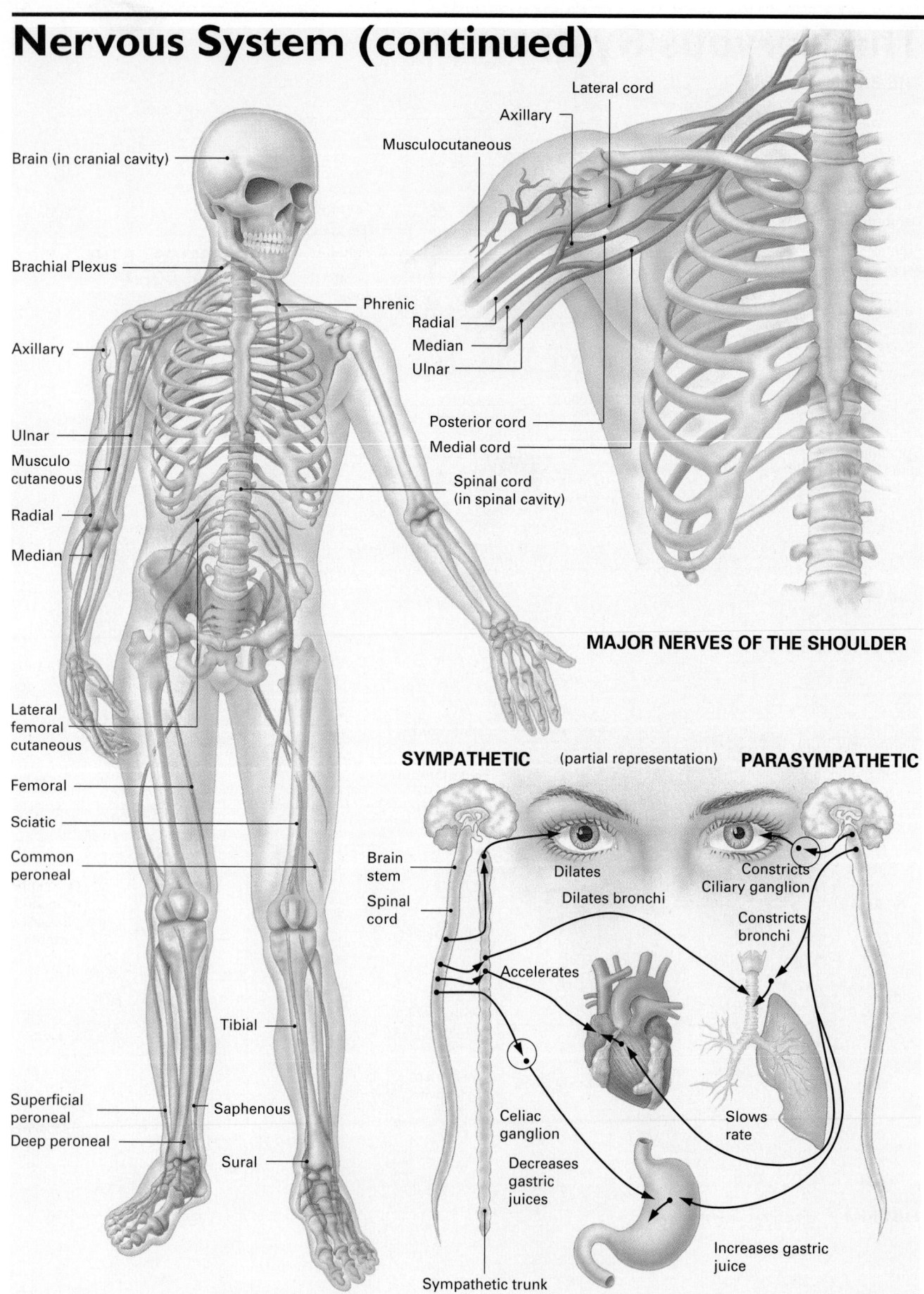

Brain (in cranial cavity)

Brachial Plexus

Axillary

Ulnar

Musculo cutaneous

Radial

Median

Lateral femoral cutaneous

Femoral

Sciatic

Common peroneal

Superficial peroneal

Deep peroneal

Tibial

Saphenous

Sural

Lateral cord

Axillary

Musculocutaneous

Phrenic

Radial

Median

Ulnar

Posterior cord

Medial cord

Spinal cord (in spinal cavity)

MAJOR NERVES OF THE SHOULDER

SYMPATHETIC   (partial representation)   **PARASYMPATHETIC**

Brain stem

Spinal cord

Dilates

Dilates bronchi

Constricts

Ciliary ganglion

Constricts bronchi

Accelerates

Celiac ganglion

Decreases gastric juices

Sympathetic trunk

Slows rate

Increases gastric juice

FIGURE 9-10   The nervous system (continued).

The Respiratory System

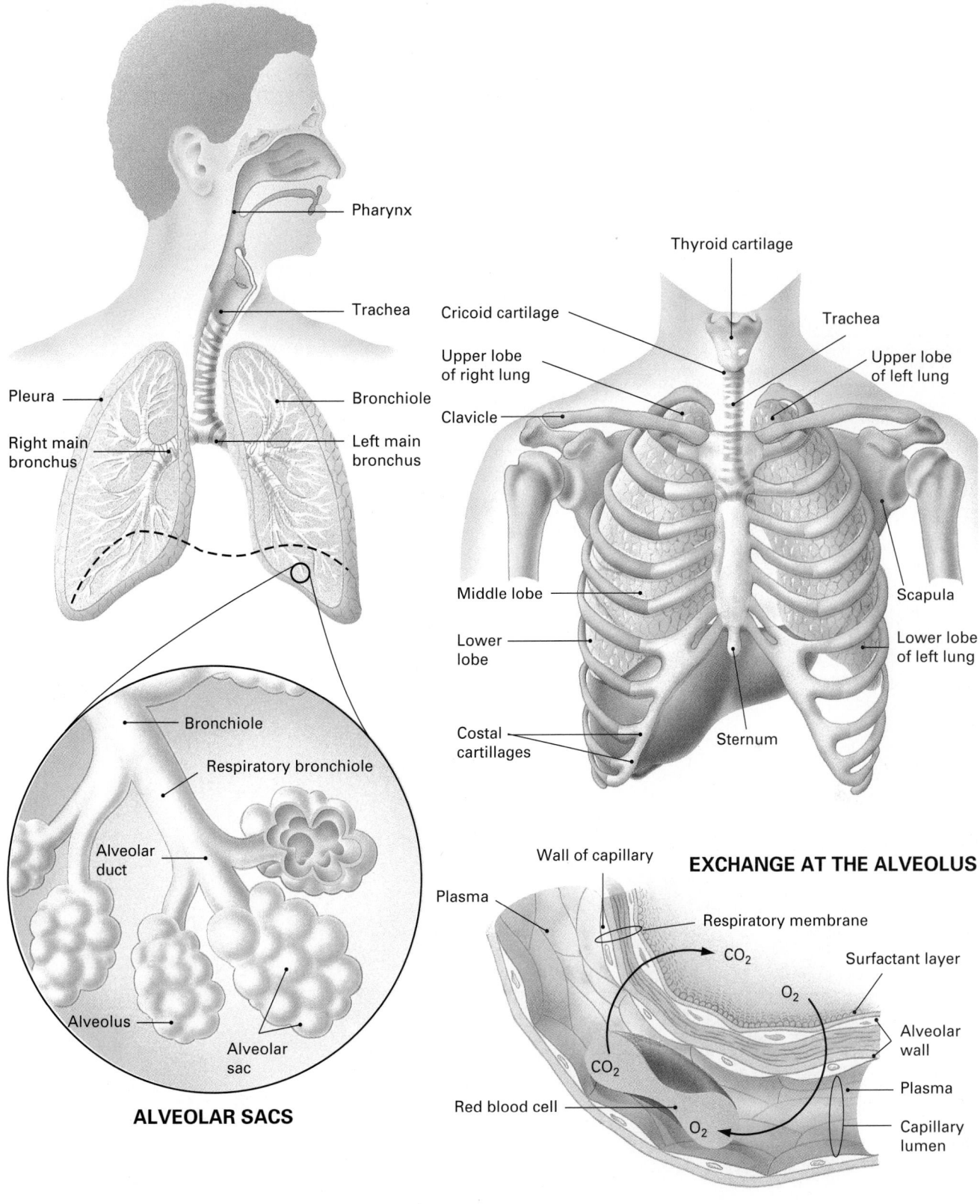

ALVEOLAR SACS

EXCHANGE AT THE ALVEOLUS

FIGURE 9-11 The respiratory system.

The Digestive System

ORGANS OF THE DIGESTIVE SYSTEM

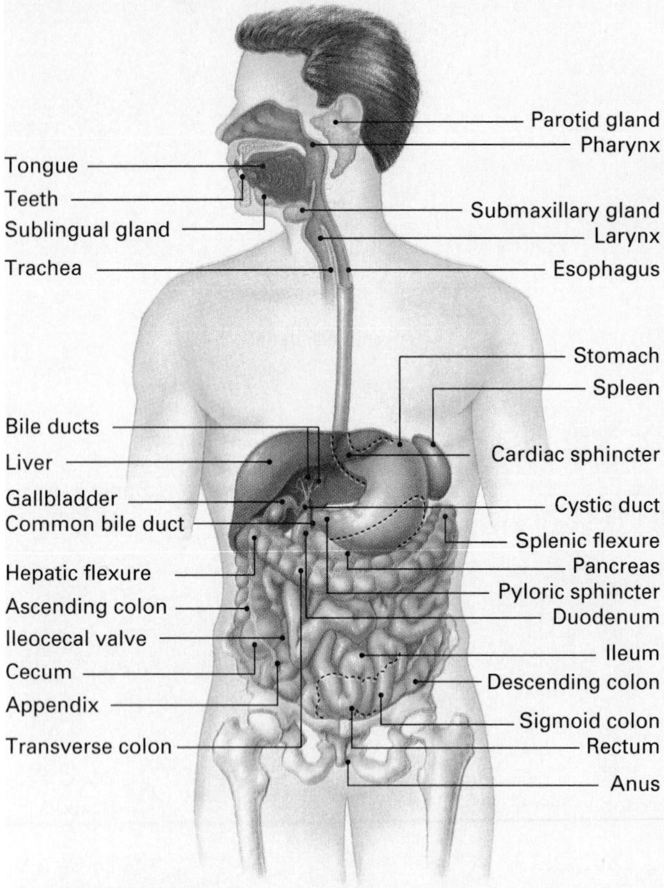

Parotid gland
Pharynx
Tongue
Teeth
Sublingual gland
Submaxillary gland
Larynx
Trachea
Esophagus
Stomach
Spleen
Bile ducts
Liver
Cardiac sphincter
Gallbladder
Cystic duct
Common bile duct
Splenic flexure
Hepatic flexure
Pancreas
Ascending colon
Pyloric sphincter
Ileocecal valve
Duodenum
Cecum
Ileum
Appendix
Descending colon
Transverse colon
Sigmoid colon
Rectum
Anus

LIVER, STOMACH, AND PANCREAS

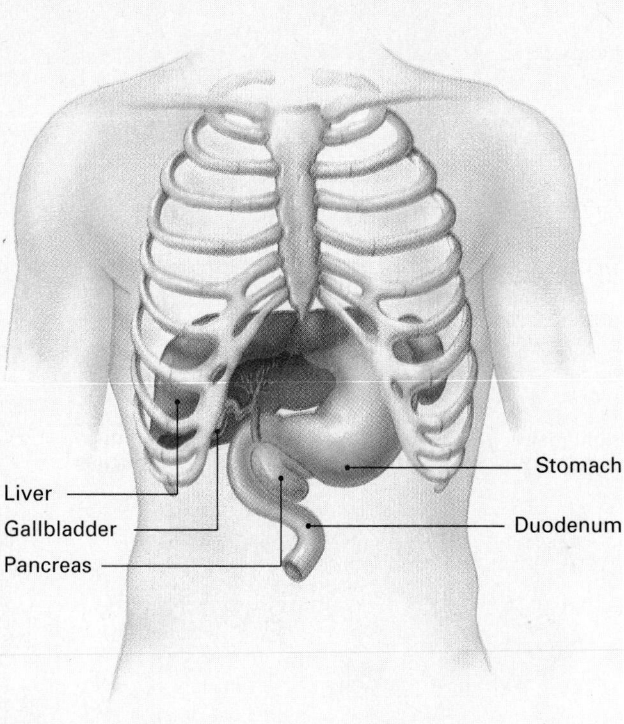

Stomach
Liver
Gallbladder
Duodenum
Pancreas

LARGE INTESTINE

Esophagus
Duodenum
Diaphragm
Hepatic flexure
Stomach
Ascending colon
Splenic flexure
Ileocecal valve
Transverse colon
Cecum
Descending colon
Appendix
Rectum
Sigmoid colon
Anus

SMALL INTESTINE

Duodenum
Transverse colon
Ascending colon
Jejunum
Cecum
Descending colon
Sigmoid colon
Ileum

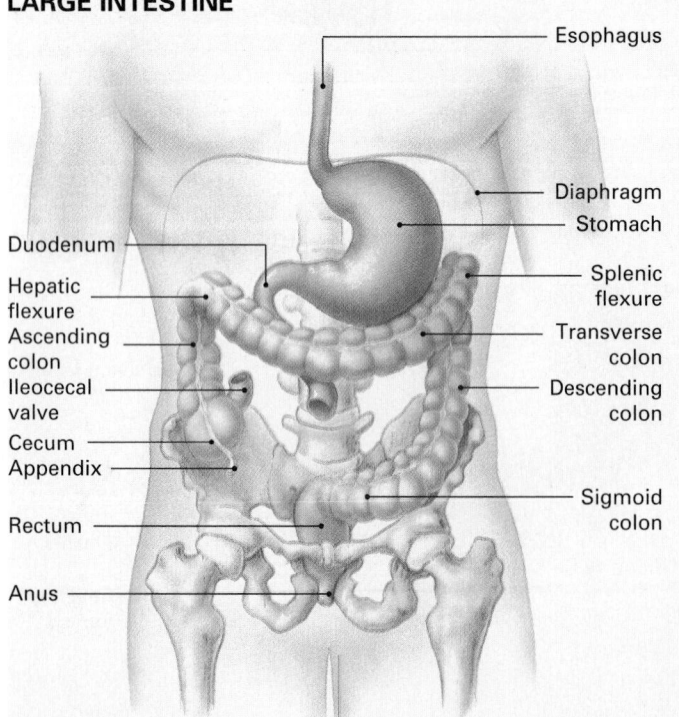
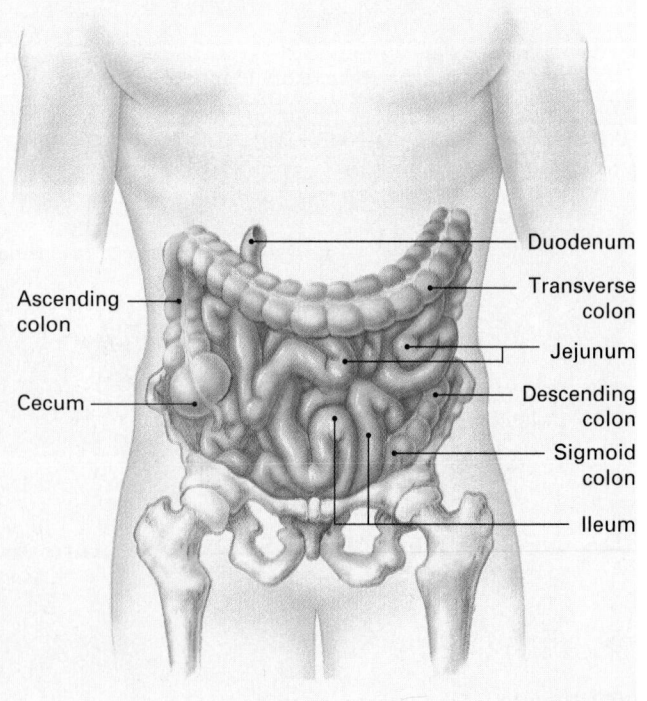

FIGURE 9-12 The digestive system.

The Urinary System

ORGANS OF THE URINARY SYSTEM

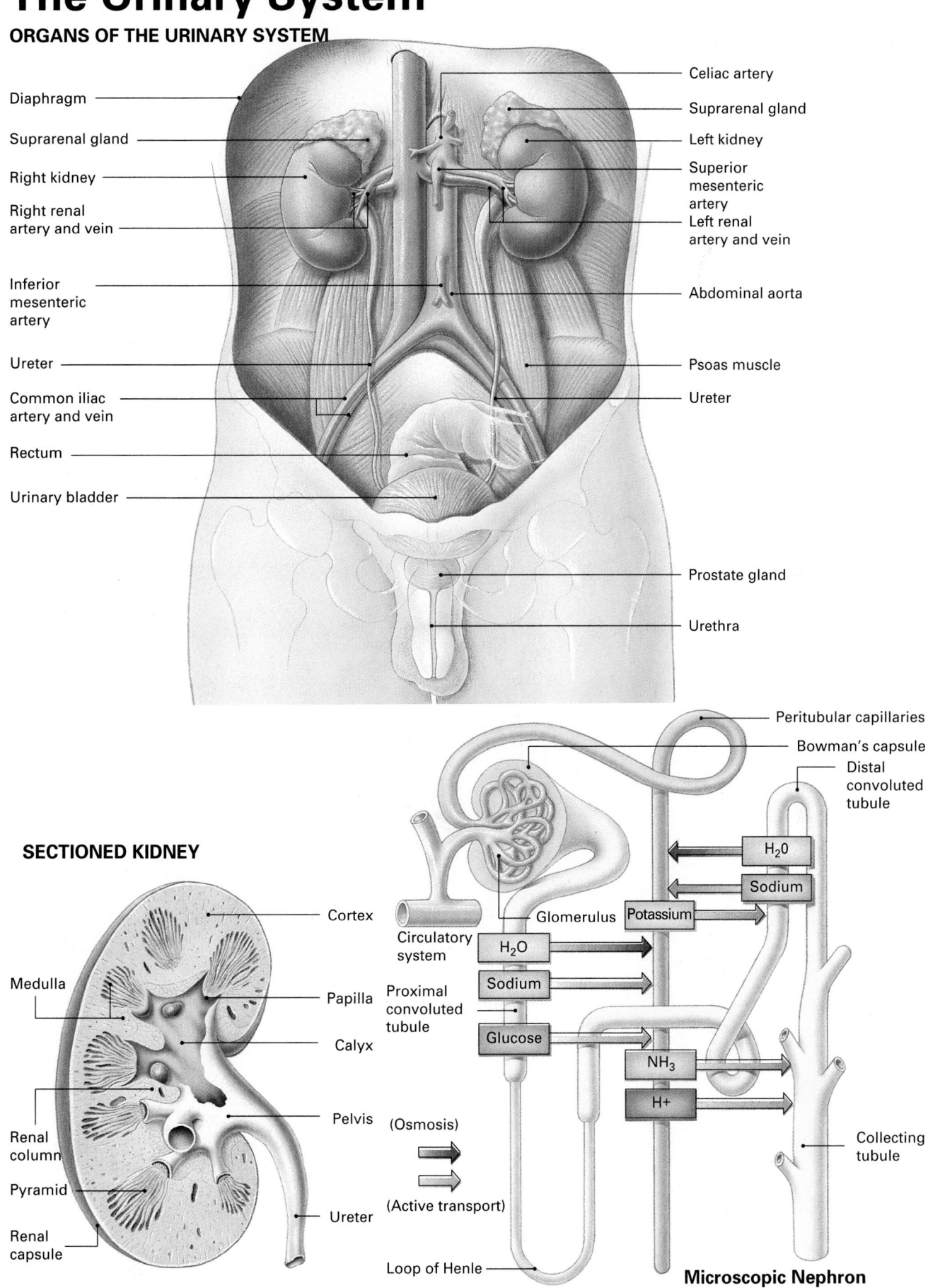

SECTIONED KIDNEY

Microscopic Nephron

FIGURE 9-13   The urinary system.

157

The Reproductive System

FEMALE   **MALE**

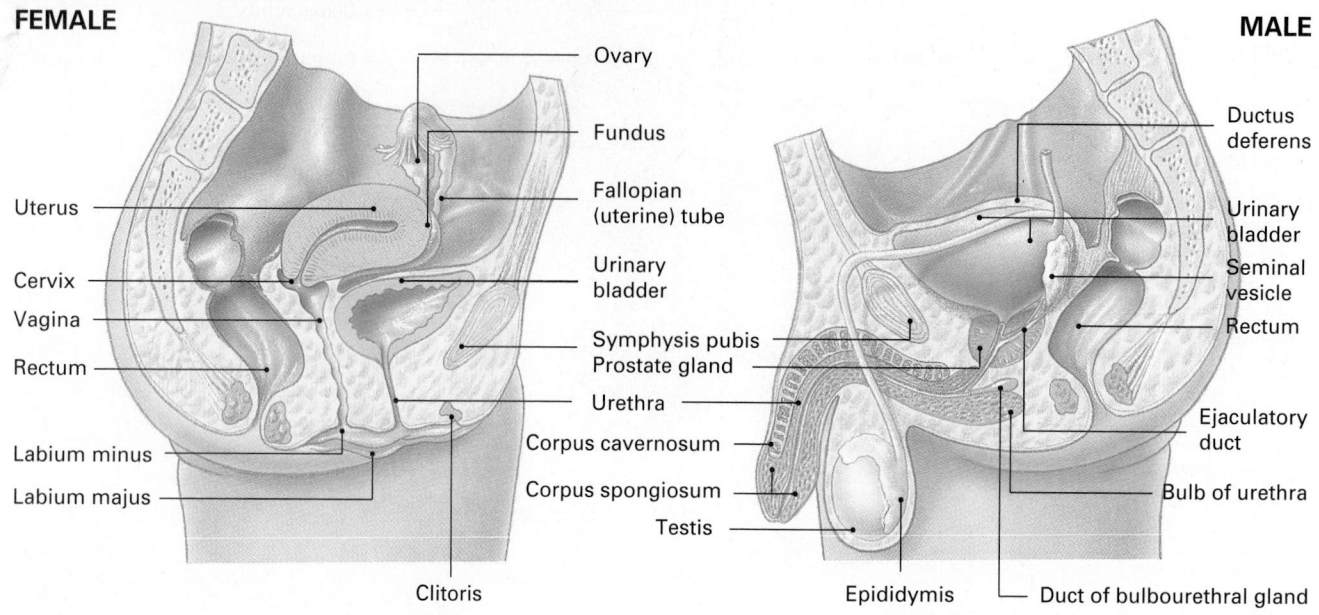

Ovary
Fundus
Fallopian (uterine) tube
Urinary bladder
Symphysis pubis
Prostate gland
Urethra
Corpus cavernosum
Corpus spongiosum
Testis

Uterus
Cervix
Vagina
Rectum
Labium minus
Labium majus

Clitoris

Ductus deferens
Urinary bladder
Seminal vesicle
Rectum
Ejaculatory duct
Bulb of urethra
Epididymis
Duct of bulbourethral gland

Labium minus (singular), Labia minora (plural)
Labium majus (singular), Labia majora (plural)

THE OVARY   **THE BREAST**

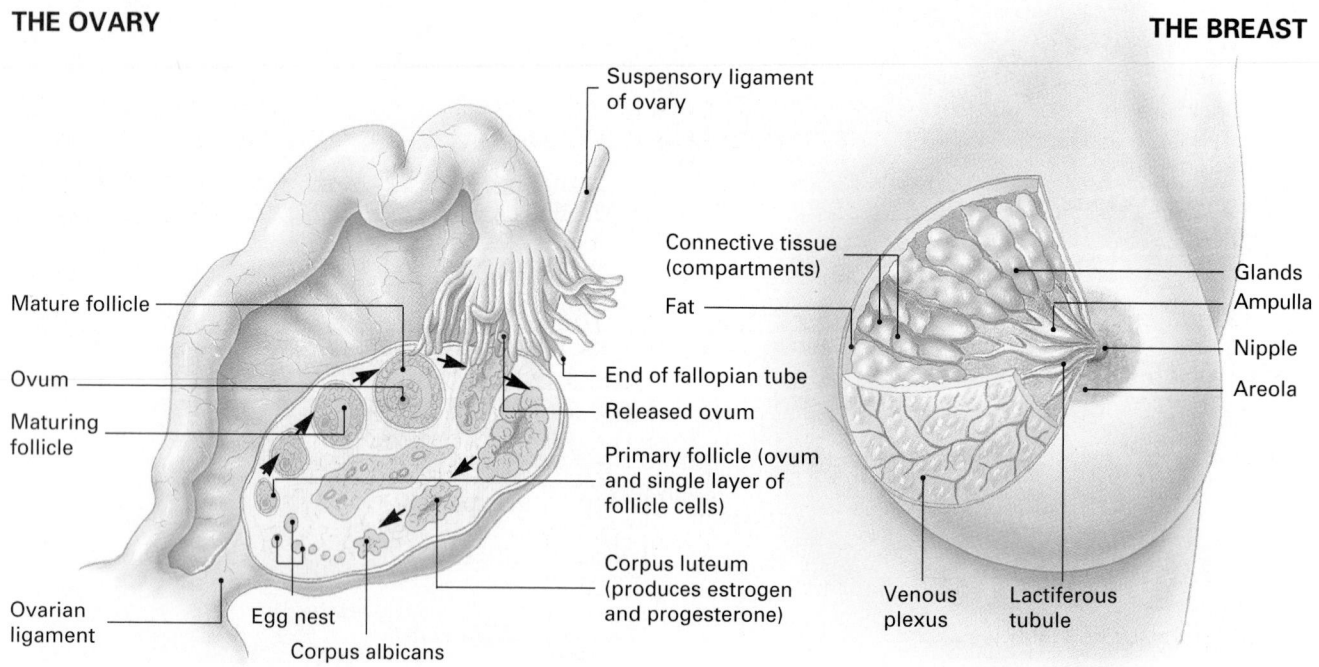

Suspensory ligament of ovary

Mature follicle
Ovum
Maturing follicle

Ovarian ligament

Egg nest
Corpus albicans

End of fallopian tube
Released ovum
Primary follicle (ovum and single layer of follicle cells)
Corpus luteum (produces estrogen and progesterone)

Connective tissue (compartments)
Fat

Glands
Ampulla
Nipple
Areola

Venous plexus
Lactiferous tubule

FIGURE 9-14   The reproductive system.

TOPOGRAPHICAL ANATOMY

As a paramedic, you will need to be familiar with topographical anatomy. You'll often have to describe certain illnesses and injuries to the medical control physician. Using topographical terms will help you to pinpoint an injury and convey other information accurately and logically.

Anatomic Terms

General topographical terms are listed and defined below.

Relating to Direction

anterior—toward the front of the body
ventral—toward the front of the body
posterior—toward the back of the body
dorsal—toward the back of the body
lateral—away from the midline of the body
medial—toward the midline of the body
craniad—toward the head
cephalad—toward the head
caudad—toward the tail
superior—toward the top of the body
inferior—toward the bottom of the body
superficial—toward the exterior of the body
deep—toward the interior of the body
internal—inside the body
external—outside the body
proximal—nearer the trunk of the body compared to another point
distal—farther from the trunk of the body compared to another point

Relating to Body Position

supine—lying horizontal with the face upward
prone—lying horizontal with the face downward
lateral recumbent—lying on the side
lithotomy position—lying with the face upward, the legs flexed, and the thighs abducted
Fowler's position—elevation of the head of the bed, usually 45 degrees or more, with the patient in a supine position
Semi-Fowler's position—elevation of the head of the bed, less than 45 degrees, with the patient in a supine position
Trendelenburg position—lying supine with the lower part of the body elevated above the head

Relating to Body Movement

abduction—a movement away from the body
adduction—a movement toward the body
flexion—the act of bending
extension—the act of straightening
pronation—the act of rotating the arm, bringing the palm of the hand to a position of facing downward
supination—the act of rotating the arm, bringing the palm of the hand to a position facing upward

Topographical Anatomy of the Chest

The exterior of the chest can be described with standard anatomical lines. (See Figures 9-15, 9-16, and 9-17.) A vertical line drawn from the mid-axilla downward separates the anterior chest from the posterior chest. This is called the *mid-axillary line*. A vertical line drawn from the center of the manubrium (the top of the sternum) to the xiphoid process (the bottom of the sternum) is called the *mid-sternal line*. It separates the right anterior chest from the left anterior chest. A vertical line drawn along the spine is the *mid-spinal line*, which separates the left posterior chest from the right posterior chest. The chest can be further divided by drawing vertical lines from the mid-clavicle and mid-scapula. Further localization can be obtained by counting the intercostal spaces (the spaces between the ribs).

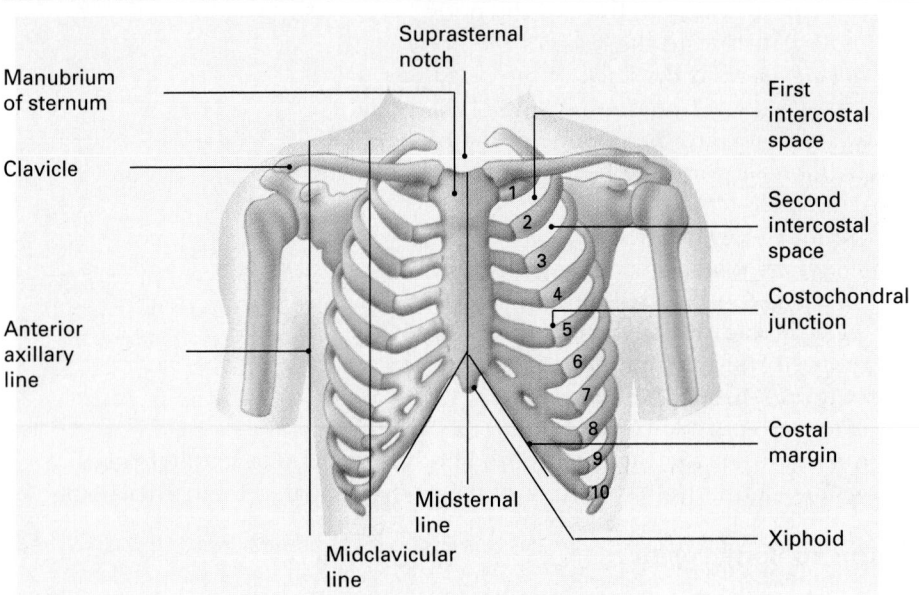

FIGURE 9-15   Topographical anatomy of the chest (anterior view).

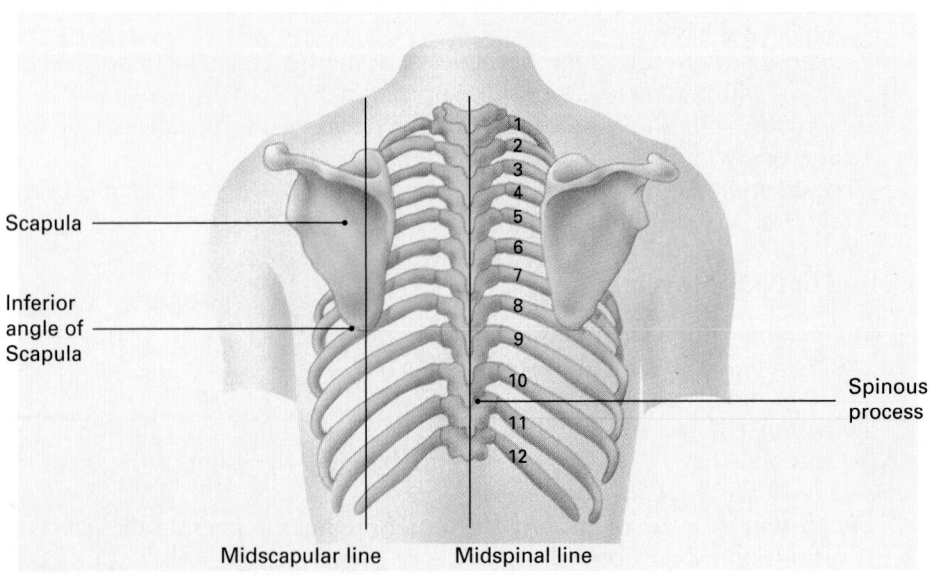

FIGURE 9-16   Topographical anatomy of the chest (posterior view).

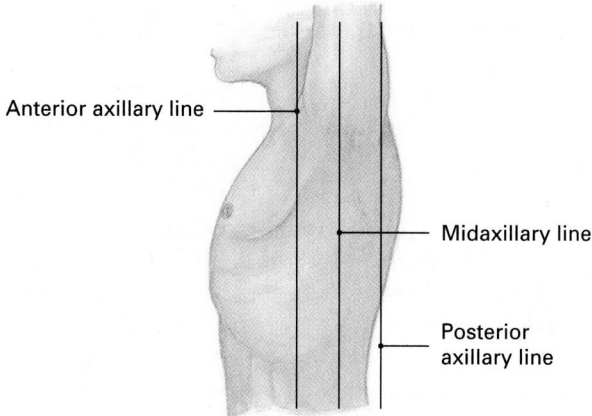

Anterior axillary line ——

Midaxillary line

Posterior
axillary line

FIGURE 9-17 Topographical
anatomy of the chest (side view).

Topographical Anatomy of the Abdomen

The abdomen is divided into four quadrants by drawing a vertical line from
the xiphoid process to the symphysis pubis. This line is then halved, and a
horizontal line drawn to separate the upper abdomen from the lower. The
back is also part of the abdomen. It should be considered when referring to
the abdomen. The point where the twelfth ribs attach to the twelfth vertebra is
called the costovertebral angle (CVA). It is an important point in physical
examination. The lateral aspect of the abdomen is often called the flank.

    Organs contained within each abdominal quadrant include the following
(see Figure 9-18):

❑ *Left Upper*: spleen, tail of the pancreas, stomach, left kidney, and part of
the colon.
❑ *Right Upper*: liver, gall bladder, head of the pancreas, part of the duodenum, right kidney, and part of the colon.

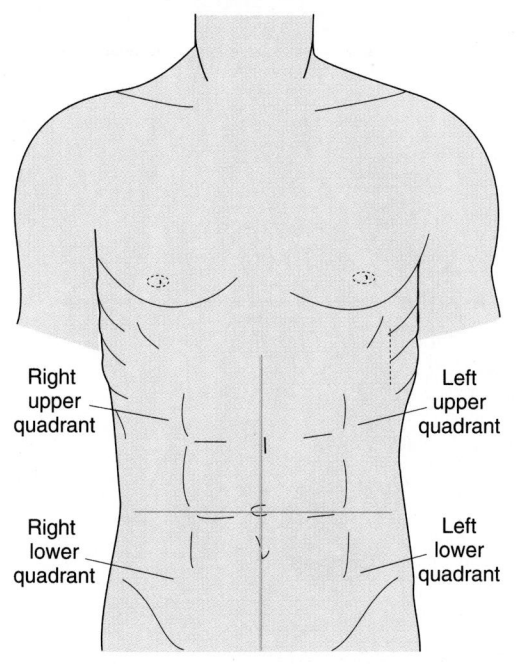

Right
upper
quadrant

Left
upper
quadrant

Right
lower
quadrant

Left
lower
quadrant

FIGURE 9-18 The four abdominal
quadrants.

❑ *Right Lower*: appendix, ascending colon, small intestine, and the right ovary and fallopian tube.
❑ *Left Lower*: small intestine, descending colon, and left ovary and fallopian tube.

BODY CAVITIES

■ **cavity** a hollow space in a larger structure; a space that holds the organs of the body.

The body contains several compartments, referred to as **cavities**. (See Figure 9-19.) The superior-most cavity is the *cranium* or *cranial vault*, which contains the brain. The *thoracic cavity* is the compartment that contains the heart, lungs, and mediastinum. It is bordered superiorly by the root of the neck and inferiorly by the diaphragm. The *abdominal cavity* is bordered by the diaphragm superiorly and the pelvic inlet inferiorly. It contains the liver, gall bladder, stomach, pancreas, spleen, intestines, kidneys, and adrenal glands. The *pelvic cavity* is bordered superiorly by the pelvic inlet and inferiorly by the pelvic floor. It contains the bladder, rectum, ovaries, fallopian tubes, and uterus. There is no anatomical division between the abdomen and the pelvis;

VENTRAL   DORSAL

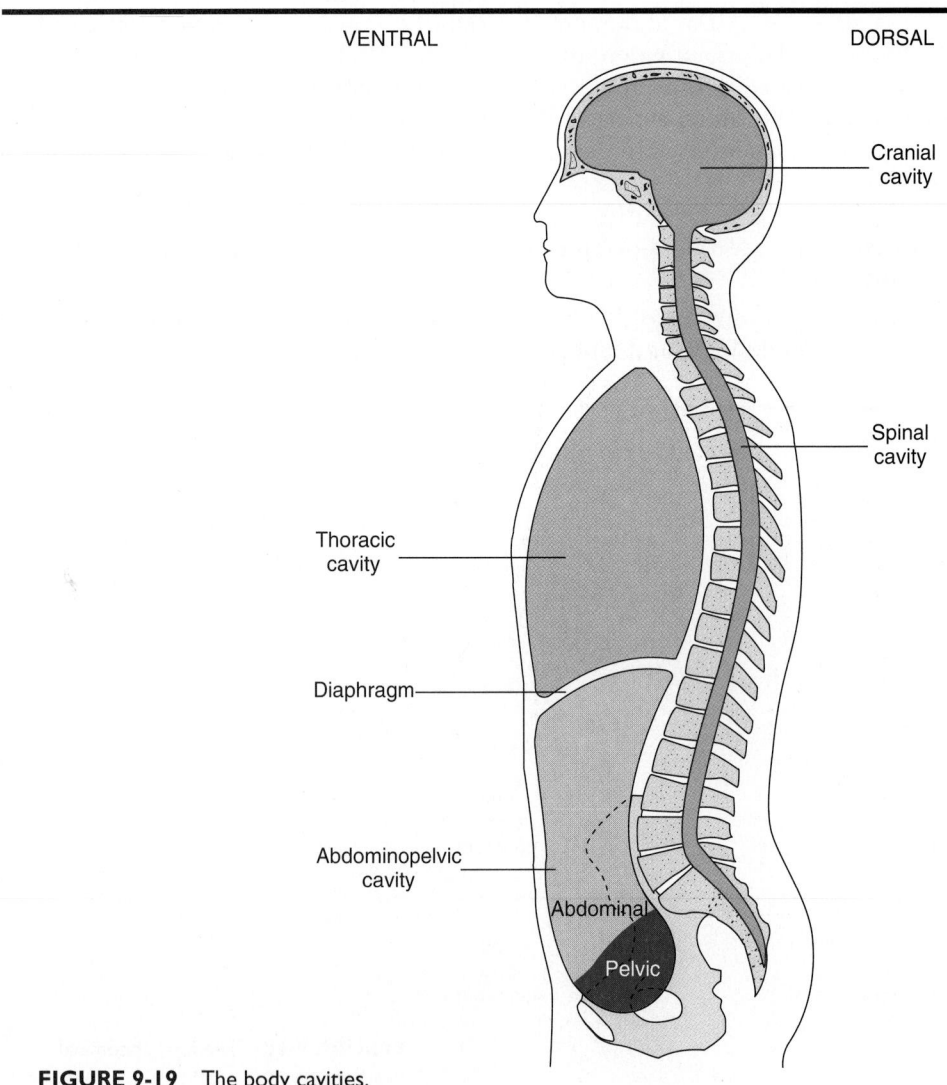

FIGURE 9-19   The body cavities.

they are often referred to as the abdominopelvic cavity. The spinal cavity extends from the base of the skull, down through the spinal canal, to the sacrum. It contains the spinal cord and associated structures.

SUMMARY

This chapter has presented the fundamentals of anatomy and physiology. Detailed discussion of each body system will appear in later chapters. At regular intervals, you should review pertinent anatomy and physiology. A thorough understanding of anatomy will often allow you to predict, with reasonable accuracy, what injuries and illnesses have occurred, based on the location of the patient's injury or complaint.

FURTHER READING

Martini, Frederic. *Fundamentals of Anatomy and Physiology*, 2nd ed. Englewood Cliffs, NJ: Prentice Hall, 1992.

Yvorra, James G. *Mosby's Emergency Dictionary: Quick Reference for Emergency Responders*. St. Louis, MO: C.V. Mosby, 1989.

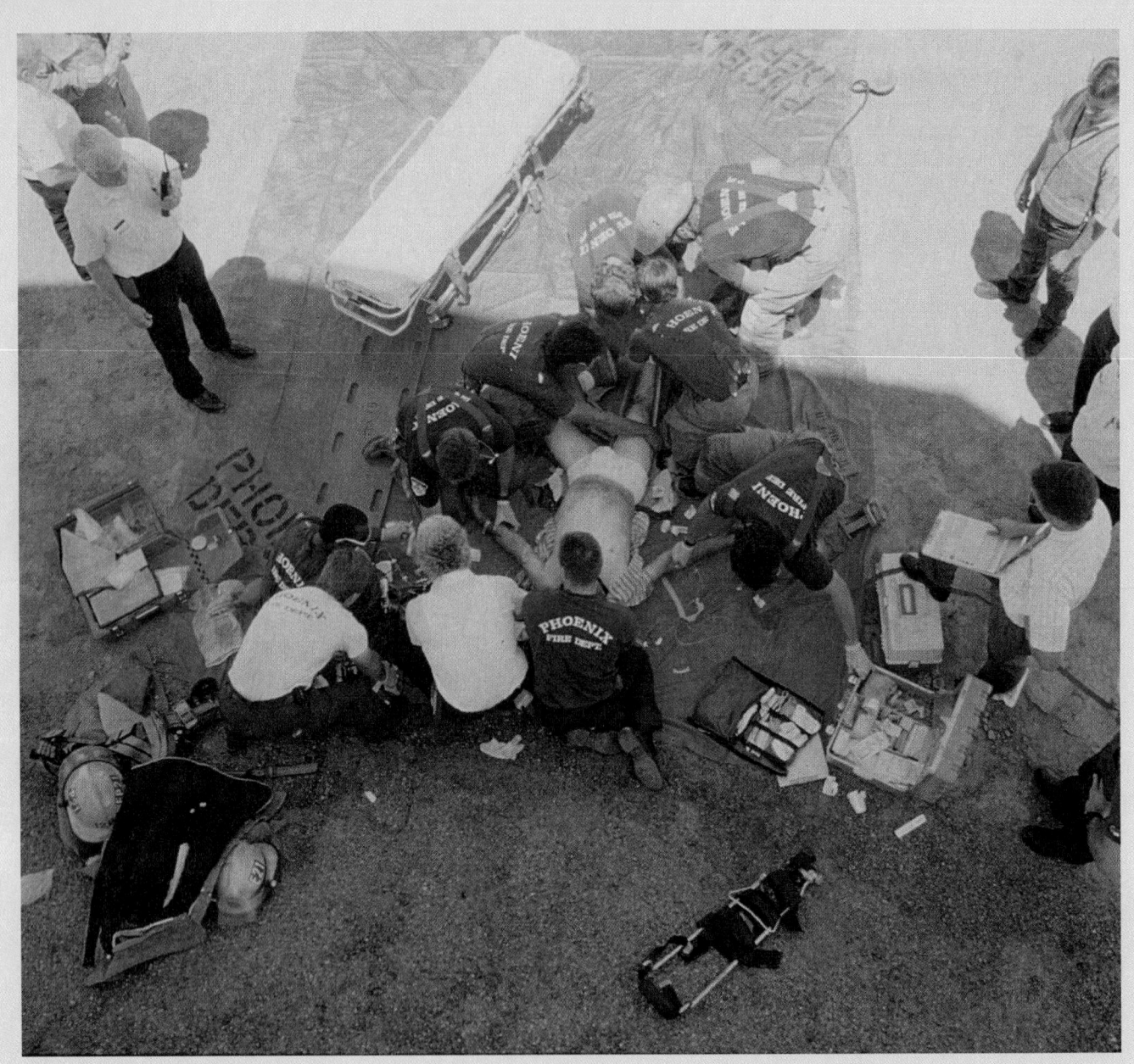

10

COMPREHENSIVE PATIENT ASSESSMENT

Objectives for Chapter 10

After reading this chapter, you should be able to:

1. Identify information gathered in each of the six phases of patient assessment. (See pp. 166–200.)

2. List some potential scene hazards to rule out before patient care can safely begin. (See p. 168.)

3. Explain the A, B, C, D, and E of the primary assessment. (See pp. 170–174.)

4. Compare and contrast the results of the primary assessment for trauma and medical patients. (See pp. 170, 174.)

5. List, by anatomical area, each of the signs evaluated during the head-to-toe physical exam. (See pp. 178–189.)

6. List the four vital signs, and explain their significance to patient evaluation. (See pp. 191–194.)

7. Identify and discuss the information that can be elicited about the patient's chief complaint by use of the OPQRST questions. (See pp. 197–198.)

8. Identify and discuss the information that can be elicited about the patient's past medical history by use of the AMPLE questions. (See pp. 198–199.)

9. Demonstrate a complete patient assessment—from scene size-up to documentation of the call. (See pp. 166–203.)

Mid day, on a warm sunny Sunday in August, the pagers sound for Riverton Rescue. There is a call at Waterfront Park for a woman down. The crew disconnects the shore power from the ambulance and heads toward the park. The dispatcher gives further information gained from a bystander via a cellular phone. It appears that the young woman was attacked by a swarm of bees. She immediately complained of shortness of breath and then collapsed.

Upon arrival at the park, John Stevens and Mary Roberts, both paramedics, are directed to a small flower garden. There they find a woman lying on her back. From a distance they can hear her stridorous respirations and notice the ashen color of her skin. John arrives at the patient's head and quickly removes the towel from under it. He then introduces himself and his partner. The patient can barely speak her name, "Denise Abbot," because of her short gasping breaths. Her respirations are about 32 per minute and shallow. The stridor is suggestive of partial airway restriction. John determines her mental status is alert, but her airway is compromised. Mary reports that Denise's radial pulse is 102 and weak and capillary refill is 3 seconds. She then administers oxygen via nonrebreather mask with a flow rate of 15 liters per minute.

John begins to question Denise about what caused her collapse and breathing problems. Denise reports that she was stung on the neck and left thigh several times by bees. John notes the skin on her neck is mottled and there are a few red welts with stingers still in place. Mary states that there is some respiratory wheezing but there is exchange in all lung fields. Denise denies any allergies but explains she has never been stung by a bee before. She is on no medications and had gall bladder surgery a year ago. She ate a hamburger and fries about an hour and a half ago.

John notices several bees swarming around him, Mary, and Denise and decides to expedite transport to the ambulance. Denise is placed on a backboard and transferred to the ambulance where an IV is started. John contacts Memorial Hospital and asks for a medical control physician. He provides the following report to Dr. Greer: "We are treating a 24 year-old, 125-pound female patient who was stung several times about the neck and left thigh by bees. She is alert but is breathing with stridorous, wheezing, and shallow respirations at a rate of 32. Her skin is ashen with mottling and capillary refill is three seconds. Her pulse rate is 102."

The on-line physician orders 0.3 mg of epinephrine 1:1,000 administered subcutaneously and 50 mg Benadryl administered intravenously. John and Mary carefully monitor Denise while she is transported uneventfully to the hospital. The stridor and wheezing disappear.

At the emergency department, the receiving physician admits the patient for observation. She goes home the next morning.

INTRODUCTION

■ **patient assessment** evaluation of a patient to detect a possible medical problem or injury.

Patient assessment is one of the most important skills that you will perform as a paramedic. It will help give you a reasonable idea of what may be wrong with the patient and will provide you with the basis for requesting, utilizing, and performing advanced life support (ALS) interventions.

Paramedic patient assessment is a straightforward skill that consumes only a few minutes. It is similar to the assessment you performed as an EMT-Basic, but it differs in depth and the kind of care you will provide as a result. Your assessment must be thorough, because many ALS procedures are potentially dangerous. Administration of drugs, defibrillation, cardioversion, pleural decompression, or advanced airway skills depend upon the probable field diagnosis. The consequences of an inaccurate assessment can be devastating.

PHASES OF PREHOSPITAL ASSESSMENT

Phases of Assessment
■ Scene size-up
■ Primary assessment
■ Secondary assessment (head-to-toe evaluation)
■ Vital Signs
■ Patient history
■ Ongoing assessment

Assessment begins with an evaluation of the patient's environment, continues with an evaluation of airway, breathing, circulatory function, and mental status, and proceeds to a comprehensive evaluation of the patient. It is a process that is never really complete, because it involves continuous re-evaluation.

A good patient assessment in a field setting can be difficult. There may be many distractions (noise, activity, etc.), and you will need to balance the need for on-scene assessment and care with the need to get the patient to the hospital without unnecessary delay. You must have a plan of assessment clearly in mind. To prioritize patient care, you need to be familiar with the six phases of patient assessment: scene size-up, primary assessment, secondary assessment, vital signs, patient history, and ongoing assessment.

Management of life threats and other problems you discover, as well as packaging and transport of the patient to the hospital and communicating and documenting relevant information, are all performed at appropriate points in the process of prehospital assessment and care.

The patient assessment process for trauma and for medical illness is similar. Any differences will be mentioned in this chapter or in the chapters on specific emergencies. Remember that trauma may have been caused by a medical problem, or vice versa. Heart attack and alcohol intoxication may result in auto accidents. Medical problems may arise from prior trauma, such as head-injury-induced epilepsy, or internal bleeding secondary to an earlier fall. Focus on what appears to be wrong, while staying alert for the unexpected.

SCENE SIZE-UP

Scene size-up is the essential first step. Review dispatch information, survey the scene and call for needed assistance, identify hazards and secure the scene, identify the mechanism of injury or nature of the illness, and locate all patients.

Review Dispatch Information

Assessment begins before you even see the patient. Start to evaluate the situation immediately upon receiving the dispatch information. (See Figure 10-1.) Dispatch information provides more data than is generally recognized. The scene location can often indicate the type of emergency and its potential seriousness. The location of a medical or trauma call, such as a response to a cardiologist's office, a particular stretch of roadway, or the home of a patient who frequently summons EMS, may help identify the nature of the call.

Modern Emergency Medical Dispatch (EMD) systems employ dispatchers who provide pre-arrival instructions to the caller and elicit information to help determine the specific nature and seriousness of the call. While you are en route, use this information to identify equipment you will need and ensure that it is operational. There is nothing more frustrating than to arrive at an acute emergency only to find that an essential piece of equipment has failed or that you must leave the patient's side to retrieve it from the ambulance.

Also use en-route time to anticipate and plan your actions. Review possible scene hazards, and mentally walk through the elements of patient assessment and care steps appropriate for the anticipated emergency. This preplanning will help you to quickly deliver appropriate care for your patient.

Survey the Scene

Upon arrival, evaluate the scene. Bystanders' faces often reveal stress levels and how they perceive the emergency. The *mechanism of injury* or *nature of the illness* may also be apparent. (Chapter 14 gives detailed information about mechanisms of injury.) If you spot hazards or patient demands beyond your capability, immediately summon additional help.

> **Scene Size-up**
> - Review the dispatch data
> - Survey the scene and call for assistance if needed
> - Identify hazards
> - Secure the scene
> - Determine mechanism of injury/nature of illness
> - Locate all patients

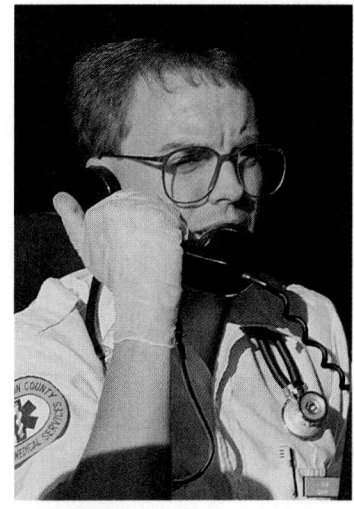

FIGURE 10-1 Review the dispatch information en route to the call. This information can help you to prepare mentally for the emergency.

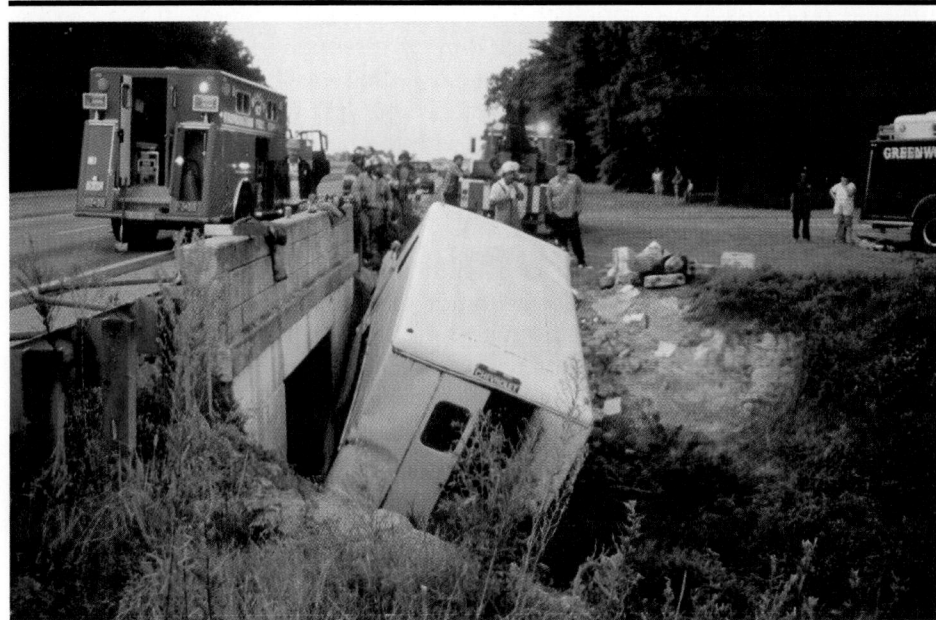

FIGURE 10-2 Look for potential hazards as you survey the scene.

Identify Potential Hazards

Actively look for hazards that may endanger you, other rescuers, or your patient—such as fire, structural collapse, toxic dust or gas, explosion, electricity, traffic problems, slippery surfaces, and broken glass or jagged metal. (See Figure 10-2.) Remember that such perils may be found at medical as well as at trauma scenes.

Body Substance Isolation Body fluids frequently contain health-threatening pathogens. The best defense against bloodborne, bodily-fluid-borne and, in some cases, airborne agents is to take **body substance isolation** precautions. Wear gloves whenever you expect to come in contact with the patient or with care equipment. Certainly this includes any physical assessment of a patient. If there is the potential for splashing of blood or vomiting, wear a face mask and protective eyewear and consider the need for a gown. Also, be aware of the increasing incidence of serious contagious airborne diseases. If a patient displays any sign of respiratory infection, mask him and consider masking yourself as well.

Secure the Scene

Safe, orderly, and controlled incident management is essential. Call for specialty personnel to stabilize wreckage or turn off electrical power. Make sure traffic is safely routed around a collision. Control bystanders and spot potential "human hazards." Make sure a hostile crowd or someone who assaulted your patient is not about to attack you. If the scene is not secure, retreat and wait for police or other expert help. You cannot help your patient if you yourself become a casualty.

Determine the Mechanism of Injury or the Nature of the Illness

Understanding the cause or nature of a patient's problem is critical. In trauma, the cause of the patient's problem is called the **mechanism of injury**. In a medical situation, the cause or signs and symptoms of the patient's problem is called the **nature of the illness**.

■ **body substance isolation** precautions taken to prevent contact with another person's blood or other body substances, based on the presumption that all such substances may be infectious.

✳ If it's wet and it's not yours, don't touch it!

■ **mechanism of injury** the strength, direction, and nature of forces that cause injury.

■ **nature of the illness** the underlying cause, or the signs and symptoms, of a medical condition.

Mechanism of Injury   The mechanism of injury is usually apparent through careful evaluation of the trauma scene. (See Figure 10-3.) Identifying the mechanism of injury can help you anticipate both the location and the seriousness of injuries. Significant mechanisms of injury include those listed below.

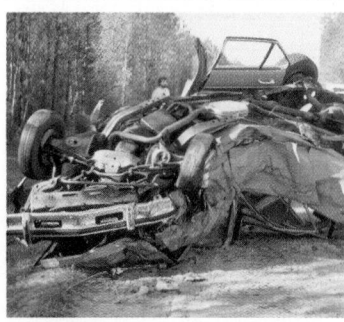

FIGURE 10-3   Evaluate the trauma scene to determine the mechanism of injury.

Significant Mechanisms of Injury

Motor Vehicle Collisions

- High-speed vehicle collision, especially with severe vehicle deformity
- Damage intruding into the passenger compartment
- Death of another occupant in the same passenger compartment
- Roll-over
- Ejection from vehicle

Other Motor Vehicle Collisions

- Motorcycle
- Motor vehicle-pedestrian
- Motor vehicle-bicycle

Other

- Falls over 20 feet (or three times body height)
- Unresponsive or altered mental status
- Penetrating injuries of the head, chest, or abdomen (including collision injuries, gunshot wounds, knife wounds, blast injuries)
- Hidden injuries that may be caused by buckled seatbelts, seatbelts not worn. Look for airbags deployed when seatbelts are not worn. Look for deformation of steering wheel, dash, or windshield even if airbags have deployed

Infants and Children

- Falls over 10 feet (or three times body height)
- Medium-speed motor vehicle collisions
- Bicycle falls or collisions

Phases of Assessment
- Scene size-up
- Primary assessment
- Secondary assessment (head to toe evaluation)
- Vital Signs
- Patient history
- Ongoing assessment

Remember that the trauma patient may suffer life-threatening internal injury without serious signs and symptoms observable at the scene.

Nature of the Illness   The nature of the illness may be determined from bystanders, family members, or the patient. Examine the environment for the patient's position, medications or drug paraphernalia, or medical-care equipment such as oxygen. This information will help determine the nature and seriousness of the emergency.

Locate Patients

The scene size-up also includes a search of the area to locate all the patients. Ask yourself: *Could there be other passengers or persons involved in the accident or affected by the medical problem?* Determine where the most seriously affected patients are likely to be found and how many patients will need transport. Evaluate the mechanism of injury; for example, a two-car accident must include at least two drivers. Clues such as diaper bags, child auto seats, clothing, or twin spider webs in the windshield should lead you to search for more patients than those who may be apparent. If the anticipated number of patients is greater than you have the capacity to care for, assure that more ambulances are directed to the scene.

✳ Always ask yourself, "Is there another patient present?"

■ **primary assessment** the first phase of patient assessment, conducted for the purpose of detecting and treating immediate threats to life.

The **primary assessment** is often called the ABCDEs (for the sequence of assessment steps: *airway, breathing, circulation, disability,* and *expose*). (See Procedure 10-1.)

The goal of the primary assessment is to detect immediate threats to life. You will treat any life-threatening conditions immediately, as you find them, before moving on to the next part of the assessment. Finally you will make priority decisions regarding this patient's need for immediate transport vs. further on-scene assessment and care. Re-employ the primary assessment frequently throughout your care—after any major intervention, whenever the patient's condition changes, or every few minutes.

The kind of life threat you are most likely to discover during the primary assessment may vary slightly between the trauma and medical patient. In the trauma patient you are more likely to find compromise of the ABCs and indications of internal head injury and/or internal bleeding. In a medical emergency, you must first rule out cardiopulmonary arrest or a respiratory emergency. In both cases, assessment targets the greatest threats to life. The initial assessment for either patient occurs quickly—the overall task consumes less than two minutes—but it provides enough information for you to determine immediate steps of care.

Begin by identifying yourself and explaining what you intend to do. (See Figure 10-4.) For example: "I'm Jane Smith, a paramedic from Ashwaubenon Rescue Squad. I'm here to help you." This establishes your level of training, authority, and reason for being at your patient's side. It also allows the patient to refuse care. As discussed in previous chapters, you cannot provide care without either implied or informed consent.

If there is a significant mechanism of injury, or the patient has any associated complaint or is unresponsive, institute manual stabilization of the head and neck on first contact with the patient. (See Figure 10-5.) Continue manual stabilization until the patient is fully immobilized to the long spine board.

Constantly reassure the patient. Listen to what he has to say. Do not trivialize a patient's complaints. All too frequently, we forget how significant an injury, even a minor one, is to a patient. With our experience, the injury or problem may seem minor. For the patient it is a real concern. The ill or injured victim may worry about the long-term consequences for work, child care, and finances. Understand these fears and support the patient psychologically, as well as physiologically.

**Primary Assessment:
The ABCDEs**

Airway
Breathing
Circulation
Disability
Expose

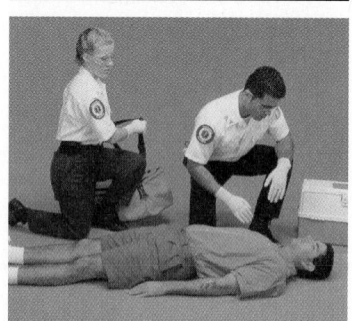

FIGURE 10-4 Identify yourself and gain the patient's consent to care.

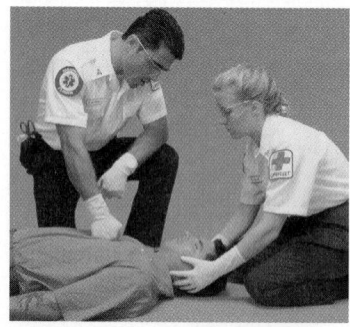

FIGURE 10-5 Initiate manual stabilization of the head and neck on first patient contact.

■ **paradoxical movement** moving in a fashion opposite to that expected. It is often seen in flail chest injuries where the flail segment moves in an opposite direction compared to the rest of the chest.

Airway and Breathing

Quickly assure a patent airway and good respiration; they are critical to a patient's survival, even in the short-term. Repeat this element of assessment often to ensure the airway remains unobstructed and breathing is adequate in rate and volume.

Though airway and breathing separately make up the A and B of the ABCDEs, evaluate them together. Breathing does not occur without an airway; conversely, a patent airway cannot be confirmed unless air moves through it. *Look, listen,* and *feel* to find out if the patient has an open airway and adequate breathing.

Look   Look at the external portions of the airway—the mouth and nose. Note any trauma, vomitus, or other mechanisms or agents that may compromise the airway. Examine for nasal flaring, fluid, or objects in the airway. Spot cyanotic (bluish) or ashen coloration of the lips. Observe for normal, smooth, and unlabored chest rise and fall. (See Procedure 10-1, Figure A.) There should be no **paradoxical movement** of the chest, and one side should not rise and fall more than the other.

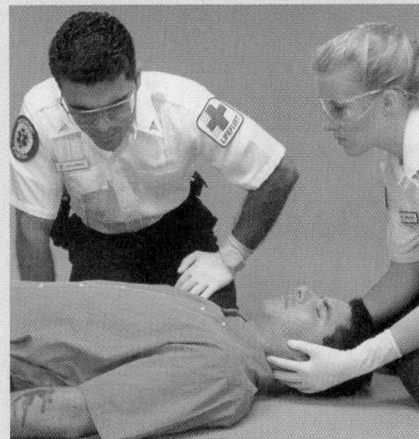

10-1A. The first step in assessing airway and breathing is to LOOK at the chest.

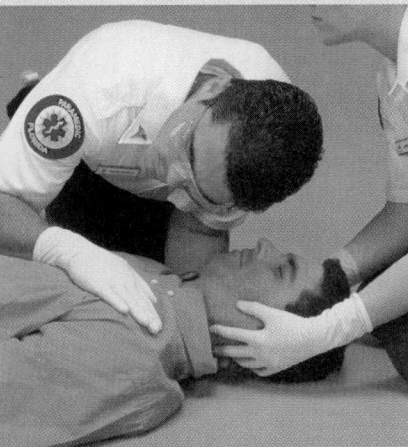

10-1B. The second step in assessing airway and breathing is to LISTEN for air movement.

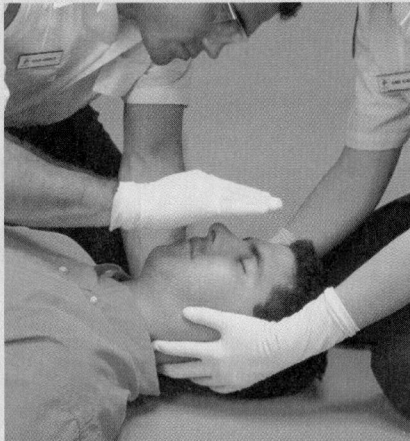

10-1C. The third step in assessing airway and breathing is to FEEL for air movement with your hand or cheek.

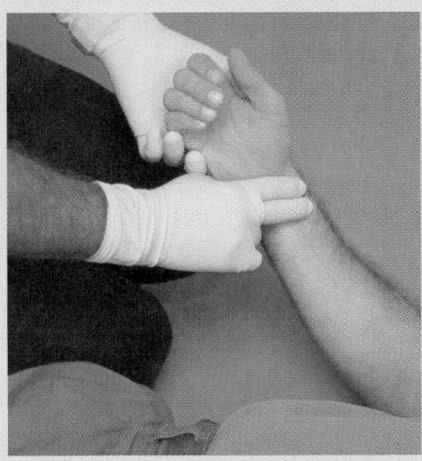

10-1D. To assess circulation, feel for a radial pulse in an adult (brachial pulse in an infant under 1 year).

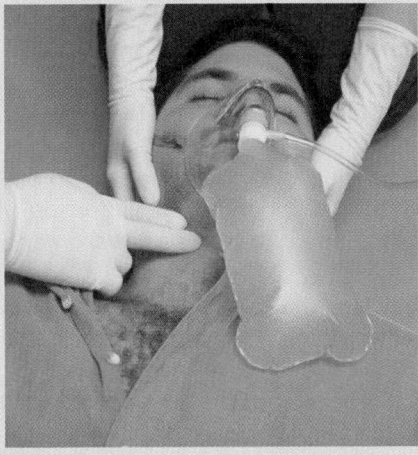

10-1E. If a radial or brachial pulse cannot be felt, palpate for the presence of a carotid pulse.

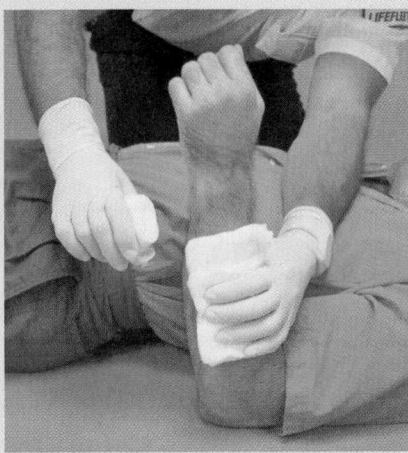

10-1F. Control major bleeding.

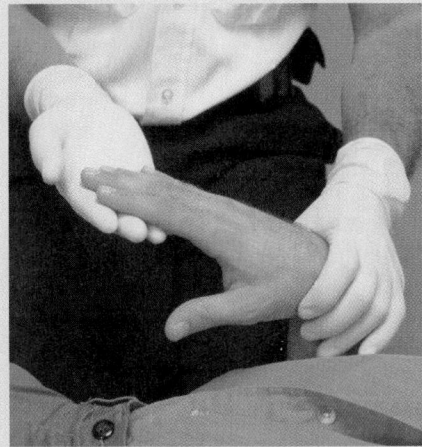

10-1G. Observe for pallor or cyanosis and a cool and clammy skin as signs of possible shock.

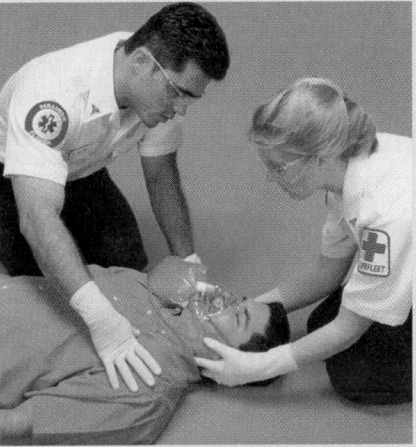

10-1H. Use the AVPU scale to assess for disability (mental status, or level of consciousness).

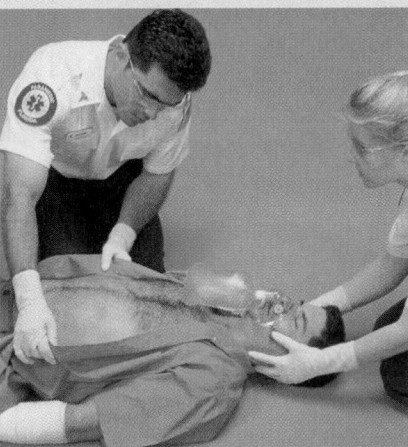

10-1I. Expose the patient's body to observe for critical injuries.

■ **retraction** the act of drawing back or inward (e.g., acute airway obstruction when the intercostal spaces and sternal notch retract).

■ **apnea** the absence of breathing.

■ **snoring** upper airway noise caused by the partial obstruction of the airway by the tongue or some similar structure or material.

■ **stridor** high-pitched "crowing" sound caused by restriction of the upper airway.

■ **wheezing** whistling-type breath sound associated with narrowing or spasm of the smaller airways.

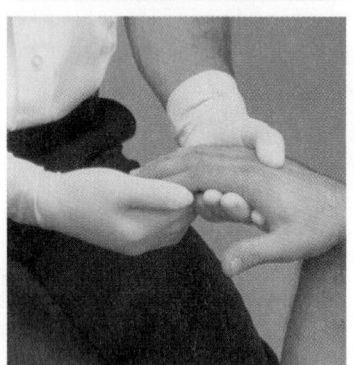

FIGURE 10-6 Assess the patient's skin color.

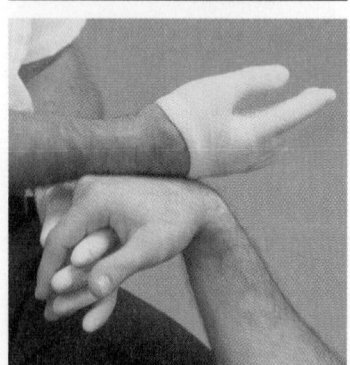

FIGURE 10-7 Assess the patient's skin temperature.

Assess the rate and volume of air being moved. Normal respiration occurs 12 to 20 times per minute. It displaces about 500 mL of air (6–12 L/min). Smaller volumes are of concern because the first 150 mL is not really used for gas exchange (dead space volume). Count the rate. If it drops below 12 breaths per minute, the total volume of inspired air may not be enough to maintain life. An abnormally fast respiration rate (more than 24 per minute) may indicate excitement, a metabolic problem, shock, or head injury.

Other respiratory characteristics should also be noted. Is abdominal movement exaggerated (suggesting spinal-cord injury and diaphragmatic breathing)? Are accessory muscles of the neck being used to move the air (indicating increased airway resistance)? Are there **retractions** between ribs or above the clavicles (signaling increased inspiratory effort caused by airway obstruction)?

Listen   Are the respirations quiet or noisy? Ensure that respirations are present but relatively quiet. (See Procedure 10-1, Figure B.) (Total silence, of course, may indicate **apnea**.) Evaluate any noisy respiration. **Snoring** is generally caused by gravity moving the relaxed tongue into the posterior pharynx. Correct it by proper head-positioning: head tilt-chin lift in the medical patient; chin lift, jaw thrust, or nasopharyngeal airway insertion in the trauma patient. (See Chapter 11.)

Stridor, or *crowing*, is an ominous sound. It commonly indicates laryngeal obstruction, which is very difficult to correct in the field. **Wheezing** suggests lower-airway constriction, which is also hard to correct in the field. You may hear gurgling—caused by fluids in the airway, mouth, or nose—which demands immediate suctioning of the airway. Gurgling may indicate congestive heart failure and a need for advanced cardiac life-support measures.

Feel   "Feel" may be the most obvious confirmation of breathing. The motion of warm, humid exhalation on your cheek or hand may indicate how much air, if any, the patient is moving. (See Procedure 10-1, Figure C.)

Management   If assessment reveals anything that threatens respiration, correct it at once. The brain, heart, and kidneys cannot survive long without oxygen. Intubate the patient who is unable to protect the airway (deeply unconscious and lacking a gag reflex). If respirations are absent, or the volume moving with each breath appears to total less than 6 liters per minute, support respiration with positive pressure ventilation supplemented with 100 percent oxygen. Confirm adequate airway and respirations before continuing your assessment.

Circulation

Oxygen delivery to the alveoli of the lungs does little good without a mechanism to circulate the oxygen to the body's cells. So once you establish adequate respiratory function, evaluate circulation, the C in the ABCDEs.

Pulse   Feel for a radial pulse, noting the general rate and character. The pulse should be between 50 and 120 beats per minute, strong and regular. If no radial pulse is felt, palpate the carotid pulse. (See Procedure 10-1, Figures D and E.)

You can use various pulse points to approximate the patient's systolic blood pressure. As the pulse wave travels away from the heart and the central circulation, it weakens. The radial pulse normally disappears when the systolic pressure drops below 80 mm Hg. Between 70 and 80 mm Hg the femoral pulse disappears. The carotid pulse usually remains until the systolic pressure drops below 60 mm Hg.

Bleeding   Once a pulse is confirmed, assess for major bleeding. (See Procedure 10-1, Figure F.)

Skin The skin is one of the first organs to lose blood flow (due to peripheral vasoconstriction) in **hypovolemia** or other types of shock. It may appear mottled (blotchy), cyanotic (bluish), pale, or ashen in color. (See Figure 10-6.) The skin may also feel cool and moist (clammy) to the touch. (See Figure 10-7.) This often indicates that warm, circulating blood has been shunted away from the skin to critical areas. If you find any of these signs, suspect a serious problem with circulation. (See Procedure 10-1, Figure G.)

You may also evaluate perfusion by looking at **capillary refill**. Compress a portion of skin or a nail bed, and it will blanch white or pale. (See Figure 10-8.) Upon release, a pink color returns within two seconds with good circulatory function. A longer capillary refill time suggests circulatory compromise. Capillary refill is most reliable as an indicator of circulatory function in infants and young children. In adults, capillary refill may be affected by factors, such as smoking, medications, cold weather, or chronic conditions in the elderly. For the adult patient, consider capillary refill as just one indicator, along with others, of circulatory function.

Management If the patient is pulseless, initiate cardiac arrest procedures including defibrillation. Control severe bleeding with techniques such as pressure, dressings, and elevation. If shock is suspected because of a significant mechanism of injury or because of indications including skin pallor or delayed capillary refill, institute shock care procedures including oxygen, splinting of fractures, keeping the patient warm, and elevating the feet if spinal or head injury is not suspected.

Disability

Disability (impaired mental status) is the D of the ABCDEs. (See Procedure 10-1, Figure H.) There are many ways to describe level of consciousness. However, terms such as obtunded, semi-conscious, and confused have different meanings for different people. A more concise and objective classification of a patient's level of consciousness is represented by the mnemonic *AVPU*, which stands for *Alert, responds to Verbal stimuli, responds to Painful stimuli,* and *Unresponsive.*

The patient's response to stimulation will tell you a great deal about his condition. An alert patient will give an organized, appropriate, coherent statement, showing that oxygenated blood is circulating to the brain and that respiration is able to support reasonable speech. A patient who appears to be unresponsive may respond to verbal stimulus by opening his eyes or by making some movement in response to a verbal command. A patient may only respond to a painful stimulus by withdrawing or a pushing away in response to a pinch or a rub of knuckles on the sternum or another infliction of pain. A truly unresponsive patient will make no response to verbal or painful stimulus.

Management A level of consciousness that is less than Alert on the AVPU scale may indicate an emergent or an already-serious problem. At a minimum, a patient with an impaired mental status may have lost, or be in danger of losing, the ability to protect his airway. Take immediate steps to protect the patient's airway by positioning, use of airway adjuncts, or intubation, as appropriate. Provide oxygen to any patient with diminished mental status, and seek out the cause.

Expose

The E of the ABCDEs refers to exposing the body to perform a quick survey for signs of critical problems. (See Procedure 10-1, Figure I.) In trauma, you expose the head, neck, chest, abdomen, and pelvis to look for significant hemorrhage, potential respiratory compromise, and other life-threatening injuries.

■ **hypovolemia** diminished blood or fluid volume, a common cause of shock.

■ **capillary refill** diagnostic sign for evaluating peripheral circulation. A capillary bed, such as one beneath a fingernail, is compressed. The time taken for a pink color to return is the capillary refill time, normally 2 seconds or less.

> **Levels of Consciousness**
> ■ **A** = **A**lert
> ■ **V** = responds to **V**erbal stimuli
> ■ **P** = responds to **P**ainful stimuli
> ■ **U** = **U**nresponsive

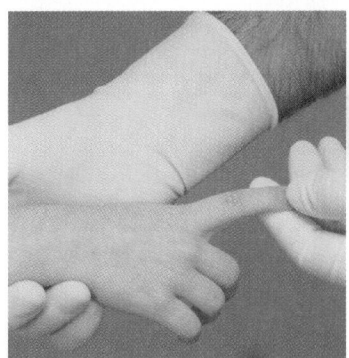

FIGURE 10-8 Compress a portion of the skin or nail bed to assess capillary refill.

Rapidly examine the head and neck for signs of injury and possible intracranial trauma. Identify facial injuries that may contribute to airway compromise. Evaluate the neck for signs of trauma, **edema**, or discoloration, suggesting vascular or airway problems to come. Examine the chest for signs of deceleration injuries or fractures or instability of the chest, such as gross deformity or flail chest. Rule out an **open pneumothorax** by observing for wounds. Remember that any penetrating wound may have an associated exit wound. Evaluate the abdomen for blunt or penetrating trauma. Observe for pulsating masses or discoloration. If there is abdominal guarding, pain, or tenderness, suspect internal bleeding.

Finally, scan the entire body for evidence of severe external bleeding. Check hidden body areas, such as behind the lower back, buttocks, inguinal region, and anywhere else that the mechanism of injury may suggest trauma.

In the medical patient, unless associated trauma is possible, rapid survey of the body need not be so aggressive. Look at patient positioning. Note any discomfort. Observe the area of the chief complaint and associated symptoms.

Management   When exposing the patient's body for examination, take steps to keep the patient warm and to protect the patient's privacy. Remove only as much clothing as necessary, use blankets or other insulating materials to maintain body temperature, and do your best to shield the patient from the gaze of bystanders.

Critical Management Priorities

Consider the priorities for different courses of action for the trauma or medical patient, as discussed in the following sections.

Trauma Patient   After completing the primary assessment, determine whether the patient requires on-scene stabilization or immediate transport with stabilization en route. Critical trauma patients are much more likely to survive if they obtain surgery within an hour of the incident. This has become known as the **Golden Hour.** The EMS system is generally given 10 minutes (1/6 of the "Golden Hour") of on-the-scene time to assess and correct immediately life-threatening problems and to prepare for transport. Should the patient show respiratory difficulties, central nervous system deficit, or any indications of developing shock, transport immediately to a definitive care facility, preferably a **trauma center**.

A **trauma score**, or trauma evaluation system, may help to prioritize severity of injury and predict outcome. One example is the Revised Trauma Score, which uses the **Glasgow Coma Scale** as well as respiratory rate, thoracic expansion, systolic blood pressure, and capillary refill. (See Figure 10-9.)

Be aware that the signs and symptoms displayed by your patient may be affected by the time between the incident and your arrival. If the patient has only been injured for a few minutes, the signs of shock and injury (like the discoloration of a **contusion**) may not yet be apparent. The patient may appear stable, only to deteriorate quickly later. If it has been some time since the accident and your arrival and the patient shows no signs of shock or serious injury, he is more likely to be stable throughout your care.

Medical Patient   The approach to a medical patient is different than for the trauma patient. Care of the cardiac arrest patient is delivered best at the scene. Many other medical emergencies, though less acute than cardiac arrest, require on-scene stabilization rather than rapid transport. However, like severe trauma, some medical conditions can require immediate transport. Hypovolemic shock, due to ruptured ectopic pregnancy or a dissecting or ruptured aneurysm, can rapidly result in exsanguination (total blood loss). The only definitive care of such cases is surgical closure of the internal wound at the hospital.

Trauma Score

Respiratory Rate	10 – 29/min	4	
	> 29/min	3	
	6 – 9/min	2	
	1 – 5/min	1	
	None	0	
Respiratory Expansion	Normal	1	
	Retractive	0	
Systolic Blood Pressure	>89 mmHg or greater	4	
	76 – 89 mmHg	3	
	50 – 75 mmHg	2	
	0 – 49 mmHg	1	
	No Pulse	0	
Capillary Refill	Normal	2	
	Delayed	1	
	None	0	
Cardiopulmonary Assessment			

Glasgow Coma Scale

Eye Opening	Spontaneous	4	
	To Voice	3	
	To Pain	2	
	None	1	
Verbal Response	Oriented	5	
	Confused	4	
	Inappropriate Words	3	
	Incomprehensible Words	2	
	None	1	
Motor Response	Obeys Commands	6	
	Locailzes Pain	5	
	Withdraw (Pain)	4	
	Flexion (Pain)	3	
	Extension (Pain)	2	
	None	1	
Glasgow Coma Score Total			

TOTAL GLASGOW COMA SCALE POINTS

13 – 15 = 5

9 – 12 = 4

6 – 8 = 3

4 – 5 = 1

Conversion = Approximately One - Third Total Value

| **Neurologic Assessment** | | |

Total Trauma Score = Cardiopulmonary + Neurologic

FIGURE 10-9 The Revised Trauma Score.

As a paramedic, you must examine the patient for subtle indications of developing problems. Be prepared to immediately transport the patient if on-scene stabilization is unsuccessful. If the decision has been made to care for the medical or trauma patient by rapid transport, move the patient quickly to the ambulance and accomplish most advanced care procedures en route. (See Figure 10-10.)

In the ambulance, the patient should receive high-flow oxygen. If respiration is not adequate, initiate positive pressure ventilation with supplemental oxygen. Consider advanced airway care, including placement of an endotracheal tube (or possible trans-tracheal jet insufflation device). If you suspect **tension pneumothorax**, medical control may request pleural decompression. Also consider fluid resuscitation, as directed by medical control. If you choose on-scene care and stabilization, provide oxygen and other supportive measures at the scene.

SECONDARY ASSESSMENT

After immediate life threats have been controlled during the primary assessment, the **secondary assessment** is undertaken to assess the patient in more detail and to determine the seriousness of the patient's condition. The elements of the secondary assessment are the head-to-toe evaluation, vital signs, and patient history.

■ **tension pneumothorax** air trapped in the thoracic cavity that has no opening to escape, thus building pressure that affects the lungs, heart, and other organs.

■ **secondary assessment** the second phase of patient assessment in which the findings of a detailed physical exam, vital signs, and patient history are evaluated to help determine the patient's traumatic or medical problem and general status.

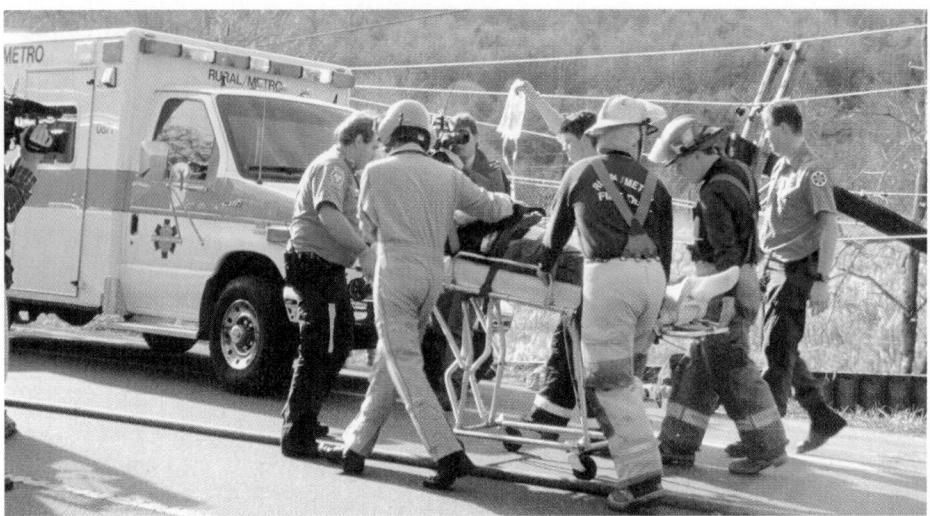

FIGURE 10-10 Expedite transport for a high priority patient and continue assessment and care en route.

Modify the secondary assessment according to patient type. For example, if the problem is trauma-related and the patient is stable enough so that expedited transport is not required, perform a complete head-to-toe evaluation at the scene. If the patient is a routine transport for direct hospital admission, limit your evaluation. A poorly performed assessment will miss significant signs and symptoms; a complete assessment will rarely cause harm unless it delays transport of the severely compromised patient.

Examining the Trauma Patient

During the physical exam for a trauma patient you will pay special attention to the areas of patient complaint and the areas of suspected injury as indicated by the mechanism of injury. In suspected serious trauma you should routinely inspect the head, neck, chest, abdomen, and pelvis. These are areas where injury can occur with limited signs and symptoms, yet they may rapidly lead to patient deterioration and death. When examining an area for injury, keep in mind that the discoloration of contusions will develop over time and may not be apparent when you first examine an injured area. Remember, your major concern may not be the injury you see but the internal injuries beneath the surface wounds.

If an area does not display visible signs of injury, palpate the region for other signs of injury. In addition to palpating for tenderness or **crepitation**, compare muscle tone and tissue compliance from one side or one limb to another. For example, is the area flaccid (without tone), normal, or tense (guarding)?

Examining the Medical Patient

The physical exam for a medical patient is intended to identify any signs and symptoms that help to support a particular reason for the patient's problem. You will concentrate your examination on the areas where the patient complains of pain or other symptoms, and those areas where you might suspect associated signs or symptoms.

Assess for the signs and symptoms associated with medical problems. These may include edema, abnormal skin color (**cyanosis**, **pallor**, **jaundice**, **erythema**, **ecchymosis**), and abnormal pulsation. Pay close attention to the examination of the chest and abdomen. Look for bilateral chest movement with respiration and listen for clear breath sounds in all lung fields, especially in the lower lobes. Palpate the abdomen to evaluate for pain, tenderness, or guarding.

■ **crepitation** a grating or crackling sensation, felt or heard in such conditions as subcutaneous emphysema or bone fracture.

■ **cyanosis** (adj. *cyanotic*) bluish color.

■ **pallor** paleness; white or gray coloration.

■ **jaundice** a yellowish coloration.

■ **erythema** reddening.

■ **ecchymosis** (adj. *ecchymotic*) black-and-blue discoloration.

Techniques for Conducting the Physical Exam

The four skills, or techniques, for conducting a physical examination include **inspection, palpation, auscultation,** and **percussion**. Each technique can reveal information essential to a complete and accurate patient assessment.

Inspection   As a non-invasive, non-endangering technique, inspection will be one of your most valuable tools in appraising patient condition. (See Figure 10-11.) Consciously evaluate each body area, looking for unusual discolorations, motions, or deformities. Pay special attention to areas where you expect to find signs and where the patient complains of symptoms. Remember the discoloration of a significant contusion may not appear until after the patient arrives at the emergency department. You will have to look carefully to observe any reddening of the skin (erythema) or other early sign of injury.

Palpation   Palpation is done with the pads of the fingers. (See Figure 10-12.) Use the same gentle, not overbearing, pressure needed to feel for a pulse. Too much pressure will dull your perception and, in some cases, injure the patient. In the case of abdominal palpation, apply pressure gently by placing the fingers of the opposite hand over the sensing fingers. This will increase your sensitivity to any masses, guarding, or other phenomenon developing within the abdomen. Honestly sense with your fingers. We often tend to "feel" with the eyes, rather than with the fingertips.

Palpate for deformity, crepitation, pulsing masses, guarding, and fluids. Sense for areas of warmth that might reflect injury before significant edema or discoloration occurs. Look to the face of a patient who is unconscious. Many patients who are unable to speak respond to pain with facial expressions and/or purposeful or purposeless motion.

Auscultation   During auscultation, you employ the stethoscope to listen to sounds generated within the body, thus determining blood pressure and assessing breath sounds. (See Figure 10-13.) Although used sparingly in the field, you will find auscultation invaluable in assessing both trauma and medical patients. However, the sounds you will hear are of very low amplitude. They may be difficult to discern against the on-scene or in-transit background noise.

Begin auscultation by warming the diaphragm of the stethoscope. Applying a cold stethoscope can startle the patient. To gain patient trust, apply the diaphragm gently. Tell the patient what you're doing, and explain why.

■ **inspection** visually examining a patient.

■ **palpation** examining a patient by touch.

■ **auscultation** listening to sounds made by the internal organs, usually associated with the use of the stethoscope.

■ **percussion** the act of striking an object or area to elicit a sound or vibration.

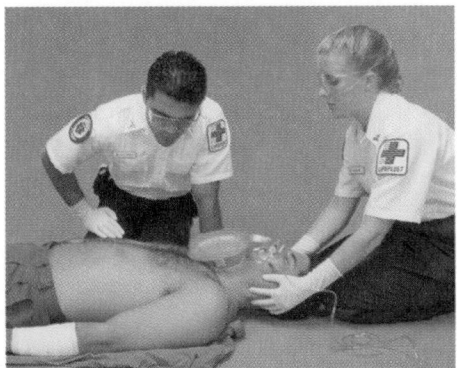

FIGURE 10-11   Inspect the patient's body for signs of illness or injury.

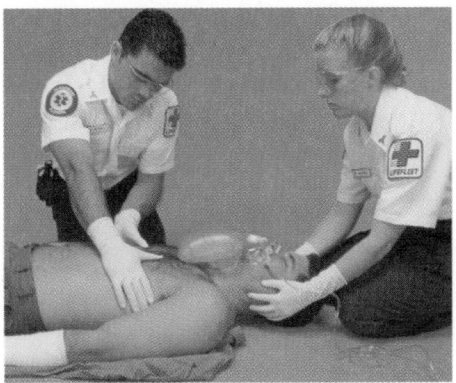

FIGURE 10-12   Palpate with the pads of your fingers.

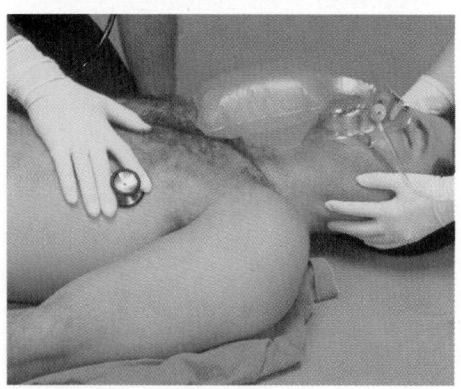

FIGURE 10-13 Auscultate body sounds with the stethoscope.

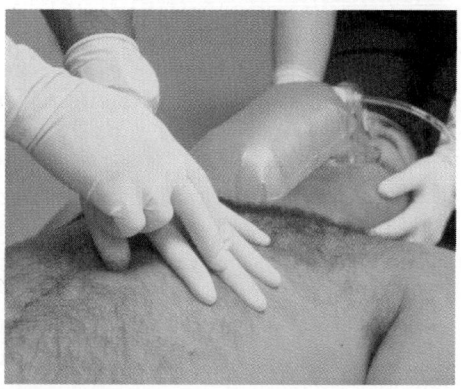

FIGURE 10-14 Percussion is the process of tapping the body to evaluate vibrations and sounds.

You may also evaluate heart sounds by auscultation. Use the bell to listen to the closing of the valves and to pick up any extraneous sounds of that process. Place the bell lightly over the heart valves at approximately the third intercostal space, just left of the sternum. Too much pressure will cause the skin beneath it to stretch and act like the diaphragm. It will then transmit high-frequency sounds, not the low-frequency sounds of the valves closing. (See Chapter 21.)

Using the stethoscope to auscultate the abdomen is of limited value in the field. Bowel sounds are difficult to hear, and proper assessment takes too much time, usually four to five minutes. Bowel sounds are a diagnostic evaluation best performed in the emergency department.

Percussion   Percussion evaluates a surface and the tissue beneath by sending a vibration through it. Accomplish percussion by transmitting the thump of one index finger impacting against the knuckle of the other over the site. (See Figure 10-14.) The resonance, or lack thereof, may tell if the underlying region is filled with air, air under pressure, fluid, or normal tissue. For example, a hollow vibrating resonance suggests a tension pneumothorax. Dull response indicates fluid or blood in the cavity. Results are most reliable when compared with sounds produced on the uninjured or unaffected side. Percussion is a skill that requires regular practice. Infrequent use will limit your ability to discern various conditions.

HEAD-TO-TOE EVALUATION

> **Secondary Assessment**
>
> ■ Head-to-toe evaluation
> ■ Vital signs
> ■ Patient history

Perform the physical assessment systematically—first head-to-toe, then the upper extremities. (See Procedure 10-2.) This approach takes into consideration that more significant injury can occur to the head, neck, chest, abdomen, and pelvis than to the extremities, and that thigh and leg pathology can be more significant than arm and forearm pathology. The following sections take you through some of the steps involved in the physical examination of most patients that you will encounter.

Head

For evaluation, divide the head into the cranium and the facial region.

Cranium   To examine the cranium, palpate the entire surface. (See Procedure 10-2, Figure A.) Sweep from the occiput to the superior surface, as well as laterally, while maintaining manual stabilization of the head and spine.

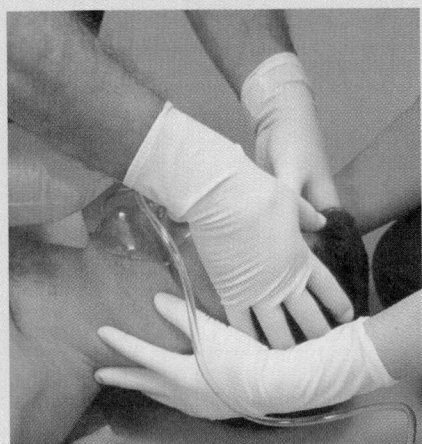

10-2A. The first step in the head-to-toe evaluation is palpation of the head.

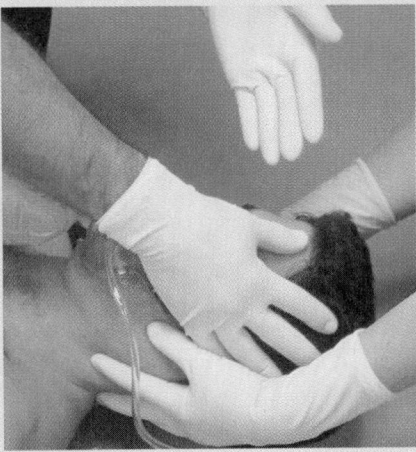

10-2B. It is important to examine your gloved fingers periodically for the presence of blood.

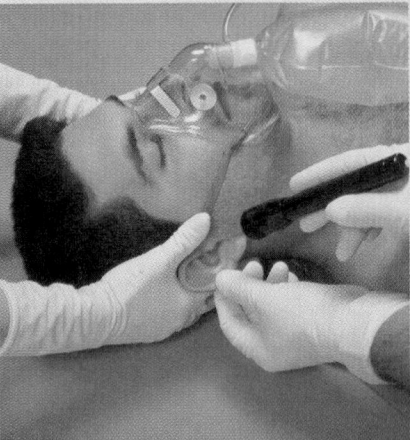

10-2C. Inspect the ears externally. Document the presence of blood or clear fluid draining from the ear.

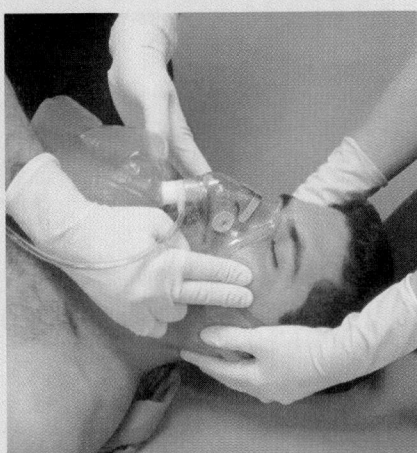

10-2D. Gently palpate the bones of the face.

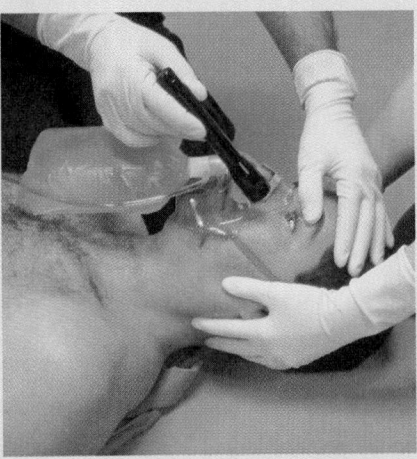

10-2E. Examine the pupils with a penlight.

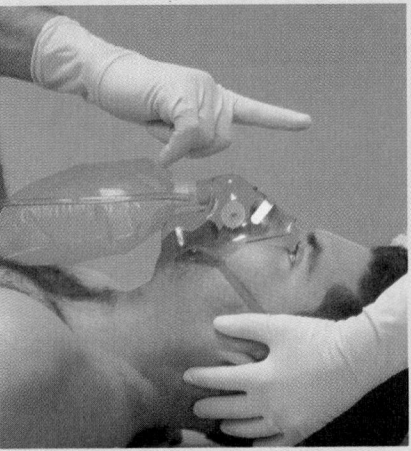

10-2F. Check extraocular eye movements by having the patient follow your finger as you draw an imaginary X.

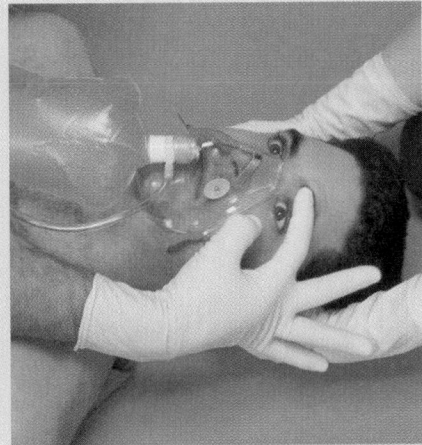

10-2G. Inspect the cornea for the presence of a contact lens or obvious ocular injury.

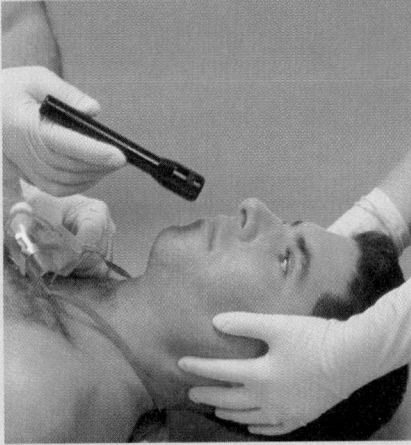

10-2H. Quickly inspect the nose for any bleeding or drainage of clear fluid.

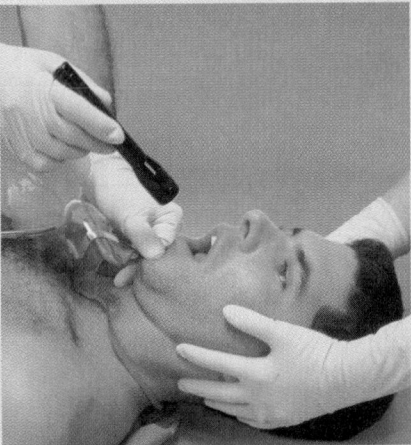

10-2I. Inspect the mouth for any signs of trauma, obstruction, or potential obstruction.

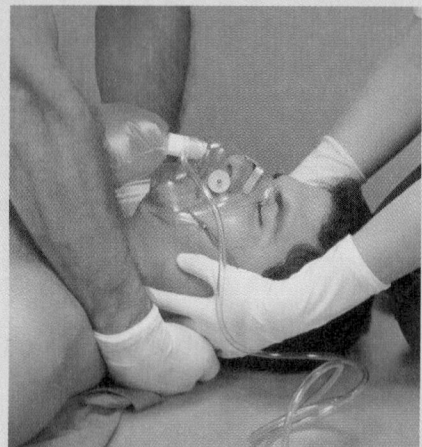

10-2J. Palpate the posterior aspect of the neck. Note any tenderness, irregularity, or edema.

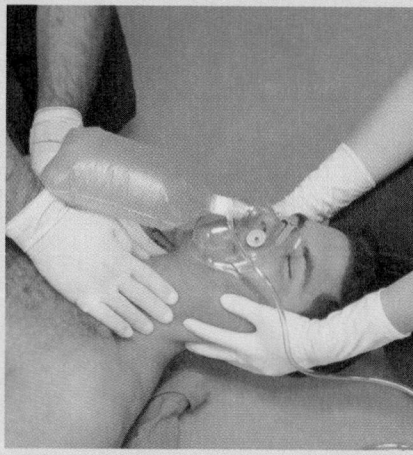

10-2K. Palpate the anterior aspect of the neck as well. Pay particular attention to tracheal deviation and subcutaneous emphysema.

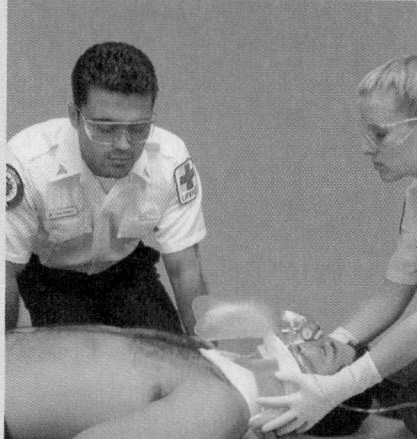

10-2L. Inspect the patient's chest for symmetry.

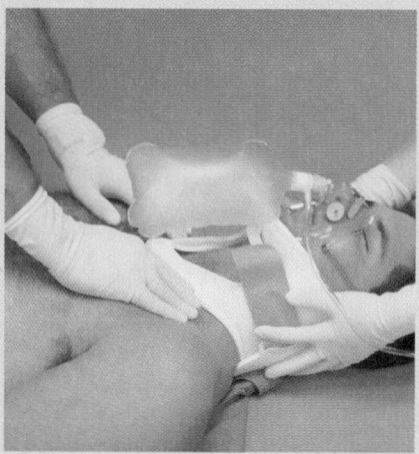

10-2M. Palpate the clavicles.

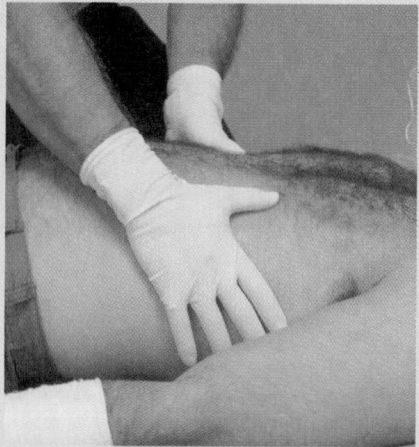

10-2N. Palpate the chest, evaluating anterior-posterior diameter, symmetry, and movement.

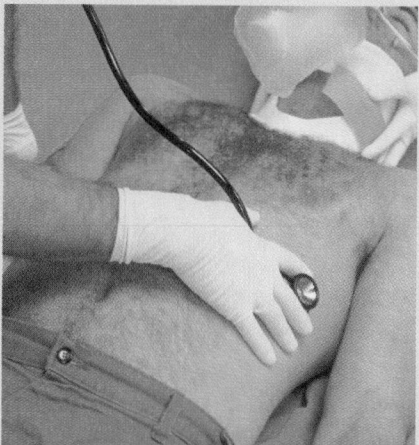

10-2O. Auscultate the chest for breath sounds.

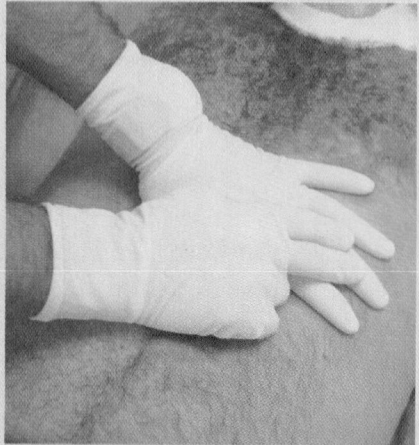

10-2P. Percussion of the chest can help determine the presence of pneumothorax or hemothorax.

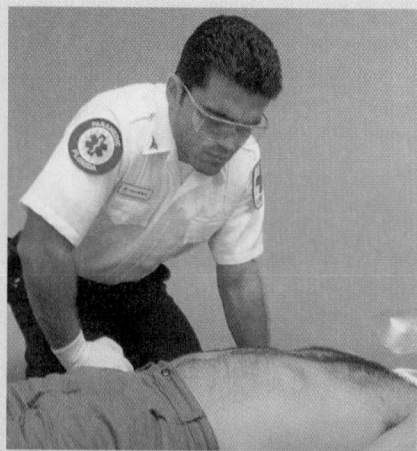

10-2Q. Examine the abdomen for swelling, discoloration, or wounds.

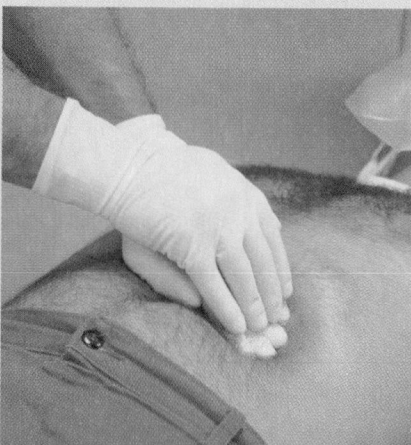

10-2R. Palpate the abdomen gently, leaving the quadrant where pain exists for last.

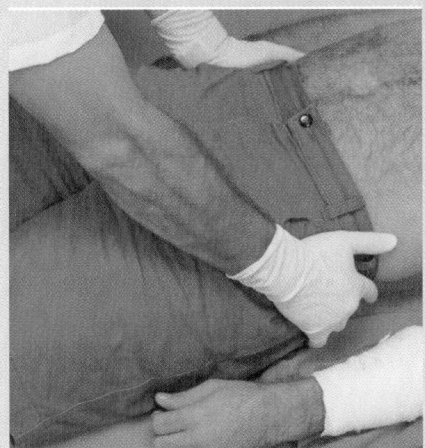

10-2S. Assess the integrity of the pelvis by gently pressing medially on the pelvic ring.

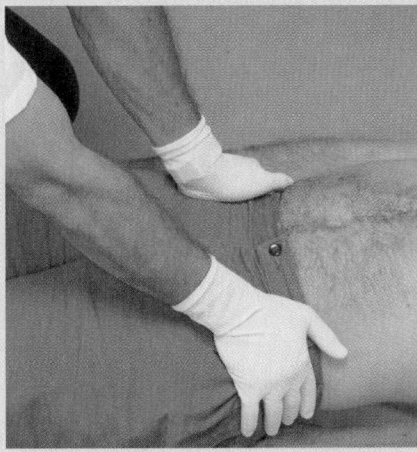

10-2T. Compress the pelvis posteriorly to complete the examination of the pelvis.

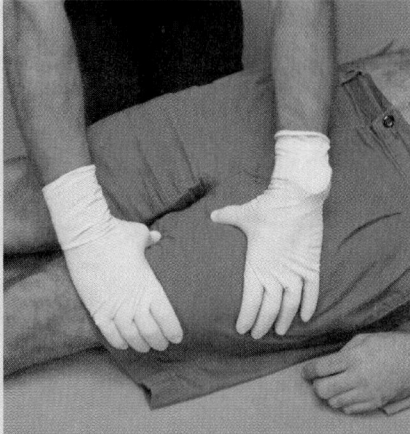

10-2U. Palpate the lower extremities.

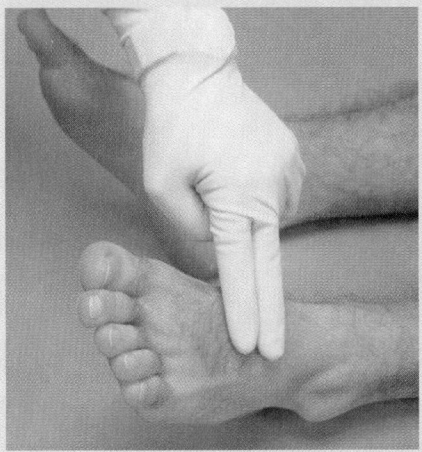

10-2V. Palpate the dorsalis pedis pulse to evaluate distal circulation in the lower extremity.

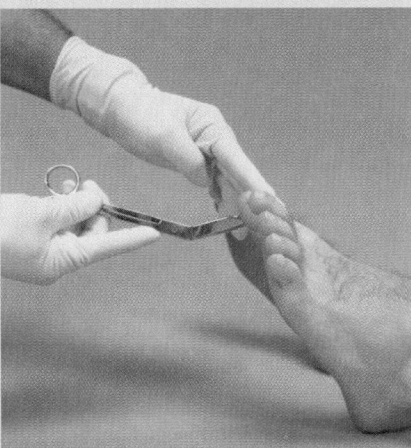

10-2W. Assess distal sensation and motor function.

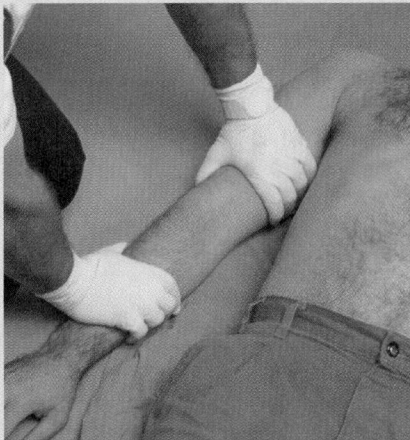

10-2X. Palpate the upper extremities.

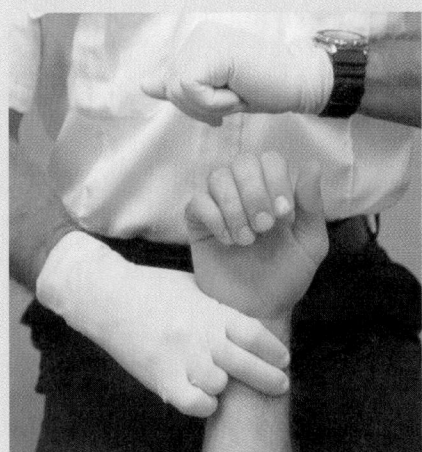

10-2Y. Palpate the radial pulse to evaluate distal circulation in the upper extremity. Assess sensation and motor function.

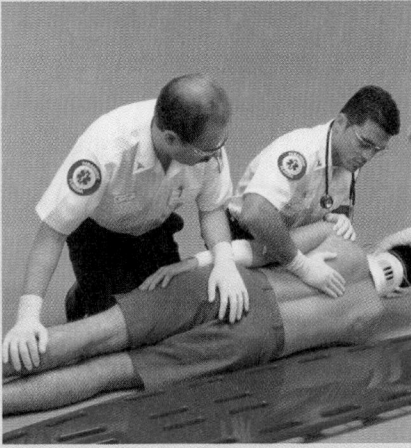

10-2Z. Inspect and palpate the posterior body.

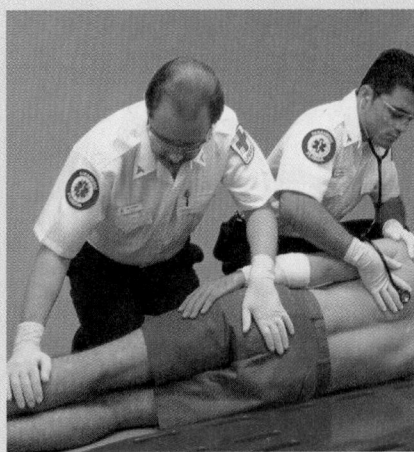

10-2ZZ. Auscultate the posterior thorax and compare breath sounds with those auscultated at the anterior thorax.

Note the general contour of the cranium and any deformities, such as depressions or protrusions. Record discoloration, unusual warmth, or lack of symmetry. Look for blood flowing into the hair, and examine your gloved fingers periodically for blood or other body fluids. (See Procedure 10-2, Figure B.)

Ears   Examine the ears for soft-tissue injury and fluid drainage from the external auditory canal. (See Procedure 10-2, Figure C.) Move your head, not your patient's, to visualize the patient's auditory canal with a penlight. Blood coming from the canal may reflect a pressure injury or skull fracture. Discharge of clear fluid (**cerebrospinal fluid, CSF**) may be secondary to fracture or infection. **Battle's sign** is an ecchymotic discoloration over the mastoid process (the bony process just posterior to the ear). It is a sign of possible basilar skull fracture that is rarely seen in the prehospital setting because of the time it takes for the discoloration to develop.

Facial Region

The facial region is one of the more important areas of your assessment. Begin evaluation by observing and then palpating the region.

Face   Palpate with the pads of the fingers over the entirety of the facial bones. (See Procedure 10-2, Figure D.) Instability or asymmetry of the orbits, nasal bones, or cartilage should lead you to suspect facial fractures. Palpate the upper jaw region to reveal deformity or instability, often due to maxillary fracture. The mandible should demonstrate mobility, as evidenced by opening and closing the mouth, as well as some slight lateral movement. Motion that elicits pain, crepitation, limited motion, or mandibular fixation indicates fracture or dislocation.

Eyes   Inspect the eyes for discoloration, pupil abnormalities, foreign bodies, or blood in the anterior chamber. **Raccoon eyes** (bilateral periorbital ecchymosis) is a discoloration surrounding and including the orbits of the eyes. It is similar to Battle's sign in appearance and in its indication of possible basilar skull fracture. As with Battle's sign, discovery of raccoon eyes in the prehospital setting should suggest the possibility of a previous injury.

During palpation, you may notice that the globes of the eyes are soft. (Do not apply pressure during palpation.) This condition is often associated with severe dehydration or possible diabetic hyperglycemia and ketoacidosis.

Examine the pupils closely. (See Procedure 10-2, Figure E.) They represent a "window into the brain" because they are controlled by some of the higher cranial nerves, and their blood supply is closely related to that of the brain itself. The rate at which the pupil of the eye reacts to light indicates cerebral perfusion. Normally, the pupils react briskly to changes in light intensity, **constricting** to increases and **dilating** to decreases. In bright indoor lighting or normal daylight, shade the eyes to check pupil reactivity, rather than shining a flashlight beam into the pupil. Additionally, pupils should respond together (consensually). That is, when you direct light at one pupil, both pupils should respond to it. Abnormal pupillary responses may reflect intracranial pathology. A sluggish pupil reaction may reflect central nervous system depression, due to **hypoxia**, **hypercarbia**, injury, or the effects of drugs. The extreme of this condition is dilated and non-reactive (fixed) pupils.

Conversely, very small or pinpoint pupils suggest intoxication from opiate derivatives (narcotics). Although pupil inequality (called **anisocoria**) is naturally present in a modest percentage of the population, it may signal head injury or stroke. This is especially true if the reactivity of the larger pupil is less brisk than that of the constricted one. The sign may reflect pathology on either the same or opposite side of the brain.

■ **cerebrospinal fluid (CSF)** the clear, watery fluid that bathes the brain and spinal cord.

■ **Battle's sign** a black-and-blue discoloration over the mastoid process (just behind the ear), characteristic of a basilar skull fracture.

■ **raccoon eyes** a black-and-blue discoloration of the area surrounding the eyes. It is associated with a basilar skull fracture.

✴ Battle's sign and raccoon eyes are not commonly seen in the prehospital setting.

✴ The evaluation of the eyes can tell much about the patient because their blood supply is closely associated with that of the brain.

■ **constrict** become smaller.

■ **dilate** become larger.

■ **hypoxia** a deficiency of oxygen in the body.

■ **hypercarbia** an increased level of carbon dioxide in the body.

■ **anisocoria** pupils of unequal size.

Carefully evaluate eye movement. If the eyes fail to move together, or seem to be looking in different directions (**dysconjugate gaze**), this may indicate a pre-existing problem, ocular muscle entrapment, or optic nerve damage. If the eyes move with the head as it is turned (known as the **doll's eye response**), instead of remaining fixed in the original direction, it may indicate severe head injury. Do not attempt this maneuver on any patient with suspected spine injury.

If the eyes are unable to follow your finger as you draw a large imaginary "X" in front of them, there may be nerve damage or orbital fracture impinging the extra-ocular muscles. (See Procedure 10-2, Figure F.) Examination will also reflect any evidence of direct eye trauma. While the orbits protect the eyes well, direct trauma can still produce serious, sight-threatening injury. If injury is found, protect the eyes and report any findings to the emergency department personnel.

The surface of the eye should sparkle in the light. If the eye is dull or lacks normal luster, suspect a circulatory deficit. Yellowish sclera (icterus) may be caused by liver dysfunction. Examine the eyes closely to detect the presence of contact lenses. (See Procedure 10-2, Figure G.) Leave them in place unless you will be transporting the unconscious patient for more than 15 minutes. If there is a chance that toxic material has contaminated the eye, remove the lenses and irrigate the eye.

Nose   Inspect and palpate for injuries, bleeding, and drainage. (See Procedure 10-2, Figure H.) Examine the **nares** for flaring and other signs of airway distress. Pay special attention to infants less than 3 months old. They are obligatory nasal breathers and need a clear, unobstructed nasal cavity for respiration. The presence of fluid may indicate internal trauma or infection. Blood and cerebrospinal fluid are signs of internal laceration, skull fracture, or both. Bleeding within the nasal cavity may be severe and very difficult to control. It may also contribute to nausea and vomiting if the patient swallows the blood.

Mouth   Gently open and examine the mouth for exterior injuries as well as damaged, loose, or dislodged teeth, materials that may obstruct the airway, a swollen or lacerated tongue, or discoloration. (See Procedure 10-2, Figure I.) Should an unresponsive patient have loose false teeth, fluids, or loose objects that might obstruct the airway, remove them with suction, **Magill forceps**, or your fingers. Use a bite block to protect your fingers any time they enter a patient's mouth.

Note any unusual odors. (See Figure 10-15.) Evaluate any odor from the patient's mouth. The odor of alcohol is a common finding and may mask other more significant odors, such as the ketones from the diabetic, or signs and symptoms of trauma or acute disease. Do not attribute any changes in the mental status of a patient who has been drinking to alcohol unless you can rule out all other causes (not likely in the field). You may also note odors that might suggest various poisonings. Fecal odor emanating from the mouth may indicate lower-bowel obstruction; the smell of gastric contents may forewarn of emesis (vomiting) and possible aspiration.

Fluids in the oral cavity or emesis can provide clues to an underlying pathology. Coffee-grounds-like material signals bleeding from the stomach, where the gastric contents begin to break down the blood. Fresh blood reflects a recent hemorrhage within the upper gastrointestinal tract. Pink-tinged sputum indicates congestive heart failure. A green or yellow phlegm suggests respiratory infection. Vomitus reflects gastrointestinal or brainstem problems, among many others. To protect the airway, immediately suction any fluids from the oral cavity

dysconjugate gaze failure of the eyes to rotate simultaneously in the same direction, or the eyes gazing in different directions.

doll's eye response the eyes turning as the head is turned. An unnatural response, indicative of head injury.

＊ Testing for doll's eye response is not typically a prehospital procedure. It should never be used in the trauma patient.

Abnormal Findings: Ears, Eyes, Nose

- Cerebrospinal fluid
- Battle's sign
- Raccoon eyes
- Anisocoria
- Dysconjugate gaze
- Doll's eye response

---

nares the openings of the nose that lead into the nasal cavity.

Magill forceps instrument used in airway management for reaching into the oropharynx to manipulate a foreign body, endotracheal tube, or similar item.

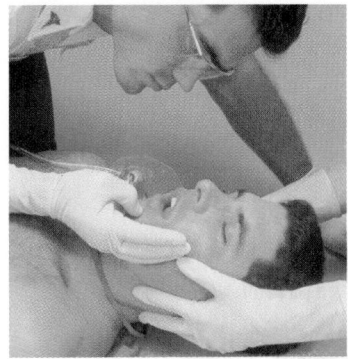

FIGURE 10-15   Note any odors on the patient's breath.

■ **embolus** (pl. *emboli*) an air bubble, clot, or other particle carried by the blood into a blood vessel. It may lodge in a smaller vessel, causing a blockage.

■ **jugular vein distention (JVD)** inflation of the jugular veins in a patient who is sitting at a 45-degree-or-greater angle, often associated with pulmonary or cardiovascular disease.

■ **tracheal deviation** position of the trachea to the right or left of its normal midline position, usually associated with tension pneumothorax or airway obstruction.

■ **contralateral** on, or referring to, the opposite side of the body.

■ **ipsilateral** on, or referring to, the same side.

■ **subcutaneous emphysema** the presence of air within the subcutaneous tissues, often associated with pneumothorax.

Neck

Palpate the lateral, anterior, and posterior neck surfaces. (See Procedure 10-2, Figures J and K.) Note, and appraise further, any apparent deformity, warmth, or discoloration. Soft-tissue injury, edema, or laceration to the neck can be rapidly life-threatening. The carotid artery, located lateral to the trachea, provides critical circulation to the brain. Penetrating injury to this large, high-pressure structure can result in massive blood loss. The jugular veins also carry high volumes of blood at relatively low pressure. During inspiration, the neck veins may maintain intravascular pressures below that of the atmosphere. An open wound may draw air in, resulting in massive air **emboli**. Evaluate any significant penetrating injury in this area for bleeding and possible air embolism.

Examine for **jugular vein distention (JVD)**. In the supine, normotensive patient, they should distend slightly. If the veins do not distend in the supine position, hypovolemia is a probable cause. (See Figure 10-16.) As the body is brought to a 45-degree angle, the jugular veins normally empty. Distention beyond 45 degrees is indicative of pathology such as pericardial tamponade (filling of the sac around the heart with fluid), tension pneumothorax, right heart failure, or cor pulmonale (right heart failure secondary to increased pulmonary vascular resistance). (See Figure 10-17.)

Palpate the anterior neck for tracheal location and movement. There should be no **tracheal deviation**; the trachea should be midline and stationary during breathing efforts. Displacement to one side indicates a tension pneumothorax on the **contralateral** (opposite) side. If the trachea tugs or moves toward one side with each inspiration, there may be an airway obstruction on the **ipsilateral** (same) side.

The neck may also display **subcutaneous emphysema**, which may cause a crackling sensation (much like crushing Rice Krispies) as the air trapped in the soft tissues moves about under your palpation. Subcutaneous emphysema is most commonly due to a developing tension pneumothorax or a tracheal tear.

If spinal injury is suspected, a cervical collar is applied as soon as examination of the neck is completed. Remember, however, that a cervical collar does not prevent all movement of the head and neck. *Therefore, even after the collar is in place, manual stabilization must be continued until the patient has been immobilized to a long spine board with a cervical immobilization device.*

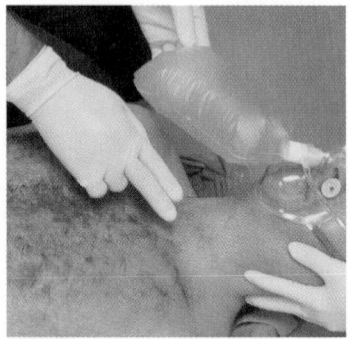

FIGURE 10-16 The jugular veins should be slightly distended when the patient is supine.

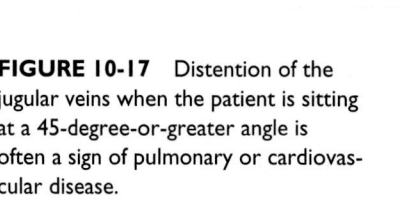

FIGURE 10-17 Distention of the jugular veins when the patient is sitting at a 45-degree-or-greater angle is often a sign of pulmonary or cardiovascular disease.

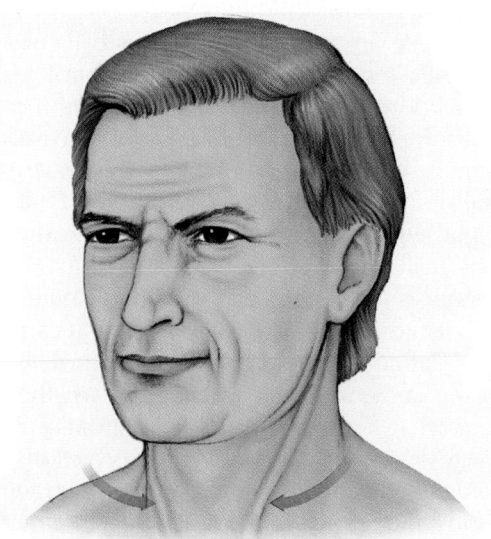

Chest

Completely expose the chest to perform the thoracic exam. Take care to protect the patient from embarrassment and the environment. First inspect the chest. (See Procedure 10-2, Figure L.) Visualize and palpate the shoulders for symmetry, muscle tone, and the absence of pain. Asymmetry or deformity suggests fracture of one of the bones composing the joint, a dislocation, or soft-tissue damage with resultant edema. Palpate the clavicles over their entire length, bilaterally. (See Procedure 10-2, Figure M.) The clavicles fracture more frequently than any other bone in the human body. They are located directly over the subclavian artery and the superior-most aspect of the lung. Fracture and displacement may disrupt the artery or lung tissue, leading to **hemothorax**, **pneumothorax**, or both.

The supraclavicular space (the region just above the clavicles), the intercostal spaces (spaces between the ribs), as well as the suprasternal notch (the notch above the sternum), may present with retraction during inspiration. This sign of partial or complete airway obstruction occurs when atmospheric pressure significantly exceeds that of inspiration. It is a serious sign that demands clearing of the airway: pharmacologically, as in asthma; physically, as in removing an airway obstruction with the laryngoscope and Magill forceps; or mechanically, with an endotracheal tube.

Examine the surface of the thorax for bilateral **excursion** with respiration. Accomplish this by placing one hand on each of the lower halves of the thorax, just below the nipple line or breast area. (See Procedure 10-2, Figure N.) Your hands will move very slightly in and out with each normal respiration. Each breath should be smooth and regular, with bilaterally symmetrical motion.

Evaluate the general shape of the chest cavity. Is the anterior-posterior dimension normal? Or is the chest large and barreled (a condition suggestive of chronic obstructive pulmonary disease)? Do any deformities appear? If so, are they congenital (something the patient was born with) or traumatic? Palpate and observe the entire thoracic surface. Are there any signs of trauma, discoloration, or edema? Once again, classical soft-tissue injury signs may not be present because the ecchymotic coloration of bruising is not likely to have had time to develop. Look for erythema caused by impact to the ribs. There may be an outline of reddened discoloration silhouetting the ribs and sternum. Inspect the chest for any penetrating trauma. If found, assess for signs of air exchange through the penetration (open pneumothorax) and a possible exit wound.

Place your hands on the lateral aspects of the thorax, and apply pressure medially. You should feel moderate resistance, yet elicit no pain or crepitation. Palpate the lateral and anterior chest surfaces. In the case of a female, your palpation should work around the breast, not directly over it. You can assess the breasts as part of the overall chest evaluation without assessing the breasts individually. This reduces the risk of offending the patient.

If, during chest palpation, you notice the crackling sensation of subcutaneous emphysema, suspect tension pneumothorax. This sensation results when air in the **pleural** space is forced into the soft tissues by increased intrathoracic pressure. Subcutaneous air will normally flow from the upper chest to the neck and head. In some cases, the patient's facial features will change drastically before your eyes.

Palpate the posterior thorax during the examination of the posterior body. Always inspect your gloves for blood following palpation.

Auscultate the lungs at the bases (the lower border of the rib cage), at the apices (just below the clavicles at their midpoint), and along the mid-axillary line (in the armpit at about the nipple line). (See Figure 10-18 and Procedure 10-2, Figure O.) Evaluate the respiratory sounds anteriorly and then laterally. (You may auscultate respiratory sounds posteriorly during examination of the

---

Abnormal Findings: Chest

- ■ Retractions
- ■ Unequal excursion
- ■ Subcutaneous emphysema
- ■ Erythema
- ■ Paradoxical motion
- ■ Abnormal breath sounds

■ **hemothorax** blood in the thoracic cavity.

■ **pneumothorax** air in the thoracic cavity. The air may enter through a tear in the lungs or from a penetrating injury to the chest.

■ **excursion** movement away from a central position, as of the chest during respiration.

✳ If a penetrating chest wound is found, suspect and search for an exit wound.

■ **pleura** a membrane covering the lungs and the interior of the thoracic cage.

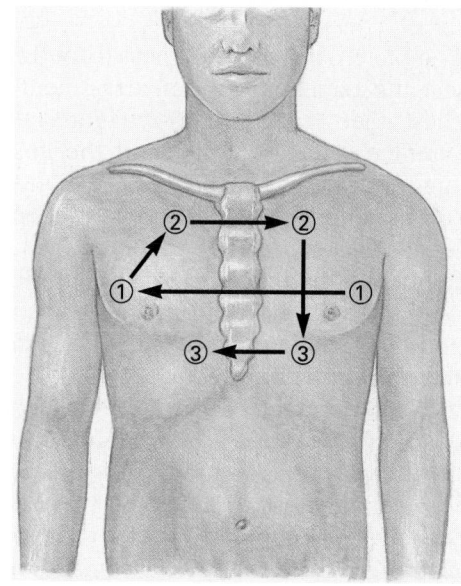

FIGURE 10-18 Method for auscultating the anterior chest.

posterior body.) The normal patient should present soft, low pitched, "sighing" sounds called **vesicular**. You should notice that inspiratory sounds last longer than expiratory sounds. If you assess the lung sounds closer to the sternum, you will hear the sounds of bronchial and tracheal passageways. They are louder, higher-pitched, and display almost equal inspiratory and expiratory phases.

Abnormal breath sounds include rales, rhonchi, wheezes, and stridor. **Rales** are fine crackling sounds, similar to the sound of hair being rolled between your fingers. They indicate fluid in the lungs and minor alveolar obstruction. **Rhonchi** are coarser sounds suggesting more significant fluid or mucus accumulation. Wheezes are prolonged, higher-pitched expiratory sounds, reflecting airway narrowing. They generally suggest bronchial constriction and asthma. The sound of stridor needs no stethoscope to be audible. It is a high-pitched sound, occurring because of laryngeal obstruction from local swelling or vocal cord spasm (**laryngospasm**). Breath sounds are hard to determine unless you listen to them frequently. Periodically auscultate your own breath sounds and those of your co-workers to keep an appreciation of the technique and quality of the sounds you listen for. In the field, listen to your own lung sounds to give you a benchmark for evaluating those of your patient.

If the respiratory sounds are not bilaterally equal, they may indicate a pneumothorax or tension pneumothorax. If respiratory or heart sounds are distant and muffled, the pathology may be hemothorax. If only heart sounds are diminished, the patient may have a pericardial tamponade. You will not be able to differentiate these conditions without other supporting signs and symptoms.

Percussion can also provide evidence regarding chest pathology. (See Procedure 10-2, Figure P.) If the region is hyperresonant, the thorax may contain air under pressure (tension pneumothorax). If the region is dull to percussion, it may be filled with blood (hemothorax) or other fluid (pleural **effusion**). Be sure to compare the sounds left-to-right and, during examination of the posterior body, front-to-back to confirm your evaluation.

Examine the patient's respiratory function. Reassess the volume of air moved and the respiratory pattern. A rapid deep pattern can be due to head injury (central neurogenic hyperventilation); metabolic problem, as in diabetic coma (**Kussmaul respirations**); extreme exertion; or hyperventilation. The **Cheyne-Stokes pattern** repeats a series of increasing, then decreasing, breaths with periods of apnea in between. Another pattern, **Biot's respirations**, consists of agonal, gasping, breaths irregular in rate and depth. Biot's and Cheyne-Stokes respirations are related to increasing intracranial pressure, severe brain stem injury, or both.

Abdomen

Inspect the abdomen and gently palpate for signs of disease or trauma. Observe for any overt motion or pulsation. (See Procedure 10-2, Figure Q.) The abdomen in the thin supine patient will pulsate with the pulsing of the abdominal aorta. Suspect an aneurysm if the pulsation is exaggerated or localized, especially if it is accompanied by "tearing" pain. Exaggerated abdominal-wall motion to assist respiration may result from spinal injury, airway obstruction, or failure of the respiratory muscles. Look for signs of injury or discoloration, especially any abrasions, contusions, open wounds, or erythema. Two characteristic abdominal ecchymotic discolorations are **Cullen's sign**, around the **umbilicus**, and **Grey Turner's sign**, along the flanks. Secondary to internal bleeding, of traumatic or medical origin, these signs often develop late and may suggest an earlier injury.

Before palpating the abdomen, determine whether any pain is generalized, regional, or limited to a specific point. Be certain to evaluate the pain carefully in the field setting. As the condition progresses (during your care and transport), the pain may become more general, while guarding (voluntary or involuntary tensing of the abdominal muscles) and increased pain may prevent effective palpation. Later, this may mask the true location of the problem from the hospital staff and slow the diagnostic process unless you accurately report the results of a good assessment.

Evaluate the four abdominal quadrants—left upper quadrant (LUQ), right upper quadrant (RUQ), left lower quadrant (LLQ), and right lower quadrant (RLQ)—for tenderness and **rebound tenderness**. Gently palpate, saving for last any quadrant with pain. (See Procedure 10-2, Figure R.) To elicit rebound tenderness, release the gentle pressure of palpation quickly. Any pain that occurs with this release is probably related to inflammation of the **peritoneum**. Gentle palpation should not elicit any muscle spasm or contraction. Such guarding reflects disease. Document any masses, painful areas, or the location of guarding. If the abdomen appears distended or feels spongy during palpation, suspect ascites. **Ascites** is an accumulation of fluid within the abdominal cavity, caused by increased pressure in the systemic circulation (right heart failure) or in the **portal system** (cirrhosis of the liver).

Palpate the flank (lateral) region of the abdomen, looking for deformity, swelling, pain, tenderness, wounds, or discoloration. During examination of the posterior body, continue the palpation underneath the small of the back from each side and to the vertebral column. This area may present with dependent edema, a fluid buildup in the lower parts of the body (the legs and lower back) due to chronic circulatory backup. The edema in the lumbar region is called **presacral edema** (swelling above the sacrum). It reflects a systemic problem, possibly due to heart failure. This sign is more commonly seen in the patient who is recumbent for prolonged periods.

Pelvis

Inspect the pelvis for signs of injury. (See Procedure 10-2, Figures S and T.) If the patient does not complain of pain or is unresponsive, gently flex and compress the pelvis to determine stability. Apply gentle pressure to the iliac crests (the bony prominences, anterior and lateral, that support the belt). Direct pressure medially, then posteriorly without rocking the pelvis. Also apply pressure posteriorly to the

■ **Biot's respirations** breathing pattern characterized by irregular periods of apnea (absent breathing) and hyperpnea (rapid breathing).

■ **Cullen's sign** a bluish discoloration of the area around the umbilicus, caused by intra-abdominal hemorrhage.

■ **umbilicus** the navel; the remnant of the umbilical cord.

■ **Grey Turner's sign** the ecchymotic discoloration of the flanks and umbilical region, associated with intra-abdominal hemorrhage, often of pancreatic origin. (retroperitoneal).

■ **rebound tenderness** pain upon sudden release of an examining hand from the abdomen, often associated with peritoneal irritation.

■ **peritoneum** the membranous lining of the abdominal cavity.

■ **ascites** the presence of fluid within the abdominal cavity, often associated with congestive heart failure and alcoholism, among other causes.

■ **portal system** part of the circulatory system consisting of the veins that drain some of the digestive organs. The portal system delivers blood to the liver.

■ **presacral edema** an accumulation of fluid in the sacral area in the recumbent patient, usually related to congestive heart failure.

Abnormal Findings: Abdomen

- ■ Pulsations
- ■ Cullen's sign
- ■ Grey Turner's sign
- ■ Guarding
- ■ Pain
- ■ Tenderness
- ■ Rebound tenderness
- ■ Ascites

symphysis pubis (the bone just above the genitalia), being careful not to trap the male genitalia. If pressure elicits pain, crepitation, or instability, suspect pelvic fracture. Be alert for severe hypovolemic shock.

Genitalia

The external male genitalia are extremely vascular and can be injured, resulting in extreme blood loss. Be careful not to overlook them during assessment. Clothing, especially denim, may contain the hemorrhage. Evaluation of the male genitalia can also reveal the presence of injury to the spinal cord. **Priapism**, a sometimes painful penile erection, results from unopposed parasympathetic stimulation. It occurs with spinal cord interruption or certain types of brain dysfunction. Follow such a finding with complete spinal immobilization and assessment.

Internal female genitalia are moderately vascular and relatively well-protected from all but penetrating injury. Trauma can occur in sexual abuse and rape. If you suspect either, have the patient assessed and treated by a member of the same sex, if possible. This may relieve any hostilities and anxiety directed toward a caregiver of the opposite gender. Encourage the patient not to bathe. Limit assessment to only that which is essential to patient stabilization. One of your most important tasks is to provide emotional support and reassurance. (For more on this subject, see Chapter 31.)

In gynecological or obstetrical emergencies, there may be discharge from the vagina. Estimate the volume and note the type of discharge (blood, amniotic fluid, or other fluid). It may be helpful for the woman to approximate the volume by indicating the number of pads or tampons needed to absorb the fluid. If the patient shows early signs of shock, transport her immediately to the hospital.

In both males and females, evaluate the pelvic region to reveal incontinence (loss of bowel or bladder control) and injury. Causes of incontinence include deep coma, stroke, seizures, or spinal injury. Either of these signs is indicative of deep central nervous system depression or interruption.

Lower Extremities

The lower extremities consist of the thigh, leg, and foot. In examining this area, palpate the surfaces anteriorly, posteriorly, laterally, and medially over the entire length of the extremity. (See Procedure 10-2, Figure U.) Look for tenderness, crepitation, or deformity. Evaluate any abnormal motion, such as jointlike characteristics where a joint shouldn't exist or resistance to normal motion.

Evaluate the distal pulse to ensure that circulation is adequate. Take the pulse using either the dorsalis pedis or medial malleolar (posterior tibial) pulse. The dorsalis pedis pulse is located on the arch of the foot, along the anterior surface about $\frac{1}{3}$ the distance from the medial to the lateral side. (See Procedure 10-2, Figure V.) This pulse is normally absent in about 10 percent of the population. You may also locate the posterior tibial pulse medially, just posterior and inferior to the inside protrusion of the ankle (medial malleolus). Because of its landmarks, the posterior tibial pulse is easier and faster to find in the field.

If you can't locate a pulse, determine the adequacy of perfusion by checking capillary refill or by assessing the temperature, color, and moisture of the skin of the foot. Assume vascular compromise if pulse is absent, the extremity is cool, capillary refill is delayed or absent, or the skin is ashen or cyanotic.

Examine the lower extremity for motor and sensory function. (See Procedure 10-2, Figure W.) Ask the patient to tell you when he feels a firm (but gentle) touch with the blunt end of a bandage scissor or similar device. (See Figure 10-19.) Do not ask "Do you feel this?" If the answer is "no," your patient will know there is a deficit and become anxious about it. Also ask the patient to push firmly against

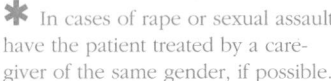

■ **priapism** a sometimes painful, prolonged erection of the penis resulting from spinal injury or disease process. (It may occur in sickle cell anemia.)

✱ In cases of rape or sexual assault, have the patient treated by a caregiver of the same gender, if possible.

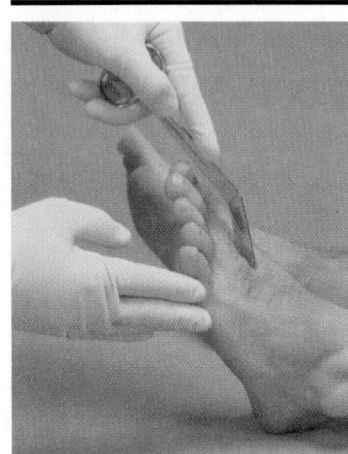

FIGURE 10-19 Assess distal sensation.

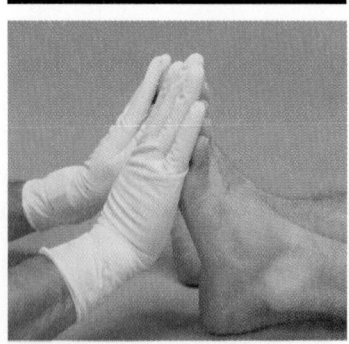

FIGURE 10-20 Assess distal motor function.

your hand with his foot, provided the extremity has been assessed as uninjured. Repeat the procedure on the opposite side and compare the results. (See Figure 10-20.) If the strength appears unequal, retry the procedure, switching hands. If the difference still remains, suspect nervous impairment or injury.

Evaluate the lower aspect of the extremity for edema. If the extremity is swollen, depress the overlying skin with your finger. If the depression remains following finger removal, it is called *pitting edema*, a sign of severe and chronic systemic fluid retention.

Upper Extremities

Palpate each upper extremity. (See Procedure 10-2, Figure X.) Use the radial pulse for circulatory assessment. (See Procedure 10-2, Figure Y.) Assess sensation and motor function, asking the patient to squeeze your first and second finger, rather than push your hand. As with the lower extremities, compare the strength and pulse bilaterally. Also examine the fingers for **clubbing**. It results from central cyanosis, a chronic hypoxic condition caused by cardiovascular or respiratory disease.

Check the neck, ankle, wrist, and the wallet for Medic Alert identification. An orange, red, or blue star of life or other medical symbol will help identify these materials. They usually contain pertinent information about the patient's medical history, allergies, or special treatment considerations. Search for this information, and use it to guide your care.

■ **clubbing** the enlargement of the distal fingers and toes, often due to chronic respiratory or cardiovascular disease.

Posterior Body

If spinal injury is suspected, carefully maintain manual stabilization of the head and spine as you log-roll the patient onto his side. Then inspect and palpate the posterior trunk. Particularly note any tenderness in the spinal area. (See Procedure 10-2, Figure Z.) Palpate the buttocks to rule out hemorrhage, contusion, or other injury. Though predominantly soft tissue, this area is a large mass and can conceal considerable internal blood loss. Auscultate the posterior thorax and compare to breath sounds noted at the anterior thorax. (See Procedure 10-2, Figure ZZ.) Place the long spine board snugly against the patient's body and maintain alignment of the head and spine as you log-roll the patient into a supine position on the spine board. The patient is now ready to be secured to the spine board.

Analysis of the Head-to-Toe Evaluation

As you complete the head-to-toe evaluation, completely analyze the results to determine if the signs support one problem or several problems occurring together. Reassess any unusual or questionable findings to ensure accuracy. Summarize the findings of the head-to-toe assessment, identify the apparent injuries, and place them in priority order from the greatest to the least severity. Keep these findings in mind as you move through the rest of the secondary assessment.

✳ At the conclusion of the head-to-toe evaluation, identify all suspected injuries and prioritize them for care.

Neurological Assessment

Continue to evaluate central nervous system (CNS) dysfunction objectively by looking at the patient's orientation and response to sensory **stimuli**. (See Figure 10-21.) Judge the patient's level of orientation through his response to questioning. As a patient moves away from a state of complete alertness, orientation diminishes in a specific order. Initially, a patient will be completely conscious and oriented to time, place, persons, and his own person. As the level of consciousness drops, the patient will often lose orientation to time, becoming unable to identify the day of the week, month, year, and time of

■ **stimulus** (pl. *stimuli*) any factor or input into the sensory system that causes an action or response.

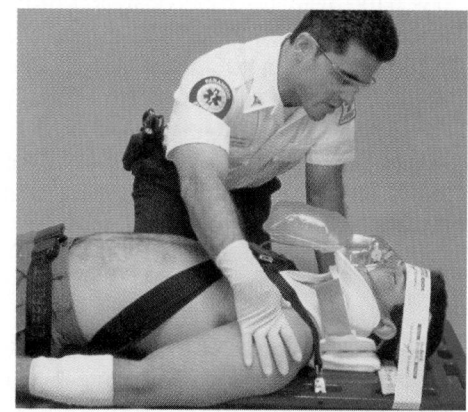

FIGURE 10-21 Evaluate the patient's neurological function.

day. (It is common for patients and bystanders to complain of long response times when you have actually arrived only minutes after the incident. This finding is normally associated with excitement or stress and is not medically significant.)

If the level of consciousness continues to slip, the patient will lose orientation to place. He may neither know where he is nor be able to recognize familiar or otherwise recognizable surroundings, such as home or the interior of an ambulance. While this can be caused by stress and excitement, it may reflect a deeper decline in cerebral function. The patient may also exhibit a decline in orientation in relation to the event. He may be unaware of how the injury took place. In addition, the patient may be unable to recall key events leading up to the incident.

The downward progression of consciousness continues with loss of orientation to person. The patient fails to recognize close friends or relatives. He is also unable to determine or remember who you are, even though you are in uniform and have introduced yourself several times.

Finally, the patient loses orientation to his own person. The patient, while still responsive to verbal commands, is not aware of his own name. He may recognize it once said, but will not be able to remember the name without hearing it. (Often orientation to person and one's own person are combined.)

As the patient moves toward unconsciousness and coma, you can further evaluate him objectively by observing physical responses to stimuli. Patients may respond by moving their extremities or opening their eyes, when you shout the patient's name or issue a loud verbal command (verbal stimuli). They may speak, but the communication is incoherent, garbled, or unintelligible.

As the level of consciousness continues to diminish, the patient who no longer responds to verbal stimulation may still respond to painful stimulation. A good location to elicit this pain is the fleshy region between the thumb and first finger (of an uninjured extremity). Squeeze the muscle in this area firmly. If the patient responds by moving away from the pain or by brushing your hand away, the response is called *purposeful*. If the hand and forearm move, but not effectively, the response is called *purposeless*. The patient who is completely unconscious and unresponsive will fail to move to any stimuli. This is identified as *unresponsive* and is reflective of deep coma.

Based on the level of orientation and responsiveness to stimuli, you can establish a continuum from complete consciousness to deep and profound coma. States of consciousness in a patient will extend from the orientations of time, place, event, person, and one's own person to the levels of response termed purposeful, purposeless, and unresponsive. You can objectively compare the results of an evaluation to an earlier evaluation. Any changes in state of consciousness will be apparent.

During the neurologic assessment, you may also notice the patient's muscle tone. Even patients in deep coma should display some muscle tone. If the tone is absent (flaccid), it may indicate severe central nervous system injury or spinal cord damage. If the flaccidity is unequal, it may suggest a head injury or stroke and hemiplegia (loss of function on one side).

In cases of severe brain injury, the patient may respond with either decerebrate or decorticate posturing. *Decerebrate posturing* is present when the arms and legs extend and the back bows forcefully. *Decorticate posturing* differs only in that the upper extremities flex rather than extend. Either posturing may be present continuously or may occur with painful stimuli.

Determine if the patient has lost consciousness or orientation at any time since the accident. If unconsciousness occurred, increase the index of suspicion for serious internal head injury. Watch any patient with this history very carefully for any change in level of orientation. Any change in the level of consciousness demands immediate transport.

Glasgow Coma Scale   The Glasgow Coma Scale provides a system to evaluate the neurologically impaired patient. It consists of three areas of assessment (eye-opening, motor response, and verbal response) and the allocation of points for the best patient response achieved. The resulting value can give an indication of the status of the patient's CNS function. A score of 15 is the maximum and most common finding. A score of 9 or above is indicative of consciousness; anything below 7 is coma. Note that the lowest score obtainable is 3. Employ this system repeatedly during your care of the patient.

Glasgow Coma Scale		
Eye Opening		
Spontaneous	4	
To Voice	3	
To Pain	2	
None	1	
Verbal Response		
Oriented	5	
Confused	4	
Inappropriate Words	3	
Incomprehensible Words	2	
None	1	
Motor Response		
Obeys Commands	6	
Localizes Pain	5	
Withdraw (Pain)	4	
Flexion (Pain)	3	
Extension (Pain)	2	
None	1	
Glasgow Coma Score Total		

VITAL SIGNS

There are four basic vital signs in medicine: blood pressure, pulse, respiration, and body temperature. (See Procedure 10-3.) The first three are of prime importance in prehospital care, while body temperature is of limited use.

Compare vital signs with the general patient condition that you observed from the primary assessment. If the vital signs suggest a more serious problem than already found, look for the cause. If the apparent patient problem should account for poorer vital signs, consider re-evaluation of the vital signs. In either case, always look for the worst and offer anticipatory patient care.

It is important to take baseline measurements of these vital signs and additional vital signs measurements periodically during patient care. Comparison of the later measurements with the baseline readings will indicate trends—improvement or deterioration—in patient condition.

Blood Pressure

Blood pressure determination is a basic and important skill. It reveals the state of the circulatory system and its compensatory mechanisms. (See Procedure 10-3, Figure A.) Its greatest shortcoming is that blood pressure drops late in the progression of shock—too late to be of much use in anticipating the problem. (See Chapter 12.) However, blood pressure is helpful in evaluating other serious conditions such as cardiac problems, head injury, stress, hypertensive crisis, and heat stroke.

The ideal adult systolic blood pressure, regardless of age, is 120 mm Hg. Females normally have a slightly lower pressure until menopause. Recognize, however, that a blood pressure of 120 mm Hg may reflect **hypotension** in one patient, **hypertension** in another. Use blood pressure with other assessment information to determine the overall status of the cardiovascular system and circulation.

Blood pressure can be difficult to determine in the field. The various sounds of blood against the arterial wall and the stethoscope can be difficult to

■ **hypotension** an arterial blood pressure that is below normal. It may be either chronic (of long duration) or acute (sudden or short term).

■ **hypertension** an arterial blood pressure that is above normal. It may be either chronic (of long duration) or acute (sudden or short term).

✱ The blood pressure must be used in concert with several factors to assess the overall state of the cardiovascular system and circulation.

distinguish, especially with extraneous scene noise. A helpful technique is to raise the patient's extremity (presuming it's uninjured), wait for a moment, then inflate the cuff rapidly. Bring the arm down to the normal position, and have the patient flex and extend the fingers a few times. Let the pressure release slowly, 3 mm Hg to 4 mm Hg per second, while you auscultate. The amplitude of the sound should increase markedly, making the values easier to hear.

If blood pressure is difficult to hear, consider taking it by palpation. Note that a blood pressure taken by this method is about 10 mm Hg lower than one taken by auscultation. If it cannot be determined by either auscultation or palpation, report that you were unable to obtain a pressure. Some circumstances that are common in the field make it nearly impossible to determine blood pressure.

A device becoming more widely used to determine blood pressure is the ultrasonic Doppler. (See Procedure 10-3, Figure B.) It is an electronic stethoscope that uses high frequency sound waves to assess blood movement through an artery. When placed over an artery, the device picks up sounds that are not otherwise audible. A small amount of conductive gel helps conduct the sound waves. Adjust the Doppler volume until you hear the "whooshing" of the artery, and then time the pulse or determine the blood pressure. It will often give readings when other more traditional approaches would not.

■ **pulse pressure** the difference between the systolic and diastolic readings.

As you evaluate the blood pressure, look to the difference between the systolic and diastolic readings. This value, called the **pulse pressure**, reflects the effectiveness of the cardiac output against the flexibility of the arterial system. Up to a point, the wider the pulse pressure, the better the state of the circulatory system. A narrow pulse pressure may indicate pericardial tamponade or tension pneumothorax. It may also be an early finding in shock.

Pulse

The pulse is a valuable indicator of circulatory function. (See Procedure 10-3, Figure C.) An increasing pulse rate signals the compensatory response to hypovolemia and is an early indication of shock. A rise of more than 15 beats per minute when the patient moves from supine to a seated position suggests significant blood loss, generally more than 500 mL. As hypovolemia becomes more profound, a rapid pulse is present in any position and the patient's pulse strength diminishes.

■ **sympathetic stimulation** a stimulus that triggers the sympathetic nervous system, increasing heart rate and blood pressure, as well as other actions of the sympathetic nervous system.

The pulse may indicate conditions other than shock. A slow and bounding pulse may reflect head injury or heat stroke. A rapid and strong pulse may indicate excitement or other **sympathetic stimulation**. An irregular pulse may indicate cardiac irritability or over-stimulation by drugs such as caffeine. As with the other vital signs, take the pulse frequently to determine any trends in patient condition.

Respiration

✱ Always determine an accurate respiratory rate.

Since oxygen and carbon dioxide exchange is essential to human life, respiration must occur continuously. You will have evaluated respiration briefly during the primary assessment, but you will reassess it to determine the exact rate, relative tidal volume, and subtle signs of distress. Determine the respiratory rate over 30 seconds by placing a hand on the chest and counting each inhalation and exhalation. (See Procedure 10-3, Figure D.) The result is the breaths per minute. The rate should be regular. Also, assure that the breaths are full and that no extraneous sounds or signs of difficult breathing exist.

Body Temperature

The body works hard at maintaining a temperature of approximately 37 degrees Centigrade (98.6 degrees Fahrenheit). This temperature reflects a balance between heat production and heat loss through the skin and respiratory

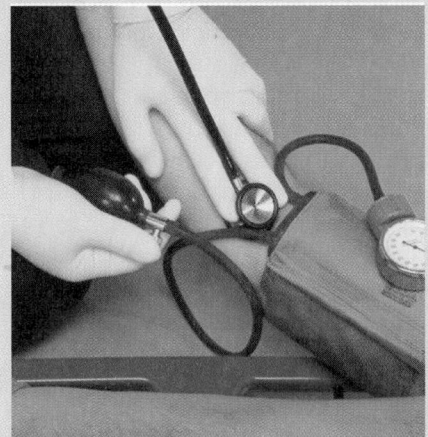

10-3A. Assess the blood pressure using a sphygmomanometer and stethoscope.

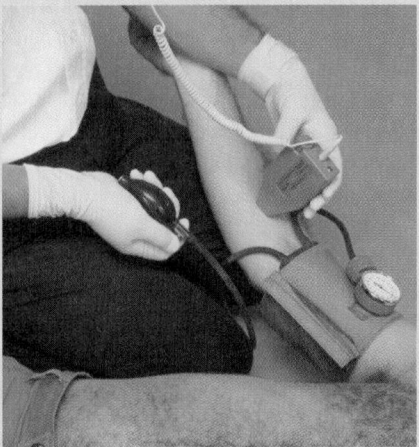

10-3B. If the blood pressure is difficult to hear, an ultrasonic Doppler may be used.

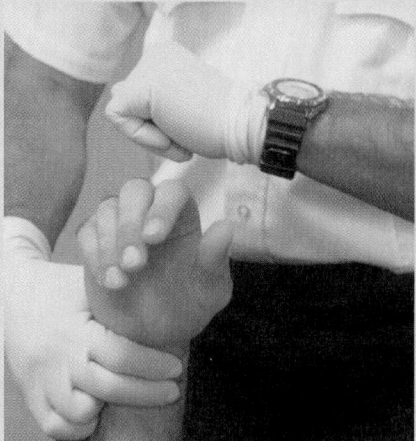

10-3C. Assess the pulse as an indicator of circulatory function.

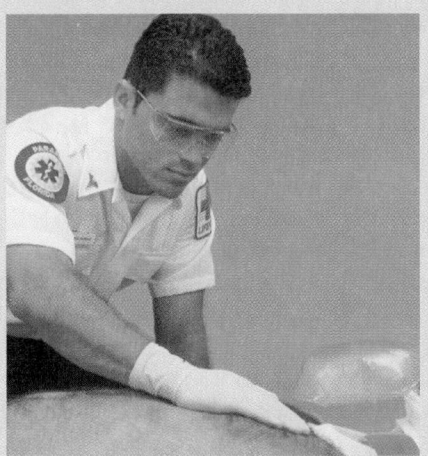

10-3D. Count the patient's respirations.

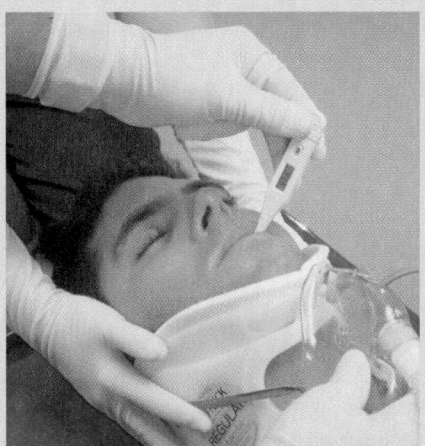

10-3E. Determine the patient's body temperature with a rectal or oral thermometer, or . . .

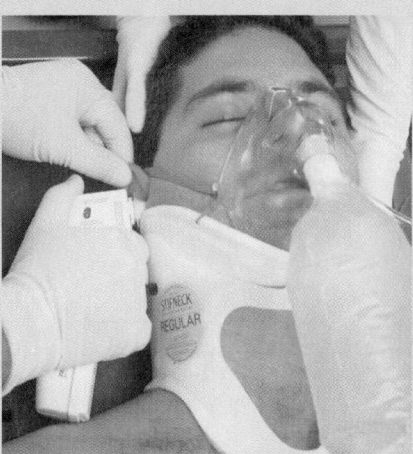

10-3F. with a thermometer that measures temperature inside the ear.

system. Any variance, even a slight one, can mean that significant events are going on within the body. Temperature is taken to approximate the internal or core environment. In emergency medical service, you normally take temperature orally or, on occasion, rectally. Some thermometers can be placed in the ear. Battery-operated thermometers are preferred to glass ones, because they reduce the danger of breakage and offer more rapid and accurate readings. (See Procedure 10-3, Figures E and F.)

An increase in body temperature indicates either the effects of environmental extremes or the body's effort to make the internal environment inhospitable to invading pathogens. Fever often presents with a history of illness and a high skin and internal temperature. The skin is relatively dry until the fever breaks and the body's cooling mechanisms begin to take effect. In a very warm environment, the body will utilize its cooling mechanisms to maintain core temperature. The temperature only rises when these mechanisms are no longer effective, as in an environment of extreme heat and humidity, or in cases like heat stroke, where the CNS control of the cooling mechanisms fail.

As the body temperature rises, it begins to threaten body processes, specifically the brain. A temperature of up to 38°C (102°F) increases metabolism markedly. As it rises above 39°C (103°F), the neurons may denature. Much above 41°C (105°F); brain cells begin to die, and seizures may occur.

Extremes of cold also affect body temperature. When peripheral vasoconstriction and shivering mechanisms can no longer balance heat production and loss, the core temperature drops. At a body temperature of 34°C (93°F), normal body warming mechanisms begin to fail. As the core temperature drops below 31°C (90°F), heart sounds diminish and cardiac irritability increases. If the temperature drops much below 22°C (70°F), the patient will present with a deathlike appearance and, possibly, irreversible asystole (absence of heartbeat). Most thermometers will not record below 36°C (96°F). Therefore, they will not be of assistance in evaluating hypothermic patients. If your service operates in areas of low environmental temperatures, equip your ambulance with a low-reading thermometer.

Other Assessment Techniques

Besides checking the four basic vital signs, you might apply the following assessment techniques to evaluate other aspects of the patient's condition.

Cardiac Monitoring Cardiac monitoring should be an element in the assessment of both the trauma and the medical patient. (See Figure 10-22.) While the analysis of an ECG is normally associated with cardiac problems, the skill is also of great value in assessing both trauma and general medical patients. In addition to cardiac problems, dysrhythmias can result from head injury, chest trauma, stroke, drugs, and respiratory and/or metabolic problems. (For more on this important aspect of assessment, see Chapter 21.)

■ **pulse oximetry** measurement of the oxygen saturation level of the blood through a noninvasive sensor placed on a finger or ear lobe.

Pulse Oximetry If available, use **pulse oximetry** with all patients. (See Figure 10-23.) The pulse oximeter is a quick and accurate tool that can objectively determine the oxygenation status of the patient. It quantifies the effect of interventions, including oxygen therapy, medication, suctioning, and ventilatory assistance. The pulse oximeter functions by measuring transmission of red and infrared light through an arterial bed, such as those present in a finger, toe, or earlobe.

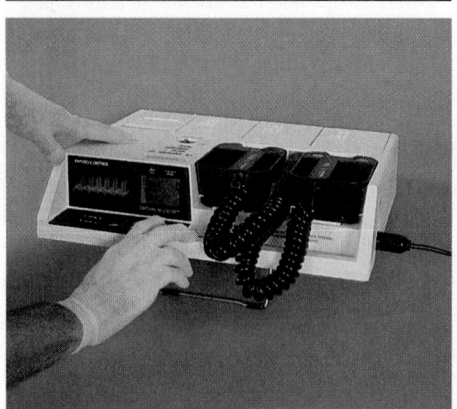

FIGURE 10-22 Cardiac monitoring should be routinely employed in prehospital care.

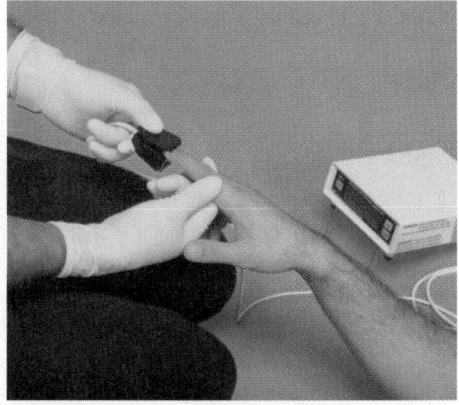

FIGURE 10-23 Pulse oximetry allows you to determine quickly and accurately the patient's oxygenation status.

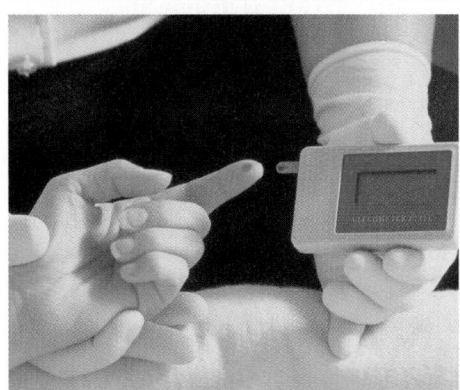

FIGURE 10-24 Determine the blood glucose with either a glucometer or Dextrostix®.

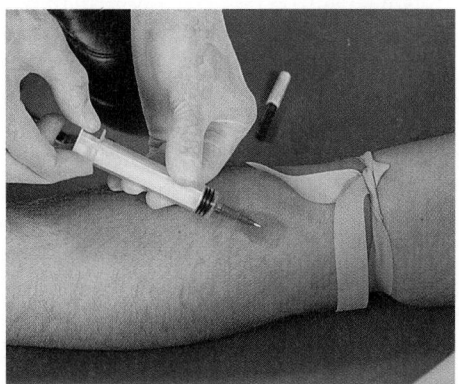

FIGURE 10-25 When performing a blood glucose test, or starting an IV, collect a sample of blood if required by local protocols.

The pulse oximeter gives a reading of 96 to 100 percent oxygen saturation in patients with effective respiration. If respirations are compromised, even slightly, oxygen saturation falls. Provide any patient whose saturation is below 90 percent with aggressive oxygenation and possibly positive pressure ventilation.

The pulse oximeter does have some shortcomings in prehospital care. In low-flow states, such as hypothermia (low body temperature) and late hypovolemia, the device may not sense accurately. The presence of carbon monoxide on the **hemoglobin** molecule tends to elevate the saturation level falsely. Be sure to rule out any possibility of carbon monoxide poisoning before placing full faith in an oximeter reading.

Be careful in using the pulse oximeter in patients with anemia and in some cases of hypovolemia. The oximeter may give a normal reading that records well-oxygenated hemoglobin. However, the *amount* of hemoglobin has been diminished. Thus, the body may not have enough hemoglobin to carry the needed oxygen supplies. In these patients, monitor the vital signs carefully, and administer high-flow oxygen regardless of the oximeter reading.

Glucose Determination   Field glucose tests, using a blood glucose test kit, provide an indication of the blood-sugar level. Currently, the tests are dependent upon proper and uniform technique. As a result, they have had only limited success. The process involves smearing a small amount of blood on a test strip and comparing the resultant color against a color scale that corresponds to blood-sugar level. Many EMS units carry electronic glucose monitors, which give relatively accurate, numeric blood-glucose readings. These are preferable to the standard reagent sticks, which may be adversely affected by heat and age. (See Figure 10-24.)

Certain drugs can assist in the patient evaluation. Naloxone, which is a narcotic antagonist, can reverse the effects of narcotic overdose, while glucose administration may bring a patient out of a hypoglycemic coma. Neither drug will generally cause harm, and a dramatic reversal in a patient's condition will support a particular diagnosis.

Venipuncture   Drawing blood from the patient may be useful for several diagnostic tests performed by emergency department personnel. Although the blood draw does not directly affect your patient assessment, it may assist the emergency physician at the hospital. Analysis of blood may reveal pre-care levels of alcohol, glucose, or narcotics, as well as the ratio of red blood cells to serum by volume (**hematocrit**). Some EMS systems draw blood during prolonged extrication and transport it to the hospital before the patient. The

■ **hemoglobin** an iron-containing compound, found within the red blood cell, that is responsible for the transport and delivery of oxygen to the body cells.

✱ Always treat the patient, not the monitoring device.

✱ Blood should be drawn, according to local protocol, to help determine the pre-care condition of the patient.

■ **hematocrit** the percentage of blood occupied by red blood cells.

Elements of the
Patient History

■ Chief complaint
■ History of present
  illness/injury
■ Past medical history

hospital staff type and cross-match it so whole blood is ready and waiting when the patient arrives. (See Figure 10-25.)

PATIENT HISTORY

As part of the secondary assessment, you should expand your knowledge of the patient's current medical problem and the patient's prior medical history by questioning the patient or, if the patient is unable to respond, by questioning the family or other bystanders. (See Figure 10-26.)

Three elements of the questioning process are essential to complete a comprehensive patient history. They are the chief complaint, the circumstances of the present illness or injury, and the past medical history. These elements of the patient history—and questioning techniques that will help you obtain this information—will be discussed in the following sections.

Questioning Techniques

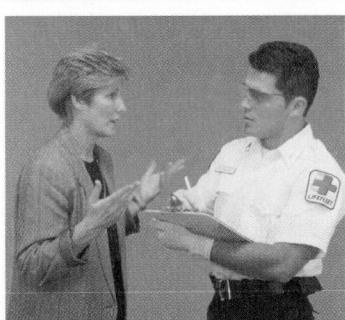

FIGURE 10-26 If the patient is unresponsive, gather information for the patient history from family members or bystanders.

To gather the patient history, you can use open-ended or closed-ended questions. Open-ended questions prompt the patient to explain how he feels in detail, rather than giving "yes" or "no" answers. An example of an open-ended question might be, "Describe the pain in your chest." Closed-ended questions limit patient response, for example, "Are you on any medications?" Select the type of question that provides you with the needed information. In any case, do not use questions that suggest answers such as, "Is your chest pain a crushing pain?" Finally, keep all questions simple and easy to understand.

Your questioning process should result in the patient feeling comfortable, confident in your care, and supportive of your control of the situation. Position yourself at the patient's eye level and focus your attention on him. Give the patient's requests and concerns a high priority, even if they are not medically significant. For example, if a patient complains of being cold, cover him with a blanket. It may not only make the patient feel warmer, but it may increase confidence in your desire and ability to help. If you cannot care for a complaint immediately, express your concern and let the patient know you will take care of it shortly. Address the patient appropriately. Ask for his name, and use it frequently during the assessment. You should also ask how a patient wants to be called—e.g., Mr. Jones, James, or Jim—and respect his wishes.

Listen carefully to what the patient says. All too often, we anticipate a problem, then suffer from tunnel vision. We fail to look for other signs, symptoms, or conditions that might account for the patient's complaint or medical problem. If we carefully listen to what the patient says, we are less likely to go wrong.

It is important to record what the patient says and not what you feel the patient meant to say. Because of our medical background, we tend to use specific words that have special meanings. It is best to record the patient's exact words. If the patient's description of a symptom changes, then it is just that—a change, not your misinterpretation of what the patient said.

The Chief Complaint

■ **chief complaint** the reason the ambulance was called.

The **chief complaint** is the pain, discomfort, or dysfunction that causes your patient to request help. In a medical case, it may be a woman calling for help because of chest pain. In a trauma case, it may be a bystander calling for assistance to a "man down," or the police reporting an injury in an auto collision.

As you interview and assess the patient, the chief complaint becomes more and more specific. The chief complaint differs from the primary problem. The chief complaint is a sign or symptom noticed by the patient or a bystander; the primary problem is the principal medical cause of the complaint. For example, a patient's chief complaint may be leg pain, while the primary problem is a tibia fracture.

Circumstances of the Present Illness or Injury

The circumstances of the present illness or injury are obtained by investigating the chief complaint. In the medical patient, especially, you must investigate the patient's symptoms carefully and identify the nature and location of the complaint. To assist you in this investigation remember the mnemonic *OPQRST*:

OPQRST
Chief Complaint
Onset
Provocation
Quality
Radiation
Severity
Time

O **O**nset: *What were you doing when the problem began?*
P **P**rovocation: *What makes the problem better or worse?*
Q **Q**uality: *How would you describe the problem or pain?*
R **R**adiation: *Does the pain radiate, or are there any associated problems?*
S **S**everity: *How intense is the pain? On a scale from 1 to 10?*
T **T**ime: *How long ago did the problem begin?*

Onset Did the problem develop rapidly or slowly? What was the patient doing when the problem started? In cases of trauma, look at the mechanism of injury, and assure that the accident was not caused by a medical problem. In cases of trauma the onset was sudden but may have been induced by a medical problem such as a seizure causing a fall. In medical emergencies, investigate the patient's activities at the time of, or shortly before, the symptoms or signs developed. Was the patient exercising or exerting himself, or at rest or sleeping? Was he eating or drinking? If so, what?

Look also at the environment where you find the patient. Examine physical conditions such as temperature, presence of odors, or airborne particles. Check the general appearance of the home and note any offending agents (e.g., medications, alcohol containers, drug paraphernalia), signs of neglect, and so on. Also notice the attitudes of the bystanders, friends, and/or family members toward the disease or emergency. These attitudes may affect how the patient perceives his infirmity. If the social environment is not supportive, the patient may feel uncomfortable about the problem and may not wish to discuss it in much detail.

Provocation In many illnesses, certain factors may increase or decrease pain, discomfort, or dysfunction. These factors include motion, pressure, jarring, ingestion of solids or fluids, and rest or sleep. Positioning may also be a factor. A patient may wish to curl up and lie on his side to reduce abdominal pain. Congestive heart failure patients will sit bolt upright to ease respiration. They may also sleep with several pillows to raise the upper body in order to relieve **paroxysmal nocturnal dyspnea**, a sleep-disturbing breathing difficulty caused by fluid that accumulates in the lungs when the patient is supine. Ask your patient how breathing affects the discomfort. Deep breathing may increase the pain of the acute abdomen patient. A patient with pleuritic or rib fracture pain will not breathe deeply, whereas breathing may not affect the pain of angina. Any patient with pain during respiration will breathe with shallower but more frequent breaths.

■ **paroxysmal noturnal dyspnea** breathing difficulty caused by fluid in the lungs while a person is supine.

If a medication is taken shortly before you arrive, its effect or lack of effect upon the patient may help determine the problem. Drugs such as bronchial dilators, hypoglycemic agents, and anti-convulsants are commonly prescribed and taken at home. Investigate any medication used to relieve a problem, and note its recent effectiveness.

■ **alleviate** to reduce or eliminate, usually with reference to a problem or discomforting feeling.

Ask for and record any activity, position, medication, or other circumstance that either **alleviates** or **aggravates** the chief complaint.

■ **aggravate** to worsen or increase in severity.

Quality Investigate how the patient perceives the pain or discomfort. Ask the patient to explain how the symptom feels, and listen carefully to the answer. Does the patient call it crushing, tearing, oppressive, gnawing, crampy, sharp, dull, or otherwise? Quote the patient's descriptors in your reports.

Radiation Identify the exact location and area of pain, discomfort, or dysfunction. Does the patient complain of pain "here," while holding a clenched fist over the sternum, or does he grasp the entire abdomen with both hands and moan? If the patient has not done so, ask him to point to the painful area. Identify the specific location, or the boundary of pain, if it is regional.

Determine if the pain is truly *pain* (occurring independently) rather than *tenderness* (pain on touch). Also determine if the pain moves or radiates. Localized pain is found in one specific area, while radiating pain travels away from the source, in one, many, or all directions. Evaluate moving pain as to initial location, progression, and factors that affect its movement.

Note any pain that may be referred from other parts of the body (felt in a part of the body away from the area that is the source of the disease or problem). The two areas that most commonly produce referred pain are the heart and the diaphragm. A cardiac problem, such as myocardial infarction or anginal pain, is most commonly referred to the left arm, with occasional referral to the neck, jaw, and back. Pain associated with irritation of the diaphragm (most commonly blood in the abdomen of the supine patient) is generally referred to the clavicular region.

Severity Severity is the intensity of pain or discomfort felt by the patient. Ask the patient how bad the pain feels, and then have him compare it to other painful problems he has experienced. Sometimes a patient can describe the severity of the pain on a scale from 1 to 10, 10 being the worst pain he has ever felt. Also notice the amount of discomfort the patient's condition causes. How easy is it to distract the patient from his concern over the pain? Is the patient very still and resistive to your touch? Or is the patient writhing about? The answers should give you a good idea of the intensity of pain felt by the patient.

Time How long has this symptom affected the patient? For several days, hours, or just a few minutes or seconds? If there were previous episodes, when did they occur? How does this one vary in length from earlier ones?

Pertinent Negatives A pertinent negative is the *absence* of a finding that might be expected to be associated with the patient's problem. For example, if a patient complains of shortness of breath but denies chest pain and cardiac history, record this as a pertinent negative finding on your report form and in radio messages. Also note any element of the history or physical assessment that does not support a suspected or possible diagnosis.

Past Medical History

If significant medical problems are recognized during your history taking, investigate in more detail. Note when the problem was first recognized and how it affected the patient. How frequently did it happen and what medical care was sought? Was the care sought effective or did the problem recur?

To obtain information about the patient's past medical history, use the acronym *AMPLE* as an aid to remembering pertinent questions to ask.

> **AMPLE**
> **Past Medical History**
> **A**llergies
> **M**edications
> **P**ast medical problems
> **L**ast oral intake
> **E**vents preceding the emergency

A   **A**llergies: *Are you allergic to any medications? foods? other substances?*

M   **M**edications: *Are you on any prescribed medications? For what? When did you last take your medication?*

P **P**ast medical problems: *Have you had recent surgery, or are you under the care of a physician for any medical problem?*

L **L**ast oral intake: *What have you had to eat or drink in the last 24 hours?*

E **E**vents preceding the emergency: *What caused the accident?* or *What were you doing just prior to the onset of your symptoms?*

Allergies Ask the patient about any known allergies, especially those to penicillin, the "caine" family (local anesthetics), or tetanus toxoid. These agents are frequently given in emergency situations. Knowledge of the patient's allergies may prevent additional complications during the emergency department visit, especially if the patient becomes disoriented or unconscious during transport.

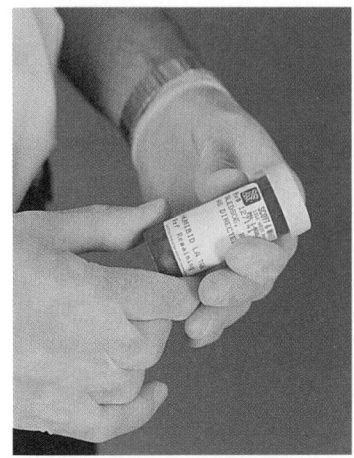

FIGURE 10-27 Note the names, dosages, and dates of any medications taken by the patient.

Medications Determine if the patient is on any medications. If so, for what reasons? (See Figure 10-27.) The patient's explanation may not be medically accurate, but it may help to determine underlying conditions. A medication not taken as prescribed may be responsible for the current medical problem—possibly by not reaching therapeutic levels or by over-medication. A recently prescribed medication may cause an allergic or untoward (severe and unexpected) reaction. It may also be out of date and no longer able to provide the desired effect. Even for a trauma patient, emergency department personnel will need to know what medications the patient is taking. Bring the patient's medications to the hospital.

✱ A patient's current medications can provide a great deal of information about his or her medical problems.

Past Medical Problems A pre-existing medical problem may contribute to a patient's current problem or influence the care that is offered in the next few hours. To discover significant pre-existing medical problems, ask if the patient has recently seen a physician or been hospitalized. If so, for what conditions? If a pre-existing medical problem is found, investigate the effects it has had on the patient. When was the patient last affected by the problem? Is the patient on any special diets, prescribed medications, or restricted in activity? Even with a trauma patient, don't forget that a medical problem may have led to an accident or may complicate the effects of the trauma. It is also helpful to obtain the patient's physician's name since it may be helpful to the ED staff.

Last Oral Intake Investigate the patient's most recent meal (anything eaten or drunk, even as a snack) and determine when and how much of what was ingested. Also determine if there was any change in eating or drinking habits. The type of food consumed may reflect a possible problem such as fatty food for a gall bladder patient or shellfish consumed by a patient with shellfish allergies. Ingestion shortly before the emergency may lead to vomiting either during your care, in the emergency department, or during surgery. Under this category you should also ask about bowel and bladder activity or irregularity. In the female patient it may be pertinent to ask questions regarding the menstrual cycle, its regularity, and any previous gynecological problems.

✱ Never allow a patient to eat or drink anything except the medications you provide.

Events Preceding the Emergency In cases of trauma, look at the mechanism of injury, and assure that the accident was not caused by a medical problem. Was the patient driving an auto when he suffered a myocardial infarction and hit a tree? Was the patient hypoglycemic when he passed out and fell down a flight of stairs? A good investigation may reveal a precipitating, and possibly a more important, medical problem. Also, has the patient undergone any change in lifestyle? Emotional or stressful events such as divorce, a recent move, job loss, recent retirement, or the death of a close friend or family member may impact the patient physiologically as well as psychologically, possibly leading to an accident, self-destructive behavior, or illness. Note the correlation of any significant life event with the beginning or progression of the illness or trauma.

✱ The information garnered from the patient history should be summarized and all pertinent findings accurately recorded.

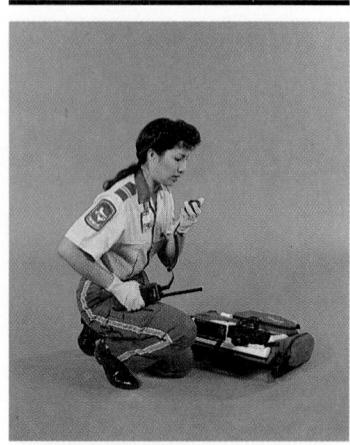

FIGURE 10-28 Report to medical direction by radio or phone.

ONGOING ASSESSMENT

During your patient care you should re-evaluate your patient frequently. The seriously ill or injured patient should be re-assessed at least every 5 minutes, including vital signs and evaluation of the chief complaint and level of consciousness. The minor trauma patient may be assessed every 10 to 15 minutes after the first few 5 minute assessments. And, the stable medical patient may be assessed every 15 minutes or so. Reassessment occurs any time you perform a patient intervention or you notice a change in any patient sign or symptom.

COMMUNICATION AND DOCUMENTATION

Communication between you and the medical control physician is extremely important. So is your written documentation of the call. The information you provide must be concise, correct, and pertinent to the patient's condition.

Radio/Phone Communication

✳ Clear communication of the results of your assessment is essential to a successful request to medical control for critical intervention.

The purpose of radio or phone communication between you and medical control or the receiving facility is to convey just enough information to support your request for approval of care and to allow the emergency department to prepare for the patient's arrival. (See Figure 10-28.) Communicate only the information that is essential to that purpose. There is rarely a need to communicate all signs and symptoms or all patient information.

Use of a standardized format for radio or phone communication of patient information assures an organized and complete report. Many hospitals and EMS systems have created pocket notebook forms to provide this format. A minimum set of data to transmit to medical direction or the receiving facility is listed below.

Radio/Phone Report Data

- Identification of your unit and level of provider
- Patient's age and sex
- Patient's chief complaint
- Brief pertinent circumstances of the present illness or injury (including mechanism of injury or nature of the illness)
- Major past illnesses or pre-existing conditions, if relevant (including medications, allergies)
- Patient's mental status
- Baseline vital signs and subsequent vital signs readings
- ECG rhythm, if relevant
- Pertinent findings of the physical exam
- Emergency care given
- Patient's response to emergency care
- Estimated time of arrival

Repeat back to the medical control physician any order for intervention to assure there is no confusion between what the physician said and what you heard. It is also appropriate to question and ultimately refuse any order from a physician that is outside your protocols or that you believe is inappropriate for the patient.

The following is an example of a radio report you might make for a moderately serious accident with a patient injured, yet stable.

> *ALS Unit 96 to United Hospital. We are at the scene of an auto/train accident with a 55-year-old male patient. He is complaining of leg and cervical pain with numbness in his hands, but not his feet. The patient has an apparent open fracture of the left femur. He is alert with a blood pressure of 136 over 88, a pulse of 110, and respirations of 18 and regular. The patient denies any previous medical history other than an allergy to Xylocaine. He is currently on oxygen at 15 Lpm by nonrebreather, cervical stabilization is being maintained, and we are awaiting extrication to apply a traction splint to the femur. We request permission to start an IV of lactated Ringer's solution and Nitronox for pain. We expect a 10-minute extrication and a 15-minute transport to your facility.*

Once you institute interventions and the patient is ready for transport, update the medical control physician as follows.

> *ALS Unit 96 to United Hospital. We have initiated an IV in the left anterior forearm and have administered Nitronox. Patient remains alert, with a blood pressure of 132 over 86, a pulse of 94, and respirations are 20 and regular. The patient reports his pain has diminished. He has been immobilized to a long spine board. A traction splint is in place, the patient has been loaded into the ambulance, and we are en route to your facility. Estimated arrival is within 10 minutes.*

Clearly communicating the results of your assessment is essential to a successful request for critical intervention. It is also very important to the continuity of care as you present your patient at the emergency department. If you present accurate information, the medical control physician will prepare the department staff physically and mentally for your arrival. They will have a picture of the patient's condition long before the doors of your ambulance open.

Emergency Department Arrival

On arrival at the emergency department, you are responsible for updating the staff on any change in the patient's condition. (See Figure 10-29.) Also supply any other pertinent information not communicated earlier. Report any patient interventions and their results. The emergency department physician will compare your communication with his or her own findings. If your assessment (and your radio-report condensation of it) was accurate, appropriate care will continue. If the condition of the patient is not what the physician envisioned from your report, he will have to reevaluate the patient, interrupting the continuity of care. Such a situation will call into question your credibility as a field care provider.

✱ The hand-off of the patient to emergency department personnel should include a brief overview of care rendered and the results of that care.

Documentation

The call ends with completion of the ambulance report form. The report must be neat, accurate, and complete, since it serves several functions. It becomes part of the patient's permanent record, which details the patient's medical care

✱ The ambulance report must be complete, neat, and accurate since it will become part of the patient's medical record and a legal document.

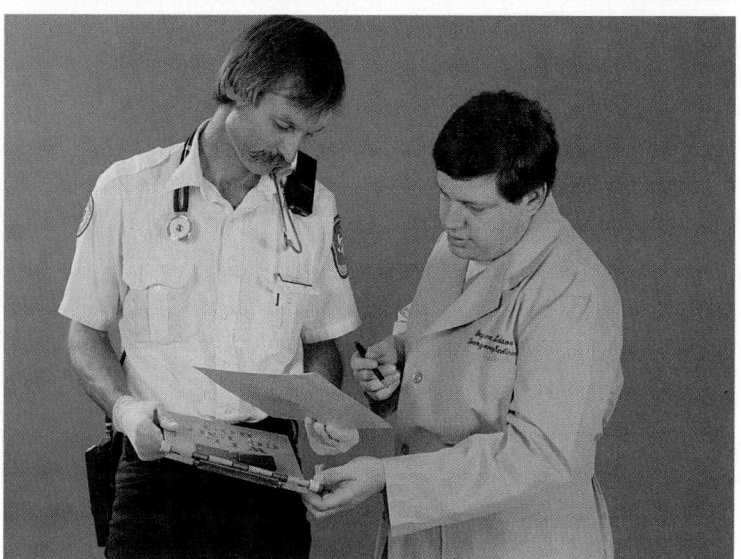

FIGURE 10-29 Provide any additional information to the emergency department physician upon arrival at the hospital.

from its beginning until discharge from the hospital. It documents any patient findings that you noted, and care offered at the scene and during transport. It may also be the documentation that comes to your defense—or incrimination—if patient care is questioned in a court of law or by medical control.

The ambulance report form should provide space to record the following data: dispatch information; findings at the scene (including medical care given before you arrived); signs, symptoms, and other patient information gained through assessment; care instituted; and impact that the care had upon vital signs and upon the patient's condition in general.

The form should be well organized so that it allows you to record information in the order in which it was obtained. It should also allow anyone reviewing the form to gain rapidly the information they need. A well-designed ambulance report form will facilitate complete and orderly documentation of the run.

SUMMARY

Patient assessment is an orderly evaluation of all information available to you, from the original dispatch to the passing of patient responsibilities to the emergency department staff. Use the senses of sight, hearing, touch, and smell to determine what is most likely wrong with your patient. Evaluate the patient in an organized and progressive fashion, from a review of dispatch information to a complete head-to-toe assessment and determination of a medical history.

Comprehensive patient assessment involves six steps: *scene size-up, primary assessment, head-to-toe evaluation* (secondary assessment), *vital signs, patient history,* and *ongoing assessment.* Remain alert to distinctions in assessment for the trauma patient and the medical patient. (See Figure 10-30.)

The results of the patient assessment steps guide patient care. They also form the basis for radio communication and requests for advanced interventions. Most of the information recorded on the ambulance report form summarizes the findings revealed by these steps. Assessment is a primary and absolutely essential skill upon which any further care or intervention is predicated.

The Patient Assessment Process

Steps	Trauma Patient	Medical Patient
Scene Size-up ■ Review dispatch information ■ Survey the scene/request aid ■ Identify potential hazards ■ Secure the scene ■ Determine the mechanism of injury or nature of illness ■ Locate all patients	**Scene Size-up** The trauma scene often presents hazards to rescuers, bystanders, and patients. Assure scene safety, request aid if needed, and locate all patients. Identifying the mechanism of injury is critical in evaluating possible injuries.	**Scene Size-up** The possibility of hazards exists at the medical as well as at the trauma scene, such as toxic fumes or substances, broken or icy steps. Be aware of how environmental conditions may affect the patient.
Primary Assessment ■ Airway and Breathing ■ Circulation ■ Disability (AVPU) ■ Expose (for critical injuries) Set priorities for immediate transport with care en route or continued care on scene.	**Primary Assessment** is identical for trauma and medical patients. With trauma, you are more likely to find compromised ABCs and indications of head or internal injury. Decision for immediate transport is more likely with a trauma patient.	**Primary Assessment** is identical for trauma and medical patients. In medical patients, cardiac arrest and respiratory emergency must be ruled out first. A decision for on-scene care (vs. transport) is more likely with a medical patient.
Secondary Assessment ■ Head-to-toe evaluation ■ Vital signs ■ Patient history	**Secondary Assessment** During the head-to-toe exam, direct special attention to areas of potential injury suggested by the mechanism of injury. Combine exam, vital signs, and patient history findings to determine the patient's general status.	**Secondary Assessment** Direct special attention to areas (and signs and symptoms) related to the chief complaint. Look for systemic findings like pitting edema or local findings like pain. Combine with vital signs and history to determine status.
Ongoing Assessment	**Ongoing Assessment** Continually monitor the trauma or the medical patient, frequently repeating assessment of airway, breathing, circulation, mental status, and vital signs and effectiveness of interventions. Reassess the patient after any major intervention or change in the patient's condition or every few minutes.	

FIGURE 10-30 The steps of patient assessment.

FURTHER READING

American College of Surgeons, Committee on Trauma. *Advanced Trauma Life Support Course: Student Manual.* American College of Surgeons, 1989.

Bosker, Gideon, and Michael Sequeira. *The 60 Second EMT.* St. Louis: The C.V. Mosby Company, 1987.

Jacobs, Donald T. *Patient Communication for First Responders and EMS Personnel.* Englewood Cliffs, NJ: Brady, 1991.

Stanford, Todd M. *EMS Report Writing—A Pocket Reference.* Englewood Cliffs, NJ: Brady, 1992.

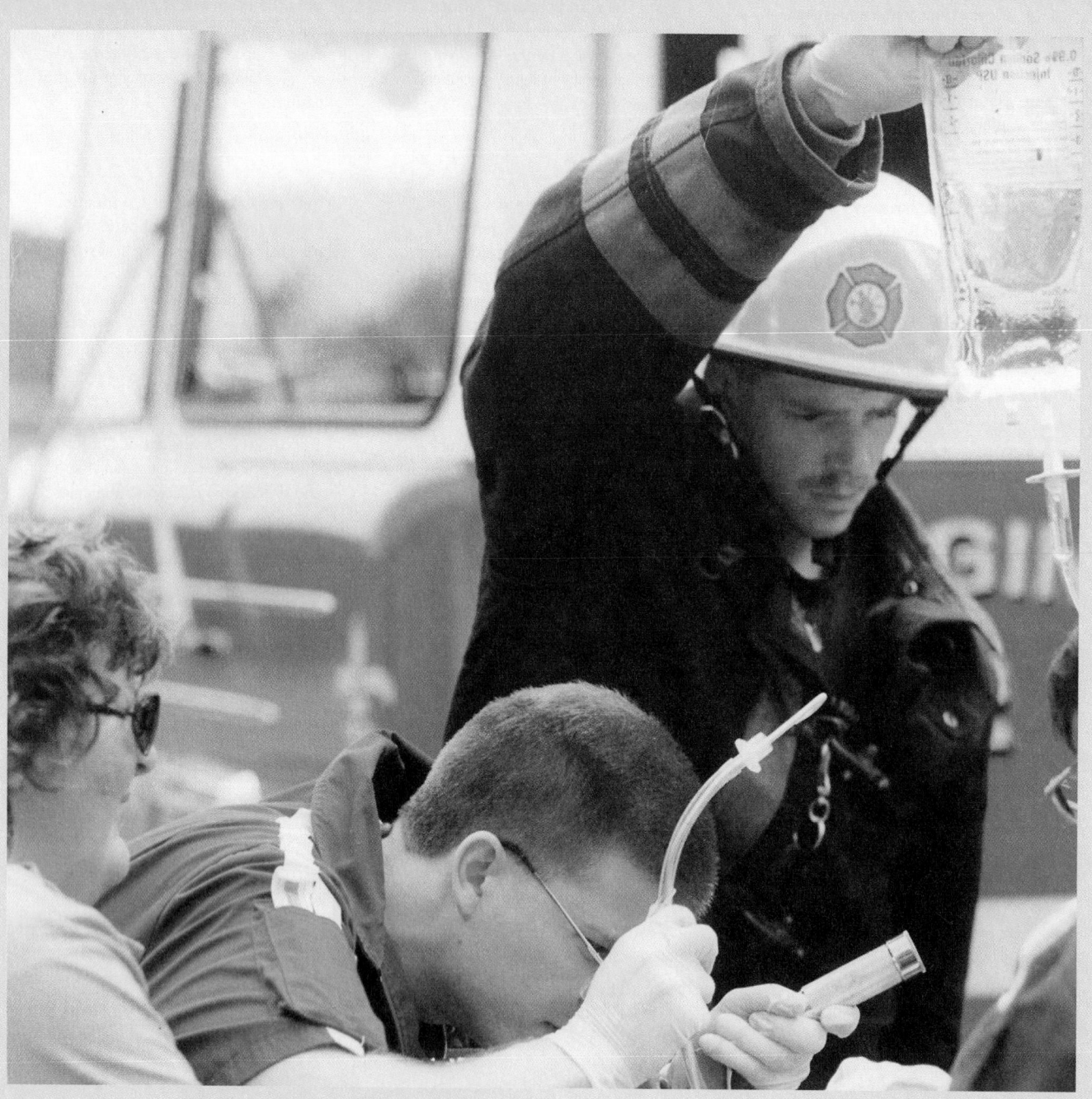

AIRWAY MANAGEMENT AND VENTILATION

Objectives for Chapter 11

After reading this chapter, you should be able to:

1. Describe the anatomy of the upper airway, including the mouth, nose, pharynx, epiglottis, and larynx. (See pp. 207–210.)

2. Name the three regions of the pharynx. (See p. 208.)

3. Identify the relationship between the larynx and the tongue, pharynx, epiglottis, esophagus, and vocal cords. (See pp. 208–209.)

4. Discuss the following functions of the respiratory system: (See below pages.)

- mechanics of ventilation (p. 212)
- pulmonary circulation (pp. 212–213)
- gas exchange in the lungs (pp. 213–214)
- diffusion of the respiratory gasses (p. 214)

5. Describe oxygen transport in the blood, and cite factors that affect it. (See pp. 214–215.)

6. Discuss carbon dioxide transport in the blood, and list factors that affect it. (See p. 215.)

7. Describe the neurological control of respiration. (See pp. 215–216.)

8. Describe the various measures of respiratory function, and give the average normal values for each. (See p. 217.)

9. Describe the common causes of airway obstruction, and detail the special considerations of each. (See pp. 218–220.)

10. Describe assessment of the airway and the respiratory system. (See pp. 220–225.)

11. Discuss pulse oximetry and capnography and describe the prehospital use of both. (See pp. 223–225.)

12. Describe the procedures used to manually open the airway. (See pp. 226–228.)

13. Discuss indications, contraindications, and methods for insertion of the following mechanical airways: (See below pages.)

- oropharyngeal airway (pp. 228–229)

- nasopharyngeal airway (pp. 230–231)
- esophageal obturator airway (EOA) (pp. 232–236)
- esophageal gastric tube airway (EGTA) (p. 236)
- Pharyngeo-tracheal Lumen (PtL) airway (pp. 265–267)
- esophageal tracheal combiTube (ETC) airway (pp. 267–269)

14. List the equipment used to perform endotracheal intubation. (See pp. 236–240.)

15. Recall the indications, contraindications, and alternatives of endotracheal intubation. (See pp. 240–242.)

16. Explain the need for rapid placement of the endotracheal tube. (See pp. 241–242.)

17. State the precautions that should be used when intubating a trauma patient. (See pp. 241–242.)

18. List and demonstrate the steps in performing endotracheal intubation. (See pp. 242–245.)

19. Describe the various methods used to assure correct placement of the endotracheal tube. (See pp. 245–246.)

20. Identify the indications, contraindications, and methods of performing a cricothyrotomy and percutaneous transtracheal catheter ventilation. (See pp. 270–274.)

21. Discuss the indications, contraindications, and methods of performing suctioning. (See pp. 275–276.)

22. Discuss and describe the various oxygen administration devices used in prehospital care and describe the advantages and disadvantages of each. (See pp. 277–279.)

23. Discuss indications, contraindications, and methods for using the following devices:

- pocket mask. (See pp. 279–280.)
- bag-valve-mask device. (See p. 280.)
- demand valve resuscitator. (See pp. 280–281.)
- automatic transport ventilator (ATV). (See pp. 281–282.)

Medic 1 responds to a call to assist a patient who has collapsed at home. Upon arrival, paramedics Al Robinson and Emma Ramirez find a 58-year-old female supine on the floor next to her living room couch. After moving a coffee table to reach the patient, they find her unresponsive. Al employs the modified jaw-thrust technique to open her airway. He then checks for respiration and finds that the patient is not breathing. The paramedics quickly insert an oropharyngeal airway and provide ventilatory support with a bag-valve-mask device and 100 % oxygen.

As resuscitative efforts continue, Emma determines that the patient is pulseless and initiates chest compressions. A "Quick-Look" ECG is obtained which reveals ventricular fibrillation. Al readies the defibrillator and delivers one 200-Joule countershock. The patient immediately regains a sinus rhythm with a palpable carotid pulse. Because of copious upper airway secretions, Emma suctions the upper airway in preparation for endotracheal intubation. Following suctioning, she applies Sellick's maneuver. Al then inserts an endo-

tracheal tube under direct visualization of the vocal cords. An end-tidal CO_2 detector is connected to the endotracheal tube, and the patient is ventilated with a bag-valve device and 100 % oxygen. Endotracheal placement of the tube is confirmed by color change on the end-tidal CO_2 detector, the presence of bilateral symmetrical breath sounds, and the absence of breath sounds over the epigastrium. After securing the tube, paramedics place a pulse oximeter and monitor the oxygen saturation.

As paramedics move the patient to the ambulance, her oxygen saturation suddenly drops. The paramedics re-evaluate the patient and note that breath sounds on the left side of the chest have disappeared. Immediately recognizing the problem, Emma slowly pulls back the endotracheal tube approximately 1 centimeter until breath sounds can once again be heard bilaterally.

Medic 1 transports the patient to the hospital emergency department without further incident. Although the patient has responded to initial treatment modalities, she later dies in the intensive care unit.

INTRODUCTION

In any patient-care situation, you must immediately establish and maintain an open airway. Many procedures and devices, varying significantly in level of sophistication, are available to assist you in this all-important step. Once you have established the airway, you must determine whether the patient is breathing. If breathing is adequate, continue to maintain the airway and administer supplemental oxygen. If breathing is inadequate, or absent, start artificial ventilation.

Chapter 11 helps you to better understand such vital, life-saving procedures. It opens with a discussion of anatomy and physiology of the respiratory system as it applies to advanced prehospital care. Next, it describes assessment of the airway and respiratory system. The chapter then discusses principles of airway management and mechanical ventilation, with emphasis on advanced airway procedures available to paramedics today.

ANATOMY OF THE RESPIRATORY SYSTEM

The respiratory system provides the body with a constant source of oxygen, while at the same time removing carbon dioxide and other waste products. *Oxygen* is the odorless, colorless, tasteless gas necessary for the conversion of essential nutrients into energy. *Carbon dioxide*, on the other hand, is a waste product of energy production that must be continuously removed. In order for this process to occur, the patient must have an open airway, intact respiratory muscles, unobstructed respiratory passages, adequate pulmonary blood flow, and appropriate neurological control.

For study, the respiratory system can be divided into two areas: the *upper airway* and the *lower airway*. The upper airway extends from the oral and nasal openings to the larynx. The lower airway extends from below the larynx to the terminal alveoli.

Anatomy of the Upper Airway

The upper airway extends from the mouth and nose to the larynx. Its components are the *nasal cavity*, *oral cavity*, and *pharynx*. (See Figure 11-1.)

Nasal Cavity   The nasal cavity is the superior-most portion of the airway. The maxillary, frontal, nasal, ethmoid, and sphenoid bones form the lateral and superior walls of the nasal cavity. The nasal cavity is divided into right and left sides by the cartilaginous nasal **septum**.

Air enters the nasal cavity through the *external nares*. The incoming air is initially filtered by nasal hairs just inside the external nares. The air then

■ **septum** a wall that divides a chamber into two cavities.

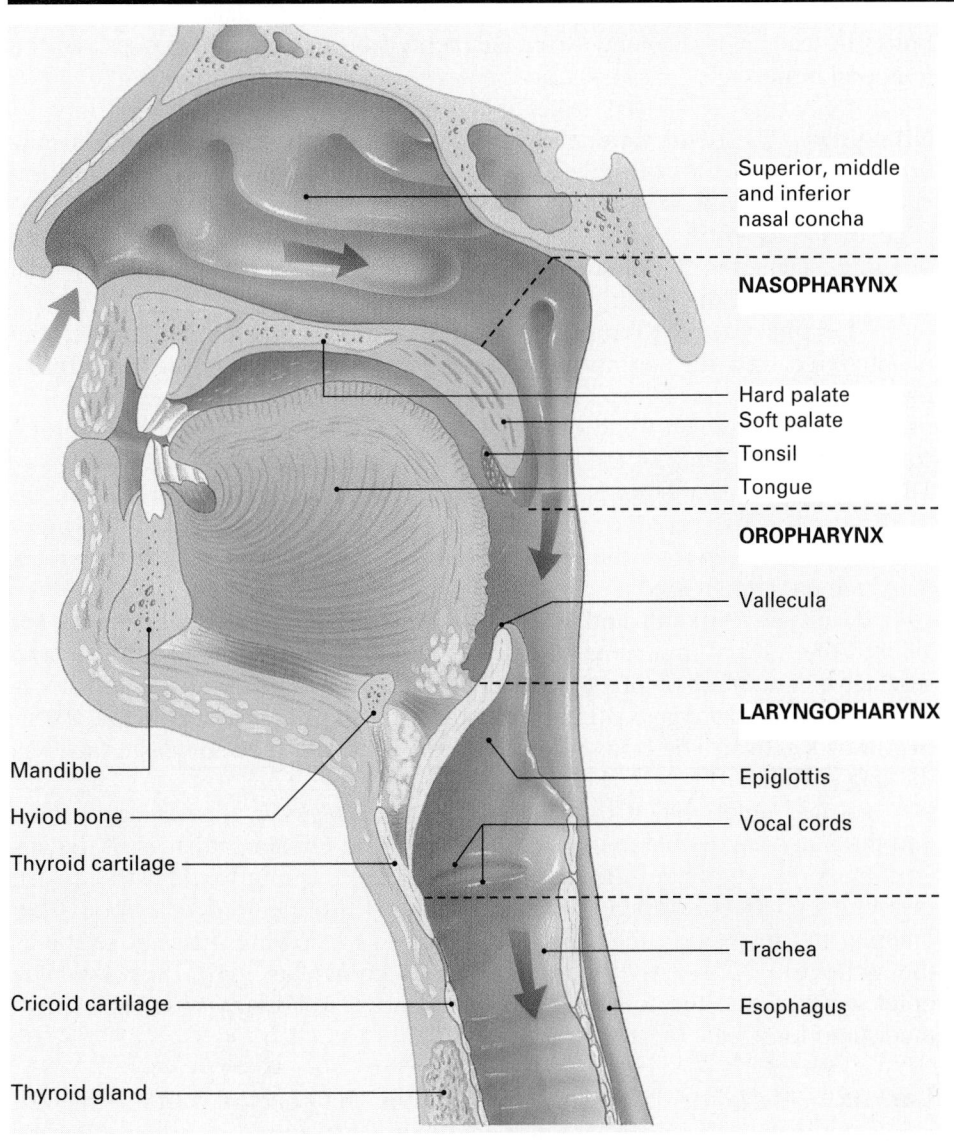

Superior, middle and inferior nasal concha

NASOPHARYNX

Hard palate
Soft palate
Tonsil
Tongue

OROPHARYNX

Vallecula

LARYNGOPHARYNX

Mandible
Hyiod bone
Thyroid cartilage

Epiglottis
Vocal cords

Cricoid cartilage

Trachea

Esophagus

Thyroid gland

FIGURE 11-1   Anatomy of the upper airway.

proceeds into the nasal cavity where it strikes three bony projections called *conchae* or *turbinates*. These shelf-like structures, called the *superior conchae*, *middle conchae*, and *inferior conchae*, cause turbulent airflow. This turbulence helps deposit any airborne particles on the *mucous membrane* that lines the nasal cavity. The **mucous membrane** is covered with **mucus** and has a rich blood supply. Because of this, air entering the nose is immediately warmed, filtered, and humidified. In fact, by the time air reaches the lower airway, it is at body temperature (37° C), 100 % humidified, and virtually free of airborne particles. The particles entrapped on the mucous membrane are then propelled to the back of the pharynx by hair-like fibers called **cilia** and subsequently swallowed. Air exits the nasal cavity through the *internal nares*. It then enters the nasopharynx.

Oral Cavity

The mouth, or *oral cavity*, is bordered by the cheeks, the hard and soft *palates*, and the *tongue*. Fleshy folds of skin called the *lips* surround the opening of the mouth. Behind the lips lie the *gums* and *teeth*.

The hard and soft palates form the top of the oral cavity. The tongue, a large mass of muscle, rests on the bottom of the cavity. It attaches to the mandible and the hyoid bone through a series of muscles and ligaments. The U-shaped *hyoid bone* is located just beneath the chin. The hyoid is unique: the only bone in the axial skeleton that does not articulate with any other bone. Instead, it is suspended by ligaments from the styloid process of the temporal bone.

Pharynx

The *pharynx*, or throat, is a muscular tube that extends vertically from the back of the soft palate to the upper end of the esophagus and trachea. It allows the flow of air into and out of the respiratory tract and the passage of foods and liquids into the digestive system. It contains several openings, including the **eustachian tubes** (from the middle ear), the internal nares, the mouth, the larynx, and the esophagus.

The pharynx is divided into three regions: the nasopharynx, the oropharynx, and the laryngopharynx. The *nasopharynx* is the uppermost part of the pharynx. It extends from the back of the nasal opening to the plane of the soft palate. The *oropharynx* is the section that extends from the soft palate in the back of the mouth to the hyoid bone below the lower jaw. The *laryngopharynx* extends from the hyoid bone at the base of the tongue to the esophagus, posteriorly, and to the trachea, anteriorly. The laryngopharynx, also known as the *hypopharynx,* is important in regard to airway management techniques.

Because the mouth and pharynx serve dual purposes (passageway for air into the trachea and lungs, for solids and liquids into the esophagus and stomach), a number of physical mechanisms help prevent accidental blockage. To prevent foreign material from entering the trachea and lungs, sensitive nerves activate the body's cough and swallowing mechanisms as well as the **gag reflex**.

Located anteriorly in the pharynx are the *epiglottis*, the laryngeal inlet, and the mucous-membrane-covered arytenoid and cricoid cartilages of the larynx. Immediately behind the laryngopharynx are the fourth and fifth cervical vertebral bodies. The epiglottis, a leaf-shaped cartilage, prevents food from entering the respiratory tract during the act of swallowing. Just above this is the **vallecula**. On either side are recesses known as *pyriform fossa*. The epiglottis is connected to the hyoid bone and mandible by a series of ligaments and muscles.

Larynx

The *larynx* is the structure that joins the pharynx with the trachea. Lying midline in the neck, inferior to the hyoid bone and anterior to the

■ **mucous membrane** a membrane lining many of the body cavities that handle air transport; it usually contains small, mucous-secreting glands.

■ **mucus** a thick, slippery secretion that functions as a lubricant and protects various surfaces.

■ **cilia** hair-like fibers projecting from the cells that propel mucus.

■ **eustachian tube** a tube connecting the pharynx and the middle ear.

■ **gag reflex** the act of retching or striving to vomit; a normal reflex triggered by touching the soft palate or the throat.

■ **vallecula** the depression between the epiglottis and the base of the tongue.

esophagus, it consists of the thyroid cartilage, cricoid cartilage, the upper end of the trachea, vocal cords, and **arytenoid folds**. The walls of the larynx are supported by cartilages that prevent it from collapsing during inhalation.

The main laryngeal cartilage is the *thyroid cartilage*, or Adam's apple. In adults, the portion of the thyroid cartilage housing the vocal cords is the narrowest part of the upper airway. The thyroid cartilage consists of two large plates that form the anterior wall of the larynx and give it its V-shaped appearance. The posterior wall of the thyroid cartilage is open and consists of muscle. The upper end of the thyroid cartilage is attached to the hyoid bone by the *thyrohyoid membrane*. The thyroid cartilage is larger in males than in females.

Beneath the thyroid cartilage is the *cricoid cartilage*. It forms the inferior walls of the larynx and is attached to the trachea's first ring of cartilage. Unlike the thyroid and tracheal cartilages, which are open on their posterior surfaces, the cricoid cartilage forms a complete ring. Just behind this lies the *esophagus*. In children, the cricoid cartilage is the narrowest part of the laryngeal airway. Connecting the inferior border of the thyroid cartilage with the superior aspect of the cricoid membrane is the **cricothyroid membrane**.

Lying on the rear surface of the cricoid cartilage are two pyramid-shaped *arytenoid cartilages*. These attach to the vocal folds and pharyngeal walls, and can open and close the vocal cords. Within the laryngeal cavity lie the true and false vocal cords. *True vocal cords* regulate the passage of air through the larynx and control the production of sound. As the muscles of the larynx contract, these cords change shape and vibrate, thus producing sounds of different pitches. The vocal cords can also close together to prevent foreign bodies from entering the airway. The space between the vocal cords is referred to as the **glottic opening**. The passage of an endotracheal tube between the vocal cords interferes not only with the creation of sound, but also with coughing. The *false vocal cords* are located above the true vocal cords. (See Figure 11-2.)

■ **arytenoid folds** cupped or ladle-shaped tissues found posterior to the vocal cords.

■ **cricothyroid membrane** the membrane located between the cricoid and thyroid cartilages of the larynx.

■ **glottic opening** the slit-like opening between the vocal cords; also known as the glottis.

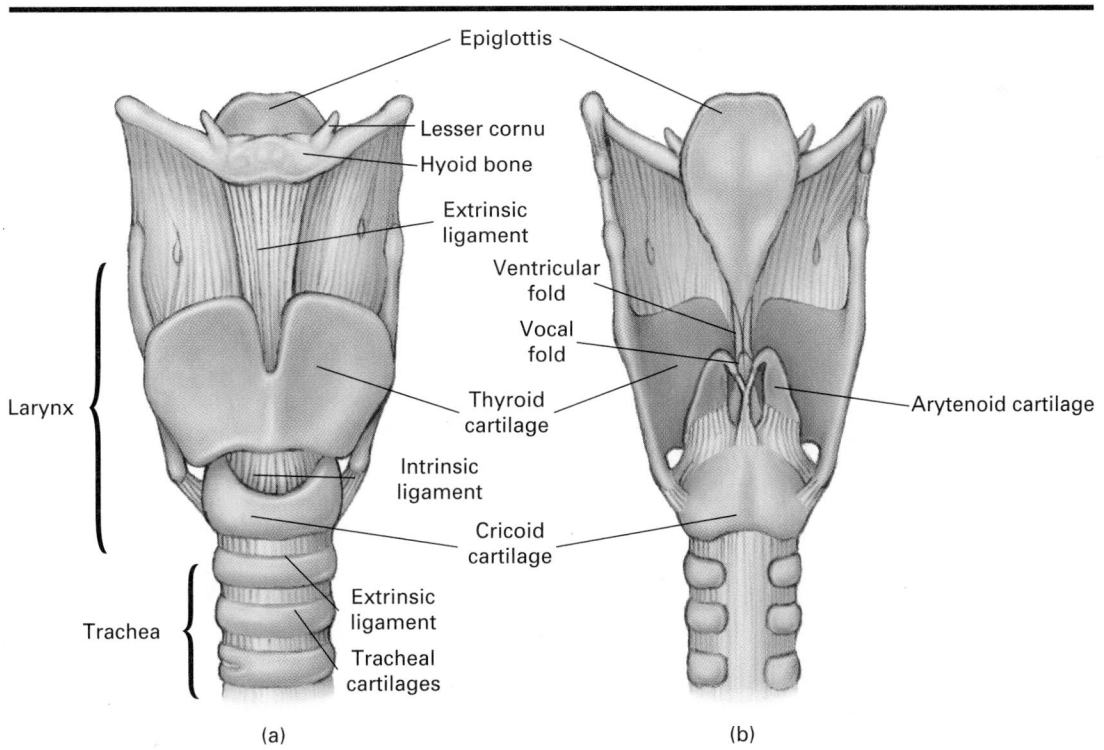

FIGURE 11-2 Internal anatomy of the upper airway: (a) anterior view; (b) posterior view.

Most of the larynx is lined with a ciliated tissue that secretes mucus. This membrane, richly lined with nerve endings from the vagus nerve, is so sensitive that any irritation sparks a cough, or forceful exhalation of a large volume of air: First, air is drawn into the respiratory passageways. Next, the glottic opening shuts tightly, trapping the air within the lungs. Then the abdominal and thoracic muscles contract, pushing against the diaphragm and increasing intrathoracic pressure. The vocal cords suddenly open, and a burst of air forces foreign particles out of the lungs. Due to the degree of vagal innervation, stimulation of the laryngeal mucous membrane (by a laryngoscope or endotracheal tube) can cause bradycardia, hypotension, and a decreased respiratory rate.

Anatomy of the Lower Airway

■ **alveoli** the microscopic air sacs where the oxygen-carbon dioxide exchange takes place.

The lower airway extends from below the larynx to the **alveoli**. It is in the lower airway that respiratory gas exchange occurs. (See Figure 11-3.)

Trachea   Air enters the lower airway from the upper airway via the *trachea*. The trachea is a tube, 10-12 centimeters long, connecting the larynx with the mainstem bronchi in the lungs. It is maintained in an open position by incomplete, C-shaped, cartilaginous rings extending throughout its length. The trachea is lined by respiratory epithelium containing cilia and mucus-producing cells. This mucus tends to trap particulate matter not filtered out in the upper airway. The cilia move the trapped particulate matter up and out of the trachea and into the mouth where it is swallowed or expelled.

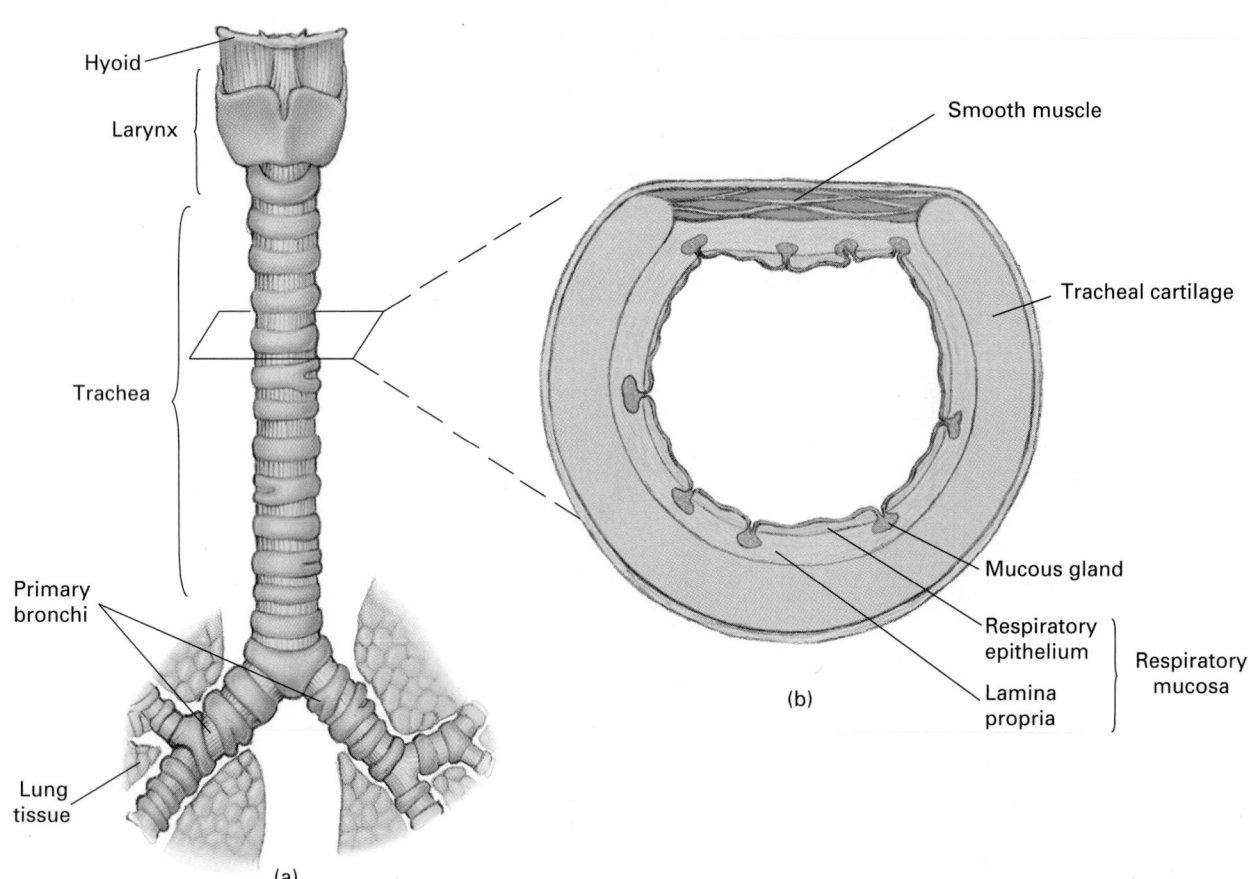

FIGURE 11-3 Anatomy of the lower airway.

Bronchi   At the **carina**, the trachea divides into the right and the left mainstem *bronchi*. The right mainstem bronchus is almost straight, whereas the left mainstem bronchus angles more acutely to the left. The mainstem bronchi then divide into the secondary bronchi. These secondary bronchi ultimately divide into the *bronchioles*, or the small airways. The bronchioles contain smooth muscle that can contract, thus reducing the diameter of the airway. This ultimately decreases the amount of respiratory gases that can be transported. After approximately 22 divisions, the bronchioles become *respiratory bronchioles*. They contain only muscular connective tissue and have a limited ability for gas exchange.

■ **carina** the point at which the trachea bifurcates into the right and left mainstem bronchi.

Alveoli   The respiratory bronchioles divide into the *alveolar ducts*. These terminate in the *alveolar sacs*. Most gas exchange takes place in the alveoli, although limited gas exchange may occur in the alveolar ducts and respiratory bronchioles.

The *alveoli* comprise the key functional unit of the respiratory system. Most oxygen and carbon dioxide gas exchanges take place here. Together, the alveoli possess more than 40 square meters of surface area (enough to cover half of a tennis court). The hollow alveoli are surrounded by a thin alveolar membrane often only one- to-two cell layers thick. They resist collapse largely because of the presence of *surfactant*—a chemical that tends to decrease the surface tension of the alveoli. (See Figure 11-4.)

Lung Parenchyma   The alveoli are the terminal end of the respiratory tree and the functional units of the lungs. However, there is additional lung tissue, called *lung parenchyma*, present. The lung **parenchyma** is composed of primary pulmonary lobules. These are the anatomic divisions of the lungs. The right lung contains three lobes, referred to as the upper lobe, middle lobe, and lower lobe. The left lung has only two lobes, the upper lobe and the lower lobe.

■ **parenchyma** the principal or essential parts of an organ.

Pleura   The lungs are covered by connective tissue called *pleura*. Unattached to the lung, except at the hilum (the point at which the bronchi enter the lungs), the pleura consists of two layers. The *visceral pleura* covers the lungs and does not contain nerve fibers. In contrast, the *parietal pleura* lines the thoracic cavity and does contain nerve fibers. A small amount of *pleural fluid* usually can be found in the pleural space, a potential space between the two layers of pleura.

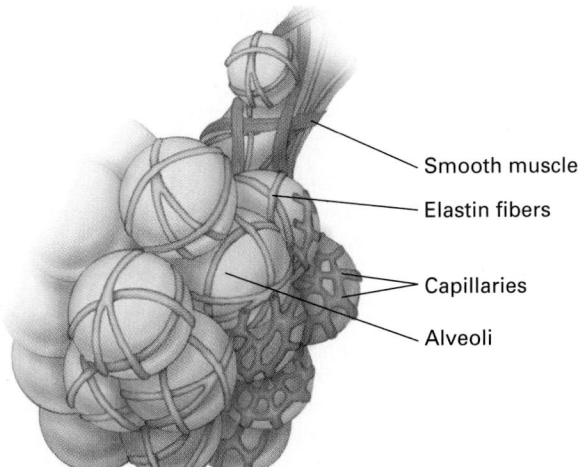

Smooth muscle

Elastin fibers

Capillaries

Alveoli

FIGURE 11-4   Anatomy of the alveoli.

PHYSIOLOGY OF THE RESPIRATORY SYSTEM

This section will detail the physiology of the respiratory system. An understanding of respiratory physiology is essential to providing competent advanced prehospital care.

Respiration and Ventilation

■ **respiration** the exchange of gases between a living organism and its environment.

Respiration is defined as the exchange of gases between a living organism and its environment. *Pulmonary respiration* occurs in the lungs when the respiratory gases are exchanged between the alveoli and the red blood cells in the pulmonary capillaries through the capillary membranes. *Cellular respiration*, on the other hand, occurs in the peripheral capillaries and is the exchange of the respiratory gases between the red blood cells and the various body tissues. **Ventilation** is the mechanical process whereby air is taken into and out of the lungs.

■ **ventilation** mechanical process that moves air in and out of the lungs.

Respiratory Cycle

The lungs have no intrinsic capability to contract or expand. Pulmonary ventilation, therefore, depends upon changes in pressure within the thoracic cavity. The *respiratory cycle* requires coordinated interaction between the respiratory system, the central nervous system, and the musculoskeletal system.

The respiratory cycle begins when the lungs have achieved a normal expiration. At this point, the pressure inside the thoracic cavity is equal to atmospheric pressure. The thoracic cavity is a closed space, with the trachea as the only opening to the external environment. The size of the thoracic cavity can be made larger by contracting the diaphragm and the intercostal muscles. Contraction of the diaphragm results in its downward movement, while contraction of the intercostal muscles results in outward expansion of the chest wall. In respiratory inadequacy, this process can be augmented by the use of *accessory respiratory muscles,* such as the strap muscles of the neck and the abdominal muscles. Both serve to increase the size of the thoracic cavity. The highly elastic lungs immediately assume the contour of the thoracic cavity. This is because of the negative pressure in the pleural space.

Increasing the size of the thoracic cavity decreases the intrathoracic pressure. As intrathoracic pressure decreases, air rushes into the lungs through the trachea (*inspiration*). When the pressure in the thoracic cavity again reaches that of atmospheric pressure, the air exchange stops. The respiratory muscles now relax, which in turn decreases the size of the chest cavity, thus increasing intrathoracic pressure. This causes air to rush out of the lungs through the trachea (*expiration*) until intrathoracic and atmospheric pressure are again equalized. Normal expiration is a passive process, while inspiration is an active, energy-utilizing process.

Pulmonary Circulation

An intact circulatory system is also required for respiration. In fact, the amount of blood pumped to the lungs is the same as pumped to the peripheral tissue. Body cells take oxygen from red blood cells in the arterial system and return carbon dioxide to red blood cells in the venous system. The venous system presents this deoxygenated blood to the right side of the heart. The right ventricle pumps blood into the *pulmonary artery*. This artery immediately divides into the right and the left pulmonary arteries, each supplying the respective lung. Both branches quickly divide into smaller vessels that end in the *pulmonary capillaries*. The pulmonary capillaries are spread across the surface of the alveoli where the blood can pick up oxygen diffusing through the *alveolar/capillary membranes*. After this occurs, the pulmonary capillaries recombine into larger veins, eventually terminating in the *pulmonary veins*. The pulmonary veins empty this oxygenated blood into the left atrium of the heart. It is then transported, via the left ventricle, to the systemic arterial system.

The lung tissue itself receives little of its blood supply from the pulmonary arteries and veins. Instead, *bronchial arteries* that branch from the aorta provide most of the blood supply. *Bronchial veins* return blood from the lungs to the superior vena cava.

Gas Exchange in the Lungs

As previously detailed, gas exchange in the lungs occurs in opposite patterns to those in the periphery. Blood presented to the lungs is low in oxygen saturation and high in carbon-dioxide saturation; blood presented to the tissues is high in oxygen saturation and low in carbon-dioxide saturation.

Measurement of Oxygen and Carbon Dioxide Levels
The amount of oxygen and carbon dioxide in the blood can be determined by measuring the **partial pressure** of those gases. Partial pressure is the pressure exerted by each of the components of a gas mixture. In others words, any partial pressure is a fractional concentration of the total gas mixture. Total gas pressure at sea level equals approximately 760 mm/Hg or 14.7 pounds per square inch. Since 1 millimeter of mercury pressure equals 1 Torr, the terms mm/Hg and Torr are interchangeable. But the latter is preferable. The partial pressure can be calculated by taking the total atmospheric pressure and multiplying it by the percentage of the desired gas present. For example, to calculate the partial pressure of oxygen at normal atmospheric pressure, multiply the percentage of oxygen present in atmospheric air (21 percent) by the atmospheric pressure (760 Torr). The computation is as follows.

■ **partial pressure** the pressure exerted by each component of a gas mixture.

$$760 \text{ Torr} \times 0.21 = 159.6 \text{ Torr}$$

Our atmosphere consists of four major respiratory gases: nitrogen (N_2), oxygen (O_2), carbon dioxide (CO_2), and water (H_2O). Although nitrogen is metabolically inert, it is necessary for the inflation of gas-filled body cavities such as the chest. These four respiratory gases are present in the environment in the following partial pressures and concentrations:

Gas	Partial Pressure	Concentration
Nitrogen	597.0 Torr	78.62%
Oxygen	159.0 Torr	20.84%
Carbon Dioxide	0.3 Torr	0.04%
Water	3.7 Torr	0.5%
TOTAL	760.0 Torr	100.00%

If you look at these same gases after the air has been taken into the alveoli, the partial pressures and concentrations are somewhat different:

Gas	Partial Pressure	Concentration
Nitrogen	569.0 Torr	74.9%
Oxygen	104.0 Torr	13.7%
Carbon Dioxide	40.0 Torr	5.2%
Water	47.0 Torr	6.2%
TOTAL	760.0 Torr	100.0%

Since alveolar partial pressure and arterial partial pressure are essentially the same, normal arterial partial pressures for oxygen and carbon dioxide may be expressed as follows:

$$\text{Oxygen } (PaO_2) = 100 \text{ Torr (Average} = 80 - 100)$$

$$\text{Carbon Dioxide } (PaCO_2) = 40 \text{ Torr (Average} = 35 - 40)$$

Alveolar partial pressures are represented by the abbreviation PA (e.g., PAO_2) while arterial partial pressures are represented by the abbreviation Pa (e.g., PaO_2). However, because these values are almost always the same, the arterial gases usually appear in shortened notations PO_2 and PCO_2.

Diffusion

Diffusion is the movement of a gas from an area of higher partial pressure concentration to an area of lower partial pressure concentration. Diffusion helps transfer gases between (1) the lungs and the blood and (2) the blood and the peripheral tissues. The rate of diffusion of a gas across the pulmonary membranes depends on its solubility in water. For example, carbon dioxide is 21 times more soluble in water than oxygen and readily crosses the pulmonary capillary membranes.

In the lungs, oxygen leaves the area of higher PO_2, the alveoli, and enters the area of lower PO_2, the arterial blood in the pulmonary capillaries. Concurrently, carbon dioxide leaves the area of higher PCO_2, the arterial blood, and enters the area of lower PCO_2, the alveoli. The blood returns via the pulmonary vein to the heart and then moves into the systemic circulation.

Oxygen Concentrations in the Blood

Oxygen diffuses into the blood plasma, where it combines with hemoglobin. Hemoglobin approaches 100% saturation when the PaO_2 reaches 50–100 Torr. Each gram of saturated hemoglobin carries 1.34 milliliters of oxygen. Oxygen saturation is the ratio comparing the actual amount of oxygen available with the oxygen-carrying capacity of the blood. This ratio is represented by the following equation:

$$\text{Oxygen Saturation} = O_2 \text{ content} / O_2 \text{ capacity} \times 100 \ (\%)$$

It is important to point out that the vast majority of oxygen in the blood is carried on the hemoglobin molecule (approximately 97%). Very little oxygen is dissolved in the plasma. Since partial pressure measurements detect only the amount of oxygen dissolved in the plasma, and do not always reflect the total oxygen saturation, these measurements can be misleading. For example, a patient who has suffered carbon monoxide poisoning cannot transport enough oxygen to the peripheral tissues since carbon monoxide displaces oxygen from the hemoglobin molecule. But, if an arterial blood gas sample were taken, it might reveal a normal or high PaO_2. This indicates that adequate oxygen is reaching the blood, yet an inadequate amount of hemoglobin is available to transport the oxygen to the peripheral tissues.

Several factors can affect oxygen concentrations in the blood.

❑ *Inadequate alveolar ventilation* is caused by many factors—low inspired-oxygen concentration, respiratory muscle paralysis, and pulmonary conditions such as emphysema, asthma, and pneumothorax.

❑ *Decreased diffusion across the pulmonary membrane* may be caused when diffusion distance increases or the pulmonary membrane changes—for example when fluid enters the space between the alveolar membrane and the pulmonary capillary membrane (pulmonary edema).

❏ *Ventilation/perfusion mismatch* can occur when a portion of the alveoli collapses, as in **atelectasis**. Blood is then shunted past these collapsed alveoli without oxygenation or without removal of carbon dioxide. Also, **pulmonary embolism**, a blood clot in the pulmonary artery, can halt blood flow through the vessel. Consequently, a significant volume of blood is prevented from reaching the alveolar/capillary membranes where gas exchange can occur.

Oxygen derangements are corrected by increasing ventilation, administering supplemental oxygen, using intermittent positive pressure ventilation (IPPV), or by administering drugs to correct underlying problems such as pulmonary edema, asthma, and pulmonary embolism. The desired **FiO_2** should be selected based on the emergency being treated.

Carbon Dioxide Concentrations in the Blood

Carbon dioxide is transported mainly in the form of bicarbonate (HCO_3^-). Approximately 66% of carbon dioxide is transported as bicarbonate, while 33% is transported combined with hemoglobin. Less than 1% is dissolved in the plasma. Carbon dioxide concentrations in the blood are influenced by several factors including increased CO_2 production and/or decreased CO_2 elimination. Causes of CO_2 derangements include:

❏ *Increased CO_2 production*—which can result from several actions including:
  • Fever
  • Muscle exertion
  • Shivering
  • Metabolic processes resulting in the formation of acids (metabolic acids)
❏ *Decreased CO_2 elimination*—which results from decreased alveolar ventilation. Common causes include:
  • Respiratory depression by drugs
  • Airway obstruction
  • Impairment of the respiratory muscles
  • Obstructive disease states such as asthma and emphysema

Increased CO_2 levels (*hypercarbia*) are usually treated by increasing the ventilation and by correcting the underlying cause.

Regulation of Respiration

Respiration falls under the control of both the voluntary and involuntary nervous systems. However, most of the body's oxygen needs are monitored by involuntary control systems—various chemical, physical, and nervous reflexes such as those noted below.

Nervous Impulses from the Respiratory Center

The main respiratory center lies in the medulla, located in the brainstem. Various neurons within the medulla initiate impulses that result in respiration. A rise in the frequency of these impulses results in an increase in respiratory rate. Conversely, a decrease in firing frequency results in a lowered respiratory rate. The medulla is connected to the respiratory muscles primarily via the vagus nerve. If the medulla fails to initiate respiration, an additional control center located in the pons, called the *apneustic center*, assumes respiratory control to ensure the continuation of respirations. Expiration, on the other hand, is controlled by a third center, the *pneumotaxic center*, also located in the pons.

■ **atelectasis** a collapse of the alveoli, which in turn decreases ventilatory effectiveness.

■ **pulmonary embolism** blood clot or other thrombus in the pulmonary circulation that adversely affects oxygenation of the blood.

■ **FiO_2** the concentration of oxygen in inspired air.

■ **hypercarbia** excessive partial pressure of carbon dioxide in the blood.

Microscopic Stretch Receptors   During inspiration, the lungs become distended, activating what are known as *stretch receptors*. As the degree of stretch increases, these receptors fire more frequently. The impulses they send to the brainstem inhibit the medullary cells, decreasing the inspiratory stimulus. Thus, the respiratory muscles relax, allowing the elastic lungs to recoil and expel air from the body. Then, as the stretch decreases, the stretch receptors stop firing. This is referred to as the *Hering-Breuer reflex*—a process that prevents overexpansion of the lungs.

Chemoreceptors   Other involuntary controls include central chemical receptors in the medulla and peripheral chemoreceptors in the carotid bodies and in the arch of the aorta. These chemoreceptors are stimulated by decreased PaO_2, increased $PaCO_2$, and decreased pH. (The pH scale expresses degree of acidity or alkalinity. A lower pH indicates greater acidity; a higher pH indicates greater alkalinity. Chapter 12 will discuss pH in greater detail.) Cerebrospinal fluid (CSF) pH is the primary control of respiratory center stimulation. A change in the CSF pH occurs very quickly in relation to arterial PCO_2. A rise in the CSF pH inhibits respiration, while a decrease in CSF pH stimulates it. Because arterial PCO_2 is inversely related to pH, including CSF pH, it is seen as the normal neuroregulatory control of respirations. Any increase in the arterial PCO_2 will stimulate the peripheral chemoreceptors. They will then send impulses to the brainstem to increase respirations. And, as indicated, any increase in $PaCO_2$ will decrease CSF pH, which will also stimulate the central chemoreceptors. The result will be increased respirations. Conversely, low $PaCO_2$ levels will decrease chemoreceptor stimulation, thereby effectively decreasing respiratory activity.

✳ Never deprive the hypoxic patient of oxygen.

Hypoxic Drive   The body also constantly monitors the PaO_2 and the pH. In fact, *hypoxemia* (decreased partial pressure of oxygen in the blood) is a profound stimulus of respiration in a normal individual. People with chronic respiratory disease such as emphysema and chronic bronchitis tend to retain CO_2 and therefore have a chronically elevated $PaCO_2$. Chemoreceptors in the periphery eventually become accustomed to this chronic condition, and the central nervous system ceases dependence upon $PaCO_2$ to regulate respiration. These individuals have to depend on changes in PaO_2 to control respiration. Such a condition is termed *hypoxic drive*. Respiratory stimulation is increased when PaO_2 falls and inhibited when it climbs. High-volume oxygen administration to people with this condition can cause respiratory arrest. Because high-flow oxygen can quickly double or even triple the PaO_2, peripheral chemoreceptors cease to stimulate the respiratory centers, causing apnea. Although this is a potential threat, it is unlikely to occur in the limited time span of the prehospital setting.

Modified Forms of Respiration

There are several modified forms of respiration. They include:

- ❑ *Coughing*—forceful exhalation of a large volume of air from the lungs. This performs a protective function.
- ❑ *Sneezing*—sudden, forceful exhalation from the nose, usually caused by nasal irritation.
- ❑ *Hiccoughing*—sudden inspiration caused by spasmodic contraction of the diaphragm. It serves no known physiological purpose.
- ❑ *Sighing*—slow, deep inspiration followed by a prolonged expiration. Sighing hyperinflates the lungs and re-expands atelectatic areas.

❏ *Grunting*—a sound that occurs primarily in neonates when the infant expires air against a partially closed epiglottis. It is usually an indication of respiratory distress.

Measures of Respiratory Function

The *respiratory rate* is the number of respirations per minute—normally 12–20 breaths per minute in adults, 18–24 breaths per minute in children, 40–60 breaths per minute in infants. Several factors affect respiratory rate:

❏ *Fever*—increases rate
❏ *Anxiety*—increases rate
❏ *Pain*—increases rate
❏ *Hypoxia* (inadequate tissue oxygenation)—increases rate
❏ *Depressant drugs*—decrease rate
❏ *Sleep*—decreases rate

The capacity of the lungs and airways has been extensively studied and is important in emergency care. Maximum lung capacity in the average adult male is approximately 6 liters and is termed the *total lung capacity (TLC)*. There are some additional respiratory capacities and measurements paramedics must be familiar with. (See Figure 11-5.) These include:

❏ *Tidal Volume ($\dot{V}_T$)*. The tidal volume is the average volume of gas inhaled or exhaled in one respiratory cycle. In the adult male this is approximately 500 mL.
❏ *Dead Space Volume ($\dot{V}_D$)*. The dead space volume is the amount of gas in the tidal volume that remains in the passageways unavailable for gas exchange. It is approximately 150 mL in the adult male.
❏ *Alveolar Volume ($\dot{V}_A$)*. The alveolar volume is the amount of gas in the tidal volume that reaches the alveoli for gas exchange. It is approximately 350 mL in the adult male. The following equation shows this relationship.

$$\dot{V}T - \dot{V}D = \dot{V}A$$

❏ *Minute Volume ($\dot{V}_{min}$)*. The **minute volume** is the amount of gas moved in and out of the respiratory tract in one minute. It is represented in the following equations.

$$\dot{V}_{min} = \dot{V}_T - \dot{V}_D \times \text{Respiratory rate}$$

or

$$\dot{V}_{min} = \dot{V}_A \times \text{Respiratory rate}$$

❏ *Functional Reserve Capacity (FRC)*. The amount of air that can be forcefully exhaled after a maximum inspiration is termed the functional reserve capacity. It is approximately 4,500 mL in an adult male.

■ **minute volume ($\dot{V}_{min}$)** the amount of air inhaled and exhaled in one minute; it equals the respiratory rate times the tidal volume.

RESPIRATORY PROBLEMS

Respiratory emergencies may result from problems in the upper or lower airway, impairment of the respiratory muscles, or a problem with respiratory control centers in the brain.

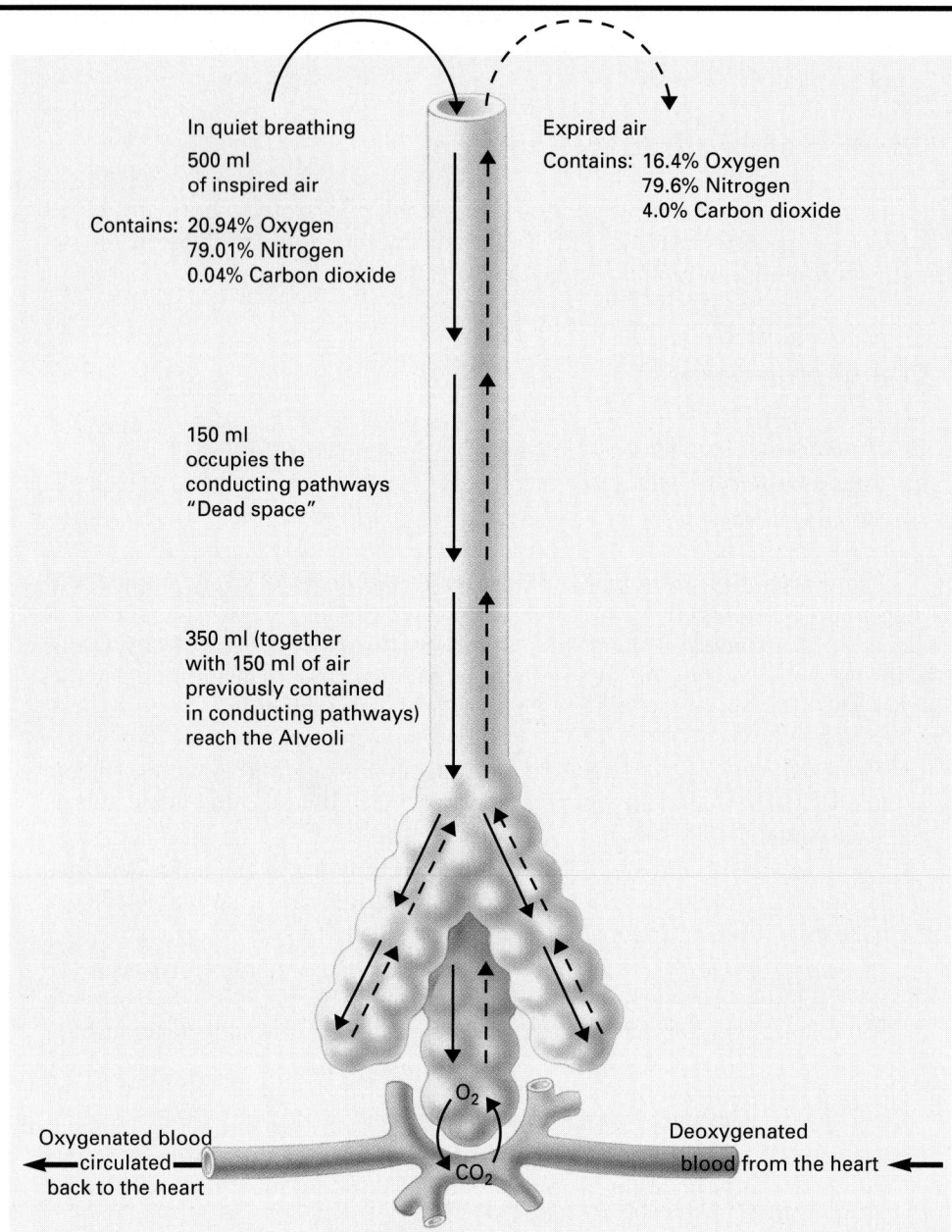

In quiet breathing
500 ml
of inspired air

Contains: 20.94% Oxygen
79.01% Nitrogen
0.04% Carbon dioxide

Expired air
Contains: 16.4% Oxygen
79.6% Nitrogen
4.0% Carbon dioxide

150 ml
occupies the
conducting pathways
"Dead space"

350 ml (together
with 150 ml of air
previously contained
in conducting pathways)
reach the Alveoli

O_2

CO_2

Oxygenated blood
circulated
back to the heart

Deoxygenated
blood from the heart

FIGURE 11-5   Gas exchange in the alveoli.

Airway Obstruction

Blockage of the airway is an immediate threat to the patient's life and a true emergency. Upper airway obstruction may be defined as "an interference with air movement through the upper airway." This interference can come from the tongue, foreign bodies, vomitus, blood, teeth, or something else.

Airway obstruction may be either "partial" or "complete." Partial obstruction allows for either adequate or poor air exchange. With adequate air exchange, the patient can cough effectively. Patients suffering poor air exchange can no longer generate an effective cough. They often emit a high-pitched noise while inhaling and may have increased breathing difficulty and cyanosis. Complete obstruction exists when airflow is not felt or heard from the nose and mouth, or when the patient cannot speak, breathe, or cough. A patient with complete airway obstruction will quickly become unconscious, and death will occur if the obstruction is not relieved. In the absence of breathing, complete airway obstruction can be recognized by the difficulty encountered when trying to ventilate the patient.

Tongue   The tongue is the most common cause of airway obstruction. (See Figure 11-6.) Normally, the submandibular muscles provide direct support of the tongue and indirect support of the epiglottis. In the absence of sufficient muscle tone, though, the relaxed tongue falls back against the rear of the pharynx, thus occluding the airway. The epiglottis may also block the airway at the level of the larynx. If the tongue and epiglottis are in this position, air-flow into the respiratory system is at least diminished, and breathing efforts may inadvertently suck the base of the tongue into an obstructing position. Airway blockage by the base of the tongue depends on the position of the head and jaw. It can occur regardless of whether the patient is in a lateral, supine, or prone position.

✳ Airway obstruction by the tongue can occur whether the patient is supine, lateral, or prone.

Foreign Body   Large, poorly chewed pieces of food can obstruct the upper airway by becoming lodged in the laryngopharynx. (Alcohol consumption and dentures are often involved in these cases.) This often occurs in restaurants and is frequently mistaken for a heart attack. It is commonly referred to as a "cafe coronary." The patient may clutch the neck between thumb and fingers, a universal distress signal. Children, especially toddlers, often aspirate foreign objects, as they have the tendency to put objects into their mouths.

Trauma   In trauma, particularly when the patient is unconscious, the air-way may be obstructed by loose teeth, facial bone fractures, tissue, and clot-ted blood. Blood contains many components—proteins, fibrin, water, and electrolytes—that may clog the alveoli, bronchioles, and bronchi if allowed to enter the lungs in large amounts. Additionally, penetrating or blunt trauma may obstruct the airway by fracturing or displacing the larynx, allowing the vocal cords to collapse into the tracheal lumen.

Laryngeal Spasm   *Laryngeal spasm* is another form of upper airway obstruction. Since the glottis is the narrowest part of an adult's airway, edema

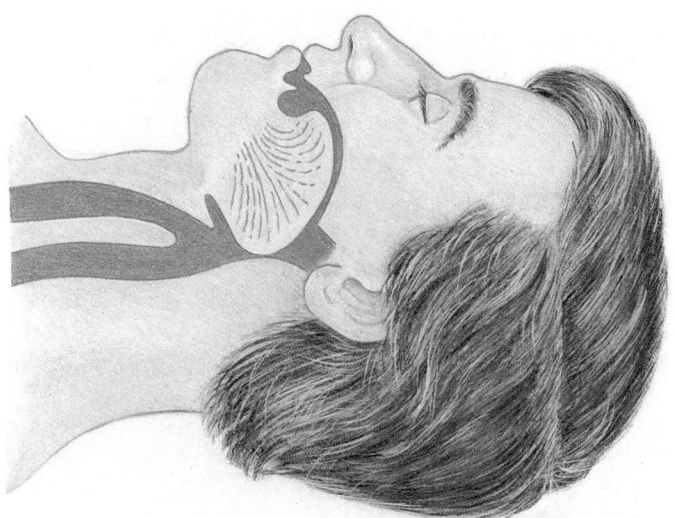

FIGURE 11-6 The tongue is the most common cause of air-way obstruction. In the unconscious patient, it can fall into the back of the throat, effectively closing the airway.

or spasm of the vocal cords is potentially lethal. Even moderate edema can severely obstruct airflow and result in asphyxia. Just beneath the mucous membrane that covers the vocal cords is a layer of loose tissue where blood or other fluids can accumulate. This tissue may swell following injury and the swelling will be slow to subside. Causes of laryngeal spasm include anaphylaxis, epiglottitis, and inhalation of super-heated air, smoke, or toxic substances.

Aspiration In adults, dentures, teeth, and vomitus are likely to obstruct the airway. Vomitus is made up of food particles, protein-dissolving enzymes, and hydrochloric acid that have been regurgitated from the stomach into the oropharynx. This mixture, if allowed to enter the lungs, can result in increased interstitial fluid and pulmonary edema, and can severely damage the alveoli. Saliva, like vomitus, contains digestive enzymes that can also damage the alveoli. Gas exchange can be seriously impaired by the marked increase in alveolar/capillary distance, thus causing **hypoxemia** and **hypercarbia**. These complications occur in 50–80% of patients who **aspirate** foreign matter. But they can usually be avoided by proper airway management and suction.

Inadequate Ventilation

As stated earlier, the adequate intake of oxygen and removal of carbon dioxide depend on sufficient minute volume respirations. A reduction of either the rate or the volume of inhalation leads to a reduction in minute volumes. In some cases, the respiratory rate may be rapid but so shallow that little air exchange takes place. This state of decreased ventilation may be brought on by depressed respiratory function, fractured ribs, a drug overdose, spinal injury, or head injury. It can lead to hypercarbia or hypoxia.

ASSESSMENT OF THE RESPIRATORY SYSTEM

Assessment of the respiratory system begins with the primary assessment followed, when practical, by a thorough secondary assessment.

Primary Assessment

The purpose of the primary assessment is to identify any immediate threats to the patient's life. First, the airway should be assessed to assure that it is **patent**. The presence of snoring or gurgling may indicate potential problems with the airway.

Second, the adequacy of breathing should be determined. If the patient is conscious and speaking without difficulty, you can assume that the airway is patent.

Patients with altered mental status warrant further evaluation. Feel for movement of air with your hand or cheek. (See Figure 11-7.) Look for rise and fall of the chest. (See Figure 11-8.) Normally, a person's chest will rise and fall with each respiratory cycle. In an adult patient, the respiratory rate generally ranges between 12 and 20 breaths per minute. Breathing should be spontaneous and regular. Irregular breathing suggests a significant problem and usually requires some ventilatory support. The chest wall should be observed for any area of asymmetrical movement. This condition, known as **paradoxical breathing**, may suggest a **flail chest**.

If the patient is not breathing, or if you suspect problems with the airway, open the airway by using the head-tilt/chin-lift or jaw-thrust maneuver, as described later. If the possibility of trauma exists, use the modified jaw-thrust method instead and maintain stabilization of the cervical spine. Once the air-

■ **hypoxemia** reduced partial pressure of oxygen in the blood.

■ **hypercarbia** increased partial pressure of carbon dioxide in the blood.

■ **aspirate** to take foreign material into the lungs during inhalation.

■ **patent** (n. *patency*) open; not obstructed.

✳ The assessment of the "A" and "B" of the primary survey will evaluate respiratory effectiveness.

■ **paradoxical breathing** an asymmetrical chest wall movement caused by a defect (flail chest) that lessens respiratory efficiency.

■ **flail chest** a defect in the chest wall that allows for free movement of a segment, causing paradoxical chest wall motion.

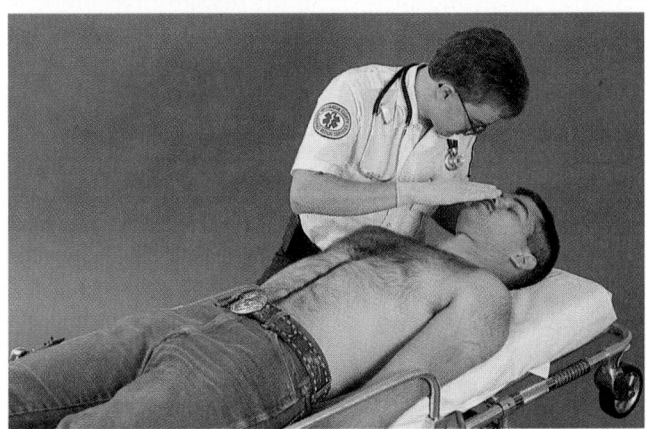

FIGURE 11-7   Feel for air movement with your hand or cheek.

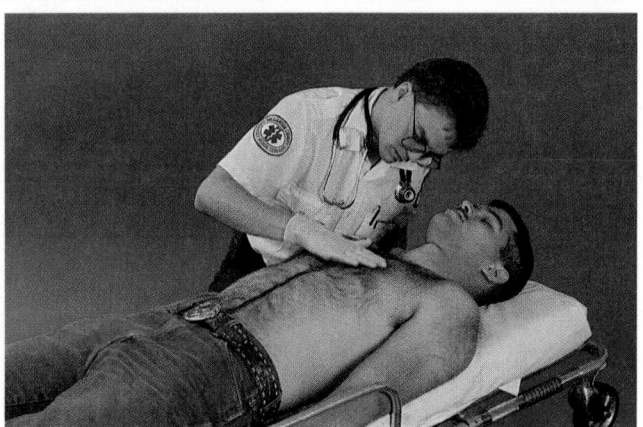

FIGURE 11-8   Assess the rise and fall of the patient's chest.

way is open, re-evaluate the status of breathing. If breathing is adequate, provide supplemental oxygen and assess circulation. If breathing is inadequate, or absent, begin artificial ventilation. (See Figure 11-9.) When assisting a patient's breathing with a ventilatory device (bag-valve-mask device or other positive-pressure device), or after placing an airway adjunct (nasopharyngeal airway, oropharyngeal airway, or endotracheal tube), monitor the rise and fall of the chest to determine correct usage and placement. (These ventilatory devices and mechanical airways will be discussed in detail later in this chapter.)

Secondary Assessment

Following completion of the primary assessment, and correction of any immediate life threats, the secondary assessment should be completed.

History   Inquire about recent trauma, food intake, and drinking. Determine whether the onset of the problem was slow or rapid. Ask about allergies and anaphylaxis. If an injury is involved, evaluate the mechanism of injury. Blunt trauma to the neck may have caused a laryngeal injury.

Physical Examination   Begin the physical assessment with inspection. Evaluate the adequacy of breathing. Note any obvious signs of trauma. Assess

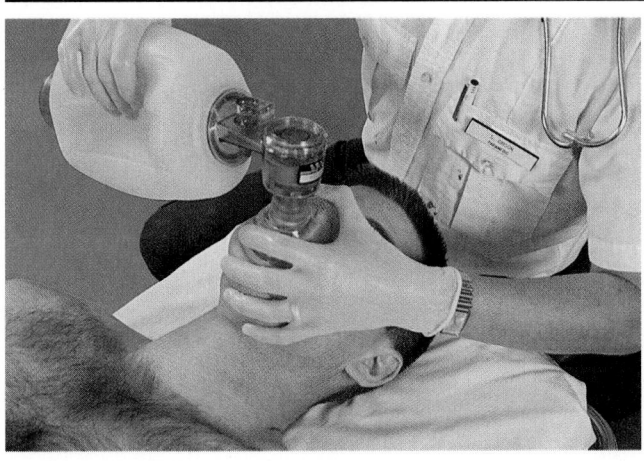

FIGURE 11-9   When ventilating with a bag-valve mask, gauge the effectiveness of airflow into the lungs by noting lung compliance and how quickly the bag empties.

skin color as an indicator of oxygenation status. Early in respiratory compromise, the sympathetic nervous system will be stimulated to help offset the lack of oxygen. When this happens, the skin will often appear pale and diaphoretic. Cyanosis is another sign of respiratory distress. When oxygen binds with the hemoglobin, the blood appears "bright red." Deoxygenated hemoglobin is blue and will give the skin a bluish color (cyanosis). However, this is not a reliable sign, since severe tissue hypoxia is possible without cyanosis. In fact, cyanosis is considered a late sign of respiratory compromise. When it does appear, cyanosis will usually affect the lips, fingernails, and skin. A red skin rash, especially if accompanied by hives, may indicate an allergic reaction. A cherry red skin discoloration may be associated with carbon monoxide poisoning.

Note any decrease or increase in the respiratory rate, one of the earliest indicators of respiratory distress. Also, look for use of the accessory respiratory muscles—intercostal retractions, suprasternal retractions, use of the abdominal muscles—another indicator of respiratory distress. In infants and children, nasal flaring and grunting indicate respiratory distress.

Following inspection, listen for the adequacy of air movement at the mouth and nose. Then listen to the chest with a stethoscope. (See Figure 11-10.) In a prehospital setting, the sites to be auscultated include the right and left apex (just beneath the clavicle), the right and left base (eighth or ninth intercostal space, midclavicular line), and the right and left mid-axillary line (fourth or fifth intercostal space, on the lateral side of the chest). There are also six locations on the posterior chest that can be monitored. When the patient's condition permits, the posterior surface is actually preferred over the anterior one. At this location heart sounds do not interfere with auscultation. However, since patients are usually supine during airway management, the anterior and lateral positions usually prove more accessible. Sounds that point to airflow compromise include:

- ❑ *Snoring*—results from partial obstruction of the upper airway by the tongue
- ❑ *Gurgling*—results from the accumulation of blood, vomitus, or other secretions in the upper airway
- ❑ *Stridor*—a harsh, high-pitched sound heard on inhalation associated with laryngeal edema or constriction
- ❑ *Quiet*—the absence of breath sounds is an ominous finding and indicates a serious problem with the airway, breathing, or both.

When assessing the effectiveness of ventilatory support or the correct placement of an airway adjunct, realize that air movement into the epigastrium may sometimes mimic breath sounds. Thus, listening to the chest should be only one of several means used to assess air movement. Another method of checking correct placement of an airway adjunct is to auscultate over the epigastrium; it should be silent during ventilation. When providing ventilatory support, watch for signs of gastric distention. This will suggest inadequate hyperextension of the head, undue pressure generated by the ventilatory device, or improper placement of airway adjuncts. Listening over the sternal notch will also confirm the presence of airflow when an endotracheal tube is correctly placed in the trachea.

Finally, palpate. First, feel for the movement of air with the back of your hand or your cheek. If an endotracheal tube is in place, the proximal end can be checked for this movement. Next, palpate the chest for rise and fall. In addition, palpate the chest wall for symmetry, abnormal motion, crepitus, and subcutaneous emphysema.

When ventilating with a bag-valve device, gauge airflow into the lungs by noting compliance. *Compliance* refers to the stiffness or flexibility of the

✱ Air movement into the epigastrium may mimic breath sounds; hence auscultation is only one of several means used to confirm proper airway placement.

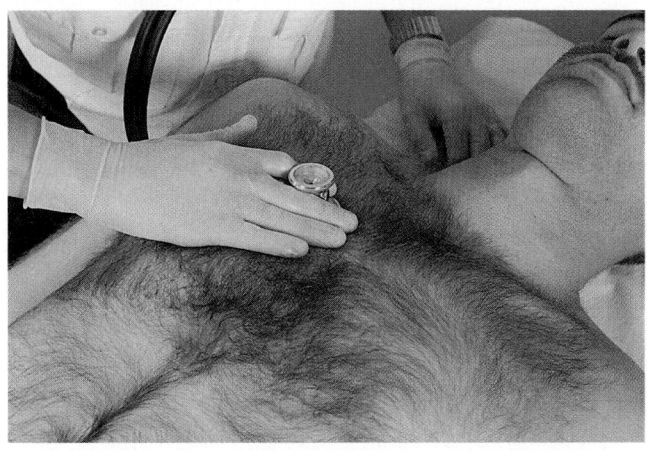

FIGURE 11-10 Auscultation of the chest provides a great deal of information about air movement through the lungs.

lung tissue, and it is determined by how easily air flows into the lungs. When compliance is good, airflow occurs with minimal resistance. When compliance is poor, ventilation is harder to achieve. Compliance is often poor in diseased lungs and in patients suffering from chest wall injuries or tension pneumothorax. It will decrease when the upper airway is obstructed by the tongue. If a patient shows poor compliance during ventilatory support, look for potential causes. Questions to aid in assessment include:

❑ Is the airway open?
❑ Is the head properly extended (non-trauma patients)?
❑ Is the patient developing tension pneumothorax?
❑ Is the endotracheal tube occluded?
❑ Has the endotracheal tube been inadvertently pushed into the right or left mainstem bronchus?

* If compliance is poor or changing, the paramedic should look for the cause.

A bag that compresses too quickly or "collapses" should arouse suspicion. It may indicate incorrect placement of the endotracheal tube into the esophagus or a defect in the bag-valve-mask device.

Pulse rate abnormalities may also suggest respiratory compromise. Tachycardia usually accompanies hypoxemia in an adult, while bradycardia hints at anoxia (absence or near-absence of oxygen) with imminent cardiac arrest.

Non-Invasive Respiratory Monitoring   Several devices are available for monitoring the effectiveness of oxygenation and ventilation. The two devices most commonly used in prehospital care are pulse oximeters and end-tidal carbon dioxide monitors.

Pulse Oximetry.   Pulse oximetry is now widely used in emergency care. A *pulse oximeter* is a device that measures oxygen saturation in peripheral tissues. It is *non-invasive* (does not require entering the body), and it is rapidly applied and easy to operate. Pulse oximetry readings are accurate and reflect, on a continuing basis, any changes in peripheral oxygen delivery. In fact, oximetry often detects problems with oxygenation before assessments of blood pressure, pulse, and respirations would detect a problem. (See Figure 11-11.)

Peripheral oxygen saturation is obtained by placing a sensor probe over a peripheral capillary bed, for example on a fingertip, toe, or ear lobe. In infants, the sensor can be wrapped around the heel and secured with tape. The sensor contains two light-emitting diodes and two sensors. The wave-

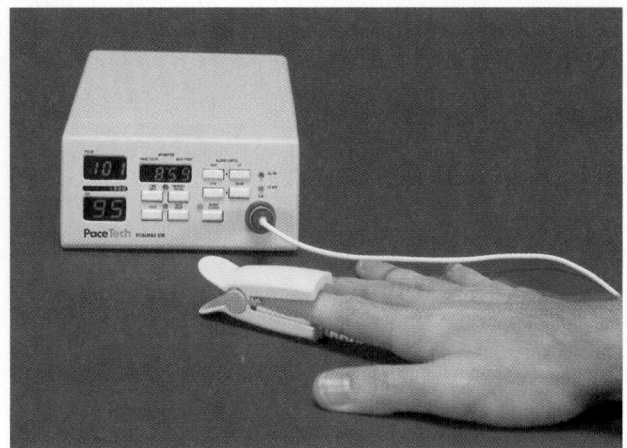

FIGURE 11-11 Pulse oximeters display the SpO_2 and pulse rate. The SpO_2 is displayed either as a number or with a visual display that also shows the wave-form of the pulse.

length of light emitted from one diode is specific for oxygenated hemoglobin (near red), while the other is specific for deoxygenated hemoglobin (infrared). Each hemoglobin state absorbs a certain amount of the emitted light, preventing it from reaching the corresponding sensor. The less light to reach the sensor, the greater the quantity of the specific type of hemoglobin present. The oximeter then compares the difference between these absorbed colors and calculates a ratio called the *oxygen saturation percentage (SpO_2)*.

Pulse oximeters display the SpO_2 and the pulse rate as detected by the sensors. The SpO_2 is displayed either as a number or with a visual display that also shows the wave-form of the pulse. The relationship between SpO_2 and the partial pressure of oxygen in the blood (PaO_2) is very complex. However, the SpO_2 does correlate with the PaO_2. The greater the PaO_2, the greater will be the oxygen saturation. It is important to remember that 98% of oxygen in the blood is carried on hemoglobin while only 2% is carried dissolved in the plasma. Thus, pulse oximetry provides an accurate analysis of peripheral oxygen delivery.

Pulse oximetry, when available, should be used in virtually any patient care situation. In fact, it is often called the "fifth vital sign." Use it during assessment to determine the patient's baseline value. Use it also to guide patient care and to monitor the patient's response to your interventions. Normal SpO_2 varies between 95% and 99%. Readings between 91% and 94% indicate mild hypoxia and warrant further evaluation and supplemental oxygen administration. Readings between 86% and 91% indicate moderate hypoxia. These patients should receive 100% supplemental oxygen. Readings of 85% or lower indicate severe hypoxia and warrant immediate intervention including the administration of 100% oxygen, ventilatory assistance, or both. The goal of therapy is to maintain the SpO_2 in the normal (95–99%) range.

The incidence of false readings with pulse oximetry is small. When it does occur, the oximeter generates an error signal or a blank screen. Causes of false readings include carbon monoxide poisoning, high-intensity lighting, and certain hemoglobin abnormalities. The absence of a pulse in an extremity will cause a false reading. In hypovolemia, and in severely anemic patients, the pulse oximetry reading may be misleading. While the SpO_2 reading may be normal, the total amount of hemoglobin available to carry oxygen may be so markedly decreased that the patient will remain hypoxic at the cellular level.

Pulse oximetry is now an important part of emergency care including prehospital care. Like the ECG monitor, it provides important information related to the patient. It is important to remember that it is only an additional tool. It does

Interpretation of Oximetry	
100–95%	normal
94–91%	mild hypoxia
91–86%	moderate hypoxia
85% or less	severe hypoxia

not replace other assessment or monitoring skills. Do not depend solely on pulse oximetry readings to guide care. Always consider and treat the whole patient.

Capnography. The measurement of exhaled carbon dioxide concentrations is called *capnography*. Devices that make such measurements are increasingly used in prehospital care. These devices, called *end-tidal carbon dioxide (ETCO$_2$) detectors*, are most commonly used to assess proper placement of an endotracheal tube. A lack of carbon dioxide in the exhaled air strongly indicates that the tube is placed in the esophagus, while the presence of carbon dioxide indicates proper tracheal placement.

End-tidal carbon dioxide detectors are available either as a disposable colorimetric device or as an electronic monitor. (See Figures 11-12 and 11-13.) The device is attached in-line between the endotracheal tube and the ventilation device. Proper tube placement is confirmed by a color change in the colorimetric device or by a light on the electronic monitor. Some devices now combine pulse oximetry, ETCO$_2$ detection, blood pressure, pulse rate, respiratory rate, and temperature monitors in one unit. (See Figure 11-14.)

As with pulse oximetry, you should use an ETCO$_2$ detector only as an adjunct to assessment of endotracheal placement. The device should be used in conjunction with other methods of assessment. It is not a replacement for actually visualizing the endotracheal tube passing through the vocal cords.

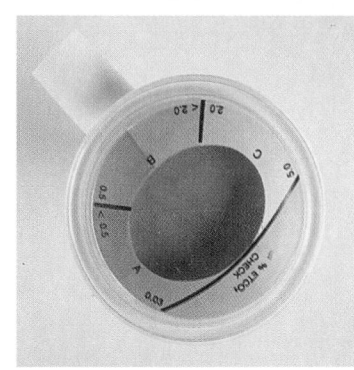

FIGURE 11-12 Colorimetric end-tidal CO$_2$ detector.

BASIC AIRWAY MANAGEMENT

The first step in the primary assessment is to determine if the patient has a patent airway. If there is a history of trauma, this must be done in conjunction with appropriate cervical spine stabilization. Any airway compromise must be rapidly corrected. Initially, manual airway maneuvers, either with or without the use of basic mechanical airways, should be applied to provide immediate ventilation and oxygenation. Shortly thereafter, advanced airway maneuvers, such as endotracheal intubation, should be carried out to maintain the airway effectively. Since airway maneuvers carry a high likelihood of contact with the patient's body fluids, wear protective gear including gloves and eyewear. (See Figure 11-15.)

✱ The endotracheal tube should be placed as soon as is practical in the non-breathing patient.

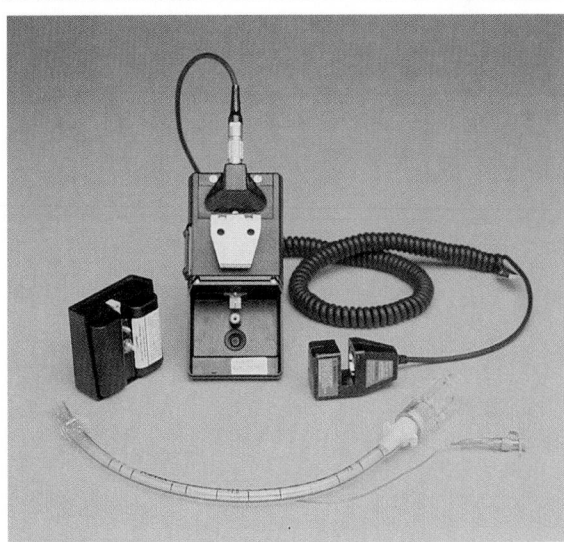

FIGURE 11-13 Electronic end-tidal CO$_2$ detector.

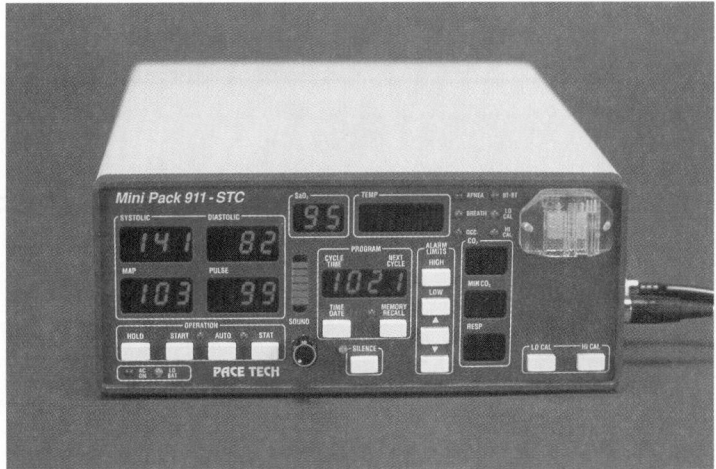

FIGURE 11-14 Prehospital monitoring device that contains pulse oximetry, ETCO$_2$ detection, blood pressure, pulse rate, respiratory rate, and temperature monitors in one unit.

Manual Airway Maneuvers

Manual airway maneuvers are highly effective and require no specialized equipment. The two common manual airway maneuvers are the head-tilt/chin-lift and the jaw-thrust. If there is a history of trauma, the modified jaw-thrust should be used as this maneuver does not involve tilting the head.

Head-Tilt/Chin-Lift Maneuver   In the absence of trauma, the preferred technique for opening the airway is the *head-tilt/chin-lift maneuver.* (See Figures 11-16 and 11-17.) To perform this maneuver:

1. With the patient supine, position yourself at his or her side.
2. Place one hand on the patient's forehead and tilt the head back by applying firm downward pressure with your palm.
3. Use your other hand to grasp the chin without applying undue pressure on the jaw. Be particularly careful to keep your fingers on the bony part of the chin. This will avoid compressing the soft tissues underneath, which may cause airway obstruction.
4. Lift the jaw anteriorly to open the airway.

Jaw-Thrust Maneuver (Non-Trauma)   The *jaw-thrust maneuver* is another useful technique for opening the airway. Because it involves some tilting of the head, it should not be used in the trauma patient. (See Figure 11-18.) To perform this maneuver:

1. With the patient supine, kneel at the top of his or her head.
2. Place the fingertips of each hand on the angles of the patient's lower jaw.
3. Forcefully displace the jaw forward, while gently tilting the patient's head backward.
4. Retract the patient's lower lip with your thumbs.

Alternatively, the *jaw-lift maneuver* can be used. With this maneuver, the jaw can be elevated by placing a gloved hand into the mouth and elevating the mandible anteriorly. This maneuver must be employed with caution as the fingers are placed inside the patient's mouth. (See Figure 11-19.)

Modified Jaw-Thrust Maneuver (Trauma)   The jaw-thrust maneuver is modified for patients who possibly have suffered a head or neck injury. The

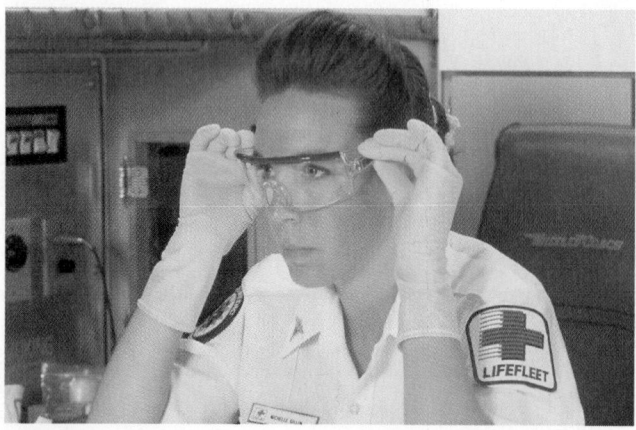

FIGURE 11-15   Protective equipment—gloves and protective eyewear—should be worn when performing airway maneuvers.

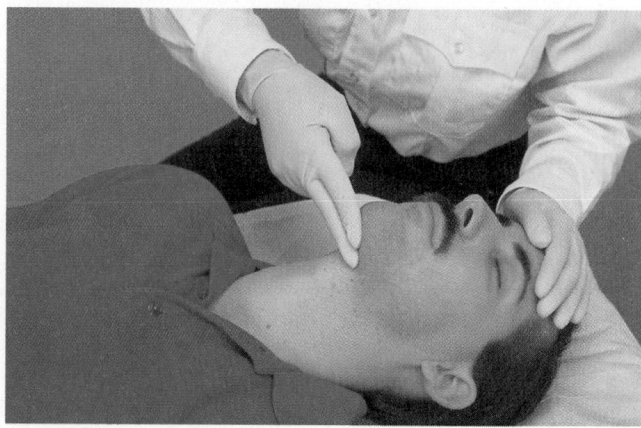

FIGURE 11-16   The head-tilt/chin-lift maneuver is effective in opening the airway if cervical spine injury is not suspected.

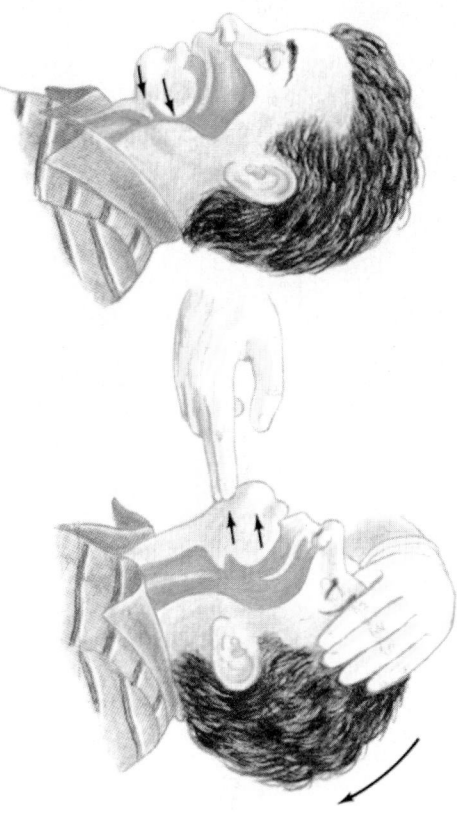

FIGURE 11-17 The head-tilt/chin-lift maneuver elevates the tongue, opening the airway.

procedure is the same except the head should be firmly supported without tilting it backward or turning it to the side. (See Figure 11-20.)

Sellick's Maneuver Gastric regurgitation occurs frequently during ventilatory support and intubation efforts. Vomitus that enters the airway can be a severe complication. To prevent regurgitation, employ a simple procedure referred to as *Sellick's maneuver*. In this procedure, slight pressure—directed posteriorly—is applied over the cricoid cartilage. Since the esophagus lies just behind the cricoid, this exertion against the cartilage at the front will close off the esophagus to pressures as high as 100 cm/H_2O. (To locate the cricoid cartilage, palpate the depression just below the thyroid cartilage, or Adam's

✱ Sellick's maneuver may be effective in preventing regurgitation during attempts at placing an endotracheal tube.

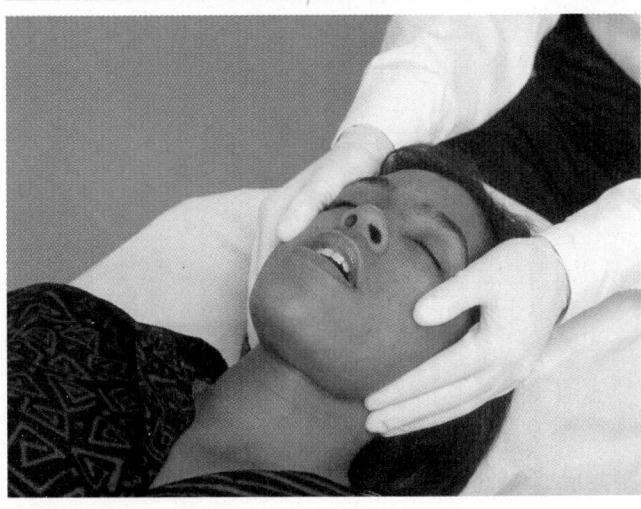

FIGURE 11-18 The jaw-thrust maneuver is also effective in opening the airway.

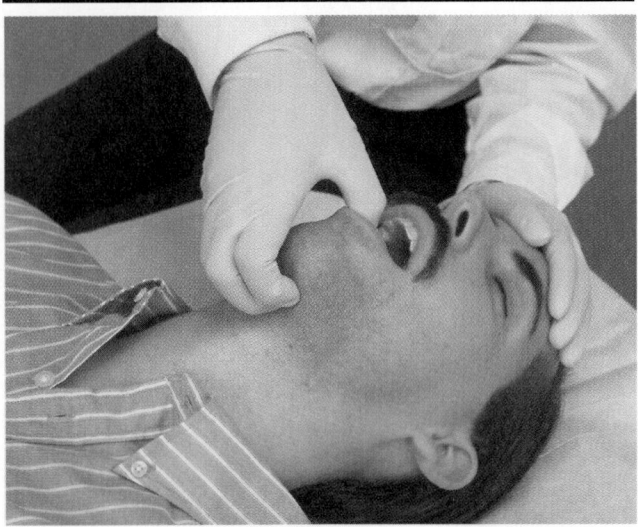

FIGURE 11-19 Use caution in performing the jaw-thrust maneuver, as it requires that fingers be placed in the patient's mouth.

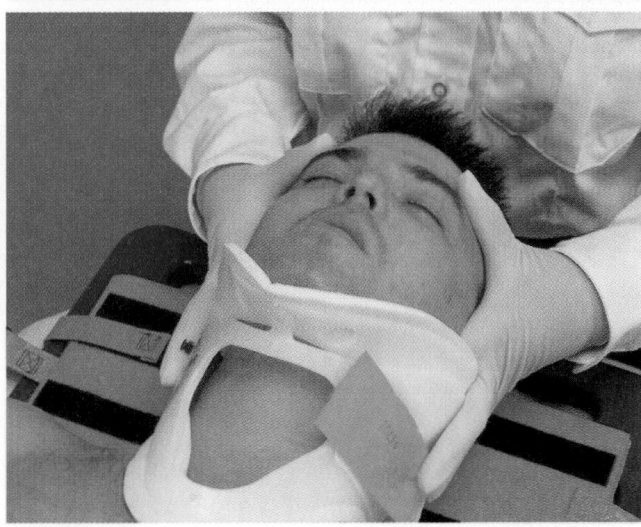

FIGURE 11-20 In cases of trauma or suspected cervical spine injury, the modified jaw-thrust maneuver should be used.

apple. This depression is the cricothyroid membrane. The prominence just below this membrane is the cricoid cartilage.)

Using the thumb and index finger of one hand, apply pressure to the anterior and lateral aspects of the cartilage just next to the midline. More pressure is required to prevent regurgitation than to prevent gastric distention.

This technique is valuable when you are providing ventilatory support (with a bag-valve-mask device or demand valve resuscitator) and during endotracheal intubation attempts. (See Figure 11-21.)

Basic Mechanical Airways

Both the oropharyngeal and nasopharyngeal airways are designed to lift the base of the tongue forward and away from the posterior oropharynx. An *oropharyngeal airway* is inserted into the mouth, while a *nasopharyngeal airway* fits into the nostril. With either airway in place, the proper head position is still important, as oropharyngeal and nasopharyngeal airways only assist with maintaining an open airway. The manual airway maneuvers described above should be attempted prior to placement of a mechanical airway.

Oropharyngeal Airway The oropharyngeal airway is a semicircular plastic and rubber device designed to conform to the curvature of the palate. It is used to hold the base of the tongue away from the posterior oropharynx. When properly positioned, this device has several advantages.

Advantages of the Oropharyngeal Airway

- ❑ It allows air to pass around and through the device.
- ❑ It helps prevent obstruction by the teeth and lips.
- ❑ It helps manage unconscious patients who are breathing spontaneously or need mechanical ventilation.
- ❑ It makes suctioning of the pharynx easier. (A large suction catheter can pass on either side.)
- ❑ It serves as an effective bite block in case of seizures or to protect the endotracheal tube.

Disadvantages of the Oropharyngeal Airway

❑ It does not isolate the trachea.

❑ It cannot be inserted when the teeth are clenched.

❑ It may obstruct the airway if it is not inserted properly.

❑ It can be dislodged easily.

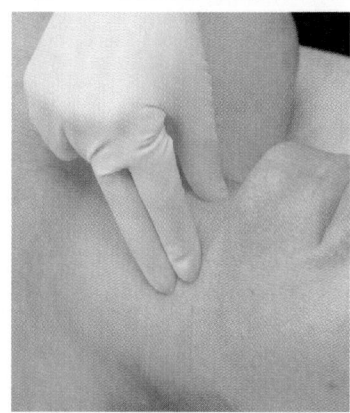

FIGURE 11-21 Sellick's maneuver (anterior cricoid pressure) is effective in preventing gastric regurgitation and gastric distention.

An oropharyngeal airway should not be used in conscious or semiconscious patients who have a gag reflex, as its insertion may stimulate vomiting (by stimulating the posterior tongue gag reflexes) or laryngospasm.

Oropharyngeal airways are available in sizes ranging from #0 (for infants) to #6 (for large adults). Selecting the proper size is important. If the airway is too long it can press the epiglottis against the entrance of the larynx, resulting in airway obstruction. (See Figure 11-22.) An airway that is too small will not adequately hold the tongue forward. The correct size is best obtained by measuring. Place the flange beside the patient's cheek, parallel to the front teeth. A properly sized airway will extend from the patient's mouth to the angle of the jaw. (See Figure 11-23.) To place the airway:

1. If no history of trauma, hyperextend the patient's head and neck.
2. Assure or maintain effective ventilatory function; if indicated, hyperventilate the patient with 100% oxygen.
3. Grasp the patient's tongue and jaw and lift anteriorly.
4. With your other hand, hold the airway at its proximal end and insert it into the mouth. Make sure the curve is reversed, with the tip pointing toward the roof of the mouth.
5. Once the tip reaches the level of the uvula, the airway should be turned 180° until it comes to rest over the tongue.
6. Verify appropriate position of the airway. (Clear breath sounds and chest rise indicate correct placement.)
7. Hyperventilate the patient with 100% oxygen (if indicated).

Make sure the airway is correctly positioned. Improper placement can obstruct the airway by pushing the tongue against the posterior oropharynx. (An indicator of improper placement is when the device advances out of the mouth during ventilatory efforts.) An alternative insertion method is to use a tongue blade to depress the tongue while pushing the airway past it.

Airway obstruction from
incorrect insertion

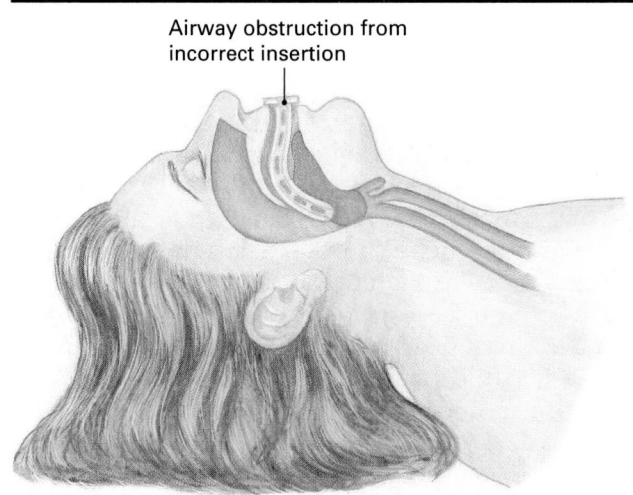

FIGURE 11-22 Improper placement of the oropharyngeal airway can cause airway obstruction.

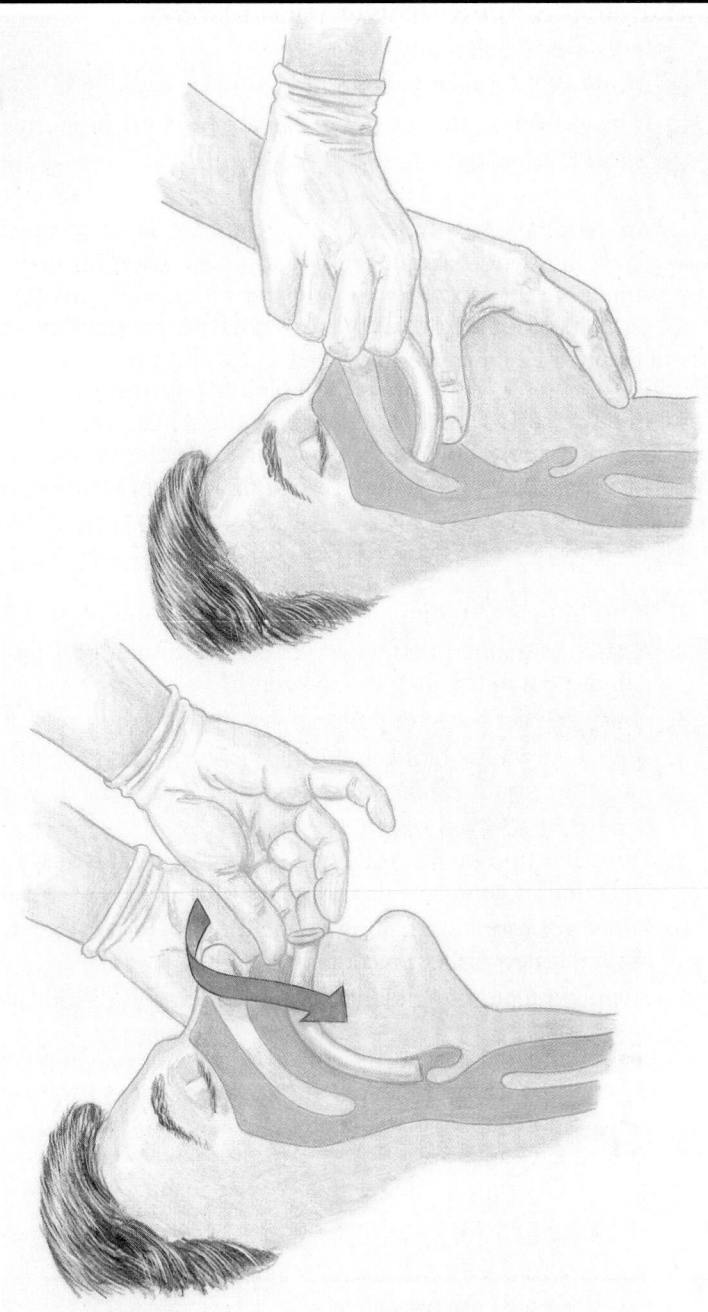

FIGURE 11-23 The oropharyngeal airway should be inserted with a twisting motion. It is an effective airway adjunct in the unresponsive patient.

Nasopharyngeal Airway   The nasopharyngeal airway is an uncuffed tube made of soft rubber or plastic. Varying from 17 to 20 cm long, its diameter ranges from 20 to 36 "french." At its proximal end is a funnel-shaped projection, which helps prevent the tube from slipping inside a patient's nose and becoming lost or aspirated. The distal end is bevel-shaped to facilitate passage. The nasopharyngeal airway is designed to follow the natural curvature of the nasopharynx, passing through the nose and extending from the nostril to the posterior pharynx just below the base of the tongue. The nasopharyngeal airway is used to relieve soft-tissue upper airway obstruction in cases where use of an oropharyngeal airway is not advised.

Advantages of the Nasopharyngeal Airway

- ❏ It can be rapidly inserted.
- ❏ It bypasses the tongue.
- ❏ It may be used in the presence of a gag reflex.
- ❏ It can be used when the patient has suffered injury to his or her oral cavity (anything from trauma to the mandible or maxilla to significant soft tissue damage to the tongue or pharynx).
- ❏ It can be used when the patient's teeth are clenched.

Disadvantages of the Nasopharyngeal Airway

- ❏ It is smaller than the oropharyngeal airway.
- ❏ It does not isolate the trachea.
- ❏ It is difficult to suction through.
- ❏ It may cause severe nosebleeds if inserted too forcefully.
- ❏ It may cause pressure necrosis of the nasal mucosa.
- ❏ It may kink and clog, obstructing the airway.
- ❏ It is difficult to insert if nasal damage (old or new) is present.
- ❏ It cannot be used if there is a basilar skull fracture.

The nasopharyngeal airway should not be used in patients who are predisposed to nosebleeds or who have a nasal obstruction. Also, it should never be used in the presence of a suspected basilar skull fracture, as the tube can inadvertently pass into the brain.

The proper-sized airway is slightly smaller in diameter than the patient's nostril and is equal to or slightly longer than the distance from the nose to the earlobe. Selecting the appropriate size is important. A tube that is too small will not extend past the tongue; one that is too long may pass into the esophagus and result in hypoventilation and gastric distention with artificial ventilation. (See Figures 11-24 and 11-25.) To insert the airway:

1. If no history of trauma, hyperextend the patient's head and neck.
2. Assure or maintain effective ventilatory function. If indicated, hyperventilate the patient with 100% oxygen.
3. Lubricate the exterior of the tube with a water-soluble gel to prevent trauma during insertion. If possible, use a lidocaine gel in the alert or responsive patient. Its anesthetic effect on the mucosa will make insertion more comfortable.
4. Push up on the tip of the nose and pass the tube into the right nostril. Avoid pushing against any resistance, as this may cause tissue trauma and airway kinking. If the septum is deviated and insertion into the right nostril cannot be accomplished, use the left nostril.
5. Verify appropriate position of the airway. (Clear breath sounds and chest rise indicate correct placement. Also, feel for airflow at the proximal end of the device on expiration.)
6. Hyperventilate the patient with 100% oxygen, if indicated.

While semiconscious patients tolerate a nasopharyngeal airway better than an oropharyngeal one, it too may cause vomiting and laryngospasm. Insertion of the nasopharyngeal airway may injure the nasal mucosa, leading to bleeding, aspiration of clots, and the need for suctioning. Forceful insertion of the airway may lacerate the adenoids, causing considerable bleeding.

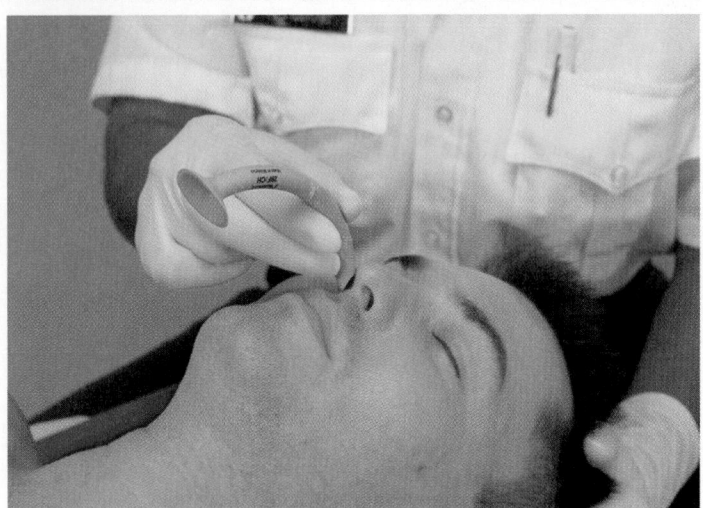

FIGURE 11-24 The nasopharyngeal airway is easy to insert and usually well-tolerated by the patient. It should not be used if basilar skull fracture is suspected.

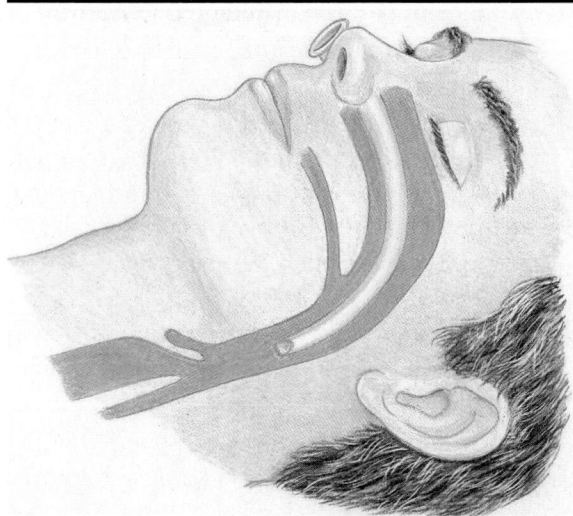

FIGURE 11-25 The nasopharyngeal airway rests between the tongue and the posterior pharyngeal wall, thus maintaining an open airway.

ADVANCED AIRWAY MANAGEMENT

✱ The preferred technique for managing the airway of an unconscious patient is by endotracheal intubation.

■ **intubation** to pass a tube into an opening of the body.

Advanced mechanical airways are devices that require special training to insert. The preferred method of airway management is endotracheal **intubation**. Endotracheal intubation is the only procedure that effectively isolates the trachea. In some EMS systems, endotracheal intubation is not available. Instead, other airway devices such as the Pharyngeo-tracheal Lumen airway (PtL), esophageal tracheal combiTube (ETC), or esophageal obturator airways are used.

Esophageal Obturator Airways

Although endotracheal intubation is preferred, the *esophageal obturator airway (EOA)* is an alternative when personnel are not trained or permitted to perform endotracheal intubation. The EOA is a large-bore flexible tube, approximately 37 cm long. The proximal end is open, while the distal end is rounded and closed. The EOA is inserted into the esophagus. Following proper insertion, a distal cuff is inflated with 30 to 35 mL of air, which effectively closes the esophagus and prevents regurgitation. Ventilations are delivered through the open end of the tube, which is housed in a detachable clear-plastic mask. When a proper seal is maintained between the patient's face and the EOA mask, air exits the tube through 16 holes located at the level of the hypopharynx. With the esophagus blocked, the air is forced into the trachea and lungs. (See Figure 11-26.)

Keep in mind that insertion of the EOA will often stimulate the gag reflex. Because of this, the device should only be used in unresponsive patients. If the patient becomes responsive, the device must be removed.

Advantages of the Esophageal Obturator Airway
❏ Insertion is easy and does not require that the paramedic see the larynx.
❏ It prevents gastric distention and regurgitation.
❏ It delivers ventilations at the level of the hypopharynx.
❏ It can be used on trauma victims who may have spinal injuries. (There is no need for hyperextension or flexion of the neck during insertion.)

Disadvantages of the Esophageal Obturator Airway

❏ Adequate mask seal is difficult to maintain.
❏ It sometimes causes esophageal trauma and rupture.
❏ It may enter the trachea if placed improperly.

Because the tube is closed at its distal end, placement in the trachea will block airflow into the lungs. Ventilatory effectiveness must be checked immediately after insertion of this device (even before inflation of the distal cuff). A rising chest and breath sounds will indicate that the tube has been placed properly in the esophagus. To prevent accidental insertion of the device into the trachea and to avoid esophageal laceration, follow these rules:

1. The patient's head and neck must be placed in a neutral position or flexed forward, because a hyperextended position may inadvertently direct the tip of the tube anteriorly into the trachea.

2. A tongue-jaw-lift should be used with one hand while the device is inserted with the other.

3. Grasp the device between the upper and middle thirds of the tube as you would grasp a pencil. This facilitates gentle maneuvering of the tube posteriorly and reduces the risk of pharyngeal trauma.

4. Never use force during insertion of the tube. Whenever you meet resistance, withdraw the device slightly, improve the jaw-lift, and re-advance the tube. This will avoid pharyngeal and esophageal trauma.

5. The amount of air used to inflate the distal cuff should be considered patient-dependent, with smaller patients needing less.

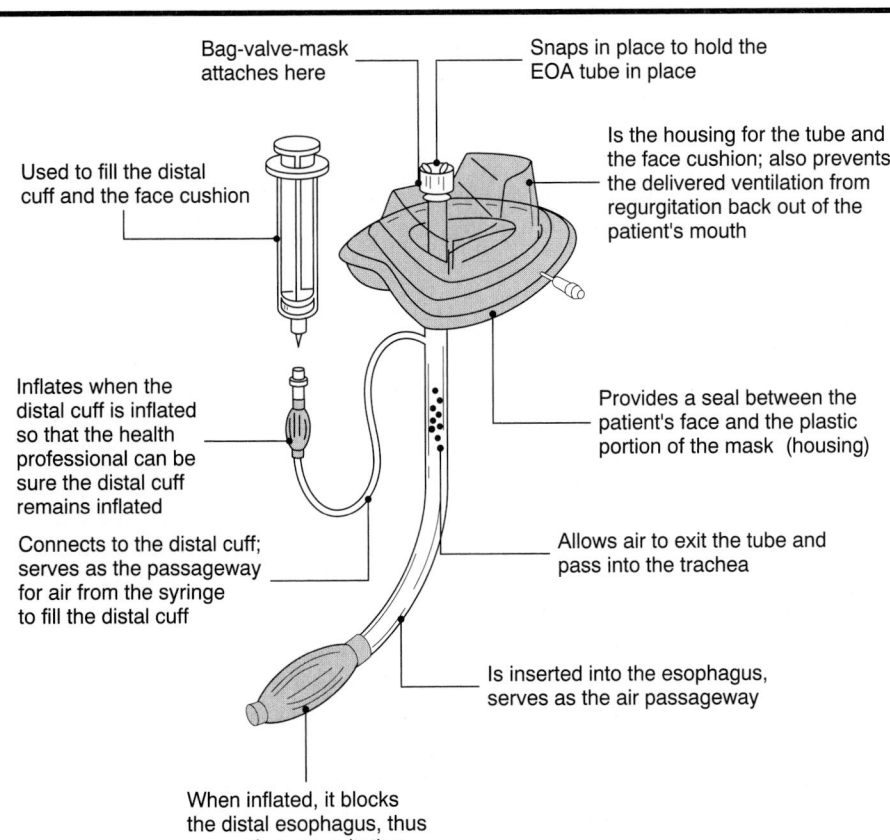

Bag-valve-mask attaches here

Snaps in place to hold the EOA tube in place

Used to fill the distal cuff and the face cushion

Is the housing for the tube and the face cushion; also prevents the delivered ventilation from regurgitation back out of the patient's mouth

Inflates when the distal cuff is inflated so that the health professional can be sure the distal cuff remains inflated

Provides a seal between the patient's face and the plastic portion of the mask (housing)

Connects to the distal cuff; serves as the passageway for air from the syringe to fill the distal cuff

Allows air to exit the tube and pass into the trachea

Is inserted into the esophagus, serves as the air passageway

When inflated, it blocks the distal esophagus, thus preventing regurgitation

FIGURE 11-26 The Esophageal Obturator Airway (EOA).

6. Finally, the tube must be stored in a natural position. Small storage compartments may inadvertently curl the tube, thus increasing the likelihood that it will aim upward into the trachea during insertion.

Use of the EOA is contraindicated in the following cases:

❑ Persons under the age of 16
❑ Persons under 5 feet or over 6 feet, 7 inches tall
❑ Persons who may have ingested caustic poisons
❑ Persons who have a history of esophageal disease or alcoholism

The esophageal obturator airway should be used with caution in patients who may be suffering from drug overdose (which can be reversed by naloxone) or hypoglycemia (which can be treated with dextrose). Improvements in mental status may activate the gag reflex and lead to vomiting. Also, the EOA does not protect the patient from aspirating foreign materials that are present in the mouth and pharynx. Appropriate suctioning techniques must be used to clear the airway. (See Procedure 11-1.) To insert the EOA:

1. While maintaining ventilatory support, hyperventilate the patient with 100% oxygen.
2. Assemble and check the equipment.
3. Connect the tube to the mask. (The tube is seated properly when its proximal end clicks into place on the mask.)
4. Pull back on the plunger of the syringe and draw in 30 to 35 mL of air. Attach the syringe to the one-way valve of the inflation tube. (It is beneficial to tape the inflation tube to the EOA tube to prevent it from being accidentally severed.) When inserting the tip of the syringe into the inflation valve, use a twisting action to seat it properly.
5. Place the patient's head in a neutral position or flexed slightly forward.
6. With your left hand, grasp the patient's jaw in your fingers. Insert your thumb deep into the subject's mouth behind the base of the tongue.
7. Lift the jaw and tongue anteriorly, away from the posterior pharynx.
8. With your right hand, grasp the esophageal obturator tube between its upper and middle thirds, holding it in a J-shaped position.
9. Insert the EOA over the patient's tongue, with the tube in the midline. Remember to follow the natural curvature of the pharynx.
10. Continue inserting the tube until the mask rests on the patient's face. If resistance is met, withdraw the tube and try again.
11. Attach a ventilatory device to the 15 mm connector and deliver a breath. Look for chest rise and listen for breath sounds. If they are absent, suspect placement into the trachea and withdraw the tube.
12. If chest rise and breath sounds are present, inflate the distal cuff with 30 to 35 mL of air. Check the pilot bulb to verify that air is inflating the distal cuff. (A filled pilot balloon indicates that the distal cuff is inflated.)
13. Remove the syringe from the one-way valve, using a reverse twisting action to prevent accidental loss of air.
14. While hyperventilating the patient, recheck the EOA's placement, chest rise, and breath sounds, and auscultate over the stomach.

Keep in mind that when the esophageal obturator is fully inserted, its distal cuff typically lies below the level of the carina. However, in some cases the cuff will lie above the level of the carina. Inflation of the distal cuff in

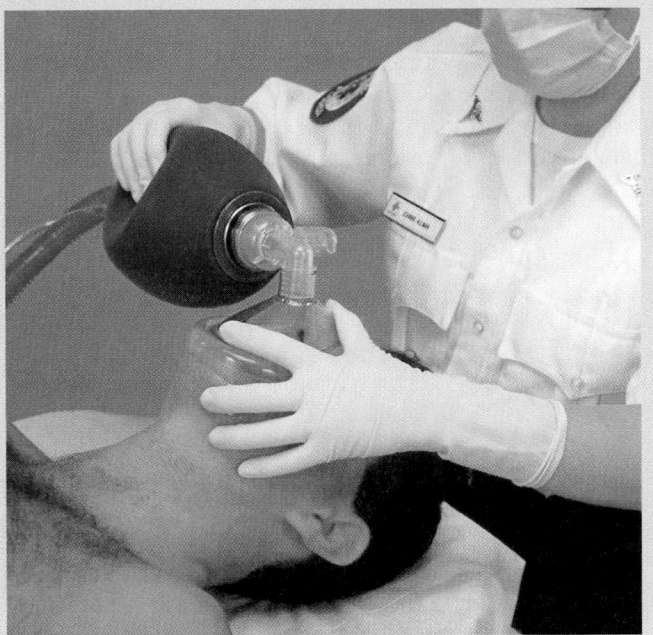

11-1A. Hyperventilate the patient.

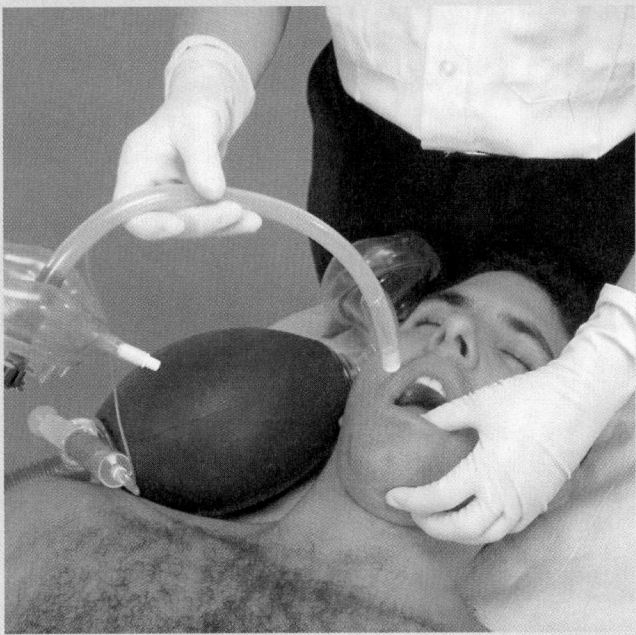

11-1B. With the head in a neutral position or slightly flexed, insert the airway.

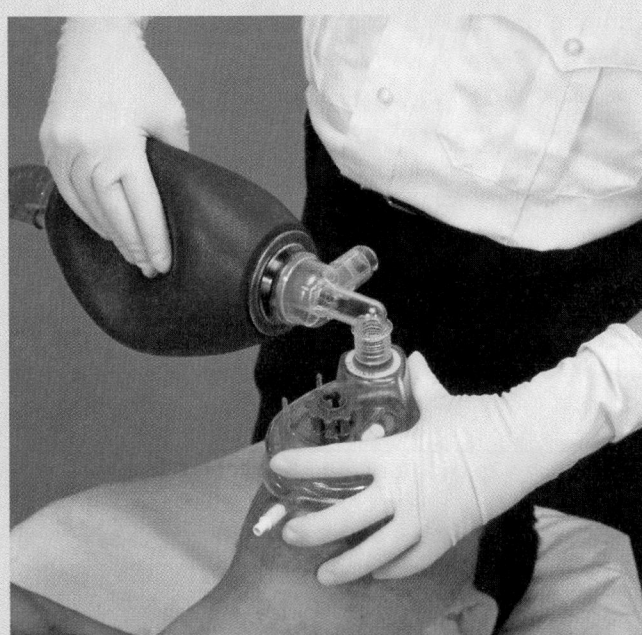

11-1C. Seal the face mask and attempt to ventilate.

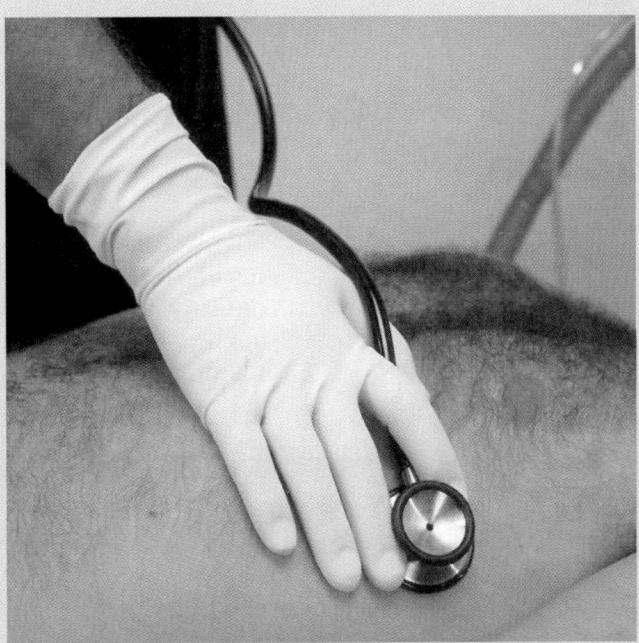

11-1D. Assess the quality of ventilations.

these cases may cause tracheal obstruction as the posterior membranous portion of the trachea is compressed. If breath sounds and chest rise, which were present prior to distal cuff inflation, disappear after 30 to 35 mL of air are introduced, withdraw air from the distal cuff until effective ventilations are restored. It may be necessary to remove the esophageal obturator airway if there is any indication that the obstruction remains.

When ventilating a patient with the EOA in place, the head should still be tilted backward to maintain an open airway, unless trauma is suspected. Use of a lubricant is usually unnecessary, as there are sufficient secretions to allow for easy passage of the device. If the patient's upper airway is dry, lubricate the distal end of the obturator with a water-soluble gel.

In some circumstances, it may be necessary to remove the EOA in the field setting. Most patients will vomit when the device is removed, so place the patient on his or her side and have suction readily available. Ideally, an endotracheal tube will be in place to prevent aspiration (as described below). To remove the EOA, deflate its distal cuff and withdraw the tube in a steady and gentle manner.

Esophageal Gastric Tube Airway

The *esophageal gastric tube airway (EGTA)* is an alternative to the EOA. An EGTA's primary advantage is that it allows for suctioning of the patient's stomach contents thus alleviating gastric distention prior to removal of the device.

The EGTA consists of an inflatable face mask and a tube, which is open throughout its length to permit passage of a gastric (Levine) tube for decompression of the stomach. The transparent face mask has two ports: one to allow for attachment of the esophageal tube; the other (a standard 15 mm connector) to serve as the ventilation port. During ventilation, air is blown into the upper port of the mask. As with the EOA, the esophagus is blocked and the air has nowhere to go but into the trachea and lungs. (See Figure 11-27.) The insertion technique and the complications for an EGTA are the same as those for the EOA.

Endotracheal Intubation

* Endotracheal intubation is the procedure of choice for advanced prehospital care.

Endotracheal intubation is the procedure where a tube is placed in the trachea for the purpose of securing a patent airway. It is the procedure of choice for advanced prehospital care. The endotracheal tube can be placed through the mouth (orotracheal route) or through the nose (nasotracheal route). Typically, the larynx is directly visualized with a laryngoscope. However, in special situations, the endotracheal tube can be placed without direct visualization. In the following sections, you will become familiar with the equipment, precautions, and various techniques involved in this advanced procedure.

Necessary Equipment   The equipment and supplies necessary for endotracheal intubation include: a laryngoscope (handle and blade); an appropriate-size endotracheal tube; a 10 mL syringe; a stylet; a bag-valve-mask device; a suction device; a bite block; Magill forceps; and tie-down tape or a commercial tube-holding device.

Laryngoscope.   The *laryngoscope* is an instrument for lifting the tongue and epiglottis out of the way so that the vocal cords can be seen. Typically, it is used in placing an endotracheal tube, but it may also be used in conjunction with Magill forceps to retrieve a foreign body obstructing the upper airway.

A laryngoscope consists of a handle and blade. The handle is made of a reusable or disposable material. It houses several batteries that power a

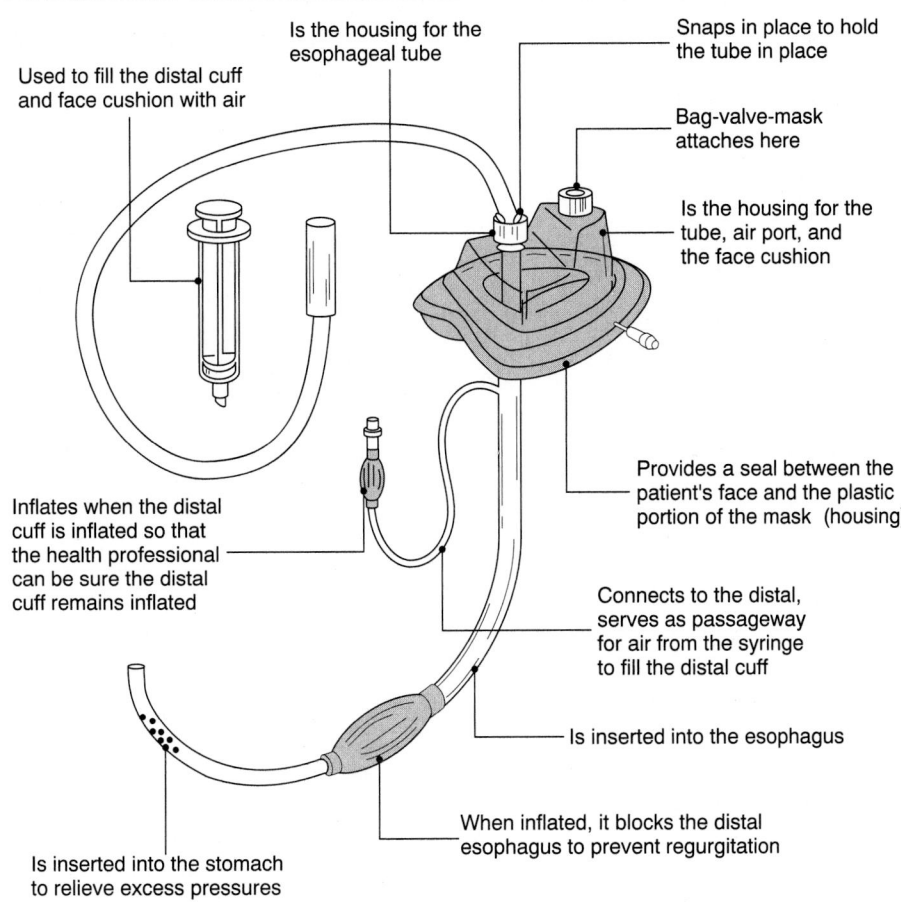

Used to fill the distal cuff and face cushion with air

Is the housing for the esophageal tube

Snaps in place to hold the tube in place

Bag-valve-mask attaches here

Is the housing for the tube, air port, and the face cushion

Provides a seal between the patient's face and the plastic portion of the mask (housing)

Inflates when the distal cuff is inflated so that the health professional can be sure the distal cuff remains inflated

Connects to the distal, serves as passageway for air from the syringe to fill the distal cuff

Is inserted into the esophagus

When inflated, it blocks the distal esophagus to prevent regurgitation

Is inserted into the stomach to relieve excess pressures and unwanted substances

FIGURE 11-27 The Esophageal Gastric Tube Airway (EGTA).

light located in the distal third of the laryngoscope blade. This light illuminates the airway, making it easier to see upper airway structures. The attachment point between the handle and blade is the "fitting." When connected, it locks the blade in place and provides electrical contact between the batteries and the bulb.

In preparing for intubation, the indentation of the laryngoscope's blade is attached to the bar of the handle. It will click into place when properly seated. To determine if the laryngoscope is functional, the blade should be elevated to a right angle with the handle. If properly positioned, the light should turn on and be bright white and steady. A yellow, flickering light will not sufficiently illuminate anatomical structures. If the light fails to go on, the problem may be either the batteries (are they dead?) or the bulb (is it loose?). Infrequently, the failure is in the contact points or the wire that travels through the blade to the bulb. (See Figures 11-28 and 11-29.)

Like the handle, the laryngoscope blade is also made of a reusable or disposable material. Two common types of blades are the *curved blade* (or MacIntosh) and the *straight blade* (often referred to as the Miller, Wisconsin, or Flagg blade). Laryngoscope blades come in a variety of sizes, ranging from 0 (for the infant) to 4 (for the large adult patient). (See Figure 11-30.)

The curved blade is designed to fit into the *vallecula*. (See Figure 11-31.) When the handle is lifted anteriorly, it elevates the tongue and indirectly elevates the epiglottis, allowing you to see the glottic opening. Because the curved blade does not touch the larynx itself, it should not traumatize or acci-

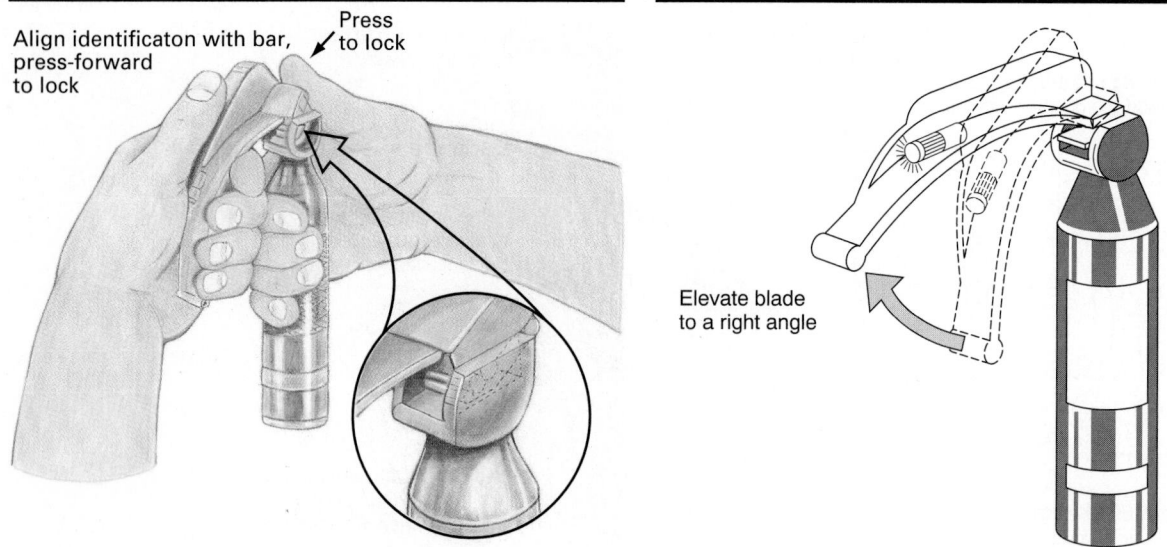

FIGURE 11-28 Engaging the laryngoscope blade.

FIGURE 11-29 Elevating the laryngoscope blade to activate the light source.

dentally stimulate the very sensitive gag receptors located on the posterior surface of the epiglottis. The curved blade also permits more room for adequate viewing and tube insertion. The straight blade, on the other hand, is designed to fit under the epiglottis. (See Figure 11-32.) When its handle is lifted anteriorly, it directly lifts the epiglottis up and out of the way. A straight blade is preferred in treating infants, since it provides greater displacement of the tongue and better visualization of the glottis.

There are advantages and disadvantages to each type of blade and use of one over the other depends largely upon individual preference. Even so, the paramedic should be skilled in the use of both blades to accommodate patient peculiarities.

Endotracheal Tubes. The *endotracheal tube* is a flexible, translucent tube approximately 35 to 37 cm long and open at both ends. (See Figures 11-33 and 11-34.) The proximal end features a standard 15/22 mm adapter that attaches to a ventilatory device. The distal end has an inflatable 5–to–10 mL cuff that is used to seal the trachea. The distal cuff is filled with air from a syringe, which is pushed through a thin inflation tube that runs the length of the main tube and into the distal cuff. A one-way valve at the proximal end of the inflation tube permits air to enter the distal cuff without allowing it to leak inadvertently. A pilot balloon, located between the valve and the distal cuff, indicates whether the distal cuff has inflated. The distal cuff should always be checked for leaks prior to insertion.

Suppliers typically prewrap an endotracheal tube in a curved shape. The reason for this shape is that the trachea lies anteriorly in the neck. In most patients, the tube must be directed upward so that it may pass through the glottic opening. Some endotracheal tubes are equipped with an O-shaped ring attached to a plastic wire. This wire runs the length of the tube and terminates distally. When the ring is pulled, the distal end of the tube bends upward, helping to redirect the angle of the distal tip into the glottic opening.

Endotracheal tubes are supplied in a variety of sizes. Markings on the tube indicate the internal diameter (i.d.) in millimeters. The typical tube sizes for average-sized patients are:

✱ The endotracheal tube may be sized to approximate the diameter of the patient's little finger.

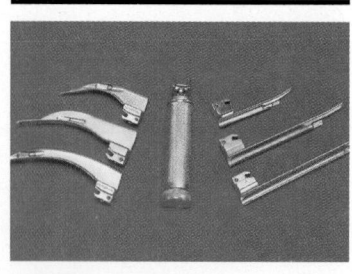

FIGURE 11-30 Laryngoscope blades.

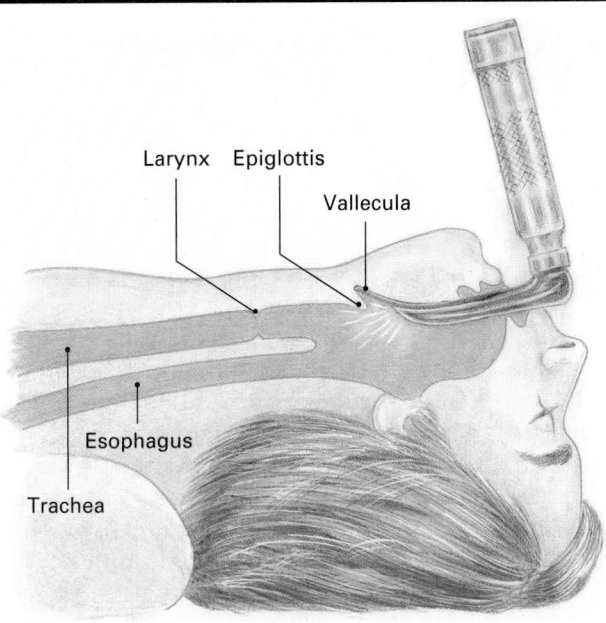

FIGURE 11-31 The curved blade should be gently guided into the vallecula so as to indirectly elevate the epiglottis.

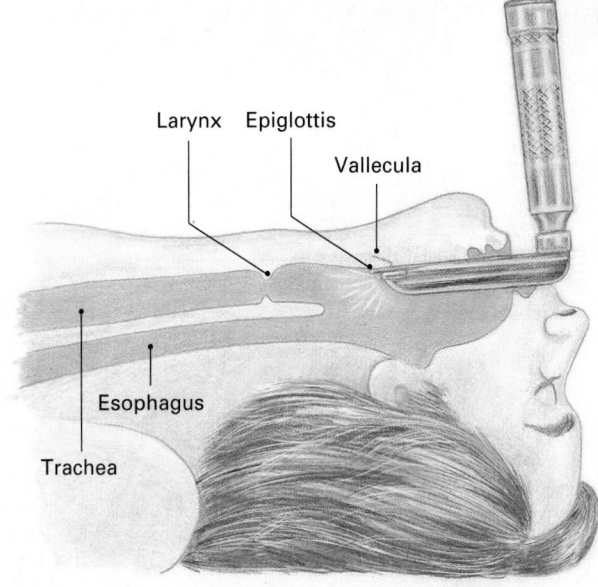

FIGURE 11-32 The straight blade should be used to elevate the epiglottis.

Newborn	2.5 to 3.5 i.d.	
Infant	3.5 to 4.0 i.d.	
Child	4.0 to 6.0 i.d.	
Adult	7.0 to 9.0 i.d.	(females 7.0 to 8.0 i.d.)
		(males 7.5 to 8.5 i.d.)

In an emergency, a good standard-size endotracheal tube for both adult female and male patients is 7.5 i.d.

Noncuffed endotracheal tubes are usually used with infants and children under the age of 8, because the round narrowing of the cricoid cartilage will

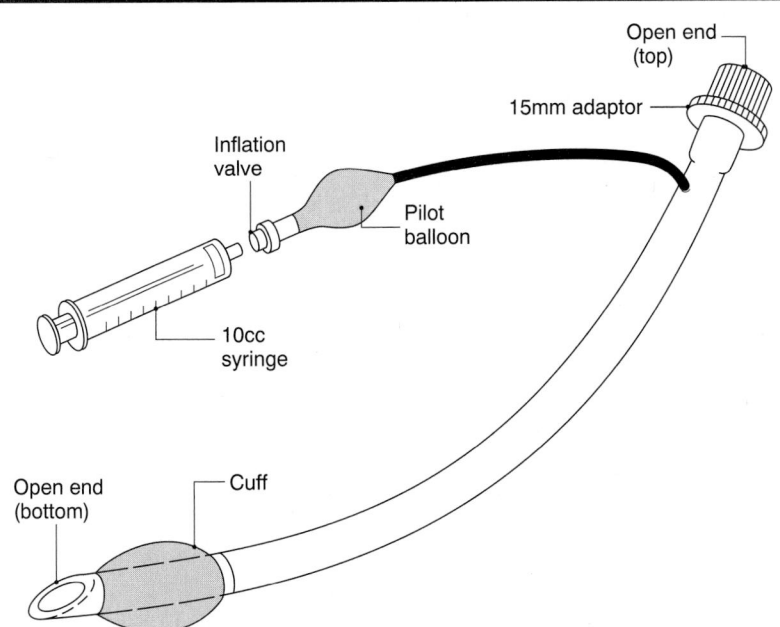

FIGURE 11-33 The endotracheal tube.

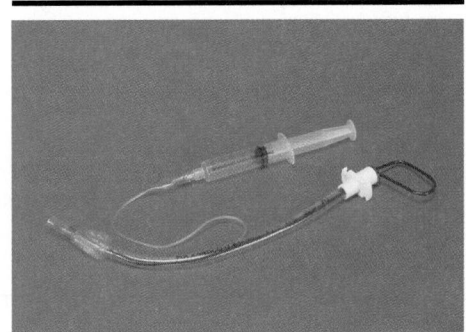

FIGURE 11-34 Cuffed endotracheal tube with the stylet in place.

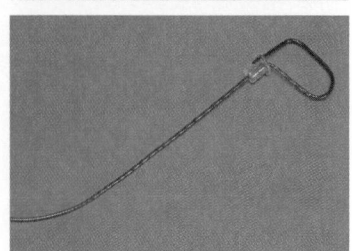

FIGURE 11-35 The stylet can be used to give the endotracheal tube a predetermined curve.

serve as a suitable cuff in those cases. Selection of the appropriate tube diameter for children is critical. Tube size can be correctly determined by measuring the outside diameter of the tube against the diameter of the child's smallest finger. A tube that is too large can cause tracheal edema and/or damage to the vocal cords; a tube that is too small may not allow for delivery of adequate ventilatory volumes. (Endotracheal intubation in children will be discussed in detail later in this chapter.)

Stylet. The *malleable stylet* is a metal wire covered with plastic. It is used to direct the endotracheal tube anteriorly when a patient's larynx and trachea lie pronouncedly forward or in cases where the patient has a short, fat neck that makes optimal positioning of the head difficult. (See Figure 11-35.) The stylet allows the endotracheal tube to be pulled into a J or hockey-stick shape. Because it is a wire, the stylet may inadvertently cause tissue damage during intubation attempts if it is allowed to extend past the distal end of the endotracheal tube. As a result, the wire's distal end should be recessed at least one-half inch from the tip of the tube when inserting the stylet into the endotracheal tube. A stylet is not employed in all cases, but it should be readily available in those where the tube needs to be directed anteriorly.

Tube-Holding Devices. A tie-down or umbilical tape is used to secure the endotracheal tube in place once it has entered the trachea. The reasons for securing the endotracheal tube are twofold. First, during the process of resuscitation and transportation, when the patient is being moved about, the tube can be dislodged easily. Even when the tube is not dislodged, movement can still cause cardiovascular stimulation, an elevation in intracranial pressure, or injury to the tracheal mucosa. Second, the person providing ventilatory support may accidentally push down on the endotracheal tube, forcing it into the right or left mainstem bronchus. Tying the tube in place prevents this accidental movement or displacement. Tying is preferred over taping, as tape tends to loosen when either the patient's face or the tube is moist. A number of commercial tube-holding devices are also available.

Magill Forceps. The *Magill forceps* are scissor-style clamps with circle-shaped tips. They are used to remove foreign materials or redirect the endotracheal tube during nasotracheal intubation. (See Figure 11-36.)

Lubricants. Water-soluble lubricants help facilitate the tube's insertion. Petroleum-based lubricants should not be used as these may damage the endotracheal tube and may cause tracheal inflammation.

Suction Units. A *suction unit* is used to remove secretions and foreign materials from the oropharynx during intubation attempts. (This is particularly important, since the patient in cardiac arrest often has large volumes of secretions.)

Additional Airways. An oropharyngeal airway should also be on hand during an endotracheal intubation. It is used as a block to prevent the patient from biting down on and collapsing the endotracheal tube.

Indications, Advantages, and Disadvantages Endotracheal intubation is used to secure an open airway when a patient is experiencing, or is likely to experience, upper airway compromise. Patients who fit into this category often exhibit the following conditions:

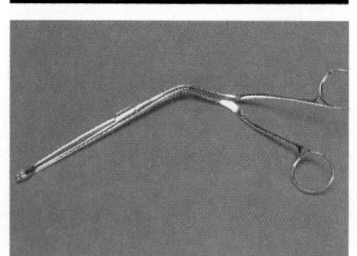

FIGURE 11-36 Magill forceps.

- ❏ Respiratory or cardiac arrest
- ❏ Unconsciousness without a gag reflex
- ❏ Decreased minute volume, due to decreased respiratory rate or volume
- ❏ Possible airway obstruction due to foreign bodies, trauma, or anaphylaxis

Endotracheal intubation should not be attempted in the presence of epiglottitis except as a last-ditch effort. Attempts at endotracheal intubation in patients suffering epiglottitis may precipitate laryngospasm. However, if the condition of such patients steadily worsens, some local protocols will permit endotracheal intubation. Check your local protocols.

In most cases, endotracheal intubation is the preferred airway management technique. As a paramedic you will be called upon to use it often.

Advantages of Endotracheal Intubation
- ❏ It isolates the trachea and permits complete control of the airway.
- ❏ It prevents gastric distention by channeling air directly into the trachea.
- ❏ It eliminates the need to maintain a mask seal.
- ❏ It offers a direct route for suctioning of the respiratory passages.
- ❏ It permits administration of medications (epinephrine, atropine, lidocaine, and naloxone) via the endotracheal tube.

While endotracheal intubation is the preferred technique for managing the airway, a number of disadvantages are associated with its use.

Disadvantages of Endotracheal Intubation
- ❏ It requires considerable training and experience in the technique.
- ❏ It demands specialized equipment, the retrieval of which can slow efforts to secure the airway.
- ❏ It requires direct visualization of the vocal cords, making it difficult to identify anatomical structures or to insert the tube as you bring your face close to the patient's face.

General Precautions   A variety of problems can arise during endotracheal intubation. Many can be eliminated or reduced by taking certain precautions.

Time is sometimes lost when equipment malfunctions—for instance, when a laryngoscope fails to light. Use of an already-assembled airway kit or "intubation wrap" reduces such time loss. To eliminate surprise equipment failures, the kit and all its contents should be inspected at the beginning of every work shift. In volunteer settings, where specific coverage is not provided, the equipment should be checked at least once a week. These inspections are effective in reducing equipment malfunction.

✱ To ensure that the equipment functions and that it is readily available, it should be tested before each shift and kept together in one kit or airway wrap.

Injury to the tissues or teeth can occur, but this hazard can be eliminated by using the laryngoscope carefully, as an instrument, not a tool. When inserting this device into the mouth and pharynx, be sure to guide it gently into place, avoiding accidental pressure on the teeth. When manipulating the jaw anteriorly, use upward traction rather than rotating and flexing your wrist, which will cause the laryngoscope to function as a lever. All levers require a fulcrum—and the only fulcrums available will be the patient's upper incisors. As a result, a rotating/flexing action may break teeth. To avoid this hazard, lift the laryngoscope's handle (exposing the epiglottis) after the blade is applied to the base of the tongue. After this, the wrist should remain straight, and any lifting should be done by the shoulder and arm.

Inadvertent delays in oxygenation result from lengthy intubation efforts or failure to provide ventilatory support between procedures. Hypoxia may occur due to the inexperience of the operator. Each patient's unique anatomy and unusual clinical situations can challenge even the most experienced paramedic. So follow one basic rule during intubation: Limit each attempt to 30 seconds. To gauge this time, some paramedics hold their breath from the point at which they stop ventilating a patient until ventilatory support is reinitiated. Note that it is seldom necessary to place the endotracheal tube on your first attempt. However, that initial effort should at least give you a "lay of the land," or some orientation to the patient's anatomy. The tube can be placed in a subsequent attempt (each of which is scheduled between hyperventilations, using a bag-valve-mask device and 100% oxygen).

A catastrophic complication associated with endotracheal intubation is accidental misplacement of the tube into the pyriform sinus, the esophagus, or one of the mainstem bronchi. If the endotracheal tube is inserted too anteriorly, it may also lodge in the vallecula.

If the tube strays from the midline, it can get hung up on either side of the epiglottis, in the pyriform sinus. These errors will cause the skin to "tent up" on either side of the laryngeal prominence. Forceful efforts can perforate these tissues, leading potentially to serious bleeding and subcutaneous emphysema. In the case of misplacement in the pyriform sinus, the problem can be resolved by slightly withdrawing and rotating the tube to the midline.

Accidental misplacement of the tube into the esophagus will cut off the patient's ventilation or oxygenation, while accidental advancement of the tube into a mainstem bronchus will greatly reduce ventilation or oxygenation. The consequences of incorrect placement may quickly be lethal.

To avoid such complications, carefully follow the insertion steps described below as well as the methods for verifying correct placement—or detecting misplacement and correcting it—in the segment that follows.

Method of Insertion: The Orotracheal Route The most common route for endotracheal intubation is through the mouth. An orotracheal procedure allows you to see the upper airway and glottic opening. Using a laryngoscope, you can then gently and accurately pass the endotracheal tube through the vocal cords. (See Procedure 11-2.) To perform orotracheal intubation, when no spinal injuries are suspected:

1. While maintaining ventilatory support, hyperventilate the patient with 100% oxygen.
2. Assemble and check your equipment. Pull back on the plunger of the syringe and draw in 5 to 10 mL of air. Attach the syringe to the one-way inflation valve on the distal cuff, using a twisting action to properly seat the syringe. Tape the inflation tube to the endotracheal tube to prevent it from being accidentally severed.
3. Position the patient's head and neck. To establish visualization of the larynx, the three axes—of the mouth, the pharynx, and the trachea—must be aligned. To achieve this, place the patient's head into a "sniffing position" by flexing the neck forward and the head backward. It may help to insert a rolled towel under the patient's shoulders or the back of the head. Establishing this position is extremely difficult in patients with short, fat necks or whose motion is limited by such conditions as arthritis.
4. Hold the laryngoscope in your left hand. Most laryngoscopes are designed for right-handed persons; that is, the right-handed person must

* Hyperventilate the patient before and after each attempt to place the endotracheal tube. Take no longer than 30 seconds for tube placement.

* Prior to performing endotracheal intubation, or any airway maneuver, always don a protective face shield, or goggles and a mask, in addition to gloves.

hold it in his or her left hand in order to use the right one for manipulating the endotracheal tube.

5. Insert the laryngoscope blade into the right side of the patient's mouth. With a sweeping action, displace the tongue to the left. This pushes the tongue out of your line of vision and allows more room to manipulate the endotracheal tube.

6. Move the blade slightly toward the midline, and advance it until the distal end is positioned at base of tongue. Simultaneously, move the patient's lower lip away from the blade using the index finger of your right hand.

7. Lift the laryngoscope handle slightly and move it forward to displace the jaw. Be careful not to put pressure on the teeth. At this point, vomitus, or secretions lying in the posterior pharynx, can usually be seen. Suctioning may be necessary to clear the airway. If suctioning fails to resolve the airway obstruction, place the patient on his or her side to facilitate drainage of the secretions.

8. Look for the tip of the epiglottis, and place the laryngoscope blade into its proper position. If you're using a curved blade, direct its tip into the vallecula. With a straight blade, extend it behind the epiglottis and lift. Frequently, the blade tip will not be perfectly positioned when the lifting maneuver is first employed. Unless the blade has been inserted too deeply, the epiglottis should come into view. If you fail to see it, withdraw the blade slightly. You might also need to advance the blade farther. To do this, place your right thumb in the patient's mouth, grasp the chin, and lift the jaw while advancing the laryngoscope.

9. With your left wrist straight, use your shoulder and arm to continue lifting the mandible and tongue at a 45-degree angle to the ground until the glottis is exposed. (See Figure 11-37.) Often the entire glottis will not be seen, but at least its posterior third or half should be visible. If the larynx lies anteriorly, another member of your team may apply firm downward pressure on the patient's neck over the cricoid cartilage (see the earlier discussion of Sellick's maneuver). This will push the larynx backward, allowing a better view. A stylet may be useful in redirecting the tube anteriorly.

10. Grasp the endotracheal tube in your right hand, holding it as you would a pencil. This permits gentle maneuvering of the tube. It may also help you to hold the tube so that the curve is in a horizontal plane (bevel sideways). Advance the tube through the right corner of the patient's mouth. Typically, you must direct the distal end up or down in order to pass it into the larynx.

11. Under direct observation, insert the endotracheal tube into the glottic opening, and pass it through until the distal cuff disappears past the vocal cords. Then advance it another half-inch or full inch.

12. Hold the tube in place with your hand to prevent its accidental displacement. Attach a bag-valve device to the 15/22 mm adapter on the tube.

13. Inflate the distal cuff with 5 to 10 mL of air. To avoid tracheal trauma due to excessive cuff pressure, use only enough air to fill the distal cuff. Determine the minimum amount of air needed by listening for air leakage around the tube prior to distal cuff inflation. The cuff should be filled just to the point where this leakage ceases. When removing the syringe, use a reverse twisting action to prevent any accidental leakage of air.

14. Check for proper tube placement. Watch to see that the chest rises and falls with each ventilation, and listen for equal, bilateral breath sounds in

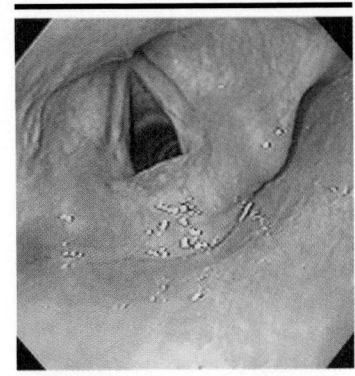

FIGURE 11-37 Open glottis visualized through laryngoscopy. Note the vocal cords on either side of the glottic opening.

✷ Always watch the tube pass through the cords.

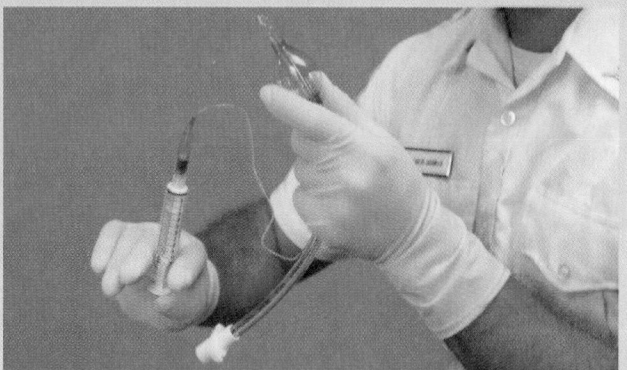

11-2A. Prepare equipment.

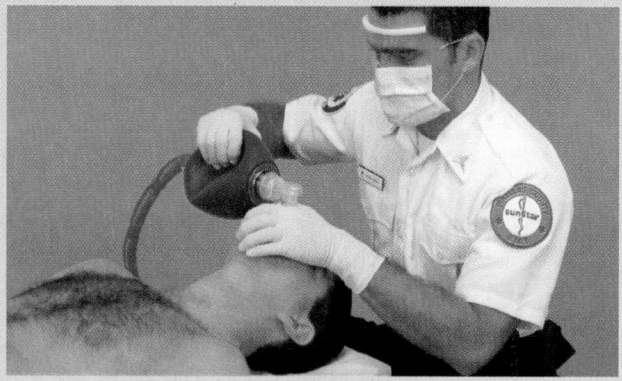

11-2B. Hyperventilate the patient.

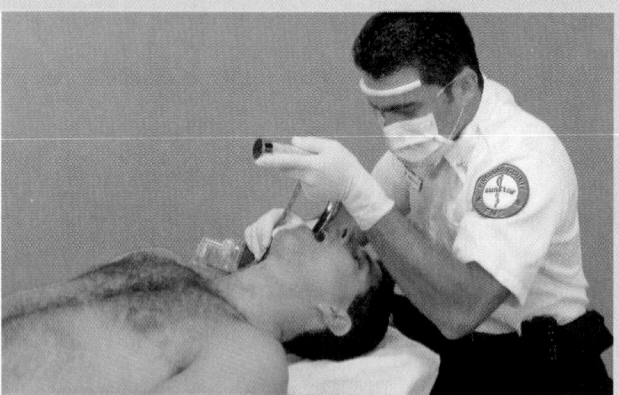

11-2C. Insert the laryngoscope.

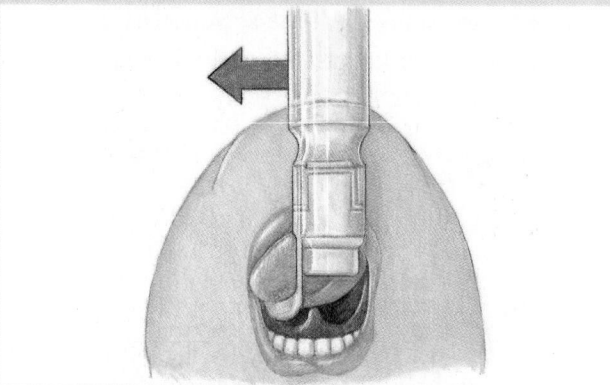

11-2D. Slide the tongue to the left.

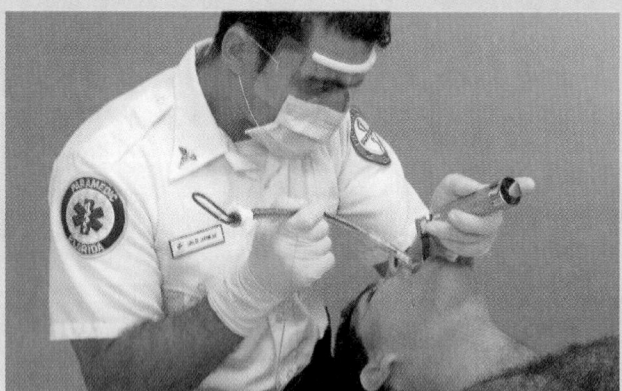

11-2E. Visualize the larynx.

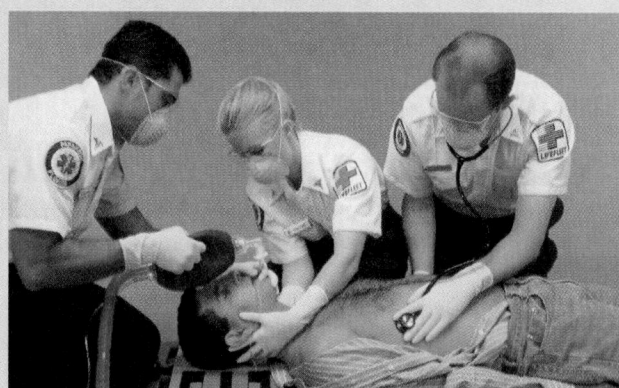

11-2F. Insert the tube, and ventilate.

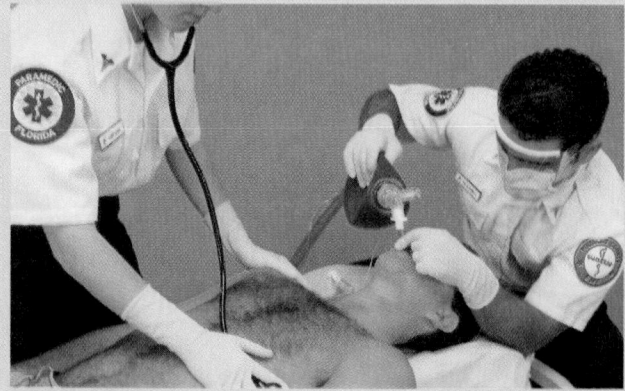

11-2G. Assess ventilations.

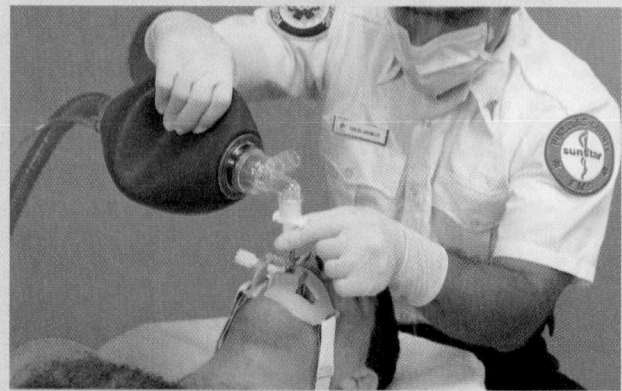

11-2H. Secure the tube.

the chest. There should an absence of sounds over the epigastrium when ventilations are delivered.

15. Hyperventilate the patient with 100% oxygen. Insert an oropharyngeal airway to serve as a bite block.

16. Secure the endotracheal tube with umbilical tape, while maintaining ventilatory support. Loop the tape around the tube at the level of the patient's teeth, attaching it tightly to the tube without kinking or pinching it. Then wrap the tape around the patient's head, and tie it at the side of the neck. Alternatively, use a commercial tube-holding device.

17. Recheck for proper tube placement. Observe the chest's rise and fall. Listen for breath sounds. Also check the proximal end of the tube for breath condensation during each exhalation. Condensation is simply the moisture present in exhaled air. It should disappear each time the patient inhales or a ventilation is delivered. The absence of breath condensation during exhalation suggests improper placement of the tube. (Recheck tube placement any time the patient is moved.)

18. Continue supporting the tube manually while maintaining ventilations.

19. Check periodically to ensure proper tube positioning.

* Always confirm proper tube placement by at least two methods, and document these in the run report.

Verification of Proper Endotracheal Tube Placement

Correct placement of the endotracheal tube should be routinely checked and rechecked. There are many ways to confirm proper placement of the endotracheal tube. Any may be used to verify proper tube placement. Remember, however, that it is important to consider the entire patient and all parameters when evaluating for proper tube placement. Do not become over-reliant on technology.

❑ *Visual Confirmation.* The best confirmation is to visualize the tube passing through the vocal cords by use of the laryngoscope. If visualization is maintained throughout intubation, there is little chance of inadvertent esophageal intubation.

❑ *Observation of Chest Rise.* Following tube placement, watch to be sure that the patient's chest rises with ventilations. If the tube has been misplaced in the esophagus, the chest will not rise.

❑ *Auscultation of Breath Sounds.* Following tube placement, breath sounds should be auscultated over both sides of the chest and the epigastrium. The presence of breath sounds over the chest, along with the absence of breath sounds over the epigastrium, confirms proper endotracheal tube placement. Likewise, the absence of breath sounds over the chest and the presence of breath sounds over the epigastrium indicates an esophageal intubation. Breath sounds present on one side but absent or diminished on the other indicate that the tube has been advanced too deeply into one of the mainstem bronchi.

❑ *End-Tidal CO_2 Detectors.* There are a number of commercially available devices which detect expired carbon dioxide. These may be electronic or colorimetric. Air expired from the lungs contains carbon dioxide. Adequate levels of exhaled carbon dioxide, as detected by an end-tidal CO_2 detector, further confirm proper endotracheal tube placement.

❑ *Esophageal Detector Device.* Esophageal detectors are simple devices that consist of a 60 mL syringe connected to the end of an endotracheal tube adapter. This device takes advantage of the anatomical differences between the esophagus (a collapsible, fibromuscular tube) and the trachea (a rigid, cartilaginous tube). The ability to withdraw air readily from the syringe confirms placement of the endotracheal tube in the trachea while resistance to air withdrawal, or the creation of vacuum, denotes esophageal intubation. In other words, suction will cause the esophagus to collapse if the endotracheal tube is placed in the esophagus whereas the cartilaginous trachea will not collapse when suction is applied to endotracheal tubes properly placed in the trachea.

❑ *Gastric Contents through Endotracheal Tube.* In some cases of esophageal intubation, vomitus will be propelled from the tube. This results from high gastric pressures brought on by resuscitation efforts, particularly by the several breaths that may have been delivered in order to check a patient for chest rise. When vomiting occurs, leave the tube in place. Removing it may cause the vomitus to travel into the pharynx and be aspirated into the trachea. Instead, move the tube to one side of the mouth and ventilate your patient with a bag-valve-mask device until the trachea can be successfully intubated. Remember, many patients will vomit and aspirate vomitus into the respiratory tree. The presence of vomitus in the tube may be due to prior aspiration. However, this also may indicate esophageal intubation and requires further evaluation.

❑ *Condensation in Endotracheal Tube.* Exhaled air approaches 100% humidity. Usually, the ambient relative humidity is less than 100%. Thus, when condensation forms on the inside of the endotracheal tube, this suggests proper endotracheal placement of the endotracheal tube.

Esophageal Intubation. If not corrected, esophageal misplacement of the tube will lead to severe hypoxia and brain death. Indications of esophageal intubation include:

❑ An absence of chest rise and breath sounds with ventilatory support
❑ Gurgling sounds heard over the epigastrium with each breath delivered
❑ An absence of breath condensation in the endotracheal tube
❑ A persistent air leak, despite inflation of the tube's distal cuff
❑ Cyanosis and progressive worsening of the patient's condition
❑ **Phonation** (any noise made by the vocal cords).

■ **phonation** the process of generating speech and other sounds.

If there is any suspicion that the tube is in the esophagus, it should be removed immediately, the patient ventilated, and another endotracheal tube placed.

Endobronchial Intubation. In addition to the possibility of misplacing an endotracheal tube in the esophagus, there is also the possibility of inserting the tube too deeply. When the tube reaches the bifurcation of the trachea, it will pass into either the right or left mainstem bronchus. Endobronchial intubation results in one-lung ventilation and possible hypoxia.

You can avoid inserting the tube too far by following a few guidelines:

1. Advance the distal cuff past the vocal cords no more than one-half inch to one full inch.
2. Once it is in this position, hold the tube in place with one hand, thus preventing it from being accidentally pushed any further.
3. Inflate the cuff and firmly secure the tube in place with umbilical tape or a commercial tube-holding device.
4. Mark the side of the endotracheal tube at the level where it emerges from your patient's mouth. This will allow you to quickly identify any changes in tube placement.

Indications of endobronchial intubation include:

❑ Breath sounds present on one side of the chest but diminished or absent on the other.
❑ Poor compliance (felt when delivering ventilations with the bag-valve device)
❑ Cyanosis, cardiac dysrhythmias, or other evidence of hypoxia

✱ If breath sounds are absent or diminished on one side, suspect that the endotracheal tube is in too far.

To resolve the problem, withdraw the tube until breath sounds are again heard equally on both sides of the chest.

Endotracheal Intubation with an EOA in Place   In addition to the normal intubation technique that has been described, you will also need to handle a number of special situations involving endotracheal intubation. As the EOA is still used in certain areas, a paramedic may be called upon to place an endotracheal tube in a patient who has already been intubated with an EOA. Since endotracheal intubation is superior to an EOA, you should do this as soon as possible. This is a cumbersome process, but the following steps will help you place an endotracheal tube correctly in a patient previously intubated with an EOA.

1. While maintaining ventilatory support, hyperventilate the patient with 100% oxygen.
2. Assemble and check the equipment.
3. Place the patient's head and neck into the appropriate positions.
4. Hold the laryngoscope in your left hand.
5. Remove the EOA mask as follows: First pinch the obturator tube where it extends through the plastic housing. (See Figure 11-38.) Then lift off the mask.
6. Insert your laryngoscope blade into the right side of the patient's mouth. With a sweeping action, displace the tongue and EOA tube to the left. (See Figure 11-39.) Proceed with intubation in the usual manner.
7. Under direct observation, insert the endotracheal tube into the glottic opening, and pass it through until the distal cuff disappears past the

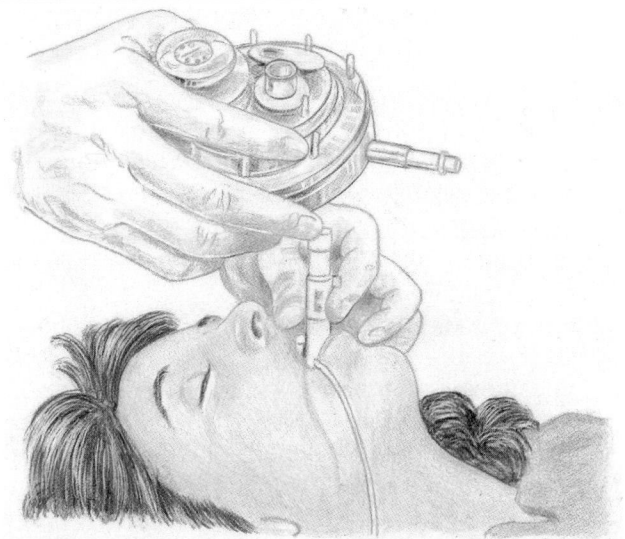

FIGURE 11-38   To perform endotracheal intubation when an EOA is already in place, remove the EOA mask.

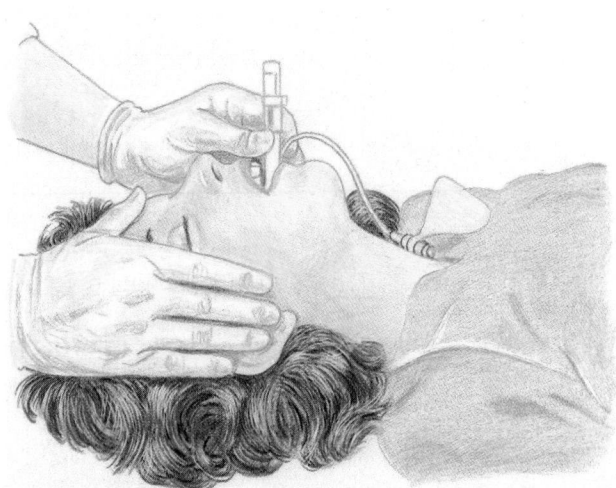

FIGURE 11-39   Move the EOA tube to the left side of the mouth.

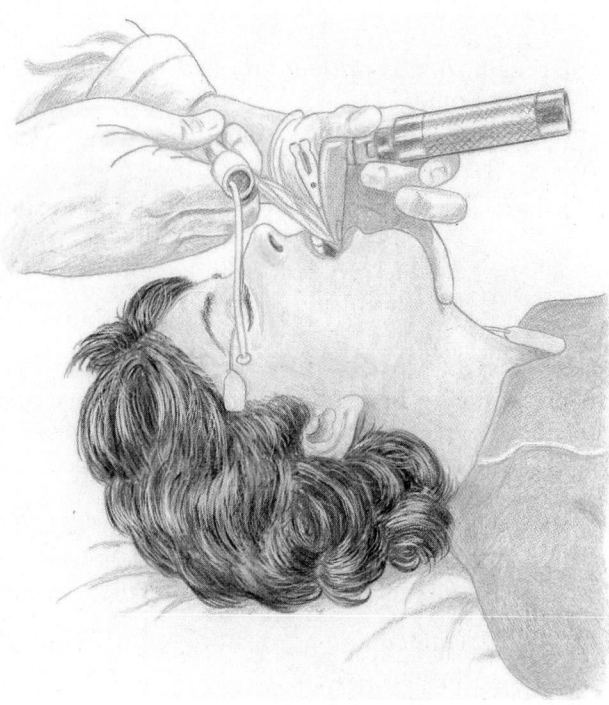

FIGURE 11-40 With the EOA tube held to the left, perform endotracheal intubation in the usual manner.

vocal cords. Then advance the tube another half-inch to full inch. (See Figure 11-40.) Appropriate precautions should be used to ensure that the tube is in the larynx, as the distensible esophagus can easily accommodate both the esophageal obturator and the endotracheal tube.

8. Hold the endotracheal tube in place with one hand to prevent displacement. Then attach a bag-valve device to the 15/22 mm adapter of the tube and deliver several breaths.

9. Check for proper tube placement by observing chest rise, breath sounds, and the absence of sounds in the epigastrium when ventilations are delivered.

10. Inflate the distal cuff with 5 to 10 mL of air, and remove the syringe.

11. Recheck for proper placement of the tube.

12. Hyperventilate the patient with 100% oxygen.

13. Secure the endotracheal tube with umbilical tape, while continuing to maintain ventilatory support.

14. With suction available, deflate the EOA's distal cuff. Then hold the endotracheal tube firmly in place while you steadily remove the EOA tube. The EOA tube must be extracted to prevent esophageal or tracheal damage, which may result from having two distal cuffs in place at the same time.

15. Maintain ventilatory support, periodically checking proper tube position.

Digital Intubation In some situations, you may be called upon to perform "digital intubation." This technique dates back to the 18th century when people performed intubations without the benefit of a laryngoscope. Instead, they used "digital" (finger) or "tactile" (touch) intubation. (See Figure 11-41.)

Today this procedure is still useful for a number of situations in the prehospital setting. Digital intubation is suggested when a patient is deeply

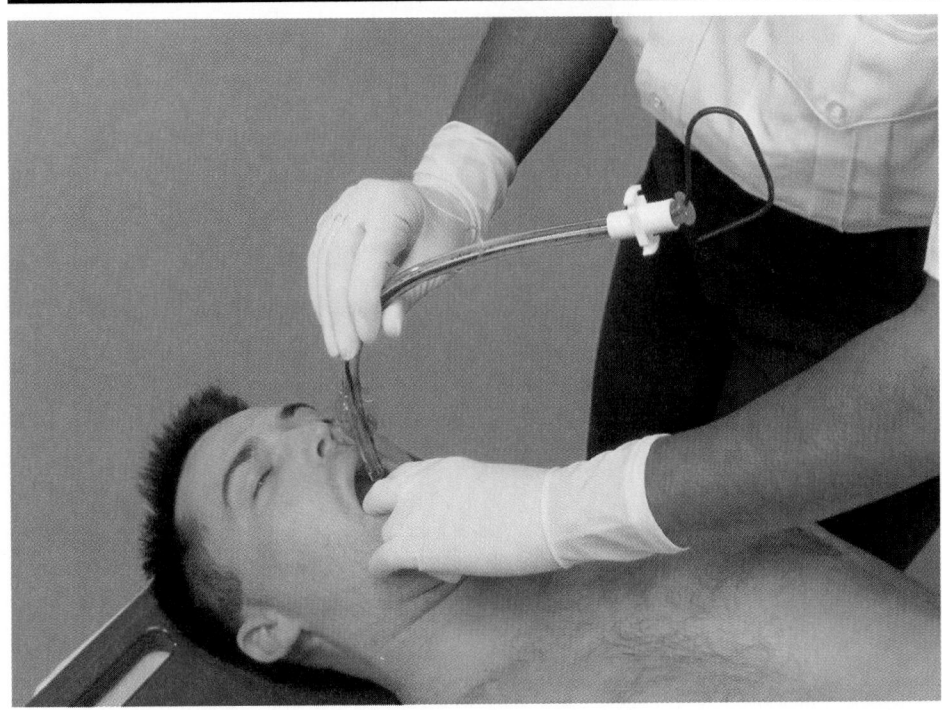

FIGURE 11-41 Blind orotracheal intubation by the digital method.

comatose or in cardiac arrest and when proper positioning is difficult to achieve. The classic example is a trauma patient with suspected cervical spine injury. Since the digital technique does not require manipulation of the head and neck, it is of great value here. It may also be useful in extrication situations where a patient cannot be properly positioned. Additionally, because this technique does not require visualization, it may be helpful when patients have facial injuries that distort the anatomy or when copious amounts of blood, vomitus, or other secretions cannot be suctioned out for a proper view of the airway. To perform digital intubation:

1. While maintaining ventilatory support, hyperventilate the patient with 100% oxygen.
2. Assemble and check your equipment. You will need the following items: an appropriately sized endotracheal tube, a malleable stylet, water-soluble lubricant, a 5 to 10 mL syringe, a bite block, and latex gloves.
3. Insert the stylet into the endotracheal tube and bend the tube/stylet into a J shape.
4. While another team member stabilizes the patient's head and neck in an in-line position, kneel at the patient's left shoulder. Be sure you are facing the patient. Place the bite block (or other such device) between the patient's molars to prevent injury to your fingers.
5. Insert the middle and index fingers of your left hand into the patient's mouth. (See Figure 11-42.) By alternating fingers, "walk" your hand down the midline, while simultaneously tugging forward on the tongue. This lifts the epiglottis up and away from the glottic opening, positioning it within reach of your probing fingers.
6. Palpate the epiglottis with your middle finger .(See Figure 11-43.)
7. Press the epiglottis forward, and insert the endotracheal tube into the mouth anterior to your fingers. (See Figure 11-44.)

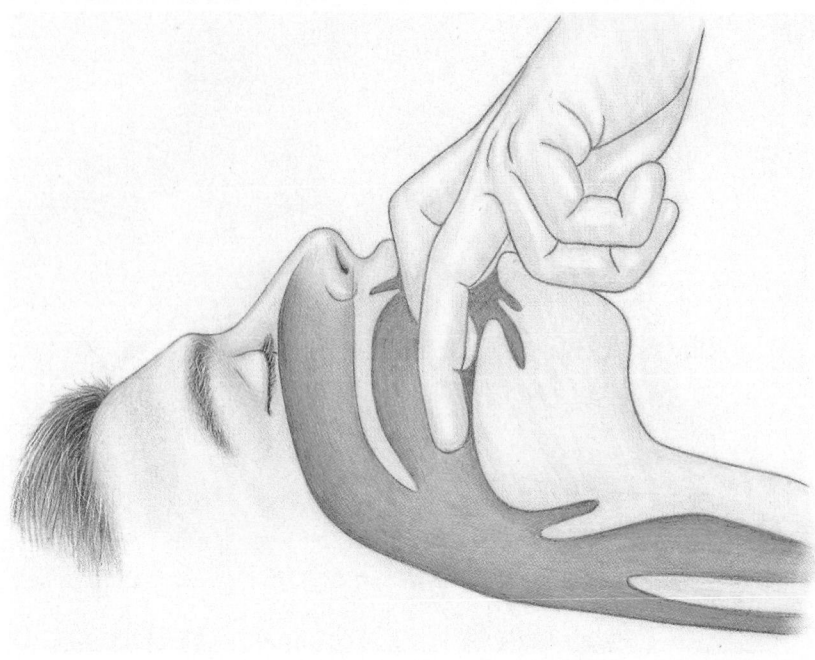

FIGURE 11-42 To perform digital intubation, insert the middle and index finger into the patient's mouth.

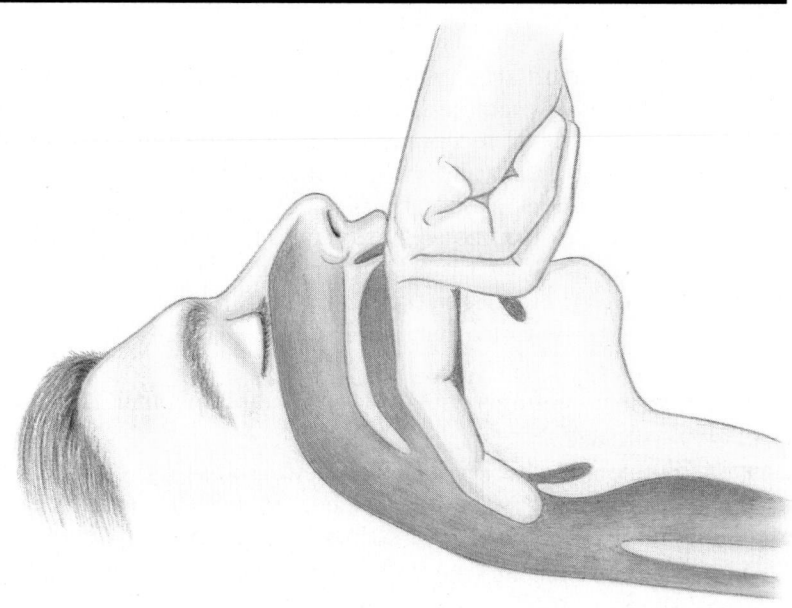

FIGURE 11-43 "Walk" the fingers down and palpate the epiglottis with the middle finger.

8. Advance the tube, pushing it with your opposite hand. Then use your index finger to maintain the tip of the tube against the middle finger. This will direct the tip to the epiglottis.

9. Use your middle and index fingers to direct the tube tip between the epiglottis (in front) and the fingers (behind). Then advance the tube through the cords while simultaneously pressing the tube forward with the index and middle fingers. This will prevent it from slipping posteriorly into the esophagus.

10. Hold the tube in place with one hand. Next, attach a bag-valve device to the 15/22 mm adapter of the tube and deliver several breaths.

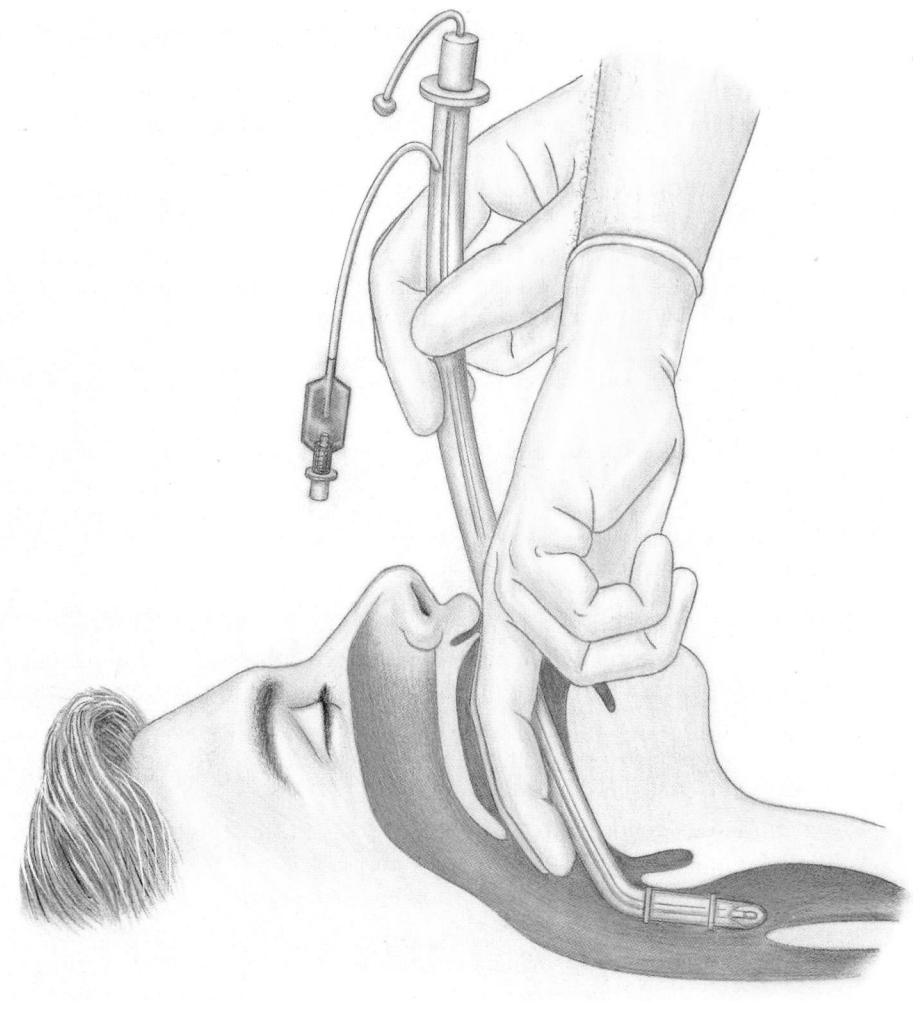

FIGURE 11-44 Insert the endotracheal tube while elevating the epiglottis.

11. Check for proper tube placement by observing chest rise, breath sounds, and the absence of sounds in the epigastrium when ventilations are delivered.

12. Inflate the distal cuff with 5 to 10 mL of air, and then remove the syringe.

13. Recheck for proper placement of the tube.

14. Hyperventilate the patient with 100% oxygen.

15. Secure the endotracheal tube with umbilical tape, while you continue ventilatory support.

16. Maintain ventilation, periodically checking proper tube position.

Transillumination (Lighted Stylet) Intubation   Another method of endotracheal intubation is the transillumination method. It is based on the fact that a bright light introduced into the larynx or trachea can be seen through the soft tissues of a patient's neck. The transillumination technique makes use of lighted stylet. (See Figure 11-45.) This stylet is a malleable, plastic-coated wire that features a small, high-intensity bulb at its distal end. Power for the device is supplied by a small battery housed at the proximal end and controlled by an on-off switch.

Since the paramedic can confirm correct placement in the trachea by observing the light from the stylet through the tissues of the neck, a transillu-

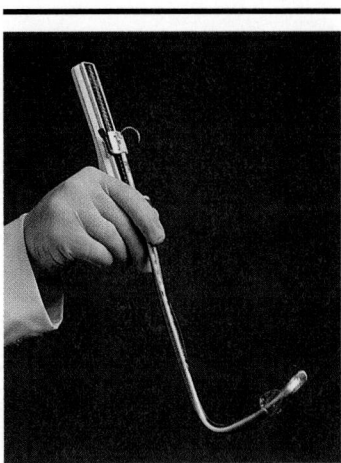

FIGURE 11-45 Lighted stylet for endotracheal intubation.

mination intubation can be safely performed without having to visualize the glottic opening directly. Endotracheal intubation can be performed in this way without manipulating the head and neck.

Several studies have shown the transillumination technique to be fast, dependable, and atraumatic. Because the head and neck do not have to be manipulated, it can be used in a trauma patient. The biggest problem associated with this method of intubation is that ambient illumination can make it difficult to see the stylet light. Therefore, when attempting this procedure, ambient light should be reduced. The method works best in a darkened room and with thin patients. In direct sun or bright daylight, the patient's neck should be shielded. To perform the transillumination technique:

1. While maintaining ventilatory support, hyperventilate the patient with 100% oxygen.

2. Assemble and check your equipment. The endotracheal tube should be 7.5 to 8.5 i.d. You will need to cut the tube to 25–27 cm in order to accommodate the stylet. Place the stylet into the tube, and bend it just proximal to the cuff.

3. Kneel on either side of the patient, facing his or her head.

4. Turn on the stylet light.

5. With your index and middle fingers inserted deeply into the patient's mouth and your thumb on the chin, lift the tongue and jaw forward. (See Figure 11-46.)

6. Insert the tube/stylet combination into the mouth and advance it through the oropharynx into the hypopharynx.

7. Use a "hooking" action with the tube/stylet to lift the epiglottis out of the way. (See Figure 11-47.)

8. When you see a circle of light at the level of the patient's Adam's apple, hold the stylet stationary. (See Figure 11-48.) Advance the tube off the stylet into the larynx approximately one-half to one full inch. A diffuse, dim, or hard-to-see light indicates that the tube/stylet combination is in

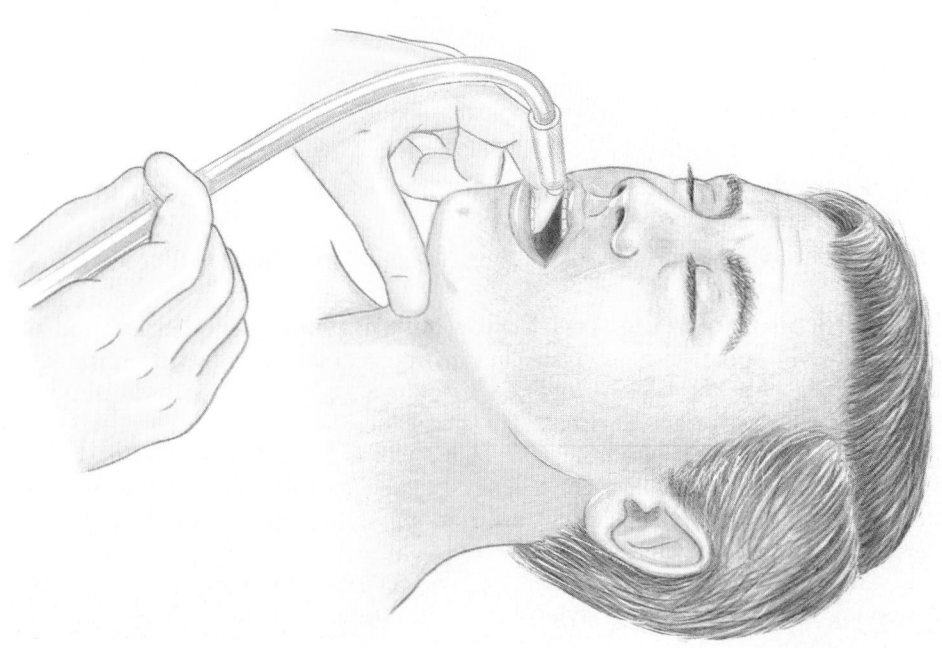

FIGURE 11-46 Insertion of the lighted stylet/endotracheal tube.

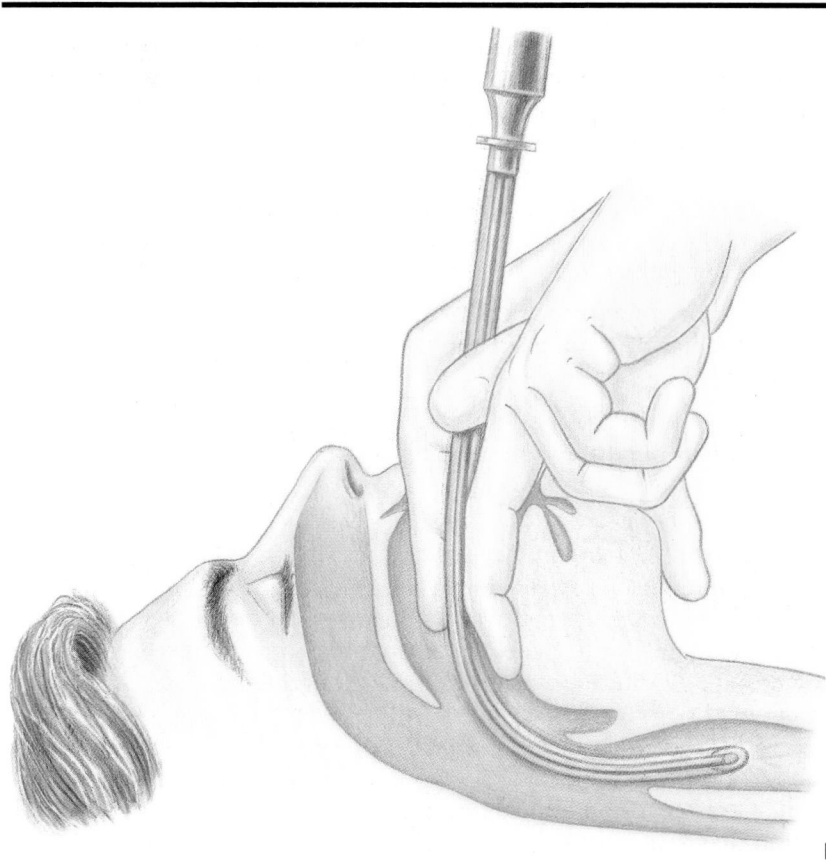

FIGURE 11-47 Lighted stylet/endotracheal tube in position.

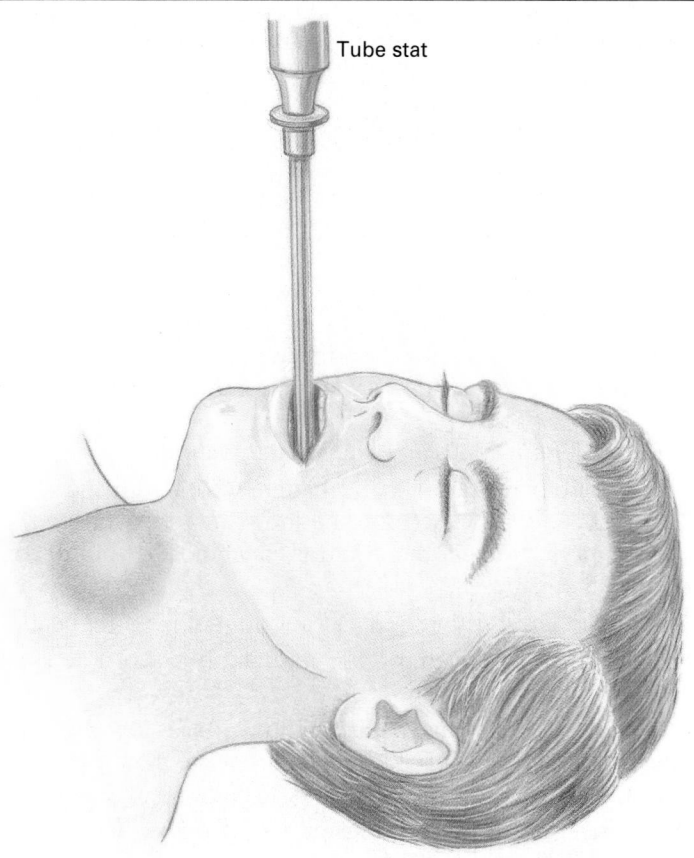

Tube stat

FIGURE 11-48 The light of the stylet, when in proper position, should be visible on the front of the patient's neck.

the esophagus. A bright light that appears laterally to the upper aspect of the laryngeal prominence indicates that it has moved into the right or left pyriform fossa. Both of these situations can be corrected by withdrawing the tube and reattempting intubation after the patient has been ventilated with 100% oxygen for several minutes.

9. Hold the tube in place with one hand, and then remove the stylet. Attach a bag-valve device to the 15/22 mm adapter of the endotracheal tube and deliver several breaths.

10. Check for proper tube placement by observing chest rise, breath sounds, and the absence of sounds in the epigastrium when ventilations are delivered.

11. Inflate the distal cuff with 5 to 10 mL of air.

12. Recheck for proper tube placement. Continue delivering ventilations while securing the tube in place.

Special Situations   There are several special situations that require variation in the technique described previously for endotracheal intubation. These include intubation of trauma patients and pediatric patients. In addition, combative patients, patients with closed head injuries, or patients with seizure activity may require modification in your approach and technique.

Endotracheal Intubation in the Trauma Patient.   Establishing and maintaining an open airway is a critical aspect of trauma care. It requires the use of special techniques, because the head and neck must be stabilized in a neutral, in-line position that will prevent spinal injuries. Endotracheal intubation is the preferred technique, so long as it can be accomplished without extension, rotation, or flexion of the neck. It must be emphasized that a cervical collar alone will not provide adequate stabilization of the cervical spine.

There are several techniques for performing endotracheal intubation in the trauma victim. These include digital intubation and lighted stylet intubation, as described earlier. You might also apply nasotracheal intubation (which will be described later in this chapter) or a technique called *orotracheal intubation using in-line stabilization.*

There are several methods for performing orotracheal intubation using in-line stabilization. One method calls for you to assume a sitting position while stabilizing the patient's head between your thighs. This immobilizes the head and cervical spine while enabling you to see the glottic opening with a laryngoscope. Another method calls for one team member to immobilize the head and spine while a second performs endotracheal intubation. (See Procedure 11-3.) To perform orotracheal intubation with in-line stabilization:

1. One team member is at the patient's side, facing the patient.

2. He or she then places both hands over the patient's ears with the little, ring, and middle fingers under the occiput, the index fingers over the tragus (the cartilaginous projection on the anterior ear), and the thumbs on the face over the maxillary sinuses.

3. Slight pressure is applied **caudally** to support and immobilize the head.

4. The paramedic charged with performing the intubation sits or kneels at the patient's head.

5. While another team member maintains manual in-line stabilization, the paramedic who will perform intubation should prepare to initiate the procedure.

6. The laryngoscope blade is inserted into the right side of the patient's mouth and, with a sweeping action, the tongue is displaced to the left. Intubation is continued in the manner described earlier.

✱ If trauma and spine injury are suspected, the head and neck must be maintained in a neutral position during intubation.

✱ All paramedics must be competent at performing endotracheal intubation with in-line stabilization.

■ **caudally** of, at, near, or toward the foot end of the body.

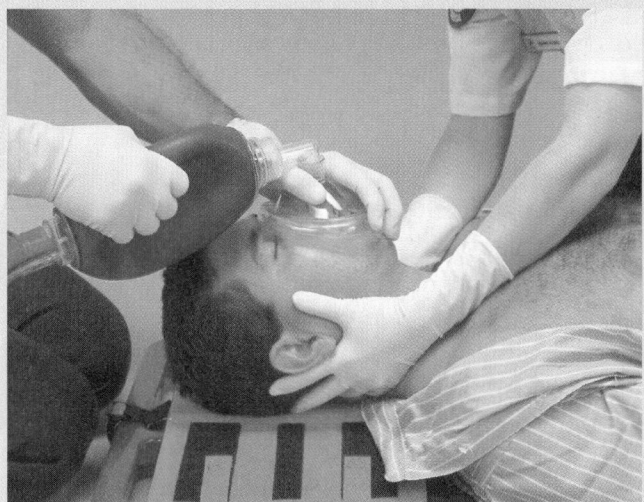

11-3A. Hyperventilate the patient with the cervical spine manually immobilized.

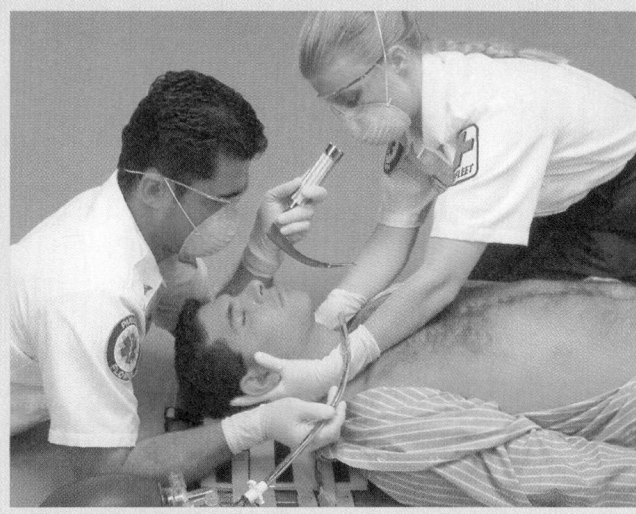

11-3B. Maintaining immobilization, prepare to visualize the patient's airway.

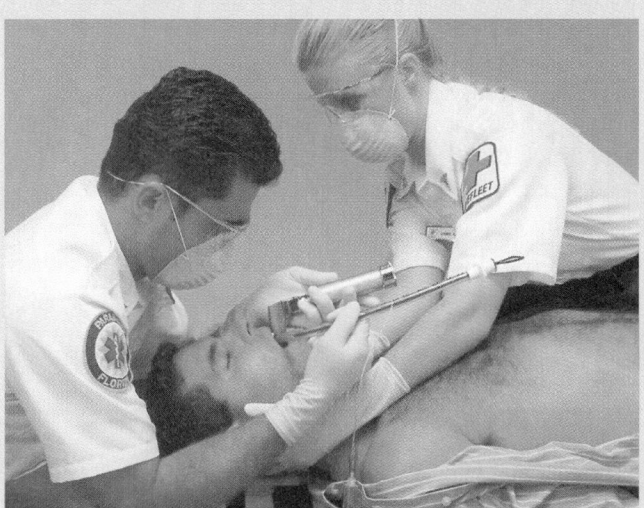

11-3C. Gently insert the laryngoscope.

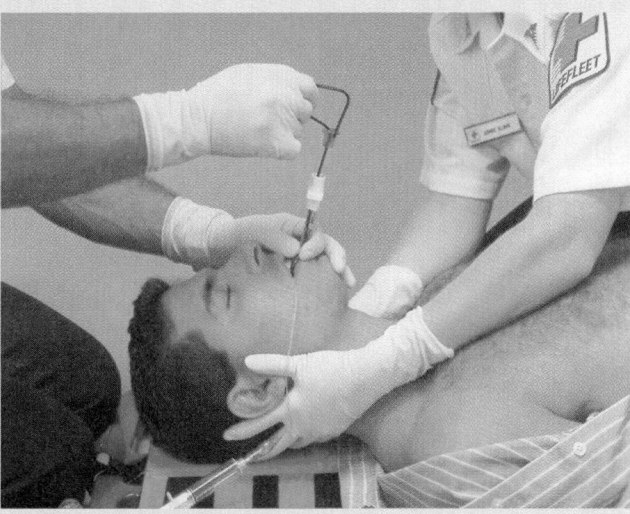

11-3D. Visualize the airway without moving the patient's neck.

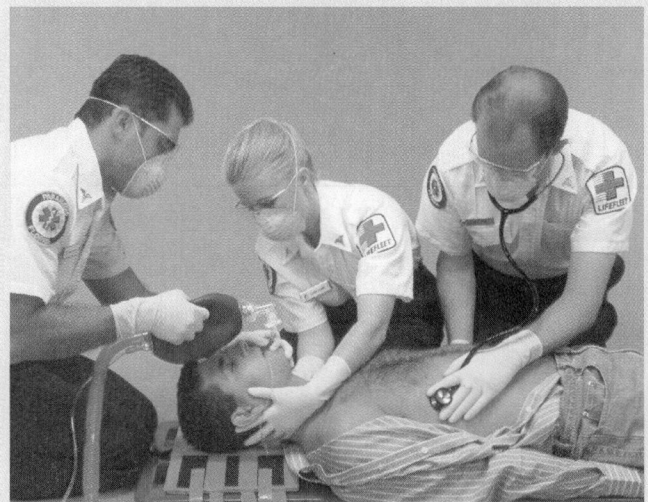

11-3E. Remove the stylet.

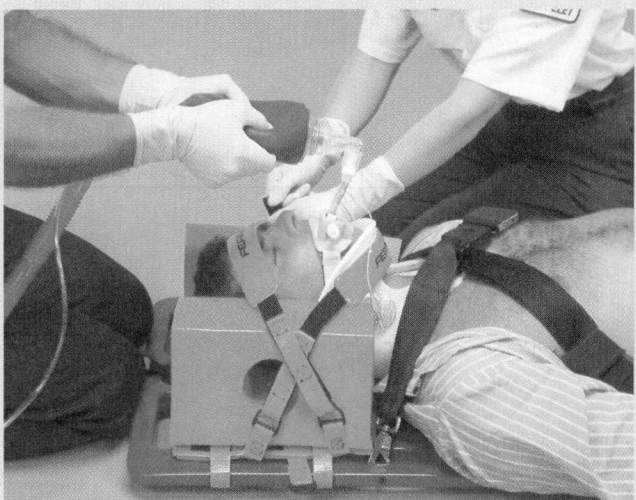

11-3F. Assess ventilations.

Endotracheal Intubation in Children. While the procedure for performing endotracheal intubation in children is similar to that used with adults, there are differences. These stem largely from differences in the anatomy of a child's airway. You should be aware of the following anatomical features of the pediatric airway. (See Figure 11-49.)

- ❏ The structures are proportionately smaller and more flexible than those of an adult.
- ❏ The tongue is larger in relation to the oropharynx.
- ❏ The epiglottis is "floppy" and narrow.
- ❏ The glottic opening is higher and more anterior in the neck.
- ❏ The vocal cords slant upward, toward the back of the head, and are closer to the base of the tongue.
- ❏ The narrowest part of the upper airway is at the cricoid cartilage, not the glottic opening as in adults.

Also remember that doctors believe infants and small children have greater vagal tone than adults. Therefore, laryngoscopy and passage of an endotracheal tube are more likely to precipitate a vagal response, dramatically slowing the child's heart and decreasing cardiac output and blood pressure. Heart rate must be monitored throughout the procedure to guard against this complication. If it falls below 60 beats per minute (or below 80 beats per minute in an infant), the procedure should be stopped and ventilations (with 100% oxygen) reinitiated.

The indications for endotracheal intubation in a pediatric patient are the same as those for adults. They include:

- ❏ Ventilatory support with a bag-valve-mask device seems inadequate.
- ❏ Cardiac or respiratory arrest.
- ❏ It is necessary to provide a route for drug administration or ready access to the airway for suctioning.
- ❏ There is a need for prolonged artificial ventilation.

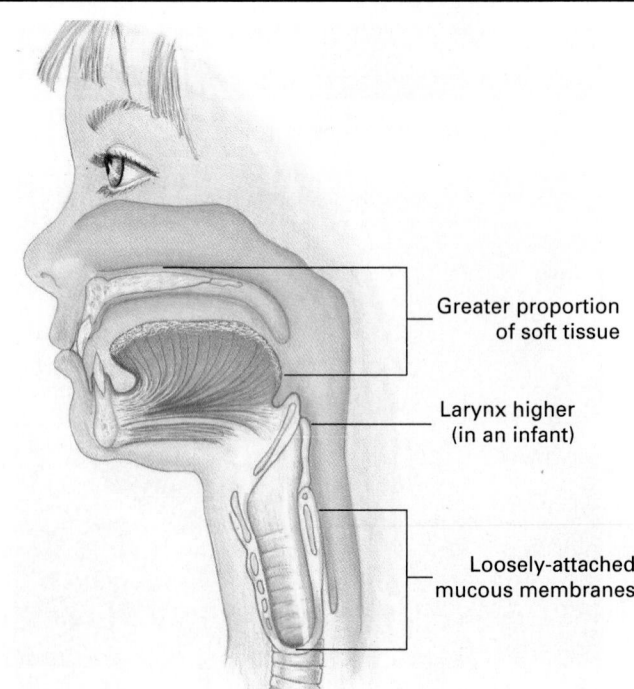

Greater proportion
of soft tissue

Larynx higher
(in an infant)

Loosely-attached
mucous membranes

FIGURE 11-49 Airway anatomy in the child.

Additionally, if local protocols allow it, endotracheal intubation may be used in a child who is suffering croup or epiglottitis and an increasingly compromised airway. (See Procedure 11-4.) To perform endotracheal intubation on a pediatric patient:

1. While maintaining ventilatory support, hyperventilate the patient with 100% oxygen. If time allows, hyperventilate for a full two minutes.
2. Assemble and check your equipment. As stated earlier, a straight blade laryngoscope is preferred with infants and small children, since it provides greater displacement of the tongue and better visualization of the relatively cephalad and anterior glottis. Also, with children younger than 8 years old, use a noncuffed endotracheal tube. Due to the distance between the mouth and the trachea, a stylet is rarely needed to position the tube properly.
3. Place the patient's head and neck into an appropriate position. With a pediatric patient, the head should be maintained in a "sniffing" position (perhaps by placing a towel under the head).

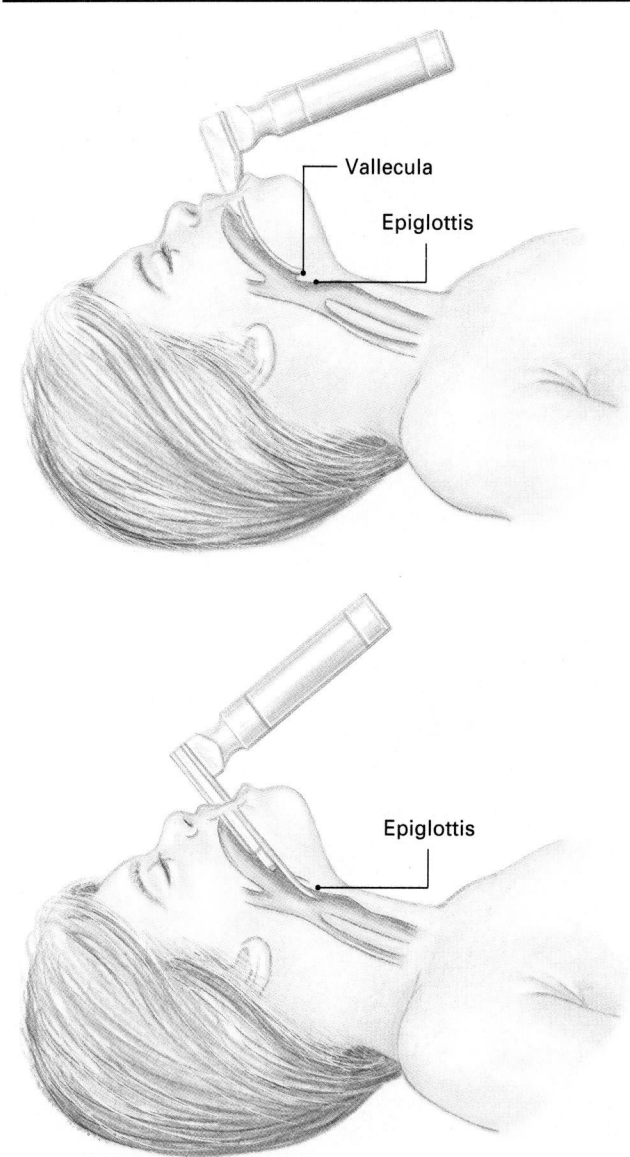

FIGURE 11-50 Proper placement of the laryngoscope blade in the pediatric patient.

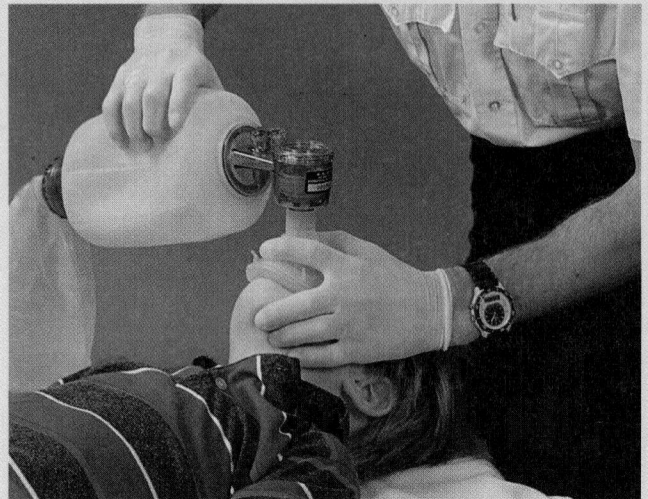

11-4A.   Hyperventilate the child.

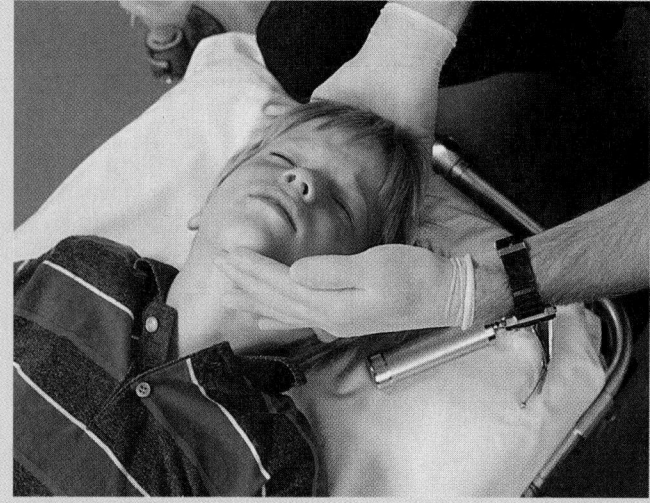

11-4B.   Position the head.

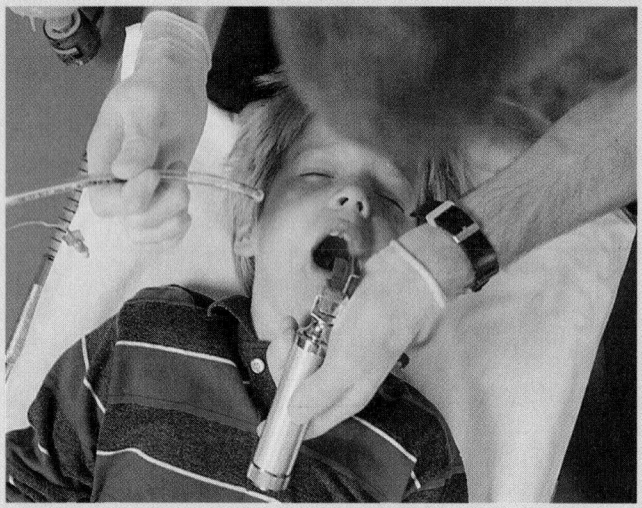

11-4C.   Insert the laryngoscope and visualize the airway.

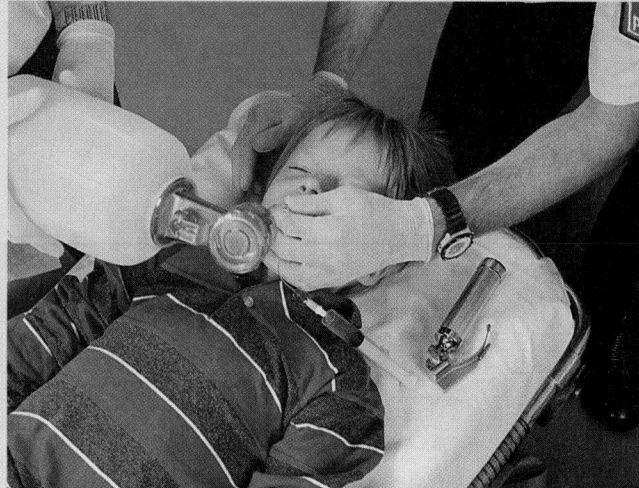

11-4D.   Insert the tube, and ventilate the child.

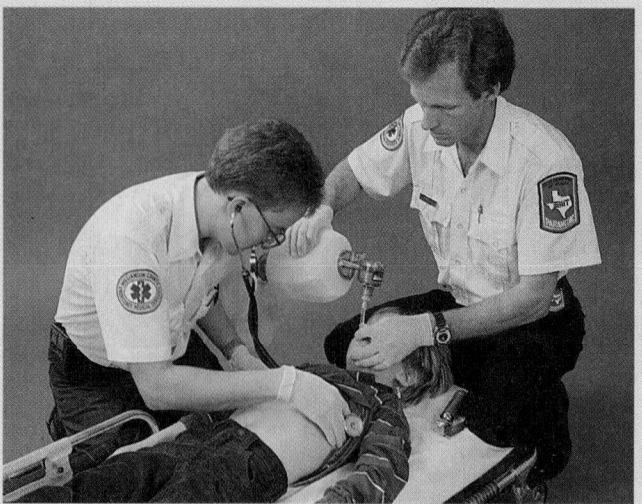

11-4E.   Confirm tube placement.

4. Hold the laryngoscope in your left hand.

5. Insert your laryngoscope blade into the right side of the patient's mouth. With a sweeping action, displace the tongue to the left.

6. Move the blade slightly toward the midline, and then advance it until the distal end is positioned at the base of the tongue. (See Figure 11-50.)

7. Look for the tip of the epiglottis, and place the laryngoscope blade into its proper position. Keep in mind that a child—particularly an infant—has a shorter airway and a higher glottis than an adult. Because of this, you'll see the cords much sooner than you may expect.

8. With your left wrist straight, use your shoulder and arm to lift the mandible and tongue at a 45-degree angle to the floor until the glottis is exposed. Use the little finger of your left hand to apply gentle downward pressure to the cricoid cartilage. This will permit easier visualization of the cords.

9. Grasp the endotracheal tube in your right hand. To pass the tube into your patient's mouth, it may be helpful to hold it so that its curve is in a horizontal plane (bevel sideways). Insert the tube through the right corner of the child's mouth.

* Always use an uncuffed tube in children less than 8 years of age.

10. Under direct observation, insert the endotracheal tube into the glottic opening and pass it through until its distal cuff disappears past the vocal cords—approximately 5 to 10 mm. As the tube is advanced, it should be rotated into the proper plane. In some cases, it will be difficult to advance an endotracheal tube at the level of the cricoid. Do not force the tube through this region, as it may cause laryngeal edema.

11. Hold the tube in place with your left hand. Attach an infant- or child-size bag-valve device to the 15/22 mm adapter and deliver several breaths.

12. Check for proper tube placement. Watch for chest rise and fall with each ventilation and listen for equal, bilateral breath sounds. There should also be an absence of sounds over the epigastrium with ventilations.

13. If the tube has a distal cuff, inflate it with the recommended amount of air.

14. Recheck for proper placement of the tube, and hyperventilate the patient with 100% oxygen.

15. Secure the endotracheal tube with umbilical tape while maintaining ventilatory support.

16. Continue supporting the tube manually while maintaining ventilations. Check periodically to ensure proper tube position. As with adults, allow no more than 30 seconds to pass without ventilating your patient.

Rapid Sequence Intubation with Neuromuscular Blockade (Optional Skill). Establishment and protection of the airway has the highest priority in emergency care. On certain occasions, patients who are still responsive may have trouble maintaining their airway and may require endotracheal intubation. This situation most commonly occurs in drug overdoses, status epilepticus, and in trauma patients with closed head injuries. Often, however, intubation is difficult because of the presence of gag reflexes, clenched teeth, or general combativeness. In these cases, endotracheal intubation can be carried out following administration of a neuromuscular blocking agent.

Neuromuscular blocking agents are drugs that cause muscle relaxation, thus facilitating endotracheal intubation. All skeletal muscles, including the muscles of respiration, respond to these drugs. Following administration, the patient will become apneic and require mechanical ventilation. Neuromuscular blocking agents have no effect on the level of consciousness or pain sensation. Neuromuscular blocking drugs are classified as *depolarizing* and *non-depolarizing,* depending on their mechanism of action. The most commonly used depolarizing drug is succinylcholine, while vecuronium and pancuronium are the most frequently used non-depolarizing agents.

❏ *Succinylcholine (Anectine).* Succinylcholine is a depolarizing neuromuscular blocker commonly used in emergency medicine. It acts in approximately 60–90 seconds and lasts approximately 3–5 minutes. Following administration, succinylcholine causes muscle **fasciculations**. This progresses to total paralysis, including the diaphragm.

❏ *Pancuronium (Pavulon).* Pancuronium is a long-acting, non-depolarizing neuromuscular blocking agent. It acts in 2–5 minutes and lasts 40–60 minutes.

❏ *Vecuronium (Norcuron).* Vecuronium is a non-depolarizing neuromuscular blocking agent with a rapid onset and short duration of action. It has fewer cardiovascular side effects than succinylcholine and does not cause fasciculations.

Before administering a neuromuscular blocking agent, you should ready equipment for airway management. Intubation should be carried out as soon as the patient becomes apneic. In addition, because a neuromuscular blocking agent has no effect on pain sensation and mental status, it should not be administered to alert patients without first administering a sedative or analgesic.

Most emergency patients have eaten or drunk something in the hours prior to the onset of the emergency. Thus, virtually every emergency patient is considered to have a full stomach. Neuromuscular blockade and endotracheal intubation may cause vomiting, which increases the risk of aspiration, so special precautions must be taken to gain rapid control of the airway as soon as the drug is administered. As a result, this procedure is often referred to as *rapid sequence intubation.* To perform a rapid sequence intubation:

1. Assemble the required equipment.
2. Assure that the IV line is functioning and secure.
3. Place the patient on a cardiac monitor and pulse oximeter.
4. Preoxygenate the patient with 100 % oxygen, using a bag-valve-mask unit.
5. Premedicate the patient, if appropriate, with one of the following drugs.
   - *Diazepam* (Valium): 5–10 milligrams intravenously
   - *Morphine sulfate:* 5–10 milligrams intravenously
   - *Atropine:* 0.01 mg/kg IV push for children and adolescents (blocks vagal effects and helps prevent muscle fasciculations)
6. Have another rescuer apply Sellick's maneuver to occlude the esophagus and maintain it until the ET tube is in place and the cuff inflated.
7. Administer 1.5 mg/kg succinylcholine IV push and continue ventilation.
8. Apnea and jaw relaxation are indications that the patient is sufficiently relaxed to proceed with endotracheal intubation.
9. Perform endotracheal intubation. If you are unable to place the tube in 20 seconds, stop. Then ventilate the patient with 100 % oxygen for 30–60 seconds before attempting the procedure again.
10. Once the tube is in place, inflate the cuff, and confirm tube placement by auscultating bilateral breath sounds and, if available, by use of an end-tidal CO_2 detector.
11. Release cricoid pressure and properly seal the endotracheal tube.

The effects of succinylcholine will wear off in 3–5 minutes. A bite block should be placed to prevent the patient from biting the endotracheal tube. Medical control may request the administration of pancuronium or vecuronium if continued paralysis is warranted.

Method of Insertion: The Nasotracheal Route The preceding techniques have largely focused on orotracheal intubation. However, certain cases will require you to use the nasotracheal route, or the passing of an endotracheal tube through the nose and into the trachea. This procedure can be accomplished either "blindly" or by using a laryngoscope. Cases in which nasotracheal intubation is called for in the field include:

❑ Patient who may have a spinal injury
❑ Patient who is not in arrest or unresponsive
❑ Patient whose mouth cannot be opened due to clenched teeth
❑ Patient with a fractured jaw
❑ Patient with oral or maxillofacial injuries
❑ Patient who has recently undergone oral surgery
❑ Severely obese patient
❑ Patient with neck arthritis that prevents placing into the sniffing position
❑ Patient who cannot be ventilated by another means

Nasotracheal intubation is *not* recommended in the following situations.

❑ Nasal fractures
❑ Basilar skull fractures
❑ A significantly deviated nasal septum
❑ Nasal obstruction.

Advantages of Nasotracheal Intubation
❑ The tube can be placed while the patient's head and neck are immobilized.
❑ It is more comfortable for the patient than insertion of an oral endotracheal tube.
❑ The tube cannot be bitten.
❑ The tube can be easily anchored.

Disadvantages of Nasotracheal Intubation
❑ It is more difficult and time-consuming to perform than orotracheal intubation.
❑ It is potentially more traumatic for patients. Passage of the tube may lacerate the pharyngeal mucosa or larynx during insertion.
❑ The tube may kink or clog more easily than an oral endotracheal tube.
❑ It poses a greater risk of infection, because the tube introduces nasal bacteria into the trachea.
❑ Improper placement is more likely when performing "blind" nasotracheal intubation as passage of the tube through the glottic opening cannot be visualized.
❑ "Blind" nasotracheal intubation requires that the patient be breathing.

Remember that nasotracheal intubation should not be attempted if a basilar skull fracture is suspected.

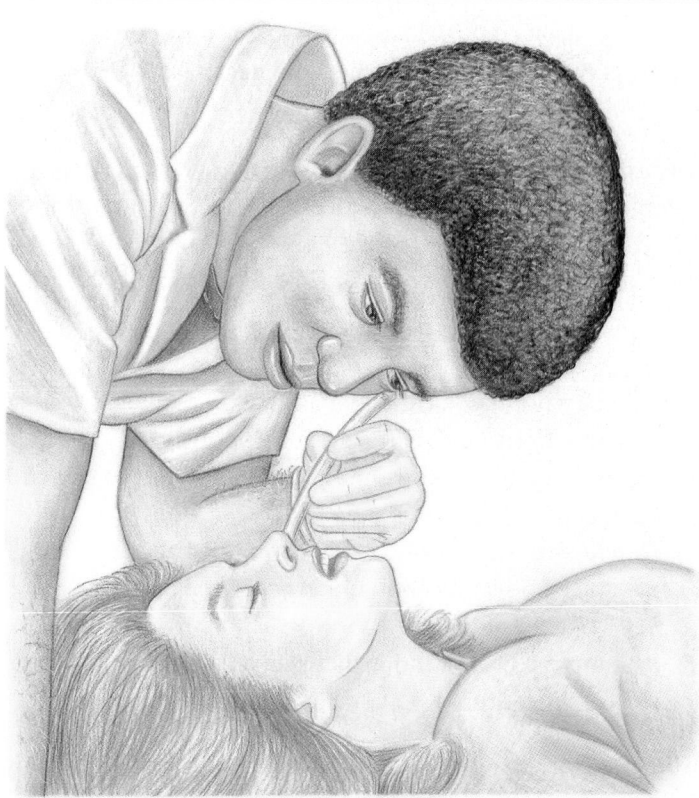

FIGURE 11-51 Blind nasotracheal intubation.

Blind Nasotracheal Intubation. Blind nasotracheal intubation is the placement of an endotracheal tube without the aid of a laryngoscope. It requires a quiet environment and a patient who is breathing. (See Figure 11-51.) To perform blind nasotracheal intubation:

1. While maintaining ventilation, hyperventilate the patient with 100% oxygen.
2. Assemble and check your equipment. Then lubricate the distal end of a proper-size tube. If time permits, apply a local spray of 4% lidocaine (a topical anesthetic) mixed with 0.25% phenylephrine (a potent vasoconstrictor) to the nasal mucosa. This will make tube insertion more comfortable to the patient and reduce the amount of possible hemorrhage.
3. Place the patient's head and neck into a relaxed position. If spinal injury is suspected, maintain the head and neck in a neutral, in-line position.
4. Inspect the nose, and select the larger nostril as your passageway.
5. Insert your tube into the nostril, with the flanged end of the tube along the floor of the nostril or facing the nasal septum. This will help avoid damage to the turbinates. Next, gently guide the tube in an anterior-to-posterior direction.
6. As the tube is felt to drop into the posterior pharynx, listen closely at its near end for the patient's respiratory sounds. These sounds are loudest when the tube is proximal to the epiglottis. Care must be taken when the tube tip reaches the posterior pharyngeal wall, because it must then be directed toward the glottic opening. At this point in the procedure, the tip of the tube may become "hung up" in the pyriform sinus. You can recognize this by the "tenting up" of skin on either side of the Adam's apple. Pyriform sinus placement is easily resolved by slightly withdrawing the tube and rotating it to the midline.

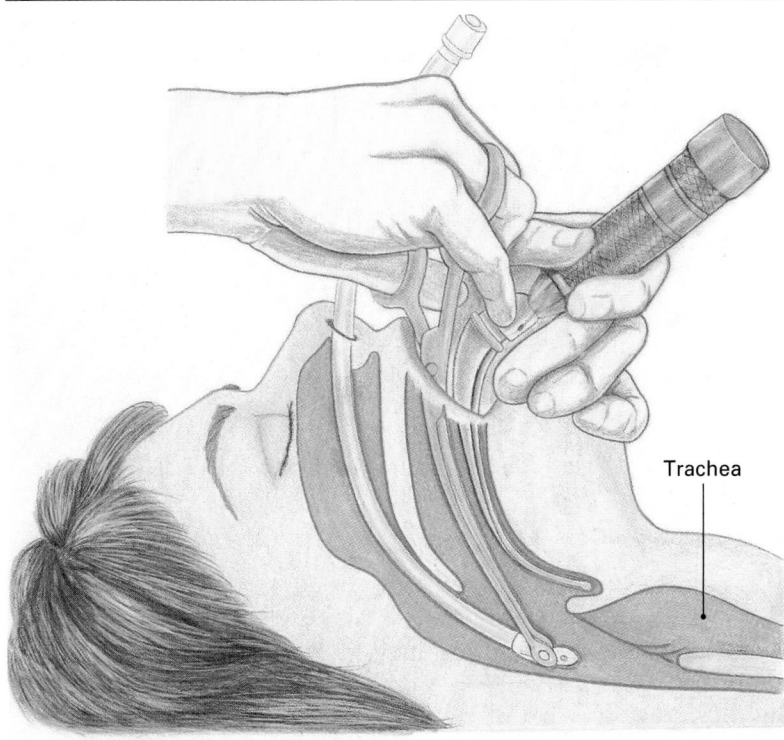

Trachea

FIGURE 11-52 The Magill forceps are useful in performing nasotracheal intubation.

7. With the patient's next inhaled breath, advance the tube rapidly into the glottic opening, and then continue passing it until the distal cuff is just past the vocal cords. At this point, the patient may cough, buck, or strain. Gagging is a sign of esophageal placement, while bulging and anterior displacement of the larynx usually indicates correct placement of the tube. When correctly placed in the trachea, the patient's exhaled air will be felt coming from the proximal end of the tube. At the same time, breath condensation should intermittently fog the clear plastic tube.

8. Hold the tube in place with one hand to prevent displacement.

9. Inflate the distal cuff with 5–10 mL of air.

10. Recheck for proper placement of the tube by observing chest rise, breath sounds, and the absence of sounds over the epigastrium.

11. Hyperventilate the patient with 100% oxygen.

12. Secure the endotracheal tube with umbilical tape, while continuing to maintain ventilatory support.

Even the most experienced paramedic will find patients in whom blind nasotracheal intubation is extremely difficult. Either tube passage is stopped in the posterior pharynx, because the tube is angled away from the middle, or it passes posteriorly into the esophagus. To correct the tube's passage into the esophagus, extend the head farther and repeat the procedure.

Nasotracheal Intubation under Direct Visualization. When performing nasotracheal intubation, the endotracheal tube can be directed into the glottic opening using a laryngoscope and Magill forceps. The procedure for this laryngoscopy is identical to that described for orotracheal intubation. With the glottic opening exposed, direct the tube tip by rotating its proximal end to position it in the mid-line. Then advance the tube between the vocal cords. If

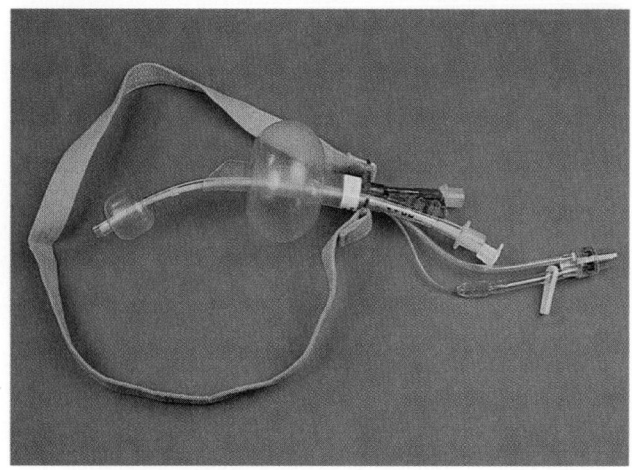

FIGURE 11-53 The Pharyngeo-tracheal Lumen (PtL) airway.

the tube falls posteriorly and cannot be directed through the glottic opening, use the Magill forceps to grasp it and direct it anteriorly. (See Figure 11-52.) While the operator holds the tube and manipulates it anteriorly, another member of the team or an assistant should carefully advance the tube by applying pressure on its proximal end. In this way, the operator is free to guide the tube without having to pull it along with the forceps.

Foreign Body Removal under Direct Laryngoscopy. Direct visualization of the larynx with a laryngoscope may also allow for removal of an obstructing foreign body. The foreign body can then be removed with Magill forceps or a suction device. Initially, basic life support maneuvers for airway obstruction should be carried out. If these fail to alleviate the obstruction, direct visualization of the airway should be attempted. The procedure for visualizing the airway is identical to that used for orotracheal intubation.

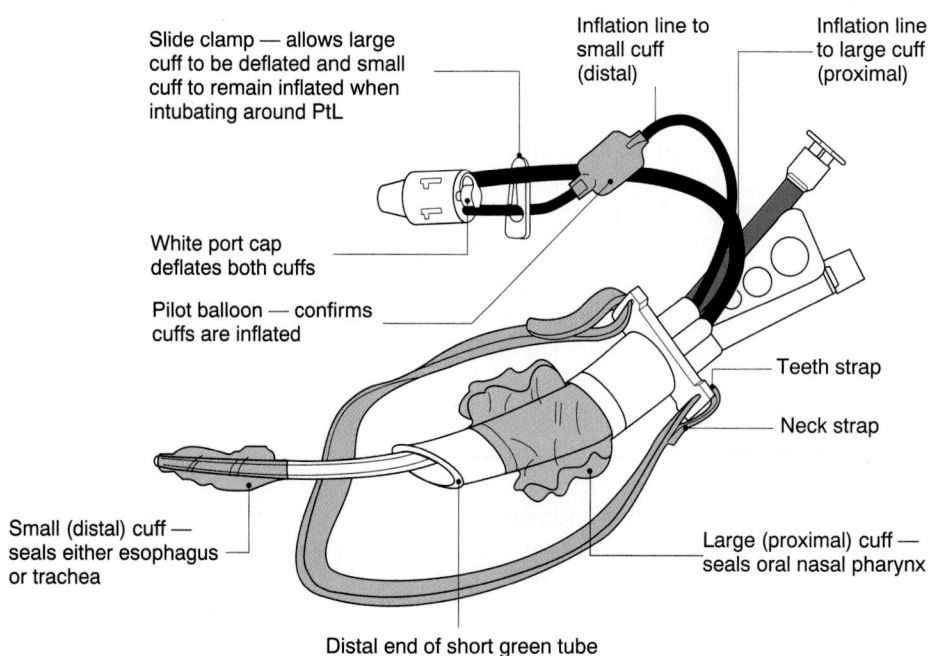

FIGURE 11-54 The PtL airway is designed for blind insertion.

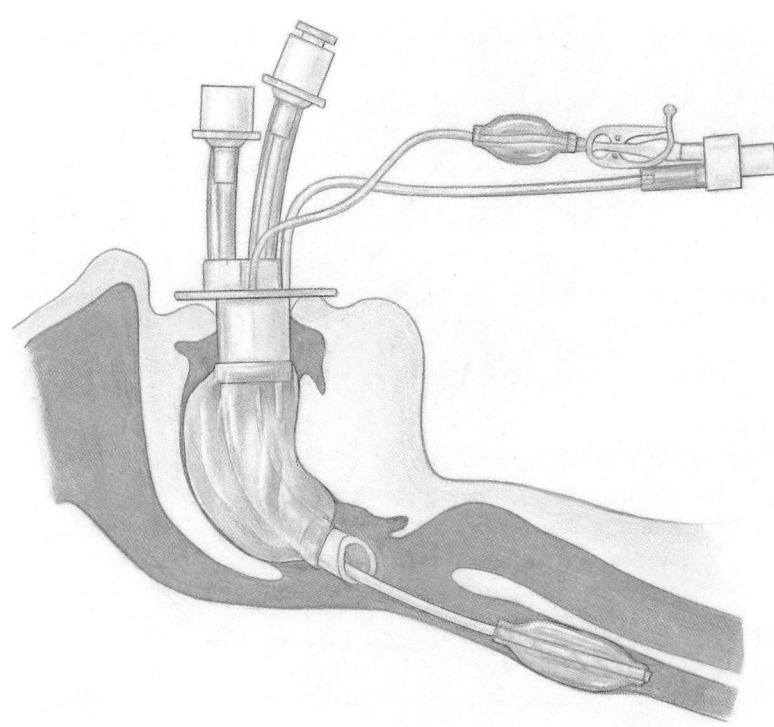

FIGURE 11-55 The PtL airway in place.

Pharyngeo-tracheal Lumen Airway

Several new devices are available to assist in airway management. Among them is the *Pharyngeo-tracheal Lumen airway (PtL)*. (See Figure 11-53.) This device is a two-tube system. The first tube is short and wide (green in color at the proximal end), with a balloon situated along its lower third. When inflated, this balloon seals the entire oropharynx. Air introduced through the tube at the proximal end will enter the pharynx. The second, clear tube travels through the first one and extends approximately 10 cm past its distal end. This second tube may be inserted into either the trachea or the esophagus. It has a distal cuff that, when inflated, can seal off whichever anatomical structure contains the tube. When the second tube is in the esophagus, the patient will be ventilated via the first tube. When the second tube is in the trachea, the patient will be ventilated through it. (See Figures 11-54 and 11-55.)

Advantages of the PtL Airway

- ❑ It can function in either the tracheal or esophageal position.
- ❑ It has no face mask to seal.
- ❑ It does not require direct visualization of the larynx.
- ❑ It does not require movement of the head or neck, thus allowing use with trauma patients.
- ❑ It helps protect the trachea from upper airway bleeding and secretions.

Disadvantages of the PtL Airway

- ❑ The oropharyngeal balloon does not totally protect the trachea.
- ❑ The oropharyngeal balloon can migrate out of the mouth anteriorly, partially dislodging the airway.
- ❑ Intubation around the PtL is difficult even with the oropharyngeal balloon deflated.
- ❑ It cannot be used in patients with a gag reflex.

The PtL includes a number of different features: a 15/22 mm connector at the proximal end of each tube, allowing for the attachment of a standard ventilatory device; a semi-rigid plastic stylet housed in the clear plastic tube, allowing for redirection of the tube; and a clamp on the inflation valve, permitting deflation of the oropharyngeal cuff while the other cuff remains inflated. The device has an adjustable, cloth neck strap that holds the tube in place. When the long, clear tube is positioned in the esophagus, deflation of the cuff in the oropharynx allows the device to be moved to the left side of the patient's mouth. This may permit endotracheal intubation while continuing esophageal occlusion. However, placement of an endotracheal tube with a PtL in place is difficult at best. To insert the PtL airway:

1. While maintaining ventilatory support, hyperventilate the patient with 100% oxygen.
2. Assemble and check the equipment.
3. Place the patient's head into the appropriate position. Use a hyperextended position if there are no potential spinal injuries. In the presence of possible spinal injury, maintain the patient's head and neck in neutral position while another team member provides in-line stabilization.
4. Insert the device using a tongue-jaw lift.
5. Once it is in place, inflate the PtL's distal cuffs simultaneously with a sustained breath fed into the inflation valve (referred to as valve number 1).
6. Deliver a breath into the green, or oropharyngeal, tube. If the patient's chest rises, the long clear tube is in the esophagus and ventilations should be continued via the green tube.

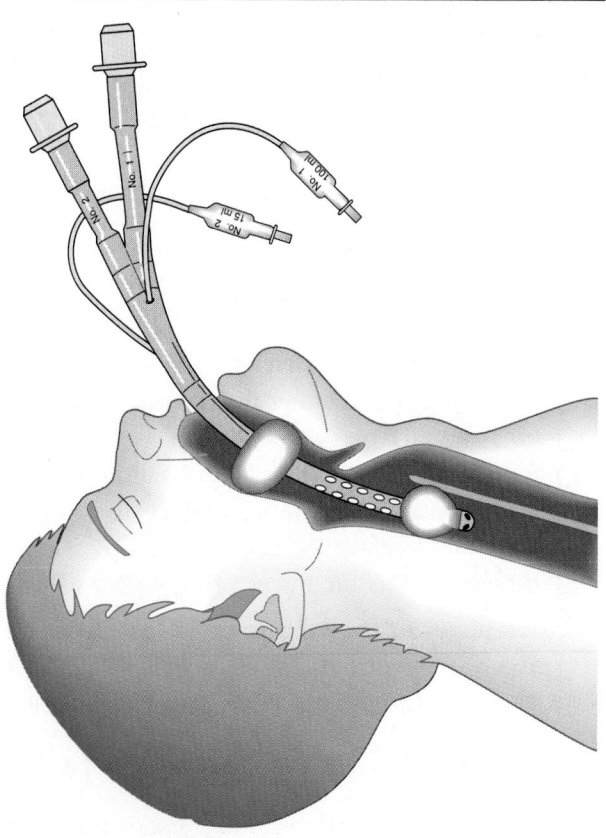

FIGURE 11-56   The esophageal tracheal combiTube (ETC) airway.

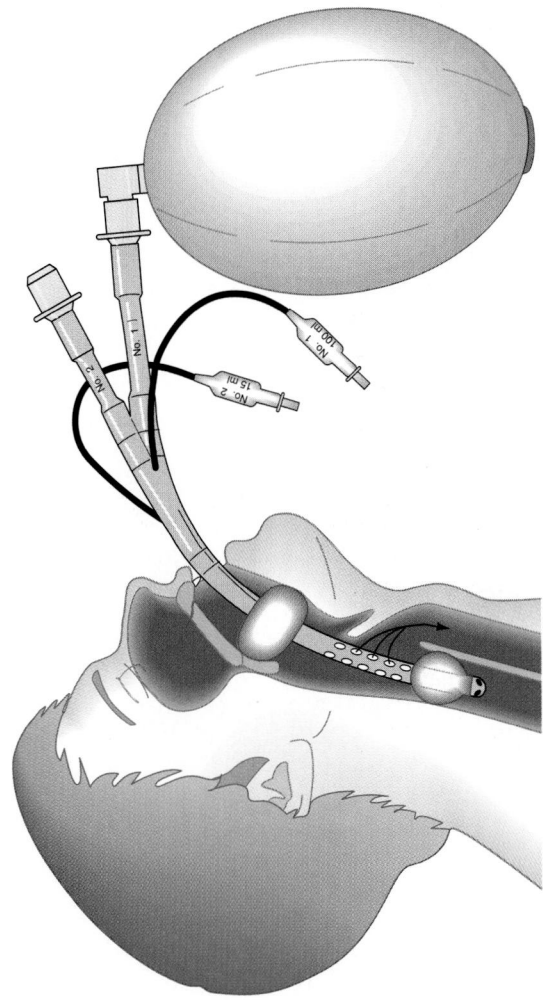

FIGURE 11-57 The ETC airway in the esophageal position.

7. If the chest does not rise, it means the long, clear tube is in the trachea. In this case, remove the stylet from the clear tube and ventilate the patient through that tube.

8. Attach a ventilatory device to the 15 mm connector, and continue delivering ventilatory support. Reassess for proper placement on an ongoing basis.

The PtL airway should be removed if the patient regains consciousness or if the protective airway reflexes return. Although an endotracheal tube can be placed with the PtL in place, it is best to go ahead and remove the PtL prior to attempting endotracheal intubation.

Esophageal Tracheal CombiTube (ETC) Airway

The Esophageal Tracheal CombiTube (ETC) airway is a two-tube system similar to the PtL airway. (See Figure 11-56.) However, the ETC tubes are combined, with their lumens separated by a partition wall. The distal end of the tube has a cuff for occluding the structure into which it is placed (esophagus or trachea). Proximally, there is a balloon that occludes the pharynx. The device is inserted blindly, entering either the esophagus or the trachea. Ventilation can be accomplished through either the esophageal or the tracheal lumen.

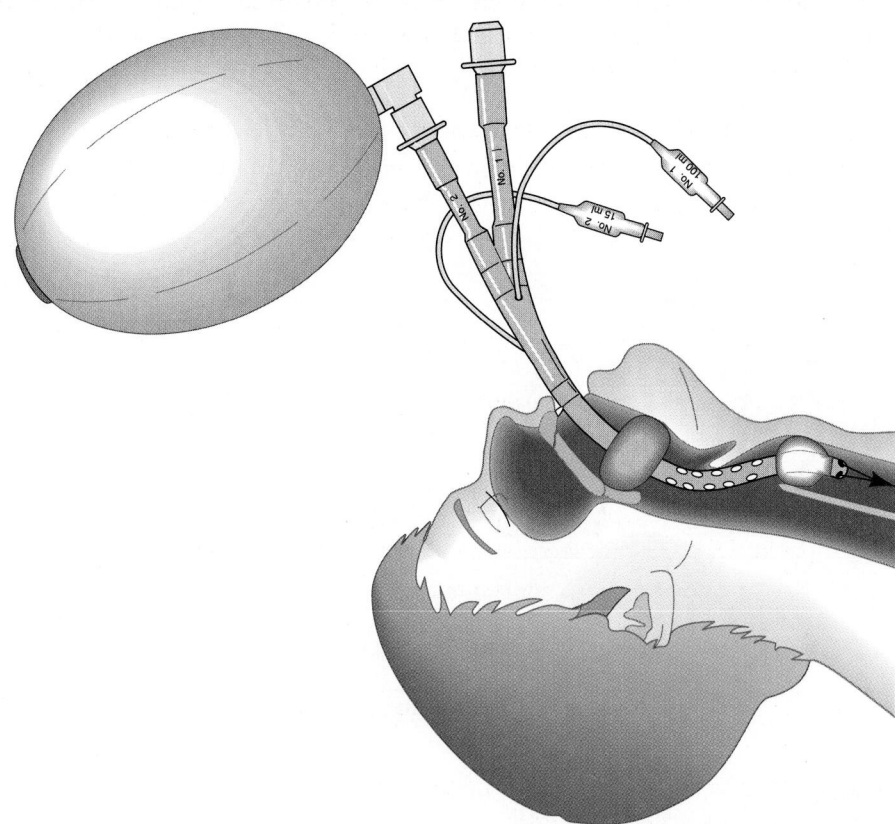

FIGURE 11-58 The ETC airway in the tracheal position.

The majority of times, the tube will enter the esophagus. In this case, ventilation is initiated through the longer blue connector (tube number 1), which leads to the esophageal lumen. (See Figure 11-57.) The distal end of this tube is closed, preventing the escape of air into the esophagus. Escape of air through the mouth is prevented through inflation of the pharyngeal balloon.

Auscultation of bilateral breath sounds, and the absence of gastric sounds, confirms placement in the esophagus. However, if you hear gastric sounds instead of breath sounds, the device is in the trachea. In this case ventilation should be performed through the shorter clear connector without changing the position of the tube. Air is now directed into the tracheal lumen and the device functions like an endotracheal tube. (See Figure 11-58.)

Advantages of the ETC Airway

❑ It can be rapidly inserted.
❑ It does not require visualization of the larynx.
❑ The airway is anchored behind the hard palate because of the pharyngeal balloon.
❑ The patient may be ventilated regardless of tube placement (esophageal or tracheal).
❑ The pharyngeal balloon can prevent aspiration of teeth and other debris.

Disadvantages of the ETC Airway

❑ It is impossible to suction tracheal secretions when the airway is in the esophageal position.
❑ Placement of an endotracheal tube is difficult with the ETC in place.
❑ It cannot be used in patients with a gag reflex.

Although endotracheal intubation is the preferred technique, an ETC can be used in any case where another mechanical airway would be used. In addition, the indications for the ETC include situations when:

❏ Immediate endotracheal intubation cannot be performed.
❏ Attempts at endotracheal intubation have proved unsuccessful.
❏ Access to the patient's head is inhibited due to entrapment.
❏ Direct visualization of the larynx is inhibited because of profuse bleeding or vomiting.

Contraindications for the ETC include cases when patients:

❏ Are less than 16 years of age
❏ Are under 5 feet tall
❏ Have an intact gag reflex
❏ Have known esophageal disease
❏ Are known alcoholics (may have esophageal varices)
❏ Have ingested a caustic substance

To place an ETC airway:

1. While maintaining ventilatory support, hyperventilate the patient with 100% oxygen.
2. Assemble and check the equipment.
3. Place the patient's head in a neutral position.
4. Insert the device, using a jaw-lift maneuver, to the depth indicated by the markings on the tube. The black rings on the tube should be positioned between the patient's teeth.
5. Once the ETC is in place, inflate its pharyngeal cuff with 100 mL of air. This firmly seals the device in the posterior pharynx behind the hard palate.
6. Inflate the distal cuff with 10–15 mL of air.
7. Begin ventilation through the longer blue connector (tube number 1).
8. Auscultate both lungs and the stomach. If you hear bilateral breath sounds instead of gastric sounds, continue ventilation through tube number 1.
9. If you hear gastric sounds instead of bilateral breath sounds, begin ventilation through the shorter clear connector (tube number 2). Confirm bilateral breath sounds and absent gastric sounds after changing the ventilation tube.
10. Continue ventilation with 100% oxygen, and periodically re-assess the airway.

Surgical Airways

A surgical airway involves placement of a catheter or similar device through the skin into the trachea. Although rarely used, these maneuvers can be life-saving when applied. As explained earlier, the larynx houses the vocal apparatus. The opening between the vocal cords—referred to as the glottic opening, or glottis—is the narrowest point along the upper airway. Foreign material, such as pieces of food, often become lodged here and obstruct the airway. Gag and other protective reflexes may restrict the airway, preventing the material from traveling deeper. Other conditions that cause laryngospasm or swelling of the vocal cords can also close the airway completely.

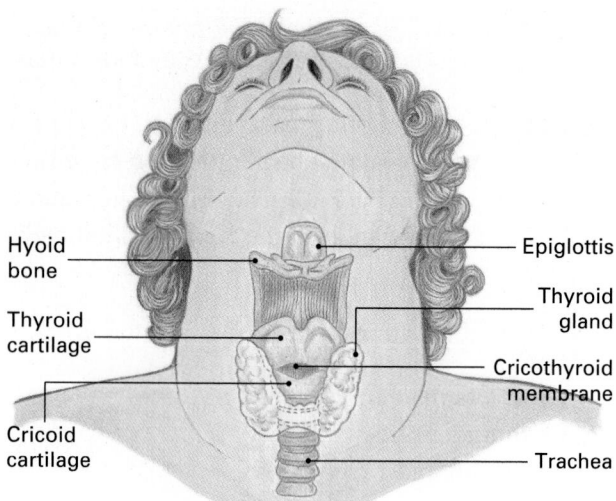

FIGURE 11-59 Anatomical landmarks associated with the cricothyroid membrane.

Hyoid bone

Thyroid cartilage

Cricoid cartilage

Epiglottis

Thyroid gland

Cricothyroid membrane

Trachea

In cases where an upper airway obstruction cannot be relieved by conventional methods, it may be necessary to open a patent airway below the vocal cords to allow ventilation. Circumstances that make this appropriate may involve severe laryngeal edema, facial or upper laryngeal trauma, and an airway obstructed by a foreign body. Because the cricothyroid membrane does not have an extensive blood supply, it can be cannulated with minimal bleeding, making it an excellent point of entry.

The cricothyroid membrane can be located by palpating the patient's neck, starting at the top. (See Figure 11-59.) The first prominence felt will be the thyroid cartilage, while the second is the cricoid cartilage. The space between these two, noted by the small depression, is the cricothyroid membrane.

Complications associated with penetrating the cricothyroid membrane to create an open airway include:

❑ Hemorrhage at the insertion site, particularly if the thyroid is perforated.
❑ Subcutaneous or mediastinal emphysema due to faulty placement of the cannula into the subcutaneous tissues rather than into the trachea.

Needle Cricothyrotomy *Cricothyrotomy* means making a puncture in the cricothyroid membrane and creating an airway tube. Cricothyrotomy allows rapid entrance to a patient's airway for temporary ventilation and oxygenation. It is used in cases where airway control is not possible by other methods.

In performing this technique, use the largest over-the-needle cannula possible. A 12- to 14-gauge cannula is desirable for adults, while a 18- or 20-gauge cannula may be adequate for children. If the catheter does not appear to be large enough, a second catheter can be inserted adjacent to the first, which will effectively double the amount of air that can be delivered. A 3.0 mm pediatric endotracheal tube adapter should be available in case transtracheal jet insufflation will be required. (Transtracheal jet insufflation will be described in the next segment.)

To perform a cricothyrotomy:

1. Place the patient on his or her back, and then hyperextend the head and neck.

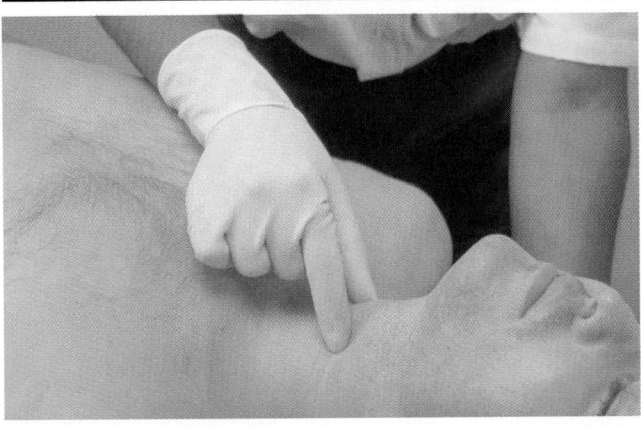

FIGURE 11-60 Locate the cricothyroid membrane by palpating inferior to the thyroid cartilage and superior to the cricoid cartilage.

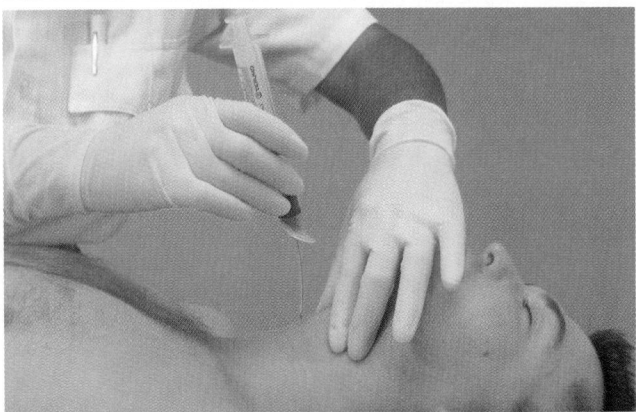

FIGURE 11-61 Perform the puncture with the 14-gauge catheter.

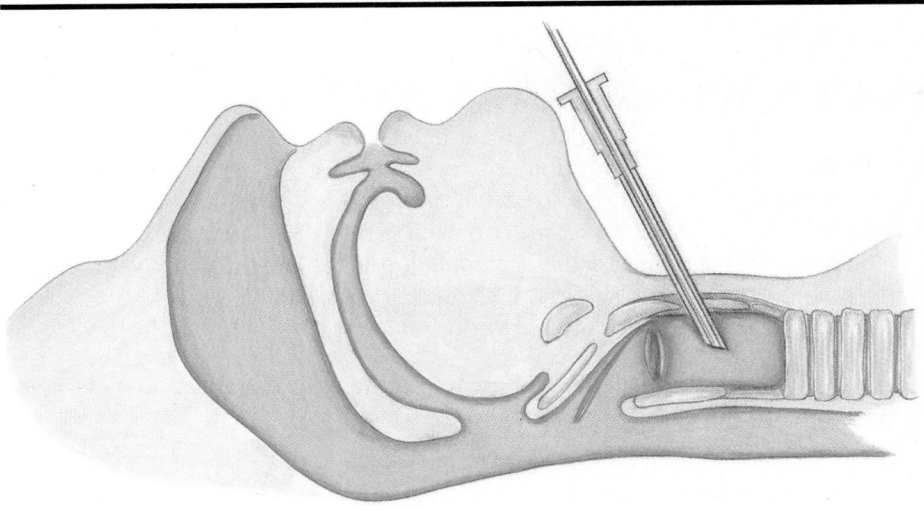

FIGURE 11-62 Cannula properly placed in the trachea.

2. Grasp the larynx with your thumb and middle finger. Locate the cricothyroid membrane with the index finger. (See Figure 11-60.)

3. Prep the area quickly with povidone-iodine swabs.

4. Attach a 14-gauge over-the-needle catheter to a syringe. Carefully insert the needle through the skin and cricothyroid membrane into the trachea. Direct the needle at a 45-degree angle caudally (toward the feet). (See Figure 11-61.) A "pop" can be felt as the needle penetrates the trachea.

5. Aspirate with the syringe. If air is returned easily, you are in the trachea. (See Figure 11-62.) If it is difficult to aspirate with the syringe, or if you obtain blood, reevaluate needle placement. (See Figure 11-62.)

6. Withdraw the stylet while gently advancing the catheter downward into position.

7. Attach the needle hub to a 3.0 mm pediatric endotracheal tube adapter.

8. Check for adequacy of ventilations. Look for chest rise with each ventilation, and listen for breath sounds in the chest. If ventilations are absent, begin transtracheal jet ventilation.

9. When the catheter or tube is correctly positioned, secure it in place.

10. Continue providing ventilatory support.

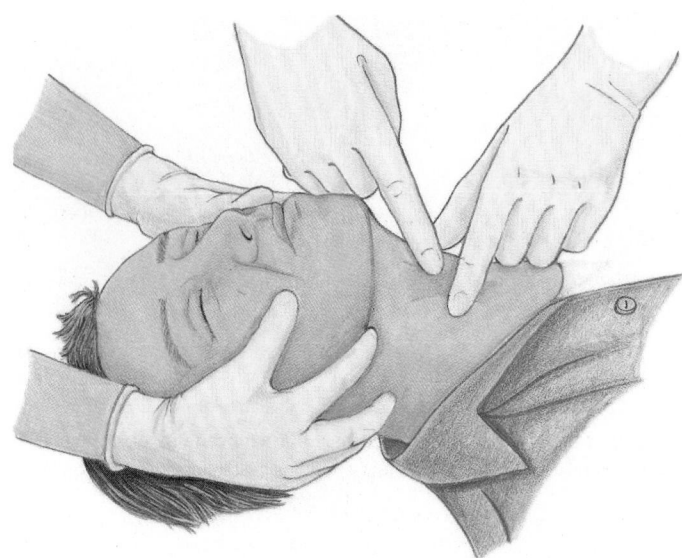

FIGURE 11-63 Palpate the cricothyroid membrane.

Transtracheal Jet Ventilation   Percutaneous transtracheal catheter ventilation is the insertion of an over-the-needle catheter into the cricothyroid membrane, followed by intermittent jet ventilation. It is a temporary, last-resort procedure that provides oxygenation in cases where the patient is experiencing asphyxia due to some unresolved upper airway obstruction. Percutaneous transtracheal catheter ventilation takes only about 30 seconds to perform and can be done without interrupting resuscitative efforts.

Equipment needed for this procedure includes:

❏ A 14-gauge (or larger) over-the-needle catheter, preferably with side holes
❏ A 5- or 10-mL syringe
❏ Manual jet ventilator device capable of delivering pressures of at least 50 psi
❏ Regulating valve attached to a high-pressure oxygen supply
❏ Povidone-iodine swabs
❏ Adhesive tape or tie

To perform percutaneous transtracheal catheter ventilation:

1. While continuing efforts to ventilate and oxygenate, place your patient into a supine position, and hyperextend the head and neck. If spinal injury is suspected, the head and neck should be maintained in a neutral, in-line position.

2. Locate the patient's cricothyroid membrane. (See Figure 11-63.)

3. Prep the area quickly with povidone-iodine swabs.

4. Attach the 14-gauge (or larger) plastic catheter with a needle to the 5- or 10-mL syringe. The syringe can be filled with 1–2 cc of saline, in order to allow easy visualization of air entry after the trachea is penetrated.

5. Carefully insert the needle and catheter in the midline, through the patient's skin and membrane. Direct it downward and caudally at a 45-degree angle to the trachea. (See Figure 11-64.) A pop can be felt as the needle penetrates the trachea.

6. Maintain negative pressure on the syringe as the needle and catheter are advanced. The needle has entered the patient's trachea when air readily fills the syringe.

✳ Percutaneous transtracheal catheter ventilation is a temporary, last-resort procedure when all other methods of obtaining an airway have been unsuccessful.

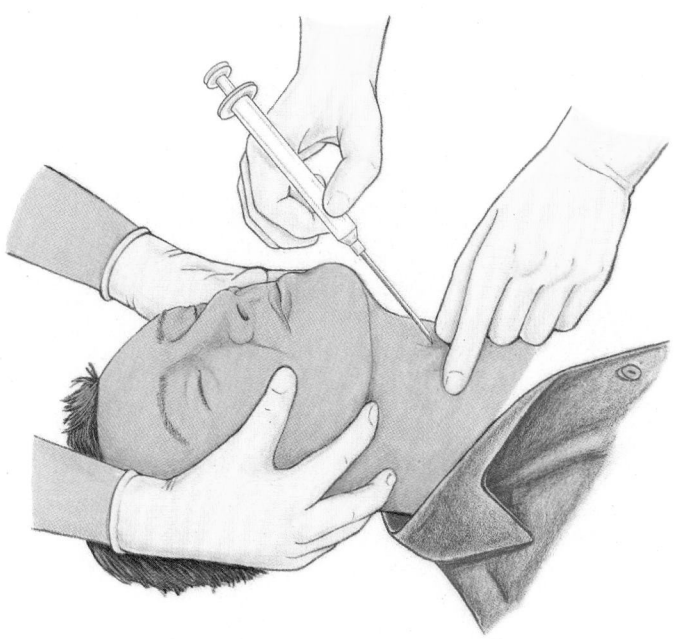

FIGURE 11-64 Position for performing a cricothyroid puncture.

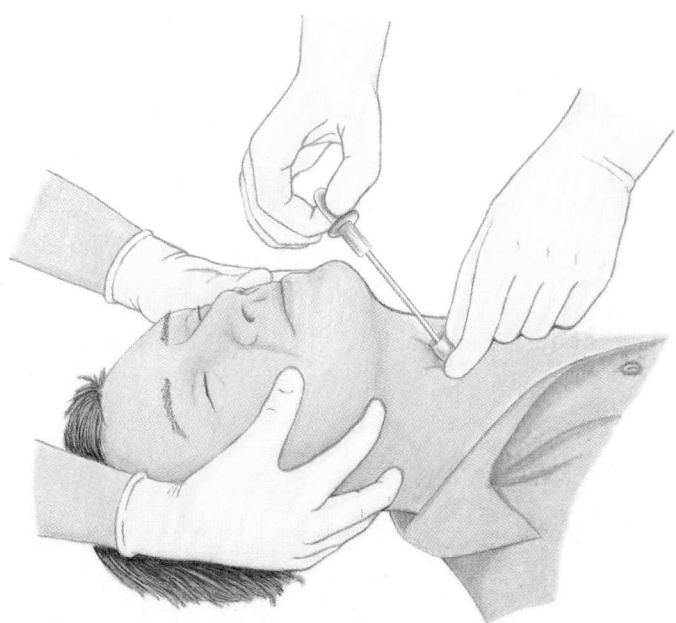

FIGURE 11-65 Advance the cannula.

7. Once in the trachea, advance the catheter over the needle until the catheter hub comes to rest against the skin. (See Figure 11-65.)
8. Hold the hub of the catheter in place to prevent accidental displacement, and then remove both the needle and the syringe.
9. Reconfirm the position of the catheter by aspirating it again with the syringe.
10. Connect one end of the flexible tubing to the catheter hub and the other to the oxygen source.

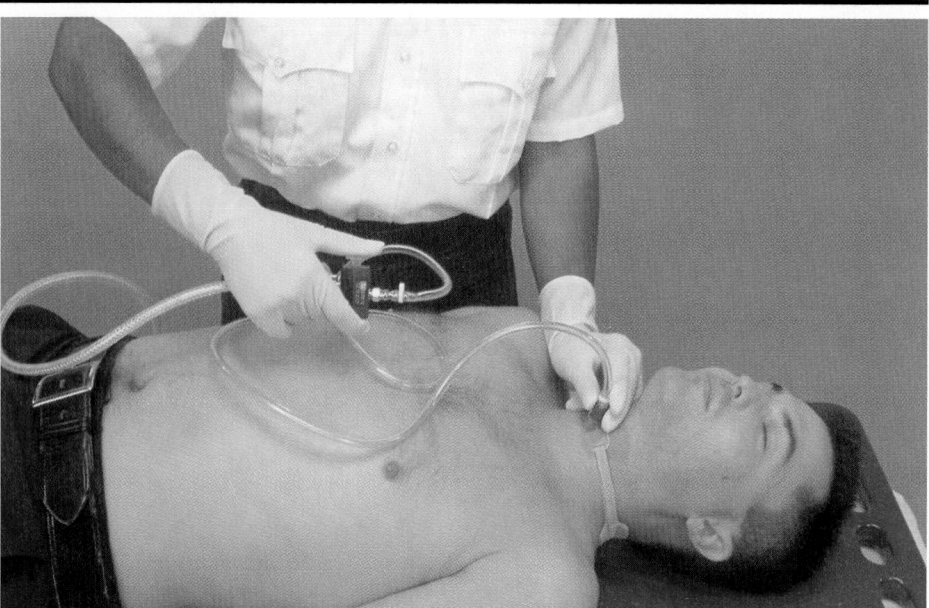

FIGURE 11-66 Ventilate the patient as shown.

11. Open the release valve to introduce an oxygen jet into the trachea. Next, adjust the pressure to allow adequate lung expansion. (See Figure 11-66.)

12. Watch the chest carefully, turning off the release valve as soon as the chest rises. Exhalation then occurs passively, due to the elastic recoil of the lungs and chest wall. A rate of at least 20 breaths per minute should be delivered. The inflation-deflation time ratio should approximate that of normal respiration, or 1:2.

13. Check for adequacy of ventilations. Look for chest rise with each ventilation, and listen for breath sounds in the chest.

14. Fasten the catheter hub securely to the skin, and continue ventilatory support.

Disadvantages of Percutaneous Transtracheal Catheter Ventilation

- ❏ It may lead to pneumothorax due to high pressures generated during ventilation.
- ❏ It may perforate the esophagus if the needle is inserted too far.
- ❏ It does not allow for direct suctioning of secretions.
- ❏ It may not allow for efficient elimination of carbon dioxide.

General Precautions   Passive exhalation is achieved through the upper airway, so it must be at least partially open to avoid lung rupture during this procedure. In cases of complete upper airway obstruction, a second large-bore tracheal catheter needle should be inserted next to the first one to accommodate exhalations. It may also be necessary to suction the catheter intermittently to promote effective expiration. If the chest remains distended, a cricothyrotomy may be called for. When performing percutaneous transtracheal catheter ventilation, neither the bag-valve device nor the demand valve resuscitator should be used, as they cannot provide sufficient driving pressures. This makes clear another disadvantage to percutaneous transtracheal catheter ventilation. It requires special equipment. Since cricothyrotomy does not require such equipment, it may be preferred in some cases.

✱ For transtracheal ventilation via a large-bore catheter to be successful, the airway must be partially open to allow for expiration.

SUCTIONING

Suctioning will prevent or alleviate airway compromise by removing vomitus, blood, and other fluids and secretions.

Equipment for Suctioning

A variety of devices are available for suctioning patients in the prehospital setting. They include portable hand-, foot-, oxygen-, and battery-powered units and stationary electrical or vacuum units (powered by the engine manifold). The ones that are most effective in an emergency situation generate vacuum levels of at least 300 mmHg when the distal end is occluded and allow a flow rate of at least 30 liters per minute when the tube is open.

A pair of recently introduced units offer tremendous portability. One is hand operated, weighs only a pound or so, and is capable of generating excellent suctioning pressures. Because it is hand powered, this device can be used without concern for a power source. The unit's small size also allows it to be stored easily in an airway kit. The other new portable suction device is powered by a rechargeable battery and offers excellent suctioning capabilities (550 mmHg with a flow rate in excess of 30 Lpm).

The most common types of suction catheters used in prehospital settings are those with "tonsil tips" and "whistle tips." The *tonsil tip*, or *Yankauer tip*, suction catheter is a rigid tube with a large tip and multiple holes at its distal end. (A newer, large-bore version is open at the tip.) It is inserted along an oropharyngeal airway or used during laryngoscopy. The tonsil tip catheter can remove larger particles and a greater quantity of secretions than the whistle tip variety. However, it can only be used to suction the upper airway, and its vigorous insertion can cause lacerations and other injuries. (See Figure 11-67.) The *whistle tip* suction catheter is a long, flexible tube that is easy to use. Because of its small size, the tube can extend into the lower respiratory tract. Unfortunately, whistle tip catheters cannot remove large volumes of secretions rapidly. They are also unable to retrieve even small food particles. The whistle tip catheter can be inserted through the nares, into the oropharynx or nasopharynx. It can also be inserted through a nasopharyngeal airway, along an oropharyngeal airway, or through an endotracheal tube. (See Figure 11-68.)

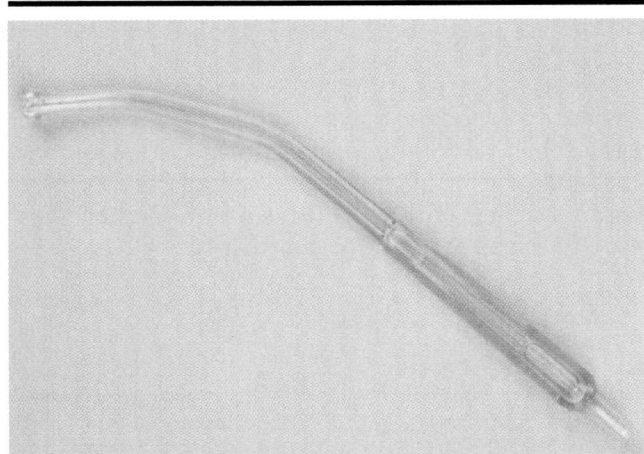

FIGURE 11-67 Yankauer "tonsil tip" suction device.

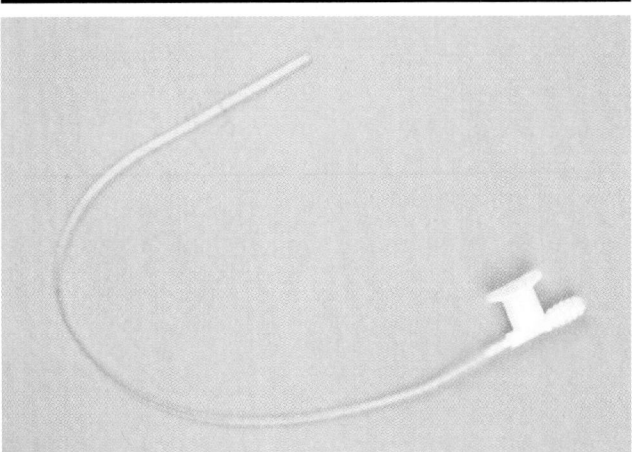

FIGURE 11-68 "Whistle-tip" suction device.

Since suctioning reduces a patient's access to oxygen, each attempt should be limited to ten seconds. If possible, hyperventilate the patient with 100% oxygen prior to and following each suctioning effort. Clear any fluids from the upper airway first, as assisted breathing may cause aspiration. Do not apply suction during insertion of the catheter. Only after the catheter is properly positioned should suction be applied as the catheter is withdrawn.

Most suction catheters have an open port or orifice at their proximal end, allowing the paramedic selectively to initiate or stop the negative pressure being generated through the catheter by uncovering or covering the orifice. When the suction device is not equipped with this orifice, you can create one by making a small slit in the catheter or suction tubing. You can also control the suction by turning the unit on and off as needed. When the fluid present in the upper airway is so great or so thick that neither the tonsil tip nor whistle tip catheter provides adequate suctioning, it may be beneficial to replace the catheter with thick-walled, wide-bore suction tubing. It may also be necessary to place your patient on his or her side and use your fingers to clear substances from the mouth.

The principal hazards associated with these procedures relate to hypoxia brought on by lengthy suctioning attempts. Serious cardiac dysrhythmias can occur during suctioning, due to decreases in myocardial oxygen supply. Suctioning can also stimulate the vagus nerve, causing hypertension and tachycardia, or bradycardia and hypotension. Finally, suctioning may stimulate the airway's mucosa and start the patient coughing. This can increase intracranial pressure and reduce cerebral blood flow.

Techniques for Suctioning

Suctioning is a basic but important skill. To suction a patient:

1. While maintaining ventilatory support, attempt to hyperventilate the patient.
2. Determine the depth of catheter insertion by measuring from the patient's earlobe to his or her lips.
3. Insert the catheter into your patient's pharynx to the predetermined depth (without the suction operating).
4. Turn on the suction unit or place your thumb over the suction control orifice, limiting suction to ten seconds.
5. Continue suctioning as you withdraw the catheter. When using a whistle tip catheter, rotate it between your fingertips.
6. While maintaining ventilatory support, hyperventilate the patient with 100% oxygen.

In many cases you will be suctioning out extremely viscous or thick secretions, which can obstruct fluid flow through the tubing. To reduce this problem, suction water through the tubing between suctioning attempts. This dilutes the secretions and facilitates flow to the suction canister. Most suction units are supplied with small water canisters that can be used for this purpose.

OXYGENATION

Oxygen administration is an important aspect of patient care. It is essential in cases that involve suspected hypoxia of any cause, chest pain due to myocardial ischemia, and cardiorespiratory arrest.

Oxygen Administration

Administering supplemental oxygen aids a hypoxic patient by:

- ❏ Increasing the percentage of inspired oxygen
- ❏ Increasing oxygen concentration at the alveolar level
- ❏ Increasing arterial oxygen levels
- ❏ Increasing the amount of oxygen delivered to the patient's cells

Oxygen administration decreases hypoxia and reduces the volume of respiration necessary to oxygenate the blood. It also reduces the myocardial work demanded to maintain a given arterial oxygen tension.

Oxygen therapy is provided through either a high-flow or low-flow system. A high-flow system uses a Venturi adapter to draw in relatively large amounts of room air for each liter of oxygen provided by the regulator. This allows for the delivery of a precise oxygen concentration, regardless of the patient's inspiratory efforts. In a low-flow system, oxygen travels directly from the regulator to the patient. If the regulator is set at 6 liters per minute, for instance, that is precisely what the patient will receive. With a low-flow system, ambient air is drawn into the respiratory passageways with each breath. This dilutes the oxygen concentration being delivered through the tube from 100%. The concentration delivered to the patient depends on the flow rate and the type of oxygen-delivery device.

With some oxygen-delivery devices, oxygen concentration can vary with variations in the respiratory minute volume (rate × depth of breathing). Patients who are hyperventilating receive less oxygen because they breathe in more room air. Conversely, barbiturate-overdose patients will receive a higher concentration of oxygen because their slow, shallow breaths take in less room air to dilute it. The devices most vulnerable to variations in the percentage of oxygen delivered to patients are the nasal cannula and simple masks. The least vulnerable are partial and nonrebreather masks.

There are no absolute contraindications to oxygen administration. However, it should be used with caution in premature infants and patients who are prone to carbon dioxide retention (hypoxic drive). It should be administered at lower flow rates with COPD patients—1 to 3 liters delivered via nasal cannula, or 24% to 28% delivered via Venturi mask. If your patient develops respiratory depression, breathing should be assisted with a bag-valve-mask device. When ventilating via a bag-valve-mask device, use 100% oxygen. When providing oxygen to a premature infant, hold the mask over the face, not directly on it.

✱ There are no absolute contraindications to oxygen therapy, although it should be used with caution in premature infants and in patients with chronic respiratory problems.

Oxygen Devices

Devices commonly used to administer oxygen in the field include the nasal cannula, the simple face mask, the nonrebreather mask, and the Venturi mask.

Nasal Cannula   The nasal cannula is a frequently used device that is comfortable and easily tolerated by the patient. It can deliver oxygen concentrations ranging from 24% to 44%. The oxygen flow rates for the nasal cannula vary from 1 to 6 liters per minute.

Liter Flow	Approx. Concentration Delivered
1	24
2	28
3	32
4	36
5	40
6	44

Flow rates of greater than 6 liters per minute do little to increase inspired oxygen concentrations, since the anatomical reserve (nasal cavity) is already filled. Higher flow rates will dry the mucous membrane and cause headaches.

Use the nasal cannula with patients who are experiencing minor to moderate hypoxia, who are prone to carbon dioxide retention, who are frightened or feeling suffocated by an oxygen mask, or who are experiencing nausea or vomiting. One benefit of the nasal cannula is that it does not stop the patient from talking, so the paramedic can continue gathering patient information during the procedure. The only contraindication for use of a nasal cannula is nasal obstruction.

Simple Face Mask   This device includes oxygen tubing and a face mask. On the outside of the mask are two inlet/outlet ports. Oxygen is delivered through the bottom of the mask via its oxygen inlet port. The simple face mask will deliver an oxygen concentration of 40% to 60%. Flow rates administered through the simple face mask range from 8 to 12 liters per minute. No fewer than 6 liters should be administered through this device, as expired carbon dioxide can otherwise accumulate in the mask. Flow rates in excess of 8 liters are needed to "wash out" any expired carbon dioxide.

The simple face mask provides oxygen to patients who are suffering from moderate hypoxia. Its disadvantages include: it may feel confining to the patient; it muffles the patient's speech; and it requires a tight face seal. Because the mask covers the patient's face, it should be used with caution in cases that involve nausea or vomiting. With the pediatric patient, a flow rate of 6 to 8 liters per minute is generally considered acceptable.

Nonrebreather Mask   This device consists of oxygen tubing and a face mask with an attached reservoir bag. On the outside of the mask are two air inlet/outlet ports, one covered with a thin rubber flap. Oxygen delivered through the oxygen tubing fills the reservoir. When the patient inhales, the 100% oxygen contained in the reservoir is drawn into the mask and the patient's respiratory passageways. Ambient air is prevented from entering the mask by the rubber flap that closes over the inlet/outlet ports during inspiration. When the patient exhales, the flapper valve is forced open to allow the expired air an exit. A one-way valve situated between the mask and the reservoir prevents the expired air from entering the reservoir bag.

The nonrebreather mask delivers the highest concentration of oxygen. When supplied with 10 to 15 liters per minute, it can deliver an 80% to 100% oxygen concentration. No fewer than 8 liters of oxygen per minute should be administered through this device. Because the nonrebreather mask is a relatively closed system, it restricts the inspiration of ambient air. Therefore, its reservoir bag should not be allowed to deflate totally. Otherwise, the patient might suffocate.

The nonrebreather mask, like the simple face mask, requires a tight seal. This may be difficult to obtain with some patients because they may find the mask confining. This device should be employed with caution in nauseated patients. Its main application is in the treatment of severely hypoxic patients—those suffering respiratory compromise, shock, acute myocardial infarction, trauma, or carbon monoxide poisoning.

Venturi Mask   This high-flow device includes oxygen tubing, a face mask, and a Venturi system. As oxygen passes through a jet orifice in the base of the mask, it entrains room air. The resulting mixture is then delivered to the patient. The same amount of ambient air is always entrained, regardless of the respiratory rate or depth. With this device, relatively precise concentrations of

＊ When using the nonrebreather mask, oxygen should be run at no less than 8 L per minute, and the reservoir bag should not be allowed to collapse.

oxygen can be provided. The Venturi mask is particularly useful for COPD patients, where careful control of inspired oxygen concentration is desirable. To control the amount of ambient air taken in, some Venturi masks are supplied with dial selection, while others come with interchangeable caps. These devices deliver oxygen concentrations of 24%, 28%, 35%, or 40%. The liter flow depends on the oxygen concentration desired.

VENTILATION

In the field, paramedics will be called upon in many cases to provide ventilatory support. Situations will range from those that involve apneic patients to less obvious cases in which patients are experiencing depressed respiratory function. Remember that when a patient is unconscious, his or her respiratory center may not function at a satisfactory level. A significant decrease in the patient's rate or depth of breathing will lead to decreased respiratory minute volume, hypercarbia, hypoxia, and a lowered pH. If not corrected, respiratory or cardiac arrest may occur. To achieve effective ventilatory support, an adequate rate and volume of oxygen must be delivered: at least 800 mL of O_2 at a rate of 12 to 20 breaths per minute.

One problem associated with ventilatory support is that you must generate enough force to overcome the elastic resistance of the lungs and chest wall as well as frictional resistance in the respiratory passageways. This can be likened to blowing up a balloon. Resistance must be overcome in order to inflate the rubber. Keep in mind that air will travel the path of least resistance. In other words, if a tight seal is not maintained between the ventilation mask and your patient's face, air will leak from the gaps rather than travel through the respiratory passageways.

Effectively ventilating a patient requires a number of conditions. First, his or her airway must be in an open position. Second, a closed system must be established and maintained between the patient and the rescuer's ventilation mask or mouth. Third, adequate ventilatory volumes must be delivered. Remember to exercise care in generating enough pressure to ventilate the lungs. Too much pressure may lead to patient regurgitation. Also, use caution in selecting devices for use in the field. Because carbon dioxide is removed during the process of expiration, the patient should always be allowed to exhale between delivered breaths.

Mouth to Mouth/Mouth to Nose

Mouth-to-mouth and mouth-to-nose breathing can provide effective ventilatory support to a patient. These techniques require no equipment and permit an effective mouth or nose seal. When applied properly, both procedures deliver sufficient ventilatory volumes. Limitations on mouth-to-mouth and mouth-to-nose breathing stem largely from the capacity of the person delivering the ventilations. Also, both methods provide only limited oxygen—expired air from the rescuer will contain only 17 percent oxygen.

The major draw-back to these techniques is the possibility of disease transmission. In addition, ventilation may be difficult due to copious secretions, bleeding, and gastric regurgitation.

Pocket Mask

The *pocket mask* is a clear plastic device that sits over a patient's mouth and nose. It prevents contact between the rescuer and the patient's mouth, thus reducing the risk of contamination and subsequent infection.

✱ When possible, the pocket mask should be used to ventilate a patient when other adjuncts are not readily available.

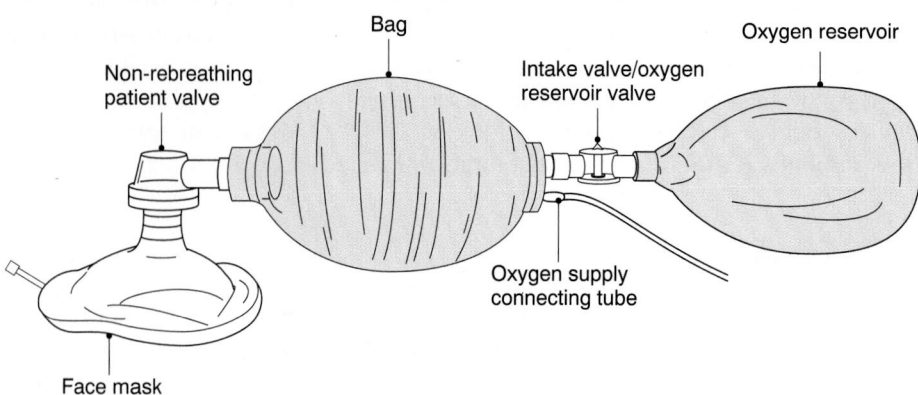

Non-rebreathing patient valve

Bag

Intake valve/oxygen reservoir valve

Oxygen reservoir

Oxygen supply connecting tube

Face mask

FIGURE 11-69 Bag-valve-mask unit.

There are a variety of pocket masks available. Some are reusable, while others are disposed of after a single use. Most are small and compact enough to store in pocket or purse and to be carried with the paramedic at all times. The device is usually designed with a one-way valve that prevents the patient's expired air from coming into contact with the rescuer. It may also provide an inlet for supplemental oxygen. With an oxygen flow rate of 10 liters per minute, combined with mouth-to-mask breathing, an inspired oxygen concentration of approximately 50 percent can be delivered through the device.

Bag-Valve Devices

✱ The bag-valve-mask can provide the patient with an oxygen-enriched mixture and can allow the paramedic to feel the compliance of the lungs.

The *bag-valve device* is used to deliver oxygen or room air to a patient who is not breathing. In addition, it will hyperexpand a patient's lungs, improving alveolar ventilation, thus preventing hypoxia. The bag-valve-mask device consists of an oblong, self-inflating silicone or rubber bag; two one-way valves (an air/oxygen inlet valve and a patient valve); and a transparent face mask. They are available in neonate, pediatric, and adult sizes. Some units are reusable. But with recent concerns over the transmission of infectious diseases, suppliers have developed a number of disposable units for prehospital use. (See Figure 11-69.)

When employed without supplemental oxygen, these devices will deliver 21% oxygen. With an oxygen source attached and the flow rate set at 12 liters per minute, the bag-valve-mask can deliver up to 60% oxygen. When a reservoir device or corrugated tubing is attached and 10 to 15 liters of oxygen is administered, the bag-valve-mask device can deliver from 90% to 95% oxygen.

Bag-valve-mask devices should not feature a pop-off valve except when used in pediatric cases. If you are providing ventilatory assistance to a patient with high airway resistance and poor lung compliance, a pop-off valve will prevent effective ventilation.

Demand Valve

The *demand valve* resuscitator, also called the "manually triggered oxygen-powered breathing device," will deliver 100% oxygen to a patient at its highest flow rates (40 liters per minute maximum). The device is rugged, compact, and easy to handle. It also includes an easy-to-locate manual control button. In addition, the entire device can be attached to a face mask or a mechanical airway.

The complete system consists of high-pressure tubing, which connects to an oxygen supply, and a valve that is activated by a push button or lever. When the valve is opened, oxygen flows to the patient. Most of these units also contain an inspiratory release valve that makes them useful in treating spontaneously breathing patients who need high oxygen concentrations. The slight negative pressure created by inhalation opens the valve. The greater the inspiratory effort, the higher the flow. When inhalation ceases, so does the oxygen flow.

The demand valve is easy to use and provides high oxygen concentrations. However, there are also negative aspects. During ventilation, the device does not provide you with a sense of chest compliance; thus, you must take care not to overinflate the lungs. Due to the high pressures generated by the device, lungs may experience pressure-related injury, which can lead to pneumothorax and subcutaneous emphysema. The demand valve resuscitator may open the esophagus, causing gastric distention in patients who have not been intubated. Since the oxygen flow rate is so high, the demand valve resuscitator will quickly drain the contents of a portable oxygen cylinder. Another means of ventilatory support will need to be employed if the cylinder requires changing during patient management.

✱ Gastric distention may reduce vital capacity, cause the patient to vomit, and lead to gastric rupture.

The demand valve resuscitator is not recommended for use with patients under the age of 16. Because of the sudden high pressures that this device can supply, it should be used with extreme caution in intubated patients or those with chest trauma. (See Figure 11-70.)

✱ The demand valve should be used with extreme caution in the intubated patient.

Automatic Ventilators

Until recently, mechanical ventilators have been limited to in-hospital use. With improved technology, however, several compact mechanical ventilators are now available for prehospital care.

Mechanical ventilators offer a number of advantages. These lightweight, compact devices are designed for convenience and easy use during patient care and transport. They have proven superior to bag-valve devices in main-

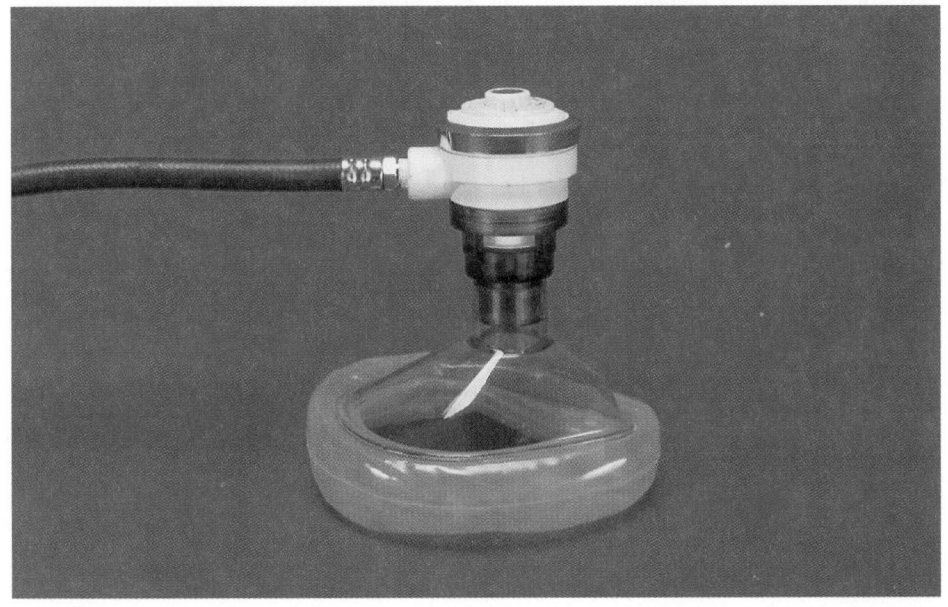

FIGURE 11-70 Demand valve.

taining minute volume. Also, they can tolerate temperature extremes—ranging from −30°F to 125°F—with great dependability. In cases of cardiac arrest, the automatic ventilator allows for chest compressions interposed between mechanical breaths.

The compact ventilator typically comes with two controls: one for the ventilatory rate, the other for tidal volume. It is also equipped with a standard 15 mm i.d./22 mm o.d. adapter, so that it can be attached to a variety of airway devices. Some of these automatic units deliver controlled ventilation only. Others function as intermittent mandatory ventilators, reverting to controlled mechanical ventilation in patients who are not breathing. Most units provide an adjustable tidal volume, while the ventilatory rate is either fixed or adjustable. The inspired oxygen concentration is usually fixed at 100%, but it may be adjustable. (See Figure 11-71.)

Many of these ventilators sport a "pop-off" valve that prevents pressure-related injury. The valve vents away some of the tidal volume when its preset level of airway pressure is exceeded (typically 60 cm H_2O). This pop-off feature can be detrimental in the presence of cardiogenic pulmonary edema, Adult Respiratory Distress Syndrome, pulmonary contusion, bronchospasm, and other disorders in which high airway pressures must be overcome.

As a rule, mechanical ventilators should not be used in children less than 5 years of age. Otherwise, when indicated, the device can prove a valuable tool. In intubated patients, use of the ventilator allows you to perform other vital tasks. In unintubated patients, use of the ventilator frees up both of your hands to maintain an adequate seal between the mask and the face.

SUMMARY

Airway management is one of the most important aspects of prehospital care. However, it is not always easy to accomplish. Effective airway management depends on continually reinforcing your skills, so that you can perform them when required. Of foremost importance in airway management is that the patient's respiratory system be able to perform its primary function—moving air in and out of the body. In order to supply the bloodstream with adequate oxygen, the patient must have a patent airway. The patient also needs adequate supplies of oxygen in the inspired air and respiratory minute volumes that are sufficient to remove appropriate levels of carbon dioxide.

Today, a number of procedures help sustain a critically ill or injured patient. All of them, however, require that the airway first be secured. Basic airway maneuvers, such as the head-tilt/chin-lift, can be used to move the tongue and epiglottis away from obstructing positions. In the presence of possible cervical spine injuries, a modified jaw-thrust maneuver should be employed. Endotracheal intubation is the preferred technique for securing an airway because it prevents aspiration of foreign materials and allows for efficient delivery of ventilatory support.

Respiratory efforts can be supported with a variety of devices. Among these, the bag-valve-mask device probably offers the most advantages, but it is difficult to use when attempting to ventilate a nonintubated patient. Only frequent practice in using the bag-valve-mask device will ensure proficiency during emergency situations. Inspired oxygen concentrations can be increased with a number of different delivery devices, each of which has specific criteria for use. Recent introductions in the area of suctioning and mechanical ventilation afford even greater portability of devices and ease of use.

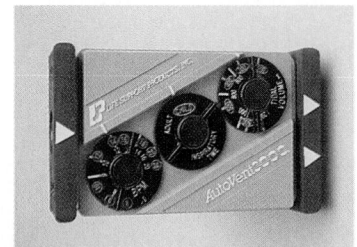

FIGURE 11-71 Portable mechanical ventilator for prehospital use.

FURTHER READING

American College of Surgeons, Committee on Trauma. *Advanced Trauma Life Support Course: Student Manual.* American College of Surgeons, 1984.

American Heart Association. *Textbook of Advanced Cardiac Life Support*, 3rd ed. Dallas: American Heart Association, 1993.

Applebaum, Edward L., and David L. Bruce. *Tracheal Intubation.* Saint Louis: W.B. Saunders Company, 1976.

Bledsoe, Bryan E. *Atlas of Paramedic Skills.* Englewood Cliffs, NJ: Prentice Hall, 1987.

Bledsoe, Bryan E., Dwayne Clayden , and Frank J. Papa. *Prehospital Emergency Pharmacology, 4th ed.* Upper Saddle River, NJ: Prentice Hall, 1996.

Campbell, John E. *Basic Trauma Life Support*, 2nd ed. Englewood Cliffs, NJ: Prentice Hall, 1988.

DeLorenzo, Robert A. and Dan Mayer. "Laryngeal Trauma: Uncovering a Hidden Injury." *J.E.M.S.* 16(9) (September, 1991): 77–83.

Johnson, John C. and Gary L. Atherton. "The Esophageal Tracheal Combitube: An Alternate Route to Airway Management." *J.E.M.S.* 16(5) (May, 1991): 29–35.

Kapsner, Christopher E., *et al.* "The Esophageal Detector Device: Accuracy and Reliability in Difficult Airway Settings." *Prehospital and Disaster Medicine* 11(1) (1996): 60–62.

Mackreth, Bill. "Assessing Pulse Oximetry in the Field." *J.E.M.S.* 15(6) (June 1990): 56–67.

McMahan, Sabina *et. al.* "Multi-Agency, Prehospital Evaluation of the Pharyngeo-Tracheal Lumen (PtL) Airway." *Prehospital and Disaster Medicine* 7(1) (January–March 1992): 13–18.

Nolan, Jerry P. and Peter J.F. Baskett. "Gas-Powered and Portable Ventilators: An Evaluation of Six Models." *Prehospital and Disaster Medicine* 7(1)(January–March 1992): 25–34.

Porter, Robert S., Mark A. Merlin, and Michael B. Heller. "The Fifth Vital Sign." *Emergency* (March 1990): 37–41.

Roberts, James R. and Jerris R. Hedges. *Clinical Procedures in Emergency Medicine*, 2nd Ed. Philadelphia: W.B. Saunders Company, 1991.

Shade, Bruce, *et. al. Advanced Cardiac Life Support: Certification, Preparation, and Review.* Englewood Cliffs, NJ: Brady Communications, 1988.

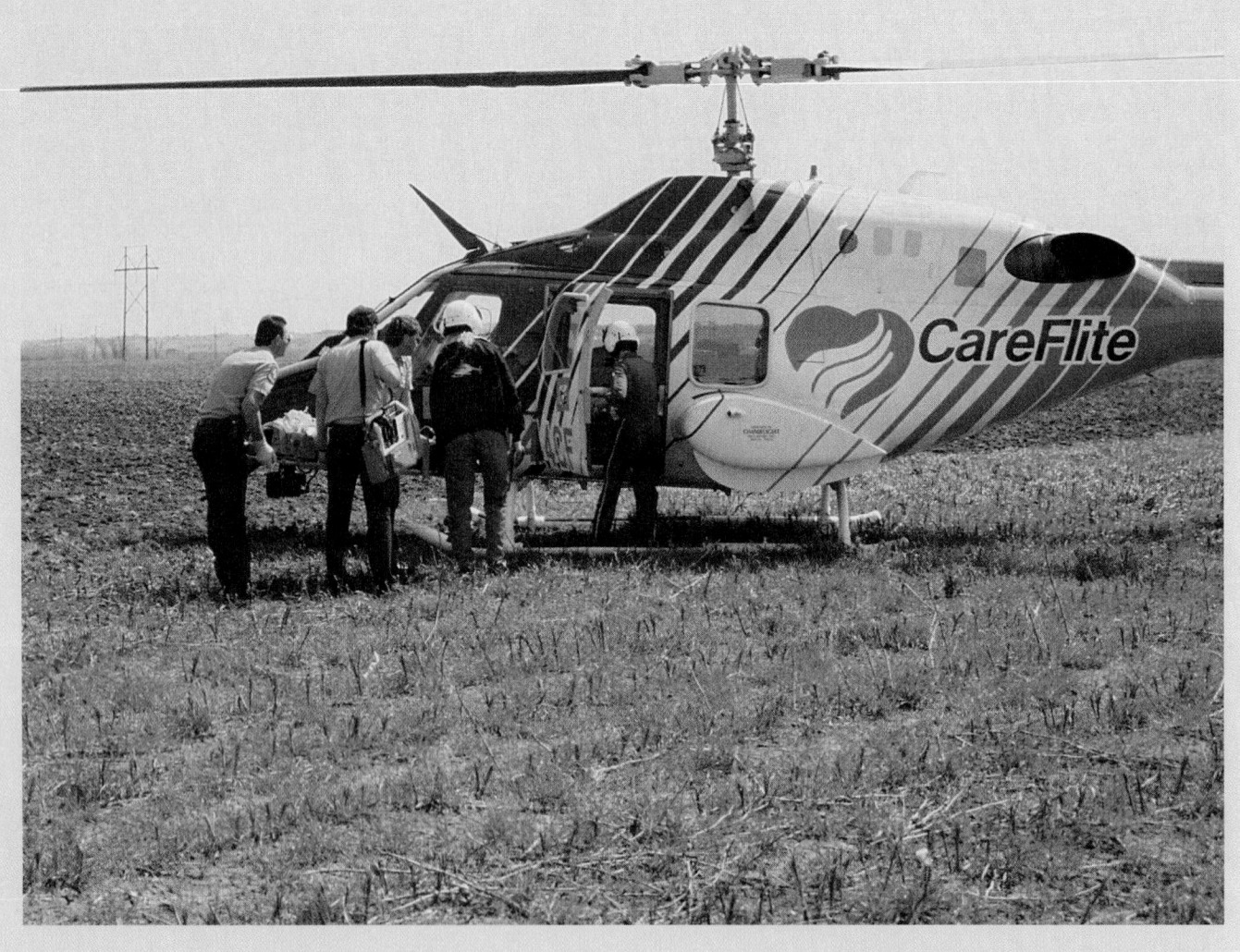

12

PATHOPHYSIOLOGY OF SHOCK

Objectives for Chapter 12

After reading this chapter, you should be able to:

1. Identify the body's major fluid compartments and the proportion of total body water they contain. (See p. 288.)

2. Name the abnormal states of hydration, and describe their common causes and effects on the human system. (See pp. 288–289.)

3. List the major electrolytes, and discuss the role they play in maintaining a fluid balance within the human body. (See pp. 289–292.)

4. Define the following terms, and explain the role each process plays in human fluid dynamics. (See below pages.)

- diffusion (p. 293)
- osmosis (p. 293)
- active transport (p. 293)
- facilitated diffusion (p. 294)

5. Identify the major elements of the blood, and describe their purpose. (See pp. 294–295.)

6. Explain the ABO blood typing system and its significance to emergency medical care. (See pp. 295–296.)

7. List the various fluid replacement products, and describe the advantages and disadvantages of field use. (See pp. 296–299.)

8. Identify the acid-base balance system, and explain its impact on the human body as it applies to shock and fluid therapy. (See pp. 299–303.)

9. Illustrate the structure and function of the cardiovascular system. (See pp. 303–308.)

10. Define shock, explain the shock process, and describe some of the body's compensatory mechanisms. (See pp. 303, 308–310.)

11. Describe the pathophysiology of hypovolemic, cardiogenic, and neurogenic shock. (See pp. 310–311.)

12. Describe the assessment of the shock patient. (See pp. 311–315.)

13. Describe the management of the shock patient. (See pp. 315–329.)

14. Identify the indications, contraindications, and application process for the PASG. (See pp. 318–320, 321.)

15. Explain the indications for, and the initiation of, intravenous therapy. (See pp. 320, 322–327.)

16. List the equipment commonly used for intravenous therapy, and explain the purpose and use of various items. (See pp. 320, 322–323.)

17. Identify the common complications of intravenous therapy, and describe the process of preventing or correcting those complications. (See pp. 325, 327.)

18. Assess the use of medications in the treatment of shock. (See p. 328.)

19. List the major steps in stabilizing a shock patient for transport. (See p. 329.)

A call comes into City Ambulance 1. The dispatcher reports a basic life support ambulance in need of assistance in another city. An overturned bulldozer has trapped a 39-year-old male.

Upon arrival at the scene, paramedics find the patient alert. His pelvis and lower extremities are pinned by the side of the dozer. The rescue crew must wait for equipment to lift the huge machine. Bob, the senior paramedic, performs the primary assessment. He detects no problem with airway, breathing, or circulation. The EMTs have already administered oxygen, using a nonrebreather mask.

Next, Bob begins the secondary assessment. The patient has good breath sounds. But he cannot feel his feet. Bob strongly suspects a pelvic fracture. Vital signs include: blood pressure 110/68, pulse 100, respirations 24, oxygen saturation 99 percent.

Paramedics quickly establish two IVs of normal saline, one infusing wide open. They also prepare the PASG and a backboard. While the rescue equipment is readied, the paramedics converse with the patient, explaining the various steps in the operation. While they talk, the paramedics recheck vital signs every four minutes or so. Bob documents that the vitals remain stable.

The extrication team slowly begins to lift off the dozer. Paramedics rush to position the patient on the waiting backboard. They apply and inflate the PASG. As the dozer eases off, it becomes apparent that the patient has suffered fractures of the pelvis, bilateral femurs, and left tibia. Both IVs are opened wide.

As the dozer is finally lifted off the patient, he reports an increase in pain. He becomes restless and attempts to get up. Then he becomes lethargic. The oximetry reveals the saturation has dropped to 94 percent and the pulse rate is up to 130 beats per minute. With time, the patient's level of consciousness improves. But the pulse rate remains elevated.

Paramedics place both IVs in pressure bags and transport the patient to the ambulance before completing any additional assessment. Upon arrival at the hospital, the patient remains stable, yet tachycardic. The ED team starts type O-negative blood and establishes a third IV. Within 20 minutes, they transport the patient into surgery with the PASG in place. The patient survives the incident. Because of multiple fractures, his rehabilitation will continue for more than a year.

INTRODUCTION

The human body is not just an inert structure of bones and cavities and tubes. In fact, the body has often been compared to a chemical laboratory or a factory because there is continual internal biochemical and physiological activity necessary to support life. **Metabolism** is the term for the totality of these ongoing biochemical and physiological processes.

When the normal metabolism is disturbed, the body will usually respond in various ways to compensate and restore normal metabolism. If the metabolism is disturbed seriously enough, or when other traumatic or medical conditions prevent it, the body's compensatory mechanisms may not function or may not be sufficient to restore normal metabolism. When metabolic disturbances are not or cannot be corrected, they may result in the death of cells, tissues, organs, and finally, the death of the person.

As a paramedic, you must understand and be able to recognize disturbances in the body's metabolism. When appropriate, you must be able to intervene with treatments aimed at correcting the problem or at sustaining enough function so that the problem can be definitively treated at the hospital. The treatments you initiate may differ from those employed by the EMT-Basic and may include advanced procedures, administration of medications, and intravenous fluid therapy.

■ **metabolism** the totality of the ongoing biochemical and physiological activity necessary to support life.

Among the metabolic disturbances your patients may be suffering are:

❏ Fluid and electrolyte abnormalities
❏ Acid-base imbalance
❏ Shock

FLUID AND ELECTROLYTES

Many medical and traumatic conditions adversely affect the fluid and electrolyte balance of the body. Severe derangements in the body's fluid and electrolyte status can result in death. Certain disease processes, such as diabetic ketoacidosis and heat emergencies, are associated with certain electrolyte abnormalities. Thus, it is prudent for paramedics to have a good understanding of the fluids and electrolytes present in the human body. In addition, as presented later in this chapter, prehospital personnel must understand, in detail, the pathophysiology and management of shock.

Water

Water is the most abundant substance in the human body. In fact, water accounts for approximately 60 percent of the total body weight. The total amount of water in the body at any given time is referred to as the *total body water (TBW)*. In a person weighing 70 kilograms (154 pounds), the amount of total body water would be approximately 42 liters (11 gallons). (See Figure 12-1.)

■ **water** the universal solvent. Approximately 60 percent of the weight of the human body is due to water.

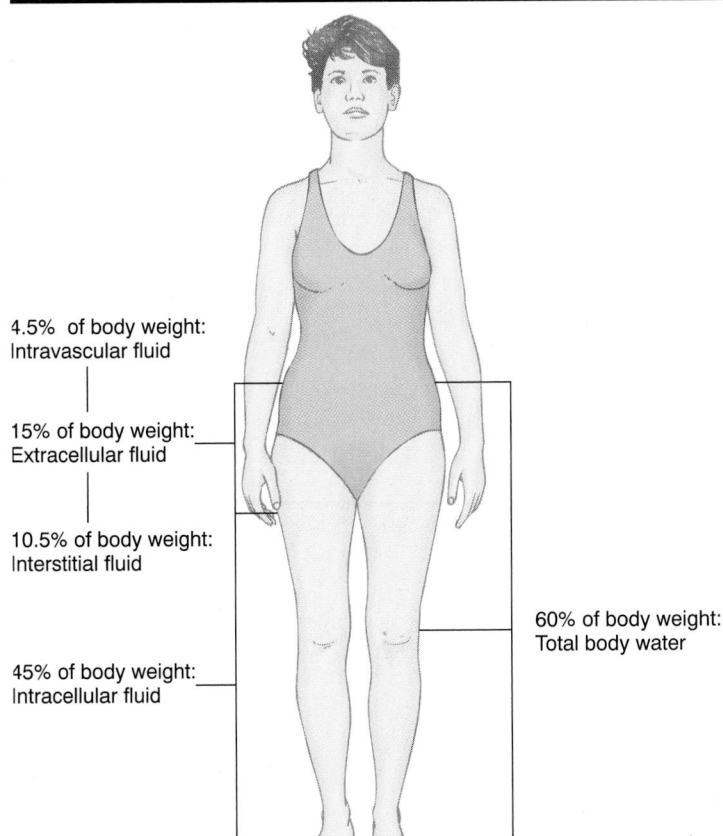

4.5% of body weight: Intravascular fluid

15% of body weight: Extracellular fluid

10.5% of body weight: Interstitial fluid

45% of body weight: Intracellular fluid

60% of body weight: Total body water

FIGURE 12-1 Percentage of total body weight due to water as distributed in the various fluid compartments.

TABLE 12-1	Body Fluid Compartments		
Compartment	**Percentage of Total Body Water**	**Volume in 70 kg Adult**	
Intracellular Fluid	75%	31.50 L	
Extracellular Fluid	25%	10.50 L	
Interstitial Fluid	17.5%	7.35 L	
Intravascular Fluid	7.5%	3.15 L	

■ **intracellular fluid (ICF)** portion of the body fluid inside the body's cells.

■ **extracellular fluid (ECF)** portion of the body fluid outside the body's cells.

■ **intravascular fluid** portion of the body's fluid outside the body's cells and within the circulatory system.

■ **interstitial fluid** portion of the body fluid found outside the body's cells, yet not within the circulatory system. Interstitial fluid is that fluid found within the interstitial space between the cells.

■ **solvent** a substance in which another substance (a **solute**) will dissolve, creating a **solution** in which the molecules of the solute are intermixed with those of the solvent. For example: water (a *solvent*) + salt (a *solute*) = saltwater (a *solution*).

■ **homeostasis** the body's natural tendency to keep the internal environment constant.

Water is usually distributed into various compartments of the body. These compartments are separated by cell membranes. The largest compartment is the *intracellular compartment*. This compartment contains the **intracellular fluid (ICF)**, which is all of the fluid found inside body cells. Approximately 75 percent of all body water is found within this compartment. The *extracellular compartment* contains the remaining 25 percent of all body water. It includes all of the fluid found outside the body cells, or **extracellular fluid (ECF)**.

There are two divisions within the extracellular compartment. The first includes the **intravascular fluid**—the fluid found outside of cells and within the circulatory system. It is essentially the same as the blood plasma. The remaining compartment includes the **interstitial fluid**—all the fluid found outside of the cell membranes, yet not within the circulatory system. (See Table 12-1.)

Hydration

Water is the universal **solvent**. That is, most substances dissolve in water. When they do, various chemical changes take place. For this reason, the water content of the body is crucial to virtually all of the body's biochemical processes. Normally, the total volume of water in the body, as well as the distribution of fluid in the three body compartments, remains relatively constant. This occurs despite wide fluctuations in the amount of water that enters and is excreted from the body on a daily basis. The water coming into the body is referred to as intake. The water excreted from the body is referred to as output. To maintain relative **homeostasis**, or balance, the intake must equal the output, as shown below.

Intake
digestive system:
    liquids   1,000 mL
    food (solids)   1,200 mL
metabolic sources: 300 mL

                   TOTAL: 2,500 mL

Output
lungs (water vapor):   400 mL
kidneys (urine):   1,500 mL
skin (perspiration):   400 mL
intestines (feces):   200 mL

                   TOTAL: 2,500 mL

Several mechanisms work to maintain a relative balance between input and output. As an example, when the fluid volume drops, the pituitary gland at the base of the brain secretes the hormone ADH (Anti-Diuretic Hormone). ADH causes the kidney tubules to reabsorb more water back into the blood and to excrete less urine. This process helps to restore the fluid volume to normal values.

Thirst also regulates fluid intake. The sensation of thirst normally occurs when body fluids decrease, stimulating the person to take in more fluids orally. On the other hand, when too many fluids enter the body, the kidneys are activated and more urine is excreted, thus eliminating excess fluid. The body also maintains fluid balance by shifting water from one body space to another.

Dehydration   **Dehydration** is an abnormal decrease in the total body water and can result from several factors. These include:

- *Gastrointestinal losses* result from prolonged vomiting, diarrhea, or malabsorption disorders.
- *Increased insensible loss* is loss of water through normal mechanisms which are difficult to detect or measure (i.e. perspiration, water vapor from the lungs, saliva). These can be increased in fever states, during hyperventilation, or with high environmental temperatures.
- *Increased sweating* (also called perspiration or diaphoresis) can result in significant fluid loss. This can occur with many medical conditions or in areas of high environmental temperatures.
- *Internal losses* (commonly called "third space" losses) are losses of fluid into various body fluid compartments. In this situation, fluid is typically lost from the intravascular compartment into the interstitial compartment, effectively taking it out of the circulating volume. This can occur with peritonitis, pancreatitis, or bowel obstruction. It can also occur in poor nutritional states where there is not enough protein in the vascular system to retain water.
- *Plasma losses* occur from burns, surgical drains and fistulas, and open wounds.

Dehydration may involve only the loss of water. However, more commonly, there is also a loss of **electrolytes**. At the hospital, fluid replacement will be based on both fluid and electrolyte deficits once the patient's electrolyte abnormalities can be determined through laboratory testing.

Clinically, the dehydrated patient will exhibit dry mucous membranes and poor skin **turgor**. There often is excessive thirst. As it becomes more severe, dehydration will be accompanied by an increased pulse rate, decreased blood pressure, and **orthostatic hypotension**. In infants, the anterior fontanelle may be sunken and the diaper may be dry or reveal the presence of highly concentrated urine. The absence of tears in a crying infant, or capillary refill time greater than two seconds, indicates severe dehydration. The treatment for dehydration is replacement of fluid.

Overhydration   **Overhydration** can occur as well. The major sign of overhydration is edema. Patients with heart disease may manifest overhydration much earlier than patients without heart disease. In severe cases of overhydration, overt heart failure may be present. Treatment is directed at removing the excessive fluid.

Electrolytes

The various chemical substances present throughout the body can be classified either as electrolytes or non-electrolytes. Electrolytes are substances that

■ **dehydration** an abnormal decrease in total body water.

■ **electrolytes** chemical substances that dissociate into electrically charged particles when placed in water.

■ **turgor** the resistance of the skin to deformation, e.g., when pinched between fingers.

■ **orthostatic hypotension** hypotension (decrease in blood pressure) that occurs when suddenly arising from a supine position.

■ **overhydration** an excess of total body water.

To describe chemical substances and reactions, scientists use chemical notation, a kind of "shorthand."

Every chemical element has a one- or two-letter abbreviation. Just four elements—hydrogen, oxygen, carbon, and nitrogen—make up over 99 % of the body's atoms. These are called the "major elements." Nine "trace elements" account for the remaining less-than-1%.

Major Element	Symbol	Percent	Trace Element	Symbol
Hydrogen	H	62%	Calcium	Ca
Oxygen	O	26%	Chlorine	Cl
Carbon	C	10%	Iodine	I
Nitrogen	N	1.5%	Iron	Fe
			Magnesium	Mg
			Phosphorus	Ph
			Potassium	K
			Sodium	Na
			Sulfer	S

An **atom** is the smallest particle of an element. A **molecule** is a combination of atoms. The notation for a molecule combines the notations of the included elements. A subscript number after an element indicates the number of atoms of that element. If there is just one atom, there is no number. For example:

NaCl (Sodium chloride, or table salt. A sodium chloride molecule has 1 sodium atom and 1 chlorine atom.)

H_2O (Water. A water molecule has 2 hydrogen atoms and 1 oxygen atom.)

H_2CO_3 (Carbonic acid. A carbonic acid molecule has 2 hydrogen, 1 carbon, and 3 oxygen atoms.)

Ions

Each atom is made up of even smaller particles: *electrons* (that have a negative electrical charge), *protons* (that have a positive electrical charge) and *neutrons* (that are uncharged). Protons and neutrons are in the inner core, or nucleus, of the atom while electrons occupy outer orbits around the nucleus. Sometimes an atom of an element can lose one or more of its outer electrons or can capture one or more extra electrons from an another element.

An **ion** is an atom that has lost one or more negatively charged electrons and now has a positive charge, or an atom that has gained one or more electrons and now has a negative charge. A superscript plus ($^+$) indicates a positively charged **cation**. A superscript minus ($^-$) indicates a negatively charged **anion**. For example:

Na^+ (A sodium ion has lost an electron and has a positive charge.)

Ca^{++} (A calcium ion has lost two electrons and has a double positive charge.)

Cl^- (A chloride ion has gained an electron and has a negative charge.)

Electrolytes are substances that form ions when they break down, or dissociate, in water. Remember that the body and its blood are mostly water. The ions formed by dissociation of electrolytes in the body's fluids is a major factor in body metabolism.

Chemical Reactions

Notations for chemical reactions use a plus sign (+) to indicate substances that are combined and an arrow (→) to show the direction of the reaction. The reactants are usually on the left, the product of the reaction on the right.

$$2H + O \rightarrow H_2O$$

(2 hydrogen atoms + 1 oxygen atom → 1 water molecule)

In some circumstances, a reaction may be *reversible*. That is, separate elements may *synthesize* (combine), or the synthesized substance may *dissociate* (break down) into separate components. A two-directional arrow (↔) shows that a reaction is reversible and can be read in either direction.

$$CO_2 + H_2O \leftrightarrow H_2CO_3$$

Read as: (carbon dioxide + water → carbonic acid) or (carbonic acid → water + carbon dioxide).

Notice that no atoms are gained or lost in a chemical reaction. In the example above, the two oxygen atoms in CO_2 and the single oxygen atom in H_2O combine to equal the three oxygen atoms in H_2CO_3. The hydrogen and carbon atoms are also equal on both sides of the reaction.

Up and down arrows (↑ ↓) are used to indicate an increase or decrease in the substance that follows the arrows. For example:

↑ H^+ (an increase in hydrogen ions)
↓ CO_2 (a decrease in carbon dioxide)

dissociate into electrically charged particles when placed into water. The charged particles are referred to as **ions**. Ions with a positive charge are called **cations**, while ions with a negative charge are called **anions**.

An example of this would be the dissociation of the drug sodium bicarbonate when placed into water. Sodium bicarbonate is a neutral salt. When placed into water, it dissociates into two charged particles, as shown below.

$$NaHCO_3 \rightarrow Na^+ + HCO_3^-$$

sodium bicarbonate → sodium cation + bicarbonate anion

neutral salt → cation + anion

Sodium bicarbonate is an example of an electrolyte that is taken into the body as a medication. However, there are many naturally occurring electrolytes present in the body.

The most frequently occurring *cations* include:

❑ *Sodium* (Na^+). Sodium is the most prevalent cation in the extracellular fluid. It plays a major role in regulating the distribution of water. In fact, it is often said that water "follows sodium." Sodium is also important in

■ **dissociate** separate, or break down.

■ **ion** an electrically charged particle.

■ **cation** (CAT-i-on) a positively charged ion. It is attracted to the negative pole of an electrode (cathode), hence the name.

■ **anion** (AN-i-on) a negatively charged ion. It is attracted to the positive pole of an electrode (anode), hence the name.

✻ Water follows sodium.

the transmission of nervous impulses. An increase in the relative amount of sodium in the body is called *hypernatremia*, while a decrease is referred to as *hyponatremia*.

❑ *Potassium* (K⁺). Potassium is the most prevalent cation in the intracellular fluid. It is also important in the transmission of electrical impulses. An abnormally low potassium level is called *hypokalemia*, while a high potassium level is referred to as *hyperkalemia*.

❑ *Calcium* (Ca⁺⁺). Calcium has many physiological functions. It plays a major role in muscle contraction as well as nervous impulse transmission. An increased calcium level is called *hypercalcemia*, while a decreased calcium level is called *hypocalcemia*.

❑ *Magnesium* (Mg⁺⁺). Magnesium is necessary for several biochemical processes that occur in the body and is closely associated with phosphate in many processes.

The most frequently occurring *anions* include:

❑ *Chloride* (Cl⁻). Chloride is an important anion. Its negative charge balances the positive charge associated with the cations. It also plays a major role in fluid balance and renal (kidney) function. Chloride has a close association with sodium.

❑ *Bicarbonate* (HCO_3^-). Bicarbonate is the principle **buffer** of the body. It neutralizes the highly acidic hydrogen ion (H⁺) and other organic acids. (Additional discussion of buffering follows later in this chapter.)

❑ *Phosphate* (HPO_4^-). Phosphate is important in body energy stores. It is closely associated with magnesium in renal function. It also acts as a buffer, primarily in the intracellular space, in much the same manner as bicarbonate.

Many other compounds carry negative charges. Among these are some of the proteins, certain organic acids, and other compounds. Electrolytes are usually measured in **milliequivalents** per liter (mEq/L).

Non-electrolytes are molecules that do not dissociate into electrically charged particles. These include glucose, urea, and similar substances.

Osmosis and Diffusion

The various fluid compartments, previously discussed, are separated by cell membranes. These membranes are unique, **semi-permeable membranes**. That is, they allow the passage of certain materials, while restricting the passage of others. Compounds with small molecules, such as water (H_2O), pass readily through the membrane; larger compounds, such as proteins, are restricted. This selective movement of fluids results from the presence of pores (openings) within the membrane. Only compounds small enough to pass through the pores can enter or exit the cell. Electrolytes do not pass as readily as water through the membrane. This is not due so much to their size as to their electrical charge.

When solutions on opposite sides of a semi-permeable membrane are equal in concentration, the relationship is said to be **isotonic**. When the concentration of a given solute is greater on one side of the membrane than on the other, it is said to be **hypertonic**. When the concentration is less on one side of the cell membrane, as compared to the other, it is referred to as **hypotonic**. This difference in concentration is known as the *osmotic gradient*.

The natural tendency of the body is to keep the balance of electrolytes and water equal on both sides of the cell membrane. This is an example of

■ **buffer** substance that neutralizes or weakens a strong acid or base.

■ **milliequivalent** weight of a substance contained in one milliliter of a normal solution.

■ **semi-permeable membrane** specialized biological membrane, such as that which encloses the body's cells, that allows the passage of certain substances and restricts the passage of others.

■ **isotonic** a state in which solutions on opposite sides of a semi-permeable membrane are in equal concentration.

■ **hypertonic** a state in which a solution has a higher solute concentration on one side of a semi-permeable membrane compared to the other side.

■ **hypotonic** a state in which a solution has a lower solute concentration on one side of a semi-permeable membrane compared to the other side.

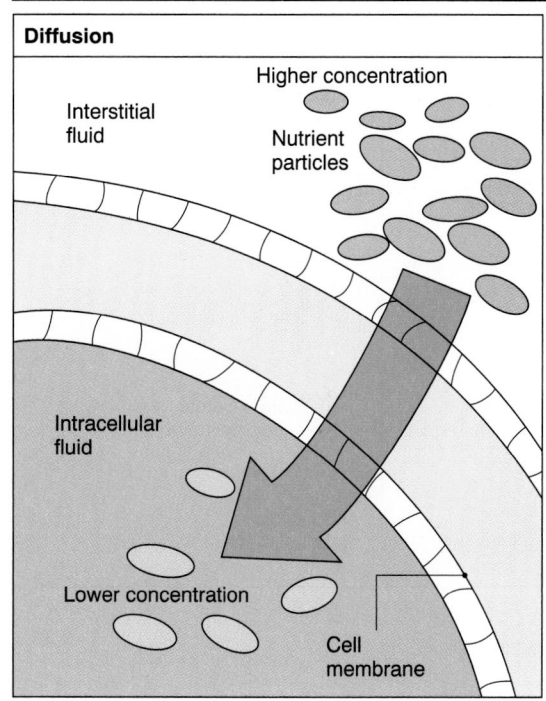

Diffusion

Interstitial fluid

Higher concentration

Nutrient particles

Intracellular fluid

Lower concentration

Cell membrane

FIGURE 12-2 Diffusion is the movement of a substance from an area of greater concentration to an area of lesser concentration.

homeostasis. If one side of a cell membrane has an increased quantity of a given electrolyte (is hypertonic), there will be a shift of the electrolyte from that side and a shift of water from the other side to restore the balanced state.

The tendency of molecules to move from an area of higher concentration to an area of lower concentration is referred to as **diffusion** and does not require energy. (See Figure 12-2) The diffusion of a solute (usually an electrolyte) across a cell membrane from the area of higher concentration to the area of lower concentration continues until the natural balance is again attained.

Water also moves across the cell membrane so as to dilute the area of increased electrolyte concentration. The movement of water is more rapid than the movement of electrolytes. This form of diffusion is referred to as **osmosis**. (See Figure 12-3.) It occurs in the opposite direction of solute movement. For example, if a semi-permeable membrane separates a solution of water and sodium, and if the concentration of sodium is two times higher on one side of the membrane as on the other, then two things will occur. Sodium will diffuse from the area of higher concentration (the hypertonic side) to the area of lesser concentration (the hypotonic side). Concurrently, water will diffuse in the opposite direction. That is, water will leave the hypotonic side and diffuse across the membrane to the hypertonic side. This will continue until both components, water and sodium, have equalized.

In addition to diffusion, two other mechanisms—active transport and facilitated diffusion—can transport substances across cell membranes. **Active transport** is the movement of a substance across the cell membrane against the osmotic gradient. For example, the body requires cells of the myocardium (heart muscle) to be negatively charged on the inside of the cells as compared to the outside. Sodium, however, tends to diffuse passively back into the cell. This would destroy the negative charge inside the cell. In order to maintain the desired gradient, sodium is actively pumped out of the cell by a mechanism known as the *sodium-potassium pump*. Active transport is faster than diffusion, but it requires the expenditure of energy. Proteins are moved across the cell membrane in a similar fashion.

■ **diffusion** the movement of solutes (substances dissolved in a solution) from an area of greater concentration to an area of lesser concentration.

■ **osmosis** the movement of a solvent (water) across a semi-permeable membrane from an area of lesser (solute) concentration to an area of greater (solute) concentration. Osmosis is a form of diffusion.

■ **active transport** biochemical process where a substance is moved across a cell membrane, often against a gradient, using energy.

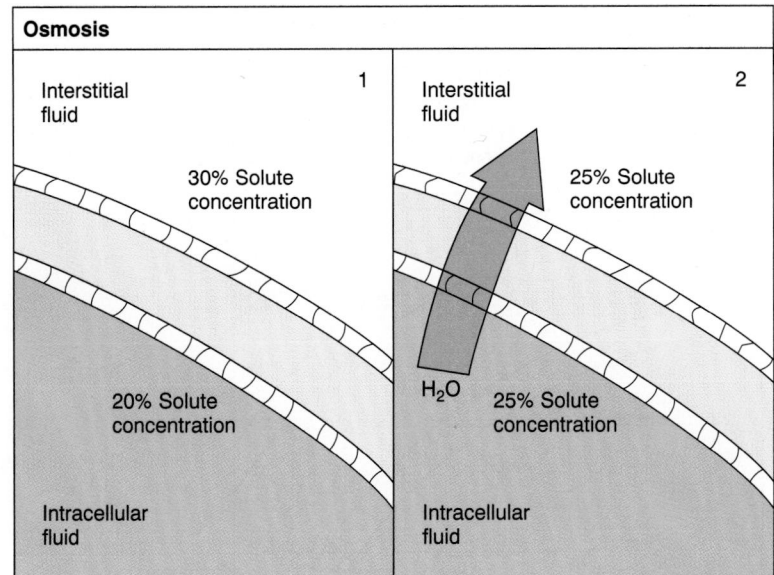

Osmosis

Interstitial fluid | 1

30% Solute concentration

20% Solute concentration

Intracellular fluid

Interstitial fluid | 2

25% Solute concentration

H_2O | 25% Solute concentration

Intracellular fluid

FIGURE 12-3 Osmosis is the movement of water from an area of higher WATER concentration to an area of lower WATER concentration. Because water is a solvent, it moves from an area of lower SOLUTE concentration to an area of higher SOLUTE concentration.

■ **facilitated diffusion** biochemical process where a substance is selectively transported across a membrane, using "helper proteins" and energy.

Certain molecules can move across the cell membrane by a process known as **facilitated diffusion**. Glucose is an example of such a molecule. Facilitated diffusion requires the assistance of "helper proteins" on the surface of the cell membrane. These proteins, once activated, bind to the glucose molecule. Following binding, the protein changes its configuration and transports the glucose molecule to the inside of the cell where it is released. Depending on the substance being transported, facilitated diffusion may or may not require energy.

Intravenous Therapy

Intravenous therapy is the introduction of fluids and other substances into the venous side of the circulatory system. It is used to replace blood lost through hemorrhage, for electrolyte or fluid replacement, and for introduction of medications directly into the vascular system.

Blood and Blood Components   To understand IV therapy, it is necessary to understand the function of blood and its components. The blood is the fluid of the cardiovascular system. An adequate amount of blood is required for the transport of nutrients, oxygen, hormones, and heat. Blood consists of the liquid portion, or plasma, and the formed elements, or blood cells. (See Figure 12-4.)

Plasma.   Plasma is made up of approximately 92 percent water, 6–7 percent proteins, and a small portion consisting of electrolytes, lipids, enzymes, clotting factors, glucose, and other dissolved substances.

Formed Elements.   The formed elements include the red blood cells, or *erythrocytes*; the white blood cells, or *leukocytes*; and the platelets, or *thrombocytes*. More than 99 percent of the cells are red blood cells. Red blood cells contain hemoglobin and are responsible for transporting oxygen to the body's peripheral cells. **Hemoglobin** is an iron-based compound that binds with oxygen in the pulmonary (lung) capillaries and transports it to the peripheral tissues where it can be unloaded. Factors such as pH (to be

■ **hemoglobin** the iron-containing substance in blood responsible for transport of oxygen.

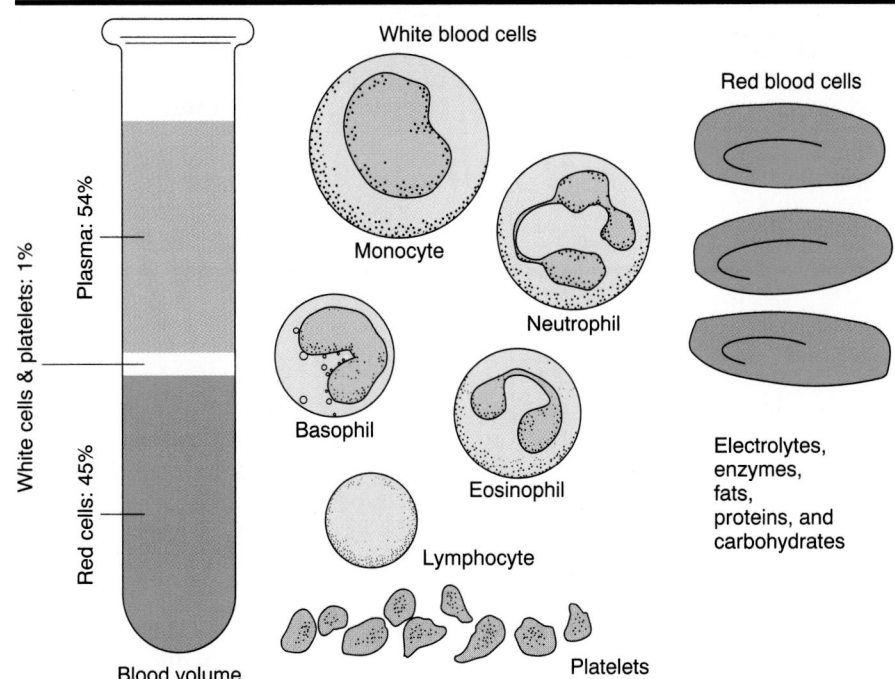

FIGURE 12-4 Blood components.

FIGURE 12-5 The percentage of the blood occupied by the red blood cells is termed the hematocrit.

discussed later in this chapter) and oxygen concentration affect the amount of oxygen that can be transported by hemoglobin.

The white cells are responsible for immunity and fighting infection. The platelets play a major role in blood clotting. The *viscosity* (thickness) of the blood is determined by the ratio of plasma to formed elements. The lesser the ratio of plasma to formed elements, the greater the viscosity.

The plasma can be separated from the formed elements by centrifugation. That is, blood can be placed in a test tube inside a centrifuge and spun at high speed. The heavier cells, the erythrocytes, will be forced to the bottom of the tube, leaving the plasma portion at the top. Usually, the red blood cells will account for approximately 45 percent of the blood volume. The percentage of blood occupied by red blood cells is referred to as the **hematocrit**. (See Figure 12-5.)

Blood Types. Blood is a type of tissue and varies from patient to patient. Blood can be categorized into various "types" as determined by the presence of proteins, known as *antigens*, on the erythrocytes. The major system of blood classification is the **ABO system**. (See Table 12-2.) This system is based on the type of antigen present on the cell.

There are two major antigen types, A and B. The patient can have either the A antigen, the B antigen, both antigens, or neither antigen. The blood type of a patient is genetically determined. With few exceptions, persons can only receive blood that is of the same type as their own. Persons with type A blood have the A antigen on the erythrocyte. Since they do not have the B antigen, they have antibody to B. If they were to receive type B blood, the immune system would determine that the blood was foreign and a reaction would occur.

There are two exceptions to this. Persons with type AB blood do not have antibody to either A or B, since they carry both antigens. Therefore, in an emergency, they can receive blood of any type. Because of this, persons with type AB blood are referred to as *universal recipients*. Type O blood does

■ **hematocrit** the percentage of the blood consisting of the red blood cells, or erythrocytes (usually 35–45 percent).

■ **ABO system** system of blood typing based on the presence of proteins on the surface of the red blood cells.

TABLE 12-2 Blood Typing—ABO System

Blood Type	Antigen Present on RBC	Antibody Present in Serum
O	None	Anti-A, Anti-B
AB	A and B	None
B	B	Anti-A
A	A	Anti-B

not contain either the A or B antigen. Therefore, in emergencies, it can be administered to a patient of any blood type. Because of this, type O is referred to as the *universal donor*. (See Table 12-3.) In addition to the ABO types, there are many additional minor blood types. In routine medical practice, blood is matched as closely as possible, considering both major and minor blood types.

RH Factor. One additional blood type worth mentioning is the *Rh factor*. Rh factor is present in approximately 85 percent of the population. Persons who are Rh negative usually do not have anti-Rh antibodies. However, if exposed to Rh positive blood through transfusion, these persons become "sensitized." Sensitization means that the patient has developed antibodies to Rh factor. If the patient were to receive an additional transfusion of Rh positive blood, then a severe or even fatal reaction could occur.

Fluid Replacement The most desirable fluid for replacement is whole blood. There are several reasons for this. First, blood contains hemoglobin, which can transport oxygen. In addition, it is the most natural replacement. However, even in the hospital setting, the routine use of whole blood is not practical. (See Table 12-4.) Blood is a precious commodity, and it must be conserved so that it can benefit the most people. Because of this, blood is often *fractionated*, or separated into parts. The red cells are packaged separately as *packed red blood cells*. The white cells are used for other purposes. Plasma is packaged as *fresh frozen plasma* for use when plasma or clotting factors are needed. Thus, with the exception of true hemorrhagic shock (resulting from blood loss), where whole blood is the fluid of first choice, packed red blood cells are now more frequently used than whole blood.

Before blood, or blood products, can be administered to a patient, they must be typed and cross-matched to prevent a severe allergic reaction. The

TABLE 12-3 Compatibility Among ABO Blood Groups

Cells of Donor	Reaction with Serum of Recipient			
	AB	B	A	O
AB	−	+	+	+
B	−	−	+	+
A	−	+	−	+
O	−	−	−	−

− = Nonagglutination
+ = Agglutination

TABLE 12-4 Resuscitation Fluids

Diagnosis	Resuscitation Fluid Used			
	1st Choice	**2nd Choice**	**3rd Choice**	**4th Choice**
Hemorrhagic Shock	Whole Blood	Packed RBC's	Plasma or Plasma Substitute	Lactated Ringer's or Normal Saline
Shock due to plasma loss (burns)	Plasma	Plasma Substitute	Lactated Ringer's or Normal Saline	
Dehydration	Lactated Ringer's or Normal Saline			

exception to this is fresh frozen plasma, which does not require cross-matching. If there is not adequate time for typing and cross-matching, O-negative blood can be administered, since it is the universal donor type.

Transfusion Reaction   For obvious reasons, blood and blood products are not used in the field. However, on occasion, you may be called upon to transport a patient with blood infusing. Because of this, you must be able to recognize the signs and symptoms of a *transfusion reaction*. Transfusion reactions occur when there is a discrepency between the blood type of the patient and the blood type of the blood being transfused. In addition to the ABO and Rh types, there are many "minor types" that can cause a transfusion reaction. Common signs and symptoms of a transfusion reaction include fever, chills, hives, hypotension, palpitations, tachycardia, flushing of the skin, headaches, loss of consciousness, nausea, vomiting, or shortness of breath.

If a transfusion reaction is suspected, IMMEDIATELY stop the transfusion and save the substance being transfused. The blood should be replaced by an electrolyte solution to keep the vein open. Quickly complete an adequate assessment of the patient's mental status. Administer oxygen and contact the medical control physician. The medical control physician may request the administration of mannitol (Osmotrol), diphenhydramine (Benadryl), or furosemide (Lasix). These drugs are used to maintain renal function, which is often severely compromised during a transfusion reaction.

In addition to overt reaction, you must always be alert for signs of fluid overload and congestive heart failure secondary to transfusion. This is evidenced by increased dyspnea, pulmonary congestion, edema, and altered mental state. If this is suspected, stop the infusion and start a crystalloid solution at a TKO ("to keep open") rate. Administer oxygen and contact the medical control physician.

Intravenous Fluids   Intravenous fluids are the most common products used in prehospital care for fluid and electrolyte therapy. Intravenous fluids occur in two general forms—colloids and crystalloids.

Colloids.   *Colloids* contain proteins, or other high-molecular-weight molecules, that tend to remain in the intravascular space for an extended period of time. In addition, colloids have **colloid osmotic pressure**, which means they tend to attract water into the intravascular space from the interstitial space and the intracellular compartment. Thus, a small amount of a colloid can be

■ **colloid osmotic pressure** pressure generated by the presence of colloids in the vascular system or interstitial space.

administered to a patient with a greater-than-expected increase in intravascular volume.. Common examples of colloids include:

❑ *Plasma protein fraction (Plasmanate)* is a protein-containing colloid. The principal protein present is **albumin**, which is suspended along with other proteins in a saline solvent.

❑ *Salt-poor albumin* contains only human albumin. Each gram of albumin holds approximately 18 milliliters of water in the blood stream.

❑ *Dextran* is not a protein, but a large sugar molecule with osmotic properties similar to albumin. It comes in two molecular weights: 40,000 and 70,000 Daltons. Dextran 40 has 2–2.5 times the colloid osmotic pressure of albumin.

❑ *Hetastarch (Hespan)*, like Dextran, is a sugar molecule with osmotic properties similar to protein. It does not appear to share many of Dextran's side-effects.

Colloid replacement therapy, at present, does not have a role in prehospital care except under rare circumstances. The colloid products are expensive and have a short shelf-life.

Crystalloids. *Crystalloids* are the primary compounds used in prehospital intravenous fluid therapy. There are multiple fluid preparations. It is often helpful to classify them according to their **tonicity** related to plasma:

❑ *Isotonic solutions* have electrolyte composition similar to the blood plasma. When placed into a normally hydrated patient, they will not cause a significant fluid or electrolyte shift.

❑ *Hypertonic solutions* have a higher solute concentration than the cells. These fluids will tend to cause a fluid shift out of the intracellular compartment into the extracellular compartment when administered to a normally hydrated patient. Later, there will be a diffusion of solute in the opposite direction.

❑ *Hypotonic solutions* have a lower solute concentration than the cells. When administered to a normally hydrated patient, they will cause a movement of fluid from the extracellular compartment into the intracellular compartment. Later, solutes will move in an opposite direction.

Replacement fluids should be chosen based on the needs of the patient and the patient's underlying problem. As a rule, hemorrhage occurs so fast that there has not been time for a significant fluid shift between the extracellular and intracellular space. Because of this, the replacement fluid should be isotonic. It is for this reason that lactated Ringer's and normal saline are often used. If the patient is dehydrated due to fluid loss from diarrhea or fever, then there is a greater deficit of water than sodium. In these cases, hypotonic fluids such as half-normal saline are chosen.

Some replacement fluids contain a single element, such as sodium chloride or dextrose, while others contain multiple elements. Solutions such as lactated Ringer's are designed so that the concentration of electrolytes is very similar to that of the plasma. As a result, these solutions are referred to as balanced salt solutions.

Three of the most commonly used solutions in prehospital care are lactated Ringer's solution, 0.9 percent sodium chloride (normal saline), and 5 percent dextrose in water (D5W).

❑ *Lactated Ringer's* is an isotonic electrolyte solution of sodium chloride, potassium chloride, calcium chloride, and sodium lactate in water.

- *Normal saline* is an electrolyte solution of sodium chloride in water. It is isotonic with the extracellular fluid.
- *D5W* is a hypotonic glucose solution used to keep a vein open and to supply calories necessary for cell metabolism. While it will have an initial effect of increasing the circulatory volume, glucose molecules rapidly diffuse across the vascular membrane with a resultant free water increase.

Both lactated Ringer's solution and normal saline are used for fluid replacement, because their administration causes an immediate expansion of the circulatory volume. However, as was noted earlier, due to the movement of the electrolytes and water, two-thirds of either of these solutions is lost to the interstitial space within one hour.

ACID-BASE BALANCE

Acid-base balance is a dynamic relationship that reflects the relative concentration of hydrogen ions (H^+) in the body. Hydrogen ions are *acidic* and the concentration of these within the body must be maintained within fairly strict limits. Any deviation in the hydrogen ion concentration adversely affects all of the biochemical events that occur in the body. The hydrogen ion concentration is dynamic, changing from second to second.

The pH Scale

The total number of hydrogen ions present in the body at any given time is very high. Because of this, the **pH** system of measurement is utilized. The pH scale is inversely related to hydrogen ion concentration. That is, the greater the hydrogen ion concentration, the lower the pH. The lower the hydrogen ion concentration, the higher the pH.

The pH scale is **logarithmic**, each number representing a value ten times that of its neighboring number, so that pH 6 represents a hydrogen ion concentration 10 times as great as that represented by pH 7. The following formula represents pH:

$$pH = \log \frac{1}{[H^+]}$$

The pH scale ranges from 1 to 14. A pH of 1 means that only hydrogen ions are present. A pH of 14 means that there are virtually no hydrogen ions present. The pH of water is 7.0, which is a neutral pH. The pH of the body is normally 7.35 to 7.45. (See Table 12-5.)

Because hydrogen ions are acidic, a pH below 7.35 is referred to as **acidosis**. A substance that produces negatively-charged ions that can neutralize the positively-charged hydrogen ions (or other acids) is called an *alkali* or a *base*. An excess of alkaline (base) substances or a deficit of acids will produce a pH above 7.45, which is referred to as **alkalosis**. A variation of only 0.4 of a pH unit in either direction (6.9 or 7.8) can be fatal.

Bodily Regulation of Acid-Base Balance

The body is constantly producing hydrogen ions (acids) through metabolism and other biochemical processes. To maintain the acid-base balance, these hydrogen ions must be constantly eliminated from the body. There are three

■ **pH** scientific method of expressing the acidity or alkalinity of a solution. It is the logarithm of the hydrogen ion concentration divided by one. The higher the pH, the more alkaline the solution. The lower the pH, the more acidic the solution.

■ **logarithm** mathematical concept that eases calculation of large numbers. The log of a number is the exponent of the power to which a given base must be raised to equal that number. For example, the log of 100 is 2 ($100 = 10^2$), and the log of 1,000 is 3 ($1,000 = 10^3$).

✻ The lower the patient's pH, the more acidic the patient.

■ **acidosis** a state in which the pH is lower than normal due to an increased hydrogen ion concentration.

■ **alkalosis** a state in which the pH is higher than normal due to a decreased hydrogen ion concentration or increased alkaline substance concentration.

TABLE 12-5   The pH Scale and Hydrogen Ion Concentrations

pH			H+ Concentrations*	
Acidic	0	Hydrochloric acid	10^0	(1.0)
	1	Stomach secretions	10^{-1}	(0.1)
	2	Lemon juice	10^{-2}	(0.01)
	3	Cola drinks	10^{-3}	(0.001)
	4	White wine	10^{-4}	(0.0001)
	5	Tomato juice	10^{-5}	(0.00001)
	6	Coffee	10^{-6}	(0.000001)
		Urine		
		Saliva		
Neutral	7	Distilled water	10^{-7}	(0.0000001)
Basic	8	Blood, semen	10^{-8}	(0.00000001)
	9	Bile	10^{-9}	(0.000000001)
	10	Bleach	10^{-10}	(0.0000000001)
	11	Milk of magnesia	10^{-11}	(0.00000000001)
	12	Ammonia water	10^{-12}	(0.000000000001)
	13	Drain opener	10^{-13}	(0.0000000000001)
	14	Lye	10^{-14}	(0.00000000000001)

* Hydrogen ion concentrations are expressed in moles per liter, a quantity based on molecular weight.

major mechanisms to remove hydrogen ions from the body. The fastest mechanism is often referred to as the *buffer system* or the *bicarbonate buffer system.*

The two components of the bicarbonate buffer system are bicarbonate ion (HCO_3^-) and carbonic acid (H_2CO_3). These two compounds are in equilibrium with hydrogen ion (H^+), as follows: In some circumstances hydrogen ion will combine with bicarbonate ion to produce carbonic acid. In other circumstances, carbonic acid will dissociate into bicarbonate ion and hydrogen ion:

$$H^+ + HCO_3^- \leftrightarrow H_2CO_3$$

Hydrogen ion + bicarbonate ion ↔ carbonic acid

For every molecule of carbonic acid, there are 20 molecules of bicarbonate ion. Any change in this 20:1 ratio is immediately corrected without significant change in the total pH. This occurs in the following manner: An increase in hydrogen ion (acidosis) is corrected as the excess hydrogen ions combine with bicarbonate ions to form carbonic acid. (Thus an increase in hydrogen ion leads to an increase in carbonic acid.) Conversely, when there is a deficit in hydrogen ions (alkalosis), carbonic acid will dissociate into bicarbonate ion and hydrogen ion. (Thus a decrease in hydrogen ion leads to a decrease in carbonic acid.) (See Figure 12-6.) For example:

$$\text{Increased Acid: } \uparrow H^+ + HCO_3^- \rightarrow \uparrow H_2CO_3$$

$$\text{Decreased Acid: } \downarrow H^+ + HCO_3^- \rightarrow \downarrow H_2CO_3$$

Carbonic acid is a weak acid that is better tolerated by the body than pure hydrogen ion. However, the body carries this reaction further. The increased carbonic acid must also be eliminated.

The elimination of excess carbonic acid takes place as follows: Carbonic acid is unstable and will eventually dissociate into carbon dioxide and water. This normally slow process is speeded by the blood's erythrocytes, which contain an enzyme called *carbonic anhydrase*. Carbonic anhydrase causes carbonic acid to be converted to carbon dioxide and water very rapidly—so rapidly that carbonic acid exists for only a fraction of a second before it is converted into carbon dioxide and water. Most buffering of acid in the body occurs in the erythrocytes.

The enzyme also works in a reverse fashion, which allows carbon dioxide and water to be quickly converted into carbonic acid. Thus, with the aid of carbonic anhydrase, there is an equilibrium between hydrogen ion and carbon dioxide. The following equation illustrates this relationship.

$$H^+ \quad + \quad HCO_3^- \quad \leftrightarrow \quad H_2CO_3 \quad \leftrightarrow \quad H_2O + \quad CO_2$$

hydrogen ion + bicarbonate ion ↔ carbonic acid ↔ water + carbon dioxide

Thus an increase in hydrogen ion (acid) would result in an increase in carbonic acid. With the aid of carbonic anhydrase, carbonic acid would quickly dissociate into water and carbon dioxide. Conversely (since the reaction can move in either direction), an increase in CO_2 causes an increase in hydrogen ion concentration and a decrease in pH (increase in acidity), as shown below.

$$\uparrow H^+ \leftrightarrow \uparrow CO_2$$

In conjunction with the bicarbonate buffer system described above, the body regulates acid-base balance by two other mechanisms, respiration and kidney function. Increased respirations cause increased elimination of CO_2, which results in a decrease in hydrogen ions and an increase in pH. Conversely, decreased respirations cause CO_2 to be retained. This causes an increase in hydrogen ions and a decrease in pH. (See Figure 12-7.)

The kidneys also can regulate the pH by altering the concentration of bicarbonate ion in the blood. Increased elimination of HCO_3^- results in a lowered pH. (There is less bicarbonate ion to combine with and eliminate hydrogen ion.) Conversely retention of HCO_3^- causes an increase in pH. (There is more bicarbonate ion to combine with and eliminate hydrogen ion.) In addition, the kidneys affect the acid-base balance by removing or retaining various chemicals. Normally, the kidneys remove larger metabolic acids, excreting them in the urine.

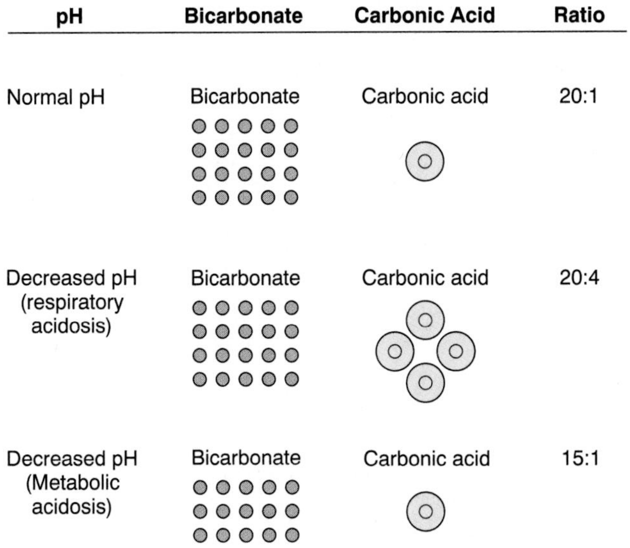

pH	Bicarbonate	Carbonic Acid	Ratio
Normal pH	Bicarbonate	Carbonic acid	20:1
Decreased pH (respiratory acidosis)	Bicarbonate	Carbonic acid	20:4
Decreased pH (Metabolic acidosis)	Bicarbonate	Carbonic acid	15:1

FIGURE 12-6 Acid-base ratios relative to pH.

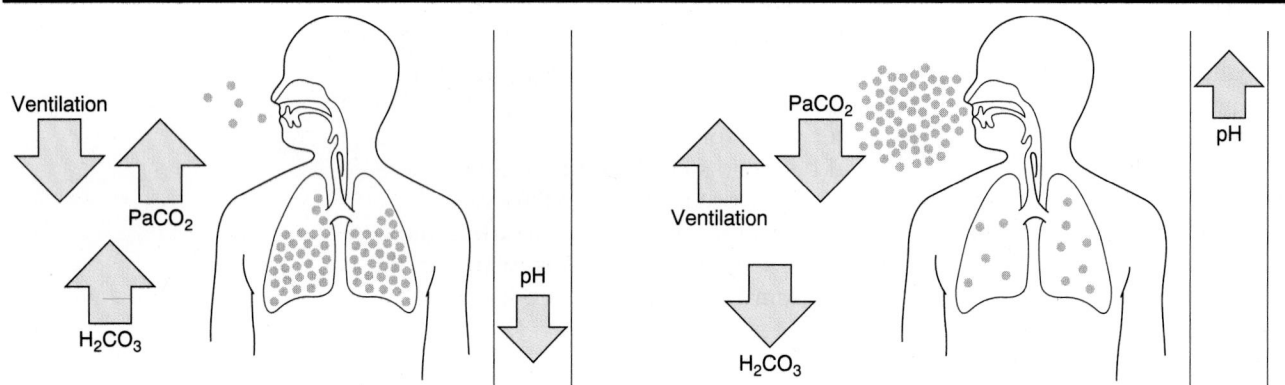

FIGURE 12-7 The respiratory component of acid-base balance.

Acid-Base Derangements

An increase in hydrogen ion (as occurs, for example, in cardiac arrest) drives the equilibrium described above to the right. Hydrogen ion is immediately combined with bicarbonate ion. This combination results in the formation of carbonic acid, which subsequently dissociates into carbon dioxide and water with the assistance of carbonic anhydrase. Carbon dioxide is eliminated by the lungs, and water is eliminated through the kidneys. Any change in a component of this equation affects the other components. For example:

$$\uparrow H^+ + HCO_3^- \rightarrow \uparrow H_2CO_3 \rightarrow H_2O + \uparrow CO_2$$

Conversely, if the amount of carbon dioxide is increased, the equation is driven the other direction, resulting in an increase hydrogen ion (acid).

$$\uparrow CO_2 + H_2O \rightarrow \uparrow H_2CO_3 \rightarrow \uparrow H^+ + HCO_3^-$$

Both types of acid-base derangements, alkalosis and acidosis, can be divided into two categories based on the underlying causes. Changes in the concentration of CO_2 result from changes in respiratory function. Thus, an acidosis caused by retained CO_2 is referred to as *respiratory acidosis*. An alkalosis caused by the excess removal of CO_2 is called *respiratory alkalosis*. However, if acidosis results from the production of metabolic acids, such as lactic acid, then *metabolic acidosis* is said to exist. If an alkalosis is caused by the excess elimination of hydrogen ion, it is termed *metabolic alkalosis*.

Respiratory Acidosis Respiratory acidosis is caused by the retention of CO_2. This can result from impaired ventilation due to problems occurring either in the lungs or in the respiratory center of the brain. The CO_2 level is increased and the pH is decreased. Treatment is directed at improving ventilation.

✱ The primary treatment for any patient suspected of acidosis is to increase ventilations.

$$\downarrow RESPIRATION = \uparrow CO_2 + H_2O \rightarrow \uparrow H_2CO_3 \rightarrow \uparrow H^+ + HCO_3^-$$

Respiratory Alkalosis Respiratory alkalosis results from increased respiration and excessive elimination of CO_2. This can occur with anxiety or following ascent to a high altitude. The CO_2 level is decreased and the pH is

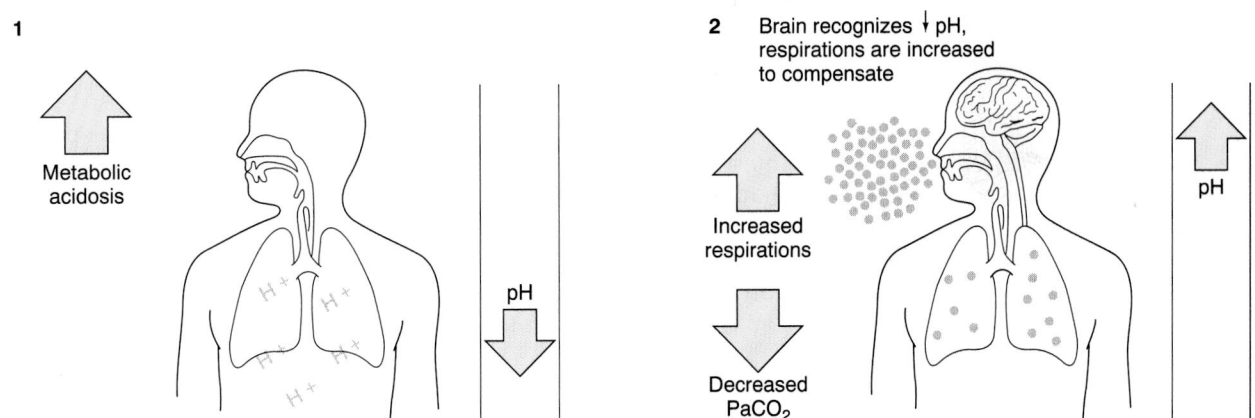

1 Metabolic acidosis

pH ↓

2 Brain recognizes ↓ pH, respirations are increased to compensate

Increased respirations

Decreased PaCO₂

pH ↑

FIGURE 12-8 Compensation for metabolic acidosis begins with an increase in respirations.

increased. Treatment, if required, consists of increasing the CO_2 level by having the patient rebreathe CO_2.

$$\uparrow \text{RESPIRATION} = \downarrow CO_2 + H_2O \rightarrow \downarrow H_2CO_3 \rightarrow \downarrow H^+ + HCO_3^-$$

Metabolic Acidosis   Metabolic acidosis results from the production of metabolic acids such as lactic acid, which consume bicarbonate ion. In addition, it can result from diarrhea, vomiting, diabetes, and medication usage. The pH is decreased, and the CO_2 level is normal. Treatment primarily consists of ventilation, which causes the elimination of CO_2 and, subsequently, hydrogen ion. (See Figure 12-8.) On rare occasions, additional bicarbonate, usually in the form of sodium bicarbonate ($NaHCO_3$), may be required.

$$\uparrow H^+ + HCO_3^- \rightarrow \uparrow H_2CO_3 \rightarrow H_2O + \uparrow CO_2$$

Metabolic Alkalosis   Metabolic alkalosis occurs much less frequently than metabolic acidosis. It is usually caused by the administration of **diuretics**, loss of chloride ions associated with prolonged vomiting, or the overzealous administration of sodium bicarbonate. The pH is increased and the CO_2 level is normal. Treatment consists of correcting the underlying cause.

■ **diuretic** a medication that stimulates the kidneys to excrete water.

$$\downarrow H^+ + HCO_3^- \rightarrow \downarrow H_2CO_3 \rightarrow H_2O + \downarrow CO_2$$

Usually, both a respiratory and a metabolic component are present. The type of acid-base derangement present can only be determined by arterial blood gas studies. These, of course, are only available in the hospital setting. Arterial blood gasses report the pH, $PaCO_2$, PaO_2, bicarbonate concentration, and oxygen saturation. Pulse oximetry is now available for field use and is quite accurate in determining oxygen saturation levels.

PHYSIOLOGICAL BACKGROUND TO SHOCK

Shock, from a medical standpoint, is defined as inadequate tissue perfusion. It can occur for many reasons such as trauma, fluid loss, heart attack, infection, spinal cord injury, and other causes. Although the causes are different, all forms of shock have the same underlying pathophysiology at the tissue level.

■ **shock** a state of inadequate tissue perfusion.

Physiology of Perfusion

All body cells require a constant supply of oxygen and other essential nutrients. At the same time, waste products, such as carbon dioxide, must be constantly removed. The circulatory system, in conjunction with the respiratory and gastrointestinal systems, provides the body's cells with these essential nutrients. Inadequate **perfusion** of body tissues results in shock. Shock occurs first at a cellular level. If allowed to progress, the tissues, organs, and ultimately the entire organism is affected.

Perfusion is dependent on a functioning and intact circulatory system. The three components of the circulatory system include:

❑ The pump (heart)
❑ The fluid (blood)
❑ The container (blood vessels)

A derangement in any one of these components can adversely affect perfusion. (See Figure 12-9.)

The Pump   The *heart* is the pump of the cardiovascular system. It receives blood from the venous system, pumps it to the lungs where it is oxygenated, and subsequently pumps it to the peripheral tissues. The amount of blood ejected by the heart in one contraction is referred to as the stroke volume. Several factors affect *stroke volume*. These include:

❑ Preload
❑ Contractile force
❑ Afterload

Preload is the amount of blood delivered to the heart during diastole. It is dependent on venous return. The venous system is a capacitance, or storage, system. That is, it can be contracted or expanded as needed to meet the physiological demands of the body. When additional oxygenated blood is required, the venous capacitance is reduced, thus increasing the amount of blood delivered to the heart. The greater the preload, the greater the stroke volume.

Preload also affects **cardiac contractile force**. The greater the volume of preload, the more the ventricles are stretched. The greater the stretch, up to a certain point, the greater will be the subsequent cardiac contraction. This is referred to as the *Frank-Starling mechanism* and can be illustrated through the example of a rubber band. The more the rubber band is stretched, the greater will be its velocity when released.

In addition, cardiac contractile strength is affected by circulating **catecholamines** (epinephrine and norepinephrine) and by sympathetic nervous system tone. Catecholamines enhance cardiac contractile strength by action on the beta-adrenergic receptors.

Finally, stroke volume is affected by **afterload**. The afterload is the resistance against which the ventricle must contract. This resistance must be overcome before ventricular contraction can result in ejection of blood. Afterload is determined by the degree of peripheral resistance. This, in effect, is due to the amount of vasoconstriction present. The arterial system can be expanded and contracted to meet the metabolic demands of the body. The greater the resistance offered by the arterial system, the less the stroke volume.

The amount of blood pumped by the heart in one minute is referred to as the **cardiac output**. It is a function of stroke volume (liters per beat) and

■ **perfusion** fluid passing through an organ or a part of the body.

■ **preload** the pressure within the ventricles at the end of the diastole.

■ **cardiac contractile force** the force generated by the heart during each contraction.

■ **catecholamine** class of hormones that act upon the autonomic nervous system. They include epinephrine, norepinephrine, and similar compounds.

■ **afterload** the resistance against which the heart must pump.

■ **cardiac output** the amount of blood pumped by the heart in one minute.

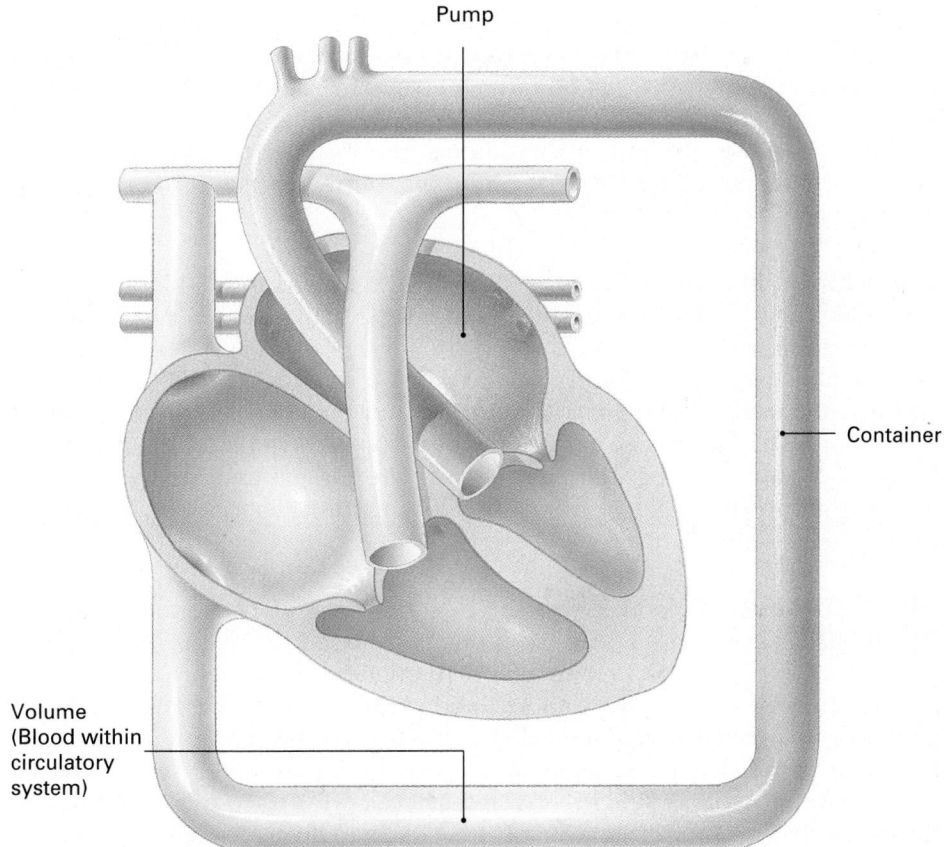

Pump

Container

Volume
(Blood within
circulatory
system)

FIGURE 12-9 Components of the circulatory system.

heart rate (beats per minute). Cardiac output is usually expressed in liters per minute. It can be defined by the below equation.

$$\text{stroke volume} \times \text{heart rate} = \text{cardiac output}$$

The equation illustrates the factors that can affect cardiac output. An increase in stroke volume or an increase in heart rate can increase cardiac output. Conversely, a decrease in stroke volume or a decrease in heart rate can decrease cardiac output. The *blood pressure* is representative of cardiac output.

$$\text{cardiac output} \times \text{peripheral vascular resistance} = \text{blood pressure}$$

Peripheral vascular resistance is the pressure against which the heart must pump. Since the circulatory system is a closed system, increasing either cardiac output or peripheral vascular resistance will increase blood pressure. Likewise, a decrease in cardiac output or a decrease in peripheral vascular resistance will decrease blood pressure.

The body strives to keep the blood pressure relatively constant through feedback mechanisms. Sensory fibers, commonly referred to as *baroreceptors*, are present in the carotid bodies—small structures that contain nerve tissue at the branch of the carotid arteries—and the arch of the aorta. These baroreceptor centers closely monitor blood pressure.

If blood pressure increases, the baroreceptors send signals to the brain that cause the blood pressure to return to its normal values. This is accomplished by decreasing the heart rate, decreasing the preload, or decreasing peripheral vascular resistance. If the blood pressure falls, the baroreceptors

■ **peripheral vascular resistance**
the resistance to blood flow due to the peripheral blood vessels. This pressure must be overcome for the heart to pump blood effectively.

are stimulated. This results in activation of the sympathetic nervous system. The heart rate is increased, as is the strength of the cardiac contractions. In addition, the peripheral blood vessels are also affected. There is arteriolar constriction, venous constriction (which results in decreased container size), and overall increased peripheral vascular resistance. Finally, the adrenal medulla (the inner portion of the adrenal gland) is stimulated. This results in the secretion of epinephrine and norepinephrine, which further enhance the response.

The Fluid   Blood is the fluid of the cardiovascular system. Blood is a viscous fluid; that is, it is thicker and more adhesive than water. As a result, it flows more slowly than water.

An adequate amount of blood is required for perfusion. The cardiovascular system is a closed system, with no major movement of fluid into or out of the system. Because of this, the volume of blood present must be adequate to fill the container. Blood, which consists of the plasma and the formed elements, transports oxygen, carbon dioxide, nutrients, hormones, metabolic waste products, and heat.

The Container   Blood vessels serve as the container of the cardiovascular system. The blood vessels can be thought of as a continuous, closed, and pressurized pipeline that moves blood throughout the body. Comprised of arteries, arterioles, capillaries, venules, and veins, the blood vessels play a significant role in maintaining blood flow. Although the heart is considered to be the pump of the circulatory system, the blood vessels—under the control of the autonomic nervous system—can regulate blood flow to different areas of the body by adjusting their size as well as by selectively rerouting blood through the large microcirculation.

While the arteries and veins, like the heart, are subject to direct stimulation from sympathetic portions of the autonomic nervous system, the microcirculation is primarily responsive to local tissue needs. The capability of some vessels in the capillary network to adjust their diameter permits the microcirculation selectively to supply undernourished tissue, while temporarily bypassing tissues with no immediate need. Capillaries have a sphincter at the origin of the capillary, called the *pre-capillary sphincter*, and another at the end of the capillary, called the *post-capillary sphincter*. The pre-capillary sphincter responds to local tissue demands, such as acidosis, and opens as more arterial blood is needed. The post-capillary sphincter opens when blood is to be emptied into the venous system.

Blood flow through the vessels occurs because of two characteristics: peripheral resistance and pressure within the system. *Peripheral resistance*, as noted earlier, is the resistance to blood flow. Vessels with larger inside diameters create less resistance, while vessels with smaller inside diameters create greater resistance. Peripheral resistance is dependent on three factors—the length of the vessel, the diameter of the vessel, and blood viscosity.

There is very little resistance to blood flow through the aorta and arteries. A significant change in peripheral resistance occurs at the arteriole level. This is because the inside diameter of the arteriole is much smaller, as compared to the aorta and arteries. Additionally, the arteriole has the pronounced ability to change its diameter as much as fivefold. It tends to do this in response to local tissue needs and autonomic nervous signals.

Contraction of the venous side of the vascular system results in decreased capacitance and increased cardiac preload. The arterial system, on the other hand, provides systemic vascular resistance. An increase in arterial tone increases resistance, which increases blood pressure.

Oxygen Transport

In addition to perfusion, oxygenation of the peripheral tissues is also essential. Oxygen is brought into the body via the respiratory system. During inspiration, approximately 500 to 800 mL of atmospheric air is taken into the lungs. Of this atmospheric air, 21% is oxygen. This air passes through the upper and lower airways, coming to rest in the *alveoli* of the lungs.

Surrounding the alveoli are capillaries perfused by the arterial side of the pulmonary circulation. The arterial blood, which has been pumped through the pulmonary circulation by the right side of the heart, is low in oxygen, approximately a 16-percent concentration. The partial pressure of oxygen in the alveoli is greater than the deoxygenated blood within the pulmonary circulation. Thus, oxygen diffuses across the alveolar-capillary membrane and into the bloodstream. The red blood cells "pick up" this oxygen while passing through the microcirculation of the pulmonary capillary bed. Oxygen binds to the hemoglobin molecule of the red blood cells, which serve as the primary carriers of oxygen within the bloodstream.

Under normal situations, between 97% and 100% of the hemoglobin is saturated with oxygen. The oxygen-enriched blood then circulates back to the heart via the venous side of the pulmonary circulation. Passing through the left atrium and into the left ventricle, the oxygen-enriched blood is pumped throughout the body via the systemic circulation.

Upon reaching the capillaries, the blood interfaces with the tissues. The tissues contain cells that are oxygen-deficient due to normal metabolic activity. Since the concentration of oxygen is greater in the bloodstream than in the tissues, oxygen will diffuse from the red blood cells into the tissues and cells. Overall, the movement and utilization of oxygen in the body is dependent upon the following conditions.

❑ Adequate concentration of inspired oxygen
❑ Appropriate movement of oxygen across the alveolar/capillary membrane into the arterial bloodstream
❑ Adequate number of red blood cells to carry the oxygen
❑ Proper tissue perfusion
❑ Efficient off-loading of oxygen at the tissue level

These conditions are collectively known as the *Fick Principle*.

Tissue Perfusion

Tissue perfusion is dependent upon each component of the circulatory system. In addition, in terms of tissue oxygenation, it is dependent upon the respiratory system. If tissue perfusion is compromised, several conditions begin to develop—conditions that ultimately can lead to shock.

Factors that can cause decreased perfusion include:

❑ Inadequate pump
  • Inadequate preload
  • Inadequate cardiac contractile strength
  • Excessive afterload
  • Inadequate heart rate
❑ Inadequate fluid
  • Hypovolemia (abnormally low circulating blood volume)
❑ Inadequate container

- Dilated container without change in fluid volume
- Inadequate systemic vascular resistance

There is some local control of tissue perfusion. When the amounts of metabolic waste products (such as lactic acid) increase, the tissues become acidotic. This local acidosis causes nearby pre-capillary sphincters to relax, thus opening the capillaries and increasing perfusion of the affected tissues.

Usually, the body is able to compensate for any of the changes described above. However, when the compensatory mechanisms fail, shock develops.

PHYSIOLOGICAL RESPONSES TO SHOCK

Shock results from many factors. However, regardless of the cause, the underlying problem remains inadequate tissue perfusion. When tissue perfusion declines, the body reacts immediately to restore and maintain blood flow to all body tissues. It accomplishes this through the activation of various *compensatory mechanisms*. These physiological mechanisms are often effective in restoring tissue perfusion. However, if the cause is not corrected, the compensatory mechanisms will eventually fail. In such cases, shock becomes irreversible, and the organism dies.

Treatment of shock is dependent upon recognizing its presence early. The initial signs and symptoms of shock are subtle. However, to prevent irreversible shock, you will need to detect these subtle signs and symptoms. In order to understand the signs and symptoms of shock, it is essential that you recognize the body's physiological response to inadequate tissue perfusion.

Systemic Response to Shock

The body's response to shock is complex, involving nearly every body system. As tissue perfusion declines, several compensatory mechanisms are activated as the body strives to maintain adequate tissue perfusion. The initial physiological response to shock is progressive vasoconstriction. This causes an increase in peripheral vascular resistance and serves to maintain blood pressure. Initially, the blood vessels in the skin, digestive organs, and skeletal muscles constrict in order to maintain blood flow to essential organs such as the kidneys, heart, and brain. In addition, cardiac output increases by increasing either the heart rate, or the stroke volume, or both. Both peripheral vasoconstriction and increased cardiac output aid in restoring tissue perfusion.

Clinically, these early physiological responses may be difficult to detect. One of the earliest detectible changes is an increase in the heart rate. As the blood vessels of the skin constrict, the skin loses its color and becomes pale. In addition, it becomes cool to touch. As vasoconstriction continues, capillary refill time will become prolonged.

Other body systems also respond to decreased tissue perfusion. The respiratory system reacts by increasing the respiratory rate and tidal volume. This serves to provide the body with increased supplies of oxygen during this period of stress. The urinary system decreases filtration of water in order to maintain intravascular fluid volume. The gastrointestinal system slows because of decreased blood supply. All of these help the cardiovascular system maintain peripheral tissue perfusion. However, when such compensatory mechanisms fail, inadequate tissue perfusion worsens.

Shock at the Cellular Level

The cell is the ultimate target of inadequate tissue perfusion. Following an interruption of oxygen supply to the cell, metabolism will switch from an

✱ One of the first signs of shock is a tachycardia and vasoconstriction of the vessels of the skin.

aerobic (with oxygen) to an *anaerobic* (without oxygen) mode. The primary energy source for the cells is glucose, taken into the cell with the aid of insulin. The initial step in glucose breakdown is called *glycolysis* and results in the formation of pyruvic acid. Glycolysis does not require oxygen, yet only yields a small amount of energy. Glycolysis alone is an inefficient utilization of glucose. Because of this, in the normal state, pyruvic acid is further degraded into carbon dioxide, water, and energy, in a process termed the *Krebs* or *citric acid cycle*. This aerobic process yields considerably more energy than glycolysis, and it requires oxygen. (See Figure 12-10.)

In poor perfusion states and in hypoxia, an inadequate amount of oxygen is presented to the cells. Thus, glucose can only complete glycolysis and cannot enter into the citric acid cycle. This causes an accumulation of pyruvic acid. In these cases, pyruvic acid is quickly degraded to lactic acid. If time elapses, lactic acid and other metabolic acids accumulate. Cellular death soon occurs under these conditions. Cellular death will ultimately lead to tissue death; tissue death will lead to organ failure; and organ failure will lead to death of the individual.

Stages of Shock

Shock can be divided into three distinct stages:

- ❏ Compensated shock
- ❏ Decompensated shock
- ❏ Irreversible shock

Compensated Shock   Following the onset of inadequate tissue perfusion, the various compensatory mechanisms of the body are stimulated. The heart rate and strength of cardiac contractions will increase. There will be an increase in systemic vascular resistance that will assist in maintaining the blood pressure. These compensatory changes will continue until the body is unable to maintain blood pressure and tissue perfusion.

Shock can be hidden by compensatory mechanisms such as generalized vasoconstriction and increases in the heart rate. During this stage of shock,

✱ Compensated shock is the most difficult stage of shock to detect. However, prompt recognition and treatment are essential.

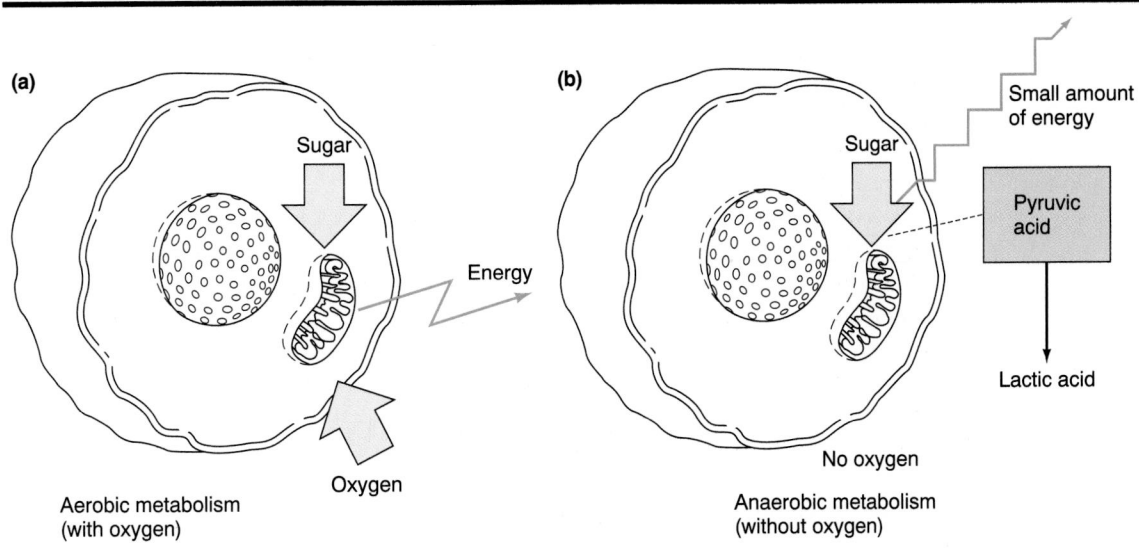

(a)

Sugar

Energy

Oxygen

Aerobic metabolism
(with oxygen)

(b)

Sugar

Small amount
of energy

Pyruvic
acid

Lactic acid

No oxygen

Anaerobic metabolism
(without oxygen)

FIGURE 12-10   Aerobic metabolism (a) requires oxygen and is most efficient. Anaerobic metabolism (b) yields much less energy and toxic by-products such as lactic acid.

you should concentrate on more subtle indicators such as tachycardia, decreased skin perfusion, and subtle alterations in mental status.

Certain medications that the patient may be taking can contribute to the problem. One example includes medications, such as propranolol, that act to block the beta receptor sites. They can initially hide the signs and symptoms of shock by hindering the compensatory increase in the heart rate and the ability of myocardial tissue to contract.

Decompensated Shock   In the later stages of shock, the blood pressure begins to fall. Prior to the fall in blood pressure, blood supply to essential organs diminishes. In addition to falling cardiac output, changes occur in the microcirculation that further interfere with oxygen delivery to the cells. The pre-capillary sphincters relax, and the post-capillary sphincters remain closed. The result is the slowing of blood flow and sludging. Ultimately, the pressure driving the erythrocytes is diminished. This renders the erythrocytes unable to bend. Under routine capillary pressures, the erythrocytes can bend to facilitate movement through the capillary. However, when inadequate capillary pressure is present, the erythrocytes do not bend and simply stack, like a roll of coins, in a formation called a *rouleaux*. This causes further stagnation of capillary blood flow.

Decompensated shock is much easier to detect than compensated shock. As the blood pressure falls, end-organ perfusion decreases. This causes prolonged capillary refill time and a marked increase in heart rate, as evidenced by a rapid and thready pulse. Eventually, mental status changes will occur. Initially, these will be in the form of agitation and restlessness. As cerebral blood flow further declines, confusion will increase, leading eventually to coma.

Irreversible Shock— Ultimately, after failure of the compensatory mechanisms, cellular death will begin. At some point, when enough cells in vital organs are disrupted, shock becomes irreversible and death is inevitable, even if vital signs are restored.

The heart is an amazing organ. With appropriate definitive care, adequate cardiac output (at least within normal values) may be restored even in a patient with no palpable blood pressure or pulse. While many patients recuperate from shock, however, others are not so fortunate.

As the initial insult of shock progresses, it becomes more deadly. Cells begin to die and so do organs. Vital organs such as the kidneys, liver, lungs and even the heart begin to falter and eventually become ineffective. A patient may be revived, only to die several days later as a result of end-organ failure—defined as the deterioration of the vital organs due to inadequate perfusion. Conditions that may occur during this phase include: adult respiratory distress syndrome (ARDS), renal failure, liver failure, and sepsis.

TYPES OF SHOCK

Although all types of shock result in inadequate tissue perfusion, the causes are different. Medical experts commonly classify shock based on the cause. The frequent types (causes) of shock are discussed below.

Hypovolemic Shock

Shock due to a loss of intravascular fluid volume is referred to as *hypovolemic shock*. Possible causes of hypovolemic shock include:

❑ Internal or external hemorrhage (This type of hypovolemic shock is also known as *hemorrhagic shock*.)

- ❑ Traumatic injury
- ❑ Long bone or open fractures
- ❑ Severe dehydration from vomiting or diarrhea
- ❑ Plasma loss from burns
- ❑ Diabetic ketoacidosis with resultant osmotic diuresis
- ❑ Excessive sweating

Hypovolemic shock can also be due to internal third-space loss. Such a condition can occur with bowel obstruction, peritonitis, pancreatitis, or liver failure resulting in ascites (accumulation of fluid within the abdominal cavity).

Cardiogenic Shock

An inability of the heart to pump enough blood to supply all body parts is referred to as *cardiogenic shock*. Cardiogenic shock is usually the result of severe left ventricular failure, secondary to acute myocardial infarction or congestive heart failure. The hypotension that accompanies this form of shock aggravates the situation by decreasing coronary perfusion. With decreased coronary perfusion, the heart muscle becomes even more damaged, thus establishing a vicious cycle that ultimately results in complete pump failure.

During cardiogenic shock, the activation of compensatory mechanisms can actually worsen the situation. When the peripheral resistance increases in an attempt to maintain blood pressure, the myocardial workload increases. This, in turn, increases the myocardial oxygen demand, further aggravating myocardial ischemia and infarction. Cardiac output is further depressed.

While the most common cause of cardiogenic shock is severe left ventricular failure, a number of other factors can have the same clinical manifestation. These include chronic progressive heart disease, such as cardiomyopathy, rupture of the papillary heart muscles or interventricular septum, and end-stage valvular disease (mitral stenosis or aortic regurgitation). Most patients who experience cardiogenic shock will have normal blood volume. However, some patients will be hypovolemic from an excessive use of prescribed diuretics or the severe diaphoresis that accompanies some acute cardiac events. Patients may also experience relative hypovolemia (neurogenic shock) from the vasodilatory (blood vessel dilation) effects of drugs such as nitroglycerin.

Neurogenic Shock

Neurogenic shock may be described as inadequate peripheral resistance due to widespread vasodilation. With this inappropriate vasodilation, a disproportionate amount of blood collects in the capillary bed. This reduces venous return, cardiac output, and arterial blood pressure. Neurogenic shock is most commonly due to an injury that results in severe spinal cord injury or total transection of the cord. Other causes of neurogenic shock include: central nervous system injury, septicemia from bacterial infection, anaphylactic reaction, insulin overdose, and Addisonian crisis (a disorder of the adrenal glands). With neurogenic shock there is an absence of the "sympathetic response."

EVALUATION OF THE SHOCK VICTIM

Shock will present itself in a variety of ways. Depending on the degree of compensation, some patients will display few signs and symptoms, while in others indications of shock will be much more obvious. Your initial approach can often yield a great deal of information. Before reaching the patient's side, you can often observe mental status, respiratory effort, and skin color. In situations where the patient is obviously in shock, you must be aggressive with your assessment and treatment.

Primary Assessment

✳ Your first action when caring for any shock patient should be the primary assessment.

As with any patient care situation, assessment should begin with the "ABCs." (See Figure 12-11.)

Airway   First, check the airway. The conscious patient who is able to speak usually has a patent (open) airway, whereas the unconscious patient is often subject to airway obstruction. In unconscious states, the tongue tends to fall back against the posterior oropharynx. Also, in trauma-related shock, bleeding in the oropharynx is often present, which can further compromise the airway.

Breathing   Once an open airway has been ensured, the adequacy of air exchange should be checked. While compensatory hyperventilation tends to occur in early shock, the unconscious shock patient will often hypoventilate. Hypoventilation occurs when the respiratory center of the brain becomes depressed due to hypoperfusion.

When evaluating the ventilatory status, be sure to check both the rate and depth of respirations. Watch for patients who exhibit rapid, shallow breathing. This type of breathing is just as ineffective as slow or irregular respirations. Rapid, shallow breathing results in severely reduced minute volumes, since an inadequate amount of air is being exchanged.

Circulation   After you have assured patency of the airway and ventilatory effectiveness, turn your attention to evaluating circulation. First, evaluate the pulse for rate and character. (See Figure 12-12.) Then examine the patient for obvious external bleeding. Because of compensatory mechanisms, a normal pulse rate may be seen even in the presence of a 10 to 15 percent volume deficit. A fast, weak, or thready pulse suggests decreased circulatory volume.

The location of the palpable pulse can also be an important indicator of circulatory status. The presence of a radial pulse indicates that the patient has a systolic blood pressure of at least 80 mm Hg. If the radial pulse cannot be palpated, the femoral pulse or carotid pulse should be checked next. A palpable femoral pulse indicates a systolic blood pressure of 70 mm Hg, while a palpable carotid pulse indicates a systolic blood pressure of 60 mm Hg. Although these are rough estimates, they can be quite helpful.

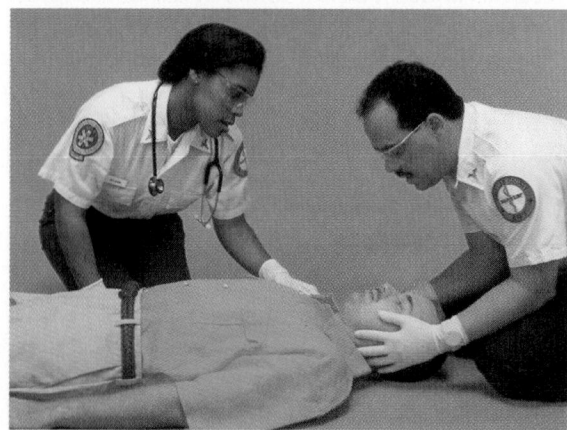

FIGURE 12-11   As with any emergency patient, assess the ABCs first.

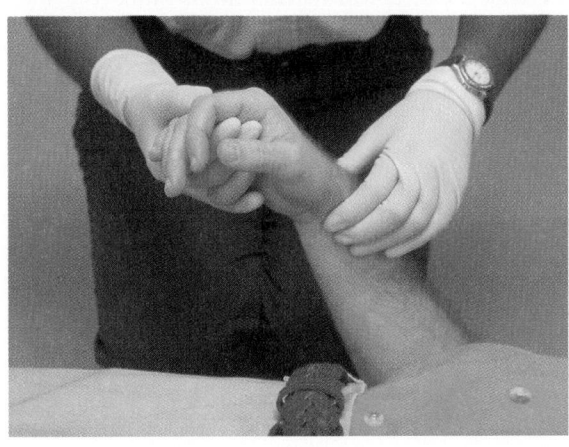

FIGURE 12-12 Evaluate the pulse for rate and character.

In the case of profound shock where severe vasoconstriction is present, you might not be able to palpate a pulse at all. Based on your findings of reduced perfusion, it would be appropriate to take immediate measures to restore circulation. In cases of obvious hypotension, as determined by using the above "rule" for checking the location of a palpable pulse, you don't need to take the time to auscultate a blood pressure before initiating immediate shock treatment.

The color, appearance, and temperature of the skin can also serve as a useful indicator of circulatory effectiveness. (See Figure 12-13.) As discussed earlier, the skin may appear normal in the initial stages of shock. However, compensatory mechanisms soon change the skin's appearance. As vasoconstriction is activated and the blood is routed to the central circulation, the skin becomes pale (decreased perfusion), cyanotic (stagnant pooling of blood with inadequate oxygenation), mottled (combination of both; a late sign of shock), as well as cool to the touch and diaphoretic. Often, the appearance of the skin will indicate shock even before there are any noticeable changes in the blood pressure.

Another method of assessing the circulation is to check the capillary refill. Capillary refill testing is performed by applying pressure to the nail bed of one of the patient's fingers. This pressure should cause a blanching of the nail bed. When the pressure is released, the nail should return to its normal pink color within two seconds. You can approximate this time period by saying "capillary refill." If the normal pink color does not return to the nail bed, it

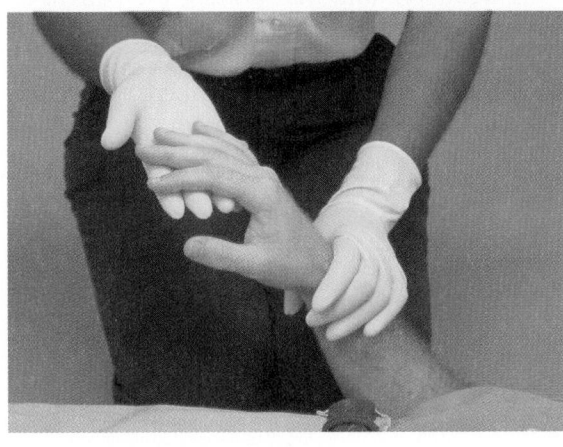

FIGURE 12-13 Examine the skin for color, temperature, and condition.

can be assumed that there is decreased perfusion to this area. Since the nail bed is the most distal part of the circulation, poor capillary refill is an early indicator of decreased perfusion to the whole body. However, use of the capillary refill test has limited value in the field setting due to poor lighting conditions and other environmental factors.

Disability   The level of consciousness should also be assessed throughout the primary survey. In fact, the level of consciousness is probably a better indicator of decreased tissue perfusion than most other signs. Because of the high energy requirements of the brain, any reduction in cerebral blood flow will be manifested by the following conditions.

❏ Agitation
❏ Disorientation
❏ Confusion
❏ An inability to respond to questions or commands appropriately
❏ Unresponsiveness

Any significant alteration in the level of consciousness must be viewed as an indication of critical hypoperfusion or hypoxia. Additionally, with an increased secretion of catecholamines, the patient often becomes anxious or apprehensive.

In evaluating trauma-related shock, remember that mind-altering substances may be involved. When alcohol and/or drugs interfere with the patient's normal thought processes, it is extremely difficult to gain an accurate view of the mental status. Your job as a health care provider can also be taxed by the fact that the intoxicated or "high" patient often behaves in a less than social manner. Keep in mind, however, that ingestion of alcohol or drugs does not rule out the possibility of a serious underlying problem. Whenever you suspect a serious trauma or medical emergency, it is probably best to assume that any altered mental status is due to decreased cerebral perfusion.

✳ Whenever you suspect a serious trauma or a medical emergency, it is probably best to assume that any altered mental status is due to decreased cerebral perfusion.

Secondary Assessment

After completion of the primary survey and initiation of the necessary treatment, a secondary survey should be performed. The thoroughness of the secondary survey is dependent upon the severity of the patient's condition. Obvious life-threatening problems that cannot be corrected in the prehospital setting warrant rapid transportation of the patient to an appropriate definitive care facility. Ideally, when assessing the seriously injured patient, you should expose and inspect the head, neck, chest, and abdomen. Throughout the secondary survey, and while providing treatment and transporting the patient to the hospital, you must continually reassess the temperature and moisture of the skin, blood pressure, pulse rate, and respiratory rate.

In shock—due to the presence of hypoxia, acidosis, and increased secretion of catecholamines—cardiac dysrhythmias must be considered a potential complication. Because of this, you should include the continual monitoring of the patient's ECG rhythm in your assessment. Look for rapid or slow heart rates as well as irregular rhythms. These conditions indicate potential life-threatening problems. Additional information can be obtained by asking your patient the appropriate questions. Find out how he or she feels. Is the patient thirsty, weak, nauseous, or dizzy? Does he or she have a history of significant medical conditions or take any medications? Such questions will give you additional information upon which to base your treatment.

Evaluation of the trauma victim for shock begins in the primary survey, where the most obvious signs of decreased tissue perfusion may be present. It is continued during the secondary survey, where more subtle clues may be found. The patient is then continually assessed for signs of developing shock until he or she is placed in the hands of emergency department personnel.

GENERAL MANAGEMENT OF SHOCK

Providing aggressive care to the shock patient begins during the resuscitation phase of the primary survey and continues until appropriate tissue perfusion and cellular oxygenation has been restored. The primary aspects of patient management include maintaining a patent airway, ensuring an adequate ventilatory rate and volume, providing supplemental oxygen, supporting circulation, and stabilizing suspected fractures or injuries.

In the classroom, you learn that patient care should always progress in a systematic fashion—first, maintain an open airway; second, ensure adequate breathing; and third, deal with circulation. In the reality of the field setting, however, you may need to provide all primary treatments at essentially the same time. To accomplish this, you and your partner (or members of your crew) must work as a team. Ideally, while some team members are stabilizing the cervical spine, maintaining a patient airway, assuring adequate ventilations, and providing supplemental oxygen, the other team members will control any significant bleeding, position the patient appropriately, apply the PASG, and establish one or more intravenous lines. As part of applying the anti-shock trousers, the patient may need to be log-rolled onto a full backboard. This way, many tasks are being performed at relatively the same time.

Maintaining a Patent Airway

As indicated earlier, the presentation of the patient in shock can range from alert to unresponsive and apneic. Usually, the appearance of the patient falls somewhere in between. If the patient is unable to maintain his or her own airway, adjuncts should be utilized to prevent the tongue from falling back against the posterior oropharynx and obstructing the airway. Additionally, fluids and other foreign objects should be removed to prevent aspiration into the trachea.

Whenever the potential exists for the patient to have sustained head or spinal injury, you must employ the appropriate cervical spine support during

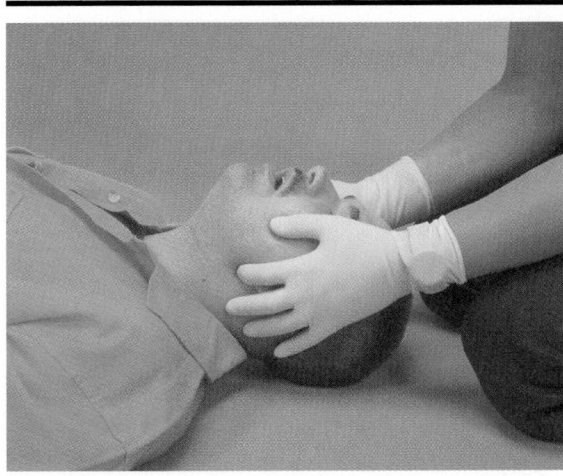

FIGURE 12-14 The airway in the shock patient should be assessed and maintained. If cervical spine injury is suspected, use the jaw-thrust maneuver.

all aspects of airway management and ventilatory support. (See Figure 12-14.) Options that can be used to prevent obstruction of airflow through the upper airway include placement of an oropharyngeal airway, nasopharyngeal airway, or endotracheal tube (ET). When dealing with the shock patient who is unresponsive, particularly in the presence of bleeding into the pharynx (as commonly occurs secondary to trauma-related shock), endotracheal intubation is the preferred airway technique. This is because the trachea can be effectively sealed off to prevent aspiration. Also, endotracheal intubation is better tolerated than adjuncts such as an EOA in cases in which the patient starts to awaken after application of the PASG or ventilation and oxygenation efforts improve cerebral blood flow and oxygenation.

Blood or fluids should be cleared with appropriate suctioning techniques, taking care not to stimulate the gag reflex or create inadvertent hypoxia. Larger foreign objects, such as teeth, should be removed utilizing the finger sweep technique. In the presence of ongoing fluid accumulation in the pharynx, it may be necessary to place the patient onto his or her side. This is an effective alternative, as fluids will seek the lowest point and drain out. Yet it is cumbersome to maintain cervical spine support and assist ventilations while the patient is in this position. Suction can help.

Maintaining Adequate Respiratory Function

Remember that an effective ventilatory volume is dependent upon two variables—adequate rate and sufficient depth of respirations. In shock, both of these may be less than normal. To complicate matters more, the patient may appear to be breathing at a sufficient rate or even display tachypnea. But, in reality, the patient may be exchanging very little air with each breath. The unconscious patient should be closely monitored to be sure that he or she is maintaining adequate respiratory minute volumes. (See Figure 12-15.)

If there is any indication of hypoventilation, you must assist the patient's breathing with a bag-valve-mask device or other ventilatory assistance adjunct. Keep in mind that inflation of the PASG can decrease thoracic capacity by forcing the abdominal organs up against the diaphragm, thus creating a situation in which the patient is moving an inadequate amount of air. Again, any indication of hypoventilation should prompt you to consider employing ventilatory assistance. Other shock-related conditions that can produce respiratory compromise must be dealt with quickly. Interventions include administration of diuretics, bronchodilators, and emergency chest decompression.

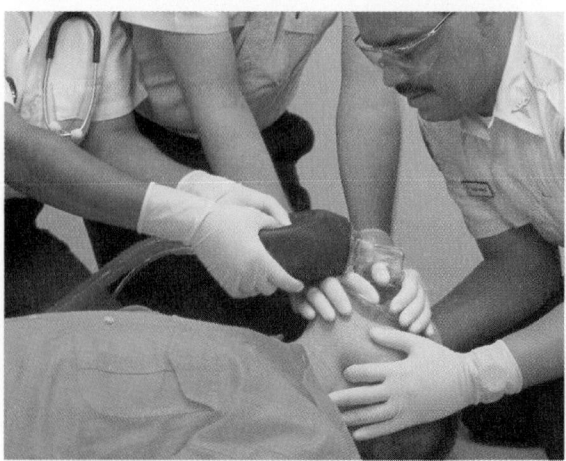

FIGURE 12-15 If necessary, assist or provide respirations and oxygenation.

Oxygenation of the Patient

Once the airway has been secured, the patient should receive as high a concentration of supplemental oxygen as possible. If the patient is breathing sufficiently, a nonrebreather mask with a liter flow of 10–15 liters per minute should be applied. Pay attention to the amount of oxygen that remains in the reservoir of the device at the end of each inspiration. Patients experiencing compensatory hyperventilation can deplete the reservoir, in which case a simple face mask should be employed to prevent suffocation. If the patient becomes nauseous or is frightened by the mask, a nasal cannula with a liter flow of 6–8 liters per minute can be employed. When there is a need to assist ventilations, as occurs in the presence of hypoventilation or when an endotracheal tube has been placed, 100 percent oxygen should be delivered via a bag-valve device, manually triggered demand-valve device, or automatic ventilator device. (See Figure 12-16.)

Control of Major Bleeding

Once breathing is assured, control any major bleeding. (See Figure 12-17.) Usually, direct pressure to sites of rapid external bleeding will be sufficient to contain blood loss. In most cases, peripheral hemorrhage can be controlled by direct pressure. If unsuccessful, other measures must be employed, including pressure points or, rarely, application of a tourniquet. Application of the pneumatic anti-shock garment may be useful in controlling intra-abdominal (aorta, liver, spleen, retroperitoneal, pelvic) and lower extremity hemorrhage.

Managing Hypotension

Hypotension can be managed in a variety of ways, including elevation of the patient's legs, applying and inflating the PASG, establishing intravenous lifelines, and administering vasopressor (vasoconstrictor) agents.

Positioning of the Patient   In shock, the preferred position for the patient is generally supine, with the legs elevated 10–12 inches. This position promotes increased venous return to the heart and increased cerebral perfusion. In some situations, elevation of the legs alone will be sufficient to raise the blood pressure. However, this position directly opposes the position best suited for easing respirations. In cases where the patient is experiencing respi-

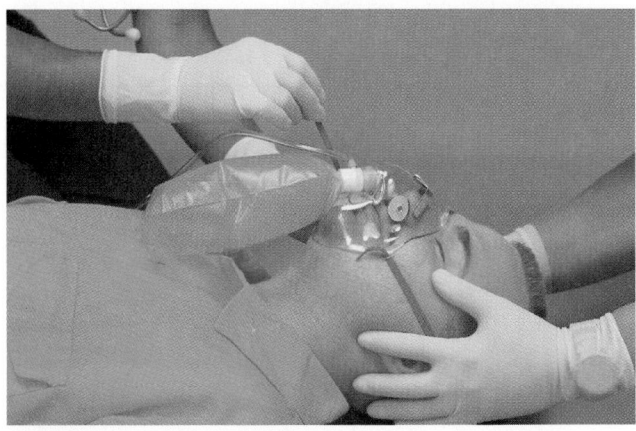

FIGURE 12-16   Provide high-flow oxygen.

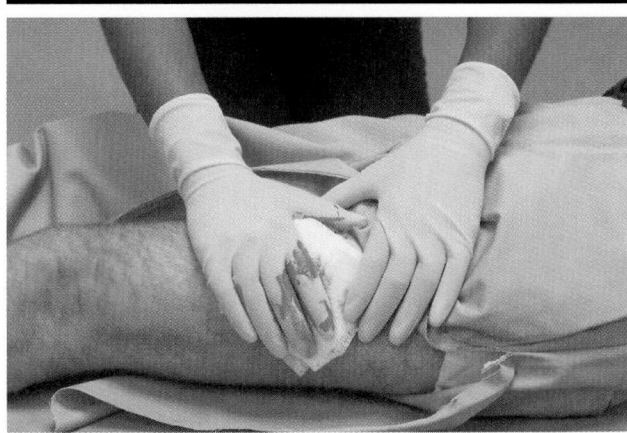

FIGURE 12-17   Control any obvious bleeding.

ratory compromise (e.g., acute pulmonary edema secondary to cardiogenic shock), an upright, sitting position is preferred. In addition, elevating the legs in patients with concomitant head injury can increase intracranial pressure and worsen an already bad situation. (See Figure 12-18.)

When attempting to determine the appropriate position for the patient experiencing shock accompanied by respiratory compromise, you must weigh the benefits of easier breathing against the disadvantages of reduced cerebral perfusion. If the respiratory compromised patient is placed in a supine position, you must take the necessary precautions to assure appropriate air exchange. It may be necessary to use a bag-valve-mask device or demand valve to assist the patient's breathing.

Pneumatic Anti-Shock Garment In special cases, the *pneumatic anti-shock garment (PASG)* may be applied and inflated. The pneumatic anti-shock garment is a three-chambered unit that is wrapped around both lower extremities and the abdomen. When inflated by use of an external pump, it applies circumferential pneumatic counter pressure to the structures beneath it. While quite a bit of controversy surrounds use of the pneumatic anti-shock garment, there does seem to be benefit to its application in the field setting. The positive effects obtained include:

❏ An increase in the blood pressure
❏ Increased blood flow to the heart, brain, and lungs
❏ Control of bleeding
❏ Stabilization of fractures of the lower limbs and pelvis

The PASG increases peripheral resistance. When circumferential pneumatic counter pressure is applied to the lower half of the body, blood vessels under the suit are compressed. This results in an elevated blood pressure and increased blood flow to the central portion of the body (heart, brain, and lungs). The PASG produces very little autotransfusion, as originally thought. Studies suggest that only a minimal amount of blood is autotransfused—as little as 300 mL in a 150-pound patient.

The garment can produce impressive changes in the patient's condition. Because of the improved cerebral blood flow, it is not uncommon for the patient's mental status to improve. Usually, this is not a problem. However,

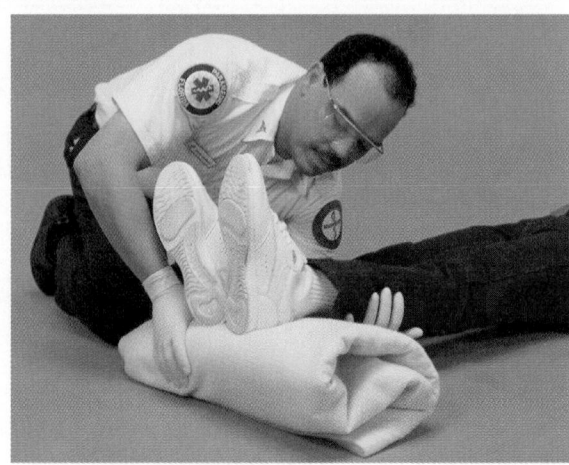

FIGURE 12-18 Elevate the feet if a head injury is not suspected.

when the patient is intubated, when there are mind-altering substances involved, or when psychiatric problems exist, it may be necessary to use restraints to prevent injury to the patient or yourself.

PASG Indications.   Indications for application of the PASG include:

❑ *Control of Bleeding.* The pneumatic anti-shock garment acts to control bleeding by applying direct pressure to the injury site. This pneumatic counter pressure creates circumferential tension, which improves hemostasis and decreases blood flow to torn vessels beneath the garment. It is also believed to exert a tamponade effect on bleeding within the abdomen.

❑ *Stabilization of Fractures.* By enclosing both the lower extremities and pelvis and by producing effects similar to a large air splint, the garment prevents movement. Application of the pneumatic anti-shock garment is indicated in cases where the hypotensive patient has sustained fractures to the lower extremities. Use of the device allows you to treat both problems at essentially the same time, thus permitting rapid packaging and transportation of the patient. Because inflation of the device can raise the patient's blood pressure, it should only be used for fracture stabilization in cases where the patient is hypotensive. Other splinting devices (traction, vacuum, and/or board splints) should be used to immobilize fractures when the patient is normotensive or hypertensive.

❑ *Blood Pressure.* Since use of the pneumatic anti-shock garment may make cannula placement easier, application of the garment should precede the placement of these lines in the severely hypotensive patient.

Contraindications and Complications.   Use of the pneumatic anti-shock garment is contraindicated in the presence of pulmonary edema occurring secondary to heart failure. This is because adding fluid volume to the central circulation may further compromise an already failing heart. Relative contraindications for inflation of the abdominal section include pregnancy beyond the second trimester, evisceration, and an impaled object in the abdomen. However, these precautions should not deter use of this device in the treatment of the severely hypotensive patient.

Potential complications associated with use of the pneumatic anti-shock garment include lower extremity compartment syndromes, metabolic acidosis after prolonged use (due to decreased lower extremity tissue perfusion), decreased renal function, and decreased respiratory vital capacity (due to compression of the abdominal organs against the diaphragm). Because of the potential for decreased diaphragmatic excursion—with resultant decreased vital capacity—caution should be exercised when using the device in the presence of any dyspnea.

Application of the PASG.   Techniques for applying the pneumatic anti-shock garment are shown in Procedure 12-1. While some people teach that the patient's clothing should be removed prior to application of the PASG, evidence has shown little real benefit to this practice. Additionally, in the field setting, many factors make this practice virtually impossible. These factors include: environmental conditions such as weather, temperature, the presence of onlookers; severity of the patient's injuries; and the patient's unwillingness to be disrobed.

You should frequently check inflation pressure on the PASG. Environmental conditions such as broken glass, splintered wood, or gasoline spills increase the chances for damage to the garment and pressure loss. The urgent conditions under which the garment is applied further increase the possibility of leaks. Additionally, changes in temperature or altitude may cause significant fluctuation in pressure within the device. This is especially true when the patient is taken from a cold environment to a warm one or when the patient is transported by air.

Once inflated, the pneumatic anti-shock garment should not be deflated without specific direction from a physician. The reason for this is that the device, by increasing the preload and/or the systemic vascular resistance, only acts to provide a temporary, interim elevation of the blood pressure. Deflation of the garment prior to restoration of adequate circulating blood volume can have life-threatening consequences as the cardiac output and blood pressure often drop precipitously.

Restoration of adequate circulating blood volume is unlikely in the field setting. Once the patient has received stabilizing care at a definitive care facility, you may be instructed to remove the pneumatic anti-shock garment. The release of air from the compartments should take place over several minutes, beginning with the abdominal section and then moving to each leg. At no time should the entire garment be deflated at once. Throughout the deflation of each compartment, the patient's blood pressure and appearance should be constantly monitored. In cases where the patient becomes hypotensive and/or symptomatic, it may be necessary to reinflate the garment.

Intravenous Fluid Therapy

Intravenous cannulation is a procedure used to directly access the venous circulation. The primary reasons for intravenous cannulation in the field setting include:

- ❑ Administration of drugs
- ❑ Replacement of fluid
- ❑ Obtaining specimens of venous blood for laboratory determinations

While many drugs can be administered subcutaneously or intramuscularly, absorption of the drug into the circulatory system is severely hampered during states of decreased cardiac output—e.g., shock. Intravenous administration of drugs usually ensures that they will reach the circulation.

Necessary Supplies. Typical supplies needed for intravenous cannulation include: protective latex gloves, eyewear, intravenous solution, administration tubing, extension set, cannulas (assorted sizes), venous constricting band, antibiotic swabs, antibiotic ointment, tape; gauze dressings (2×2's, 4×4's), 35 mL syringe, and a padded arm board. (See Figure 12-19.) Keep in mind the following considerations when selecting supplies.

- ❑ *Intravenous Solutions.* Intravenous solutions, as discussed earlier in the chapter, are divided into two groups: colloids and crystalloids. Colloid solutions contain molecules that are too large to pass easily through the capillary membranes. Thus, these solutions tend to remain in the vascular space for a considerable period of time.

  On the other hand, crystalloid solutions contain electrolytes and water, but they lack proteins and larger molecules. Therefore, without larger molecules to keep the fluid in the vascular space, crystalloid solutions easily move across the capillary walls into the tissues. Because crystalloid solutions often have a transitory effect, there is a need to administer crystalloids at two or three times the amount of blood lost when treating patients who have experienced hemorrhagic shock.

  Although colloids are particularly useful in maintaining the vascular volume, their use is prohibitive in the field setting due to the cost and special requirements for storage. However, you may be asked to assist with their administration in the emergency department or during a lengthy entrapment or disaster scene, where medical personnel are

✱ The PASG should not be removed in the field setting.

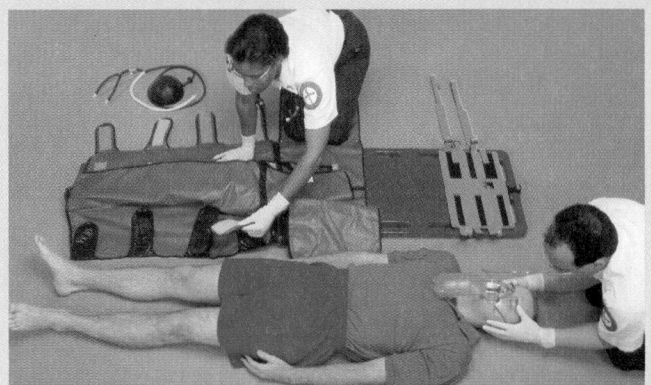

12-1A. Prepare the PASG.

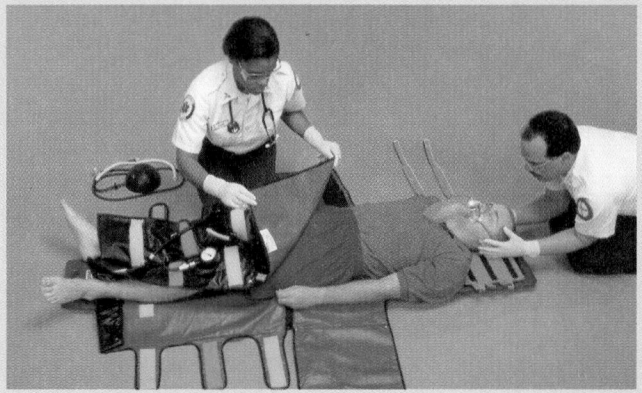

12-1B. Position the patient.

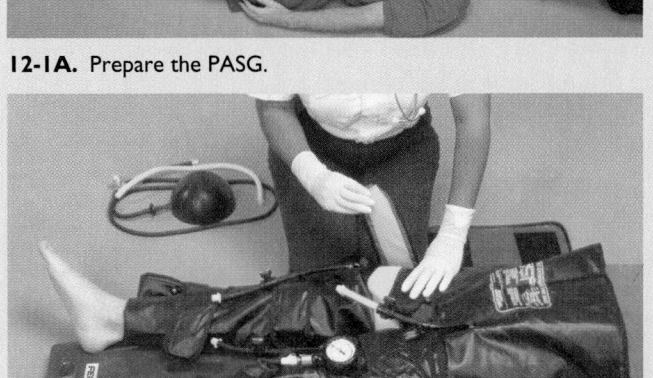

12-1C. Wrap the legs, following the manufacturer's recommendations.

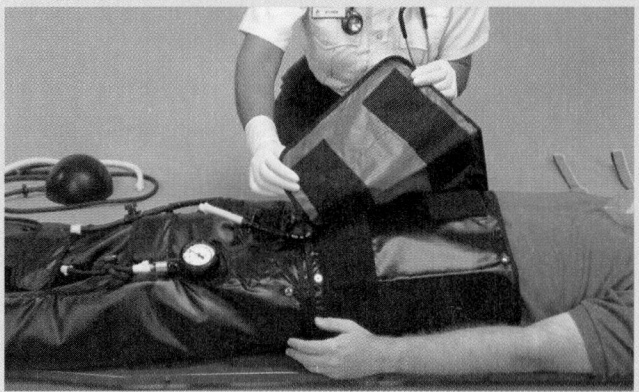

12-1D. Wrap the abdomen last.

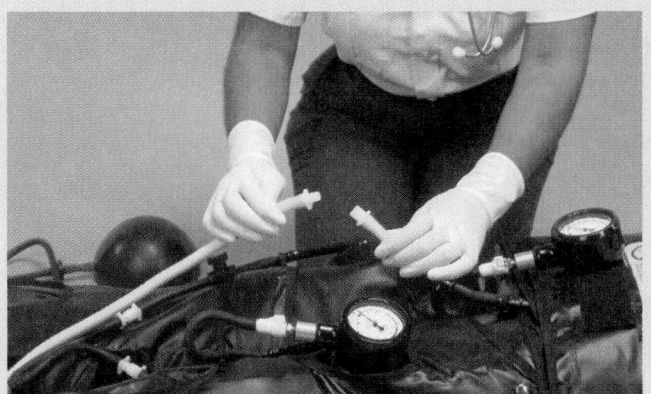

12-1E. Connect the tubing.

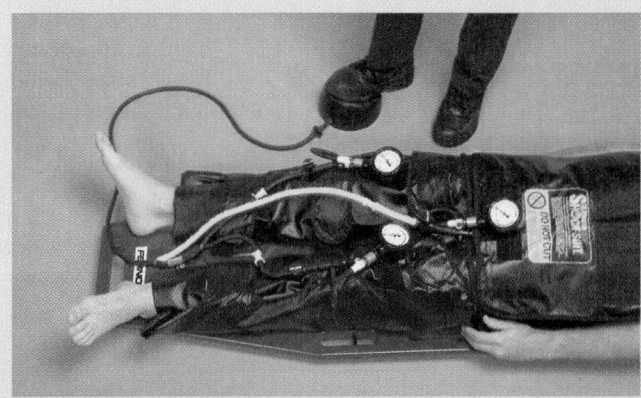

12-1F. Inflate the PASG, both legs first.

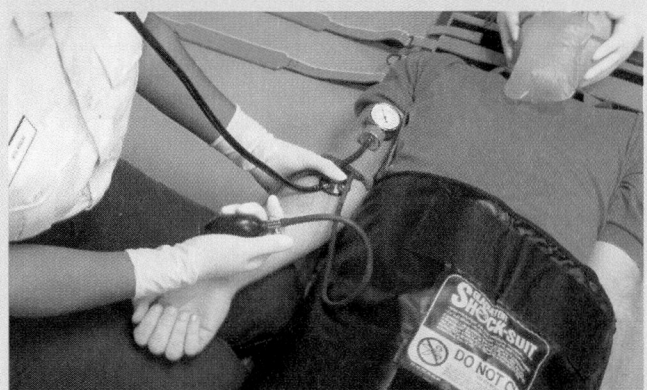

12-1G. Monitor the patient.

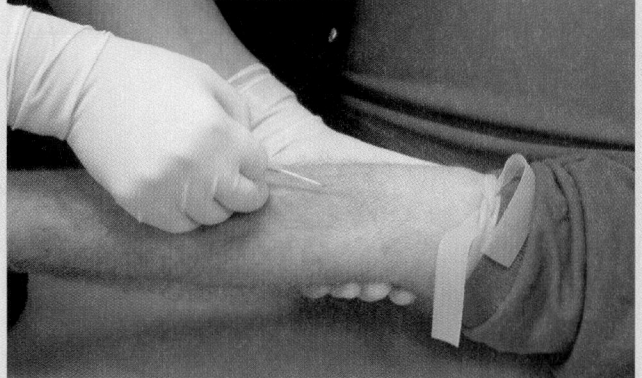

12-1H. Establish an IV.

brought in to assist. You should therefore be familiar with the more common types.

❑ *Administration Set.* Intravenous solutions are almost always administered through clear plastic tubing. This allows for easy detection of air bubbles or precipitation of certain medications administered through the tubing. There are two primary types of intravenous administration sets: the *microdrip* and the *macrodrip* (standard). (See Figure 12-20.) The microdrip is typically used in situations where it is necessary to restrict the amount of fluids administered—e.g., cardiac, medical, and pediatric emergencies. When administering solutions through the microdrip administration set, 60 drops are equal to 1 milliliter. The macrodrip is used in situations where large amounts of fluid are to be administered—e.g., shock, fluid replacement, etc. With the macrodrip administration set, 10 drops are equal to 1 milliliter. However, it is important to note that, depending on the manufacturer, the drop size may vary. Be sure to read the box in which the administration set comes.

❑ *Cannulas.* There are three types of cannulas:

1. Hollow needles, e.g., butterfly, or winged, needles
2. Plastic catheters inserted over a hollow needle, e.g., Angiocath
3. Plastic catheters inserted through a hollow needle, e.g., Intracath

In the field setting, the over-the-needle catheter is generally preferred, since it can be anchored better and permits freer movement of the patient. Additionally, the puncture in the vein is exactly the same size as the plastic catheter. Thus, there is less chance for bleeding around the venipuncture site.

The outside diameter of the needle is called a gauge. The larger the gauge number, the smaller the diameter of the shaft. For example, a 22-gauge cannula is small, whereas a 14-gauge cannula is large. A large diameter catheter (14-gauge) provides a much greater fluid flow than does a small diameter catheter (22-gauge). Cannulas used for prehospital care come in a variety of sizes:

• 22-gauge (used for fragile and/or small veins such as in pediatric patients)
• 20-gauge (used for average-sized adult patients)
• 18-gauge, 16-gauge, and 14-gauge (used for volume replacement or the administration of viscous medications such as glucose)

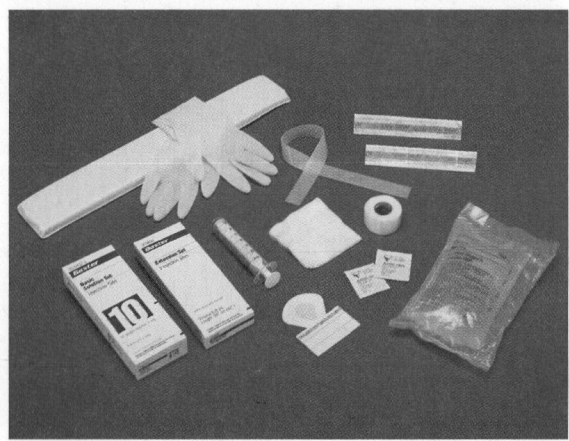

FIGURE 12-19 Supplies for initiating IV therapy.

The other variable that should be considered when selecting an intravenous cannula is its length. The longer the cannula, the less the flow rate will be. The flow rate through a 14-gauge, 5 cm catheter (approximately 125 mL/minute) is twice the flow rate as through a longer, 16-gauge, 20 cm catheter. For cannulation of a peripheral vein, a needle and catheter length of 5 cm is adequate, while the cannulation of a central line requires a needle length of 6–7 cm and catheter length of at least 15–20 cm.

Venous Access. As discussed earlier, use of peripheral veins is preferred for field use over central vein cannulation. The technique is relatively easy to master; it provides an effective route for administration of fluids and medications; and it does not interfere with other life-sustaining measures, such as cardiopulmonary resuscitation and airway management. Cannulation of central veins often takes longer, requires the use of sterile procedures (gloves, drapes, prep, solution), has a higher complication rate (pneumothorax, arterial injury, abnormal placement), and usually necessitates that a chest X-ray be taken immediately after placement to ensure correct positioning. However, central veins are useful in situations where peripheral veins have collapsed.

For peripheral cannulation, the veins of the dorsal aspect of the hand, forearm, and antecubital fossa are the most convenient. The veins on the back of the hand offer the advantage of permitting the patient to freely move his or her arm. Additionally, if a problem develops with these more distal veins, another site higher up on the arm can be selected. The disadvantage of the

✳ The shorter the length of an IV catheter, and the greater the diameter, the greater will be the volume that can be delivered through it.

✳ Central line placement is not normally indicated in prehospital care.

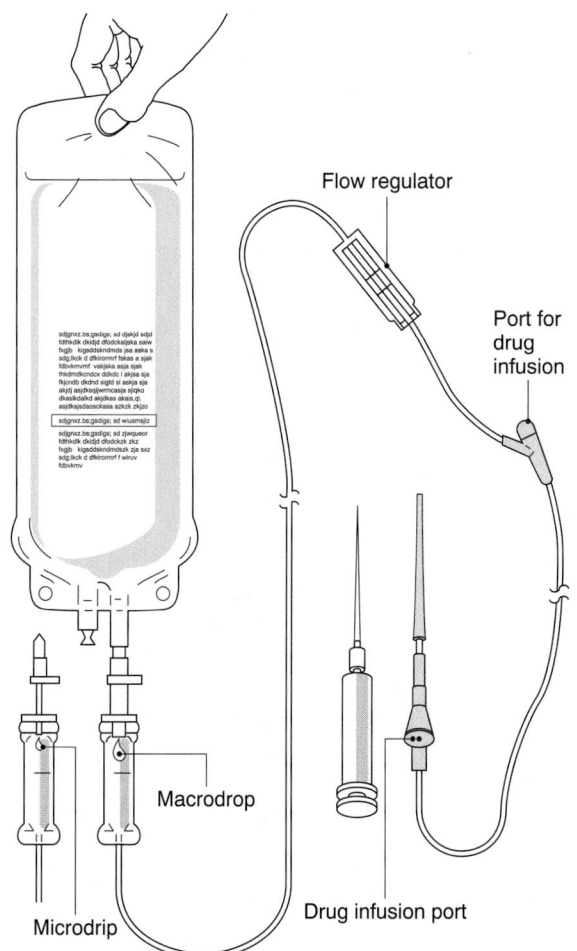

Flow regulator

Port for drug infusion

Macrodrop

Microdrip

Drug infusion port

FIGURE 12-20 Comparison of macrodrip and microdrip IV administration sets.

more distal veins is that they are sometimes fragile and difficult to cannulate. In addition, in states of decreased cardiac output, medications administered through these vessels take longer to reach the central circulation.

The veins of the forearm and antecubital fossa offer the advantage of being larger and easier to cannulate. Additionally, because they are closer, medications will reach the central circulation quicker. In cardiac arrest and other states of decreased perfusion, the forearm or the antecubital fossa is the preferred site for cannulation. In selected cases of hypovolemia, application of the pneumatic anti-shock garment can precede venous cannulation, as the garment can potentially make it easier to find and cannulate the vein.

An alternative to central line placement is the external jugular vein. This vein is easily accessed and relatively free of complication. The external jugular vein is generally considered a peripheral vein. (See Figure 12-21.)

In children, several veins are available. In addition to the veins of the arm and leg, the external jugular vein is available as well as several scalp veins.

While repeated practice makes starting IVs easier, there are some patients in whom cannulating a vein is particularly difficult. These include obese patients, patients experiencing shock and cardiac arrest, chronic "main line" IV drug users, elderly patients with "fragile" or "rolling" veins, and small children. The following guidelines will help you to insert IVs correctly. (Also, see Procedure 12-2.)

* Always use appropriate personal protective equipment when attempting IV cannulation.

Intravenous Cannulation.   Ready equipment and explain the procedure to the patient. Tear several pieces of tape, and set up the administration set and IV solution. Arrange the equipment so that it is easily accessible.

1. Locate a suitable venipuncture site. The back of the hand, forearm, antecubital fossa, leg, thigh, or neck are often considered.

2. Place the constricting band to halt venous return without obstructing arterial flow. Leave one end of the slip knot exposed to assure rapid release when the procedure is complete.

3. Locate a suitable vein. Palpate one that is well fixed (not rolling) and that does not have valves (firm nubs of tissue) proximal to the intended site of entry.

4. Cleanse the venipuncture site. Employ alcohol or betadine in an expanding circular pattern, using a firm pressure.

5. Insert the needle and catheter. With the bevel up, enter the skin at about a 30–45 degree angle until you feel the needle pop into the vein and see a flashback of blood. Then reduce the angle with the skin and ease the catheter about 1 centimeter farther.

6. While holding the needle hub, advance the catheter with a gentle twisting motion. Continue advancement until the catheter hub is about 1 centimeter from the venipuncture site.

7. Place one finger firmly on the vein just above the end of the catheter to occlude venous flow while you hold the catheter hub firmly in place and withdraw the needle.

8. Hold the catheter hub firmly, attach the IV administration set, and allow the fluid to run.

9. Apply a small amount of antibiotic solution to the site and secure the catheter with a small piece of tape.

10. Loop the first few inches of administration tubing, and tape it to prevent tugging on the venipuncture site.

In some cases, the IV will not flow as it should. Consider the following corrective questions and actions:

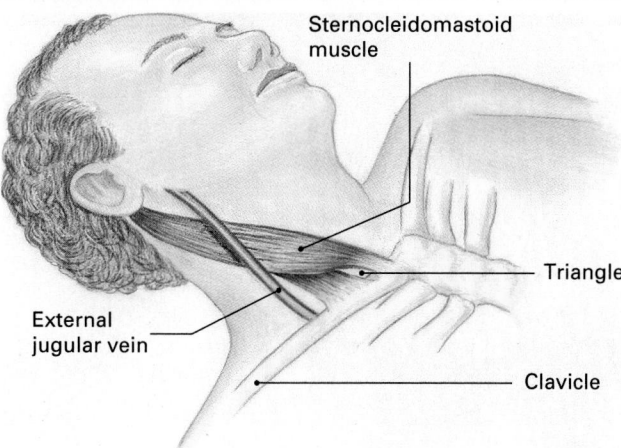

Sternocleidomastoid muscle

Triangle

External jugular vein

Clavicle

FIGURE 12-21 Anatomy of the external jugular vein.

1. Has the venous constricting band been removed? This is probably the most common mistake made in both the hospital and field settings. Additionally, check to make sure that the patient is not wearing restrictive clothing that may be interfering with venous flow.

2. Is there swelling at the cannulation site? This indicates infiltration into the tissues.

3. Are the tubing control valves open? Be sure to check both the primary control valve and any control valves that are part of the extension set.

4. Is the cannula up against a valve or wall of the vein? This can be checked by slightly repositioning the cannula. It may be necessary to untape the cannula and retape it after a good flow rate has been achieved by repositioning. It may be necessary to use a padded armboard to keep the patient's hand or arm in the appropriate position.

5. Is the IV bag high enough? Sometimes, when moving the patient, the cannulation site is raised higher than the bag. It subsequently interferes with gravity, which is required to move the fluid.

6. Is the drip chamber completely filled with solution? This can be easily corrected by simply inverting the bag and squeezing the drip chamber to return some of the fluid to the bag. If the flow is still slow or absent, lower the IV bag below the level of the insertion site. If blood return is seen in the IV tubing, the site is patent. If problems still persist, the IV should be removed and reestablished on another extremity.

Complications of Intravenous Therapy. Complications that can occur with intravenous therapy include:

❑ *Pain.* Pain at the puncture site may be due to penetration of the skin with the needle or **extravasation**. Pain can lead to increased anxiety, which can predispose the patient to cardiac dysrhythmias. Pain can be minimized by using a smaller gauge catheter, anesthetizing the overlying skin using one percent lidocaine (without epinephrine) prior to penetration, or by using the sharp tip of a smaller needle to make an incision in the skin through which a larger cannula can pass more easily.

❑ *Hematoma or Infiltration.* Hematoma or infiltration at the puncture site results either from injury to the blood vessel or from dislodging of the catheter from the vein. Fluid then accumulates in the interstitial space. In the presence of a hematoma or infiltration at the puncture site, the catheter should be removed and the IV reestablished at another site.

■ **extravasation** the leakage of fluid or medication outside a blood vessel.

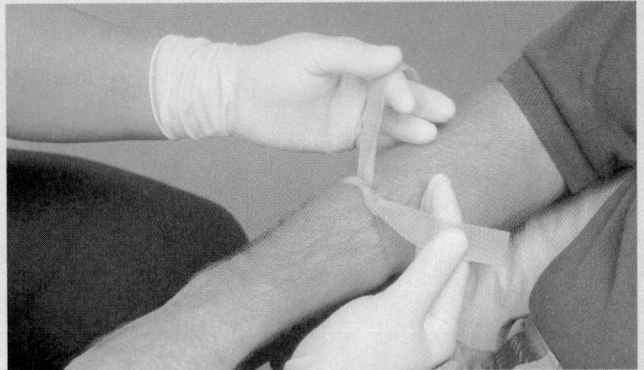

12-2A. Apply the tourniquet, and select a suitable vein.

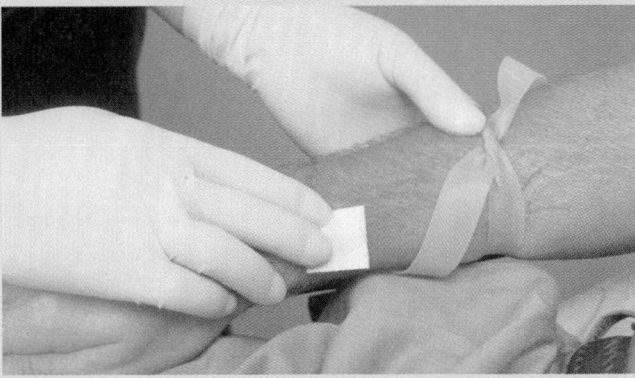

12-2B. Prep the site with an anti-bacterial solution.

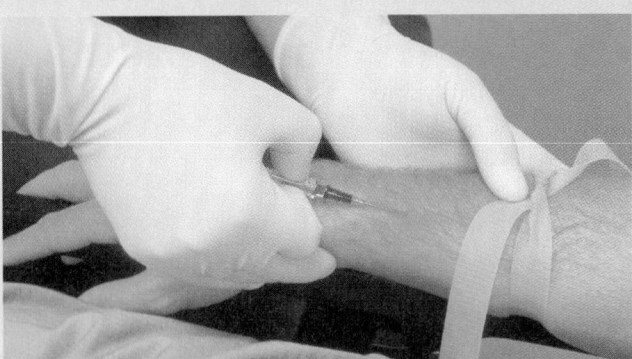

12-2C. Insert the needle into the vein.

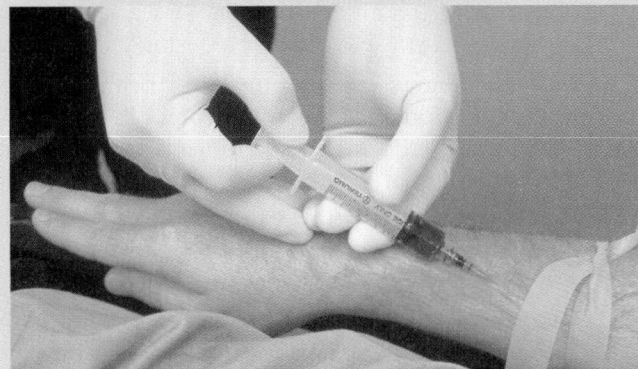

12-2D. Withdraw any blood samples needed.

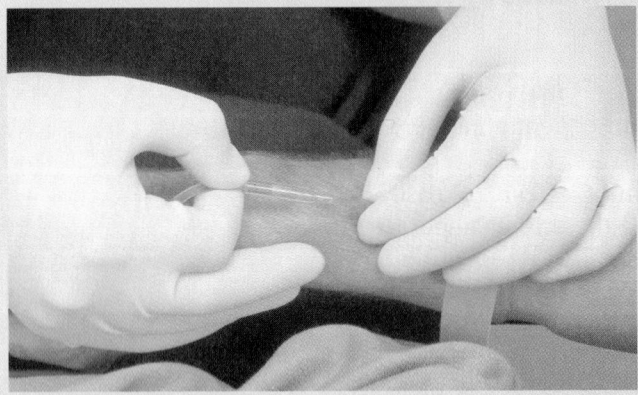

12-2E. Connect the IV tubing.

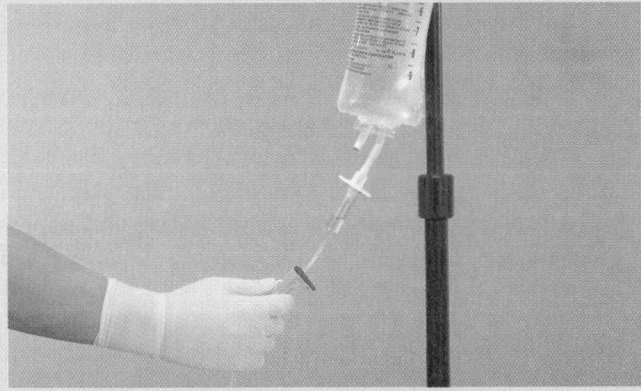

12-2F. Turn on the IV and check the flow.

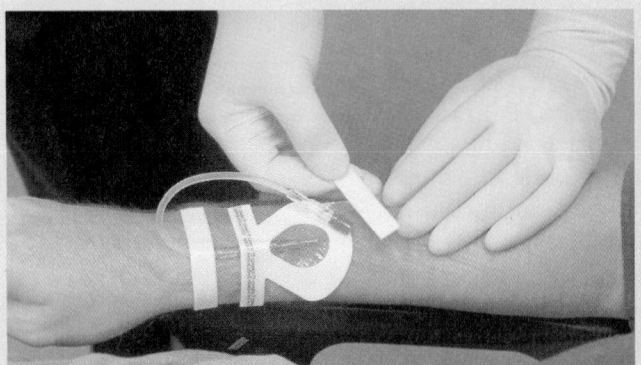

12-2G. Secure the site.

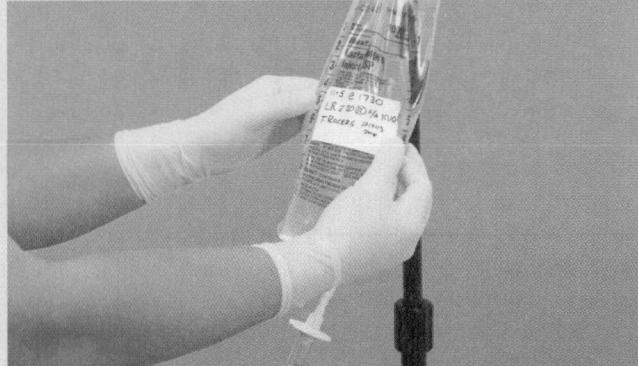

12-2H. Label the bag.

❏ *Local Infection*. Local infection occurs when appropriate cleansing techniques are not utilized and bacteria are introduced into the puncture site.

❏ *Pyrogenic Reaction*. A pyrogenic reaction occurs when **pyrogens** (foreign proteins capable of producing fever) are present in the administration set or intravenous solution. It is characterized by the abrupt onset of fever (100–106° F), chills, backache, headache, nausea, and vomiting. Cardiovascular collapse may also result. A reaction usually occurs within one-half to one hour following initiation of IV therapy. If a pyrogenic reaction is suspected, the IV should be immediately terminated and established in the other arm using a new administration set and solution. The potential for this complication to occur emphasizes the need to discard any IV bag that shows leakage or cloudiness.

❏ *Catheter Shear*. A catheter shear occurs when the catheter is pulled back through or over the needle after it has been advanced forward. Since the catheter is plastic, it easily snags on the sharp edge of the needle and is sheared off, becoming a plastic embolus. For this reason, the catheter should never be drawn back over or through the needle. Always withdraw the needle first, and then withdraw the catheter.

❏ *Inadvertent Arterial Puncture*. Because of its sometimes close proximity to veins, an artery may be inadvertently punctured. Arterial puncture is recognized by the appearance of spurting, bright red blood. When arterial puncture occurs, immediately withdraw the catheter, and apply direct pressure to the site for at least 5 minutes or until the bleeding has stopped.

❏ *Circulatory Overload*. Circulatory overload occurs when too much intravenous solution is administered for a given patient's condition. This emphasizes the need to monitor the IV flow rate closely, particularly in patients prone to heart failure. Constantly watch the patient for signs of developing congestive heart failure—rales, tachypnea, external jugular vein distention—in which case the IV flow rate should be significantly reduced or terminated.

❏ *Thrombophlebitis*. Inflammation of the vein is particularly common when intravenous therapy is long-term. Thrombophlebitis is manifested by redness and edema at the puncture site. It also presents as pain along the course of the vein, which is sometimes accompanied by inflammation and tenderness. Typically, thrombophlebitis does not occur immediately but is more common after several hours of intravenous therapy. When thrombophlebitis is suspected, terminate the IV and apply warm compresses to the site.

❏ *Air Embolism*. Air embolism occurs when air is allowed to enter the vein. It is more likely to occur during central vein cannulation or when air has not been cleared from the IV administration set appropriately.

Flow Rates. In the field setting, there are typically two rates for administering intravenous solutions. In medical emergencies, where intravenous lines are placed prophylactically or for the purpose of administering medications, the flow is usually maintained at a "to keep open" rate. In trauma or other situations where intravenous fluids are being used to replace circulatory volume, the flow rate should be based on the patient's response (improvements in pulse, blood pressure, capillary refill, and cerebral function). In the severely hypovolemic patient, the solution should be administered at a rapid flow rate. The maximum amount of intravenous fluids that should be administered to an adult in the field setting is about 2–3 liters. When treating the patient with severe blood loss, the flow rate can be increased three to four times normal by wrapping a blood pressure cuff around the IV bag and inflating it to 300 mm Hg or by using a commercial pressure infuser.

■ **pyrogen** any substance capable of causing fever.

✱ Do not remove the tourniquet if a catheter shear occurs. Splint the arm and start an IV in the opposite arm. Transport immediately.

■ **extravasation** the leakage of fluid or medication outside a blood vessel.

Maintaining Body Temperature

In the course of treating the patient for shock, the body temperature should be maintained as close to normal as possible. (See Figure 12-22.) Pay attention to factors that affect body temperature, including environmental/weather conditions, temperature of the oxygen and intravenous fluids, and the location where the patient is found, to name but a few. Persons lying on the ground, particularly during inclement weather, are prone to hypothermia. Body temperature can be maintained by protecting the patient from the elements and by removing any wet clothing. Cover the patient to avoid heat loss, but be careful not to overbundle. Too much heat produces vasodilation, which counteracts the body's compensatory mechanism of vasoconstriction and increases fluid loss by perspiration.

Use of Medications in the Treatment of Shock

Medications that may be used in the treatment of some forms of shock include alpha-and beta-stimulating catecholamines, vasodilators, corticosteroids, diuretics, anti-dysrhythmics, and naloxone. Suggested guidelines follow.

* Medications are never used in the treatment of hypovolemic shock unless fluid replacement has been carried out. Thus, they are very rarely used in the prehospital management of hypovolemic shock.

❑ *Hypovolemic Shock.* In the field setting, medications are rarely used in the treatment of hypovolemic shock. The primary efforts are directed toward replacing circulatory volume and improving cellular oxygenation.

❑ *Cardiogenic Shock.* When cardiogenic shock is caused by severe myocardial depression, sympathetic stimulating agents such as dopamine, dobutamine, and norepinephrine may be used to improve the pumping action of the heart and cardiac output. The exact doses of these medications are based on patient response and must be administered with great care. Typically, when dopamine is used, it should be titrated to maintain a systolic blood pressure of 80–100 mm Hg. Use the lowest dose consistent with the desired result. When cardiac dysrhythmias result in depressed cardiac output, antidysrhythmic agents such as lidocaine, bretylium, procainamide (ventricular origin), atropine (bradycardia), and verapamil and adenosine (supraventricular tachycardia) may be used to restore normal cardiac output.

❑ *Neurogenic Shock.* Vasopressors such as dopamine or norepinephrine may be used to treat some forms of inappropriate systemic vascular resistance seen with neurogenic, septic, or anaphylactic shock. Definitive therapy is directed toward correction of the underlying cause.

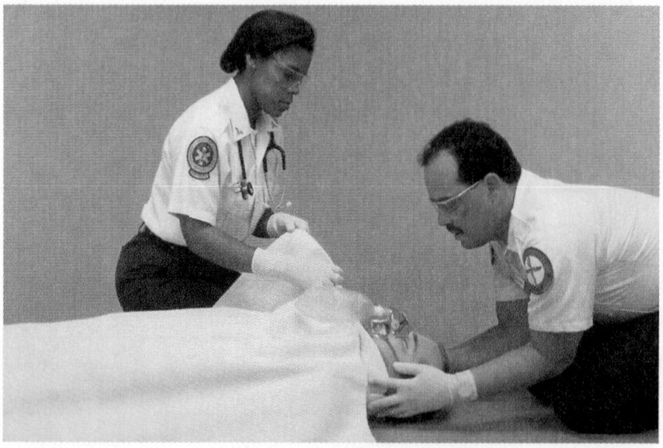

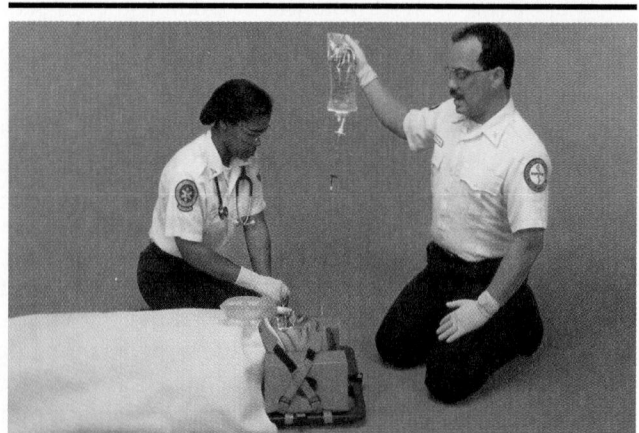

FIGURE 12-22 Always maintain the patient's body temperature.

FIGURE 12-23 The packaged patient.

RAPID PACKAGING AND TRANSPORT

Shock patients should be transported to the hospital as rapidly as possible, under constant monitoring. Packaging is a skill that should be repeatedly practiced. (See Figure 12-23.) The severely injured patient requires definitive, often surgical, in-hospital care. Field stabilization should be rapid, with many procedures initiated en route. The steps in field management of the severely injured patient include:

- ❑ *Stabilization.* Brief stabilization of the airway, breathing, and circulation should be completed. In addition, any major sources of hemorrhage should be controlled.
- ❑ *Extrication.* The patient should be removed as rapidly as possible, utilizing rapid-movement techniques and methods of stabilization.
- ❑ *PASG.* The PASG should be readily available. Even if the patient appears stable, the PASG should be in place. Should the patient deteriorate, it can be inflated en route.
- ❑ *Load for Transportation.* The patient should be placed in the ambulance and prepared for transport.
- ❑ *IV Therapy.* While the IV is being prepared, transport should be initiated. While en route, the venous constricting band should be applied, the vein identified, the tape prepared, the IV prepared, and the skin prepped. Then, the driver should pull to the side of the road for cannula placement. As soon as the cannula is in place, transport should resume. The cannula is subsequently stabilized and the flow rate adjusted.

SUMMARY

This chapter has presented fundamental physiology, pathophysiology, and management of fluid and electrolyte disorders, acid-base balance, and shock. Shock is the final, common denominator of a large variety of disease processes and represents a life-threatening decompensation of vital functions. It demands immediate recognition and treatment

FURTHER READING

American College of Surgeons, Committee on Trauma. *Advanced Trauma Life Support Course: Student Manual.* American College of Surgeons, 1989.

Bledsoe, Bryan E. *Atlas of Paramedic Skills.* Englewood Cliffs, NJ: Prentice Hall, 1987.

Bledsoe, Bryan E., Dwayne Clayden, and Frank J. Papa. *Prehospital Emergency Pharmacology,* 4th ed. Upper Saddle River, NJ: Prentice Hall, 1995.

Butman, Alexander et. al. *Comprehensive Guide to Pre-Hospital Skills.* Akron, Ohio: Emergency Training, 1995.

Campbell, John E. *Basic Trauma Life Support,* 3rd ed. Upper Saddle River, NJ: Prentice Hall, 1995.

Prehospital Trauma Life Support Committee of the National Association of Emergency Medical Technicians. *Prehospital Trauma Life Support: Basic and Advanced:* Saint Louis, MO: Mosby Year Book, 1994.

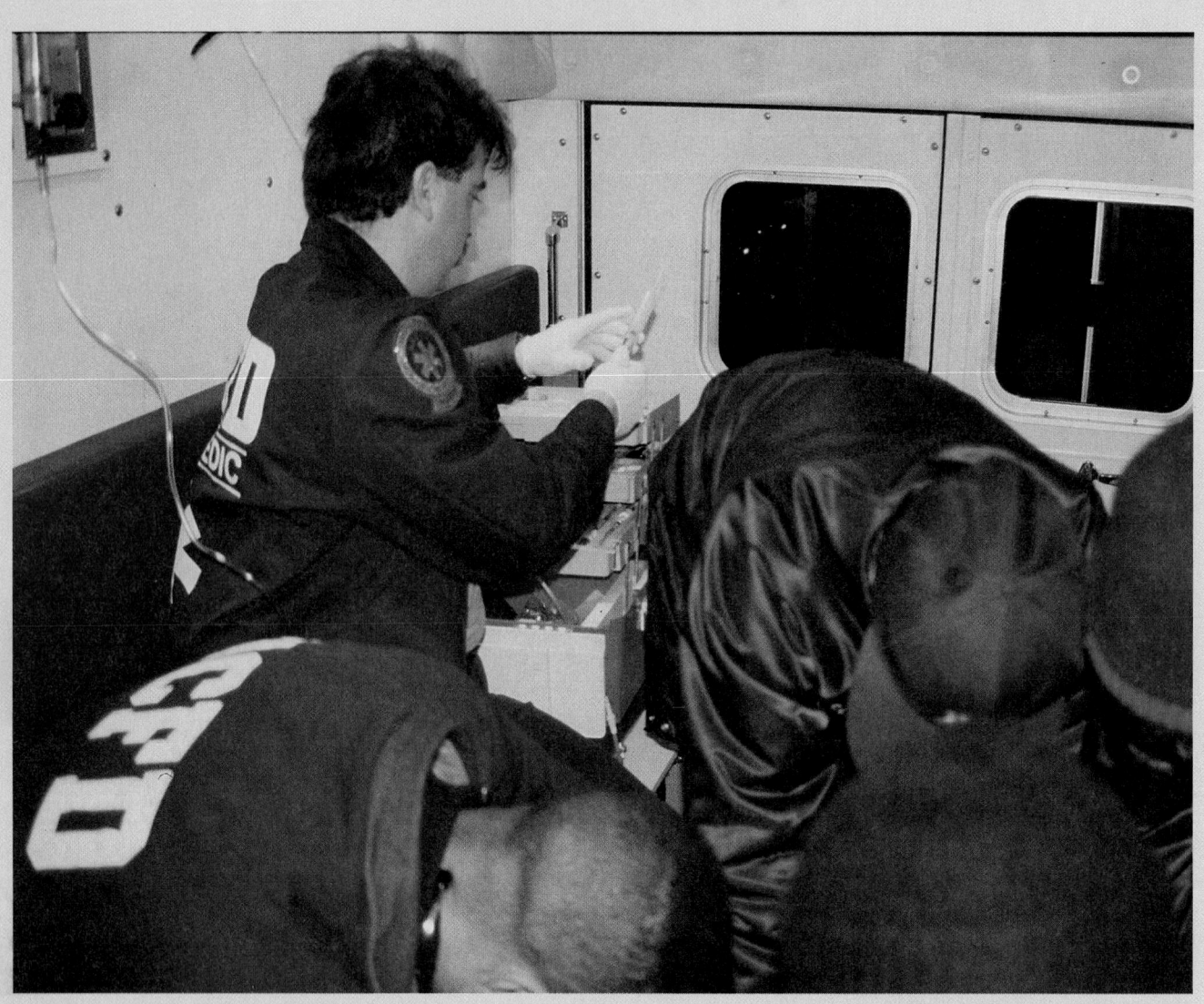

13

EMERGENCY PHARMACOLOGY

Objectives for Chapter 13

After reading this chapter, you should be able to:

1. Define the following terms. (See below pages.)
   - pharmacology (p. 332)
   - drug (p. 332)
   - pharmacokinetics (p. 337)
   - pharmacodynamics (p. 337)

2. List four drug sources, and give an example of a drug derived from each source. (See p. 332.)

3. Name three federal legislative acts that regulate drugs. (See p. 333.)

4. List the five addictive drug schedules, and give an example of a medication from each. (See pp. 333–334.)

5. List four names that can be used to identify a drug. (See p. 334.)

6. Describe three common references, and know how to find a medication in one of these references. (See p. 334.)

7. List several examples of both liquid and solid drugs. (See pp. 334–335.)

8. Define "parenteral drugs." (See p. 335.)

9. Define the following terms. (See below pages.)
   - ampule (p. 335)
   - vial (p. 335)
   - prefilled syringe (p. 335)

10. Define important pharmacological terminology. (See pp. 335–336.)

11. Define a drug's mechanism of action. (See p. 337.)

12. List four factors that influence the concentration of a drug at its site of action. (See pp. 337–338.)

13. List two factors that slow drug absorption and two factors that enhance it. (See p. 337.)

14. Define "blood brain barrier." (See p. 338.)

15. Describe the theory of drug receptors, and give an example of one such receptor. (See p. 339.)

16. Describe the principles of "therapeutic threshold," "therapeutic index," and "minimum effective concentration." (See pp. 339–340.)

17. Define the following terms. (See below pages.)
   - agonist (p. 339, 345)
   - antagonist. (p. 339, 345)
   - sympathomimetic (p. 345)
   - sympatholytic (p. 345)
   - parasympathomimetic (p. 347)
   - parasympatholytic (p. 347)

18. Describe the autonomic nervous system, and explain its role in pharmacology. (See pp. 340–347.)

19. Describe the location and action of α and β adrenergic receptors. (See p. 345.) .

20. Define "metric system." (See p. 348.)

21. Demonstrate the ability to do routine calculations and conversions using the metric system. (See pp. 348–352.)

22. Be able to calculate any given drug dose for all medications used in your EMS system. (See pp. 348–352.)

23. List ten routes of medication administration, and assess the advantages and disadvantages of each. (See pp. 352–360.)

24. Describe and list the indications, contraindications, and dosages for the drugs used in your EMS system. (See pp. 361–399.)

Engine 21 and EMS 28 respond to a "chest pain" call at 4817 West Fuller. As the ambulance pulls up, a sheriff's deputy runs to the emergency unit. The deputy states: "This guy looks bad."

The paramedics grab the drug kit, airway bag, monitor/defibrillator, and the stretcher. They then race into the residence. Seated in a recliner is a male in his late 50s. He is pale, diaphoretic, and short of breath. When asked what is wrong, he states: "I'm having chest pain. I've never had anything like this in my life. I think I'm gonna die."

The senior paramedic quickly completes the primary assessment while his partner places a nonrebreather mask to administer oxygen. The airway is patent, the patient is moving air, and the pulse is present, yet weak. The patient's mental status is alert. One of the EMTs from Engine 21 begins to take the vital signs while a second paramedic carries out the secondary assessment. The paramedic places the ECG electrodes and sets up the monitor. The patient's wife reports that he was watching baseball on television when the pain started. He has a history of diabetes but controls it with oral medication. The patient is hypertensive and has an appointment with his family doctor next week for a stress test. He is not allergic to any medications.

The EMT reports the blood pressure as 150/90, the pulse rate 100, and the respiratory rate 20. An oximeter is placed which reveals an SpO_2 of 100% on supplemental oxygen. The ECG reveals a sinus rhythm with occasional premature ventricular contractions. A paramedic starts an IV of normal saline in the left forearm at a "to keep open" rate. Following standing orders, the senior para-

INTRODUCTION

■ **pharmacology** the study of drugs and how they affect the body.

■ **drugs** chemical agents used in diagnosis, treatment, and prevention of disease.

This chapter presents the fundamentals of pharmacology as it applies to prehospital care. **Pharmacology** is the study of drugs and how they affect the body. **Drugs** are defined as chemical agents used in diagnosis, treatment, and prevention of disease. The medications frequently used in prehospital emergency care will also be covered in this chapter. Additional clinical correlation will be presented in the clinical chapters.

BASIC PHARMACOLOGICAL BACKGROUND

Most of the drugs used in prehospital care are for cardiovascular emergencies. The medications used in an EMS system will vary from system to system. Paramedics are able to administer a far wider range of medications than EMT-Basics. As a paramedic, you will need to become familiar with all the medications used in your system. The following sections provide some basic background to help orient you to emergency pharmacology.

Drug Sources

Drugs derive from four primary sources: *plants, animals, minerals,* and *synthetics.* Emergency medications derived from plants include atropine, morphine, and digitalis. Insulin and glucagon are examples of medications derived from animals. Two medications derived from minerals are calcium chloride and sodium bicarbonate. The majority of emergency medications, however, are synthetic, or made by humans. Synthetic medications include bretylium tosylate, lidocaine, and procainamide.

medic administers 0.4 mg of nitroglycerin sublingually. After 3 minutes, there is no change in the patient's pain and a second dose of 0.4 mg nitroglycerin is administered sublingually. Like the first, the second dose does not afford any pain relief. The medical control physician is contacted and requests the administration of morphine sulfate intravenously in 2 milligram increments until the pain is improved. The paramedics recall that nitroglycerin reduces cardiac work and can alleviate chest pain associated with angina pectoris. Morphine is a narcotic that helps to alleviate pain and decreases anxiety.

Shortly thereafter, an EMS supervisor arrives with a prehospital 12 lead monitor. The monitor is placed and a 12 lead ECG tracing is obtained. The 12 lead ECG indicates an acute inferior wall myocardial infarction based on ST segment elevation in Leads II, III, and a VF. The ECG is telemetered to the medical control hospital to begin screening the patient for possible thrombolytic therapy.

The transport to the hospital goes without problem. Upon arrival, the patient is alert and calm with good respiratory effort. In the emergency department, the patient is found to meet criteria for thrombolytic therapy. He receives tissue plasminogen activator (tPA) via a front-loaded protocol and is moved to the ICU. In the ICU he develops reperfusion dysrhythmias which are treated with intravenous lidocaine. Shortly after receiving the last of the tPA, the patient becomes pain-free and his ST segments return to normal, suggesting successful thrombolysis.

Drug Laws

Governmental agencies strictly control medications used in the United States. Most of these agencies resulted from several landmark pieces of drug legislation. The most sweeping legislation was the *Federal Food, Drug, and Cosmetic Act of 1938*. This act required manufacturers to print the names of all ingredients on the labels used to package foods and medications. It also required companies to identify any habit-forming ingredients and to cite the percentages of such drugs on the labels.

Narcotics, because of their addictive nature, have always been a problem. In 1914, the federal government enacted the *Harrison Narcotic Act*. This act regulated the sale, importation, and manufacture of the opium plant and its derivatives. Opium is a primary source of narcotic products. In 1970, the government further regulated addictive medications through the *Controlled Substances Act*. This act classified addictive medications into five schedules, summarized below:

1. *Schedule I.* These drugs have a high potential for abuse and offer no accepted medical indications. Examples include heroin, LSD, "crack," and marijuana.

2. *Schedule II.* These drugs have a high potential for abuse, yet also have accepted medical indications. Emergency medications in this class include morphine, meperidine, and dilaudid.

3. *Schedule III.* These drugs have a lesser potential for abuse as well as a number of accepted medical indications. An example is the fixed combination acetaminophen with codeine (Tylenol #3).

4. *Schedule IV.* This group of drugs has a low potential for abuse, but may cause physical or psychological dependence. An example is the anticonvulsant, diazepam (Valium).

5. *Schedule V.* Schedule V drugs have a low potential for abuse, yet contain small quantities of narcotic preparations. Several cough preparations and anti-diarrheal agents fall under this classification.

In addition to establishing drug classifications, the Controlled Substances Act prohibits the refilling of prescriptions for Schedule II drugs and requires that the original prescription be filled within 72 hours. Enforcement of the Controlled Substances Act rests with the federal Drug Enforcement Administration (DEA).

Drug Names

Drugs can be identified by four names. The most elemental name is the *chemical name*, which identifies the drug's chemical structure. The *generic name* is usually an abbreviated version of the chemical name and is frequently used. The *trade name* is the name given to a drug by its manufacturer. A medication may appear under several trade names if it is made by a number of manufacturers. Finally, the *official name* is the name published in the United States Pharmacopeia. The official name is followed by the letters U.S.P. The following example gives the four names of the analgesic preparation known as meperidine.

- ❑ *Chemical Name*: *ethyl-1-methyl-4-phenylisonipecotate hydrochloride*
- ❑ *Generic Name*: meperidine hydrochloride
- ❑ *Trade Name*: Demerol Hydrochloride
- ❑ *Official Name*: meperidine hydrochloride, U.S.P.

Drug References

Several valuable sources of information provide easy-to-use medication guides. These include:

- ❑ *AMA Drug Evaluations.* This manual, published by the American Medical Association, provides information on all drug groups. It covers dosages, side effects, indications, and contraindications.
- ❑ *Physicians' Desk Reference (PDR).* The Physicians' Desk Reference (PDR) is a standard that should be on board every paramedic unit. It contains a very useful Product Identification Guide, with photographs of various medications showing actual size and color, as well as information on most drugs currently on the market. The PDR is published yearly by the Medical Economics Data Production Company.
- ❑ *Drug Inserts.* The written literature packaged with most drugs provides a good source of information. These inserts can be collected in a notebook for personal use.

Drug Forms

Drugs come in many forms. Each form has advantages and disadvantages. The following are some common drug preparations.

Liquid Drugs   Liquid drugs usually consist of a powder dissolved in a liquid. The drug is referred to as the solute. The liquid part is called the *solvent*. In liquid drug preparations, it is primarily the *solute* that distinguishes one preparation from another.

- ❑ *Solutions.* Solutions are preparations in which the drugs are dissolved in a solvent, usually water (for example, 5 percent dextrose in water).

- *Tinctures.* Tinctures are drug preparations in which the drug was extracted chemically with alcohol. They will usually contain some dilute alcohol (for example, tincture of iodine).
- *Suspensions.* Suspensions are liquid drug preparations that do not remain mixed. After sitting for even a short time, these preparations will tend to separate. They must always be shaken well before use (for example, amoxicillin preparations).
- *Spirits.* Spirit solutions contain volatile chemicals (chemicals that quickly vaporize) dissolved in alcohol (for example, spirit of ammonia).
- *Emulsions.* Emulsions are preparations in which an oily substance is mixed with a solvent that will not dissolve it. After mixing, globules of fat form and float in the solvent. These preparations are similar to what occurs in a mixture of oil and vinegar.
- *Elixirs.* Elixirs are preparations that contain the drug in an alcohol solvent. Flavoring, frequently cherry, is added to improve the taste (for example, Nyquil).
- *Syrups.* Often drugs are dissolved in sugar and water to improve the taste. These are referred to as syrups (for example, cough syrup).

Parenteral Drugs   Liquid drugs administered into the body through intramuscular, subcutaneous, or intravenous routes are called **parenteral drugs**. These drugs are introduced through routes outside of the digestive tract (also called the *enteral tract*). Most drugs used in emergencies are parenteral. These preparations must be sterile because they are introduced into the body.

Parenteral medications are packaged in several types of containers. *Ampules* are sterile parenteral containers designed to carry a single patient dose. (See Figure 13-1.) Generally, ampules are broken and the drug is drawn into a syringe for administration.

For most emergency situations, drugs are provided in *prefilled syringes* to save time. (See Figure 13-2.) Containers of parenteral medications that contain more than one dose are called *vials*. (See Figure 13-3.) A few of the drugs used in emergencies are provided in vials. Today, single-dose vials are available that do not require breakage in order to withdraw the drug.

Solid Drugs   Solid drugs are usually administered orally, but can be administered rectally or vaginally as well. They include:

- *Pills.* Pills are drugs that are shaped into a form that's easy to swallow. They are often coated to improve taste and to ease swallowing.
- *Powders.* Powders are drugs in powdered form. They are not as popular as pills, yet some are still in use (for example, B.C. Powder).
- *Capsules.* Capsules are gelatin containers into which a powder has been placed. The gelatin dissolves, liberating the powder into the gastrointestinal tract (for example, Dalmane capsules).
- *Tablets.* Tablets are similar to pills. They are composed of a powder that has been compressed into an easily swallowed form.
- *Suppositories.* Suppositories are mixed into a base that is solid at room temperature (approximately 70° F). But, when placed into the body (rectally or vaginally), they dissolve and are absorbed into the surrounding tissue.

Pharmacological Terminology

There are several important pharmacological terms with which prehospital personnel should be familiar. They include:

■ **parenteral drugs** drugs administered into the body without going through the digestive tract.

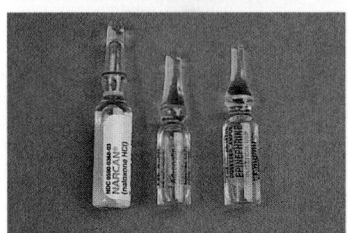

FIGURE 13-1   Ampules.

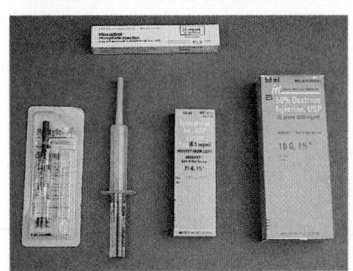

FIGURE 13-2   Prefilled syringes.

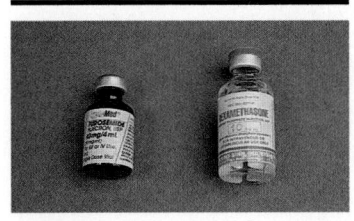

FIGURE 13-3   Vials.

- *Antagonism.* Antagonism signifies the opposition between two or more medications; that which counteracts something else (for example, between naloxone and morphine).
- *Bolus.* A bolus is a single, often large dose of medication (for example, lidocaine bolus, which is often followed by a lidocaine infusion).
- *Contraindications.* Contraindications are the medical or physiological conditions present in a patient that may cause harm when an otherwise appropriate medication is administered.
- *Cumulative action.* A cumulative action occurs when a drug is administered in several doses, causing an increased effect. This is usually due to a buildup of the drug in the blood.
- *Depressant.* A depressant is a medication that decreases a bodily function or activity.
- *Habituation.* Habituation is physical or psychological dependence on a drug.
- *Hypersensitivity.* Hypersensitivity is a state of altered reactivity to some foreign substance (including medications), with an exaggerated immune response.
- *Idiosyncrasy.* An idiosyncrasy is an individual reaction to a drug that is unusual, or different from that normally seen.
- *Indication.* An indication refers to the medical condition or conditions in which a drug has proven to be of therapeutic value.
- *Potentiation.* Potentiation is the enhancement of the effects of one drug by another (for example, barbiturates and alcohol).
- *Refractory.* Patients who do not respond to a drug are said to be refractory to the drug (for example, a patient with premature ventricular contractions who does not respond to lidocaine).
- *Side effects.* Side effects are undesired effects that a drug may cause, even in therapeutic doses.
- *Stimulant.* A stimulant is a drug that increases a bodily function or activity (for example, caffeine in coffee).
- *Synergism.* Synergism is the combined action of two drugs that is much stronger than the effects of either one.
- *Therapeutic action.* A therapeutic action is the intended action of a drug given in the appropriate medical condition.
- *Tolerance.* When a patient has been on a drug for a long time, he or she may require larger dosages to achieve a therapeutic effect. This increased requirement is termed tolerance.
- *Untoward effect.* An untoward effect is a side effect harmful to the patient.

Studying Medications

You can begin to compile your own background data on drugs by using this simple technique. Whenever you study a medication, ask yourself the following questions.

- What is the usual dose of the medication?
- What, if any, is the required dilution?
- What is the drug's action?
- What are the prehospital indications and uses?
- What precautions should you take when administering the drug?
- What are the contraindications to administering the medication?

- ❑ What are the drug's compatibilities and incompatibilities with other medications?
- ❑ What are the common side effects?
- ❑ What, if any, antidotes exist for the medication?

Learn the answers to all of these questions for the medications in your EMS system. You might want to carry this information on cards, thus making your own ready reference.

ACTIONS OF DRUGS

For a drug to exert its desired effects upon the body, it must reach its targeted tissue in suitable form and in sufficient concentration. The study of how drugs enter the body, reach their site of action, and eventually are eliminated is called **pharmacokinetics**. Once drugs reach their targeted tissue, they begin a chain of biochemical events that ultimately lead to the desired physiological changes. These biochemical and physiological events are called the drug's *mechanism of action*. The study of a drug's action upon the body is called **pharmacodynamics**. The following section covers the fundamentals of pharmacokinetics and pharmacodynamics as they apply to prehospital emergency care.

■ **pharmacokinetics** the study of how drugs enter the body, reach their site of action, and eventually are eliminated.

■ **pharmacodynamics** the study of a drug's action upon the body.

Pharmacokinetics

Several factors influence the concentration of a drug at its site of action. These factors include *absorption* of the drug into the circulatory system, *distribution* of the drug throughout the body, *biotransformation* of the drug into its active form, and, finally, *elimination* of the drug from the body. It is important to understand that not all of these factors are involved in every medication used in prehospital care. However, a fundamental understanding of each factor is essential.

Absorption   Most medications used in prehospital care are given by the intravenous, intramuscular, or subcutaneous route. A drug administered into a muscle or into subcutaneous tissue must be absorbed into circulation through the walls of the capillaries. The drug can then be transported to its sites of action. Several factors may affect the rate of absorption. Factors that delay absorption from parenteral sites include shock, acidosis, and hypothermia that results in peripheral vasoconstriction. Factors that can increase the rate of absorption include hyperthermia and fever, which can cause peripheral vasodilation. Muscles, as a rule, are more richly supplied with blood vessels than subcutaneous tissue. Therefore, a drug should be absorbed more rapidly from muscle than from subcutaneous tissue. Other factors that can affect drug absorption include the size, age, and general medical condition of the patient.

Drug absorption delays may be avoided by injecting the medication directly into the circulatory system through the veins. (See Figure 13-4.) The desired effects are seen much sooner and the eventual blood levels of the medication are much more predictable. Because of this, most critical-care medications are administered intravenously.

Distribution   Once in the circulatory system, a drug is distributed throughout the body tissues. Most medications pass easily from the intravascular compartment, through the interstitial spaces, to the target cells. These drugs tend to have a rapid onset of action and short duration of effect. Some drugs, on the other hand, are immediately bound to serum proteins after entering the circulation.

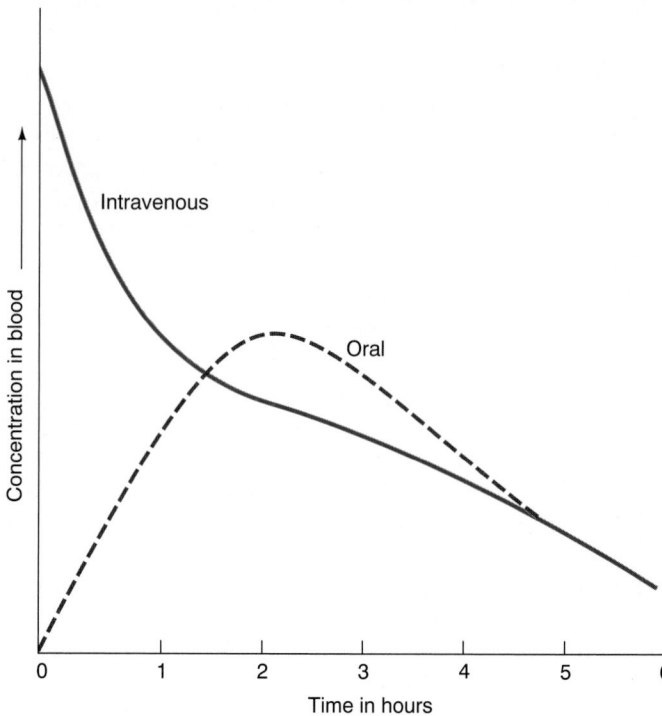

FIGURE 13-4 Comparison of intravenous and oral administration of the same drug.

There drugs tend to have a delayed onset of action and remain in the circulatory system for a prolonged time.

Generally, drugs will concentrate in tissues with good blood supplies, such as the heart, brain, liver, and kidneys. It is important to remember that in critical situations, such as shock, the tissues receiving the most blood are the heart and brain. Delivery of blood to the brain is limited by a protective mechanism called the **blood brain barrier**. It selectively allows the entry of only a limited number of compounds into the brain. Drugs that are protein-bound, or drugs in an ionized form, are weak penetrators of the blood brain barrier.

■ **blood brain barrier** a protective mechanism that selectively allows the entry of only a limited number of compounds into the brain.

Biotransformation Many drugs are inactive when administered. Once absorbed, they are converted into an active form, either in the blood or by the target tissue. The process of changing a drug to another form, either active or inactive, is called *biotransformation*. It results in chemical variations of the drugs, which are called *metabolites*.

Several drugs used in prehospital care must be converted into an active form to take effect. Diazepam, for example, is relatively inactive as administered. Once in the body, it is biotransformed into an active metabolite. Other drugs are active as administered, but are biotransformed into an inactive metabolite before elimination. Epinephrine is an example of a medication that is quickly biotransformed to an inactive metabolite. Because of this rapid biotransformation, epinephrine must be readministered approximately every three to five minutes in certain situations.

Elimination Drugs are eventually eliminated from the body in either their original form or as metabolites. Drugs may be excreted by the kidneys into the urine, by the liver into the bile, by the intestines into the feces, or by the lungs into the expired air. The rate of elimination varies with the medication and the condition of the body. During shock states, the kidneys are poorly perfused, and drugs may remain in the body longer. The slower the rate of elimination, the longer the drug stays in the body.

Pharmacodynamics

Once a drug has reached its target tissue, it must induce the desired biochemical or physiological response. To do so, most drugs bind to drug receptors. (See Figure 13-5.) *Drug receptors* are proteins present on the surface of cell membranes. Think of these receptors as locks with drugs serving as the keys. Once the drug has bound to the receptor—i.e., the key is in the lock—biochemical actions begin that lead to the desired biochemical response. Drugs that bind to a receptor and cause a response are referred to as *agonists*. Certain drugs, however, may bind to a receptor and block a biochemical response. Their presence on the receptor may prevent other drugs from binding. These drugs are known as *antagonists*. (See Figure 13-6.)

Classic illustrations of these principles are the drugs epinephrine and propranolol (Inderal). Epinephrine is transported to the target tissues—namely the heart, lungs, and peripheral blood vessels. Once there, it binds to its receptors, alpha (α) and beta (β) adrenergic receptors. (See "Adrenergic Receptors" later in this chapter.) If the drug binds to these receptors, the desired physiological response will be seen. However, there are several inactive drugs that can bind to the β receptors in much the same manner as epinephrine. These medications are referred to as beta blockers. The prototype of this group is propranolol. If the beta blocker is already bound to the receptor, then epinephrine cannot bind and its β effects are effectively inhibited.

To be effective, a medication must reach a certain concentration in the target tissues. The minimal concentration of a drug necessary to cause the desired response is referred to as the *therapeutic threshold* or *minimum effective concentration*. A concentration below this threshold will not induce a clinical response. Conversely, there is a point at which the drug concentration can get high enough to be toxic or even fatal. The general goal of pharmacological therapy is to give the minimum concentration of a drug necessary to obtain the desired response.

The difference between the minimum effective concentration and the toxic level varies widely between drugs. The difference between effective and toxic concentrations is called the *therapeutic index*. (See Figure 13-7.) It is usually determined in the laboratory. With certain drugs, digoxin (Lanoxin) among them, there is little difference between effective and toxic doses. These drugs are said to have a *low therapeutic index*. Drugs such as naloxone (Narcan), a narcotic

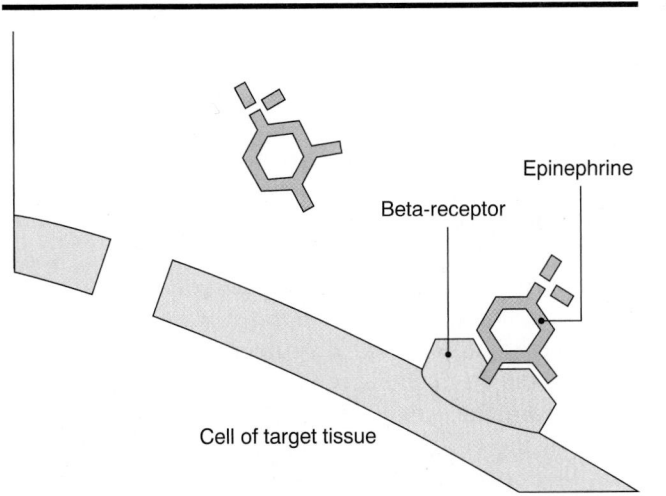

FIGURE 13-5 Example of drug (epinephrine) interacting with a drug receptor (β receptor).

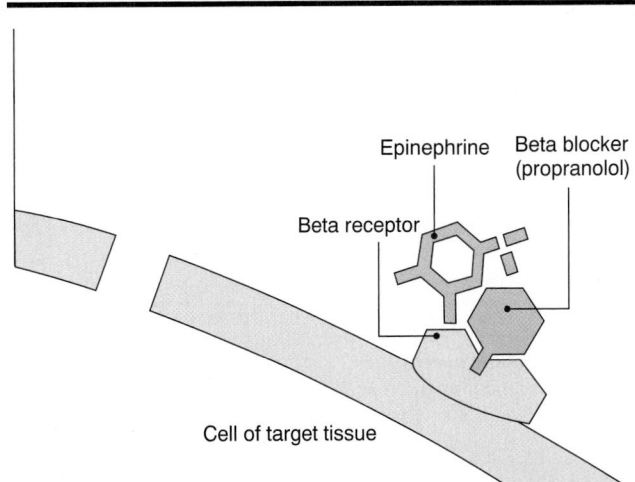

FIGURE 13-6 Drug receptor blocked by antagonist (β blocker).

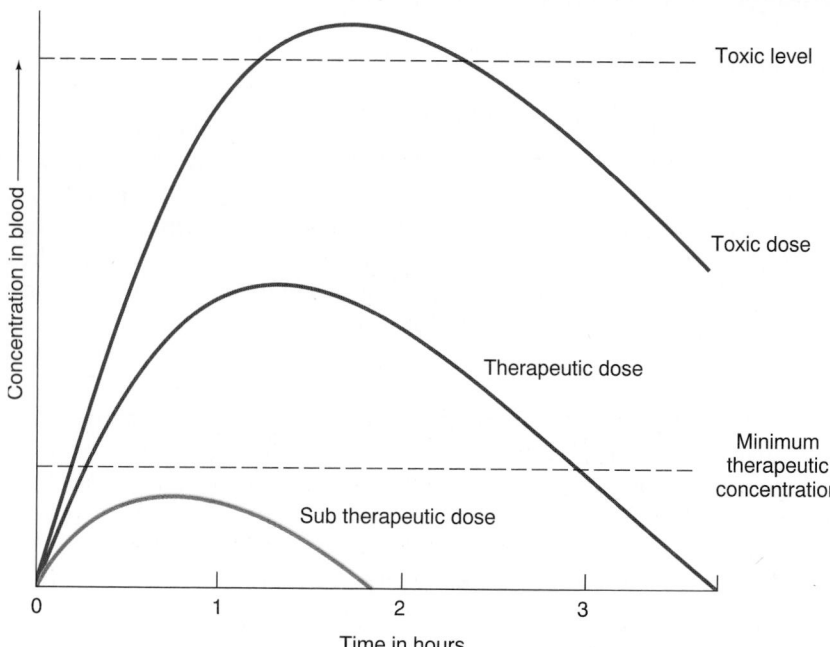

FIGURE 13-7 Comparison of subtherapeutic, therapeutic, and toxic doses of the same drug.

antagonist, have a significant margin between effective and toxic doses. Drugs of this kind are said to have a *high therapeutic index.* As a paramedic, you must be familiar with the therapeutic indices of medications used in your system.

THE AUTONOMIC NERVOUS SYSTEM

■ **autonomic nervous system** the part of the nervous system responsible for control of involuntary actions.

The **autonomic nervous system** is the part of the nervous system responsible for control of involuntary "automatic" actions. Many medications used in prehospital care directly affect the autonomic nervous system. It is essential that prehospital personnel have a good understanding of this aspect of the nervous system and the ways in which emergency medications affect it.

The two functional divisions of the autonomic nervous system are the *sympathetic nervous system* and the *parasympathetic nervous system.* (See Figure 13-8.) The sympathetic nervous system allows the body to function under stress. It is often referred to as the "fight-or-flight" aspect of the nervous system. The parasympathetic nervous system, on the other hand, primarily controls vegetative functions such as digestion of food. It is often referred to as the "feed-or-breed" or "rest-and-repose" aspect of the autonomic nervous system. The parasympathetic nervous system is in constant opposition with the sympathetic nervous system.

Basic Anatomy and Physiology

■ **autonomic ganglia** groups of autonomic nerve cells located outside the central nervous system.

■ **pre-ganglionic nerves** nerve fibers that extend from the central nervous system to the autonomic ganglia.

■ **post-ganglionic nerves** nerve fibers that extend from the autonomic ganglia to the target tissues.

The autonomic nervous system arises from the central nervous system. The nerves of the autonomic nervous system exit the central nervous system and subsequently enter specialized structures called **autonomic ganglia**. In the autonomic ganglia, the nerve fibers from the central nervous system interact with nerve fibers that extend from the ganglia to the various target organs. Autonomic nerve fibers that exit the central nervous system and terminate in the autonomic ganglia are called **pre-ganglionic nerves**. Autonomic nerve fibers that exit the ganglia and terminate in the various target tissues are called **post-ganglionic nerves**. The ganglia of the sympathetic nervous system are

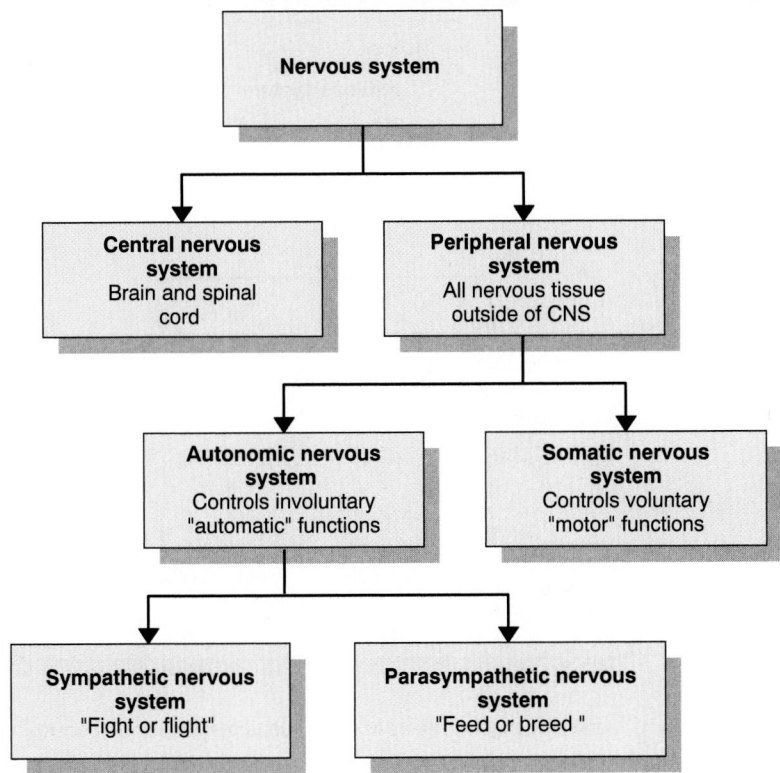

FIGURE 13-8 Functional organization of the autonomic nervous system.

located close to the spinal cord, while the ganglia of the parasympathetic nervous system are located close to the target organs. (See Figure 13-9.)

No actual physical connection exists between two nerve cells or between a nerve cell and the organ it innervates. Instead, there is a space between nerve cells called a **synapse**. The space between a nerve cell and the target organ is called a **neuroeffector junction**. Specialized chemicals called **neurotransmitters** are used to conduct the nervous impulse between nerve cells or between a nerve cell and its target organ.

Neurotransmitters are released from pre-synaptic **neurons** and subsequently act on post-synaptic neurons or on the designated target organ. When released by the nerve ending, the neurotransmitter travels across the synapse and activates membrane receptors on the adjoining nerve or target tissue. The neurotransmitter is then either deactivated or taken back up into the pre-synaptic neuron.

The two neurotransmitters of the autonomic nervous system are *acetylcholine* and *norepinephrine*. Acetylcholine is utilized in the pre-ganglionic nerves of the sympathetic nervous system and in both the pre-ganglionic and post-anglionic nerves of the parasympathetic nervous system. Norepinephrine is the post-ganglionic neurotransmitter of the sympathetic nervous system. Synapses that use acetylcholine as the neurotransmitter are called **cholinergic** synapses. Synapses that use norepinephrine as the neurotransmitter are called **adrenergic** synapses.

The Sympathetic Nervous System

The sympathetic nervous system arises from the thoracic and lumbar regions of the spinal cord. Pre-ganglionic nerves leave the spinal cord through the spinal nerves and end in the sympathetic ganglia. There are two types of sympathetic ganglia: *sympathetic chain ganglia* and *collateral ganglia*. (See Figure 13-10.) In addition, special pre-ganglionic sympathetic nerve fibers innervate the

■ **synapse** a space between nerve cells. Electrical impulses are transmitted across the synaptic cleft by special messenger chemicals called neurotransmitters.

■ **neuroeffector junction** a specialized synapse between a nerve cell and the organ or tissue that it innervates.

■ **neurotransmitter** chemical messenger that conducts a nervous impulse across a synapse.

■ **neuron** nerve cell.

■ **cholinergic** pertaining to the neurotransmitter acetylcholine.

■ **adrenergic** pertaining to the neurotransmitter norepinephrine.

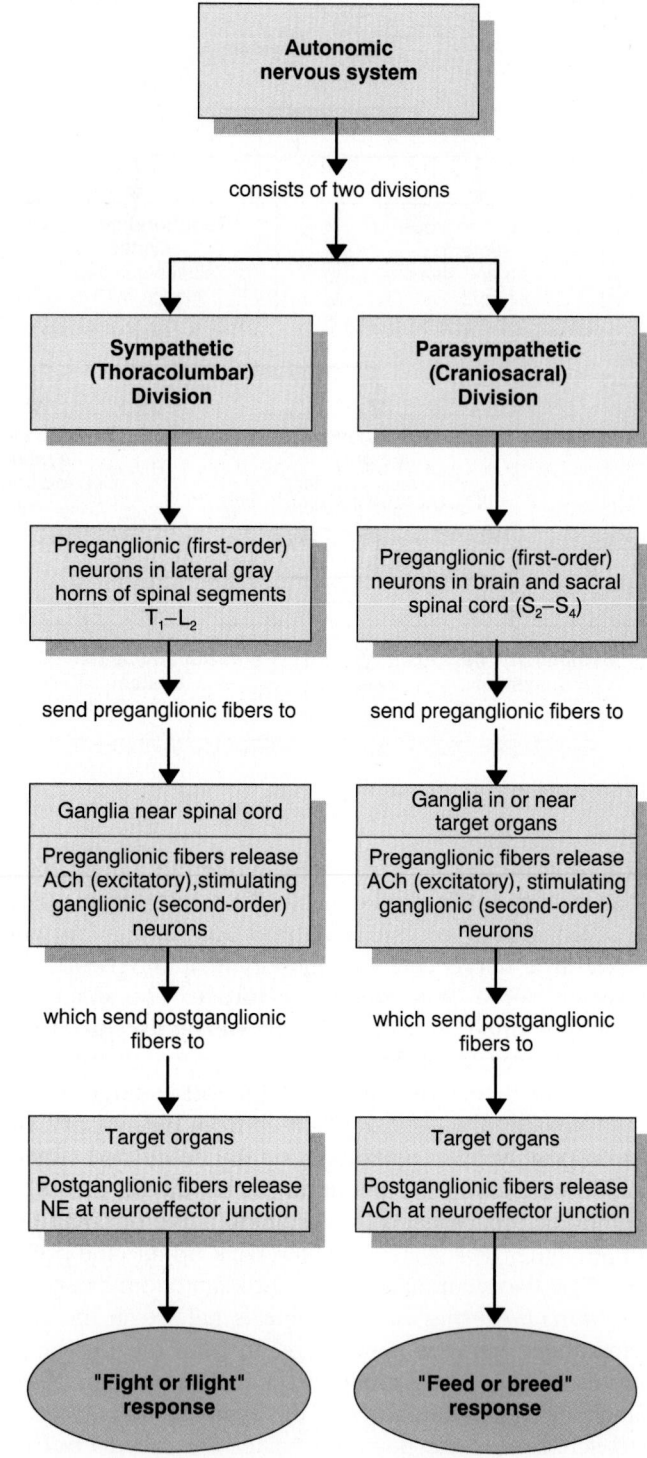

FIGURE 13-9 Components of the autonomic nervous system.

adrenal medulla. Post-ganglionic nerves that exit the sympathetic chain ganglia extend to several peripheral target tissues of the sympathetic nervous system. When stimulated, these fibers have several effects. These include:

❏ Stimulation of secretion by sweat glands
❏ Constriction of blood vessels in the skin
❏ Increase in blood flow to skeletal muscles

- Increase in the heart rate and force of cardiac contractions
- Bronchodilation
- Stimulation of energy production

The collateral ganglia are located in the abdominal cavity. Nerves leaving the collateral ganglia innervate many of the organs of the abdomen. Stimulation of these fibers causes several conditions. These include:

- Reduction of blood flow to abdominal organs
- Decreased digestive activity
- Relaxation of smooth muscle in the wall of the urinary bladder
- Release of glucose stores from the liver

Sympathetic nervous system stimulation also results in direct stimulation of the *adrenal medulla*, the inner portion of the adrenal gland. (See Figure 13-11.) The adrenal medulla in turn releases the hormones **norepinephrine** (noradrenalin) and **epinephrine** (adrenalin) into the circulatory system. Approximately 80% of the hormones released by the adrenal medulla are epinephrine, while norepinephrine constitutes the remaining 20%. Once released, these hormones are carried throughout the body where they cause their intended effects by acting on hormone receptors. The release of norepinephrine and epinephrine by the adrenal medulla stimulates tissues that are not

■ **norepinephrine** neurotransmitter of the post-ganglionic sympathetic nerves and a hormone secreted by the adrenal medulla.

■ **epinephrine** major hormone secreted by the adrenal medulla in response to sympathetic stimulation; a major mediator of the sympathetic response.

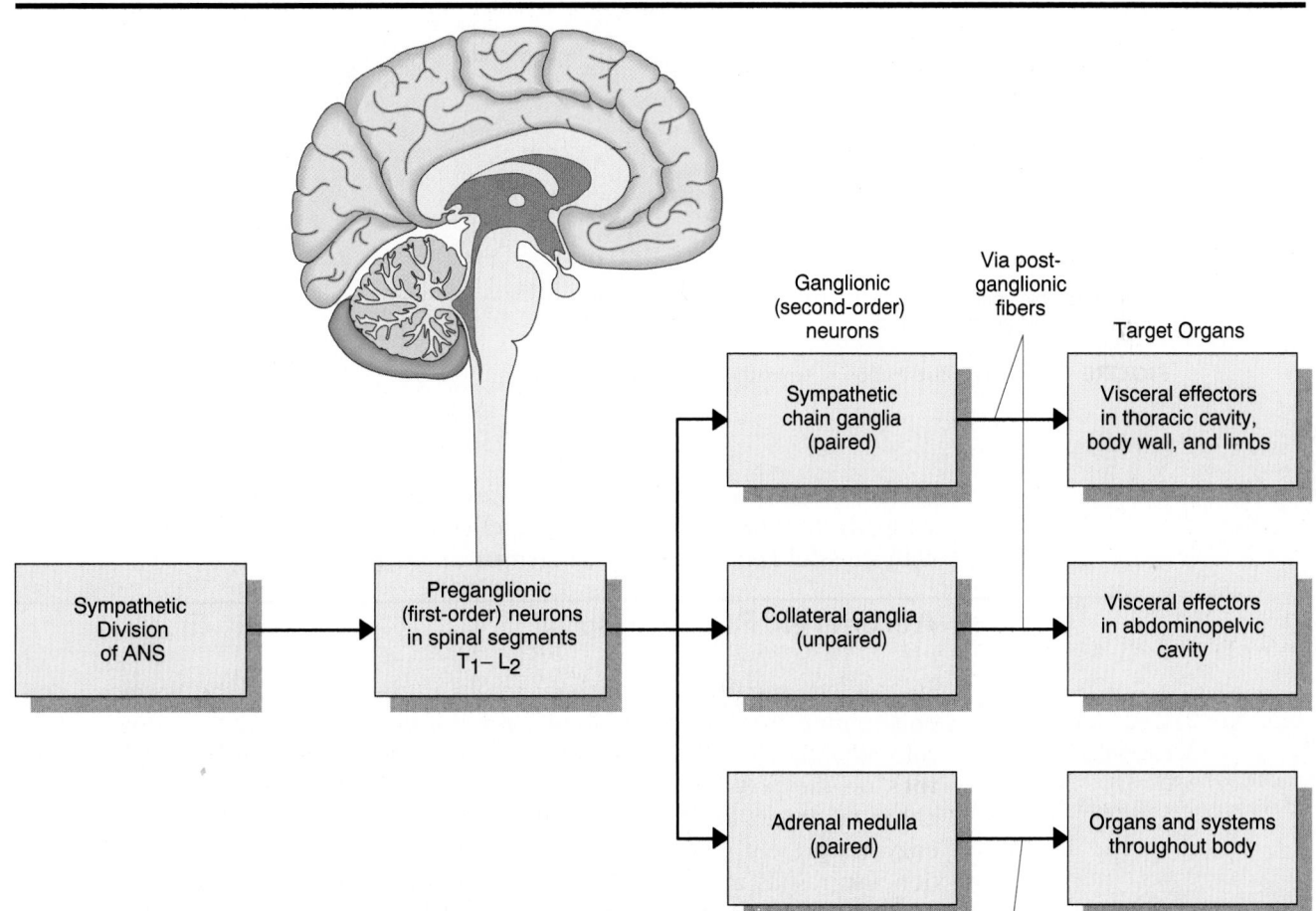

FIGURE 13-10 Organization of the sympathetic division of the autonomic nervous system.

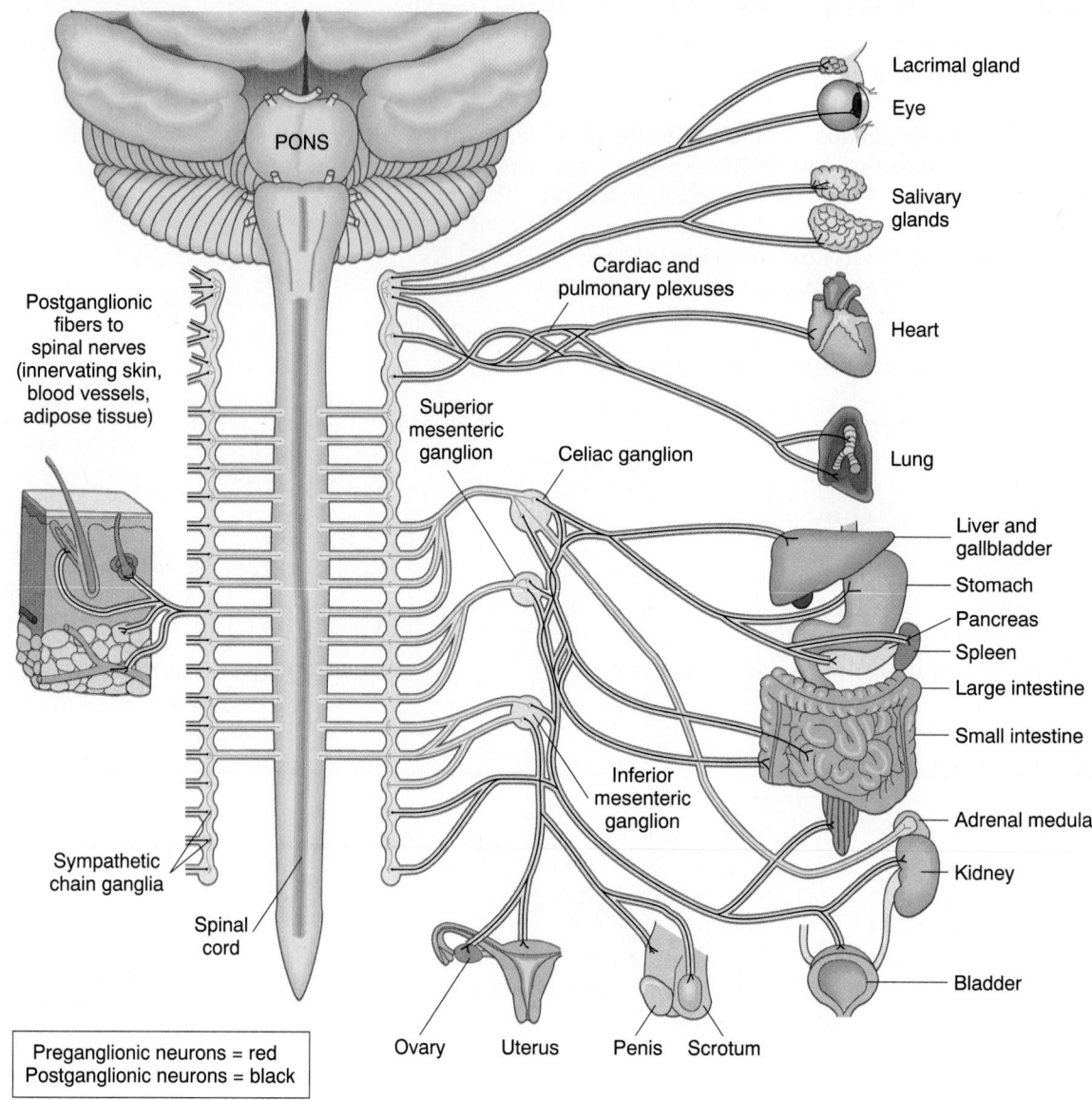

PONS

Lacrimal gland

Eye

Salivary glands

Cardiac and pulmonary plexuses

Heart

Postganglionic fibers to spinal nerves (innervating skin, blood vessels, adipose tissue)

Lung

Superior mesenteric ganglion

Celiac ganglion

Liver and gallbladder

Stomach

Pancreas

Spleen

Large intestine

Small intestine

Inferior mesenteric ganglion

Adrenal medula

Kidney

Sympathetic chain ganglia

Spinal cord

Bladder

Ovary   Uterus   Penis   Scrotum

Preganglionic neurons = red
Postganglionic neurons = black

FIGURE 13-11   The distribution of sympathetic post-ganglionic fibers.

innervated by sympathetic nerves. In addition, it prolongs the effects of direct sympathetic stimulation. All of these effects serve to prepare the body to deal with stressful and potentially dangerous situations.

Adrenergic Receptors

Sympathetic stimulation ultimately results in the release of the hormone norepinephrine from post-ganglionic, *pre-synaptic* nerves. The norepinephrine subsequently crosses the synaptic cleft and interacts with **adrenergic receptors** on the *post-synaptic* nerves. Shortly thereafter, the norepinephrine is either taken up by the pre-synaptic neuron for reuse or broken down by enzymes present within the synapse. (See Figure 13-12.) Sympathetic stimulation also results in the release of the hormones epinephrine and norepinephrine from the adrenal medulla. In addition, both epinephrine and norepinephrine interact with specialized adrenergic receptors on the mem-

■ **adrenergic receptors** receptors specific to norepinephrine and epinephrine-like substances.

branes of the target organs. These receptors are located throughout the body. Once stimulated by the appropriate hormone, they cause a response in the organ or organs they control.

The two known types of sympathetic receptors are the adrenergic receptors and the dopaminergic receptors. The *adrenergic receptors* are generally divided into four types. These four receptors are designated *alpha 1 (α_1)*, *alpha 2 (α_2)*, *beta 1 (β_1)*, and *beta 2 (β_2)*. The α_1 receptors cause peripheral vasoconstriction, mild bronchoconstriction, and stimulation of metabolism. The α_2 receptors are found on the pre-synaptic surfaces of sympathetic neuro-effector junctions. Stimulation of α_2 receptors is inhibitory. These receptors serve to prevent over-release of norepinephrine in the synapse. When the level of norepinephrine in the synapse gets high enough, the α_2 receptors are stimulated and norepinephrine release is inhibited. Stimulation of β_1 receptors causes increases in heart rate, cardiac contractile force, and cardiac automaticity and conduction. Stimulation of β_2 receptors causes vasodilation and bronchodilation. *Dopaminergic receptors*, although not fully understood, are believed to cause dilation of the renal, coronary, and cerebral arteries.

Medications that stimulate the sympathetic nervous system are referred to as **sympathomimetics**. Medications that inhibit the sympathetic nervous system are called **sympatholytics**. Some medications are pure α **agonists**, while others are pure α **antagonists**. Some medications are pure β agonists, while others are pure β antagonists. Medications such as epinephrine stimulate both alpha and beta receptors. Other medications, such as the bronchodilators, are termed β selective, since they act more on β_2 receptors than upon β_1.

The Parasympathetic Nervous System

The parasympathetic nervous system arises from the brainstem and the sacral segments of the spinal cord. The pre-ganglionic neurons of the parasympathetic nervous system are typically much longer than those of the sympathetic nervous system, because the ganglia are located close to the target tissues. Parasympathetic nerve fibers that leave the brainstem travel within four of the cranial nerves including the oculomotor nerve (III), the facial nerve (VII), the glossopharyngeal nerve (IX), and the vagus nerve (X). These fibers synapse in the *parasympathetic ganglia* with short post-ganglionic

■ **sympathomimetics** drugs or other substances that cause effects like those of the sympathetic nervous system (also called adrenergic).

■ **sympatholytics** drugs or other substances that block the actions of the sympathetic nervous system (also called antiadrenergic).

■ **agonists** drugs or other substances that cause a physiological response.

■ **antagonists** drugs or other substances that block a physiological response or the action of another drug or substance.

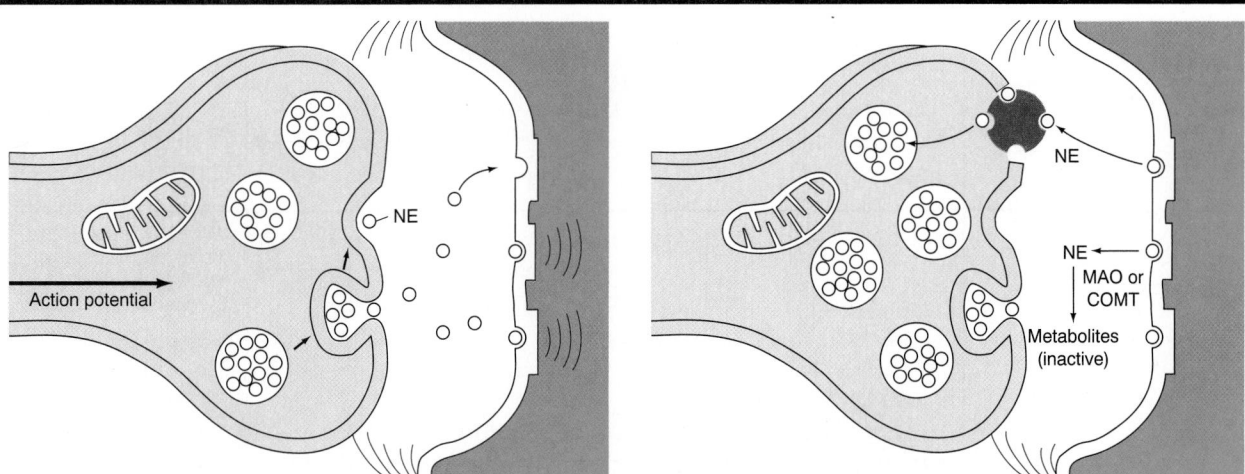

FIGURE 13-12 Physiology of an adrenergic synapse. Norepinephrine is released from the pre-synaptic nerve and stimulates receptors on the post-synaptic nerve. Subsequently, the norepinephrine is either taken up by the pre-synaptic nerve or deactivated by enzymes present in the synapse.

fibers that then continue to their target tissues. Post-synaptic fibers innervate much of the body, including the intrinsic eye muscles, the salivary glands, the heart, the lungs, and most of the organs of the abdominal cavity. The sacral segment of the parasympathetic nervous system forms distinct pelvic nerves that innervate ganglia in the kidneys, bladder, sex organs, and the terminal portions of the large intestine. (See Figure 13-13.) Stimulation of the parasympathetic nervous system results in the following conditions.

❑ Pupillary constriction
❑ Secretion by digestive glands
❑ Increased smooth muscle activity along the digestive tract
❑ Bronchoconstriction
❑ Reduction in heart rate and cardiac contractile force

These and other functions facilitate the processing of food, energy absorption, relaxation, and reproduction. (See Figure 13-14.)

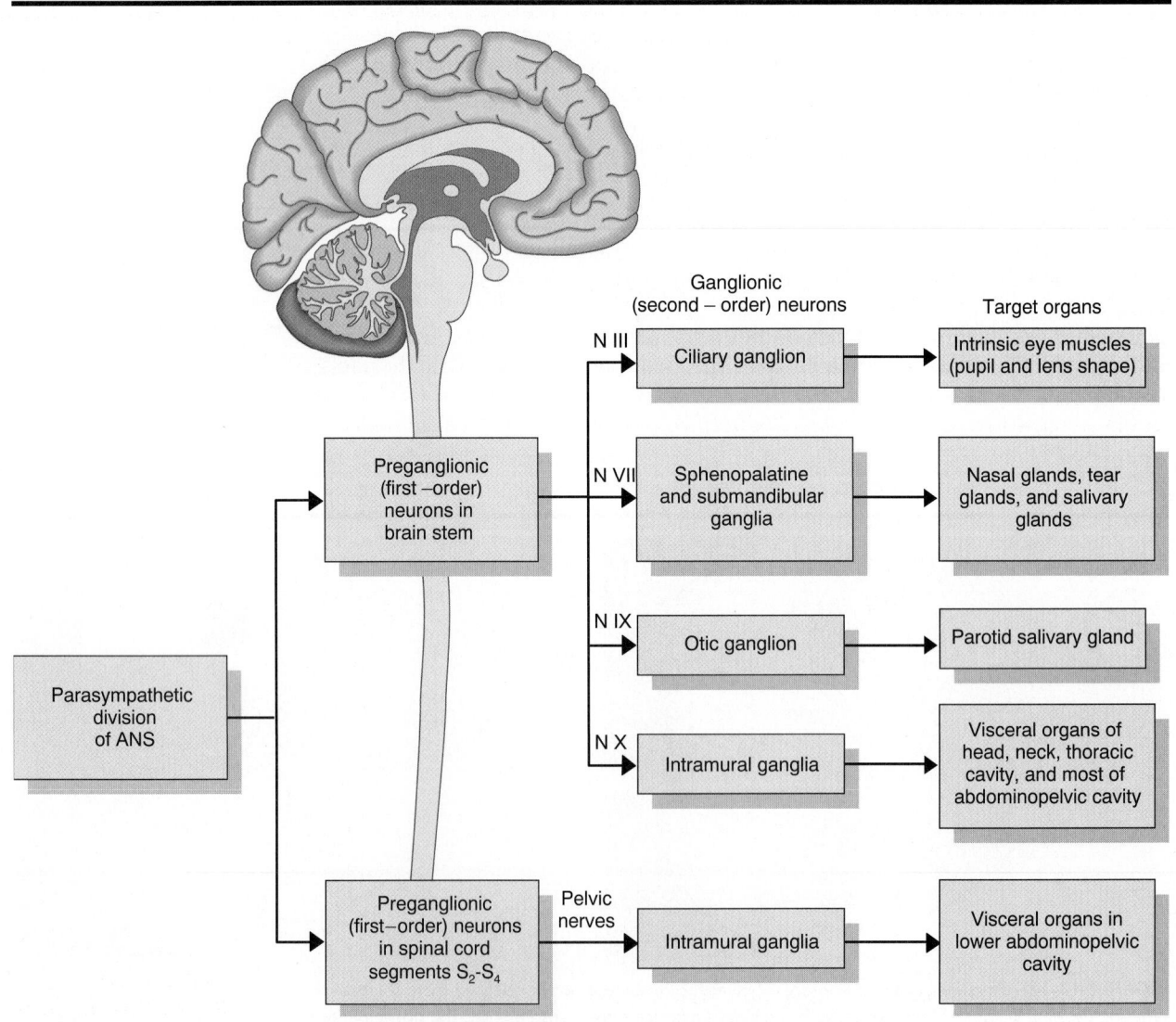

FIGURE 13-13 Organization of the parasympathetic division of the autonomic nervous system.

All pre-ganglionic and post-ganglionic parasympathetic nerve fibers use *acetylcholine* as a neurotransmitter. Acetylcholine, when released by presynaptic neurons, crosses the synaptic cleft and activates receptors on the post-synaptic neurons or on the neuroeffector junction. Acetylcholine is also the neurotransmitter for the somatic nervous system and is present in the neuromuscular junction. Acetylcholine is very short-lived. Within a fraction of a second after its release, acetylcholine is deactivated by another chemical called *acetylcholinesterase*. *Acetic acid* and *choline*, which are produced when acetylcholine is deactivated, are taken back up by the pre-synaptic neuron. (See Figure 13-15.)

The emergency medication atropine is an antagonist to the parasympathetic nervous system and is used to increase heart rate. Atropine binds with acetylcholine receptors, thus preventing acetylcholine from exerting its effect. Medications like atropine, which block the actions of the parasympathetic nervous system, are referred to as **parasympatholytics** or anticholinergics. Medications that stimulate the parasympathetic nervous system are referred to as **parasympathomimetics** or cholinergics.

■ **parasympatholytics** drugs or other substances that block or inhibit the actions of the parasympathetic nervous system (also called anticholinergics).

■ **parasympathomimetics** drugs or other substances that cause effects like those of the parasympathetic nervous system (also called cholinergics).

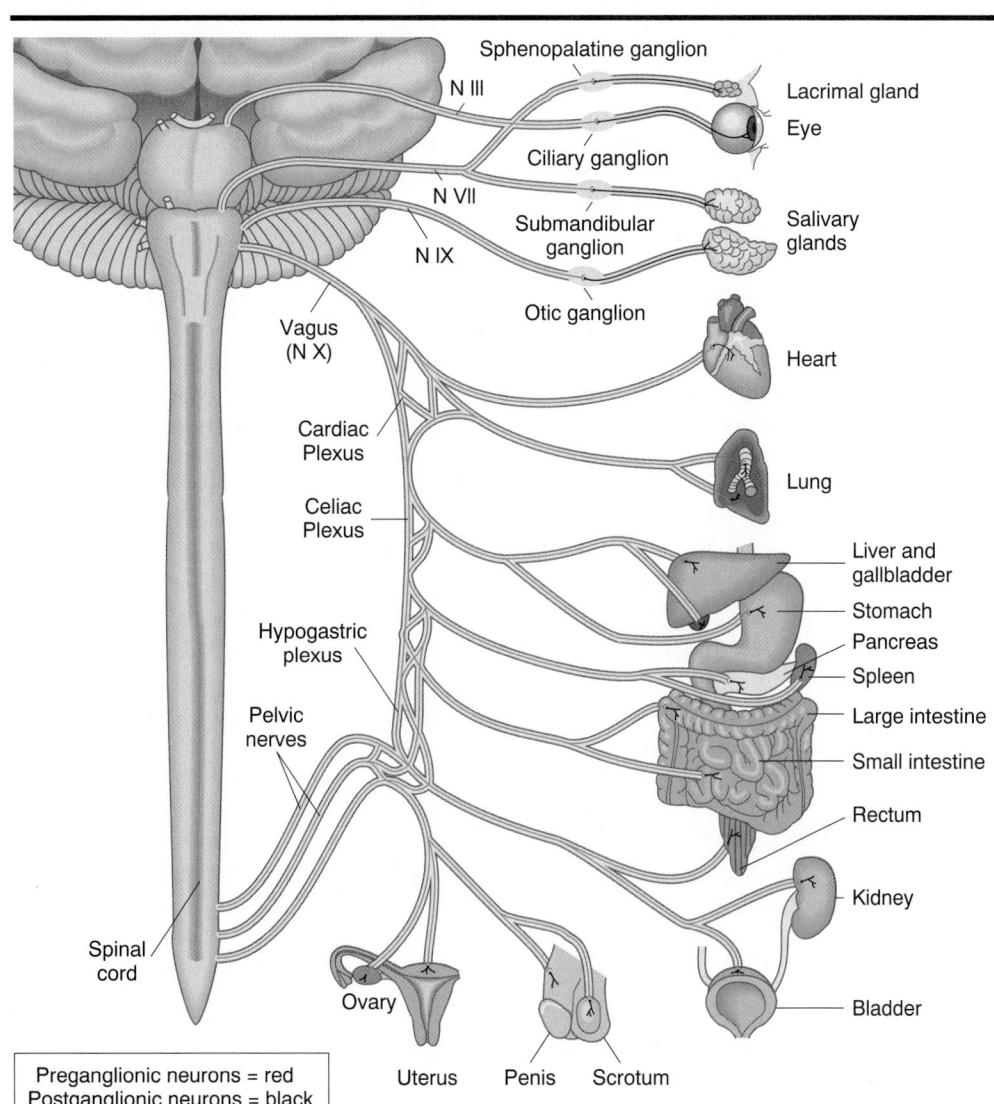

Preganglionic neurons = red
Postganglionic neurons = black

FIGURE 13-14
Distribution of the parasympathetic nerves.

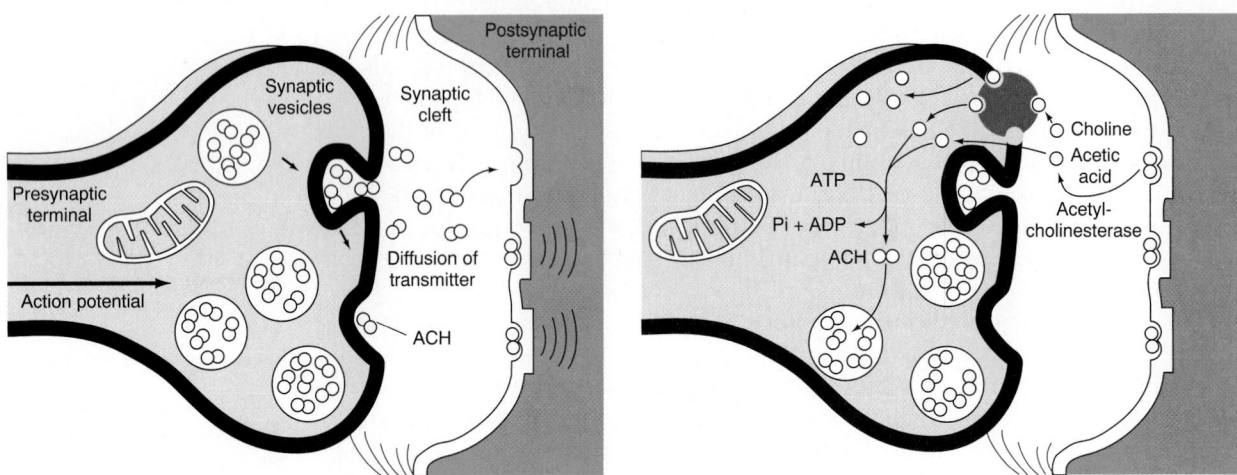

FIGURE 13-15 Physiology of a cholinergic synapse. Acetylcholine is released from the pre-synaptic nerve and stimulates receptors on the post-synaptic nerve. Subsequently, the acteylcholine is broken down by acetylcholinesterase and the products are taken up by the pre-synaptic nerve fiber.

ADMINISTRATION OF DRUGS

Once you understand some of the mechanics of the autonomic nervous system, you can begin to think about some of the practical aspects of drug administration. One step involves mathematic computations based upon the metric system. Another step involves selection of the most appropriate route of entry (based upon assessment of the patient's medical condition).

Weights and Measures

■ **metric system** a system of weights and measures widely used in science and medicine. It is based on a unit of 10.

■ **apothecary's system** an antiquated system of weights and measures used widely in early medicine.

The **metric system** is used worldwide as the standard system of weights and measures in science and medicine. It is the principal system of weights and measures used in pharmacology. However, because of tradition, the mostly antiquated **apothecary's system** of weights and measures remains in occasional use.

The metric system was devised by the French and is based on the unit 10. All units are 10 times larger than, or 1/10 as large as, the next unit. Because the metric system is based on the unit 10, conversion from one unit to another is simple. The change from one set of units to another requires only moving a decimal point.

Physical descriptions in science and medicine rest upon three measurements: mass, length, and volume. *Mass* is the quantity of matter in a substance. *Length* is the distance between two points. *Volume* is the space occupied by a substance. The metric system has three fundamental units for these measurements. The fundamental unit for measuring mass is the gram (G). The fundamental unit for measuring length is the meter (M). The fundamental unit for measuring volume is the liter (L). All other metric units used to describe mass, length, and volume are derivatives of these three fundamental, or base, units. Instead of using a lot of zeros in metric conversions, simply change the prefix. Common metric system prefixes include:

$$
\begin{aligned}
\text{kilo} &= 1000 \text{ (k)} \\
\text{hecto} &= 100 \text{ (h)} \\
\text{deka} &= 10 \text{ (D)} \\
\text{Fundamental Unit} &= 1 \text{ (gram, liter, or meter)} \\
\text{deci} &= 1/10 \text{ or } 0.1 \text{ (d)} \\
\text{centi} &= 1/100 \text{ or } 0.01 \text{ (c)}
\end{aligned}
$$

$$\text{milli} = 1/1000 \text{ or } 0.001 \text{ (m)}$$
$$\text{micro} = 1/1,000,000 \text{ or } 0.000001 \text{ (µ)}$$

The most common prefixes in prehospital care include: kilo-, centi-, milli-, and micro-.

Metric Conversions   To change a prefix, move the decimal point the indicated number of places left or right. The following are common examples of metric conversions.

$$1,000 \text{ liters} = 1 \text{ kiloliter}$$
$$1,000 \text{ grams} = 1 \text{ kilogram}$$
$$1/1000 \text{ gram} = 1 \text{ milligram } (0.001 \text{ gram} = 1 \text{ milligram})$$
$$1/100 \text{ meter} = 1 \text{ centimeter } (0.01 \text{ meter} = 1 \text{ centimeter})$$

Multiplication of decimals is easily accomplished by moving the decimal point. For example, when multiplying a decimal by 10, move the decimal one place to the right (see below).

$$10 \text{ milliliters} \times 10 = 100 \text{ milliliters}$$
$$0.1 \text{ centimeter} \times 10 = 1 \text{ centimeter}$$

When multiplying a decimal by 100, simply move the decimal point two places to the right (see below).

$$10 \text{ liters} \times 100 = 1,000 \text{ liters}$$
$$0.01 \text{ milliliter} \times 100 = 1 \text{ milliliter}$$

To divide a decimal, simply move the decimal point the indicated number of places to the left. For example, to divide a decimal by 10, move the decimal point one place to the left (see below).

$$1 \text{ liter} \div 10 = 0.1 \text{ liter}$$
$$100 \text{ centimeters} \div 10 = 10 \text{ centimeters}$$

To divide by 100, simply move the decimal point two places to the left. For example:

$$1000 \text{ milligrams} \div 100 = 10 \text{ milligrams}$$
$$10 \text{ milliliters} \div 100 = 0.1 \text{ milliliter}$$

Conversion between cubic centimeters and milliliters is often used in medicine. One milliliter of water occupies 1 cubic centimeter of space. The conversion appears as follows. [Milliliter (mL) is replacing "cubic centimeter" (cc) as the preferred term.]

$$1 \text{ cubic centimeter } (cm^3) = 1 \text{ milliliter (mL)}$$

Occasionally, orders will be received for certain drugs in the old apothecary's system. The most common apothecary measure likely to be seen is the grain. Some physicians still prescribe certain medications, such as analgesics, in grains. The conversion appears as follows.

$$1 \text{ grain} = 60 \text{ milligrams}$$
$$\text{thus}$$
$$1/4 \text{ grain} = 15 \text{ milligrams}$$

The English system of weights and measures is generally used by the lay public. To bring the metric system into perspective, below are some common conversions.

$$
\begin{aligned}
1 \text{ centimeter} &= 0.39 \text{ inches} \\
1 \text{ meter} &= 39.37 \text{ inches} \\
1 \text{ liter} &= 1.05 \text{ quarts} \\
1 \text{ kilogram} &= 2.2 \text{ pounds} \\
2.54 \text{ centimeters} &= 1 \text{ inch}
\end{aligned}
$$

Drug Dosage Calculations   Most medications are provided in stock solutions. Paramedics, as well as other health care workers, must calculate the quantity of medication to be administered. There are several methods for accomplishing this. This text will present a simple method that works for all prehospital applications.

When preparing to administer a medication to a patient, you will usually have the following information available.

1. *The desired dose.* The desired dose is the quantity of medication or fluid the medical control physician wants administered to the patient. This is usually expressed in milligrams, grams, or grains.
2. *The concentration of the drug on hand.* The concentration of the drug on hand is the amount of the drug present in the ampule or vial. This is usually expressed in milligrams, grams, or grains. It is found on the label.
3. *The volume of the drug on hand.* The volume of the drug on hand is the amount of fluid within the ampule or vial in which the drug is dissolved. This is usually represented in milliliters. It is also found on the label.

Based on these three pieces of information, you can calculate the volume of the drug to be administered. The following formula represents this relationship.

$$
\text{Volume administered } (X) = \frac{(\text{Volume on hand}) (\text{Desired dose})}{\text{Concentration on hand}}
$$

Example 1. A physician wants 5 milligrams of a medication administered to a patient. The ampule contains 10 milligrams of the drug in 2 milliliters of solvent. The following calculation can then be made.

$$
\text{Volume administered} = \frac{\text{Volume on hand (2 mL)} \times \text{Desired dose (5 mg)}}{\text{Concentration on hand (10 mg)}}
$$

To solve, multiply:

$$
X = \frac{(2 \text{ mL})(5 \text{ mg})}{(10 \text{ mg})}
$$

Thus:

$$
X = \frac{10}{10}
$$

Then:

$$
X = 1 \text{ mL}
$$

Example 2. A physician wants a patient to receive 75 milligrams of lidocaine administered in a bolus. The drug is supplied in prefilled syringes that contain 100 milligrams of the drug in 5 milliliters of solvent. To calculate the number of milliliters to be administered, perform the following computations.

$$X = \frac{(5 \text{ mL}) (75 \text{ mg})}{100 \text{ mg}}$$

Thus:

$$X = \frac{375}{100}$$

Then:

$$X = 3.75 \text{ mL}$$

This formula works for all drug calculations routinely used in prehospital care, but it only works if all measurements are in the same units.

Variations on a Theme. The above formula is useful for calculating the infusion rate of IV drips. All you must do is multiply X, the volume to be administered, by the drops per milliliter delivered by the set that you are using. The result will be the number of drops per minute that must be delivered.

Example 3. A physician wants 2 milligrams per minute of lidocaine administered to a patient. She orders 2 grams of lidocaine to be placed in 500 milliliters of 5 percent dextrose in water. A minidrip administration set that delivers 60 drops per milliliter is being used. The problem can be solved as follows.

$$\frac{(500 \text{ mL}) (2 \text{ mg/minute})}{2000 \text{ mg}} \times 60 \text{ drops/mL} = X \text{ drops/minute}$$

$$\frac{1000}{2000} = 0.5 \times 60 \text{ drops/mL} = 30 \text{ drops/minute}$$

Other Calculations. Occasionally, an order will be received to administer a medication based on the patient's weight. The drug dosage must be calculated based upon the patient's weight. It can then be plugged into the formula.

Example 4. A physician wants a patient to receive 5 milligrams per kilogram of a medication. The patient weighs 220 pounds. The medication is supplied in an ampule containing 500 milligrams of the drug in 10 milliliters of solvent. How many milliliters of the drug should be administered?

In order to solve this problem, you must make two preliminary calculations. First, convert the patient's weight to kilograms. Second, multiply the number of milligrams per kilogram to be administered. The calculation appears as follows.

1. *Convert the patient's weight to kilograms:*
   220 pounds ÷ 2.2 pounds/kilogram = 100 kilograms
2. *Calculate the desired dose:*
   100 kilograms × 5 milligrams/kilogram = 500 milligrams
3. *Calculate the volume to be administered:*

$$X = \frac{(10 \text{ mL})(500 \text{ mg})}{500 \text{ mg}}$$

Then:

$$X = \frac{5000}{500}$$

Thus:

$$X = 10 \text{ mL}$$

Frequent practice is essential to mastering drug dosage calculations. You should practice these computations routinely during paramedic training and after graduation. There are sample problems in the accompanying workbook. Review them periodically.

Medication Administration Routes

In prehospital care, medications must be administered promptly, in the correct dose, and by the correct route. If given by an inappropriate route, many drugs can be fatal. This section will detail the common methods of medication administration used in prehospital care.

✱ Remember the five "Rights" of correct medication administration:
• The *Right* drug
• The *Right* dose
• The *Right* route
• The *Right* patient
• The *Right* time

General Administration Routes
The two primary channels for getting medications into the body are through the digestive tract and by parenteral routes. Most critical-care medications are administered parenterally because the onset of action is much quicker and more predictable.

Parenteral Routes.   Any method of drug administration that does not involve passage through the digestive tract is termed parenteral. Parenteral routes include:

❑ *Intradermal.* Drugs can be injected into the dermal layer of the skin. The amount of medication that can be administered by this route is limited and systemic absorption is very slow. Generally, this route is reserved for diagnostic skin testing, such as allergy testing or tuberculin skin tests.

❑ *Transdermal.* Several medications are now available that can be placed on the skin and absorbed into the circulatory system through the skin. Medications available in this form include nitroglycerin, blood pressure medications, and hormone preparations.

❑ *Subcutaneous.* With subcutaneous administration, medications are injected directly into the fatty, subcutaneous tissue under the skin that overlies the muscle. Absorption from this route is slow, resulting in a delayed onset of action and prolonged effect. (See Procedure 13-1.)

❑ *Intramuscular.* The most commonly used route of parenteral medication administration in general medical practice is the intramuscular route. The drug is injected into the muscle tissue, from which it is absorbed into the bloodstream. (See Figure 13-16.) This method of administration has a predictable rate of absorption, but its onset of action is considerably slower than with intravenous administration. (See Procedure 13-2.)

❑ *Intravenous.* The majority of medications used in prehospital care are administered by the intravenous route. Injection can be in the form of an intravenous bolus (see Procedure 13-3) or as a slow intravenous infusion, sometimes referred to as a "piggyback" infusion (see Procedure 13-4). The rate of absorption is rapid and predictable. However, of the routes frequently employed, intravenous administration of drugs has the most potential for causing adverse reactions.

❑ *Endotracheal.* When an IV cannot be started, it is often possible to administer emergency medications through an endotracheal tube, which permits absorption into the pulmonary capillaries of the lungs. It has been documented that this route of medication administration has a rate of absorption almost as fast as the intravenous route for certain drugs.

   The dose of medications administered by the endotracheal route should be 2 to 2.5 times the recommended IV dose. In addition, the medication should be diluted in 10 mL of normal saline and sprayed quickly down the endotracheal tube. Several quick ventilations should be given to aerosolize the medication and enhance absorption. Ideally, a small catheter should be passed beyond the tip of the endotracheal tube and the medication administered through the catheter. If CPR is underway, compressions should be stopped before administration of the medication and resumed after ventilation and nebulization of the medication.

Drugs that can be administered endotracheally include naloxone, atropine, epinephrine, and lidocaine. Diazepam (Valium) is not water soluble and thus cannot be diluted in the field. Because of this, endotracheal administration of diazepam is not recommended. (See Procedure 13-5.)

❑ *Intraosseous injection.* Placement of intraosseous (into the bone) lines, particularly in critically-ill pediatric patients, has become a common practice when IV access is not readily available. Fluids and drugs administered by the intraosseous route quickly enter the circulatory system. Thus, the intraosseous administration of emergency medications is an alternative when IV access cannot be obtained. The intraosseous dose of a medication is the same as the intravenous dose. (See Procedure 13-6.)

❑ *Inhalation.* Many modern respiratory medications can be administered by inhalation. This is advantageous because inhalation delivers the medication directly to the site of action. Inhaled medications can be administered by metered-dose inhalers, small volume nebulizers, or Rotohalers. The inhalational administration of medications is detailed in Chapter 20.

❑ *Sublingual injection.* In the rare instance when neither an IV nor an endotracheal tube can be used, certain drugs can be injected into the vast capillary network immediately under the tongue. Lidocaine and epinephrine are the most common examples.

❑ *Intracardiac.* Injection of medication directly into the ventricle of the heart is referred to as intracardiac injection. It is seldom used because there are inherent complications, such as pericardial tamponade and laceration of the coronary vessels, as well as a lack of documented effectiveness of the procedure.

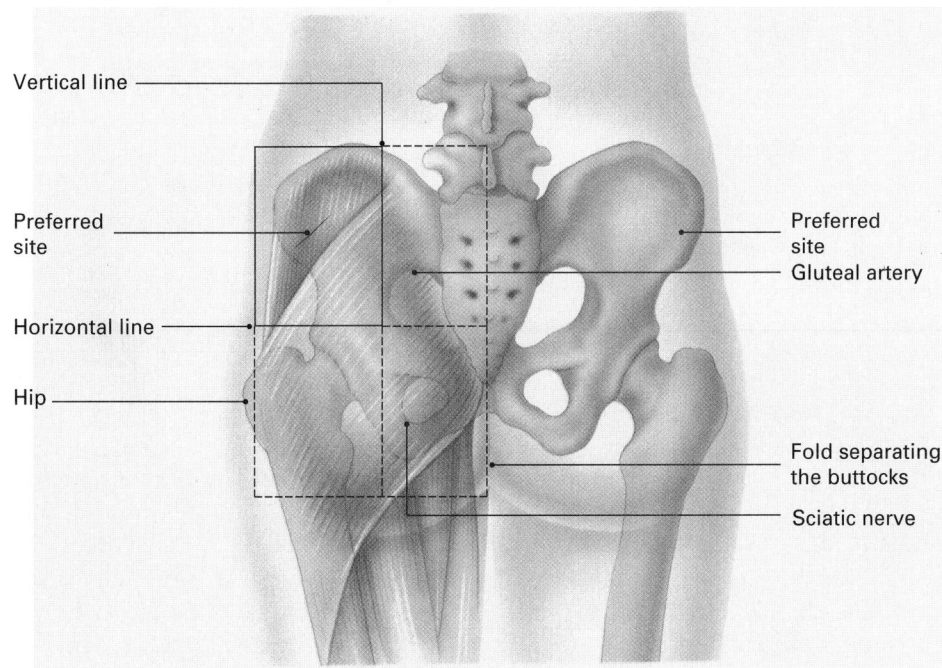

Vertical line

Preferred site

Horizontal line

Hip

Preferred site
Gluteal artery

Fold separating the buttocks

Sciatic nerve

FIGURE 13-16 Desired placement for intramuscular medications in the prehospital setting.

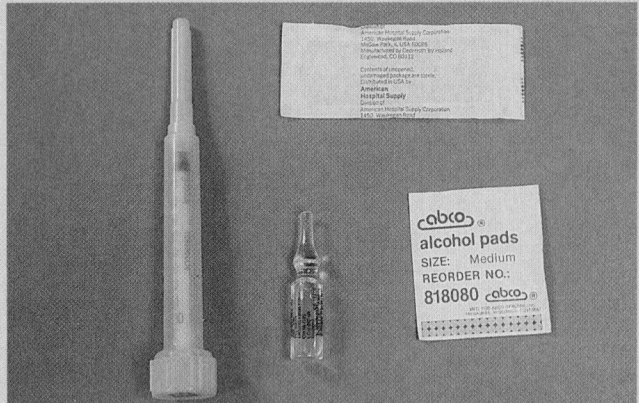

13-1A.   Prepare the equipment.

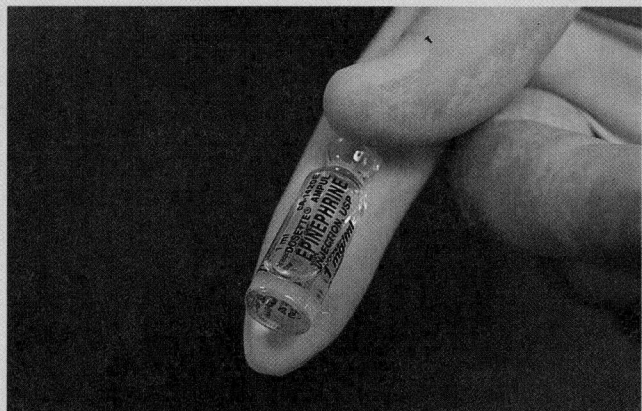

13-1B.   Check the medication.

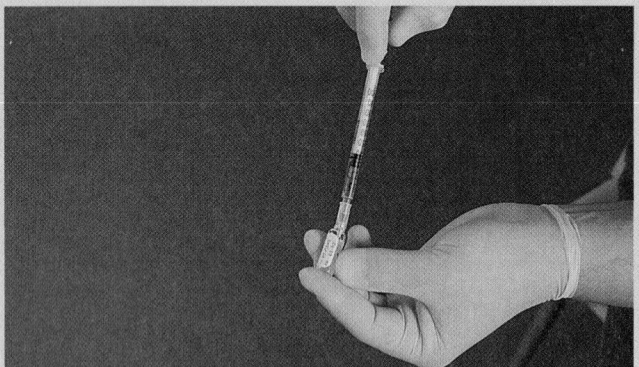

13-1C.   Draw up the medication.

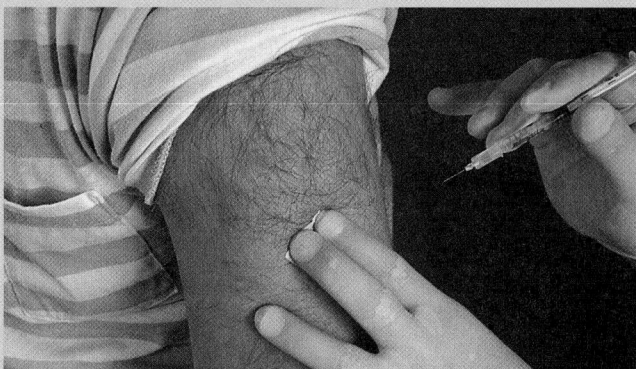

13-1D.   Prep the site.

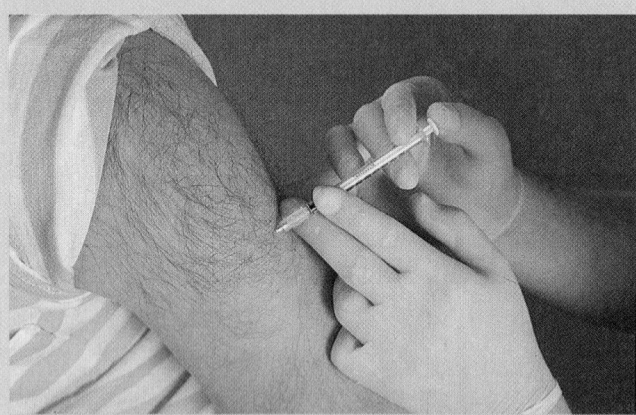

13-1E.   Insert the needle at a 45-degree angle.

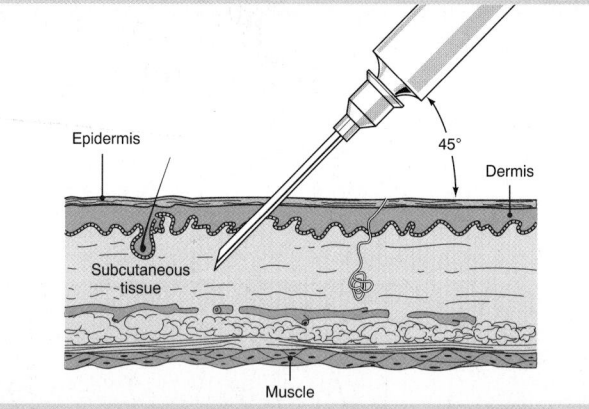

13-1F.   The needle should enter the subcutaneous tissue.

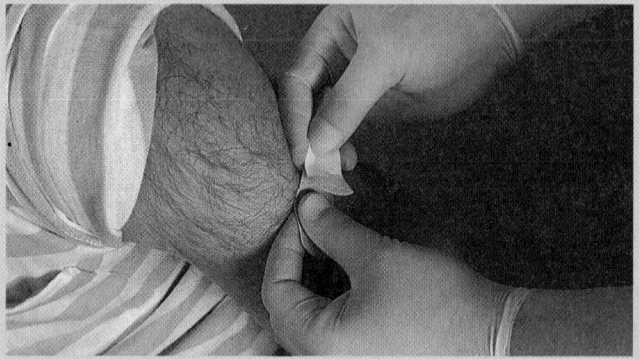

13-1G.   Remove the needle and cover the puncture site.

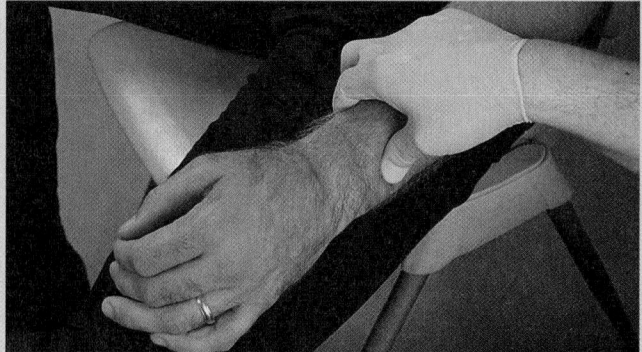

13-1H.   Monitor the patient.

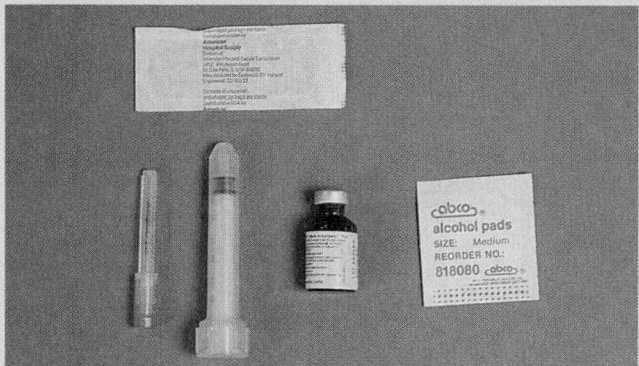

13-2A. Prepare the equipment.

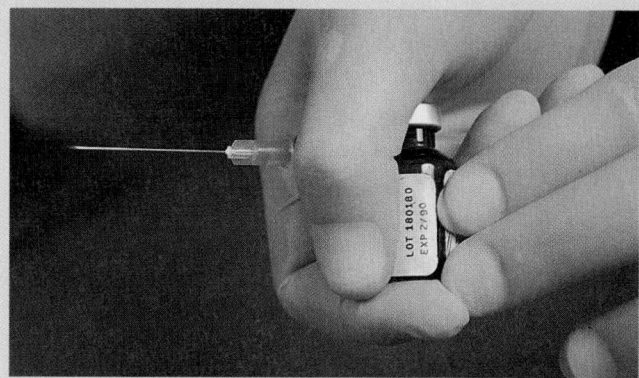

13-2B. Check the medication.

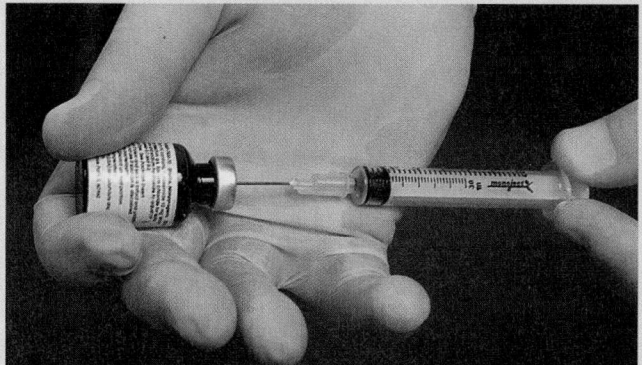

13-2C. Draw up the medication.

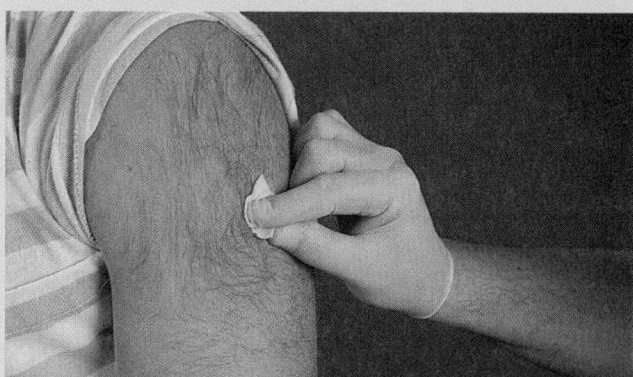

13-2D. Prep the site.

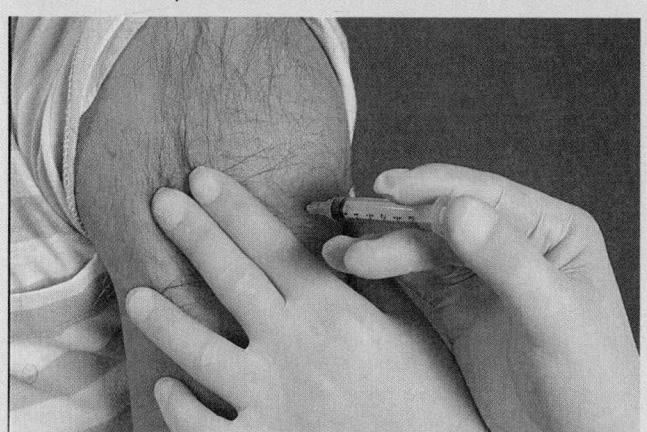

13-2E. Insert the needle at a 90-degree angle.

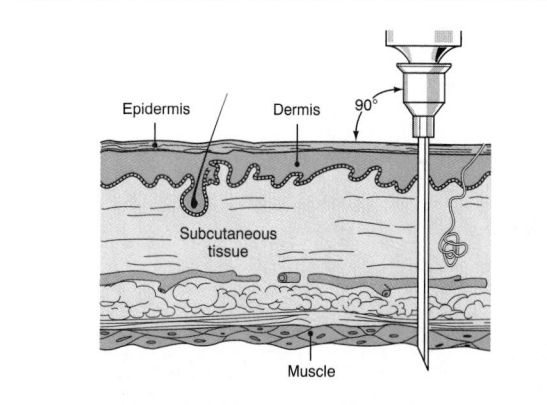

13-2F. The needle should enter muscle tissue. Aspirate to ensure that a blood vessel has not been entered. Inject medication.

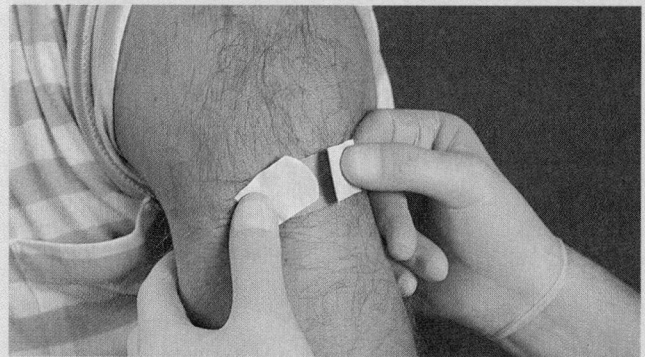

13-2G. Remove the needle, and cover the puncture site.

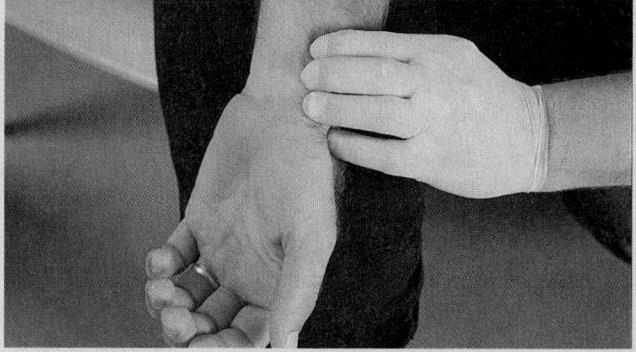

13-2H. Monitor the patient.

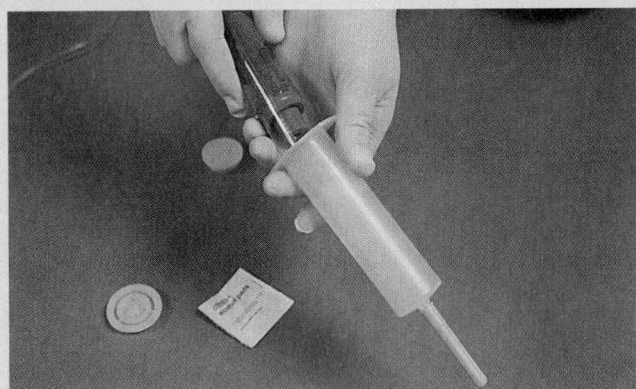

13-3A. Prepare the equipment.

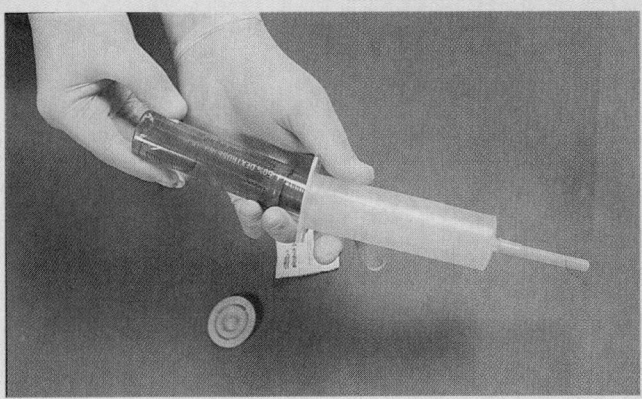

13-3B. Prepare the medication.

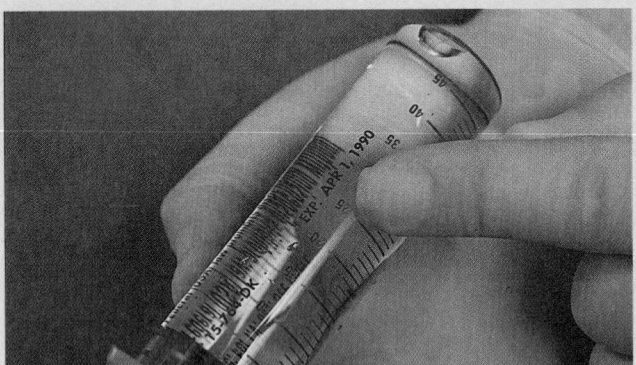

13-3C. Check the label.

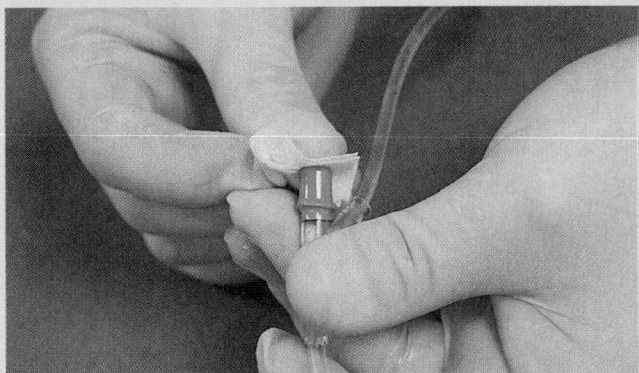

13-3D. Select and clean an administration port.

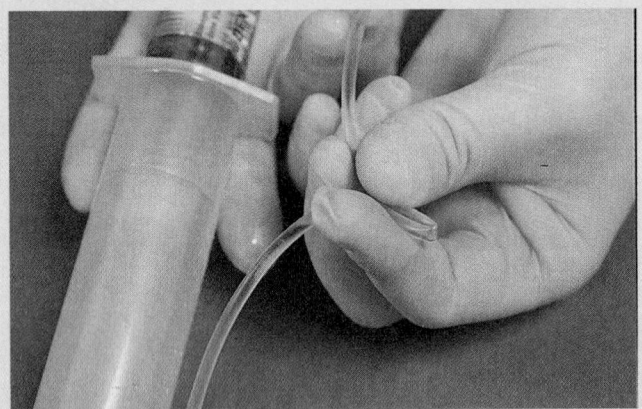

13-3E. Pinch the line.

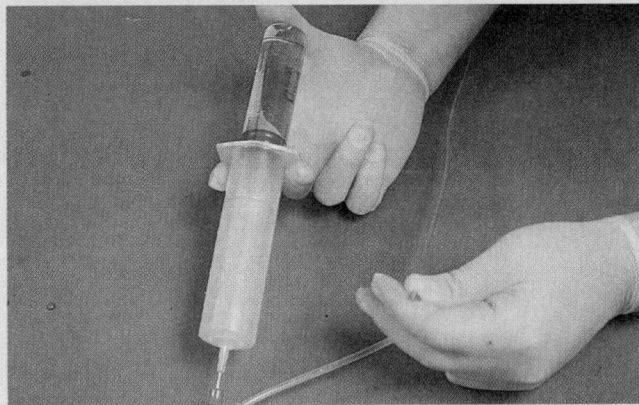

13-3F. Administer the medication.

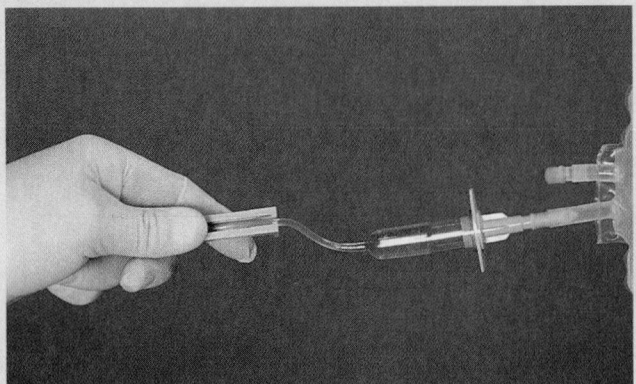

13-3G. Adjust the IV flow rate.

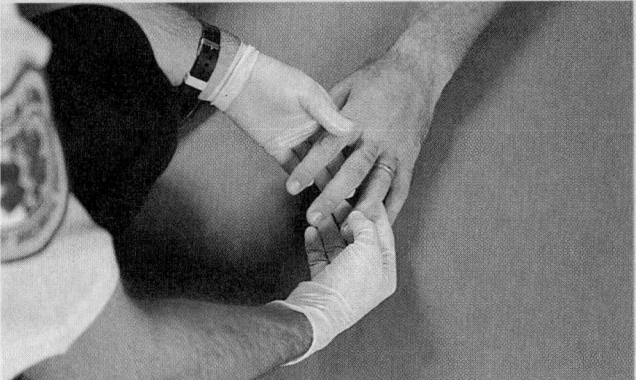

13-3H. Monitor the patient.

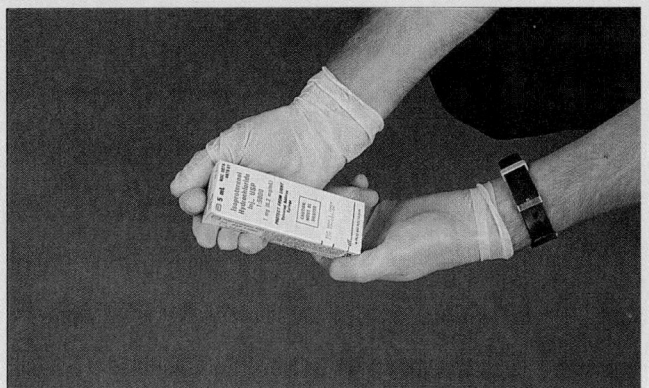

13-4A. Select the drug.

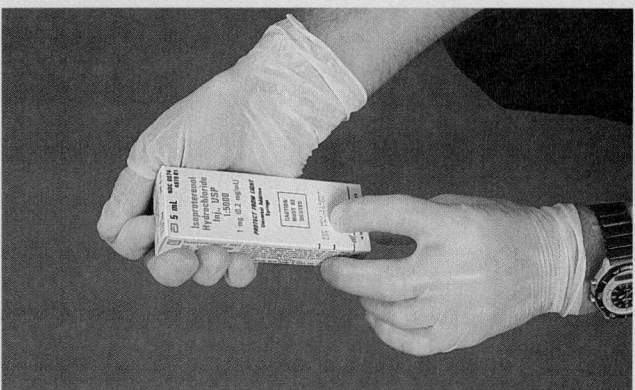

13-4B. Check the label.

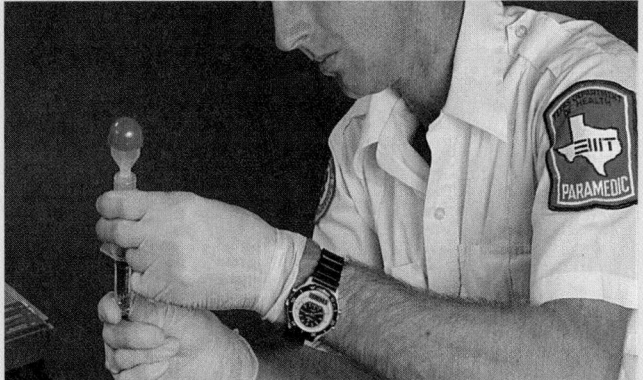

13-4C. Draw up the drug.

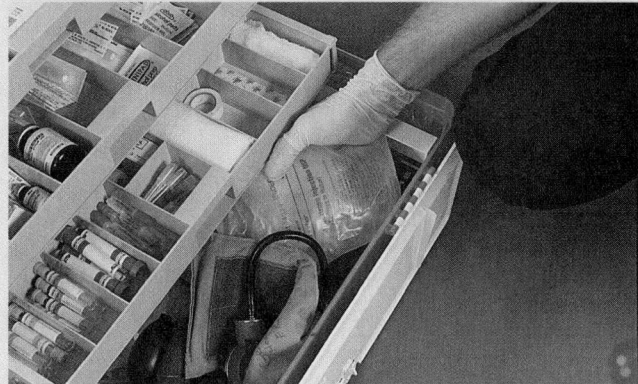

13-4D. Select IV fluid for dilution.

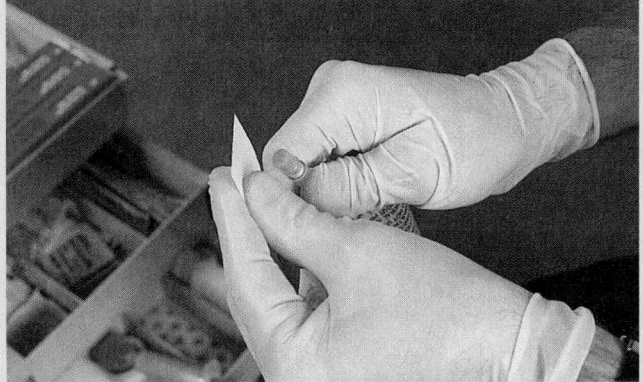

13-4E. Clean the medication addition port.

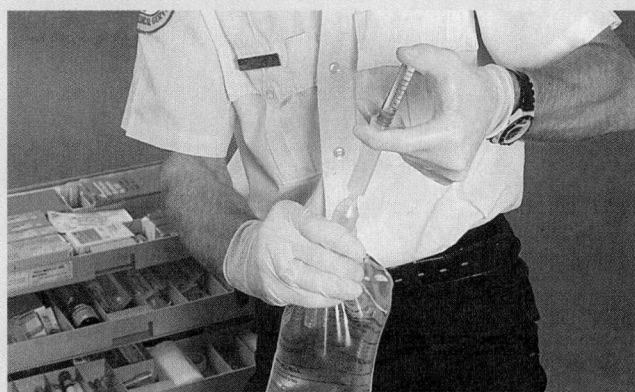

13-4F. Inject the drug into the fluid.

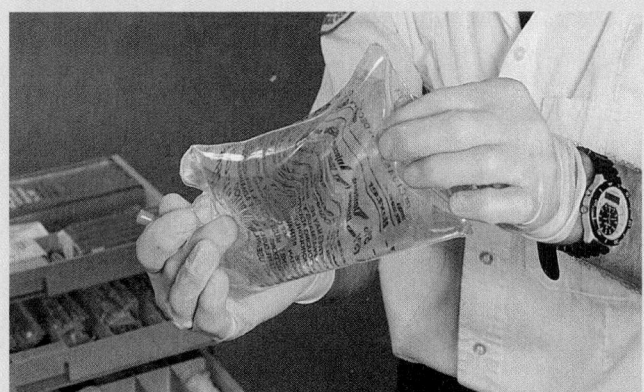

13-4G. Mix the solution.

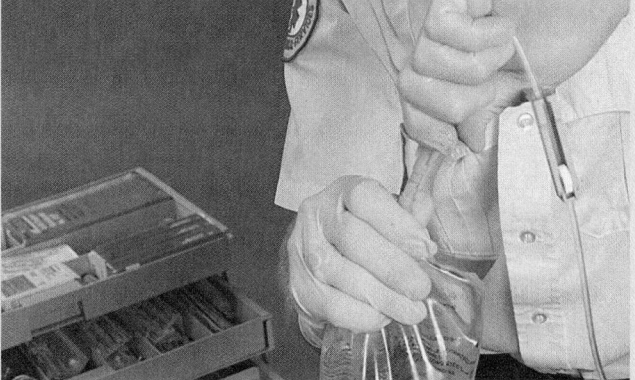

13-4H. Insert an administration set, and connect to main IV line with needle.

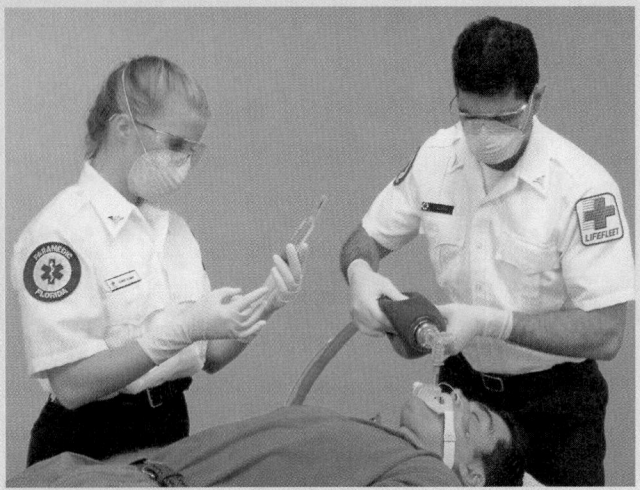

13-5A. Hyperventilate the patient.

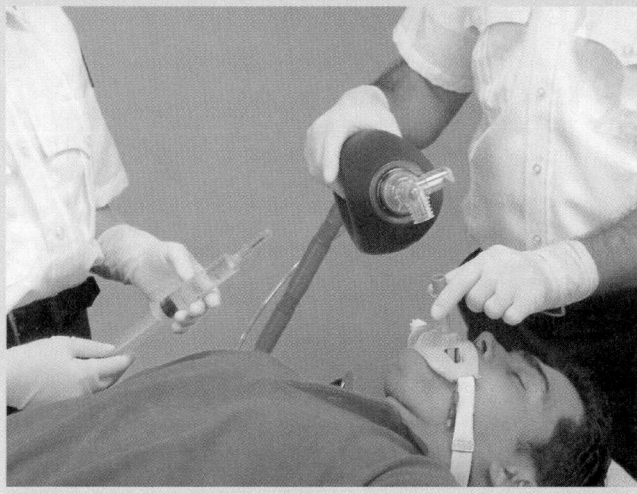

13-5B. Disconnect the ventilation device.

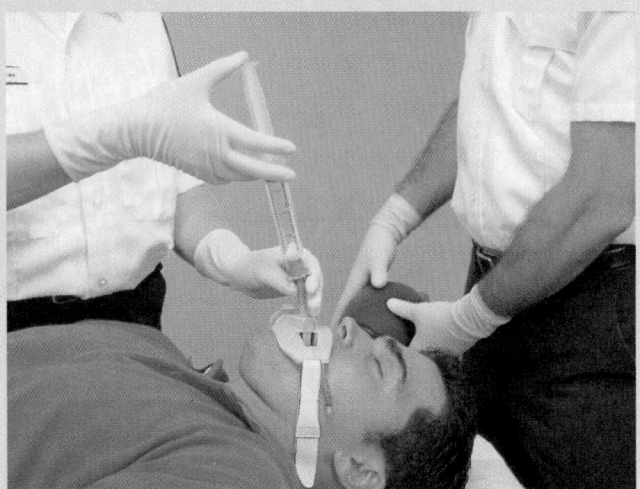

13-5C. Administer the drug.

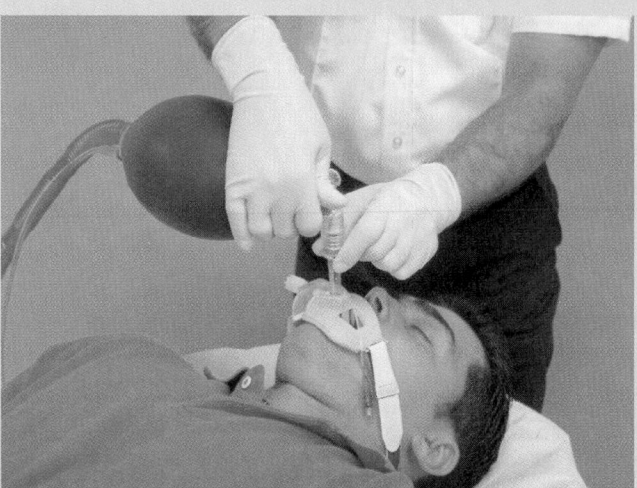

13-5D. Reconnect the ventilation device.

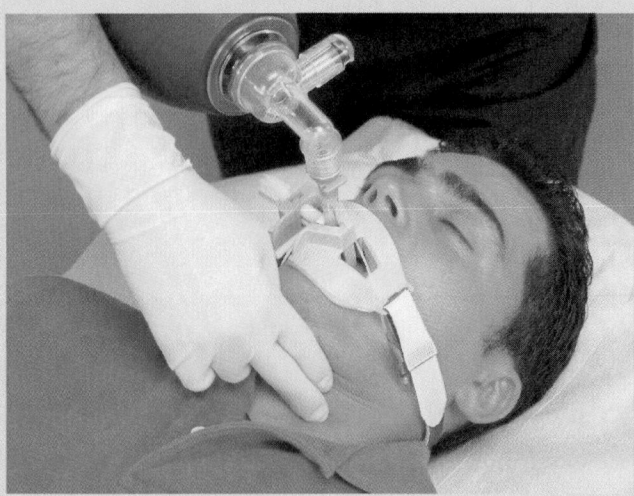

13-5E. Monitor the patient.

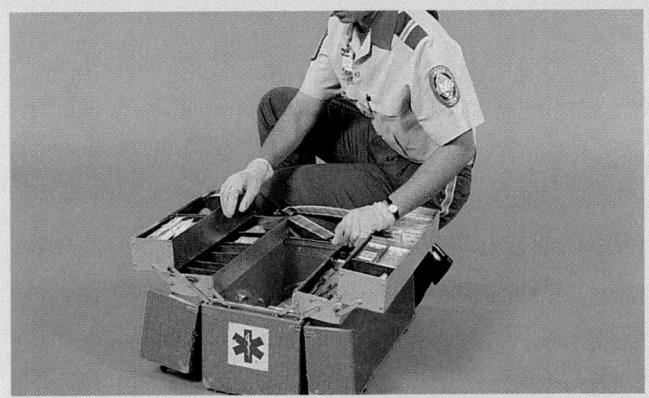

13-6A. Select the medication, and prepare equipment.

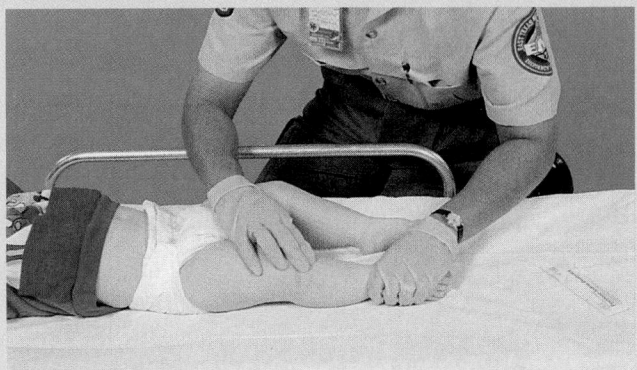

13-6B. Palpate the puncture site, and prep with an antiseptic solution.

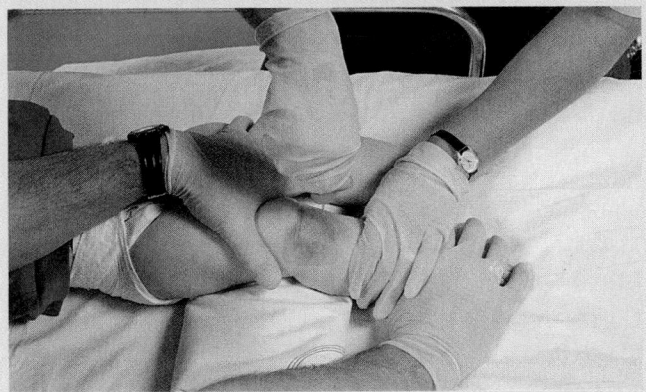

13-6C. Make the puncture.

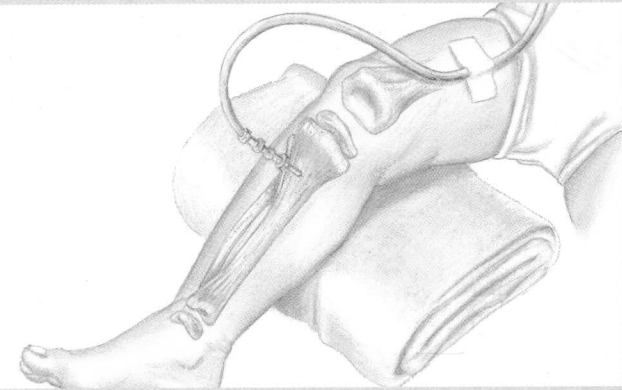

13-6D. Intraosseous needle properly placed.

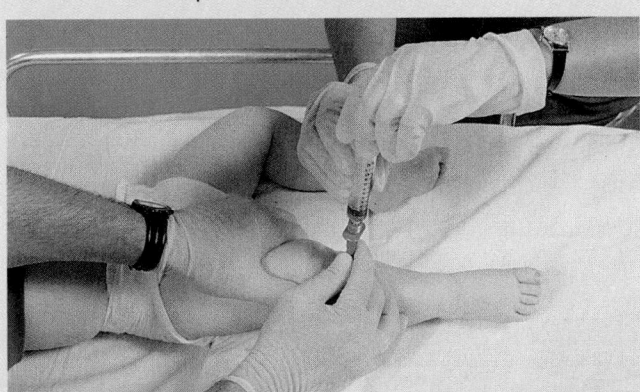

13-6E. Aspirate to confirm proper placement.

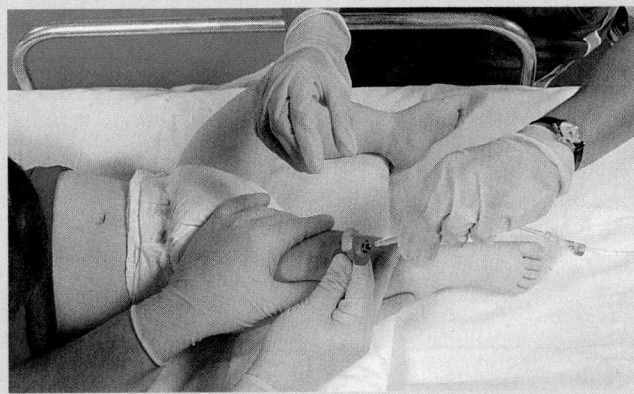

13-6F. Connect the IV fluid tubing.

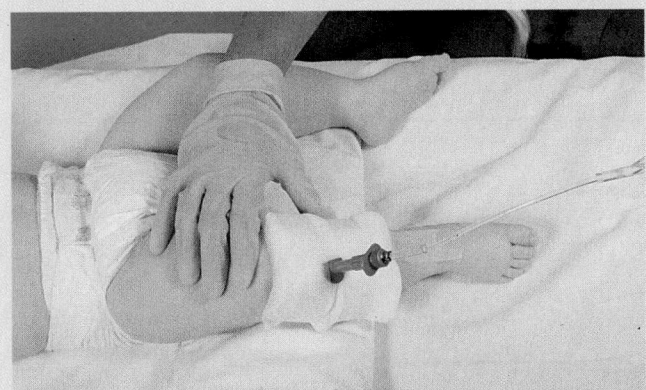

13-6G. Secure the needle appropriately.

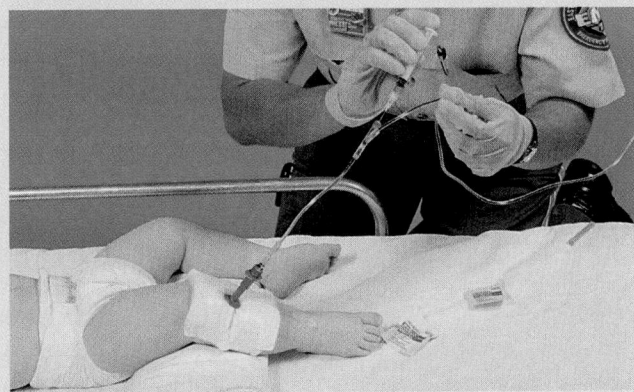

13-6H. Administer the medication. Monitor the patient for effects.

Enteral Routes. Very few medications used in prehospital care are administered into the digestive tract. Common methods of enteral medication administration include:

❑ *Sublingual.* Certain emergency medications, such as nitroglycerin and nifedipine (Procardia), can be placed under the tongue for rapid absorption into the capillary bed. The sublingual route is better for these medications, because intravenous nitrates are difficult to administer and nifedipine is not available in parenteral form.

❑ *Oral.* The most convenient way of administering medication is by mouth. Medications used in prehospital care that are administered orally include syrup of ipecac and activated charcoal.

❑ *Rectal.* Several emergency medications can be administered rectally. The medications are absorbed from the rectum into the circulatory system. The anticonvulsant medications diazepam and lorazepam can be administered rectally to a seizure patient if an IV cannot be established nor an endotracheal tube placed.

General Precautions When preparing medications for administration, keep the following precautions in mind.

❑ Concentrate on the task.
❑ Assure that the medical control physician understands the situation.
❑ Assure that the medical control physician's orders are clearly understood.
❑ Repeat orders back to the medical control physician to confirm them before administering the medication.
❑ Read drug labels carefully.
❑ Check the expiration date of the medication.
❑ Double-check all calculations before administration.
❑ Use correct, properly operating equipment.
❑ Adhere to body substance isolation precautions.
❑ Use aseptic techniques.
❑ Check for incompatibility problems.
❑ Monitor the patient for the desired effects, as well as any unexpected side effects.

DRUGS USED IN PREHOSPITAL CARE

Many medications are available for use in prehospital care to treat a great variety of emergencies. This section will detail the common emergency medications used in prehospital care.

Drug Index

activated charcoal, p. 396
adenosine (Adenocard), p. 374
albuterol (Proventil) (Ventolin), p. 387
aminophylline (Somophyllin), p. 385
atropine sulfate, p. 376
bretylium tosylate (Bretylol), p. 372
calcium chloride, p. 383
dextrose, 50 percent in water, p. 389

diazepam (Valium), p. 391
diphenhydramine (Benadryl), p. 395
dobutamine (Dobutrex), p. 366
dopamine (Intropin), p. 365
epinephrine 1:1,000, p. 384
epinephrine 1:10,000, p. 362
furosemide (Lasix), p. 380
glucagon, p. 390

haloperidol (Haldol), p. 398
ipratropium (Atrovent), p. 388
labetalol (Trandate) (Normodyne),
    p. 368
lidocaine (Xylocaine), p. 369
magnesium sulfate, p. 394
methylprednisolone (Solu-Medrol),
    p. 392
morphine sulfate, p. 378
nalaxone (Narcan), p. 397
nifedipine (Procardia) (Adalat), p. 382
nitroglycerin (Nitrostat), p. 381
nitrous oxide (Nitronox), p. 379

norepinephrine (Levophed), p. 363
oxygen, p. 361
oxytocin (Pitocin), p. 393
procainamide (Pronestyl), p. 371
promethazine (Phenergan), p. 398
racemic epinephrine (microNEFRIN)
    (Vaponefrin), p. 386
sodium bicarbonate, p. 377
syrup of ipecac, p. 395
thiamine, p. 390
terbutaline (Brethine) (Bricanyl), p. 387
verapamil (Isoptin) (Calan), p. 375

Drugs Used in Cardiovascular Emergencies

By far, the majority of medications used in prehospital care involve the treatment of cardiovascular emergencies. These medications include oxygen, sympathomimetics, antidysrhythmics, parasympatholytics, analgesics, and others.

oxygen

Class: Gas

Description. Oxygen is an odorless, tasteless, colorless gas necessary for life.

Mechanism of Action. Oxygen enters the body through the respiratory system and is transported to the cells by hemoglobin, found in the red cells. Oxygen is required for the efficient breakdown of glucose into a usable energy form. Its onset of action following administration is immediate. The administration of enriched oxygen increases the oxygen concentration in the alveoli, which subsequently increases the oxygen saturation of available hemoglobin.

Indications

❑ *Hypoxia.* Oxygen is indicated whenever hypoxia is suspected or possible. This includes all forms of trauma, medical emergencies, chest pain that may be due to cardiac ischemia, any respiratory difficulty, during labor and delivery, and in any critical patient.

✱ Never withhold oxygen from a hypoxic patient.

Contraindications. There are no contraindications to oxygen. NEVER DEPRIVE THE HYPOXIC PATIENT OF OXYGEN FOR FEAR OF RESPIRATORY DEPRESSION.

Precautions. Oxygen should be used cautiously in patients with chronic obstructive pulmonary disease (COPD). In these patients, respirations may be regulated by the level of oxygen in the blood (hypoxic drive) instead of carbon dioxide. In some cases, COPD patients may suffer respiratory depression if high concentrations of oxygen are delivered.

The administration of high concentrations of oxygen to neonates for a prolonged period of time can damage the infant's eyes (retrolental fibroplasia). Although this is rarely a problem in prehospital care, it is a consideration in long distance and prolonged transport.

Oxygen delivered at a flow rate of 6 liters per minute or greater should be humidified to prevent drying of the mucous membranes of the upper respiratory system.

When possible, oxygen administration should be monitored by use of pulse oximetry. The pulse oximeter is a non-invasive device that accurately measures the oxygen saturation of hemoglobin. It is relatively inexpensive, easy to apply, and quite accurate in detecting oxygen delivery problems.

Side Effects. There are few, if any side effects associated with oxygen administration. Prolonged administration of high-flow, non-humidified oxygen may result in drying of the mucous membranes resulting in irritation and possibly nose bleeds.

Interactions. There are no interactions associated with oxygen administration. However, oxygen may increase the toxicity of certain herbicides (e.g., paraquat, diaquat) in patients who have ingested these poisons. These chemicals are sometimes sprayed on illicit agricultural products such as marijuana. Poisoning by these agents is uncommon.

Dosage. The dosage of oxygen is based on the patient's underlying problems. In the prehospital setting, oxygen should be administered at the highest concentration available. Pulse oximetry, if available, should be used to guide care. General guidelines follow:

❑ *Cardiac arrest and other critical patients*—100%
❑ *Chronic obstructive pulmonary disease*—35% (increase as needed)

Pediatric Dosage. 24–100% as required

How Supplied. Oxygen is supplied in pressurized cylinders of varying size. Liquid oxygen is becoming more common in prehospital care. The sizes and types of liquid oxygen containers varies.

The Sympathomimetics
The term *sympathomimetic* means to mimic the actions of the sympathetic nervous system. Drugs in this group will either act directly on receptors of the sympathetic nervous system or indirectly by stimulating the release of endogenous catecholamines. *Catecholamine* is the name used to describe several chemically similar drugs that act upon the sympathetic nervous system.

---

epinephrine 1:10,000

Class: Sympathetic agonist

Description. Epinephrine is a naturally occurring catecholamine. It is a potent α and β adrenergic stimulant, however its effect on β receptors is more profound.

Mechanism of Action. Epinephrine acts directly on α and β adrenergic receptors. Its effect on β receptors is much more profound than its effect on α receptors. The effects of epinephrine include:

❑ Increased heart rate
❑ Increased cardiac contractile force
❑ Increased electrical activity in the myocardium
❑ Increased systemic vascular resistance
❑ Increased blood pressure
❑ Increased automaticity

> ✱ Epinephrine increases the rate and force of the cardiac contraction and causes peripheral vasoconstriction.

Epinephrine can stimulate spontaneous firing of myocardial conductive cells. In the emergency setting, it is used to convert fine ventricular fibrillation to coarse ventricular fibrillation. This change significantly increases the chances of successful electrical defibrillation. In asystole, it is used to initiate electrical activity in the myocardium. Once initiated, electrical defibrillation may be attempted.

Epinephrine's effects usually appear within 90 seconds of administration, and they are usually of short duration. Therefore, it must be administered every 3–5 minutes to maintain therapeutic levels.

Indications

❑ Cardiac arrest (asystole, ventricular fibrillation, pulseless ventricular tachycardia, pulseless electrical activity)
❑ Severe anaphylaxis
❑ Severe reactive airway disease

Contraindications. Epinephrine 1:10,000 is contraindicated in patients who do not require extensive cardiopulmonary resuscitative efforts. With simple allergic reactions and asthma, the 1:1000 dilution should be used and is administered subcutaneously.

Precautions. Epinephrine, like all catecholamines, should be protected from light. It can be deactivated by alkaline solutions such as sodium bicarbonate. Because of this, it is essential that the IV line is adequately flushed between the administration of epinephrine and sodium bicarbonate.

Side Effects. Epinephrine can cause palpitations, anxiety, tremulousness, headache, dizziness, nausea and vomiting. Because of its strong **inotropic** and **chronotropic** properties, epinephrine increases myocardial oxygen demand. Even in low doses it can cause myocardial ischemia. When administering epinephrine in the emergency setting, these effects should be kept in mind. Like most of the other drugs used in emergency medicine, epinephrine is only effective when the myocardium is adequately oxygenated.

■ **inotropic** affecting the contractile force of the heart.

■ **chronotropic** affecting heart rate.

Interactions. Epinephrine is pH dependent and can be deactivated when administered with highly alkaline solutions such as sodium bicarbonate. The effects of epinephrine can be intensified in patients who are taking anti-depressants.

Dosage. Epinephrine 1:10,000 can be administered intravenously, intraosseously, or endotracheally. Common doses include:

❑ *Cardiac arrest (adults)*. The dose of epinephrine in cardiac arrest is 0.5 to 1.0 milligram of a 1:10,000 solution intravenously. This can be repeated every 3–5 minutes as required. Higher dosages may be ordered by medical control and are potentially helpful in the cardiac arrest setting. If an IV cannot be started, epinephrine can be administered endotracheally. The endotracheal dose should be increased at least 2 to 2.5 times the intravenous dose.

❑ *Cardiac arrest (children)*. The initial dose of epinephrine in pediatric cardiac arrest is 0.01 mg/kg of a 1:10,000 solution intravenously (0.1 ml/kg). Second and subsequent doses should be 0.1 mg/kg of a 1:1,000 solution intravenously (0.1 ml/kg). The second and subsequent dose is ten times the initial dose. The total volume of drug administered remains the same, as epinephrine 1:1,000 is used instead of epinephrine 1:10,000.

❑ *Severe anaphylaxis/severe asthma (adult)*. Intravenous epinephrine should only be used for life-threatening, severe anaphylaxis and severe asthma. Less severe cases should be treated with epinephrine 1:1,000 subcutaneously or another β agonist. In severe anaphylaxis/asthma the initial dose should be 0.3–0.5 milligram intravenously. The dose may be repeated every 5–15 minutes as required. An epinephrine drip may be required in severe cases.

❑ *Severe anaphylaxis/severe asthma (children)*. Intravenous epinephrine should only be used for life-threatening, severe anaphylaxis and severe asthma. Less severe cases should be treated with epinephrine 1:1,000 subcutaneously or another agonist. In severe anaphylaxis/asthma the initial dose should be 0.01 mg/kg intravenously. The dose may be repeated every 5–15 minutes as required. An epinephrine drip may be required in severe cases.

Pediatric Dosage. 0.01 mg/kg

How Supplied. Epinephrine 1:10,000 comes in prefilled syringes containing 1 milligram of the drug in 10 milliliters of solvent.

norepinephrine (Levophed)

Class: Sympathetic agonist

Description. Norepinephrine is a naturally occurring catecholamine. It acts on both α and β adrenergic receptors. However, its action on α receptors is more profound.

✱ Norepinephrine is primarily a vasoconstrictor with mild to moderate cardiac effects.

Mechanism of Action. Because of its action on α receptors, norepinephrine is a potent peripheral vasoconstrictor. This vasoconstriction serves to increase blood pressure in cardiogenic shock and other hypotensive emergencies. Because norepinephrine also tends to constrict the renal and mesenteric blood vessels, it is reserved for emergencies where dopamine may not be effective. As a rule, dopamine, which maintains renal and mesenteric perfusion, is the preferred vasopressor for treating cardiogenic shock.

Indications

❑ Hypotension (systolic blood pressure < 70 mmHg) refractory to other sympathomimetics
❑ Neurogenic shock

Contraindications. Norepinephrine should not be given to patients who are hypotensive from hypovolemia.

Precautions. Because of the powerful effects of norepinephrine, it is essential to measure the blood pressure every 5 to 10 minutes to prevent dangerously high blood pressures. Norepinephrine should be given through the largest vein readily available because it may cause local tissue necrosis if it extravasates. Phentolamine (Regitine) can be diluted in saline and infiltrated into the area of extravasation to help minimize necrosis and sloughing.

Like the other sympathomimetics, norepinephrine can increase myocardial oxygen demand. It should be used with caution in persons suffering from cardiac ischemia.

Side Effects. Norepinephrine can cause anxiety, tremulousness, headache, dizziness, nausea, and vomiting. It can also cause bradycardia as a reflex response to increased peripheral vasoconstriction. Because of its inotropic and chronotropic properties, norepinephrine increases myocardial oxygen demand. Even in low doses it can cause myocardial ischemia. When administering norepinephrine in the emergency setting, these effects should be kept in mind.

Interactions. Norepinephrine can be deactivated by alkaline solutions such as sodium bicarbonate. Concomitant administration with beta blockers can result in markedly elevated blood pressure.

Dosage. The current dosage recommended by the American Heart Association for norepinephrine is 0.5 to 30 micrograms per minute. Higher doses may be required to maintain adequate blood pressure. The best dilution is attained by placing 8 milligrams in 500 milliliters of D5W. This will give a concentration of 16 micrograms per milliliter. The same concentration can be attained by placing 4 milligrams in 250 milliliters of D5W. (See Figure 13-17.)

Because of its potency, norepinephrine is given only in extremely diluted IV infusions. To control its administration, it should be "piggybacked" into an already established IV line.

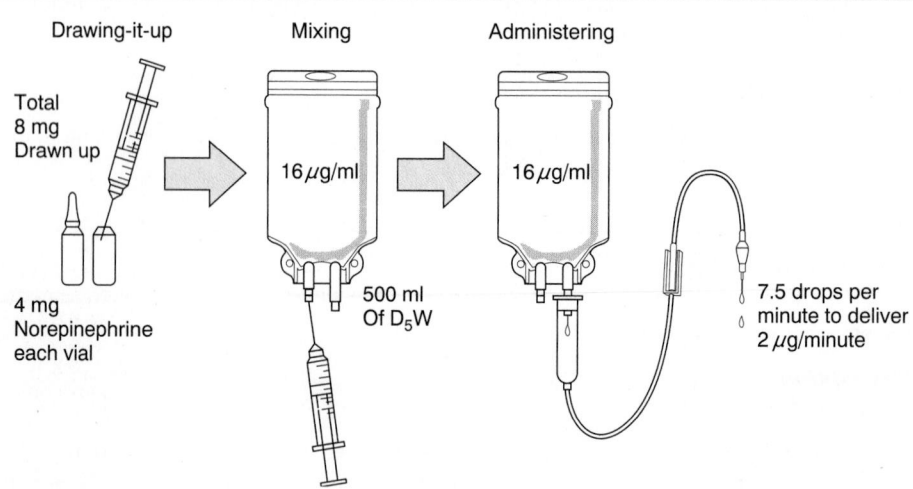

Drawing-it-up   Mixing   Administering

Total
8 mg
Drawn up

16 µg/ml   16 µg/ml

4 mg
Norepinephrine
each vial

500 ml
Of D₅W

7.5 drops per
minute to deliver
2 µg/minute

FIGURE 13-17 Preparation of norepinephrine infusion.

Pediatric Dosage. 0.01–0.5 µg/kg/min (rarely used)

How Supplied. Norepinephrine is supplied in 4-milliliter ampules containing 4 milligrams of the drug.

dopamine (Intropin)

Class: Sympathetic agonist

Description. Dopamine is a naturally occurring catecholamine. It is a chemical precursor of norepinephrine. It acts on α, β₁, and dopaminergic adrenergic receptors. Its affects on α receptors is dose-dependent.

Mechanism of Action. Dopamine is one of the most frequently used agents in the treatment of hypotension associated with cardiogenic shock. It is chemically related to both epinephrine and norepinephrine and increases blood pressure by acting on both α and $β_1$ adrenergic receptors. Dopamine's effect on $β_1$ receptors causes a positive inotropic effect on the heart. It does not increase myocardial oxygen demand as much as isoproterenol and epinephrine and does not have the same powerful chronotropic effects. Dopamine also acts on α adrenergic receptors causing peripheral vasoconstriction. Unlike norepinephrine, when used in therapeutic dosages, dopamine maintains renal and mesenteric blood flow because of its effect on the dopaminergic receptors. For these reasons, dopamine is the most commonly used vasopressor. Dopamine will increase both the systolic blood pressure and the pulse pressure (the difference between the systolic and diastolic blood pressures), but as a rule, there is usually less effect on the diastolic pressure.

✱ Dopamine increases cardiac contractile force and thus cardiac output. It is the drug of choice for the management of cardiogenic shock.

Indications

- ❑ Hemodynamically significant hypotension (systolic blood pressure of 70–100 mmHg) not resulting from hypovolemia.
- ❑ Cardiogenic shock

Contraindications. Dopamine should not be used as the sole agent in the management of hypovolemic shock unless fluid resuscitation is well under way. Dopamine should not be used in patients with pheochromocytoma (a tumor of the adrenal gland).

Precautions. Dopamine will increase the heart rate and can induce or worsen supraventricular and ventricular arrhythmias. Whenever the dosage of dopamine surpasses 20 micrograms/kilogram/minute, its α effects predominate and it functions very much like norepinephrine. Dopamine, like the other catecholamines, should not be administered in the presence of tachyarrhythmias or ventricular fibrillation.

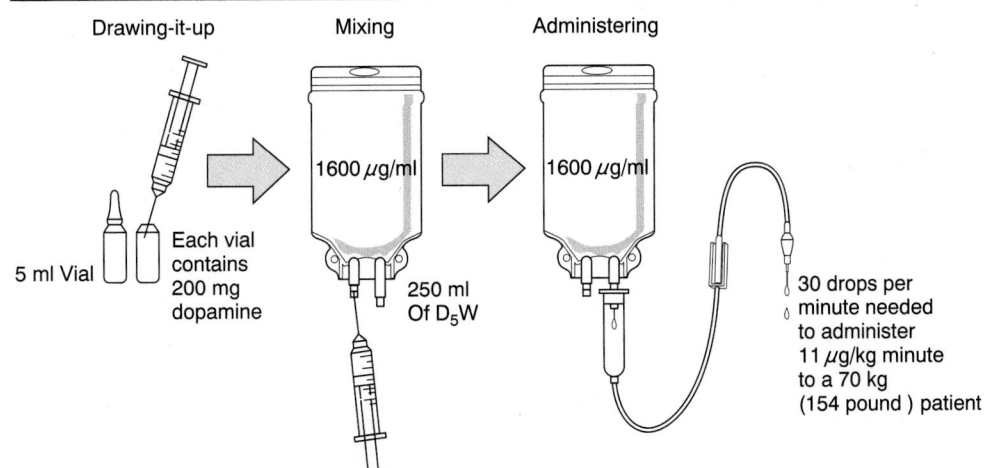

FIGURE 13-18 Preparation of dopamine infusion.

TABLE 13-1 Intropin (Dopamine HC) Dosage Phenomena

The Effects of Intropin at Three Dose Ranges	2–5 mcg/kg/min	5–20 mcg/kg/min	>20 mcg/kg/min
Cardiac output	no change	increase	increase
Stroke volume	no change	increase	increase
Heart rate	no change	there is an initial increase followed by a decrease toward normal rates as infusion continues	
Myocardial contractility	no change	increase	increase
Potential for excessive myocardial oxygen demands	low* coronary blood flow increased	low* coronary blood flow increased	data unavailable
Potential for tachyarrhythmias	low*	low*	moderate
Total systemic vascular resistance	slight decrease to no change	no change to slight increase	increase
Renal blood flow	increase	increase	decrease**
Urine output	increase	increase	decrease**

* Low but needs monitoring
** Relative to peak values achieved at lower dosages.
© 1981 American Critical Care, Division of American Hospital Supply Corporation
(Courtesy of American Critical Care, Division of American Hospital Supply Corporation, McGaw Park, Illinois, 1983)

Side Effects. Dopamine can cause nervousness, headache, dysrhythmias, palpitations, chest pain, dyspnea, nausea, and vomiting. Many of these side effects are dose-related.

Interactions. Like all of the catecholamines, dopamine can be deactivated by alkaline solutions such as sodium bicarbonate. If the patient is taking monoamine oxidase inhibitors (a type of antidepressant), the dose should then be reduced. Dopamine may cause hypotension when used concomitantly with phenytoin (Dilantin).

Dosage. The standard method of preparing a dopamine infusion is to place 800 milligrams in 500 milliliters of D5W. This dilution can be attained by adding 400 milligrams to 250 milliliters of D5W. This gives a concentration of 1600 micrograms per milliliter. The effects of dopamine are dose dependent. Table 13-1 illustrates effects based on common dosages.

The initial infusion rate is from 2 to 5 micrograms per kilogram per minute. This may be increased until blood pressure improves. (See Figure 13-18.) Dopamine is administered only by IV drip, which should be piggybacked into an already established IV infusion.

Pediatric Dosage. 2–20 μg/kg/min

How Supplied. Dopamine comes in prefilled syringes, ampules, and pre-mixed bags. The standard preparation is 200 milligrams in 5 milliliters of solvent; 400 milligram preparations in 5 milliliters of solvent are also available.

dobutamine (Dobutrex)

Class: Sympathetic agonist

Description. Dobutamine is a synthetic catecholamine. It acts primarily on β_1 receptors but is less of a β agonist than isoproterenol.

Mechanism of Action. Dobutamine increases the force of the systolic contraction (positive inotropic effect) with little chronotropic activity. For these reasons, it is useful in the management of congestive heart failure when an increase in heart rate is not desired.

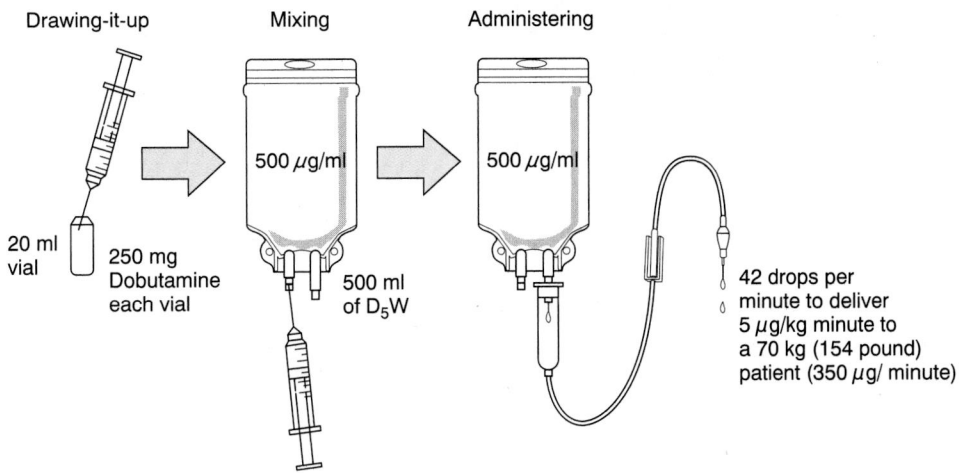

Drawing-it-up

Mixing

Administering

20 ml
vial

250 mg
Dobutamine
each vial

500 μg/ml

500 ml
of D₅W

500 μg/ml

42 drops per
minute to deliver
5 μg/kg minute to
a 70 kg (154 pound)
patient (350 μg/ minute)

FIGURE 13-19   Preparation of dobutamine infusion.

Indications

❑ Short-term management of congestive heart failure when an increased cardiac output, without an increase in cardiac rate, is desired

Contraindications.   Dobutamine should not be used as the sole agent in hypovolemic shock unless fluid resuscitation is well under way. To increase cardiac output in severe emergencies like cardiogenic shock, dopamine is the preferred agent.

Precautions.   Tachycardia and an increase in the systolic blood pressure are common following the administration of dobutamine. Increases in heart rate of more than 10 percent may induce or exacerbate myocardial ischemia. Premature ventricular contractions (PVCs) can occur in conjunction with dobutamine administration. Lidocaine should be readily available. As with any sympathomimetic, blood pressure should be monitored.

Side Effects.   Dobutamine can cause nervousness, headache, hypertension, dysrhythmias, palpitations, chest pain, dyspnea, nausea, and vomiting. Many of these side effects are dose-related.

Interactions.   Dobutamine may be ineffective when administered to patients on beta blockers as these medications can block the β receptors on which dobutamine acts. Patients taking tricyclic antidepressants are at increased risk of hypertension with dobutamine administration.

Dosage.   The desired dosage range for dobutamine is between 2 and 20 micrograms per kilogram per minute. Dobutamine should be administered according to the patient's response. (See Figure 13-19.)

Dobutamine should be diluted in either 500 milliliters or 1 liter of D5W and administered via IV infusion.

Pediatric Dosage.   2–20 μg/kg/min

How Supplied.   Dobutamine is supplied in 20-milliliter ampules containing 250 milligrams of the drug. 250 milligrams are usually placed in 500 milliliters of solvent to give a concentration of 0.5 milligram (500 micrograms) per milliliter.

The Sympathetic Blockers

Sympathetic blockers are a unique class of drugs that antagonize (block) adrenergic receptor sites. Certain drugs will block only α receptors, while others block only β receptors. Some of the β blockers are so selective that they block only $β_1$ or $β_2$ receptors. The drugs that block the β receptors are used the most.

labetalol (Trandate) (Normodyne)

Class: Non-selective beta blocker

Description.   Labetalol is a non-selective β blocker and a selective α_1 blocker.

Mechanism of Action.   Labetalol differs considerably in its action from the β blockers previously presented. Like propranolol, labetalol is a nonselective β adrenergic antagonist showing no preference for either β_1 or β_2 receptors. However, unlike the other β blockers, labetalol also blocks α_1 adrenergic receptors. Blockage of α_1 receptors inhibits peripheral vasoconstriction, thus causing peripheral vasodilatation. Because of these properties, labetalol is a potent agent for lowering blood pressure in cases of hypertensive crisis. It does this by decreasing cardiac output through its β_1 blocking properties and by causing peripheral vasodilation through its α_1 blocking properties.

Indications.   Labetalol is indicated for the acute management of hypertensive crisis.

Contraindications.   Labetalol is contraindicated in patients with bronchial asthma, congestive heart failure, heart block, bradycardia, or cardiogenic shock.

Precautions.   As with all β blockers the blood pressure, pulse rate, ECG, and respiratory status should be continuously monitored. Prehospital personnel should be alert for signs and symptoms of congestive heart failure, bradycardia, shock, heart block, or bronchospasm when administering labetalol. The appearance of any of these signs or symptoms is an indication for discontinuing the drug.

Because of the effects of labetalol on β_1 receptors, postural hypotension might occur and should be anticipated. The patient should be supine at all times during drug administration.

Side Effects.   Labetalol may cause bradycardia, hypotension, lethargy, congestive heart failure, dyspnea, wheezing, and weakness.

Interactions.   Labetalol should not be administered to patients who have received intravenous verapamil. It should be administered with caution to patients on antihypertensive agents.

Dosage.   The following are two accepted methods of administering labetalol in the treatment of hypertensive crisis:

1. Twenty milligrams of labetalol can be administered by slow IV injection over 2 minutes. Immediately before the injection and at 5 and 10 minutes after the injection the supine blood pressure should be recorded. Additional injections of

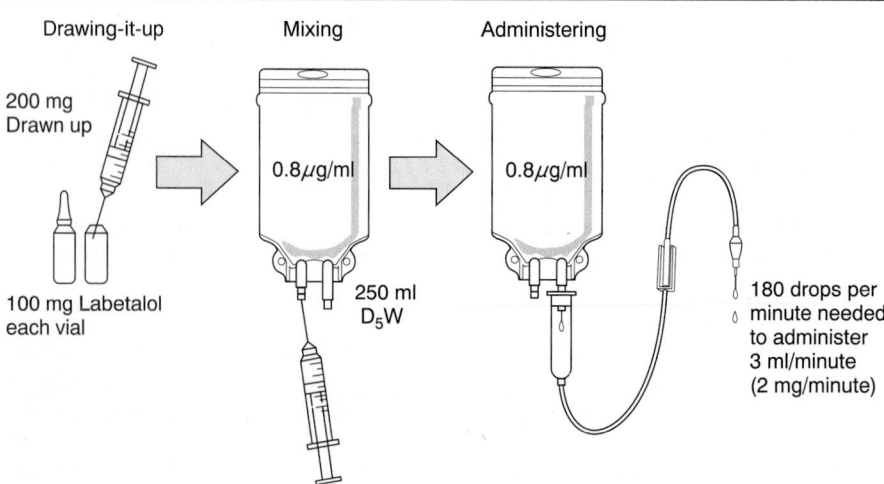

FIGURE 13-20   Preparation of labetalol infusion.

40 milligrams can be given every 10 minutes until a desired supine blood pressure is achieved or 300 milligrams of the drug has been given.

2. Two ampules (200 milligrams) of labetalol can be added to 250 milliliters of D5W. This gives a concentration of 0.8 milligram per milliliter. This solution should be administered at a rate of 2 milligrams per minute (2.5 milliliters per minute). The blood pressure should be continuously monitored. (See Figure 13-20.)

Labetalol should be administered by slow IV injection or infusion as described above.

Pediatric Dosage. Safety in children has not been established.

How Supplied. Labetalol (Trandate, Normodyne) is supplied in ampules containing 100 milligrams in 20 milliliters of solvent (5 milligrams per milliliter).

The Antidysrhythmics
Many drugs are useful in the treatment and prevention of cardiac dysrhythmias. Some are useful in the treatment of atrial dysrhythmias, while others are useful in the treatment of ventricular dysrhythmias. It is essential to distinguish between ventricular and atrial dysrhythmias.

lidocaine (Xylocaine)

Class: Antiarrhythmic

Description. Lidocaine is an amide-type local anesthetic. It is frequently used to treat life-threatening ventricular dysrhythmias.

Mechanism of Action. Lidocaine is probably the most frequently used antiarrhythmic agent in the treatment of life-threatening cardiac emergencies. Moreover, it has been shown to be effective in suppressing premature ventricular contractions, treating ventricular tachycardia and some cases of ventricular fibrillation, and in increasing the fibrillation threshold in acute myocardial infarction.

✱ Lidocaine suppresses ventricular ectopic activity and is thus useful in the treatment of many ventricular dysrhythmias.

Lidocaine depresses depolarization and automaticity in the ventricles. It has very little effect on atrial tissues. In therapeutic doses it does not slow AV conduction and does not depress myocardial contractility. The most common cause of ventricular arrhythmias is acute myocardial infarction. Lidocaine suppresses ventricular ectopy in the setting of myocardial infarction and increases the ventricular fibrillation threshold. This prevents PVCs from inducing ventricular fibrillation. After acute myocardial infarction, the ventricular fibrillation threshold is often significantly reduced. Moreover, because electrical defibrillation tends to cause ventricular irritability, patients who have been successfully defibrillated should be treated with lidocaine.

Lidocaine is most apt to suppress ventricular arrhythmias only when the level of the drug in the blood is between 1.5 and 6.0 micrograms per milliliter of blood. A 75-milligram to 100-milligram bolus of lidocaine will maintain adequate blood levels for only 20 minutes. (See Figure 13-21.) Therefore, once an arrhythmia is suppressed, the lidocaine bolus should be followed by a 2- to 4-milligrams-per-minute infusion to assure therapeutic blood levels. (See Figure 13-22.) It is important to distinguish patterns of premature ventricular contractions that are likely to lead to serious arrhythmias. Premature ventricular contractions that may lead to life-threatening arrhythmias are called "malignant premature ventricular contractions." These include the following:

❑ More than six unifocal PVCs per minute
❑ PVCs that appear to be coming from more than one ectopic focus (for example, multifocal PVCs)
❑ PVCs that occur in couplets (two PVCs together without a normal QRS complex in between)
❑ Runs of more than two PVCs, or ventricular tachycardia PVCs falling in the vulnerable period of the preceding normal complex (R on T phenomena)

The aforementioned premature ventricular contractions, as well as ventricular tachycardia and ventricular fibrillation, must be treated vigorously with lidocaine.

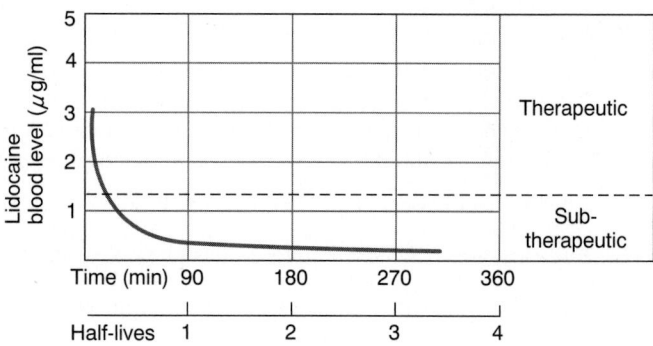

FIGURE 13-21 Blood levels of lidocaine following bolus alone.

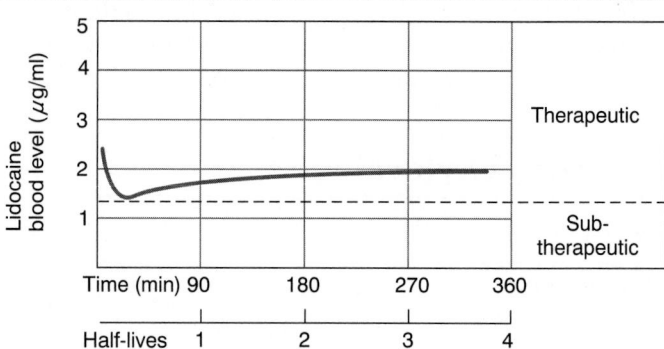

FIGURE 13-22 Blood levels of lidocaine following bolus and continuous infusion.

Indications

❑ Ventricular tachycardia
❑ Ventricular fibrillation
❑ Malignant premature ventricular contractions

Contraindications. Lidocaine is usually contraindicated in second-degree Mobitz II and third-degree blocks. Lidocaine slows conduction of the electrical impulse from the atria to the ventricles. Decreased ventricular rates may accompany high-grade heart block, resulting in escape beats that are premature ventricular contractions. Whenever premature ventricular contractions occur in conjunction with bradycardia (heart rate less than 60), the bradycardia should be treated first. The drug of choice is atropine sulfate followed by external pacing if atropine is not effective. If PVCs are still present after increasing the rate, lidocaine should be administered.

Precautions. Central nervous system depression may occur when the dosage exceeds 300 milligrams per hour. Symptoms of central nervous system depression include a decreased level of consciousness, irritability, confusion, muscle twitching, and, eventually, seizures. Exceedingly high doses can result in coma and death.

Routine prophylactic (preventive) lidocaine therapy in patients with acute myocardial infarction is no longer recommended. However, it may be used in conjunction with thrombolytic therapy to suppress expected reperfusion dysrhythmias.

Side Effects. Lidocaine may cause drowsiness, seizures, confusion, hypotension, bradycardia, heart blocks, nausea, vomiting, and respiratory and cardiac arrest.

Interactions. Lidocaine should be used with caution when administering concomitantly with procainamide, phenytoin, quinidine, and β blockers as drug toxicity may result.

Dosage.

❑ *Refractory ventricular fibrillation and pulseless ventricular tachycardia.* The initial dose of lidocaine should be 1.0–1.5 milligram per kilogram body weight. Lidocaine can be repeated every 3–5 minutes at a dose of 0.5–0.75 mg/kg to a

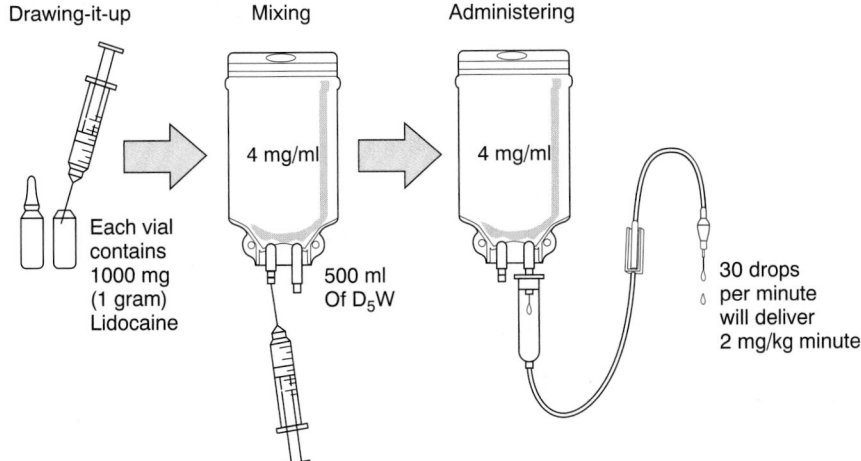

Drawing-it-up   Mixing   Administering

Each vial
contains
1000 mg
(1 gram)
Lidocaine

4 mg/ml

500 ml
Of D$_5$W

4 mg/ml

30 drops
per minute
will deliver
2 mg/kg minute

FIGURE 13-23 Preparation of lidocaine infusion.

maximum of 3.0 mg/kg. A single bolus dose of 1.5 mg/kg in cardiac arrest is generally acceptable, as plasma lidocaine levels will remain therapeutic because of reduced drug elimination during CPR. Only bolus therapy should be used during CPR. Once a patient has been resuscitated, IV infusion therapy can be started to maintain therapeutic blood levels of the drug.

❑ *Ventricular tachycardia with a pulse and malignant PVCs.* The initial dose of lidocaine should be 1.0–1.5 milligram per kilogram. Repeat boluses of 0.5–0.75 mg/kg can be repeated every 5–10 minutes as required to a maximum dose of 3.0 mg/kg. Once the arrhythmia has been suppressed, a lidocaine drip should be initiated at 2–4 mg/minute. The dosage of lidocaine should be reduced 50% in patients over 70 years of age, and in those with known liver disease, heart failure, bradycardias, and conduction disturbances.

Lidocaine is generally given in an IV bolus followed by an infusion. (See Figure 13-23.) It can also be given endotracheally, however, when an IV line cannot be established. The dose should be increased 2 to 2.5 times the intravenous dose when administering it endotracheally. A preparation of lidocaine is also available that can be given intramuscularly for ventricular arrhythmias. This should be reserved for times when an IV line cannot be established, and the patient is not intubated.

Pediatric Dosage. 1 mg/kg

How Supplied. Lidocaine is supplied in the following dosages:

❑ *Prefilled syringes*—100 milligrams in 5 milliliters of solvent 1- and 2-gram additive syringes

❑ *Ampules*—100 milligrams in 5 milliliters of solvent 1- and 2-gram vials (in 30 milliliters of solvent)

❑ *Premixed bags*—Premixed bags containing 1 to 2 grams in 500 milliliters of 5% dextrose.

procainamide (Pronestyl)

Class: Antiarrhythmic

Description. Procainamide is an ester-type local anesthetic. It is frequently used to treat life-threatening ventricular dysrhythmias refractory to lidocaine.

Mechanism of Action. Procainamide is effective in suppressing ventricular ectopy. It may be effective in cases where lidocaine has not suppressed life-threatening ventricular arrhythmias. Procainamide reduces the automaticity of the various pacemaker sites in the heart. Procainamide slows intraventricular conduction to much greater degree than lidocaine.

Indications

❑ Persistent cardiac arrest due to ventricular fibrillation and refractory to lidocaine.

❑ Premature ventricular contractions refractory to lidocaine

❑ Ventricular tachycardia refractory to lidocaine

Contraindications. Procainamide should not be administered to patients with severe conduction system disturbances, especially second- and third-degree heart blocks.

Precautions. Procainamide must not be administered to patients demonstrating PVCs in conjunction with a bradycardia. The heart rate should be first increased with atropine or transcutaneous pacing. Only after increasing the heart rate can the PVCs be treated with lidocaine or procainamide if they persist.

Hypotension is common with intravenous infusion. Constant blood pressure monitoring is essential.

Side Effects. Procainamide may cause drowsiness, seizures, confusion, hypotension, bradycardia, heart blocks, nausea, vomiting, and respiratory and cardiac arrest.

Interactions. The hypotensive effects of procainamide may be increased if administered with antihypertensive drugs. The chances of neurological toxicity by both lidocaine and procainamide increases when the medications are administered together.

Dosage. In treating PVCs or ventricular tachycardia, 100 milligrams should be administered every 5 minutes at a rate of 20 milligrams per minute. This should be discontinued if any of the following occur:

❑ Arrhythmia is suppressed.

❑ Hypotension ensues.

❑ QRS complex is widened by 50 percent of its original width.

❑ A total of 17 mg/kg of the medication has been administered.

The maintenance infusion of procainamide is 1 to 4 milligrams per minute. The duration of procainamide's effect is shorter than lidocaine requiring a more rigorous approach.

Procainamide should be administered by slow IV bolus (20 milligrams per minute) followed by a maintenance infusion. Generally, one gram of procainamide is placed in 500 ml of D5W. This gives a final concentration of 2 mg/ml.

Pediatric Dosage. Rarely used

How Supplied. Procainamide is supplied in the following: 10-milliliter vials containing 1000 milligrams of the drug; 2-milliliter vials containing 1000 milligrams of the drug (for infusion).

bretylium tosylate (Bretylol)

Class: Antiarrhythmic

Description. Bretylium is an antiarrhythmic that exhibits both adrenergic and direct myocardial effects.

* The pharmacological effects of bretylium are often delayed 3–5 minutes or more following administration. Other resuscitative measures should be carried out in the interim.

Mechanism of Action. Bretylium tosylate causes two effects on adrenergic nerve endings. Once administered, bretylium causes release of norepinephrine from adrenergic nerve endings. This causes a slight increase in heart rate, blood pressure, and cardiac output. These sympathomimetic effects last approximately 20 minutes in the non-cardiac-arrest setting. Then, norepinephrine release is inhibited which results in an adrenergic blockade. At this time, hypotension may develop (particularly orthostatic hypotension). Adrenergic blockade usually begins 15–20 minutes after drug administration and lasts for several hours. (See Figure 13-24.) The antiarrhythmic effect of bretylium is poorly understood but it appears that it elevates the ventricular fibrillation threshold much like lidocaine. Bretylium will *sometimes* convert ventricular fibrillation

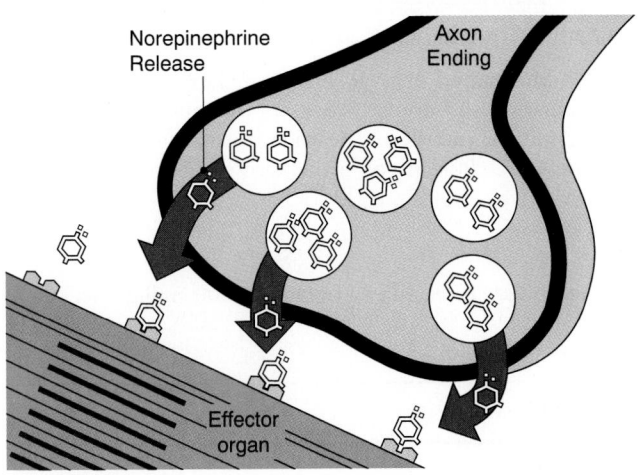

A. Bretylium provokes the release of norepinephrine from the axon ending

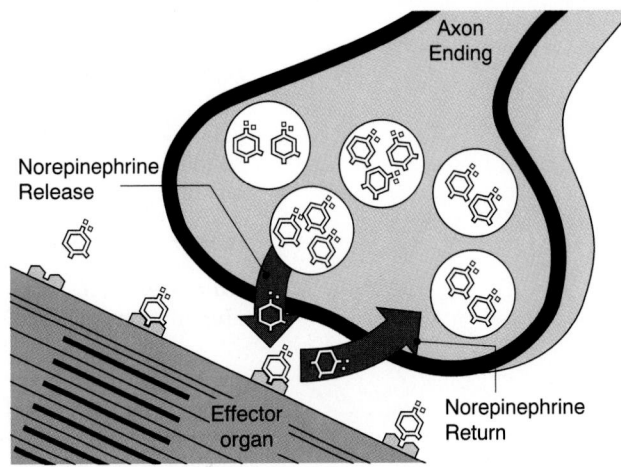

B. Normally norepinephrine is released and then taken back up to the axon ending

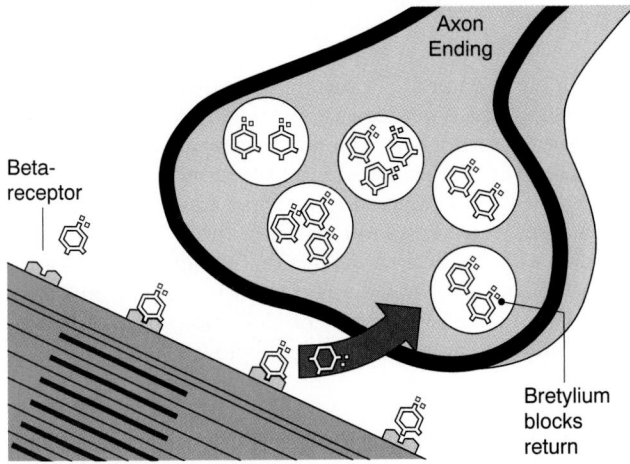

C. Bretylium blocks the return of norepinephrine to axon ending

FIGURE 13-24 Pharmalacological actions of bretylium.

or ventricular tachycardia to a supraventricular rhythm. Because of this action, bretylium is sometimes referred to as a "chemical defibrillator."

Indications

- ❏ Ventricular fibrillation refractory to lidocaine
- ❏ Ventricular tachycardia refractory to lidocaine

At present, bretylium is not considered a first-line antiarrhythmic.

Contraindications. There are no contraindications to bretylium when used in the treatment of life-threatening ventricular arrhythmias.

Precautions. Postural hypotension occurs in approximately 50 percent of the patients receiving bretylium. This side effect should be anticipated, and the patient should be kept in a supine position.

Side Effects. Bretylium may cause dizziness, syncope, seizures, hypotension, hypertension, angina, nausea, and vomiting.

Interactions. Arrhythmias caused by digitalis toxicity may be worsened by the initial release of norepinephrine which accompanies bretylium usage. Bretylium can interact with other antiarrhythmic agents causing antagonistic or additive effects. The hypotensive effects of bretylium may be worsened if administered with Class IA antiarrhythmics such as procainamide, quinidine, or disopyramide.

Dosage. Bretylium should be administered at a dose of 5 milligrams per kilogram body weight. If the arrhythmia persists, subsequent doses of 10 milligrams per kilogram can be administered at five-minute intervals. The total dose should not exceed 30 milligrams per kilogram. Because bretylium is somewhat slow in its onset, it should be administered by IV bolus.

Pediatric Dosage. 5 mg/kg

How Supplied. Bretylium is supplied in ampules containing 500 milligrams of the drug in 10 milliliters of solvent.

adenosine (Adenocard)

Class: Antiarrhythmic

* Adenosine is the drug of choice for treating narrow complex paroxysmal supraventricular tachycardia.

Description. Adenosine is a naturally occurring nucleoside that slows AV conduction through the AV node. It has an exceptionally short half-life and a relatively good safety profile.

Mechanism of Action. Adenosine is a naturally occurring substance (purine nucleoside) that is present in all body cells. Adenosine decreases conduction of the electrical impulse through the AV node and interrupts AV re-entry pathways in paroxysmal supraventricular tachycardia (PSVT). It can effectively terminate rapid supraventricular arrhythmias such as PSVT. The half-life of adenosine is approximately 5 seconds. Because of its rapid onset of action, and very short half-life, the administration of adenosine is sometimes referred to as "chemical cardioversion." A single bolus of the drug was effective in converting PSVT to a normal sinus rhythm in a significant number (90%) of patients in the initial drug studies. Adenosine does not appear to cause hypotension to the same degree as does verapamil (described below).

Indications

■ **Wolff-Parkinson-White** a disorder of the heart characterized by early depolarization of the heart muscle.

❏ PSVT (including that associated with **Wolff-Parkinson-White** syndrome) refractory to common vagal maneuvers.

Contraindications. Adenosine is contraindicated in patients with second- or third-degree heart block, sick sinus syndrome, or those with known hypersensitivity to the drug.

Precautions. Adenosine will typically cause arrhythmias at the time of cardioversion. These will generally last a few seconds or less, and may include PVCs, premature atrial contractions, sinus bradycardia, sinus tachycardia, and various degrees of AV block. In extreme cases, transient asystole may occur. If this occurs, appropriate therapy should be initiated. Adenosine should be used cautiously in patients with asthma.

Side Effects. Adenosine can cause facial flushing, headache, shortness of breath, dizziness, and nausea, among others. Because the half-life of adenosine is so brief, side effects are generally self-limited.

Interactions. Methylxanthines (aminophylline, theophylline) may decrease the effectiveness of adenosine thus requiring larger doses.

Dosage. The initial dose of adenosine is 6 milligrams given as a rapid intravenous bolus over a 1- to 2-second period. To be certain that the drug rapidly reaches the central circulation, it should be given directly into a vein or into a proximal medication port of a functioning IV line. It should be followed immediately by a rapid saline flush.

    If the initial dose does not result in conversion of the PSVT within 1 to 2 minutes, a 12-milligram dose may be given as a rapid IV bolus. The 12-milligram dose may be repeated a second time if required. Doses greater than 12 milligrams should not be administered.

* Adenosine should be administered by rapid IV bolus in the medication port closest to the patient.

    Adenosine should only be given by rapid IV bolus, directly into the vein, or into the medication administration port closest to the patient.

Pediatric Dosage. Safety in children has not been established.

How Supplied. Adenosine (Adenocard) is supplied in vials containing 6 milligrams of the drug in 2 milliliters of saline solvent.

verapamil (Isoptin) (Calan)

Class: Calcium channel blocker

Description. Verapamil is a calcium-ion antagonist (calcium channel blocker). Calcium channel blockers cause a relaxation of vascular smooth muscle and slow conduction through the AV node. Verapamil has a greater effect on conduction and lesser effect on vascular smooth muscle than other agents in the same class.

Mechanism of Action. Verapamil causes vascular dilation and slows conduction through the atrioventricular (AV) node. The advantages of this are twofold. First, verapamil will inhibit arrhythmias caused by a reentry mechanism such as with paroxysmal supraventricular tachycardia. Second, it will decrease the rapid ventricular response seen with atrial tachyarrhythmias such as atrial flutter and fibrillation. Verapamil also reduces myocardial oxygen demand because of its negative inotropic effects and causes coronary and peripheral vasodilation.

> ✳ Verapamil slows AV conduction and is effective in treating supraventricular tachydysrhythmias.

Indications

- ❏ Paroxysmal supraventricular tachycardia (PSVT) refractory to adenosine

Contraindications. Verapamil should not be administered to any patient with severe hypotension or cardiogenic shock. In addition, verapamil should not be administered to patients with ventricular tachycardia in the prehospital setting.

   Before attempting to treat a patient suffering atrial flutter or atrial fibrillation, it is essential that the paramedic assure that the patient does not suffer from Wolff-Parkinson-White syndrome.

Precautions. Verapamil can cause systemic hypotension. Because of this it is essential that the blood pressure be constantly monitored following verapamil administration. Calcium chloride can be used to prevent the hypotensive effects of calcium channel blockers and in the management of calcium channel blocker overdosage.

Side Effects. Verapamil can cause nausea, vomiting, dizziness, headache, bradycardia, heart block, hypotension, and asystole.

Interactions. Verapamil should not be administered to patients receiving intravenous β blockers because of an increased risk of congestive heart failure, bradycardia, and asystole.

Dosage. In the treatment of paroxysmal supraventricular tachycardia, a 2.5- to 5-milligram IV dose should be given initially during a 2- to 3-minute interval. A repeat dose of 5 to 10 milligrams can be given in 15–30 minutes if PSVT persists and there have not been any adverse responses to the initial dose. The total dose of verapamil should not exceed 30 milligrams in 30 minutes.

Pediatric Dosage. *0–1 year:* 0.1–0.2 mg/kg (maximum 2.0 mg) administer slowly; *1–15 years:* 0.1–0.3 mg/kg (maximum 5.0 mg) administer slowly

How Supplied. Verapamil (Isoptin) is supplied in 2-milliliter ampules containing 5 milligrams of the drug.

The Parasympatholytics

Drugs that inhibit the actions of the parasympathetic nervous system are known as parasympatholytics. Sometimes they are referred to as anticholinergics. The parasympathetic nervous system plays a major role in the maintenance of homeostasis. The primary nerve of the parasympathetic nervous system is the vagus nerve, also called the tenth cranial nerve. When stimulated, it causes acetylcholine to be released from the presynaptic nerve endings. Acetylcholine then activates acetylcholine receptors, either on the post-synaptic membrane or on the target organ, such as the heart. This results in slowing of the heart rate and other activities. However, a second compound—*acetylcholinesterase*—is released almost immediately, which deactivates acetylcholine, terminating its effect.

Several medications affect this mechanism. Atropine binds to acetylcholine receptors, blocking the action of acetylcholine. Organophosphates, a common class of insecticides, bind irreversibly to acetylcholinesterase, prolonging the effect of acetylcholine. Pralidoxime (2-PAM), an antidote for organophosphate poisoning, reactivates acetylcholinesterase.

atropine sulfate

Class: Anticholinergic

Description. Atropine is a parasympatholytic (anticholinergic) that is derived from parts of the *Atropa belladonna* plant.

Mechanism of Action. Atropine sulfate is a potent parasympatholytic and is used to increase the heart rate in hemodynamically significant bradycardias. Hemodynamically significant bradycardias are those slow heart rates accompanied by hypotension, shortness of breath, chest pain, altered mental status, congestive heart failure, and shock.

Atropine acts by blocking acetylcholine receptors thus inhibiting parasympathetic stimulation. Although it has positive chronotropic properties, it has little or no inotropic effect. It plays an important role as an antidote in organophosphate poisonings.

Atropine has shown to be of some use in asystole, presumably because some cases of asystole may be caused by a sudden and tremendous increase in parasympathetic tone. The mechanism by which atropine is effective in asystole is not clear. However, despite no definite proof of its value in asystole, there is little evidence that its use is harmful in this setting.

Indications

❑ Hemodynamically significant bradycardia
❑ Asystole

Contraindications. None in emergency situations.

Precautions. Atropine may actually worsen the bradycardia associated with second-degree Mobitz II and third degree AV blocks. In these cases, go straight to transcutaneous pacing instead of trying atropine.

A maximum dose of 0.04 milligrams per kilogram body weight of atropine should not be exceeded except in the setting of organophosphate poisoning. If the heart rate fails to increase after a total of 0.04 mg/kg has been given, then transcutaneous pacing is indicated.

Side Effects. Atropine sulfate can cause blurred vision, dilated pupils, dry mouth, tachycardia, drowsiness, and confusion.

Interactions. Few in the prehospital setting.

Dosage

❑ *Hemodynamically-significant bradycardia.* An initial dose of 0.5 milligram should be administered intravenously. This can be repeated every 3–5 minutes until a maximum dose of 0.04 mg/kg has been administered.
❑ *Asystole.* In the treatment of asystole, the dose should be increased to 1.0 mg. When an IV cannot be placed, atropine can be administered endotracheally. However, the dose should be increased to 2–2.5 times in the intravenous dose.

Atropine should be given as an IV bolus in emergency situations or endotracheally when an IV cannot be placed.

✱ Atropine blocks the action of the parasympathetic nervous system and the vagus nerve. It is effective in the treatment of symptomatic bradycardias.

Pediatric Dosage. *Bradycardia* 0.02 mg/kg (minimum dose of 0.1 mg)
Maximum single dose (child 0.5 mg) (adolescent 1.0 mg)
Maximum total dose (child 1.0 mg) (adolescent 2.0 mg)

How Supplied. Atropine is supplied in prefilled syringes containing 1.0 milligrams in 10 milliliters of solution.

The Alkalinizing Agents

Alkalinizing drugs, such as sodium bicarbonate, are used to buffer the acids present in the body during and after severe hypoxia. Normal body pH is 7.4 (7.35–7.45). During hypoxia, serum pH may fall quickly. Sodium bicarbonate will help correct metabolic (usually lactic acid) acidosis until hypoxia is corrected. The following reaction illustrates the role of sodium bicarbonate in acid-base balance.

$$H^+ \quad + \quad HCO_3^- \quad \leftrightarrow \quad H_2CO_3 \quad \leftrightarrow \quad H_2O \ + \ CO_2$$

$$\text{Hydrogen} + \text{Bicarbonate} \leftrightarrow \text{Carbonic} \leftrightarrow \text{Water} + \text{Carbon}$$
$$\text{ion} \qquad\qquad \text{ion} \qquad\qquad \text{acid} \qquad\qquad\qquad \text{Dioxide}$$

Bicarbonate combines with strong acids, such as lactic acid, and forms a weak, volatile acid. This acid is subsequently degraded to carbon dioxide and water. The end products are removed via the kidneys or lungs.

Excessive administration of sodium bicarbonate can cause metabolic alkalosis, which can be worse than the metabolic acidosis being treated. Sodium bicarbonate delivers 50 mEq of sodium with each prefilled syringe, which can cause additional problems.

The primary treatment of metabolic acidosis in the setting of hypoxia or cardiac arrest is adequate oxygenation and blood-pressure support.

sodium bicarbonate

Class: Alkalinizing agent

Description. Sodium bicarbonate is a salt that provides bicarbonate to buffer metabolic acidosis, which can accompany several disease processes.

Mechanism of Action. For many years sodium bicarbonate was the cornerstone of advanced cardiac life support care. However, controlled studies have shown that sodium bicarbonate was ineffective in the treatment of cardiac arrest. It many instances it has actually been associated with many adverse reactions.

Sodium bicarbonate is occasionally used in the treatment of certain types of drug overdose. The most common example is drugs in the tricyclic class of antidepressants. Overdosage of these drugs has serious effects including life-threatening cardiac arrhythmias. Tricyclic antidepressant excretion from the body is enhanced by making the urine more alkaline (raising the pH). Sodium bicarbonate is sometimes administered to increase the pH of the urine to speed excretion of the drug from the body.

* The role of sodium bicarbonate in advanced cardiac life support is questionable due to the absence of proven effectiveness and numerous adverse reactions.

Indications

- ❏ Late in the management of cardiac arrest, if at all. Hyperventilation, prompt defibrillation, and the administration of epinephrine and lidocaine should always precede use of sodium bicarbonate. Because these therapies take at least 10 minutes to carry out, sodium bicarbonate should rarely be administered in the first 10 minutes of a resuscitation.
- ❏ Tricyclic antidepressant overdose
- ❏ Phenobarbital overdose
- ❏ Severe acidosis refractory to hyperventilation
- ❏ Known hyperkalemia

Contraindications.   When used in the management of the situations described earlier, there are no absolute contraindications.

Precautions.   Sodium bicarbonate can cause metabolic alkalosis when administered in large quantities. It is important to calculate the dosage based on patient weight and size.

Side Effects.   Few when used in the emergency setting.

Interactions.   Most catecholamines and vasopressors (i.e. dopamine and epinephrine) can be deactivated by alkaline solutions like sodium bicarbonate. Sodium bicarbonate should not be administered in conjunction with calcium chloride. A precipitate can form, which may clog the IV line.

Dosage.   The usual dose of sodium bicarbonate is 1 milliequivalent per kilogram of body weight initially, followed by 0.5 milliequivalent per kilogram body weight every 10 minutes. When possible, the dosage of sodium bicarbonate should be based on the results of arterial blood gas studies. Sodium bicarbonate should be administered only as an IV bolus.

Pediatric Dosage.   1 mEq/kg initially, followed by 0.5 mEq/kg every 10 minutes as indicated by blood gas studies

How Supplied.   Sodium bicarbonate comes in prefilled syringes containing 50 milliequivalents of the drug in 50 milliliters of solvent.

The Analgesics   Drugs that have proven effective in alleviating pain are referred to as analgesics. Although they may be administered in many types of emergencies, they are usually reserved for the treatment of emergencies involving the cardiovascular system, especially myocardial infarction.

morphine sulfate

Class: Narcotic analgesic

Description.   Morphine is a central nervous system depressant and a potent analgesic. Although morphine sulfate is one of the most potent analgesics known to humans, it also has hemodynamic properties that make it extremely useful in emergency medicine.

Mechanism of Action.   Morphine sulfate is a central nervous system depressant that acts on opiate receptors in the brain, providing both analgesia and sedation. It increases peripheral venous capacitance and decreases venous return. This effect is sometimes called a "chemical phlebotomy." Morphine also decreases myocardial oxygen demand. This action is due to both the decreased systemic vascular resistance and the sedative effects of the drug. Patient apprehension and fear can significantly increase myocardial oxygen demand and, in some cases, can conceivably increase the size of myocardial infarction. The hemodynamic properties of morphine make it one of the most important drugs used in the treatment of pulmonary edema. Morphine is frequently administered to patients with signs and symptoms of pulmonary edema who are not having chest pain.

Indications

❑ Severe pain associated with myocardial infarction, kidney stones, etc.
❑ Pulmonary edema either with or without associated pain

Contraindications.   Morphine should not be used in patients who are volume depleted or severely hypotensive because of the hemodynamic effects described earlier. Morphine should not be administered to any patient with a history of hypersensitivity to the drug, or to patients with undiagnosed head injury or abdominal pain.

Precautions.   Morphine is a narcotic derivative of opium. It has a high tendency for addiction and abuse and is thus covered under the Controlled Substances Act of 1970. It is classified as a Schedule II drug. Because of this, there are special considerations involved in the handling of the drug. Many emergency medical services (EMS) systems have opted to use the synthetic analgesics, like nalbuphine and pentazocine, instead of morphine and meperidine because of these problems.

Morphine causes severe respiratory depression in higher doses. This is especially true in patients who already have some form of respiratory impairment. The narcotic antagonist naloxone (Narcan) should be readily available whenever the drug is administered.

Side Effects. Morphine can cause nausea, vomiting, abdominal cramps, blurred vision, constricted pupils, altered mental status, headache, and respiratory depression.

Interactions. The CNS depression associated with morphine can be enhanced when administered with antihistamines, antiemetics, sedatives, hypnotics, barbiturates, and alcohol.

Dosage. There are many different approaches to the administration of morphine. An initial dose in the range of 2 to 10 milligrams intravenously is standard. This can be augmented with additional doses of 2 milligrams every few minutes and can be continued until the pain is relieved or until signs of respiratory depression occur.

Intramuscular injection usually requires 5 to 15 milligrams based on the patient's weight to attain desired effects. However, morphine is routinely given intravenously in emergency medicine and is often administered with an anti-emetic agent such as promethazine (Phenergan). This helps prevent nausea and vomiting which often accompanies morphine administration. The anti-emetics also tend to potentiate morphine's effects. Morphine can also be given intramuscularly and subcutaneously.

Pediatric Dosage. 0.1–0.2 mg/kg IV

How Supplied. Morphine comes in tamper-proof ampules and Tubex prefilled cartridges. To ease administration, the 10 milligrams in 1-milliliter dilution is preferred.

✳ A common method of dosing morphine in the prehospital phase is in 2 milligram increments until pain is relieved ("2 + 2").

nitrous oxide (Nitronox)

Class: Analgesic/anesthetic gas

Description. Nitronox is a blended mixture of 50 percent nitrous oxide and 50 percent oxygen, which has potent analgesic effects.

Mechanism of Action. Nitrous oxide is a CNS depressant with analgesic properties. In the prehospital setting it is delivered in fixed mixture of 50% nitrous oxide and 50% oxygen. When inhaled, it has potent analgesic effects. These quickly dissipate, however, within 2 to 5 minutes after cessation of administration.

The Nitronox unit consists of one oxygen and one nitrous oxide cylinder. The gases are fed into a blender that combines them at the appropriate concentration. The mixture is then delivered to a modified demand valve for administration to the patient.

Nitronox must be self-administered. It is effective in treating many varieties of pain encountered in the prehospital setting, including pain from many types of trauma. The high concentration of oxygen delivered along with the nitrous oxide will increase the oxygen tension in the blood, thus reducing hypoxia.

Indications

❑ Pain of musculoskeletal origin, particularly fractures
❑ Burns
❑ Suspected ischemic chest pain
❑ States of severe anxiety including hyperventilation

Contraindications. Nitronox should not be used in any patient who cannot comprehend verbal instructions or those intoxicated with alcohol or other drugs. It should not be administered to any patient with a head injury who exhibits an altered mental status. Nitronox should not be administered to any patient with COPD where the high concentration of oxygen (50 percent) might result in respiratory depression. Nitrous oxide tends to diffuse into closed spaces more readily than either carbon dioxide or oxygen. Many COPD patients have air-containing blebs in their lungs, and nitrous oxide can concentrate in these blebs, causing them to swell. Swollen blebs may rupture, causing a pneumothorax.

Nitronox should not be administered to patients with a thoracic injury suspicious of pneumothorax, as the gas may accumulate in the pneumothorax increasing its size. Also, patients with severe abdominal pain and distention suggestive of bowel obstruction should not receive Nitronox. Nitrous oxide can concentrate in pockets of obstructed bowel, possibly leading to rupture.

Precautions. Nitronox should only be used in areas that are well ventilated. When the gas is used in the patient compartment of an ambulance, it is recommended that a scavenging system be in place.

Nitrous oxide exists in a liquid state inside the gas cylinder. Heat present in the air, the cylinder wall, or the various regulators and lines causes the liquid to vaporize. This vaporization process makes the cylinder tank and lines cool to touch. Following prolonged use, frost may develop on the cylinder, regulator, or lines. In very cold environments, generally less than 21°F (6°C), the liquid may be slow to vaporize, and administration may be impossible.

Side Effects. Nitrous oxide/oxygen mixture can cause dizziness, light-headedness, altered mental status, hallucinations, nausea, and vomiting.

Interactions. Nitrous oxide can potentiate the effects of other CNS depressants such as narcotics, sedatives, hypnotics, and alcohol.

Dosage. Nitronox should only be self-administered. Continuous administration may take place until the pain is significantly relieved or the patient drops the mask. The patient care record should document the duration of drug administration.

Pediatric Dosage. Self-administered only

How Supplied. Nitrous oxide/oxygen mixture is supplied in a cylinder system where both gasses are fed into a blender, which delivers a fixed 50%/50% mixture to the patient. The blender is designed to shut off if the oxygen cylinder becomes depleted. It will allow continued administration of oxygen if the nitrous oxide cylinder becomes depleted.

In several countries (England, Canada, Australia), the nitrous oxide/oxygen mixture (Entonox, Dolonox) is premixed and supplied in a single cylinder. This setup is much lighter than the system used in the United States.

The Diuretics
One of the more common cardiovascular emergencies is congestive heart failure. Congestive heart failure occurs when the heart loses its ability to pump blood effectively. In congestive heart failure, the veins leading to the heart become engorged. Failure of the left side of the heart causes a buildup of blood in the pulmonary circulation. Failure of the right side of the heart results in congestion of the peripheral circulation, which often manifests as peripheral edema. Common signs of right-heart failure include jugular venous distention, ascites, and pedal (ankle or pretibial) edema.

Drugs that cause the elimination of fluid from the body, via the kidneys, are referred to as diuretics. Furosemide is the most commonly used diuretic in prehospital care.

furosemide (Lasix)

Class: Diuretic

Description. Furosemide is a drug used to treat pulmonary edema and to lower blood pressure.

Mechanism of Action. Furosemide is a potent diuretic that inhibits sodium and chloride reabsorption in the kidney. It also causes venous dilation. It is extremely useful in the treatment of congestive heart failure and pulmonary edema. Its effects are usually evident within five minutes of administration.

* Nitronox should only be self-administered in the field.

* Furosemide promotes venous pooling and stimulates the kidneys to excrete water. It is a mainstay in the treatment of congestive heart failure.

Indications

- ❏ Congestive heart failure
- ❏ Pulmonary edema

Contraindications. Usage in pregnancy should be limited to life-threatening situations. Furosemide has been known to cause fetal abnormalities.

Precautions. Dehydration and electrolyte depletion can result from excessive doses of potent diuretics. Furosemide should be protected from light.

Side Effects. Furosemide can cause hypotension, ECG changes, chest pain, dry mouth, hypochloremia, hypokalemia, hyponatremia, and hyperglycemia.

Interactions. Furosemide administration may cause potassium depletion potentially resulting in digitalis toxicity, and sodium depletion potentially resulting in lithium toxicity.

Dosage. The standard dosage of furosemide is 40 milligrams. It is given by slow IV push in patients already on chronic oral furosemide therapy and 20 milligrams IV in patients who are not regularly taking the drug orally. Dosages as high as 80 milligrams IV may be indicated in severe cases.

Furosemide should be given intravenously in emergency situations.

Pediatric Dosage. 1 mg/kg

How Supplied. Furosemide is supplied in 2mL ampules (10 mg/ml) and 10 mL vials (10 mg/ml).

The Antianginal Agents

A common manifestation of advanced cardiovascular disease is *angina pectoris*. It results from a narrowing of the coronary arteries, due to the buildup of atherosclerotic plaques, or coronary artery vasospasm. In exercise and other stressful situations, the amount of blood that can be carried by the coronary arteries may not be sufficient to meet the oxygen demands of the myocardium. This results in myocardial hypoxia, causing the classic pain syndrome called angina pectoris. Sublingual nitroglycerin usually gives immediate relief by causing a decrease in cardiac work, and, to a lesser degree, dilatation of the coronary arteries.

In recent years, nitroglycerin has been tried with patients suffering myocardial infarction in the hope of decreasing the extent of myocardial damage. Nitroglycerin is often administered to patients complaining of chest pain to rule out angina as the cause. When cardiac pain is not relieved by nitroglycerin, morphine and other potent analgesics are administered.

Nitroglycerin is generally administered sublingually. A nitroglycerin intravenous infusion is often used in the treatment of unstable angina and acute myocardial infarction.

Calcium-ion antagonists, such as diltiazem (Cardizem) and nifedipine (Procardia), have proven effective in the management of angina, especially if it's due to coronary artery vasospasm. In certain areas, these two agents may be on prehospital drug lists.

nitroglycerin (Nitrostat)

Class: Nitrate

Description. Nitroglycerin is a potent smooth muscle relaxant used in the treatment of angina pectoris.

Mechanism of Action. Nitroglycerin is a rapid smooth-muscle relaxant that reduces cardiac work, and to a lesser degree, dilates the coronary arteries. This results in increased coronary blood blow and improved perfusion of the ischemic myocardium. Relief of ischemia causes reduction and alleviation of chest pain. Pain relief following nitroglycerin administration usually occurs within 1 to 2 minutes, and therapeutic effects can be observed up to 30 minutes later. Nitroglycerin also causes vasodilation which decreases preload. Decreased preload leads to decreased cardiac work. This feature, in conjunction with coronary vasodilation, reverses the effects of angina pectoris.

Indications

- ❏ Chest pain associated with angina pectoris
- ❏ Chest pain associated with acute myocardial infarction
- ❏ Acute pulmonary edema (unless accompanied by hypotension)

Contraindications. Nitroglycerin is contraindicated in patients who are hypotensive or who may have increased intracranial pressure. It should not be administered to patients in shock.

Precautions. Patients taking nitroglycerin may develop a tolerance for the drug, which necessitates increasing the dose. Headache is a common side effect of nitroglycerin administration and results from vasodilation of cerebral vessels. Nitroglycerin deteriorates quite rapidly once the bottle is opened. When a bottle of nitroglycerin is opened, it should be dated. Nitroglycerin should also be protected from light.

Always monitor the blood pressure and the other vital signs during nitroglycerin administration.

Side Effects. Nitroglycerin can cause headache, dizziness, weakness, tachycardia, hypotension, orthostasis, skin rash, dry mouth, nausea, and vomiting.

Interactions. Nitroglycerin can cause severe hypotension when administered to patients who have recently ingested alcohol. It can cause orthostatic hypotension when used in conjunction with beta blockers.

Dosage. One tablet (0.4 milligram) sublingually for routine angina pectoris. This can be repeated in 3–5 minutes as required. Usually, more than three tablets should not be administered in the prehospital setting. Nitroglycerin should be administered sublingually. Care should be taken to assure that it is not swallowed. IV nitroglycerin is used in the emergency department and intensive care units, but the sublingual route is adequate for most prehospital situations. Nitroglycerin is also available in patches and in ointment form for transdermal administration.

Pediatric Dosage. Not indicated

How Supplied. Nitroglycerin is supplied in bottles containing 0.4 milligram tablets (1/150 grain). The tablets must be protected from light and air to prevent deterioration.

---

nifedipine (Procardia) (Adalat)

Class: Calcium channel blocker

Description. Nifedipine is a calcium channel blocker that is widely used in emergency medicine in the treatment of hypertension.

Mechanism of Action. Nifedipine causes relaxation of the smooth muscles that encircle the peripheral blood vessels, principally the arterioles. This relaxation results in peripheral vasodilation, decreased peripheral vascular resistance, and a decrease in both the systolic and diastolic blood pressure. Nifedipine is also effective in reducing coronary artery spasm in angina. Nifedipine can be used in hypertension associated with pregnancy if hydralazine is not available.

Indications

- ❏ Severe hypertension
- ❏ Angina pectoris

Contraindications. Nifedipine is contraindicated in patients with known hypersensitivity to the drug. It should not be administered to patients who are hypotensive.

Precautions. Nifedipine can cause a significant drop in blood pressure. Thus, the blood pressure should be frequently monitored. Nifedipine should be used with caution in patients with heart failure. Nifedipine should not be administered to patients receiving IV β blockers.

Side Effects. Nifedepine can cause nausea, vomiting, dizziness, headache, bradycardia, heart block, hypotension, and asystole.

Interactions. Nifedepine should not be administered to patients receiving intravenous blockers because of an increased risk of congestive heart failure, bradycardia, and asystole.

Dosage. One 10-milligram capsule should have several small puncture holes placed in the capsule and then should be placed under the tongue where it can be absorbed. Alternatively, the capsule can be bitten by the patient and swallowed with approximately the same rate of onset. In severe hypertension, the medical control physician may order an initial dose of 20 milligrams. Nifedipine should only be administered orally or sublingually as described earlier.

Pediatric Dosage. 0.25–0.50 mg/kg

How Supplied. Nifedipine is supplied in 10- and 20-milligram tablets.

Other Cardiovascular Drugs There are several other cardiovascular agents that you may be called upon to administer in the field. One of these is calcium chloride. Note its indications and limitations.

calcium chloride

Class: Calcium supplement (calcium salt)

Description. Calcium chloride provides elemental calcium in the form of the cation (Ca^{++}). Calcium is required for many physiological activities.

Mechanism of Action. Calcium chloride replaces calcium in cases of hypocalcemia. Calcium chloride causes a significant increase in the myocardial contractile force and appears to increase ventricular automaticity. Although frequently used for many years in the management of cardiac arrest, especially that resulting from asystole and electromechanical dissociation, recent studies have presented data that seriously question the role of calcium chloride, even in these situations. Calcium chloride is an antidote for magnesium sulfate and can minimize some of the side effects of calcium channel blocker usage.

Indications

- ❏ Acute hyperkalemia (elevated potassium)
- ❏ Acute hypocalcemia (decreased calcium)
- ❏ Calcium-channel-blocker toxicity (nifedipine, verapamil, etc.)

✱ Calcium chloride is rarely indicated in prehospital care.

Contraindications. Caution is warranted when calcium chloride is administered to patients receiving digitalis, as it may precipitate digitalis toxicity.

Precautions. It is extremely important to flush the IV line between administration of calcium chloride and sodium bicarbonate to avoid precipitation. Calcium chloride can cause tissue necrosis at the injection site. It should always be administered through an IV that is patent and running well.

Side Effects. Calcium chloride can cause bradycardia, arrhythmias, syncope, nausea, vomiting, and cardiac arrest.

Interactions. Calcium chloride will interact with sodium bicarbonate and form a precipitate. In addition, calcium chloride can cause elevated digoxin levels, and possibly digitalis toxicity, when administered to patients receiving digitalis preparations.

Dosage. The standard dose for calcium chloride is 2 to 4 milligrams per kilogram intravenously. This may be repeated every 10 minutes as required. Calcium chloride should only be given intravenously in the emergency setting.

Pediatric Dosage. 5–7 mg/kg of a 10-percent solution

How Supplied. Calcium chloride comes in prefilled syringes containing 1 gram of the drug in 10 milliliters of solvent (10 milliliters of a 10% solution).

Drugs Used in the Treatment of Respiratory Emergencies

Oxygen is the most commonly used drug in the management of respiratory emergencies. In addition to oxygen, however, several pharmacologic agents have proven effective in the prehospital phase of emergency medical care.

Another agent frequently used in the management of respiratory emergencies is aminophylline. Aminophylline, chemically unrelated to the catecholamines, belongs to a class of drugs called *xanthines*. A commonly encountered drug in the xanthines class is caffeine. Aminophylline causes relaxation of the bronchiolar smooth musculature, which in turn relieves bronchospasm.

In addition to oxygen and aminophylline, the β agonists play a major role in the treatment of respiratory emergencies. Drugs are now available that act predominantly on β_2 receptors. These agents are preferred to non-selective agents because of the decreased incidence of side effects, such as rapid heart rate.

---

epinephrine 1:1,000

Class: Sympathetic agonist

Description. Epinephrine is a naturally occurring catecholamine. It is a potent and adrenergic stimulant, however its effect on β receptors is more profound.

Mechanism of Action. Epinephrine acts directly on α and β adrenergic receptors. Its effect on β receptors is much more profound than its effect on α receptors. The effects of epinephrine include increased heart rate, cardiac contractile force, systemic vascular resistance, and blood pressure. It also causes bronchodilation due to its effects on β_2 adrenergic receptors. It is occasionally used to treat the bronchoconstriction accompanying asthma and COPD, and is also effective in treating bronchoconstriction associated with anaphylaxis.

Epinephrine's effects usually appear within 90 seconds of administration, and they are usually of short duration. Occasionally it must be readministered in 15–30 minutes if needed. Epinephrine 1:1,000 is given subcutaneously to ensure a steady and prolonged action. Inhaled β agonists are preferred over epinephrine in the treatment of bronchospasm, as they have fewer undesirable side effects.

Indications (Respiratory)

- ❏ Bronchial asthma
- ❏ Exacerbation of some forms of COPD
- ❏ Anaphylaxis

Contraindications. Because of the cardiac effects seen with the administration of epinephrine, it should not be administered to patients with underlying cardiovascular disease or hypertension. Patients with profound anaphylactic reactions, characterized by hypotension and shock, are usually peripherally vasoconstricted which will delay absorption of the drug from the subcutaneous site of injection. In these cases, epinephrine 1:10,000 should be administered intravenously.

Precautions. Epinephrine should be protected from light. Also, as with the other catecholamines, it tends to be deactivated by alkaline solutions. Any patient receiving epinephrine 1:1,000 should be carefully monitored for changes in blood pressure, pulse, and ECG. Palpitations, anxiety, nausea, and headache are fairly common side effects.

Side Effects.   Epinephrine can cause palpitations, anxiety, tremulousness, headache, dizziness, nausea, and vomiting. Because of its strong inotropic and chronotropic properties, epinephrine increases myocardial oxygen demand. Even in low doses it can cause myocardial ischemia. These effects should be kept in mind when administering epinephrine in the emergency setting.

Interactions.   The effects of epinephrine can be intensified in patients who are taking antidepressants.

Dosage.   The standard dose of epinephrine 1:1,000 ranges from 0.3 to 0.5 milligram subcutaneously depending on the patient's weight and overall medical condition. Typically, 0.3 milligram is the starting dose for adults. In the prehospital phase of emergency medical care, epinephrine 1:1,000 should only be administered subcutaneously (except in the case of pediatric cardiac arrest).

✳ Epinephrine 1:1,000 is for subcutaneous administration only, except in cases of pediatric cardiac arrest.

Pediatric Dosage.   0.01 mg/kg up to 0.3 mg

How Supplied.   Epinephrine 1:1,000 is supplied in ampules and prefilled syringes containing 1 milligram of the drug in 1 milliliter of solvent.

aminophylline (Somophyllin)

Class: Xanthine

Description.   Aminophylline is a xanthine bronchodilator that sometimes proves effective in cases in which sympathomimetics have not been effective.

Mechanism of Action.   Aminophylline achieves its bronchodilation effects via a different mechanism than the sympathomimetics. It relaxes bronchial smooth muscle, but does not act on adrenergic receptors. Aminophylline also stimulates the respiratory center in the brain. This effect is particularly useful in the treatment of infants with apnea. In addition to bronchodilation, aminophylline has mild diuretic properties, increases the heart rate and the cardiac output, and may precipitate arrhythmias. Owing to its mild diuretic and inotropic effects, aminophylline is also used in the management of congestive heart failure and pulmonary edema. In prehospital emergency care, aminophylline is usually given by slow IV infusion. Some systems also carry aminophylline suppositories for use in special situations.

Indications

- ❏ Bronchial asthma
- ❏ Reversible bronchospasm associated with chronic bronchitis and emphysema
- ❏ Congestive heart failure
- ❏ Pulmonary edema

Contraindications.   Aminophylline should not be administered to any patient with a history of hypersensitivity to the drug. It should not be used in patients who have uncontrolled cardiac dysrhythmias.

Precautions.   Extreme caution should be used when administering aminophylline to any patient with a history of cardiovascular disease or hypertension. Any patient receiving aminophylline should have a cardiac monitor. One should be alert for any signs of cardiac irritability, especially PVCs and tachycardia. Hypotension can occur following rapid administration.

Side Effects.   Aminophylline can cause tachycardia, arrhythmias, palpitations, chest pain, nervousness, headache, seizures, nausea, and vomiting.

Interactions.   Aminophylline should not be administered to patients who are on chronic theophylline therapy (Slo-Bid, Theo-Dur, etc.) until the amount of drug in the blood has been obtained (theophylline level). Concomitant use with β blockers and drugs of the erythromycin class of antibiotics may lead to theophylline toxicity.

Dosage. Two major regimens are used in administering aminophylline. The first is for use in patients in whom fluid overload or edema does not appear to be present (that is, acute bronchial asthma):

❑ Place 250 or 500 milligrams in 90 or 80 milliliters of 5% dextrose, respectively. This can be done with a 100-milliliter IV bag or with a Buretrol or Volutrol-type administration set. This is then infused during 20 to 30 minutes. This mechanism of slow infusion tends to reduce the chances of arrhythmias.

In patients with congestive heart failure, or in patients in whom any additional fluid might be dangerous, a more concentrated infusion is prepared:

❑ Place 250 or 500 milligrams (2 to 5 milligrams per kilogram) in 20 milliliters of 5% dextrose in water. This is then infused during 20 to 30 minutes using a Buretrol or Volutrol-type administration set.

Parenteral aminophylline should only be given by slow IV infusion by one of the regimens discussed above.

Pediatric Dosage. 6 mg/kg loading dose to be infused over 20–30 minutes; maximum dose not to exceed 12 mg/kg/24 hrs

How Supplied. Aminophylline is supplied in ampules containing 250 milligrams in 10 milliliters of solvent or containing 500 milligrams in 20 milliliters of solvent.

racemic epinephrine (microNEFRIN) (Vaponefrin)

Class: Sympathetic agonist

Description. Racemic epinephrine is slightly different chemically from the epinephrine compounds that have been discussed previously. Compounds that differ only in their chemical arrangement are called *isomers*. This particular form is frequently used in children to treat croup.

Mechanism of Action. Racemic epinephrine stimulates both α and β adrenergic receptors. However, racemic epinephrine has a slight preference for β_2 adrenergic receptors and causes bronchodilation. It also has some effect in relieving the subglottic edema associated with croup. Racemic epinephrine should only be administered by inhalation.

Indications

❑ Croup (laryngotracheobronchitis)

Contraindications. Racemic epinephrine should not be used in the management of epiglottitis.

✱ Always be alert for "rebound worsening" of croup when using racemic ephinephrine.

Precautions. Racemic epinephrine can result in tachycardia and possibly arrhythmias. Vital signs should be monitored. Many patients will develop "rebound worsening" 30–60 minutes after the initial treatment and the effects of racemic epinephrine have worn off. Because of this, all children who receive racemic epinephrine should be transported to the hospital. Most hospitals have an institutional policy that requires all children who have received racemic epinephrine to be admitted for at least 24 hours in case rebound worsening occurs.

Side Effects. Racemic epinephrine can cause tachycardia and dysrhythmias.

Interactions. MAO inhibitors and bretylium may potentiate the effect of epinephrine. The bronchodilating response may be blunted by β adrenergic antagonists. Sympathomimetics and phosphodiesterase inhibitors may exacerbate dysrhythmia response.

Dosage. A standard dose is 0.25–0.75 ml racemic epinephrine diluted with 2 ml normal saline (2.25%) and administered via a standard aerosol nebulizer. It should only be used initially and not repeated. Racemic epinephrine should be given only by inhalation, generally by small-volume nebulizer, diluted with 2 to 3 milliliters of normal saline.

Pediatric Dosage.   0.25–0.75 ml of a 2.25-percent solution in 2.0 ml of normal saline

How Supplied.   Racemic epinephrine is supplied in inhaler or nebulizer bottles containing either 7.5, 15, or 30 milliliters.

terbutaline (Brethine) (Bricanyl)

Class: Sympathetic agonist

Description.   Terbutaline is a synthetic sympathomimetic that is selective for β_2 adrenergic receptors.

Mechanism of Action.   Terbutaline, because of its effects on β_2 adrenergic receptors, causes immediate bronchodilation with minimal cardiac effects. Its onset of action is similar to that of epinephrine. Terbutaline is also used to suppress preterm labor.

Indications

- ❑ Bronchial asthma
- ❑ Reversible bronchospasm associated with chronic bronchitis and emphysema

Contraindications.   Terbutaline should not be administered to any patient with a history of hypersensitivity to the drug.

Precautions.   As with any sympathomimetic, the patient's vital signs must be monitored. Caution should be used when administering terbutaline to elderly patients and those with cardiovascular disease or hypertension. Lung sounds should be auscultated before and after each treatment. Ideally, the patient's peak flow rate should be measured both before and after drug administration.

Side Effects.   Terbutaline can cause palpitations, anxiety, dizziness, headache, nervousness, tremor, hypertension, arrhythmias, chest pain, nausea, and vomiting.

Interactions.   The possibility of developing unpleasant side effects increases when terbutaline is used with other sympathetic agonists. β blockers may blunt the pharmacological effects of terbutaline.

Dosage.   The standard dose is two inhalations, 1 minute apart, from a metered-dose inhaler. Terbutaline can also be administered by subcutaneous injection. The usual dose is 0.25 milligram. This can be repeated in 15 to 30 minutes if needed. Terbutaline should only be administered by inhalation or by subcutaneous injection as described herein.

Pediatric Dosage.   0.01 mg/kg subcutaneously

How Supplied.   Terbutaline is supplied in aerosol canisters. Each spray delivers approximately 0.20 mg of the drug. Terbutaline for subcutaneous injection is supplied in vials containing 1 milligram of the drug in 1 milliliter of solvent.

albuterol (Proventil) (Ventolin)

Class: Sympathetic agonist

Description.   Albuterol is a sympathomimetic that is selective for β_2 adrenergic receptors.

Mechanism of Action.   Albuterol is a selective β_2 agonist with a minimal amount of side effects. It causes prompt bronchodilation and has a duration of action of approximately 5 hours.

Indications

- ❑ Bronchial asthma
- ❑ Reversible bronchospasm associated with chronic bronchitis and emphysema

✳ The aerosolized β agonists are the drug of choice for the emergency management of bronchospasm associated with asthma and COPD.

Contraindications. Albuterol should not be administered to any patient with a known history of hypersensitivity to the drug.

Precautions. As with any sympathomimetic, the patient's vital signs must be monitored. Caution should be used when administering albuterol to elderly patients and those with cardiovascular disease or hypertension. Lung sounds should be auscultated before and after each treatment. Ideally, the patient's peak flow rate should be measured both before and after drug administration.

Side Effects. Albuterol can cause palpitations, anxiety, dizziness, headache, nervousness, tremor, hypertension, arrhythmias, chest pain, nausea, and vomiting.

Interactions. The possibility of developing unpleasant side effects increases when albuterol is administered with other sympathetic agonists. β blockers may blunt the pharmacological effects of albuterol.

Dosage. Albuterol can be administered by metered-dose inhaler or small-volume nebulizer. A common initial dose is two sprays when using a metered-dose inhaler. Each spray delivers 90 micrograms of albuterol. When using a small-volume nebulizer the standard adult dose is 2.5 milligrams (0.5 milliliter of a 0.5% solution diluted in 2.5 milliliters of normal saline). This amount is typically delivered during 5 to 15 minutes.

Albuterol (Ventolin) is also available in the Rotohaler form. A special 200-microgram Rotocap is placed in the device and inhaled by the patient. Albuterol should only be administered by inhalation.

Pediatric Dosage. 0.15 mg (0.03 ml)/kg in 2.5 ml of normal saline by nebulizer

How Supplied. Albuterol is supplied in metered dose inhalers that contain approximately three hundred 90-microgram sprays. The solution for inhalation is supplied in single-patient vials containing 0.5 milliliter of the drug in 2.5 milliliters of normal saline. Rotocaps for inhalation are supplied in special 200-microgram capsules.

ipratropium (Atrovent)

Class: Anticholinergic

Description. Ipratropium is an anticholinergic (parasympatholytic) bronchodilator which is chemically related to atropine.

Mechanism of Action. Ipratropium is a parasympatholytic used in the treatment of respiratory emergencies. It causes bronchodilation and dries respiratory tract secretions. Ipratropium acts by blocking acetylcholine receptors, thus inhibiting parasympathetic stimulation.

Indications

- ❑ Bronchial asthma
- ❑ Reversible bronchospasm associated with chronic bronchitis and emphysema

Contraindications. Ipratropium should not be used in patients hypersensitive to the drug. It is not indicated for the acute treatment of bronchospasm where rapid response is required.

Precautions. The patient's vital signs must be monitored during therapy with ipratropium. Caution should be used when administering it to elderly patients and those with cardiovascular disease or hypertension. Lung sounds should be auscultated before and after each treatment. Ideally, the patient's peak flow rate should be measured both before and after drug administration.

Side Effects. Ipratropium can cause palpitations, anxiety, dizziness, headache, nervousness, rash, nausea, and vomiting.

Interactions. Few in the prehospital setting.

Dosage. Ipratropium is usually administered with a β agonist. Typically, 500 micrograms of Atrovent is placed in a small volume nebulizer. A β agonist can be added if desired. This solution is then administered by small volume nebulizer with or without a β agonist. Atrovent is also available in a metered dose inhaler.

Pediatric Dosage. Safety in children has not been established.

How Supplied. Atrovent is supplied in unit dose vials containing 500 micrograms (0.02% inhalation solution) of the drug already diluted in 2.5 ml saline.

Drugs Used in the Treatment of Endocrine and Metabolic Emergencies

Glands that secrete hormones directly into the blood, without the aid of ducts, are called *endocrine glands*. With the exception of the pancreas, they rarely cause emergency disorders. Occasionally the thyroid, the endocrine gland that controls the metabolic rate, will begin secreting excess thyroid hormones. This disorder, called "thyroid storm," is characterized by increased heart rate, loss of body weight, and congestive heart failure. Fortunately, it is rare and probably would not be diagnosed in prehospital emergency medical care.

50% dextrose in water (D50W)

Class: Carbohydrate

Description. "Dextrose" is used to describe the six-carbon sugar *d-glucose*, which is the principal form of carbohydrate used by the body.

Mechanism of Action. 50% dextrose in water supplies supplemental glucose in cases of hypoglycemia. Serious brain injury can occur if hypoglycemia is prolonged. Thus, in hypoglycemia the rapid administration of glucose is essential. When the hypoglycemic patient is unresponsive, glucose cannot be given by mouth and should be given as IV D50W solution.

Indications

- ❏ Hypoglycemia
- ❏ Coma of unknown origin

Contraindications. There are no major contraindications to the IV administration of D50W to a patient with suspected hypoglycemia. Even if a patient was suffering from ketoacidosis, the amount of glucose present in 50 milliliters of 50% dextrose would not adversely affect the clinical outcome. 50% dextrose should be used with caution in patients with increased intracranial pressure as the dextrose load may worsen cerebral edema.

Precautions. It is important to perform a Dextrostix or obtain a Glucometer reading and draw a sample of blood before initiating an IV infusion and giving 50% dextrose. Localized venous irritation may occur when smaller veins are used. Infiltration of 50% dextrose may result in tissue necrosis.

Side Effects. 50% dextrose can cause tissue necrosis and phlebitis at the injection site.

Interactions. None in the emergency setting.

Dosage. The standard dosage of 50% dextrose in hypoglycemia is 25 grams (50 milliliters of a 50% solution) intravenously. If an initial dose is ineffective, a second dose of 25 grams can also be given.

Fifty percent dextrose is only given intravenously. Concentrated glucose solutions can cause venous irritation if administered for an extended period.

Pediatric Dosage. 0.5 g/kg slow IV; should be diluted 1:1 with sterile water to form a 25% solution (D25W)

How Supplied.   Fifty percent dextrose is supplied in prefilled syringes containing 25 grams of *d-glucose* in 50 milliliters of water.

thiamine

Class: Vitamin

Description.   Thiamine is an important vitamin commonly referred to as vitamin B_1. It is required for the conversion of pyruvic acid to acetyl-coenzyme-A.

Mechanism of Action.   A vitamin is a substance that the body cannot manufacture but that is required for metabolism. Most of the vitamins required by the body are obtained through the diet. Thiamine is required for the conversion of pyruvic acid to acetyl-coenzyme-A. Without this step, a significant amount of the energy available in glucose cannot be obtained. The brain is extremely sensitive to thiamine deficiency.

Chronic alcohol intake interferes with the absorption, intake, and use of thiamine. A significant percentage of alcoholics have thiamine deficiency. During extended periods of fasting, neurological symptoms owing to thiamine deficiency can occur. These include Wernicke's syndrome and Korsakoff's psychosis. Wernicke's syndrome is an acute and reversible encephalopathy characterized by an unsteady gait, eye muscle weakness, and mental derangement. Korsakoff's psychosis is a significant memory disorder and may be irreversible. Any comatose patients, especially those who are suspected to be alcoholic, should receive IV thiamine in addition to the administration of 50% dextrose or naloxone.

Indications

- ❑ Coma of unknown origin, especially if alcohol may be involved
- ❑ Delirium tremens

Contraindications.   There are no contraindications to the administration of thiamine in the emergency setting.

Precautions.   A few cases of hypersensitivity to thiamine have been reported.

Side Effects.   Few side effects are reported with thiamine usage. However, hypotension, dyspnea, and respiratory failure have been reported with its use.

Interactions.   None in the emergency setting.

Dosage.   The emergency dose of thiamine is 100 milligrams intravenously or intramuscularly. The intravenous route is preferred in emergency medicine.

Pediatric Dosage.   Rarely indicated

How Supplied.   Thiamine is supplied in 1-milliliter ampules containing 100 milligrams of the vitamin.

glucagon

Class: Hormone/antihypoglycemic

Description.   Glucagon is a protein secreted by the α cells of the pancreas. Glucagon for parenteral administration is extracted from beef and pork pancreas. It is used to increase the blood glucose level in cases of hypoglycemia where an IV cannot be immediately placed.

✳ Glucagon can be used to increase blood glucose levels in cases where an IV cannot be started.

Mechanism of Action.   Glucagon is a hormone secreted by the pancreas. When released, it causes a breakdown of stored glycogen to glucose. It also inhibits the synthesis of glycogen from glucose. Both actions tend to cause an increase in circulating blood glucose. In hypoglycemia, the administration of glucagon increases blood glucose levels. The drug of choice in the management of insulin-induced hypoglycemia is still D50W. A return to consciousness is seen almost immediately following the administration of glucose. A return to consciousness following the administration of glucagon usually takes from 5 to 20 minutes. Glucagon is only effective if there are sufficient stores of glycogen in the liver.

Glucagon exerts a positive inotropic action on the heart and decreases renal vascular resistance.

Indications

❑ Hypoglycemia

Contraindications. Because glucagon is a protein, hypersensitivity may occur. Do not administer glucagon to patients with a known hypersensitivity to the drug.

Precautions. Glucagon is only effective if there are sufficient stores of glycogen within the liver. In an emergency situation, intravenous glucose is the agent of choice. Glucagon should be administered with caution to patients with a history of cardiovascular or renal disease.

Side Effects. Although side effects are rare, glucagon can cause hypotension, dizziness, headache, nausea, and vomiting.

Interactions. Few interactions with glucagon are reported in the emergency setting.

Dosage. A standard initial dose is 0.25 to 0.5 units intravenously. If an IV cannot be obtained, 1 milligram of glucagon can be administered intramuscularly. Glucagon can be administered intravenously, intramuscularly, or subcutaneously.

Pediatric Dosage. 0.03 mg/kg

How Supplied. Glucagon must be reconstituted before administration. It is supplied in rubber-stoppered vials containing 1 unit of powder and 1 milliliter of diluting solution. It must be used or refrigerated after reconstitution.

Drugs Used in the Treatment of Neurological Emergencies

Emergencies involving the nervous system can be devastating. In addition, they are notoriously difficult to manage. Signs and symptoms of neurological disorders can range from slight headache to coma. Prompt recognition and treatment of neurological emergencies is essential.

diazepam (Valium)

Class: Anti-convulsant/sedative

Description. Diazepam is a benzodiazepine which is frequently used as an anticonvulsant, sedative, and hypnotic.

Mechanism of Action. In emergency medicine, diazepam is principally used for its anticonvulsant properties. It suppresses the spread of seizure activity through the motor cortex of the brain. It does not appear to abolish the abnormal discharge focus, however.

Diazepam, one of the most frequently prescribed medications in the United States, is used in the management of anxiety and stress. It is effective in treating the tremors and anxiety associated with alcohol withdrawal. It is also an effective skeletal muscle relaxant, which makes it an effective adjunct in orthopedic injuries. It is a good premedication for minor operative procedures and cardioversion because it induces amnesia, which diminishes the patient's recall of such procedures.

✻ Valium may effectively suppress the source of seizure activity in the brain, making it an effective medication in the acute management of seizures.

Indications

❑ Major motor seizures
❑ Status epilepticus
❑ Premedication before cardioversion
❑ Skeletal muscle relaxant
❑ Acute anxiety states

Contraindications. Diazepam should not be administered to any patient with a history of hypersensitivity to the drug.

Precautions. Because diazepam is a relatively short-acting drug, seizure activity may recur. In such cases, an additional dose may be required. Flumazenil (Romazicon), a benzodiazepine antagonist, should be available to use as antidote if required.

Injectable diazepam can cause local venous irritation. To minimize this, it should only be injected into relatively large veins and should not be given faster than 1 milliliter per minute.

Side Effects. Diazepam can cause hypotension, drowsiness, headache, amnesia, respiratory depression, blurred vision, nausea, and vomiting.

Interactions. Diazepam is incompatible with many medications. Any time diazepam is given intravenously in conjunction with other drugs, the IV line should be adequately flushed. The effects of diazepam can be additive when used in conjunction with other CNS depressants and alcohol.

Dosage. In the management of seizures, the usual dose of diazepam is 5 to 10 milligrams IV. In many instances it may be necessary to give diazepam directly into the vein, as the seizure activity will prevent the insertion of an indwelling catheter. When given directly into a vein, it is essential that a large vein, preferably in the antecubital fossa, is used.

In acute anxiety reactions, the standard dosage is 2 to 5 milligrams intramuscularly or intravenously.

To induce amnesia prior to cardioversion, a dosage of 5 to 15 milligrams of diazepam is given intravenously. Peak effects are seen in 5 to 10 minutes.

Diazepam should be given intravenously by slow IV push. It can be injected intramuscularly, but absorption via this route is variable. When an IV line cannot be started, parenteral diazepam can be administered rectally with a similar onset of action.

Pediatric Dosage. 0.1–0.2 mg/kg

How Supplied. Valium is supplied in ampules and prefilled syringes containing 10 milligrams in 2 milliliters of solvent.

methylprednisolone (Solu-Medrol)

Class: Corticosteroid/anti-inflammatory

Description. Methylprednisolone is an intermediate-acting corticosteroid related to the natural hormones secreted by the adrenal cortex.

Mechanism of Action. Methylprednisolone is an intermediate-acting steroid. In general medical practice, steroids have a wide range of uses. Effective as anti-inflammatory agents, they are used in the management of allergic reactions and occasionally as an adjunctive agent in the management of shock. The role of steroids in the management of neurological emergencies remains controversial.

It is generally agreed that a large single dose of steroids has little harmful effect. Consequently, it is used in patients with spinal cord injury both in the emergency department and in the prehospital setting.

Indications

- ❑ Spinal cord injury
- ❑ Anaphylaxis
- ❑ Asthma
- ❑ Exacerbation of COPD

Contraindications. There are no major contraindications to the use of methylprednisolone in the emergency setting.

Precautions. A single dose of methylprednisolone is all that should be given in the prehospital phase of care. Long-term steroid therapy can cause gastrointestinal bleeding, prolonged wound healing, and suppression of adrenocortical steroids.

Side Effects. Methylprednisolone can cause fluid retention, congestive heart failure, hypertension, abdominal distention, vertigo, headache, nausea, malaise, and hiccups.

Interactions. Few in the prehospital setting.

Dosage

- ❏ *Spinal cord injury.* High-dose methylprednisolone is used in treating spinal cord injuries. An initial bolus of 30 mg/kg is administered intravenously over a 15-minute period. This is followed 45 minutes later by a maintenance infusion of 5.4 milligrams/kilogram/hour.
- ❏ *Asthma/COPD/allergic reactions.* For other emergencies, 80–125 milligrams is usually administered intravenously or intramuscularly.

Pediatric Dosage. 30 µg/kg

How Supplied. Methylprednisolone is supplied in vials containing 125 and 250 milligrams of the drug. The drug must be reconstituted prior to administration.

Drugs Used in the Treatment of Obstetrical and Gynecological Emergencies

Prehospital care for most obstetric and gynecologic emergencies is supportive. However, there are two complications that necessitate intervention with pharmacological agents. These include toxemia of pregnancy and severe postpartum vaginal bleeding. Magnesium sulfate has proven effective in controlling the convulsions associated with toxemia of pregnancy. Pitocin, a drug chemically identical to the hormone oxytocin, is effective in causing uterine contraction. In many cases, it will slow postpartum vaginal bleeding.

oxytocin (Pitocin)

Class: Hormone/uterine stimulant

Description. Oxytocin is a naturally occurring hormone that is secreted by the posterior pituitary.

Mechanism of Action. Oxytocin causes contraction of uterine smooth muscle and lactation. Oxytocin is used to induce labor in selected cases and is also effective in inducing uterine contractions following delivery, thereby controlling postpartum hemorrhage.

When a baby is placed on the breast, the sucking action causes the posterior pituitary to release oxytocin. It is important to remember this inherent mechanism whenever confronted by a patient suffering moderate to severe postpartum bleeding.

Indications

- ❏ Postpartum hemorrhage

Contraindications. In the prehospital setting, oxytocin should be administered only to patients suffering severe postpartum bleeding. Before administration it is essential to verify that the baby and the placenta have been delivered and that there is not an additional fetus in the uterus.

Precautions. Excess oxytocin can cause overstimulation of the uterus and possible uterine rupture. Hypertension, cardiac arrhythmia, and anaphylaxis have been reported in conjunction with the administration of oxytocin. Vital signs and uterine tone should be monitored.

Side Effects. Oxytocin can cause hypotension, arrhythmias, tachycardia, seizures, coma, nausea, and vomiting in the mother. When administered prior to delivery, oxytocin can cause fetal hypoxia, fetal asphyxia, fetal arrhythmias, and possibly fetal intracranial bleeding.

Interactions. Oxytocin can cause hypertension when administered in conjunction with vasoconstrictors such as norepinephrine.

Dosage. The following are two regimens for the administration of oxytocin in the management of patients with postpartum hemorrhage:

■ **titrate** estimate by slowly changing the dose.

❏ 3 to 10 units can be administered intramuscularly following delivery of the placenta.

❏ 10 to 20 units can be placed in either 500 or 1000 milliliters of D5W or lactated Ringer's. This should be **titrated** (estimated by slowly changing the dose) according to the severity of the bleeding and the uterine response.

Oxytocin should only be administered intramuscularly or by slow IV infusion.

Pediatric Dosage. Not indicated

How Supplied. Pitocin is supplied in 0.5- and 1-milliliter ampules containing 10 milligrams per milliliter. A 1-milliliter prefilled syringe containing the same concentration is also available.

magnesium sulfate

Class: Electrolyte

Description. Magnesium sulfate is a salt that dissociates into the magnesium cation (Mg^{++}) and the sulfate anion when administered. Magnesium is an essential element in numerous biochemical reactions that occur within the body.

Mechanism of Action. Magnesium sulfate is a central nervous system depressant effective in the management of seizures associated with eclampsia. It is used for the initial therapy of convulsions associated with pregnancy. After cessation of seizure activity, other anticonvulsant agents may be administered.

Indications

❏ Eclampsia (seizures accompanying pregnancy)
❏ Pre-term labor

Contraindications. Magnesium sulfate should not be administered to any patient with heart block or recent myocardial infarction. It should not be administered to patients in shock, who have persistent severe hypertension, who routinely undergo dialysis, or who are known to have a decreased calcium level (hypocalcemia).

Precautions. Magnesium sulfate, like other central nervous system depressants, can cause hypotension, circulatory collapse, and depression of cardiac and respiratory function. The most immediate danger is respiratory depression. Calcium chloride should be readily available for IV administration as an antidote in case respiratory depression occurs. Magnesium sulfate should be administered slowly to minimize side effects. Any patient receiving intravenous magnesium sulfate should have continuous cardiac monitoring as well as frequent monitoring of vital signs. If possible, the knee and biceps deep tendon reflexes should be checked prior to magnesium therapy.

Side Effects. Magnesium sulfate can cause flushing, sweating, bradycardia, decreased deep tendon reflexes, drowsiness, respiratory depression, arrhythmias, hypotension, hypothermia, itching, and a rash.

Interactions. Magnesium sulfate can cause cardiac conduction abnormalities if administered in conjunction with digitalis.

Dosage. The standard dosage for the management of convulsions associated with eclampsia is 2–4 grams intravenously. If an IV cannot be started, magnesium sulfate can be administered intramuscularly. Because of the volume of the drug (5–10 ml), the dose should be divided in half and each half administered intramuscularly at a separate site (usually each gluteus).

Pediatric Dosage. Not indicated

How Supplied. Magnesium sulfate is supplied in prefilled syringes containing 5 and 10 milliliters of a 50% solution.

Drugs Used in the Management of Toxicological Emergencies

Toxicological emergencies account for a high percentage of EMS calls (see Chapter 26). Therefore, you should be familiar with the following medications. Remember to always consult with the local Poison Control Center.

diphenhydramine (Benadryl)

Class: Antihistamine

Description. Diphenhydramine is a potent antihistamine that blocks both H1 and H2 histamine receptors.

Mechanism of Action. Histamine is released from Mast cells following exposure to an antigen to which the body has been previously sensitized. When released into the circulation following an allergic reaction, histamine acts on two different receptors. The first type of receptor, called H1, when stimulated, causes bronchoconstriction and contraction of the gut. The second type of receptor, called H2, when stimulated, causes peripheral vasodilation and secretion of gastric acids.

Antihistamines are administered after epinephrine in the treatment of anaphylaxis. Epinephrine causes immediate bronchodilation by activating β_2 adrenergic receptors, whereas diphenhydramine inhibits histamine release.

Diphenhydramine is also useful in the treatment of dystonic reactions accompanying phenothiazine use. A *dystonic* or **extrapyramidal reaction** is characterized by an unusual posture, change in muscle tone, drooling, or uncontrolled movements. It is occasionally seen following the administration of antipsychotic medications (Haldol, Thorazine, Mellaril) as well as certain medications used for nausea and vomiting (Phenergan, Compazine, Reglan). Diphenhydramine, when administered, causes marked improvement, if not total resolution of the symptoms.

■ **extrapyramidal (EPS) reaction** a response to a drug marked by uncontrolled movements, changes in muscle tone, and abnormal posture.

Indications

❑ Anaphylaxis
❑ Allergic reactions
❑ Dystonic (extrapyramidal) reactions

Contraindications. Diphenhydramine should not be used in the management of lower respiratory diseases such as asthma.

Precautions. The primary drug for the treatment of severe allergic reactions, anaphylaxis, and urticaria is epinephrine. Epinephrine will reverse many of the effects of histamine. Diphenhydramine will block histamine receptors preventing subsequent stimulation by circulating histamine.

Side Effects. Diphenhydramine can cause hypotension, headache, palpitations, tachycardia, sedation, drowsiness, and disturbed coordination.

Interactions. The sedative effects of diphenhydramine can be potentiated by the administration of CNS depressants, other antihistamines, narcotics, and alcohol.

Dosage. The standard dosage of diphenhydramine is 25 to 50 milligrams, either intravenously or intramuscularly. Diphenhydramine should be administered intravenously or intramuscularly.

Pediatric Dosage. 2–5 mg/kg

How Supplied. Diphenhydramine is supplied in ampules and prefilled syringes containing 50 milligrams of the drug in 1 milliliter of solvent.

syrup of ipecac

Class: Emetic

Description. Syrup of ipecac is a potent and effective emetic used in the management of poisonings where the induction of vomiting is indicated.

Mechanism of Action. Syrup of ipecac is used to remove the stomach contents in cases of poisoning. Syrup of ipecac acts as a local irritant on the enteric tract and on emetic centers within the brain, thus causing emesis. To assure complete evacuation of the stomach, the administration of ipecac is usually followed by several glasses of warm water. Recently, some studies have advocated the use of carbonated beverages instead of warm water. Carbonated beverages may cause emesis sooner. Emesis, following administration, usually occurs within 5 to 10 minutes.

Indications

- ❑ Poisoning
- ❑ Overdose

Contraindications. Vomiting should not be induced in any patient with impaired consciousness. It should also not be induced when the ingested substance is a strong acid base (that is, caustic ingestion) or petroleum distillate.

In addition, administration of syrup of ipecac is not indicated when the ingested agent was an antiemetic, especially of the phenothiazine type.

The trend in the management of toxicological emergencies has been to use activated charcoal alone without ipecac. This is primarily because of the increased risk of aspiration associated with ipecac usage.

Precautions. It is important to monitor constantly the patient's airway during and following emesis. Activated charcoal should only be administered after vomiting has occurred. Ipecac should be used with caution in patients with heart disease.

Side Effects. Ipecac can cause arrhythmias, hypotension, diarrhea, depression, and bleeding from Mallory-Weiss tears and esophageal varices.

Interactions. Syrup of ipecac should not be given with activated charcoal as the activated charcoal can nullify the effects of the ipecac.

Dosage. The standard dose of syrup of ipecac is 15 to 30 milliliters orally, followed by several glasses of warm water or carbonated soda. Syrup of ipecac should only be administered orally.

Pediatric Dosage. *Less than 1 year:* 10 ml; *1-12 years:* 15 ml; *Greater than 12 years:* 30 ml

How Supplied. Syrup of ipecac is supplied in bottles containing 1 ounce (approximately 30 milliliters).

activated charcoal

Class: Adsorbent

Description. Activated charcoal is a fine black powder that binds and adsorbs ingested toxins still present in the gastrointestinal tract following emesis or in lieu of emesis.

Mechanism of Action. Activated charcoal has a tremendous surface area. It binds and adsorbs ingested toxins present in the gastrointestinal tract. Once bound to the activated charcoal, the combined complex is excreted from the body.

Indications

- ❑ Poisoning

Contraindications. There are no major contraindications to the use of activated charcoal in severe poisoning.

Precautions. Activated charcoal should not be administered to the patient who has an altered level of consciousness unless administered by nasogastric tube and the airway protected by an endotracheal tube. If emesis is to be induced with ipecac, it is often best to wait until the patient has vomited to administer activated charcoal.

Side Effects. Activated charcoal can cause nausea, vomiting, abdominal cramping, abdominal bloating, and constipation.

Interactions.   Activated charcoal should not be given with syrup of ipecac as the activated charcoal can nullify the effects of the ipecac.

Dosage.   The standard dosage in the management of poisoning is 50–75 grams mixed with a glass of water to form a slurry. This is administered orally or through a nasogastric tube. Activated charcoal is often mixed with a cathartic, commonly sorbitol, to promote elimination of the ingested poison from the GI tract and to prevent the constipation associated with activated charcoal usage. Activated charcoal should only be administered orally in a slurry solution made with water as described earlier.

Pediatric Dosage.   1 g/kg mixed in water to form a slurry

How Supplied.   Activated charcoal is supplied in bottles containing 25 and 50 grams of the drug.

naloxone (Narcan)

Class: Narcotic antagonist

Description.   Naloxone is an effective narcotic antagonist. It has proved effective in the management and reversal of overdoses caused by narcotics or synthetic narcotic agents.

Mechanism of Action.   Naloxone is chemically similar to the narcotics. However, it has only antagonistic properties. Naloxone competes for opiate receptors in the brain. It also displaces narcotic molecules from opiate receptors. It can reverse respiratory depression associated with narcotic overdose.

Indications

❑ For the complete or partial reversal of depression caused by narcotics including the following agents:

morphine	Demerol	heroin
paregoric	Dilaudid	codeine
Percodan	Fentanyl	methadone

❑ For the complete or partial reversal of depression caused by synthetic narcotic analgesic agents including the following drugs:

Nubain	Talwin	Stadol	Darvon

❑ Treatment of coma of unknown origin

Contraindications.   Naloxone should not be administered to a patient with a history of hypersensitivity to the drug.

Precautions.   Naloxone should be administered cautiously to patients who are known or suspected to be physically dependent on narcotics. Abrupt and complete reversal by naloxone can cause withdrawal-type effects. This includes newborn infants of mothers with known or suspected narcotic dependence.

Side Effects.   Side effects associated with naloxone are rare. However, hypotension, hypertension, ventricular arrhythmias, nausea, and vomiting have been reported.

Interactions.   Naloxone may cause narcotic withdrawal in the narcotic-dependent patient. In cases of suspected narcotic dependence, administer only enough of the drug to reverse respiratory depression.

Dosage.   The standard dosage for suspected or confirmed narcotic or synthetic narcotic overdoses is 1 to 2 milligrams IV. If unsuccessful, then a second dose may be administered 5 minutes later. Failure to obtain reversal after 2 to 3 doses indicates another disease process or overdosage on non-opioid drugs. Larger-than-average doses (2 to 5 milligrams) have been used in the management of Darvon overdoses and alcoholic coma.

An intravenous infusion can be prepared by placing 2 milligrams of naloxone in 500 milliliters of D5W. This gives a concentration of 4 micrograms per milliliter. One hundred milliliters per hour should be infused, thus delivering 0.4 milligrams per hour. In the emergency setting, naloxone should be administered intravenously only. When an IV line cannot be established, intramuscular or subcutaneous administration can be performed.

Naloxone can be administered endotracheally. The dose should be increased to 2.0–2.5 times the intravenous dose. Furthermore, naloxone should be diluted in enough normal saline to provide a total of 10 milliliters of fluid.

Pediatric Dosage. *Less than 5 years:* 0.1 mg/kg; *Greater than 5 years:* 2.0 mg

How Supplied. Naloxone is supplied in ampules and prefilled syringes containing 2 milligrams in 2 milliliters of solvent. In addition, vials containing 10 milliliters of the 1 milligram per milliliter concentration are also available.

Drugs Used in the Management of Behavioral Emergencies

In behavioral emergencies, remember the rule "safety first." In cases in which a psychologically disturbed patient must be quieted, consider haloperidol (or other medication suggested by medical control).

haloperidol (Haldol)

Class: Major tranquilizer

Description. Haloperidol is a frequently used major tranquilizer.

Mechanism of Action. Haloperidol is a major tranquilizer that has proved effective in the management of acute psychotic episodes. It has pharmacological properties similar to those of the phenothiazine class of drugs (for example, Thorazine). Haloperidol appears to block dopamine receptors in the brain associated with mood and behavior. However, its precise mechanism of action is not clearly understood. Haloperidol has weak anticholinergic properties.

Indications

❏ Acute psychotic episodes

Contraindications. Haloperidol should not be administered in cases in which other drugs, especially sedatives, may be present. Haloperidol should not be used in the management of dysphoria caused by Talwin, as it may promote sedation and anesthesia.

Precautions. Haloperidol may impair mental and physical abilities. Occasionally, orthostatic hypotension may be seen in conjunction with haloperidol use. Caution should be used when administering haloperidol to patients on anticoagulants.

Extrapyramidal, or Parkinson-like, reactions have been known to occur following the administration of haloperidol, especially in children. Diphenhydramine (Benadryl) should be readily available.

Side Effects. Haloperidol can cause extrapyramidal symptoms (EPS), insomnia, restlessness, sedation, seizures, respiratory depression, dry mouth, constipation, increased salivation, hypotension, and tachycardia.

Interactions. Antihypertensive medications may increase the likelihood of a patient developing hypotension with haloperidol administration. Haloperidol should be used with caution in patients taking lithium, as irreversible brain damage (encephalopathic syndrome) has been reported when these two drugs are used together.

Dosage. Doses of 2 to 5 milligrams intramuscularly are fairly standard in the management of an acute psychotic episode with severe symptoms. Haloperidol should be given intramuscularly only.

Pediatric Dosage. Rarely used

How Supplied. Haloperidol is supplied in 1-milliliter ampules containing 5 milligrams of the drug.

Other Medications

In certain cases, such as those detailed below, you may find it useful to administer promethazine.

promethazine (Phenergan)

Class: Antihistamine/antiemetic

Description.   Promethazine is a phenothiazine derivative with potent antihistamine properties and anticholinergic properties.

Mechanism of Action.   Promethazine possesses sedative, antihistamine, antiemetic, and anticholinergic properties. It competitively blocks histamine receptors. The duration of action of promethazine is 4–6 hours. It is an effective and frequently used antiemetic. Promethazine, unlike hydroxyzine, can be given intravenously. It is often administered with analgesics, particularly narcotics, to potentiate their effect.

Indications

- ❑ Nausea and vomiting
- ❑ Motion sickness
- ❑ To potentiate the effects of analgesics
- ❑ Sedation

Contraindications.   Promethazine is contraindicated in unresponsive states and in patients who have received a large amount of depressants. Also, it should not be administered to any patient with a history of hypersensitivity to the drug.

Precautions.   Promethazine may impair mental and physical abilities. Care must be taken to avoid accidental intra-arterial injection. It should never be administered subcutaneously. Extrapyramidal symptoms (EPS) have been reported following promethazine use. Diphenhydramine (Benadryl) should be available.

Side Effects.   Promethazine can cause drowsiness, sedation, blurred vision, tachycardia, bradycardia, and dizziness.

Interactions.   The CNS-depressant effects of narcotics, sedative/hypnotics, and alcohol is potentiated by promethazine. An increased incidence of extrapyramidal symptoms has been reported when promethazine is administered to patients taking monamine oxidase inhibitors (MAOI).

Dosage.   The standard dosage of promethazine in the management of nausea and vomiting is 12.5 to 25 milligrams either intravenously or intramuscularly. The standard dosage in adjunctive use with analgesics is 25 milligrams. Promethazine should be given by IV or deep intramuscular injection only. Care must be taken to avoid accidental intra-arterial injection.

Pediatric Dosage.   0.5 mg/kg

How Supplied.   Promethazine is supplied in ampules and Tubex syringes containing 25 milligrams of the drug in 1 milliliter of solvent.

SUMMARY

This chapter has presented the fundamental aspects of pharmacological therapy as it applies to prehospital care. The medications used in prehospital care vary among EMS systems. As a paramedic, it is your responsibility to be familiar with all medications in your EMS system. Infrequently used medications should be periodically reviewed. Overall, it is important to appreciate the inherent dangers of emergency medications and to use them properly. The rule to remember is "When in doubt, do no harm."

✳ When in doubt, do no harm.

FURTHER READING

American Heart Association. *Textbook of Advanced Cardiac Life Support*, 3rd ed. Dallas: American Heart Association, 1993.

American Heart Association and American Academy of Pediatrics. *Textbook of Pediatric Advanced Life Support.* Dallas: American Heart Association, 1993.

Bledsoe, Bryan E., Dwayne Clayden, and Frank J. Papa. *Prehospital Emergency Pharmacology,* 4th ed. Upper Saddle River, NJ: Prentice Hall, 1992.

Goodman, L.S., and A. Gillman. *The Pharmacological Basis of Therapeutics.* 7th ed. New York: MacMillan, 1985.

Martini, Fredric. *Fundamentals of Anatomy and Physiology,* 2nd ed. Englewood Cliffs, NJ: Prentice Hall, 1992.

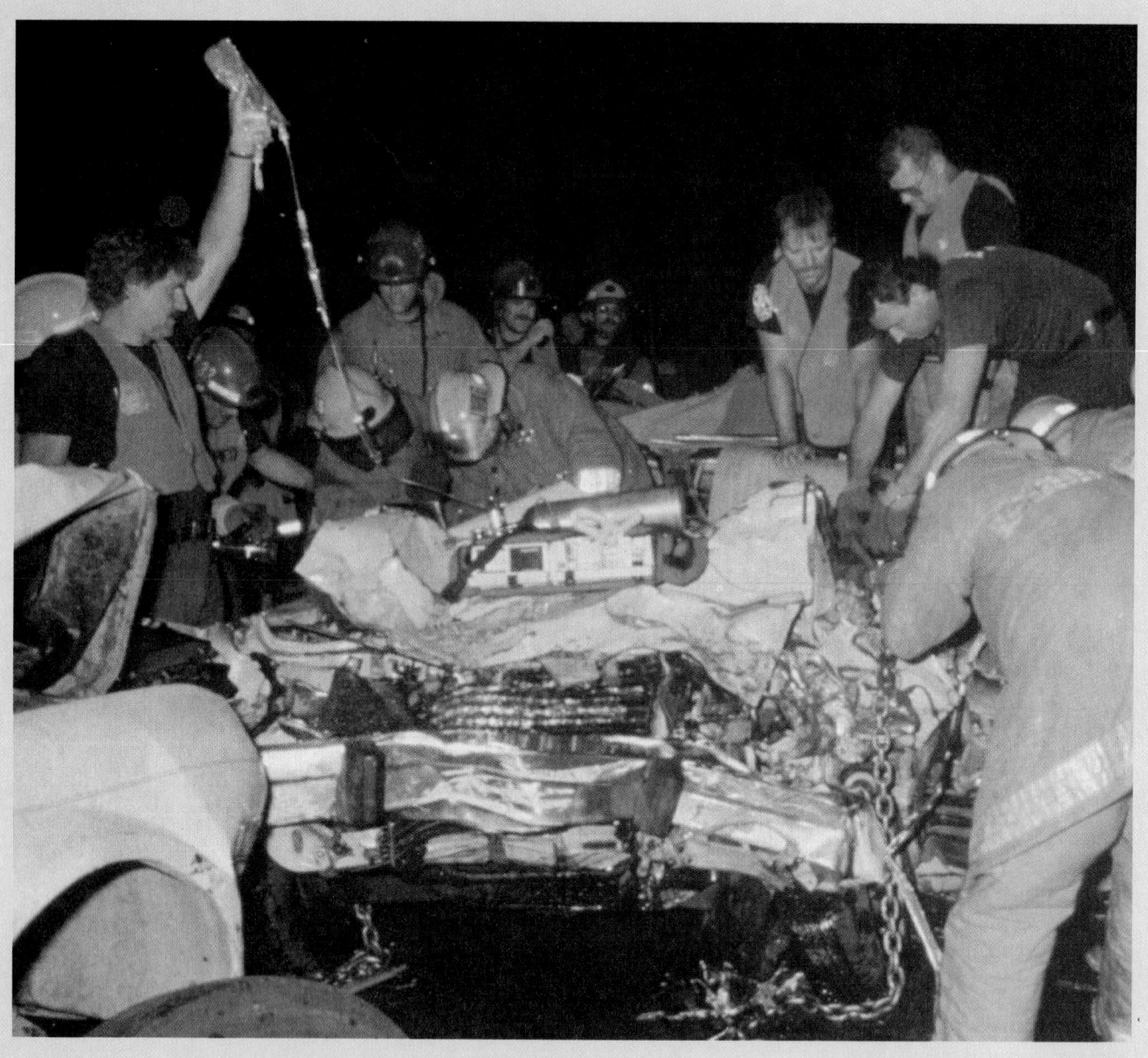

14

THE KINETICS OF TRAUMA

Objectives for Chapter 14

After reading this chapter, you should be able to:

1. Describe the prevalence and significance of trauma. (See p. 402.)

2. Explain the "Golden Hour" concept, and describe how it applies to prehospital emergency medical service. (See p. 404.)

3. Identify, and explain by example, the laws of inertia and conservation of energy. (See p. 406.)

4. Apply the principles of kinetic energy and force to various types of trauma. (See pp. 406–407.)

5. Compare and contrast the types of impact associated with auto and motorcycle accidents. (See pp. 408–420.)

6. Predict injuries expected from various types of auto impacts and other blunt and penetrating trauma. (See pp. 411–418.)

7. Discuss the benefits and disadvantages of the use of auto restraint and motorcycle helmets. (See pp. 410–420.)

8. Describe the significance and meaning of the terms velocity, cavitation, and profile as they relate to penetrating trauma. (See pp. 426–429.)

9. Associate various types of penetrating trauma with the extent of injury they can involve. (See pp. 429–431.)

10. Describe how the environment and mechanism of injury can alert you to specific types of injury. (See pp. 402–431.)

A call comes into City Ambulance. The dispatcher reports multiple people injured in a two-car accident at the freeway interchange. Because of backed-up traffic, the dispatcher tells the unit to use the exit ramp.

Police arrive at the scene and update the en route ambulance. A green auto traveling at freeway speed has plowed into a red car stalled at the interchange. The wreck involves three injured parties—one in the red car and two in the green.

When the ambulance crew reaches the scene, they note that about 100 yards separate the two vehicles. The green car has severe front-end damage. Two "spider web" cracks run across the windshield, and the steering column is deformed. The police officer in charge reports that both people failed to wear seatbelts. The red car has severe rear-end damage, but the windshield is intact. The driver in this vehicle wore a seatbelt and the headrest is in the up position. Before acting, the paramedics call for another unit to back them up and secure the scene. They proceed to the green car, where they expect to find the worst injuries.

The crew assesses the two victims. The driver has suffered chest trauma caused by impact with the steering wheel. Although she is experiencing difficult and painful breathing, the airway is clear. She is oriented to time and place and denies any period of unconsciousness. Her pulses are strong, regular, and at a moderate rate. A physical exam reveals a forehead contusion, a reddened anterior chest with crepitation, and clear breath sounds bilaterally. The passenger is unresponsive and cannot be aroused. The paramedics note shallow rapid breaths and a rapid, barely palpable pulse. Her forehead is badly contused and with moderate bleeding. Her thighs appear noticeably shortened and physical assessment reveals instability of the pelvis and both femurs.

A first-responder-trained police officer indicates that the driver of the other car is conscious and alert. Although "shaken up," he has a blood pressure of 126/84 and a pulse of 86. He is breathing normally at a rate of 20. The paramedic in charge asks the officer to stay with him until the second ambulance arrives.

The paramedics tell the driver of the green car not to move. They stabilize the passenger's

INTRODUCTION

The three most frequent causes of death in the United States include: cardiovascular disease, cancer, and **trauma**. Trauma is the leading cause of death for persons under age 34. It claims more than 140,000 lives each year, approximately 44,000 of which are lost on the nation's highways. These statistics clearly reveal the prevalence and importance of trauma in prehospital emergency care.

Although trauma poses a serious threat to life, the form in which it appears often masks the patient's true condition. Extremity injuries, for example, rarely cause death. Yet they are frequently obvious and grotesque. Life-threatening problems, such as internal bleeding and shock, often occur with only subtle signs and symptoms. In trauma, assessment must look beyond obvious injuries for evidence that suggests life-threatening situations.

As emergency medical service evolved in the late 1960s, a new emphasis was placed upon care at the auto accident—care that had not been provided before. Experts later found, however, that many seriously injured patients received care for obvious injuries, while they bled to death internally. Some patients reached the emergency department and surgery too late to survive. In recent years, the approach to treating trauma patients has been modified to ensure quick identification and rapid transportation of seriously injured patients. The result has been a reduction in trauma deaths (*mortality*) and disability (*morbidity*).

head manually and apply a cervical collar. Next, they prepare a long spine board with straps and a PASG. They place the patient on the board, strap her securely, and affix the head with a cervical immobilization device. They then load her into the ambulance.

When the second ambulance arrives, the paramedics brief the crew and assign the remaining patients. They rush the most critical victim to a nearby trauma center. En route, vital signs are taken quickly and reveal a blood pressure of 82 by palpation and a weak radial pulse of 130. The legs look ashen, feel cool to the touch, and show no palpable pulses. Capillary refill time is three seconds in the upper extremities and longer in the lower ones.

Paramedics give a brief report to medical control and receive orders. They inflate the PASG, start two large-bore IVs, and run fluids using pressure infusers. Next, they administer oxygen by nonrebreathing mask. They ready intubation equipment and hyperventilate the patient using the bag-valve-mask. The ambulance stops briefly while paramedics attempt nasotracheal intubation. When the effort proves unsuccessful, they withdraw the tube, hyperventilate the patient, and try digital intubation. The technique works. Lung sounds are clear, chest excursion improves, and oximetry readings begin to rise.

The patient arrives at the trauma center with just under 2,000 mL of fluid infused, the PASG fully inflated, and the operating room ready. Doctors clear the C-spine by X-ray, repair vascular injuries associated with the pelvic fracture, and infuse six units of typed and cross-matched whole blood. The patient recovers after a few weeks of hospitalization and will walk again with only slight reminders of the injuries and care she received.

The second ambulance crew decides to transport the other two patients to the trauma center based on the speed of impact and vehicle damage. The driver of the green car has two fractured ribs, a C-spine cleared by X-ray, and no neurologic deficit. She stays overnight for observation and is released the next afternoon with some medication for rib fracture pain. The other driver has a clear C-spine and returns home shortly after the emergency department evaluation.

TRAUMA TRIAGE PROTOCOLS

You will assess trauma through the use of what is known as **trauma triage protocols**. These criteria include two elements. First, they identify the mechanisms of injury that can cause serious internal trauma. Second, they establish the physical or clinical findings that reflect internal injury. By applying these criteria, patients with a high likelihood of internal injury can be sent quickly to a trauma center. The first step in using trauma triage protocols is analysis of the mechanism of injury.

■ **trauma triage protocols** guidelines to aid prehospital personnel in determining which patients will require urgent transportation to a trauma center.

Mechanism of Injury

To help determine the **mechanism of injury**, you mentally recreate the accident from evidence available at the scene. That is, you identify the forces involved, the direction from which they came, and the bodily locations affected by these forces. In the auto accident, the mechanism of injury is the process by which forces are exchanged between the auto and what it struck, the patient and the auto interior, and the various tissues and organs as they collide, one with another, within the patient. Close inspection of the auto and the forces, or various collisions, can lead to an index of suspicion for possible injuries.

■ **mechanism of injury** the strength, direction, and nature of forces that cause injury to a patient.

✳ The mechanism of injury is the exchange of forces that results in injury to the victim.

Index of Suspicion

■ **index of suspicion** the anticipation of injuries based on analysis of the mechanism of injury.

The **index of suspicion** is an anticipation of possible injuries based upon analysis of the event. A pedestrian struck by a car is expected to have fractures of the lower extremities. Further, if the auto was moving at 20 miles per hour, fracture severity would be less than if it were moving at 55 miles per hour. Also, there is less probability of internal injury at lower speeds than at higher speeds. By evaluating the strength and nature of impact, you can anticipate the organs damaged and the degree to which they have been damaged. This analysis provides the *index of suspicion*.

If your primary assessment rules out any immediate life threat, examine the suspected area of trauma. Physical signs of trauma such as abrasions or contusions confirm the index of suspicion. If you do not identify any physical evidence, re-examine the mechanism of injury and evaluate the vital signs. Many serious injuries will be missed if the index of suspicion is too low.

The Golden Hour

■ **Golden Hour** the one-hour time period following a severe injury. Based on research, it has been demonstrated that severe trauma patients who reach surgery within this period have a higher survival rate.

Time is an important consideration when caring for trauma patients. The **Golden Hour** has been greatly publicized by the Maryland Institute for Emergency Medical Services and is well accepted as the standard for emergency intervention. (See Figure 14-1.) The institute's research has shown that if severely injured patients can undergo surgery within one hour, their chances of survival are greatly enhanced.

Of that hour, prehospital care accounts for about ten minutes of on-the-scene time. You will use this time to assess, stabilize (in an emergent sense), package, extricate, and begin transporting critical or potentially critical patients. With such a short period for patient care, you must assess trauma patients quickly and provide only the most essential care. As a paramedic, the care you provide will be extremely effective if you distinguish quickly between those patients that need on-the-scene stabilization and those that need rapid transport.

Decision to Transport

The decision either to transport a patient immediately or to attempt more extensive on-the-scene care is among the most difficult decisions you must

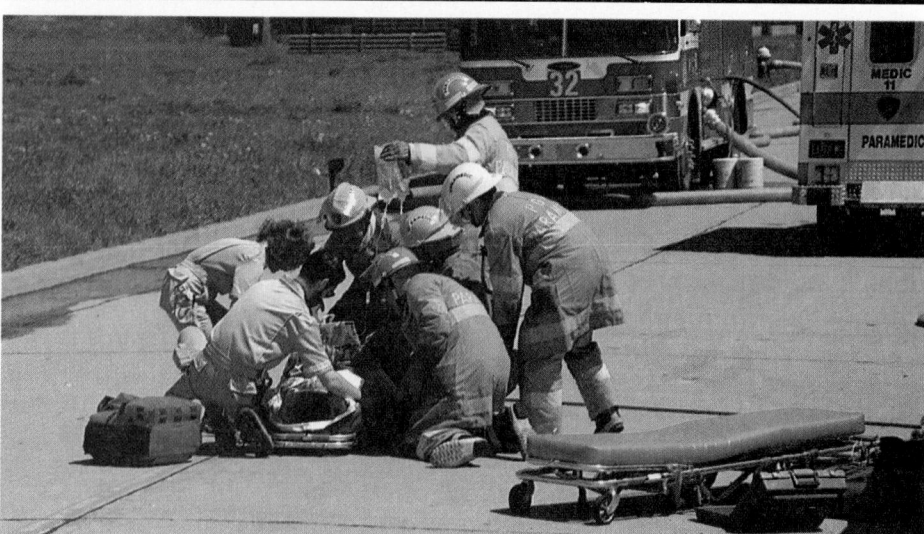

FIGURE 14-1 Victims of severe trauma have enhanced chances of survival if they can be delivered to the operating room within one hour after their accident (the "Golden Hour").

make. Application of the trauma triage protocols guide you in this decision. As a rule, patients who experience certain mechanisms of injury, or display distinct clinical findings, should be transported quickly with intravenous access and other procedures attempted en route. (See Figure 14-2.) Indicators include:

Mechanism of Injury

Fall greater than 20 feet
Death of a car occupant
Struck by a vehicle traveling over 20 MPH
Ejected from the vehicle
Severe vehicle deformity
Rollover with signs of impact

Physical Findings

Pulse greater than 120 or less than 50
Systolic blood pressure less than 90
Respiratory rate less than 10 or greater than 29
Glasgow Coma Scale less than 13
Penetrating trauma (except extremities)
Greater than two proximal long bone fractures
Flail chest
Burns to greater than 15 percent of B.S.A.
Burns to face or airway

In applying trauma triage protocols, it is best to err on the side of precaution. If a patient does not fit the above criteria, be suspicious. Remember, you often arrive at the patient's side only minutes after the accident. He or she may not yet have lost enough blood internally to demonstrate signs of shock or progressive head injury. If in doubt, transport to a trauma center without delay.

✳ When applying the trauma triage protocols, it is best to err on the side of precaution.

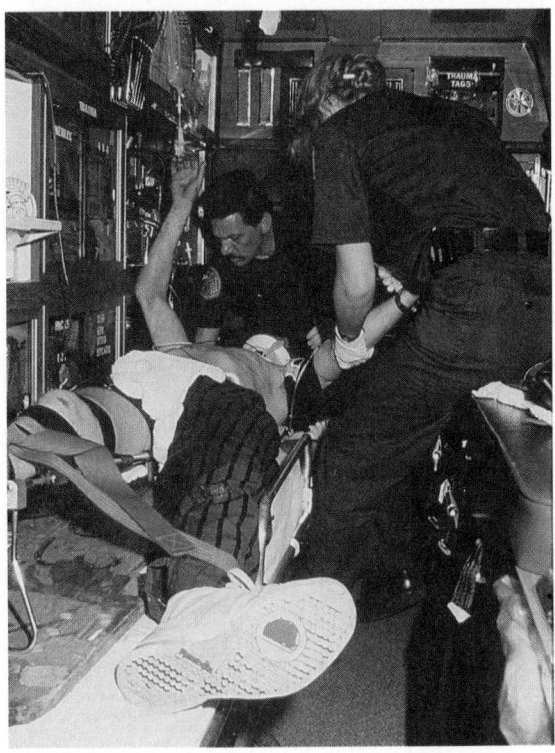

FIGURE 14-2 Victims of major trauma should be transported immediately with stabilization procedures, such as IV therapy, attempted en route.

KINETICS OF TRAUMA

Trauma results from the collision of two or more bodies in motion. As a result, the study of trauma is related to a branch of physics known as **kinetics**. To grasp the kinetics of trauma, you need to understand two basic principles of physics—the law of inertia and the law of conservation of energy. Application of these principles can help you identify the mechanism of injury and the probable effects of **impact**, or collision, upon the victim or victims. A grasp of these principles can help you better analyze trauma.

Inertia

The law of **inertia**, as described by Sir Isaac Newton, helps explain what happens during an accident. The first part of his first law states: "A body in motion will remain in **motion** unless acted upon by an outside force." As an example, think of identical autos moving at 55 miles per hour. One car brakes for a red light; the other rams into a bridge abutment. An "outside force" stops the motion of both vehicles, but with very different results. In the first case, the energy of motion is absorbed by the brakes. In the second, the energy is absorbed by the front end of the auto, the frame, and eventually the occupant.

The second part of the law states: "A body at rest will remain at rest unless acted upon by an outside force." Examples of this include an auto accelerating from a stop sign or a stopped vehicle being propelled forward by a rear-end collision. In the first case, the auto engine provides the force to initiate movement. In the second, the energy of the moving vehicle provides the force as the stopped car absorbs the energy and jolts ahead.

Conservation of Energy

The Law of Conservation of Energy states: "**Energy** can neither be created nor destroyed. It is only changed from one form to another." In an auto crash, as in other trauma, identification of probable energy changes will help you to assess the impact of various collisions. Kinetic energy, the energy possessed by a moving car and its passengers, is transformed into other forms of energy whenever a car stops.

If an auto slows down gradually for a stop sign, the brakes develop friction against the turning wheels, producing heat. During an auto crash, however, the energy of motion is converted at a much faster rate. The transmission of energy is manifest in the sound of impact, heat in the twisted steel, and injury to the passengers as they collide with the vehicle interior. When all the kinetic energy converts to other energy forms, the auto and its passengers come to a stop.

Kinetic Energy

Kinetic energy is the energy of motion. It is a function of an object's mass and its **velocity**. (While mass and weight, and velocity and speed, are not identical, we will consider them as such for these discussions.) Kinetic energy of an object while in motion can be measured by the following formula.

$$\text{Kinetic Energy} = \frac{\text{Mass (weight)} \times \text{Velocity (speed)}^2}{2}$$

The formula illustrates that if you double the weight of an object, kinetic energy is doubled. It is twice as damaging to be hit by a two-pound baseball as to be hit by a one-pound ball. It is three times as damaging to be hit by a three-pound ball, and so on.

As speed (velocity) increases, there is a larger (squared) increase in kinetic energy. Being hit with a one-pound baseball traveling at 20 miles per hour is four times as injurious as being hit with it at 10 miles per hour. If speed is increased to 30 miles per hour, trauma is nine times worse. This concept plays a key role in understanding the devastating effects of a gunshot wound. A very small object (the bullet) traveling very fast causes great harm.

Kinetic energy is the measure of how much energy an object in motion has, not necessarily how much injury will occur. Two autos traveling at 55 miles per hour have about the same kinetic energy. The same two autos would have equal kinetic energy once they have stopped, even if one came to rest by hitting a bridge. The difference between these two events is the rate of slowing. This rate is proportional to the accident force.

Force

The Law of Inertia is known as Newton's first law of motion. Newton's second law of motion explains the forces at work during an accident. It is summarized by the formula below.

Force = Mass (weight) × Acceleration (or Deceleration)

The formula emphasizes the importance of the rate at which an object changes speed, either increasing (**acceleration**) or decreasing (**deceleration**). Slow changes in speed are usually uneventful. Normal deceleration, such as slowing for a stop sign, covers about 120 feet (from 55 miles per hour to 0 miles per hour at a braking rate of 22 feet/10 miles per hour). It therefore rarely results in injury. On the other hand, colliding with a bridge abutment and slowing from 55 miles per hour to 0 miles per hour in a matter of inches produces tremendous force and devastating injuries.

■ **acceleration** the rate at which speed or velocity increases.

■ **deceleration** the rate at which speed or velocity decreases.

KINDS OF TRAUMA

When kinetic energy is applied to human anatomy, we call it trauma. Trauma is defined as a wound or injury that is externally or violently produced by some outside force. The wounds may be either blunt (closed) or penetrating (open).

Blunt trauma occurs when a body area is struck by, or strikes, an object. The transmission of energy, rather than the object, damages the tissues or organs beneath the skin as they collide with each other. An example of this is hitting your thumb with a hammer. The thumb is compressed between the hammer (which pushes the tissue) and the board (which resists the motion). Tissue injury results as flesh and bone become trapped between these two forces (acceleration and deceleration). Muscle cells stretch, blood vessels tear, and bone may fracture.

Blunt trauma can also induce internal injury deep within the body cavity. Forces of compression cause hollow organs like the bladder or bowel to rupture, spilling their contents and hemorrhaging. In the thorax, alveoli or small airways may burst, permitting air to enter the pleural space. Solid organs, such as the spleen, liver and kidney, may contuse or lacerate, leading to swelling, blood loss, or both.

Further trauma may result from the effects of rapid speed change and organ attachment. An example includes the liver, which is suspended by

✱ Trauma can be classified as either blunt or penetrating.

the *ligamentum teres*. During severe deceleration, the liver may be sliced by the ligament similar to cheese when cut by a wire cheese cutter. Similarly, the aorta may be injured as the chest slows and the heart, which is suspended from this great vessel, twists upon impact. Layers of the vessel are torn apart, and blood enters the injury with the force of the systolic blood pressure. The aorta balloons like a defective tire, leading to a tearing chest pain, circulatory compromise, and immediate or delayed exsanguination (severe blood loss).

Wounds that break the skin are classified as penetrating trauma. Penetrating trauma occurs when the energy source (such as a knife) progresses into the body. Energy may also be transmitted to surrounding body tissue, thus extending the trauma beyond the open wound. This frequently happens with gunshot wounds.

As a paramedic, you will encounter both blunt and penetrating trauma. The rest of this chapter will present examples of each category of injury.

BLUNT TRAUMA

Blunt trauma most commonly results from motor vehicle accidents involving automobiles, motorcycles, pedestrians, or recreational vehicles. It also can be caused by falls, sports injuries, and blasts.

Automobile Accidents

Auto accidents account for a large proportion of paramedic responses. Each year, over 100,000 serious accidents occur on the nation's highways. Some 44,000 people lose their lives in these accidents, while many more are seriously injured or permanently disabled. As a paramedic, you must be prepared to offer rapid assessment and appropriate care to victims. To this end, you must recognize the various types of auto accidents, identify possible mechanisms of injury, and form a reasonable index of suspicion.

Events of Impact   There are basically five vehicle impacts—frontal, lateral, rotational, rear-end, and rollover. Each progresses through a series of four events. These events include:

1. *Vehicle Collision.* Vehicle collision begins when the auto strikes an object. Energy of motion is converted to vehicle damage or transferred to the object hit by the auto. (See Figure 14-3.) The force developed in the accident depends upon the stopping distance. If the auto slides into a

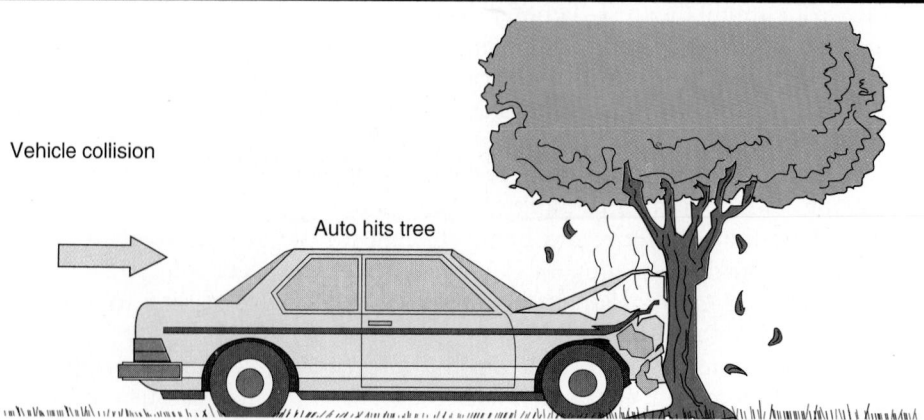

Vehicle collision

Auto hits tree

FIGURE 14-3   Step 1—Vehicle Collision. The vehicle strikes an object.

snow bank, damage is limited. If the auto strikes a concrete retaining wall, the damage is much greater. The degree of auto deformity is a good indicator of forces experienced by its occupants.

2. *Body Collision.* Body collision occurs when the passenger strikes the vehicle interior. The vehicle and its interior have slowed dramatically during the crash, yet an unrestrained occupant remains at the initial speed. As the passenger contacts the interior, energy is transferred to the vehicle or is transformed into tissue deformity, compression, stretching, and trauma. (See Figure 14-4.) If vehicle collision causes intrusion into the passenger compartment, displacement may physically injure occupants or otherwise worsen the injury process.

3. *Organ Collision.* Organ collision results from compression or deceleration. These forces produce blunt trauma as organs or tissues press into each other or the wall of the body cavity. As an organ twists or decelerates, it can tear attachments such as ligaments or rupture blood vessels. (See Figure 14-5.)

4. *Secondary Collisions.* Secondary collisions occur when the patient is either thrown about the vehicle after initial impact or is struck by flying debris. (See Figure 14-6.) These collisions may induce, or increase, the seriousness of patient injuries. Consider someone who has sustained a femur fracture. It took a great deal of energy to break the bone initially. However, the energy now needed to displace bone-ends and cause further, possibly more severe, injury might be small. It is important to consider what effect any secondary impact may have upon the initial injuries and patient condition.

✻ Secondary collisions may be the cause of the patient's injuries or may increase the seriousness of other injuries.

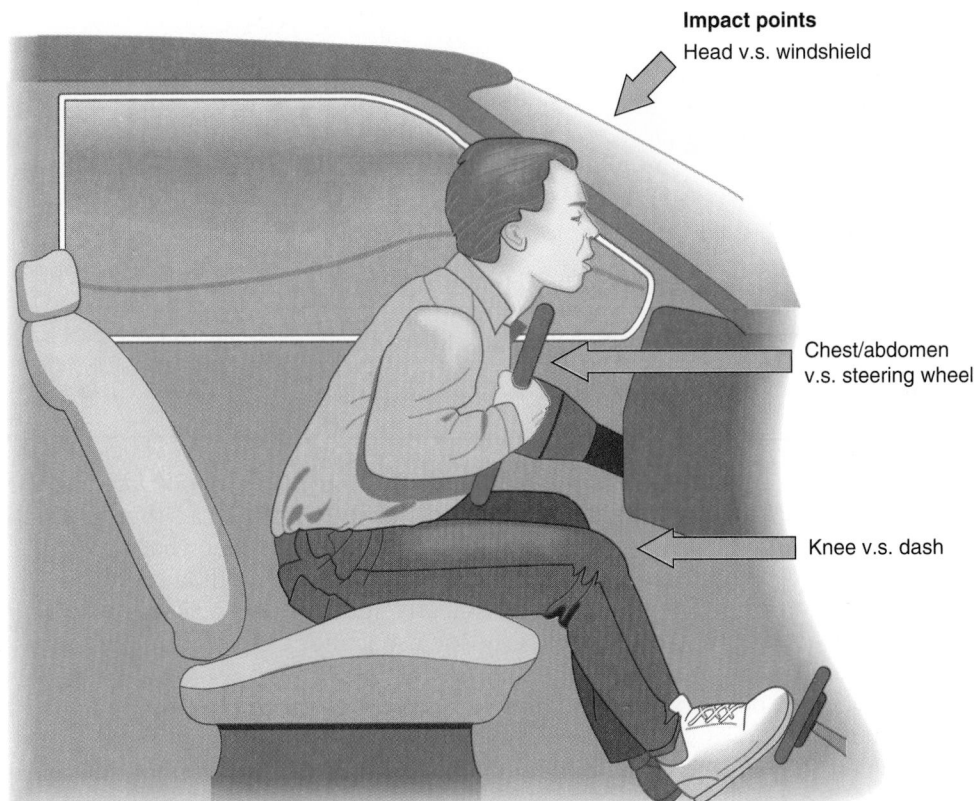

Impact points
Head v.s. windshield

Chest/abdomen v.s. steering wheel

Knee v.s. dash

FIGURE 14-4 Step 2— Body Collision. The occupant continues forward and strikes the inside of the automobile.

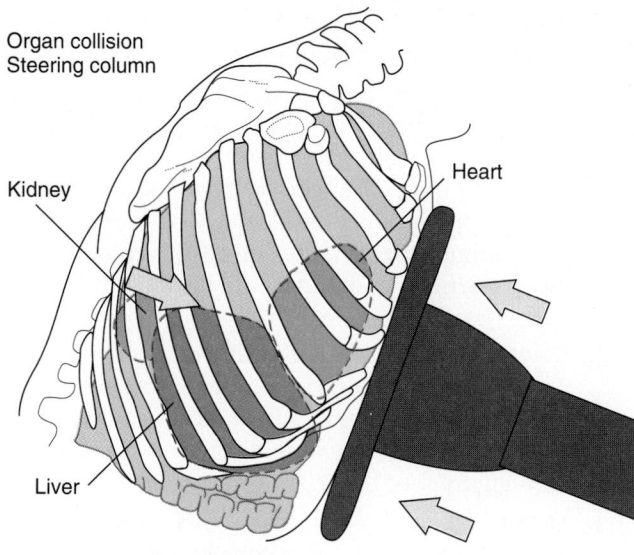

Organ collision
Steering column

Kidney

Heart

Liver

Body hits steering wheel
causing myocardial
contusion

FIGURE 14-5 Step 3—Organ Collision. The organs continue to move forward and strike the inside of the chest or other organs.

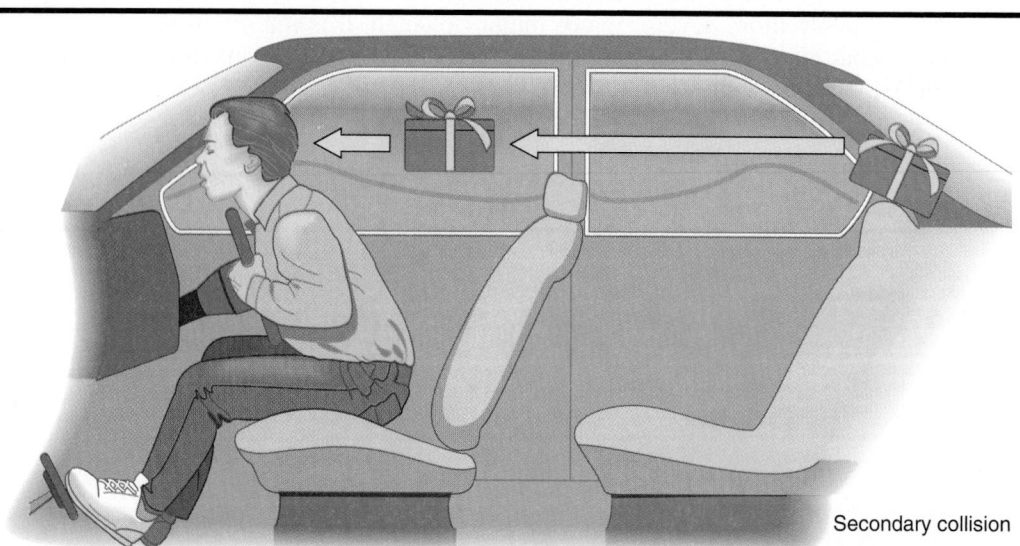

Secondary collision

FIGURE 14-6 Step 4—Secondary Collision. Secondary impact results when the occupant is struck by loose objects within the vehicle.

Restraints Seatbelts and shoulder straps can affect events of impact. Use of these safety devices slows the occupants along with the car, thus preventing them from colliding with the interior. Air bags work somewhat differently. They explosively inflate upon auto impact, producing a cushion to absorb the energy exchange. Both mechanisms clearly reduce auto-related death and injury. However, if worn improperly, or used under certain circumstances, these devices may account for injuries.

The lap belt worn alone will not restrain the torso, neck, or head from continuing forward. These body parts may impact the dash or steering wheel, resulting in chest, neck, and head injury. Abdominal compression and spinal (T12 to L2) fractures may result if the lap belt is worn too high. If worn too low, it may cause hip dislocations. If the shoulder strap is worn alone, it may cause severe neck injury, or even decapitation in more violent accidents. If worn as intended, the lap belt and shoulder strap may account for contusions and rib fractures.

Air bags (supplemental restraint systems) are extremely effective for frontal impacts. They provide a cushion to slow the body much like the inflated bag used by pole vaulters and movie stuntmen. If an impact is lateral or from the rear, no protection is offered. Since the bag deflates immediately after initial inflation, the same holds true for any subsequent collision.

The value of seat belts is demonstrated frequently. They should be required of all EMS personnel, especially while driving. The lap belt provides positive positioning so the driver is not so affected by the gravitational forces (G forces) sometimes associated with emergency driving.

✳ Seatbelt use should be required of all EMS personnel.

Types of Impact   As you have read, there are five general types of auto impacts. They include:

❑ Frontal
❑ Lateral
❑ Rotational
❑ Rear-end
❑ Rollover

The nature and severity of potential injuries can be anticipated by looking carefully at the vehicle and analyzing the impact it received. The angle of impact will suggest possible injuries that the patient may have sustained. The extent of deformity will give you an idea of the strength of impact and forces experienced by the patient. Together, these elements of evaluation will help you to develop an index of suspicion for various injuries. (See Figure 14-7.)

The following is a breakdown of motor vehicle impacts. Figures reflect an urban setting. In a more rural area, anticipate a greater percentage of frontal impacts with corresponding reductions in other categories.

✳ The visual examination of the auto accident can tell you a good deal about what happened to the patient and what injuries should be suspected.

Frontal:	32 percent
Lateral:	15 percent
Rotational:	38 percent
Rear End:	9 percent
Rollover:	6 percent

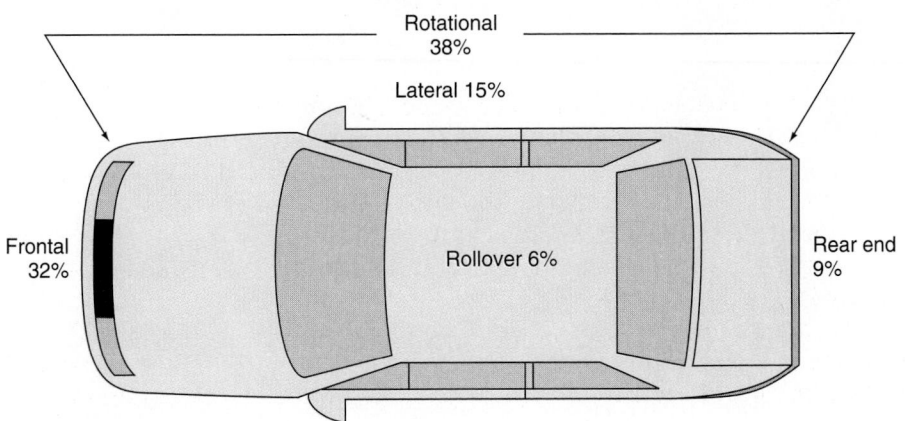

FIGURE 14-7 Motor vehicle trauma based upon the type of impact.

Rotational impact includes four sub-categories: left front, right front, left rear, and right rear.

Frontal Impact. Frontal impact is most common and produces three pathways of patient travel. (See Figures 14-8 and 14-9 for examples of injury mechanisms associated with frontal impact.) They include:

1. *Down-and-Under Pathway.* In the down-and-under pathway the occupant slides downward as the vehicle comes to a stop. The knees contact the fire wall, under the dash, and absorb the initial impact. Knee, femur, and hip dislocations or fractures are common. Once the lower body slows, the upper body is brought forward, pivoting at the hip, and crashing against the steering wheel or dash. Chest injuries like flail chest, myocardial contusion (see Figure 14-10), and aortic tears result. If the neck contacts the steering wheel, tracheal and vascular injury may occur. A frequent injury process associated with steering wheel impact is the "paper bag" syndrome. (See Figure 14-11.) The driver takes a deep breath in anticipation of the collision. Lung tissue (alveoli, bronchioles, and larger airways) rupture when the chest impacts the steering wheel, much like an inflated paper bag caught between clapping hands. Pneumothorax and pulmonary contusion may result.

2. *Up-and-Over Pathway.* In the up-and-over pathway, the occupant tenses his or her legs in preparation for impact. With vehicle slowing, the upper half of the body pivots forward and upward. The steering wheel impinges the femurs, causing bilateral fractures. In addition, it compresses and decelerates the abdominal contents, causing hollow-organ rupture and liver laceration. Traumatic compression may also force abdominal contents against the diaphragm, causing it to rupture and allowing organs to enter the thoracic cavity. As the body continues forward, the lower chest impacts the steering wheel and may account for the same thoracic injuries seen with the down-and-under pathway.

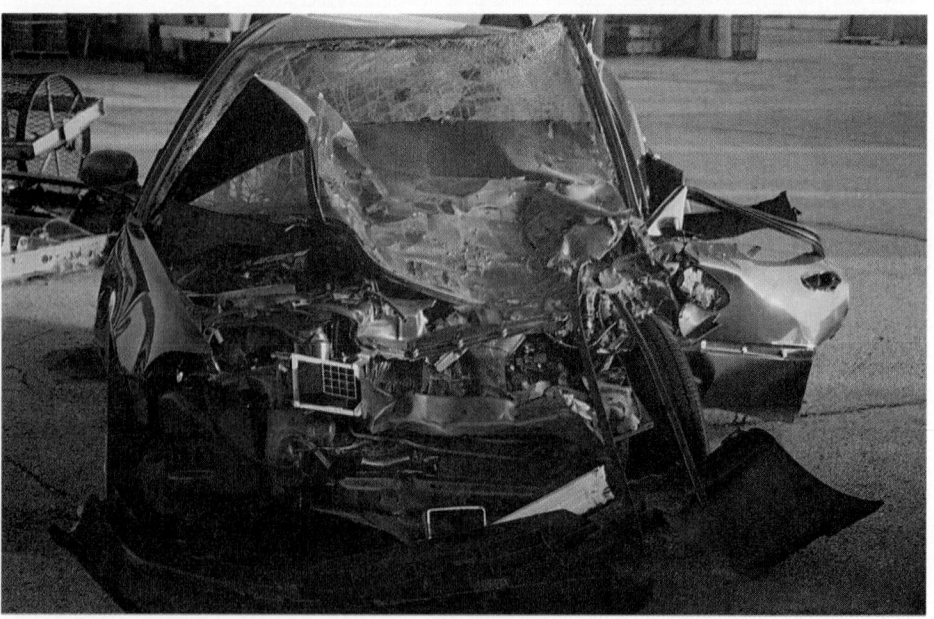

FIGURE 14-8 Frontal impact.

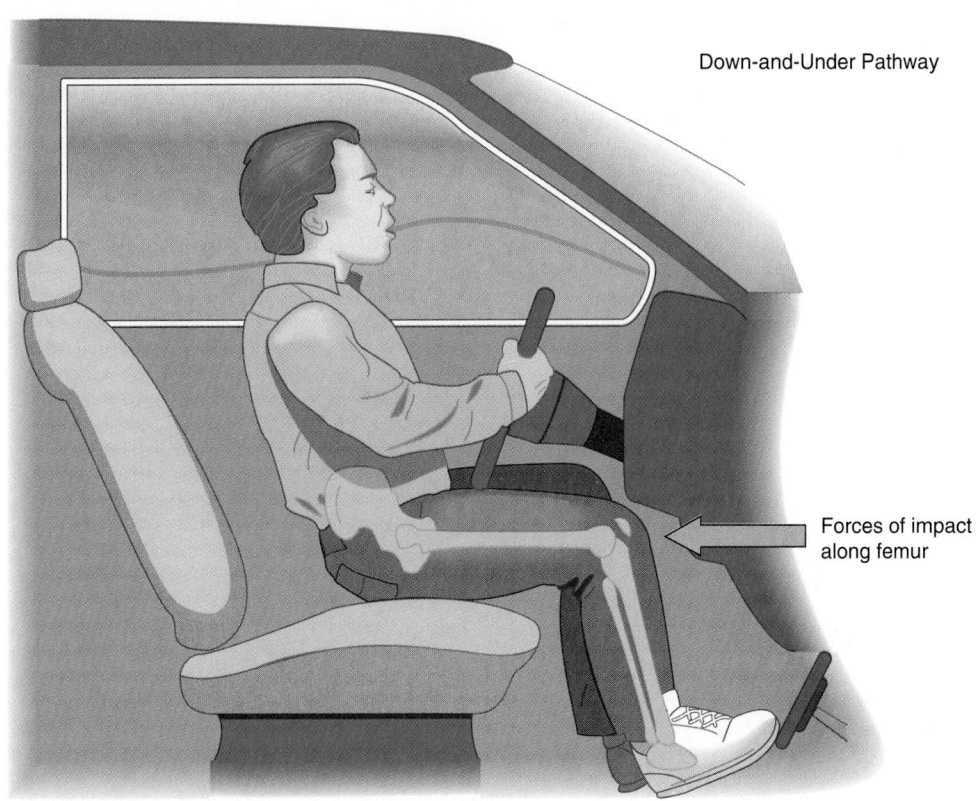

Down-and-Under Pathway

Forces of impact
along femur

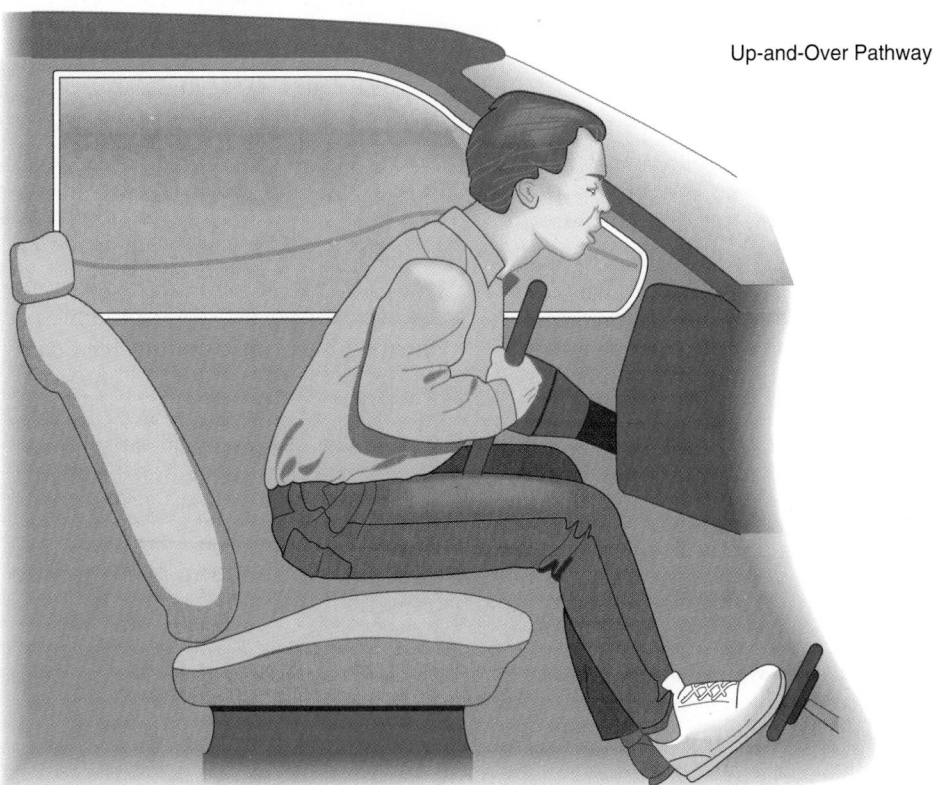

Up-and-Over Pathway

FIGURE 14-9 Examples of injury mechanisms associated with frontal impact.

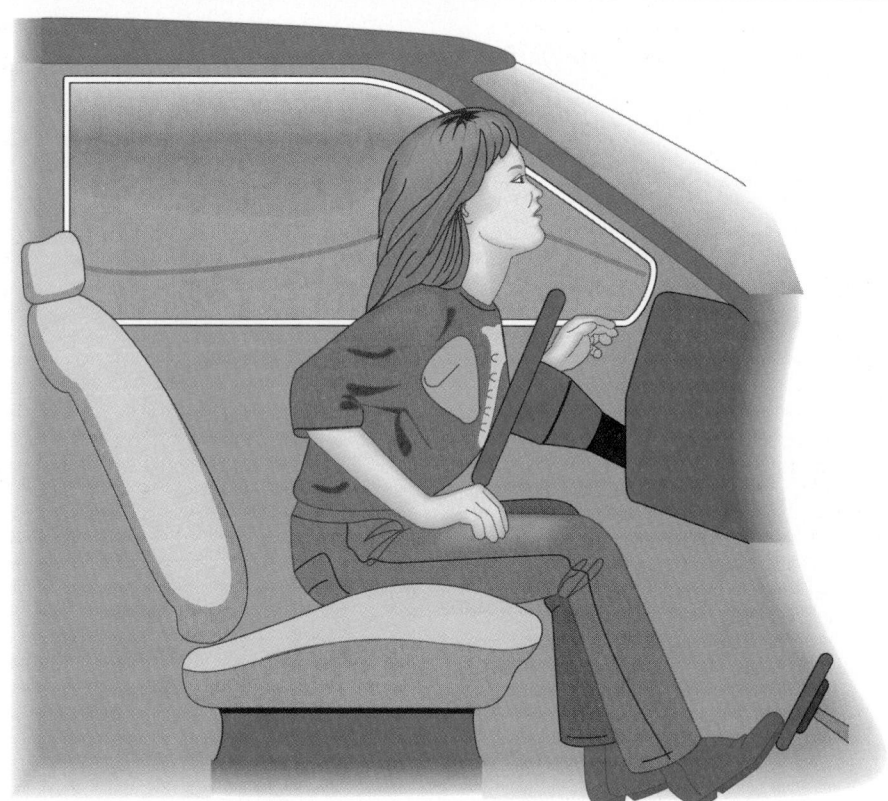

FIGURE 14-10 Myocardial contusion can result from impact with the steering wheel.

■ **axial loading** application of the forces of trauma along the axis of the spine. This often results in compression fractures of the vertebra.

The same forward motion, propels the head into the windshield, leading to skull or facial fractures or soft-tissue or internal head injury. Neck injury may result from hyperextension, hyperflexion, or compressional forces of windshield impact. As the body is thrown upward and forward, the head contacts the windshield. The rest of the body tries to push the head through the windshield. The result is a compressional force on the cervical spine called **axial loading**. It may result in collapse of the vertebral column support elements. Over half of vehicular deaths are attributed to the up-and-over pathway.

3. *Ejection.* The up-and-over pathway may lead to ejection of an unrestrained occupant. Victims experience two impacts: contact with the vehicle interior and windshield and impact with the ground, tree, or other object. This mechanism of injury is responsible for about 27 percent of vehicular fatalities. While ejection may occur from other types of impact, it is most commonly associated with frontal impact.

Lateral Impact. The kinetics of lateral impact are the same as for frontal impact with two exceptions. First, occupants present a different profile (turned 90 degrees) to collision forces. Second, the amount of structural steel between the impact site and the vehicle interior is greatly reduced. (See Figure 14-12.) Lateral impacts account for 15 percent of all auto accidents, yet they are responsible for 22 percent of vehicular fatalities. When a lateral impact occurs, the index of suspicion for serious internal injury should be higher than vehicle damage alone suggests.

✱ The lateral impact accident is associated with a higher index of suspicion for serious injury than vehicle damage alone would otherwise indicate.

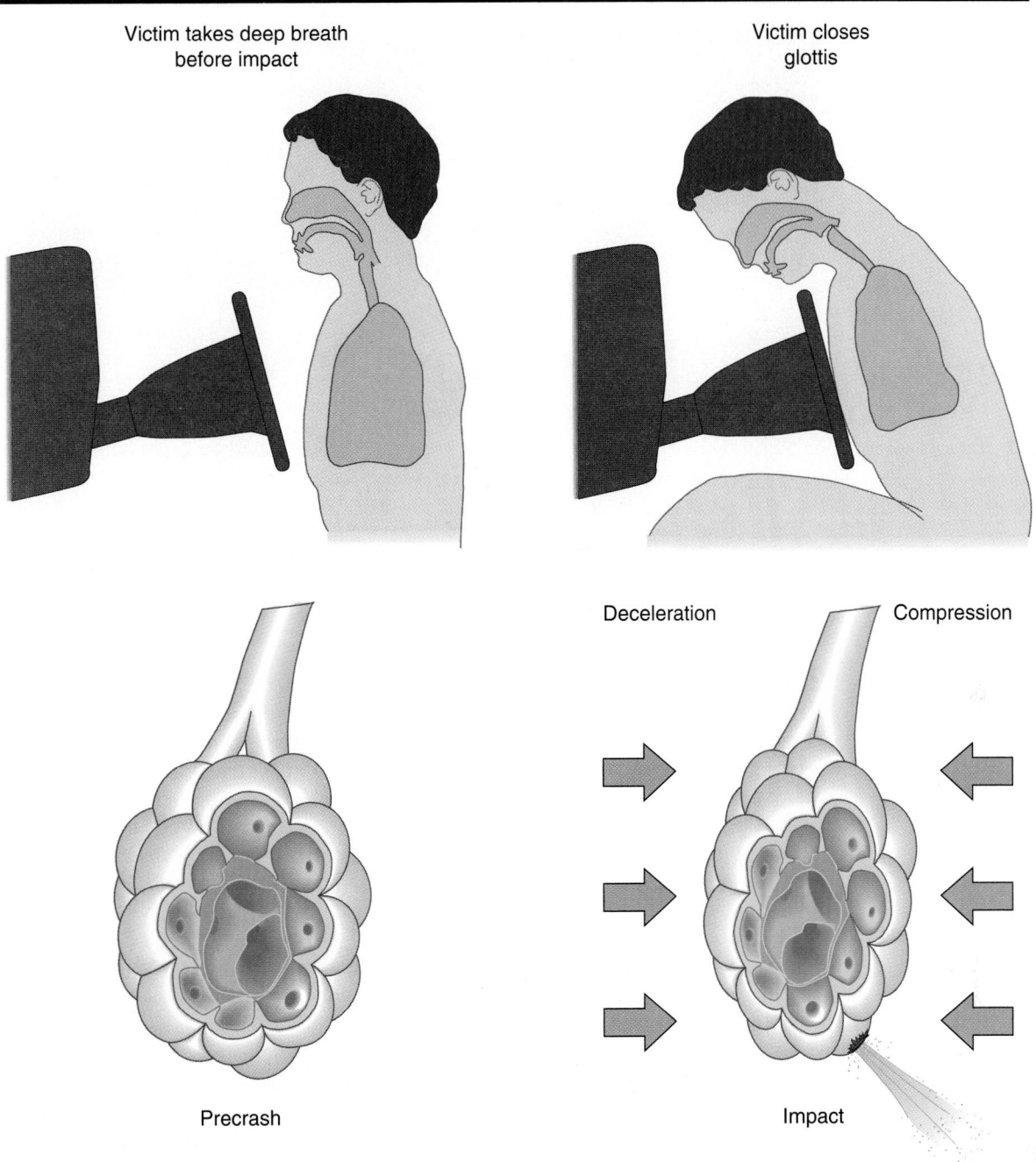

Victim takes deep breath
before impact

Victim closes
glottis

Deceleration

Compression

Precrash

Impact

FIGURE 14-11 The "paper bag" syndrome results from compression of the chest against the steering column.

In lateral impact, there is an increase in upper extremity injuries and a reduced incidence of rib fractures (although they still occur). The clavicle, pelvis, and femur may fracture on the impacted side. Cervical spine injury is common, as are skull fractures and internal head injuries. Lateral compression, effecting the body cavity, may give rise to diaphragm rupture, pulmonary contusion, aortic tear, and much more.

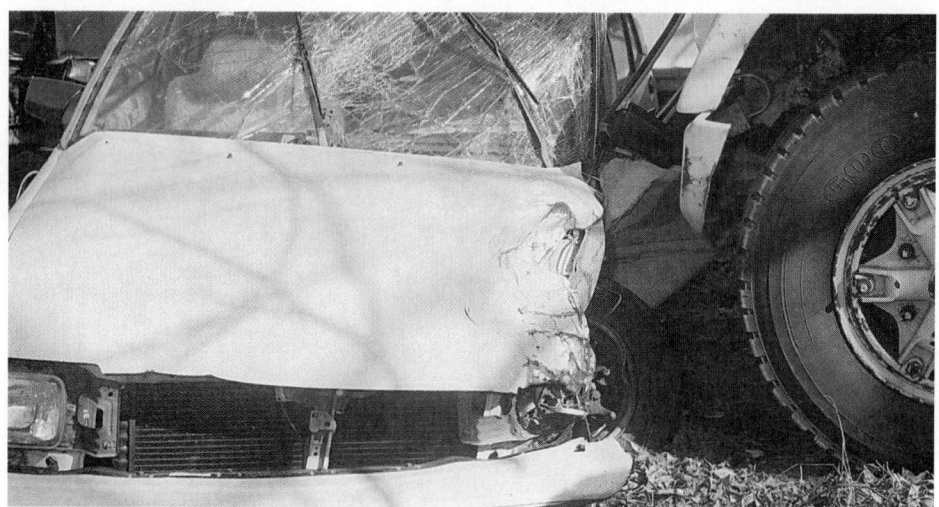

FIGURE 14-12 Lateral impact.

Accident evaluation should take into consideration an unrestrained passenger opposite the impact site. If the driver's side is struck and the passenger is not belted, he or she will become an object striking and injuring the driver shortly after initial impact.

■ **oblique** having a slanted position or direction.

Rotational Impact. In rotational impact, the auto is struck at an **oblique** angle. The vehicle rotates as forces of collision are expended. (See Figure 14-13.) Acceleration (or deceleration) is greatest further from the center of the auto and closest to impact. Ensuing rotation can cause injuries similar to frontal and lateral impacts. While injuries sustained can be serious, they are often less than vehicle damage might suggest. Autos involved are deflected from their paths rather than being stopped abruptly. Stopping distance for the occupant is much greater, deceleration is more gradual, and less serious injuries can be expected.

Rear-end Impact. In rear-end impact, the auto is pushed forward by the collision force. (See Figure 14-14.) The occupant is propelled forward by the

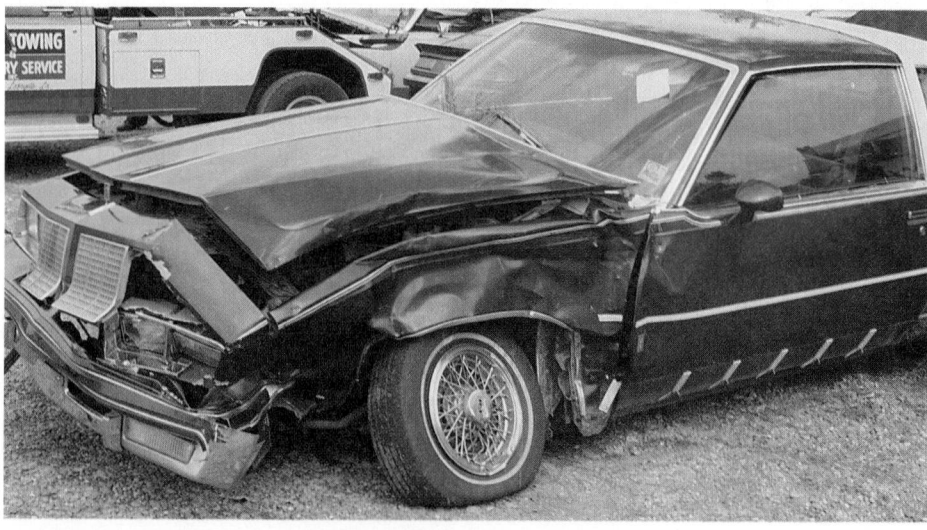

FIGURE 14-13 Rotational impact.

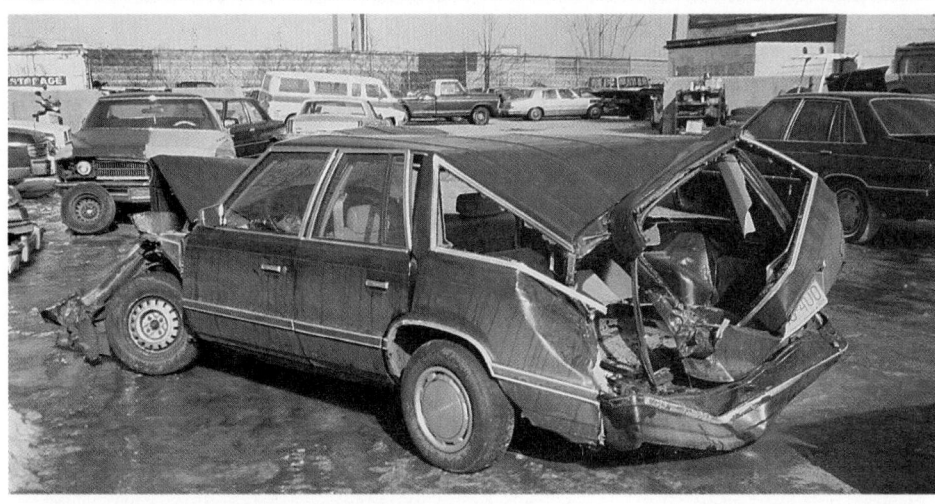

FIGURE 14-14   Rear-end impact.

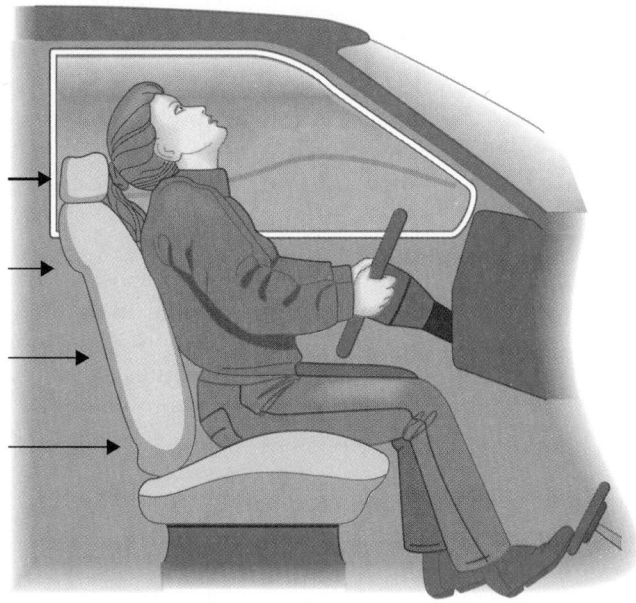

A. Victim moves ahead while head remains stationary. Head rotates backward. Neck extends.

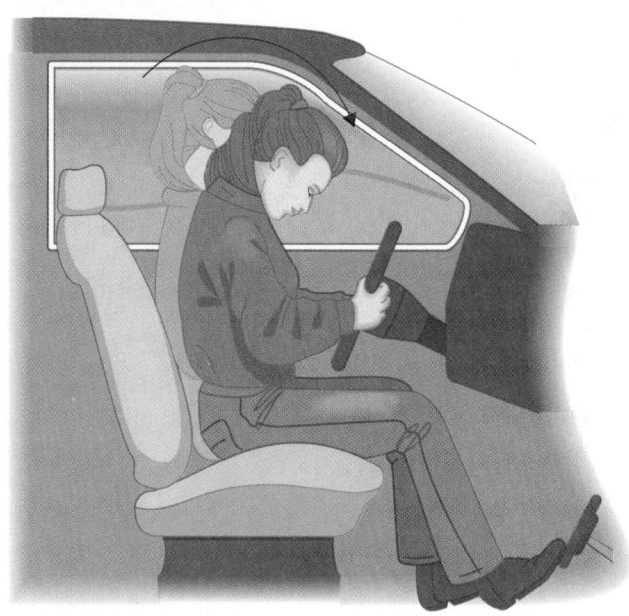

B. Head snaps forward. Head rotates forward. Neck flexes.

FIGURE 14-15   Movement in rear-end collision.

vehicle seat. If the head rest is not up, the head is unsupported and remains stationary. The neck extends severely, while the head rotates backward. Once acceleration ceases, the head snaps forward and the neck flexes. This rapid and extreme hyperextension followed by hyperflexion may result in connective tissue and skeletal neck injuries. (See Figure 14-15.) There is also risk of injury when the auto finally ends its acceleration and the occupant is thrown forward.

Rollover. Auto rollover is normally caused by a change in elevation and/or a vehicle with a high center of gravity. (See Figure 14-16.) As the vehicle rolls, it impacts the ground at various locations. The occupant experiences impacts

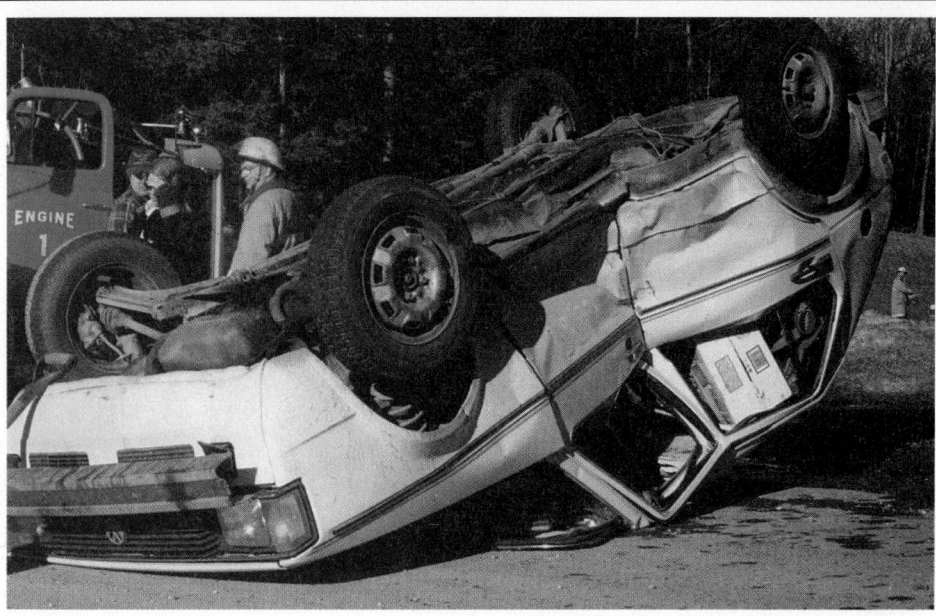

FIGURE 14-16 Rollover.

associated with each vehicle impact. The type of injuries expected would be related to the specific vehicle impacts involved. Remember, any injury occurring with the first collision can be compounded with subsequent impacts. A common result of rollover is ejection or partial ejection with a limb or head trapped between the vehicle and the ground.

Intoxication Whenever you examine motor vehicle trauma, consider the possibility of alcohol intoxication. Figures from states requiring mandatory alcohol level testing after fatal auto accidents reveal that more than 50 percent of the drivers were legally intoxicated. Alcohol also contributes to many recreational-vehicle accidents, boating accidents, and accidental drownings.

    If you suspect alcohol intoxication, remember that it interferes with the patient's level of consciousness, masking injury as well as neurologic status. Intoxication mimics the signs of head injury, lowers the level of orientation, and anesthetizes trauma pain. These factors make the mechanism of injury analysis and the resultant index of suspicion even more important. Otherwise, significant injuries may be overlooked or brushed off as symptoms of alcohol intoxication.

Vehicular Mortality Examination of motor vehicle trauma on the human anatomy shows certain areas prone to life-threatening injury. A study of the incidence of mortality and the associated location of trauma is identified in the table below.

✳ Alcohol intoxication is associated with most serious accidents.

Motor Vehicle Fatalities
(incidence by body area)

Head	47.7 %
Internal (chest/abdominal/pelvic)	37.3 %
Spinal and Chest Fracture	8.3 %
Fractures to the Extremities	2.0 %
All other	4.7 %

✳ Head and body cavity injuries account for 85 percent of total auto fatalities.

    Trauma to the head and body cavity accounts for 85 percent of vehicular mortality. For this reason, primary assessment is directed at the head, neck, thorax, abdomen, and pelvis. Once you have assured the airway, breathing, and circulation, you can proceed to the physical assessment. Examine the head, chest, and abdomen first to identify any evidence of life-threatening injuries.

Accident Evaluation   Because of the high incidence of deaths by auto, it is necessary to be thoroughly practiced in trauma assessment. By way of review, keep in mind the following tips or questions. Whenever you respond to an accident, analyze the four types of collision. In each case, ask yourself these questions. How did the objects collide? From what direction did they come? At what speed were they traveling? Were the objects similarly sized or grossly different? (For example, did a car and a semi-truck collide?) Were any secondary collisions or additional transfers of energy involved?

In analyzing the mechanisms of injury, also consider the cause of the accident. Did wet pavement or poor visibility contribute to the accident? Was alcohol involved? Is there an absence of skid marks? If so, what happened to the driver to prevent him or her from braking?

Do not forget to examine the auto interior—the mass struck by the moving occupant. Does the windshield show evidence of impact by the victim's head? Is it bloody or broken in the characteristic spider web or star shape? Has it been penetrated by the patient's head or body? Is the steering wheel deformed or collapsed? Is the dash indented where the knees or head hit it? Has the damage of impact extended so there is intrusion into the passenger compartment? Answers to such questions will complement your mechanism of injury analysis and help you to develop accurate indices of suspicion.

Motorcycle Accidents

In addition to auto accidents, you will probably respond to many motorcycle accidents. Because of the lack of protective devices, motorcycle accidents often result in severe trauma, even at low speeds. The rider, rather than the structural steel, absorbs much of the crash energy. (See Figure 14-17.) Injury

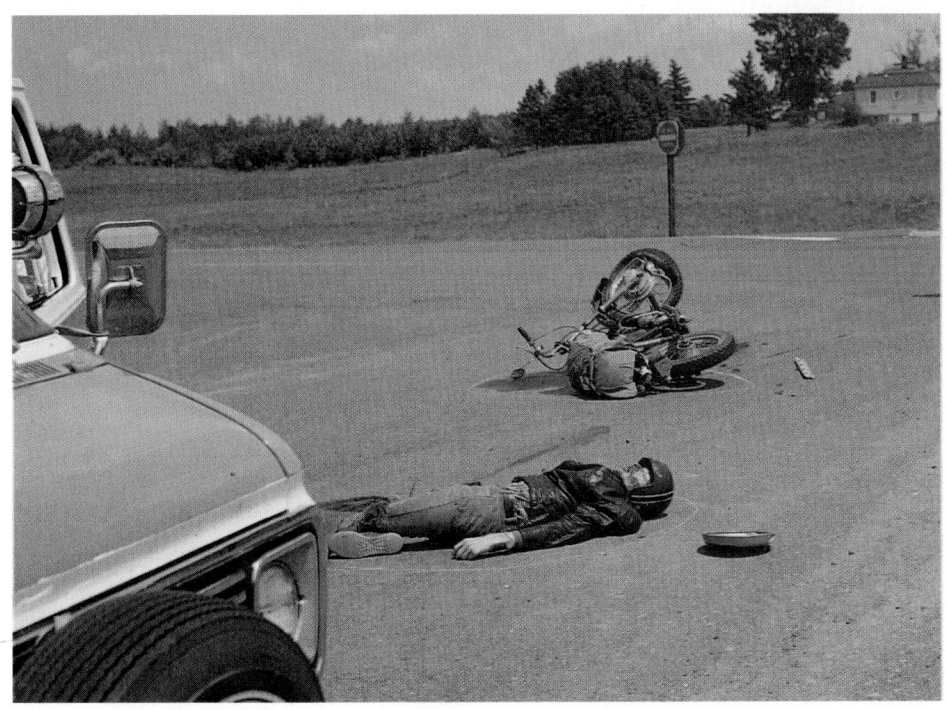

FIGURE 14-17 Motorcycle accidents can result in many types of trauma due to lack of protection of the rider.

can be severe, with an especially high incidence of head trauma. The impact of a motorcycle accident differs somewhat from that of an auto. The four types of impact include: frontal, angular, ejection, and sliding.

In a frontal, or head-on impact, the bike dips downward, causing the rider to be propelled upward and forward. The lower abdomen or pelvis is caught by the handle bars, resulting in abdominal and/or pelvic injury. Occasionally, the rider is propelled through a higher trajectory. Femurs are trapped by the handle bars, often resulting in bilateral fractures.

An angular impact occurs when the bike strikes an object at an oblique angle. The rider's lower extremity is trapped between the bike and the object struck. This may fracture or crush the foot, ankle, knee, and femur. Open wounds often occur.

Ejection during a motorcycle accident is common and usually results in serious injury. It may occur with either mechanism previously described, resulting in the following impacts.

❑ Initial bike/object collision
❑ Rider/object impact
❑ Rider/ground impact

Likely injuries include skull fracture and/or head injury, spinal fractures and paralysis, internal thoracic or abdominal injury, and extremity fractures.

Sliding impact occurs when an experienced rider, faced with an imminent crash, "lays the bike down." The rider slides the bike sideways into another object, reducing the chances of ejection. The result is an increase in lacerations, abrasions, and minor fractures, with a decrease in more serious injuries.

In assessing a motorcycle accident, remember that protective equipment affects injury patterns. A helmet considerably reduces the incidence and severity of head injury. However, it neither increases nor decreases the incidence of spinal trauma. Leather clothing protects the rider against open soft-tissue injury, but it can also hide underlying contusions and fractures.

✳ A helmet considerably reduces the incidence and severity of head injury in motorcycle accidents. However, it neither increases nor decreases the incidence of spinal trauma.

Pedestrian Accidents

Some vehicular accidents involve pedestrians. Injuries differ between adults and children because of their different anatomical size and because of their different responses to the impending accident. (See Figure 14-18.) Recognition of these differences will help you anticipate injuries and necessary treatment.

In the case of adults, pedestrians generally turn away from oncoming vehicles and present a lateral surface to impact. Anatomically, impact is low. The bumper strikes the lower leg first and fractures the tibia and fibula. Transmitted energy to the opposing knee can lead to ligament injury. As the lower extremities are propelled forward with the car, the upper and lateral body crashes into the hood causing femur, lateral chest, or upper extremity fractures. The victim then slides into the windshield, leading to head, neck, and shoulder trauma. The adult may be further injured when thrown to the ground. This collision may cause additional injury or compound those already present. (See Figure 14-9.)

In contrast to adults, children turn toward an oncoming vehicle. Because they are smaller, injury is located anatomically higher. The bumper impacts the femur or pelvis, causing fracture. Children are frequently thrown in front of the vehicle because of their smaller size and lower center of gravity. They may then be run over or pushed to the side. If a child is thrown upward, the injuries expected are similar to those of an adult.

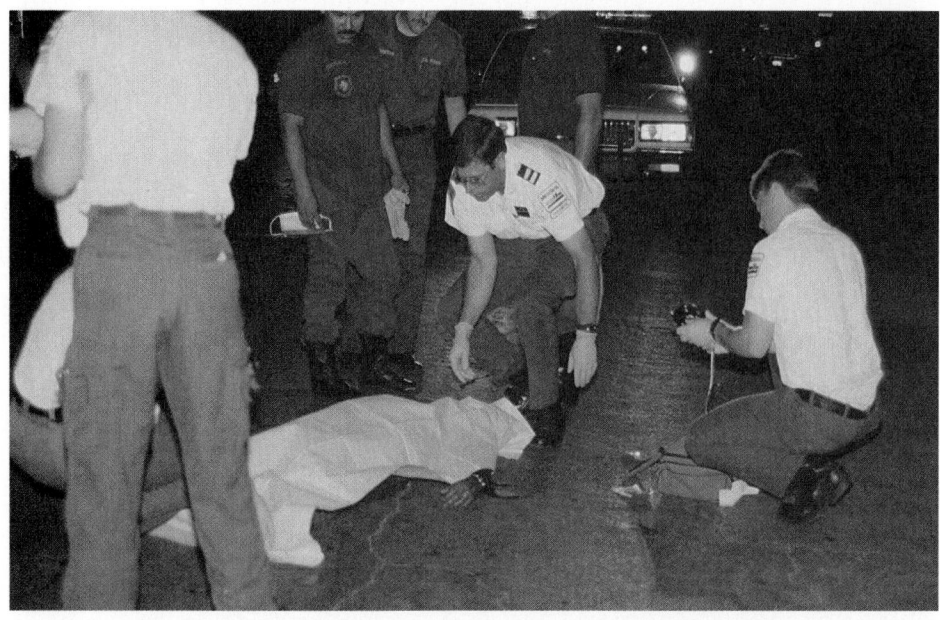

FIGURE 14-18 The injuries associated with pedestrian accidents will vary based on the size of the patient, the velocity of the vehicle, and the part of the body struck.

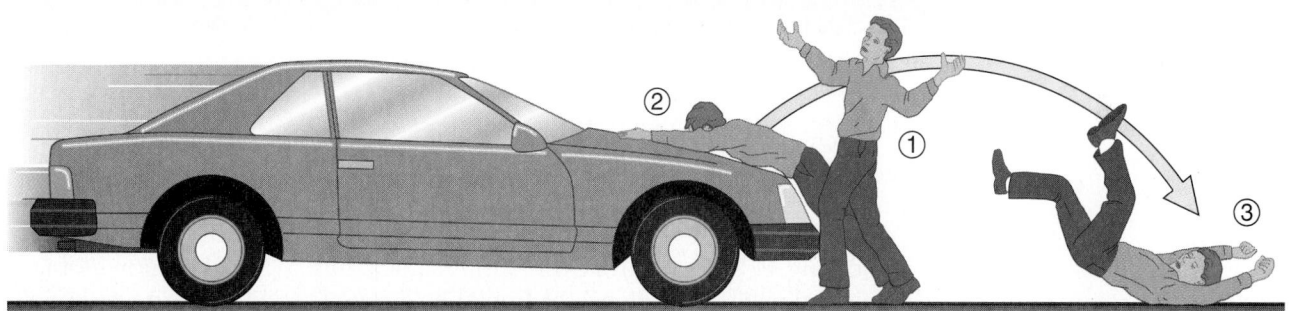

FIGURE 14-19 Typically in pedestrian injuries: (1) the leg is struck first by the bumper, (2) then the head and chest strike the hood and grill, and (3) finally the pedestrian's head hits the ground.

Recreational Vehicle Accidents

Over the past few years, recreational vehicle usage has increased, and with it, the incidence of related trauma. Recreational vehicles often cause injuries similar to those associated with the auto. However, drivers and passengers are not afforded the same structural protection. Because these vehicles travel off road, there is often difficulty in reaching and retrieving the victims once accidents are detected. The two major types of recreational vehicles most often involved in accidents are snowmobiles and all-terrain vehicles (ATVs).

Snowmobile accidents commonly result in crush injuries secondary to rollover and glancing blows against obstructions in the snow. Riders also experience severe head and neck injuries due to collisions with other vehicles, including autos, other snowmobiles, or with stationary objects such as trees. Snowmobile trauma may include severe neck injury when the rider runs into an unseen wire fence. The anterior neck is deeply lacerated, yielding airway compromise, severe bleeding, and, in some cases, complete decapitation. Snowmobile injuries may be compounded by the effects of cold exposure and hypothermia.

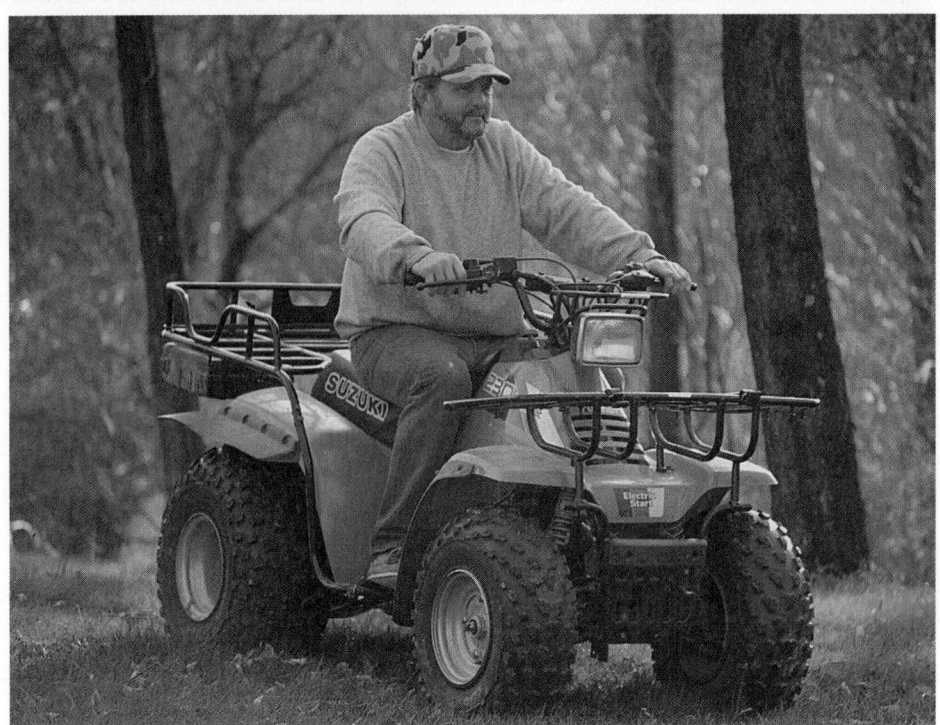

FIGURE 14-20 All-terrain vehicles (ATV) can cause a multitude of injuries due to their speed and instability.

There are two types of ATVs: the three- and four-wheel versions. The three-wheeled ATV is notoriously unstable, especially when ridden by children, young adults, persons of lower body weight, or those with limited vehicle experience. (See Figure 14-20.) The center of gravity is relatively high, contributing to frequent rollover during quick turns. As with snowmobiles, there is a significant incidence of frontal collision. The injuries expected might include upper and lower extremity fracture and head and spine injury.

Other Blunt Trauma

Blunt trauma can be caused by other mechanisms. These include falls, sports injuries, and blast injuries.

Falls In terms of physics, falls are a release of stored gravitational energy. The greater the height, the greater the impact velocity, the greater the exchange of energy, and the greater the resultant trauma. As with auto accidents, stopping distance may be more important than velocity of impact. A person may dive pleasurably from a 12-foot platform into deep water, but a fall from a second story window to a concrete sidewalk results in serious injury. Newton's Second Law—Force = Mass × Acceleration (or Deceleration)—illustrates that the more rapid the deceleration (the shorter the stopping distance), the greater the force and injury.

Trauma resulting from a fall is dependent upon the area of contact and the pathway of energy transmission. If the victim lands feet first, energy is transmitted up the skeletal structure through the calcaneus, femur, and lumbar spine. (See Figure 14-21.) Fractures along this skeletal pathway are common. The lumbar spine is especially prone to compression injury because it supports the entire upper body. As the victim continues the collision, he or she will fall forward or backward. In forward falls, an outstretched arm may attempt to break the impact, resulting in shoulder, clavicle, and wrist fractures. Pelvic, thoracic,

✱ The potential for injury from a fall depends on the height and the stopping distance.

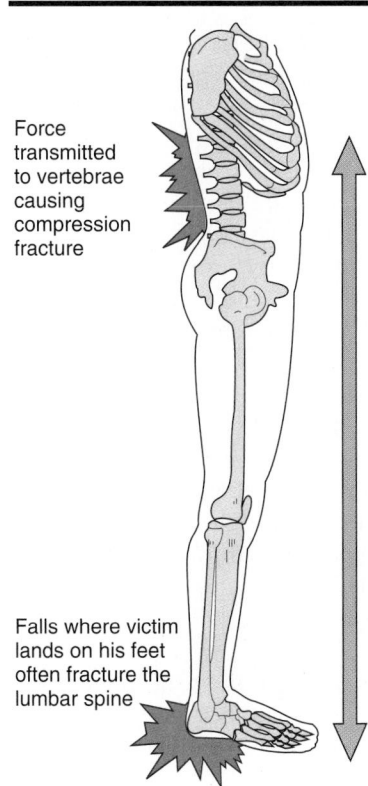

Force transmitted to vertebrae causing compression fracture

Falls where victim lands on his feet often fracture the lumbar spine

FIGURE 14-21   In falls, energy is transmitted up the skeletal system.

and head injury may result from a backward fall. In some cases, the fall will progress with the patient continuing a straight impact. The tongue may be bitten deeply as the weight of the cranium pushes the maxilla against the mandible.

The initial impact may involve other body surfaces with kinetic energy transmitted from the contact point toward the body's center of mass. In diving injuries, the patient's head meets with the lake bottom, while the rest of the body compresses the cervical spine between the head and shoulders. Axial loading crushes the vertebra, disrupts the spinal cord, and paralyzes the patient. This may result even from a very shallow dive, as from pool side or from within the water.

In severe falls, with a person dropping more than 20 feet, focus your attention on potential internal injuries. Rapid deceleration causes many organs to be compressed, displaced, and twisted. The heart, for example, is held in the center of the thorax by the aorta, the vena cavae, and the *ligamentum arteriosum.* When the victim contacts the ground, the heart is pulled downward with such force that it may tear the aorta in two, thus leading to immediate exsanguination.

Sports Injuries   Sports medicine is growing very rapidly. It is an extensive field, which certainly cannot be covered completely in this chapter. However, some basic principles will help you to better understand and care for athletic injuries.

Sports injuries are most commonly produced by extreme exertion, fatigue, or by direct forces of trauma. Injuries can be secondary to acceleration, deceleration, compression, rotation, and hyperextension or hyperflexion. These forces leave behind soft-tissue damage to skin and muscle, connective tissue injury to tendons and ligaments, skeletal trauma to long bones or the spinal column, as well as internal damage to either hollow or solid organs.

When a debilitating sports-related injury occurs, the athlete should be transported to an emergency department and examined before further participation is allowed. Injuries that display minimal pain may be significantly worsened by the stress of further competition. Such stress may cause complete rupture of ligaments or other soft-tissue injury and increase the potential for permanent disability.

In some contact sports, athletes may experience severe impact. If collision leads to any period of unconsciousness, neurologic deficit, or lowered level of orientation, the individual should be evaluated by emergency department personnel. There is a strong desire by coaches and players alike to return to the game. However, until a head and cervical spine injury can be ruled out, discourage such action.

Protective gear reduces the chance for, and significance of, injury. However, gear can sometimes be a contributing factor in sports injuries. In major contact sports, for example, shoes are designed to give maximum traction, using cleats to lock the foot firmly in position. In football, a player might be struck, forcing the body to turn on an immobile foot. Ligaments may tear in the knee, resulting in a severe and disabling leg injury. In other cases, protective gear may hinder your complete assessment and patient stabilization. Therefore, it is important to remove all gear from the area of injury.

Blast Injuries   Blast injuries are not uncommon in prehospital emergency care. Natural gas, gasoline, fireworks, and even dust within a grain elevator, can give rise to violent explosions and a specific scenario of trauma.

The blast induces injury through a series of events. First, an explosion creates intense heat, which in turn causes combustion gases to expand rapidly. The expansion sends a wave of pressure outward from the blast center. It violently compresses, then decompresses, anything in its path. As the wave contacts objects, they become projectiles, flying outward with great speed and energy. A person, caught in the pressure wave path, may become a projectile and be thrown against objects or the ground. The following data summarizes the three main phases of a blast.

Primary. The primary phase is the initial air blast and pressure wave. Injuries resulting from the compression of air-containing organs include:

- ❏ Auditory injuries (usually involving ruptured tympanic membranes)
- ❏ Sinus injuries
- ❏ Lung injuries (may include pneumothorax, parenchymal hemorrhage, and alveolar rupture)
- ❏ Stomach injuries
- ❏ Intestinal injuries

The blast may also induce burns if the victim is in close proximity to the source. These are usually flash burns and occur at the instant of the explosion. More extensive thermal burns may occur due to smoldering clothing or fire subsequent to the blast.

Secondary. In the second phase of the blast, the victim is struck by debris propelled by the force of the air-pressure wave. Impacting debris may produce blunt or penetrating trauma.

Tertiary. In the third phase, the victim is thrown away from the blast and into objects or the ground. Injuries are similar to those found in auto ejection. (See Figure 14-22.)

✱ If a collision leads to any loss of consciousness, neurological deficit, or altered level of consciousness, the athlete should be evaluated by emergency department personnel.

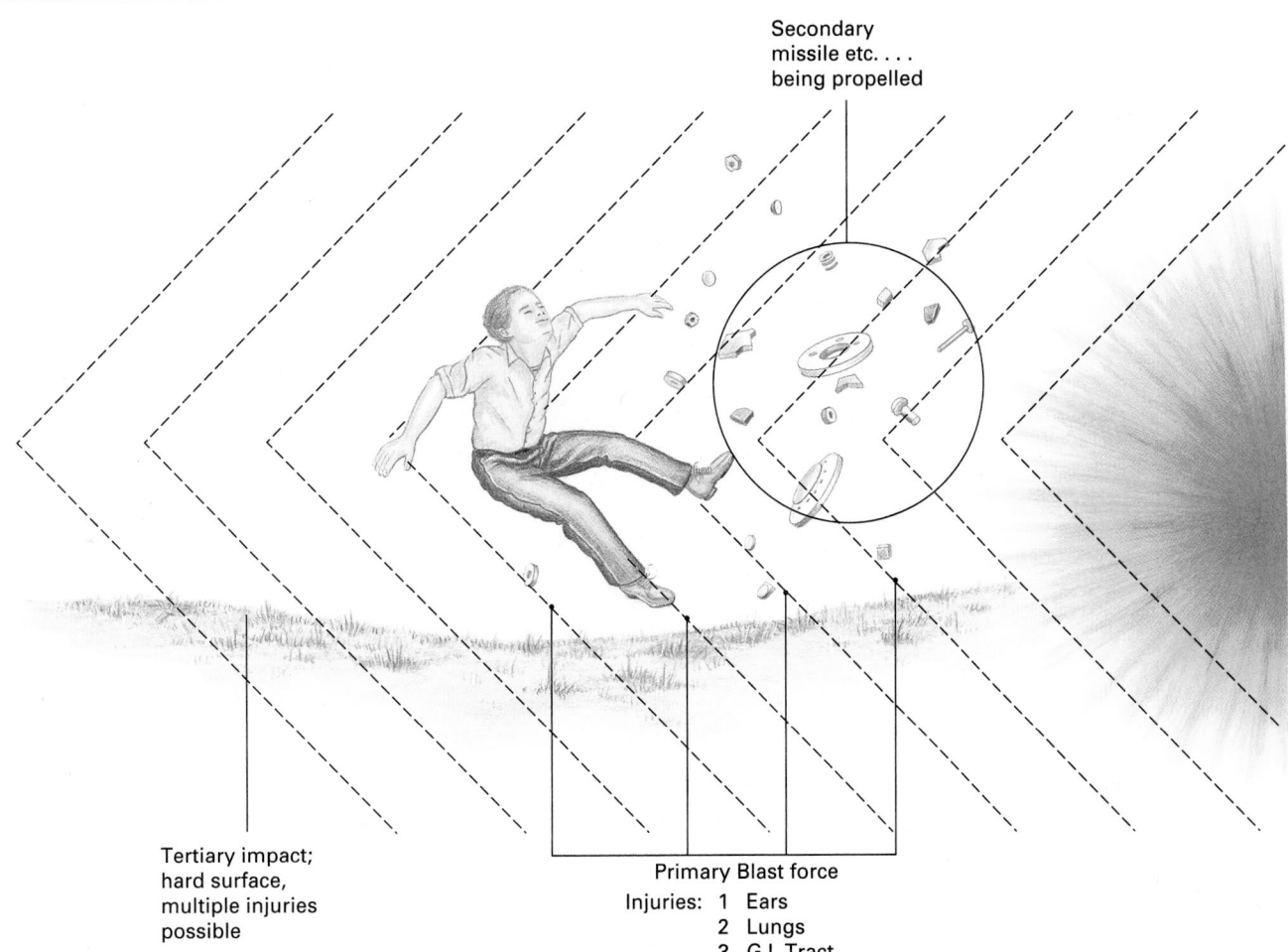

Secondary
missile etc. . . .
being propelled

Tertiary impact;
hard surface,
multiple injuries
possible

Primary Blast force
Injuries: 1 Ears
2 Lungs
3 G.I. Tract

FIGURE 14-22 Blast injuries can cause injury with the initial blast, when the victim is struck by debris, or when the victim is blown away from the site of the blast.

Be careful to assess the victim of an explosion completely. Many injuries are internal and difficult to recognize, especially in the minutes immediately after an incident. You are well advised to transport the patient for extensive evaluation at a trauma center, even if there appears to be minimal apparent injuries.

PENETRATING TRAUMA

Penetrating trauma is caused by many mechanisms, most commonly, knives, arrows, and bullets. The extent of damage depends upon Newton's laws of motion and the kinetic energy formula. If you recall, kinetic energy is equal to an object's mass times the square of its velocity. This is then divided by two. Remember, as the mass of an object is doubled, its energy is doubled. However, if the speed is doubled, the energy increases fourfold. Hence a very small and light bullet traveling at a very high speed can do tremendous damage within the human body.

The Law of Conservation of Energy (energy can neither be created nor destroyed, only changed) explains that projectile kinetic energy is transformed into damage as it slows. If a bullet remains within the object struck, then all

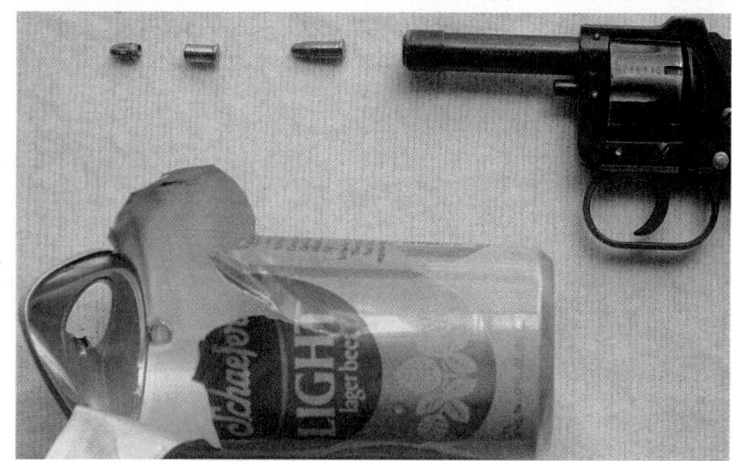

FIGURE 14-23 Destructive effect of .22 caliber hand gun.

energy is expended. If it passes through, then energy expended is equal to the energy just prior to entering the body, minus the energy remaining as it leaves.

Ballistics

Ballistics is the study of projectile properties and characteristics. One aspect of this study is **trajectory**, or the curved path that a bullet follows once fired from a gun. As it travels through the air, the bullet is constantly pulled downward by gravity. The faster the bullet, the flatter its curve of travel, and the straighter its trajectory.

A second, more significant, aspect of projectile travel is energy dissipation. Factors that affect energy dissipation include drag, expansion, profile, and cavitation. As a bullet passes through the air, it experiences wind resistance, or drag. The faster it travels, the more drag it experiences and the greater the slowing effect. Since this represents a reduction in bullet speed, it also means, if all else is equal, that the damage caused by a bullet fired at close range will be more severe than one fired from a distance.

Damage done within the body is dependent upon a number of elements. The first is the bullet's **profile**, or surface through which it exchanges energy. The larger the diameter of the projectile, the more tissue it contacts, and the more rapidly it exchanges energy. A small .22 caliber bullet (about 1/4 inch in diameter) loses energy less rapidly than a .45 caliber bullet (about 1/2 inch in diameter). As the diameter doubles from 1/4 inch to 1/2 inch, the surface transmitting energy increases fourfold. (See Figures 14-23 to 14-26.)

To increase the rate of energy release, some bullets expand upon entry. Such is the soft-point, hollow-tipped bullet (dum-dum or wad cutter) that mushrooms and/or fragments upon impact. Rotation or tumble will also present a wider bullet profile and increase the energy transfer rate. Whatever the mechanism, any increase in the bullet profile will increase the rate of energy exchange and damage inflicted upon the victim.

The speed of a penetrating object determines the energy that can be expended. With a knife or arrow, speed is relatively low and damage is limited to the actual path. However, with a high-speed, high-energy projectile, such as a rifle bullet, the damage is many times larger. (See Figure 14-27.)

Pathway expansion is an important concept in understanding the pathology of bullet wounds. As a bullet contacts the patient's semi-fluid body, it generates a **cavitation** wave. The bullet pushes tissue in front of, and lateral to, its travel. This causes a wave of pressure to move in front of and along

■ **ballistics** the study of projectile motion and its effects upon any object it impacts.

■ **trajectory** the path a projectile follows. It is typically curved because of the effect of gravity.

■ **profile** the size and shape of a projectile as it contacts a target.

■ **cavitation** formation of a partial vacuum, and subsequent cavity, within a liquid. This describes the action of a high-velocity projectile on the human body, which is 60 percent water.

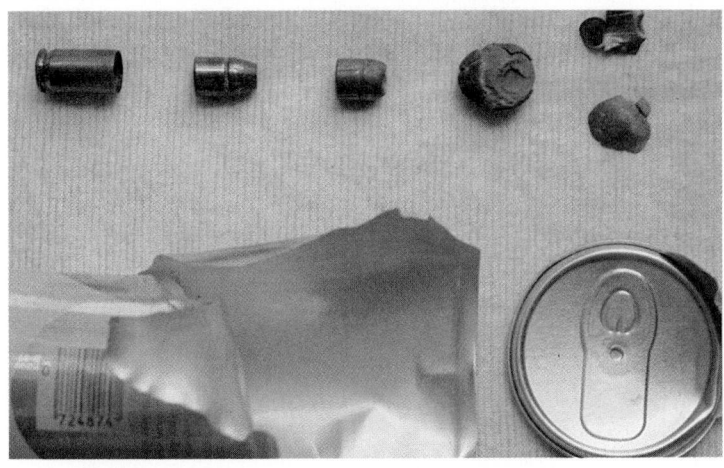

FIGURE 14-24 Destructive effect of .32 caliber hand gun.

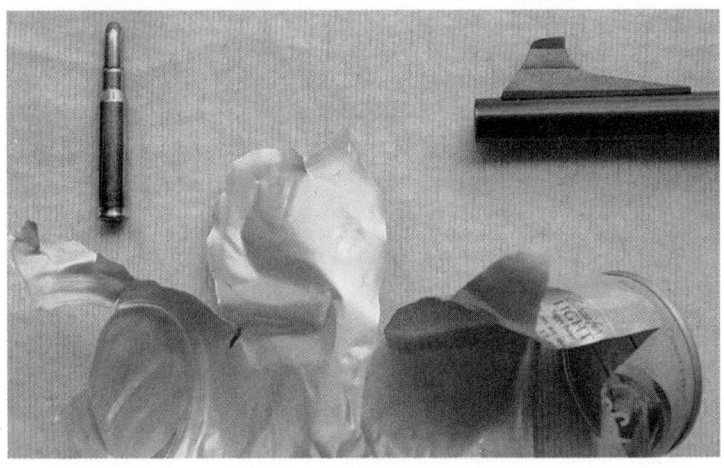

FIGURE 14-25 Destructive effect of .308 caliber rifle.

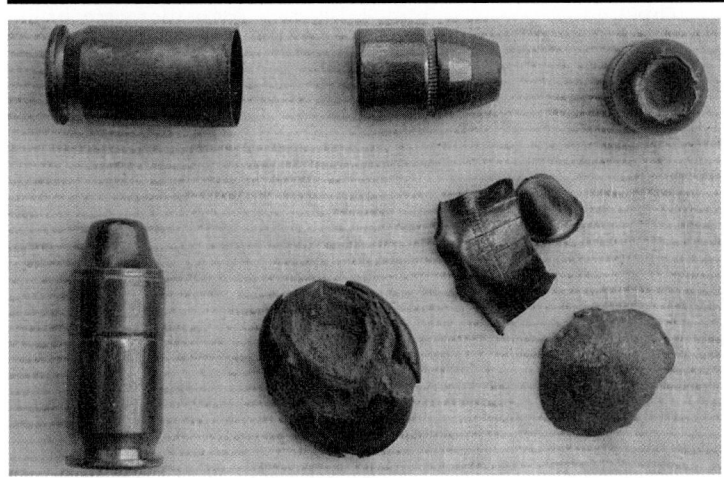

FIGURE 14-26 The profile of a bullet will vary based on its design.

side the projectile, leaving a cavity in its wake. Organs and tissues are compressed drastically, causing contusion, rupture, and fracture. The faster the bullet travels, and the greater its profile, the greater the energy exchange, the greater the cavitation wave, and the greater the resultant damage.

✳ The faster the bullet travels and the greater the profile it presents, the greater will be the rate of energy transfer and the larger the cavitational wave and the resultant damage.

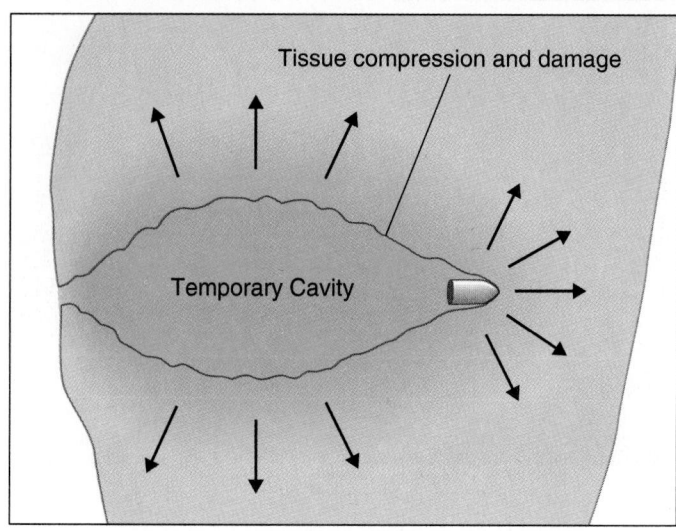

FIGURE 14-27 The severity of injury associated with penetrating trauma is, in many ways, related to the velocity of the penetrating object.

Cavitational Wave

There are three categories of projectile injury. They include:

❑ Low velocity
❑ High velocity/medium energy
❑ High velocity/high energy

Low Velocity   Low-velocity injury is caused by weapons such as a knife, ice pick, or arrow or by flying objects such as blast debris or a wire thrown by a lawn mower. In either case, the kinetic energy is limited by the relatively slow speed of the object when it enters the body. A common example would be a stabbing in which an individual weighing about 150 pounds strikes another at 50 mph. The knife's speed is noticeably less than that of a bullet, although the mass behind the penetration is significant.

In low-velocity penetration, remember that entrance wounds may not reflect the extent of injury. In the case of a stabbing, the expectant trauma is limited to the pathway of the knife. However, it may have plunged deep into the body. It may also have been twisted, moved about, or shoved in at an oblique angle. As a result, the entrance wound may not indicate the depth of entry, nor the actual organs involved.

The physical characteristics of the attacker are also important. Knife-wielding males, for example, will strike with a forward, outward, or crosswise stroke. Females usually strike with an overhand and downward blow. Initially, victims attempt to protect themselves by using the arms. Deep upper extremity lacerations (commonly called *defense wounds*) result. As the attack continues, injuries are directed to the chest, abdomen, or back.

If an object causing a low-velocity wound lodges in the body, it may be dangerous to remove. If the object bent as it hit a bone upon entry, attempts at removal may cause further injury. If the object is held firmly by soft tissue, it may obstruct blood vessels, thereby reducing potential blood loss. The only impaled objects that you should remove on the scene are those lodged in the cheek so that they interfere with the airway or those that you must remove to provide CPR.

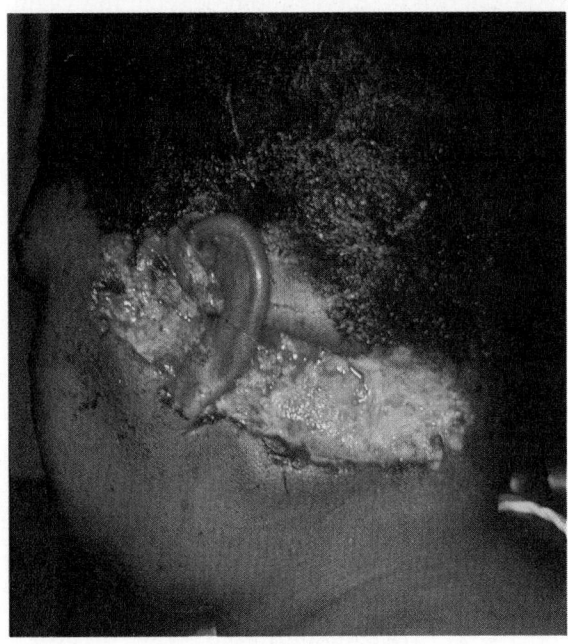

FIGURE 14-28 Wound resulting from close-range shotgun blast. Note the tattooing of the skin from gun powder.

High Velocity High-velocity injuries, most commonly caused by bullets, are classified as medium-energy or high-energy wounds. Medium-energy wounds result from shotgun pellets or handgun bullets. High-energy wounds are usually caused by high-power, high-speed rifle bullets. These wounds are of great concern because high kinetic energy creates the potential for immense injury. A bullet with a muzzle velocity of 1,000 feet per second travels at about 720 miles per hour. At this rate of speed, the kinetic energy is tremendous. Because the bullet is light, it may transfer its energy very rapidly, resulting in extensive destruction.

Examination of an entrance wound may reveal residue from the blast, abrasion from muzzle exhaust, and powder burns (tattooing), if the gunshot was delivered at close range. (See Figure 14-28.) The exit wound is commonly larger and appears more severe. Cavitation increases the pathway of damage as the bullet exits, thus accounting for the increase in wound size. If all the energy is expended within, no exit wound exists and the projectile remains lodged inside the patient.

Pathologies of Penetrating Trauma.

Stabbings, gunshot blasts, and other penetrating trauma can affect vital structures within the head, neck, thorax, and abdomen. Anticipating the seriousness of these injuries is important to proper assessment and care.

Head Injuries Penetrating head injuries can be divided into two areas of discussion. The first area involves facial trauma. Penetrating facial trauma may endanger the airway and some of the body's sensory organs. It can also induce heavy bleeding. Frequently, this area is severely damaged in attempted suicide. When a rifle or shotgun is used, the victim places the barrel under the chin or in the mouth, while reaching for the trigger. As the trigger is squeezed, the head tilts back and the blast impacts the mandible, maxilla, and nasal bones. The bullet, however, may not penetrate the cranium, leaving the victim alive. In such cases, the resultant injuries seriously threaten the airway, causing severe hemorrhage and difficult-to-manage wounds.

The second area of penetrating head injuries involves the cranium. The cranium is a container of fixed volume and inflexible shape. When penetrated by a bullet, contents are trapped, with no room to absorb the energy of the cavitational wave. In addition to direct injury from the passing bullet, the brain is severely compressed, contused, and may be lacerated as it moves against the rough surface of the base of the skull. The rich vasculature of this area is damaged, resulting in intracerebral hemorrhage, edema, and increasing intracranial pressure. Ricochet, or deflection, may permit the projectile to expend all of its energy within the cranium. Therefore, most penetrating gunshot wounds to the cranium are fatal.

✳ Most gunshot injuries in which the projectile enters the cranium are fatal.

Neck Injuries
Neck wounds risk airway compromise and severe hemorrhage. The trachea lies at the anterior aspect of the neck, exposing it to any frontal injury. It may collapse due to damaged cartilaginous rings or pressure from nearby tissue swelling or hemorrhage. Large venous and arterial vessels traverse the neck, creating the potential for life-threatening blood loss. Additionally, neck veins, at times, carry pressures less than those present in the atmosphere (relatively negative). An open wound may draw air into a large vein, leading to massive air emboli—a serious life threat.

✳ An open neck wound may draw air into a large vein, leading to massive air emboli and cardiac arrest.

In examining neck injuries, some concern should be directed toward possible spinal cord injury. Although very well protected by the vertebra, the importance of the spinal cord to survival and bodily function make it a critical structure. Penetrating injury may damage the spinal column integrity or cause direct injury to the cord. Hence, penetrating injury to this region must be treated as a spinal injury until ruled out by X-ray and in-hospital evaluation. Penetrating neck injuries are cared for by spinal stabilization, hemorrhage control, airway protection, and prevention of air embolization from venous injury.

Thoracic Injuries
The thorax is a large, relatively common target for both low- and high-velocity projectiles. The lungs are rather tolerant to injury. Their spongy structure, created by air-filled alveoli, is better able to absorb and withstand the energy of cavitation than other tissues. Structures of the mediastinum (heart, great vessels, trachea, esophagus and nerves), for example, are not so tolerant. Pulmonary contusions or pneumothorax may occur as well as esophageal injury, rupture of great vessels, and rapid exsanguination.

Pericardial tamponade may result if a bullet passes through the heart. Both the ventricle and the pericardium are perforated. As the chamber contracts, blood enters the pericardial sac. It does not escape the pericardium as rapidly as it enters, thus creating a pressure. This pressure limits ventricular filling, cardiac output, and may rapidly lead to heart failure and death.

An open pneumothorax, or sucking chest wound, is of concern in any penetrating chest injury. However, the size of a wound needed to allow air in and out of this cavity is rather large. Such a wound does not routinely occur with a knife or gunshot injury unless the wound is extensive. A shotgun blast fired at close range may induce an open pneumothorax, but most other gunshot wounds only rarely do so.

If a rib is subjected to high-energy impact, it may fracture, allowing for a more rapid energy exchange, bullet deflection, and fragmentation of the projectile. This will increase the size of the damage pathway and the significance of injury. It is also important to remember that abdominal and thoracic contents move up and down with respiration. If the entrance wound is in an area close to the rib margin, structures involved may be either abdominal, thoracic, or both.

✳ Remember that the abdominal and thoracic organs move up and down with respiration. If the entrance wound is near the rib margin, either abdominal or thoracic organs may be involved, or both.

Abdominal Injuries   Passage of a projectile or other object into the abdomen may rupture hollow organs, tear vascular tissue, and damage solid organs. The large and small bowel, pancreas, gall bladder, and urinary bladder may perforate with bullet passage or rupture due to cavitation. Massive abdominal inflammation (peritonitis) will result, though often well after pre-hospital care providers have examined the patient. Pancreatic damage may also affect metabolism of glucose and digestion. Solid organs, such as the liver, kidneys, and spleen will bleed heavily.

Other Considerations   Penetrating extremity trauma is rarely a life-threatening concern. These injuries can be very extensive. The long bones are large and strong, and projectile impact provides a quick exchange of energy. Yet the lack of critical structures reduces concern, except where significant bleeding occurs. Control hemorrhage, and if no other life-threatening injury exists, assess and protect distal circulation and neurologic function in the extremity.

In penetrating injury, you will not be able to determine exactly which organs are effected and to what degree. Use the mechanism of injury to determine the nature and extent of injury. Then provide care for the worst-case scenario. Penetrating trauma to the head, chest, or abdomen indicates that the patient should be treated with limited scene care and transported to a trauma center as quickly as possible.

SUMMARY

As a paramedic, you will be called upon to decide what care a trauma patient receives and whether it will be delivered at the scene or en route. To make the most appropriate choice, you must understand the mechanisms of injury experienced by your patient and the indices of suspicion that they suggest. Carefully recreate the accident in your mind, determining what forces may have been experienced and what anatomical locations may have been impacted. Determine which organs are most likely injured, to what degree, and what level of life threat their injury suggests. Based on this analysis, decide whether to provide scene care or rapid transport with care en route.

FURTHER READING

AMERICAN COLLEGE OF SURGEONS, COMMITTEE ON TRAUMA. *Advanced Resources for Optimal Care of the Injured Patient.* American College of Surgeons, 1990.

AMERICAN COLLEGE OF SURGEONS, COMMITTEE ON TRAUMA. *Advanced Trauma Life Support Course: Student Manual.* American College of Surgeons, 1989.

BAXT, WILLIAM G. *Trauma, The First Hour.* 1st ed. Englewood Cliffs, NJ: Prentice-Hall, Inc., 1985.

BUTMAN, ALEXANDER M. AND JAMES L. PATURAS. *Pre-Hospital Trauma Life Support.* Akron, OH: Emergency Training, 1990.

CAMPBELL, JOHN E. *Basic Trauma Life Support.* 2nd ed. Englewood Cliffs, NJ: Prentice-Hall, Inc., 1988.

MAULL, KIMBALL KIRBY, JACKIE AND DENNIS ROWE. *Trauma Update for the EMT.* 1st ed. Englewood Cliffs, NJ: Prentice-Hall, Inc., 1992.

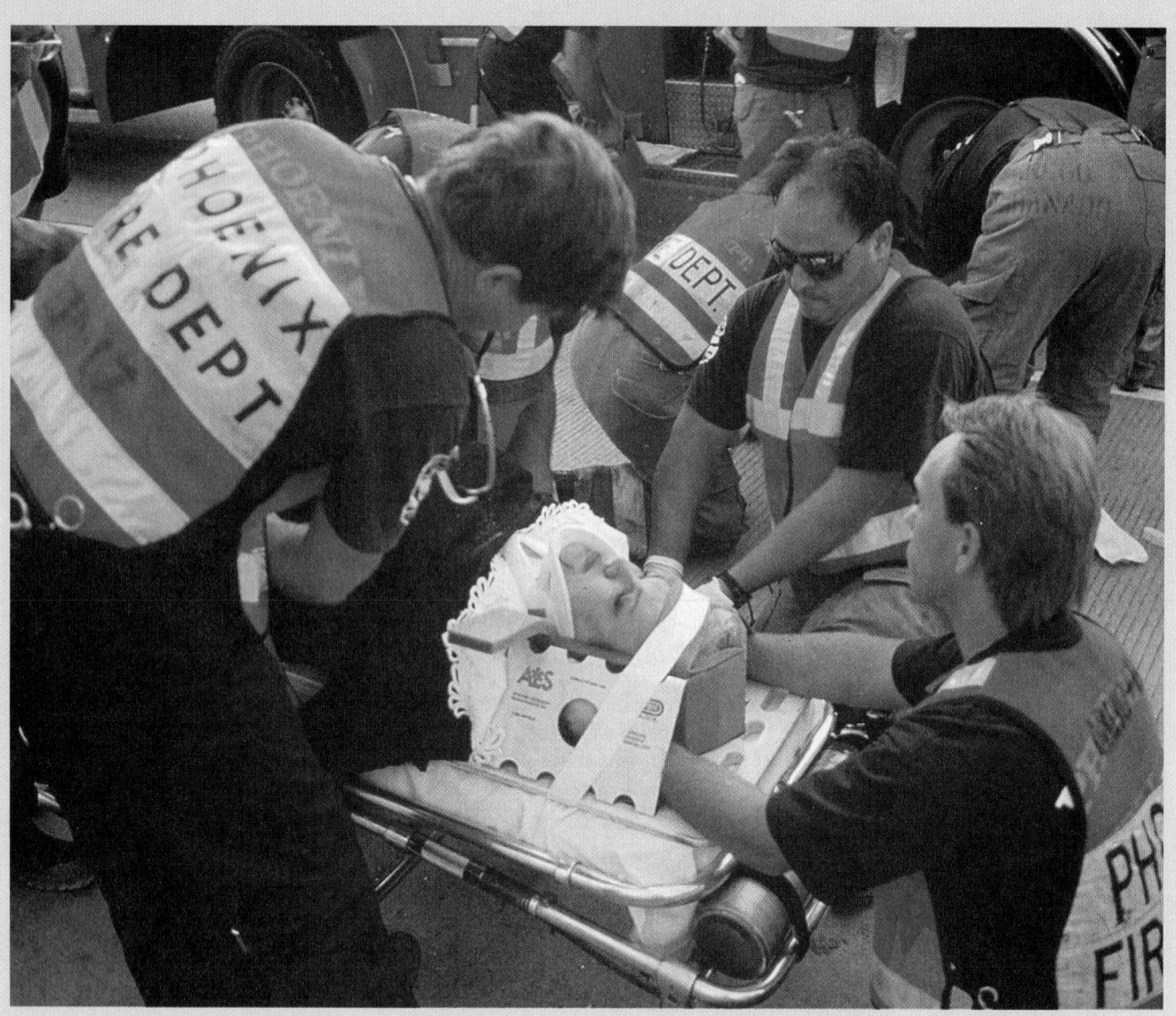

15

HEAD, NECK, AND SPINE INJURY

Objectives for Chapter 15

After reading this chapter, you should be able to:

1. List the structures that protect the central nervous system from trauma, and describe how they accomplish this function. (See pp. 435–439.)

2. List the components of the central nervous system, and explain how they help control the human body. (See pp. 439–442.)

3. List the signs and symptoms for the following conditions. (See below pages.)

- Soft-tissue injury to the scalp, face, and neck (pp. 444–447.)
- Skull fracture (pp. 445–447.)
- Central nervous system injury (pp. 447–452.)
- Special sense organ injury (pp. 452–453.)

4. Identify the various head, neck, and spine injuries, and explain the progression of their respective injuries. (See pp. 444–453.)

5. Explain the significance of the primary assessment as it relates to CNS injury. (See pp. 453–456.)

6. Identify the proper care steps for the following conditions. (See below pages.)

- Central nervous system injury (pp. 460–467.)
- Soft-tissue injury to the scalp, face, and neck (pp. 464–465.)
- Special sense organ injury (pp. 465–466.)

7. Describe the assessment of a patient with a head, neck, or spinal injury, and list the care steps required for each finding named. (See pp. 453–467.)

Unit 765 responds to a report of a one-car accident with a single victim. Arriving at the scene, the two paramedics observe an auto against a tree. The frontal impact has greatly deformed the vehicle and severely bent the frame. The driver's side windshield is broken in a "spider web" configuration, and the driver's door is ajar. No wires are down, and there does not appear to be any leaking gas or ignition source. Police at the scene have already taken control of traffic. A police officer tells paramedics that the patient was initially unconscious but woke up a few minutes ago.

When the paramedics approach the vehicle, they discover a conscious 31-year-old male who is disoriented to time and event. He doesn't know what happened nor what day it is. One paramedic manually stabilizes his head, while the other applies a cervical collar. The paramedics note a contusion on his left forehead. They note too that the patient complains of moderate chest pain that varies with respiration. The patient denies any pain prior to the accident and rules out any history of heart problems.

As the patient complains of pain, one crew member palpates the chest region and feels some crepitus. Lung sounds are clear, and the monitor shows a normal sinus rhythm. Vital signs include: blood pressure of 130/88, a distal pulse of 70, rapid capillary refill, and deep respirations at a rate of 20. During further patient questioning, the patient denies any previous medical history, prescribed medications, or allergies.

As assessment continues, the patient becomes agitated and then combative. The crew applies oxygen, but the patient's condition worsens. He becomes unresponsive and his left pupil dilates noticeably. The patient now only responds to deep pain and then only with ineffective motion. The paramedics move him rapidly to a long spineboard and begin transport.

En route to the hospital, paramedics start an IV with normal saline running at a rate to keep the vein open. They call medical command, give a short report, and receive orders to intubate. The on-line physician diverts the ambulance to the regional neurocenter. One paramedic intubates the patient orally, while the other firmly immobilizes the head. They hyperventilate the patient with 100 percent oxygen. They apply pulse oximetry, which now reads 97 percent.

Upon arrival at the receiving hospital, the staff quickly assesses the patient and sends him off to X-ray and the CAT scan. Although they find no cervical spine injury, they do note a epidural hematoma. They now rush the patient into surgery, where a neurosurgeon evacuates blood from the skull. Surgery is successful. When the EMS crew does a 24-hour follow-up, they find the patient conscious, alert, and doing well.

INTRODUCTION

Trauma commonly affects the head, neck, and spine. Head injury is the most frequent cause of vehicular death, while spinal injury accounts for a high incidence of serious disability. Despite the frequency and danger of these injuries, they are often difficult to recognize in the prehospital setting. As a result, subtle and unforeseen problems relating to these areas of the body quietly allow a patient to deteriorate, while we direct our attention toward more gruesome and visually apparent injuries. Even if a life-threatening injury is found, there is little definitive care you can provide in the field. To lessen the chances of death, you must recognize the signs and symptoms of head, neck, and spinal injury early in your assessment. This will allow you to provide rapid transport to a facility that can properly care for the patient, offering whatever care you can at the scene and/or while en route.

✱ Despite the frequency and danger of these injuries, they are often difficult to recognize in the prehospital setting.

ANATOMY AND PHYSIOLOGY

To gain an adequate understanding of the pathology, assessment, and care of head, neck, and spinal injury, it is first necessary to understand the anatomy and physiology of the central nervous system and these regions of the body. This will provide the basis to explain the injury process, the resulting signs and symptoms, and the appropriate care for these injuries.

The *central nervous system* (CNS) consists simply of the brain (cerebrum, cerebellum, pons, and medulla oblongata) and spinal cord. The central nervous system regulates all body functions, maintains consciousness, and permits our awareness of the environment. Additionally, it controls all our voluntary movements and many of our involuntary bodily functions.

The nervous system is made up of very specialized cells called neurons. CNS neurons, which may extend up to three feet in length, differ from peripheral neurons in that they have no protective sheath. Because of this, injury to a neuron makes repair or regeneration of cells in the central nervous system unlikely.

Central Nervous System Protection

Several protective layers prevent injury to the central nervous system in all but the most extreme circumstances. The scalp and hair fend off the effects of external temperature and trauma. The hard plate of the skull and the rigid support of the vertebral column withstand rigorous kinetic forces. The final layer of protection, the **meninges** and the **cerebrospinal fluid** (CSF), surround the brain and spinal cord to further absorb shock and suppress injury. (The brain and spinal cord actually "float" in CSF.)

■ **meninges** three membranes that surround and protect the brain and spinal cord. They are the dura mater, the arachnoid membrane, and the pia mater.

■ **cerebrospinal fluid** fluid surrounding and bathing the brain and spinal cord (the elements of the central nervous system).

The Scalp   The scalp protects the brain from both the effects of trauma and the extremes of weather. It is a strong and flexible mass of skin and fascia (bands of connective and muscular tissue) able to withstand and absorb tremendous kinetic energy. The scalp is also extremely vascular in order to help maintain the brain at the proper temperature. Hair further insulates the brain from environmental temperatures and, to a lesser degree, trauma.

The Skull   Under the soft tissue of the scalp are the bones making up the skull. (See Figure 15-1.) These include the facial bones and the cranium. The facial bones provide support and form for the nose, mouth, orbits, and jaw. The **cranium** is the protective container housing the brain.

Facial bones make up the anterior and inferior structures of the head and include the zygoma, maxilla, mandible, and nasal bones. The *zygoma* is the prominent bone of the cheek. It protects the eyes and the muscles controlling eye and jaw movement. The *maxilla* comprises the upper jaw and supports the *nasal bones*. These bones form the attachment for the nasal cartilage and the shape of the nose. The last of the facial bones is the *mandible*, or jawbone. It resembles two horizontal "L's," which join anteriorly and hinge underneath the posterior zygomatic arch. Besides forming the beginning of the airway and the alimentary canal, the protective facial bones form support structures for several sense organs, including the tongue, eye, and olfactory nerve.

■ **cranium** vault-like portion of the skull encasing the brain.

The cranium, or cranial vault, encapsules and protects the brain. It is quite strong, light, and rigid. It actually consists of several bones (the *frontal, sphenoid, occipital, parietal,* and *temporal* bones) fused together at pseudo-joints called **sutures**. These bony plates consist of two layers of hard compact bone, separated by a layer of spongy, or **cancellous**, bone. Such a configura-

■ **sutures** pseudo-joints that join the various bones of the skull to form the cranium.

■ **cancellous** having a lattice-work structure, as in the spongy tissue of the bone.

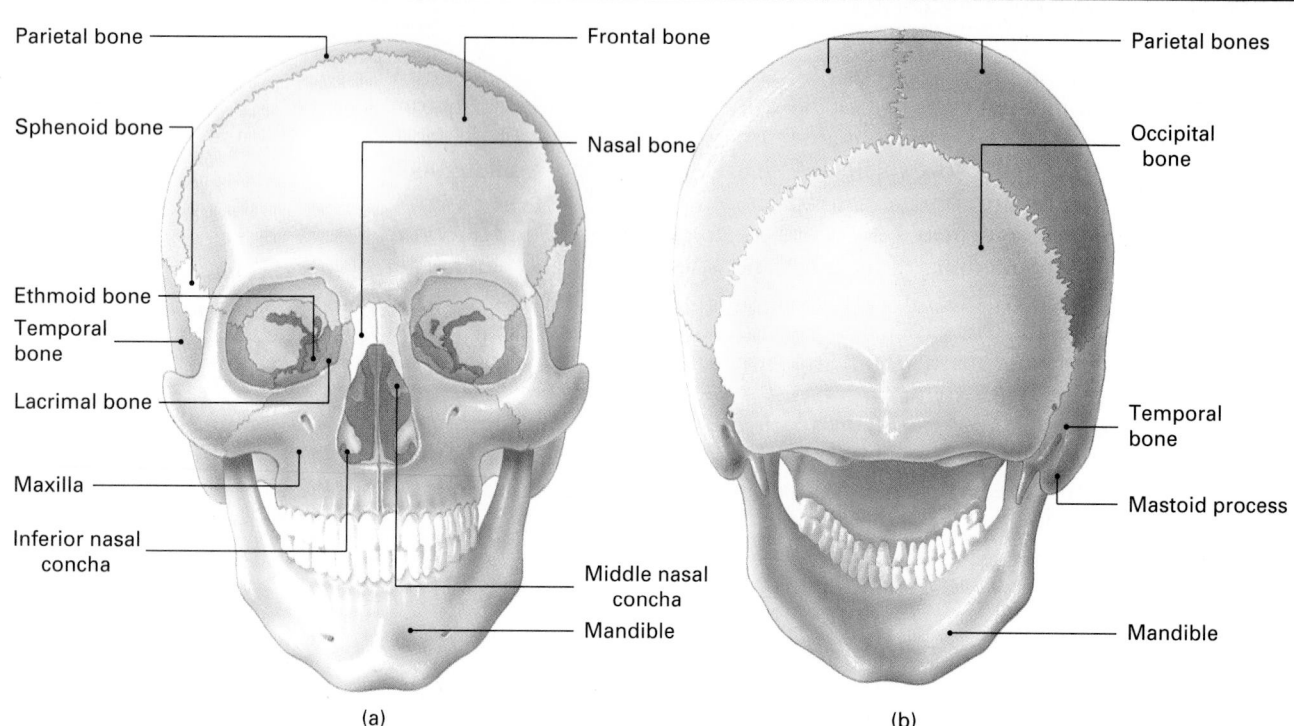

Parietal bone

Sphenoid bone

Ethmoid bone

Temporal bone

Lacrimal bone

Maxilla

Inferior nasal concha

Frontal bone

Nasal bone

Middle nasal concha

Mandible

Parietal bones

Occipital bone

Temporal bone

Mastoid process

Mandible

(a)   (b)

FIGURE 15-1   The human skull.

tion makes the skull strong yet light. The skull is, therefore, quite effective in protecting its contents from the direct impact of trauma. However, the cranial vault allows little space for swelling or bleeding. The result is increased intracranial pressure that can severely damage the brain.

The Vertebral Column   At its base, the skull connects with the *vertebral column*. (See Figure 15-2.) This column protects the spinal cord and allows for the mobility of the head and upper body. The column, composed of 32–34 separate and irregular bones, is divided into the five spinal regions. These include the *cervical, thoracic, lumbar, sacral*, and *coccygeal* regions.

The cervical spine consists of seven vertebrae numbered C1 through C7. The first, called the *Atlas*, supports the skull and allows for a large range of motion as the head turns from left to right. The second cervical vertebra, the *Axis*, has a small finger-like upward projection that forms the pivot point for this motion. This protrusion, the **odontoid process** (or dens), is the primary structure keeping the upper reaches of the spinal column in line while the head turns. Because of its small size and fragile nature, minor forces can cause fracture of the odontoid. Movement of the neck following this fracture can lead to injury or severance of the spinal cord. The cervical spine ends with the seventh cervical body. You can palpate this vertebra at the level of the shoulders. It is the first bony prominence you will feel as you work your fingers down the posterior surface of the neck.

The next 12 vertebrae are *thoracic*, with one connected to each pair of ribs. This relationship, as well as the overlying scapulae and back muscles, serve to protect the thoracic spinal cord from injury.

The *lumbar spine* is located between the chest and sacrum. It is made up of five of the largest vertebral bodies. The lumbar vertebrae support the entire upper torso, neck, head, and upper extremities. They are susceptible to compression fracture and injury to the intervertebral discs.

■ **odontoid process** fingerlike projection of the second cervical vertebra, around which the first cervical vertebra rotates.

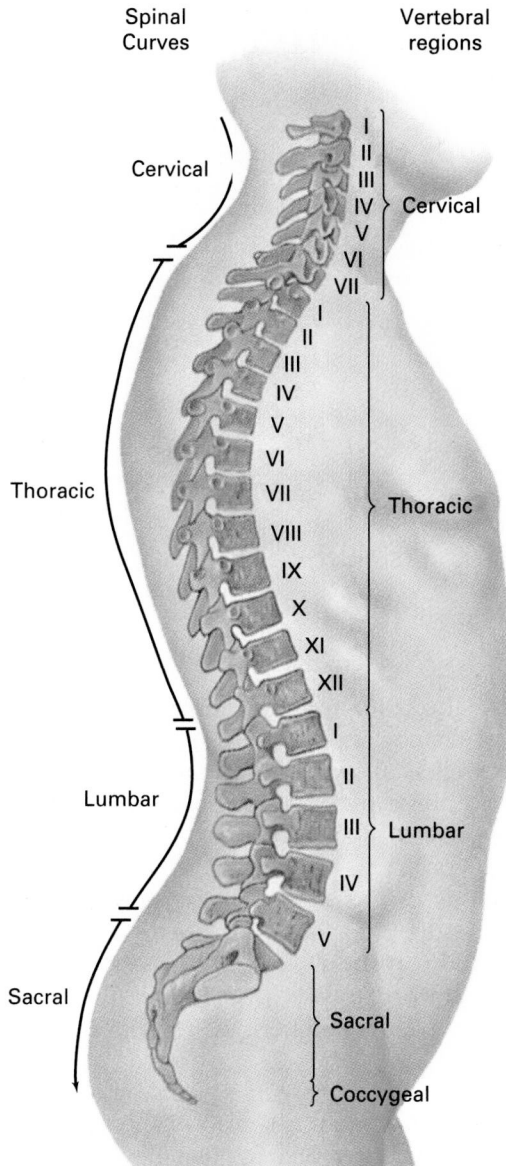

Spinal
Curves

Vertebral
regions

Cervical

Thoracic

Lumbar

Sacral

Cervical
I
II
III
IV
V
VI
VII

Thoracic
I
II
III
IV
V
VI
VII
VIII
IX
X
XI
XII

Lumbar
I
II
III
IV
V

Sacral

Coccygeal

FIGURE 15-2 The vertebral column.

The *sacrum* forms the posterior aspect of the pelvis and is composed of five fused vertebra. The pseudo-joint between the pelvis and the sacrum (called the sacroiliac joint) is an area of possible fracture. If fracture occurs, it is painful and may be unstable.

The final region of the vertebral column is the *coccyx*. It is a series of three, four, or five small vertebrae that, early in life, fuse into one or two bones. Although the coccyx provides little support or function, it is often fractured in falls where the patient lands on the buttocks.

Each vertebra is made up of several components. (See Figure 15-3.) The major weight-bearing aspect is the *body*. It is a round cylinder that supports the structures above and allows rotational movement. Between the vertebral bodies are cartilaginous *discs*. The discs protect articular and weight-bearing surfaces for the spinal column. Their resilient outer capsule and inner semi-

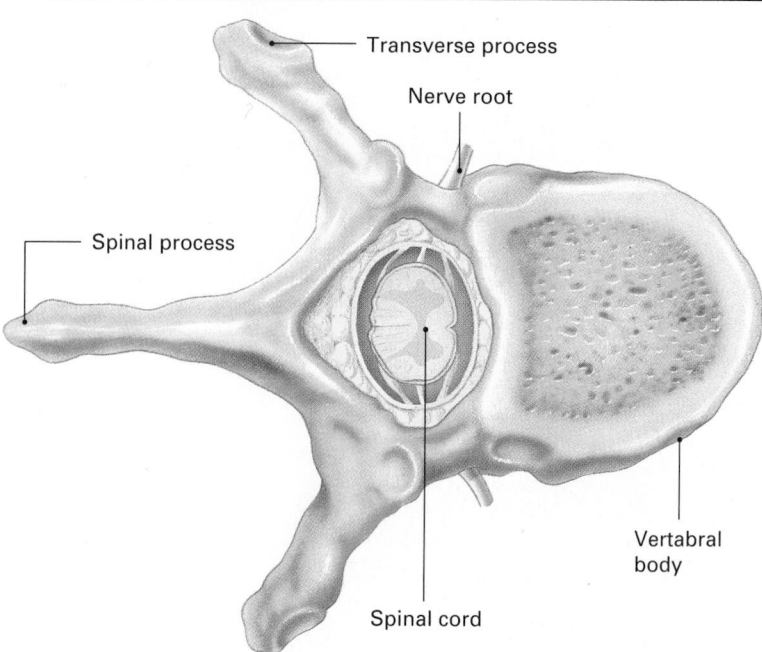

Transverse process

Nerve root

Spinal process

Vertabral body

Spinal cord

FIGURE 15-3 Although relatively well protected in the spinal canal, the spinal cord is subject to injury during accidents.

■ **spinal foramen** the opening in the vertebrae through which the spinal cord passes.

■ **dura mater** tough outermost layer of the meninges firmly attached to the interior of the skull.

■ **periosteum** the exterior covering of a bone.

■ **pia mater** inner and most delicate layer of the meninges. It covers the convolutions of the brain and spinal cord.

■ **arachnoid membrane** middle layer of the meninges.

■ **arachnoid** web-like in appearance.

liquid center enables them to cushion the column and the upper body from the jarring effects of walking and other minor impact. They also give the column its flexibility in lateral motion as well as allowing flexion and extension.

Posterior to the vertebral body are three processes—two lateral and one directly posterior. They provide for muscular and ligamentous attachment and provide some protection for the spinal cord. You can palpate the distal end of the posterior process (called the spinous process) from the seventh cervical vertebra to the sacrum. Central to the body and spinal processes is the opening for the spinal cord, called the **spinal foramen**, or canal. This space provides a tube through which the spinal cord travels from the skull to the second lumbar vertebra where the cord ends. This tube must remain in alignment to prevent injury to the spinal cord.

The share of weight each vertebra bears varies with its location. Moving from the top of the vertebral column to the bottom, the size of the vertebral body increases. This occurs because the amount of body weight the spine supports increases as you move down the column to the pelvis.

The Meninges   The final protective mechanism for the brain and the spinal cord is the meninges. (See Figure 15-4.) It is a group of three tissues between the skull and the brain and between the inside of the spinal foramen and the cord. The outermost layer is the **dura mater**. It is a tough layer and a major source of central nervous system protection. The dura mater is actually the inner **periosteum** of the skull and is attached to the interior surface of the cranium as well as to the spinal column.

The layer of the meninges closest to the brain and spinal cord is the **pia mater**. It is a delicate tissue, covering all the convolutions of the brain and the cord. Although more delicate than the dura mater, the pia mater is still much more substantial than brain and spinal cord tissue.

Separating the two layers of mater is a strata of connective tissue called the **arachnoid membrane**. It suspends the brain in the cranial cavity and the cord in the spinal foramen. The arachnoid membrane gets its name from its web-like appearance. Beneath the **arachnoid** membrane is the subarachnoid

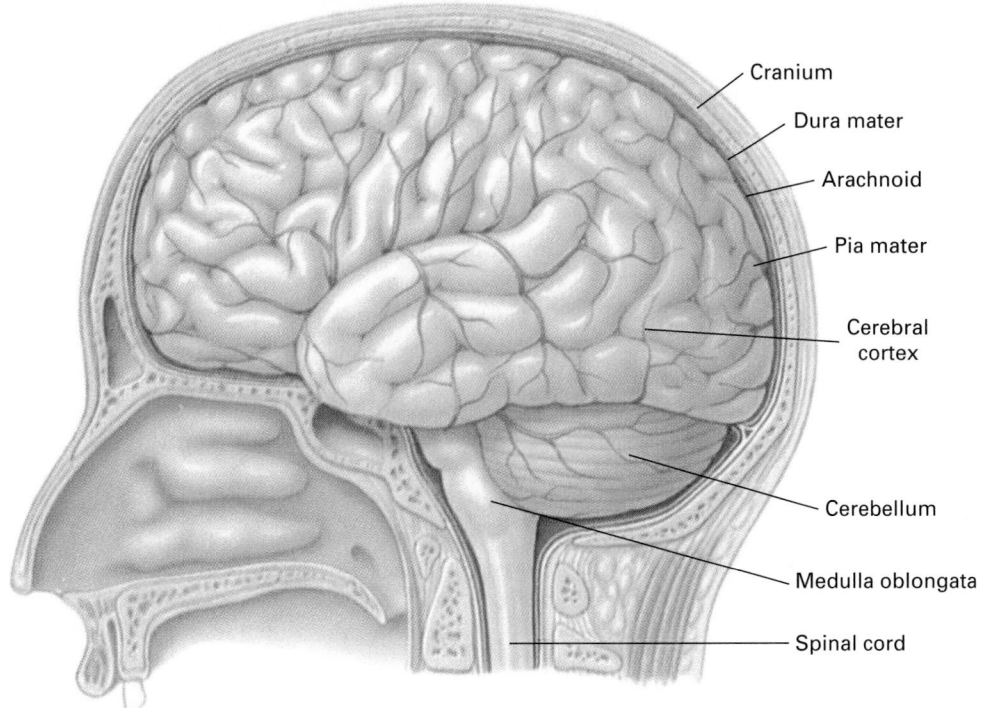

Cranium

Dura mater

Arachnoid

Pia mater

Cerebral cortex

Cerebellum

Medulla oblongata

Spinal cord

FIGURE 15-4 The meninges and skull.

space, which is filled with cerebrospinal fluid. Cerebrospinal fluid is the medium that surrounds the central nervous system and acts to absorb shocks of minor deceleration. The brain constantly generates cerebral spinal fluid, which in turn circulates throughout the brain and spinal cord before being reabsorbed.

The Central Nervous System

The functional unit of the central nervous system is the *neuron.* As you have read, CNS neurons differ in structure from the peripheral neurons. They do not have the protective protein sheath (called **neurilemma**) along their long arm, or *axon.* This subtle difference is important when considering trauma and regenerative repair. When injured, peripheral nerves may regenerate along the pathway provided by the neurilemma. In the central nervous system, however, injury that either interrupts the axon or kills the cell is generally permanent.

■ **neurilemma** thin, fibrous sheath surrounding the peripheral nerve fiber.

The Brain The brain consists of several regions that are essential to human function. They include the cerebrum, cerebellum, pons, and medulla oblongata. The *cerebrum* is the largest and occupies most of the cranial cavity. It is the center of conscious thought, personality, speech, motor control, and visual, auditory, and tactile (touch) perception. The cerebrum is regionalized into lobes roughly lying beneath the bones of the skull (and given the same names). The frontal region is anterior and controls personality. The parietal region, which is superior and posterior, directs motor and sensory activities. The occipital region, which is posterior and inferior, is responsible for sight. Laterally, the temporal region controls hearing and speech.

A structure called the *falx cerebri* divides the cerebrum into right and left hemispheres. A ligamentous partition, the falx cerebri extends into the cranial cavity from the interior and superior surface of the skull. Corresponding to the falx cerebri is a fissure in the brain called the *central sulcus.* This fissure physically divides the cerebrum into the left and right hemispheres, each of which controls (for the most part) the activities of the opposite side of the body. The **tentorium** is a similar fibrous sheet within the occipital region, running at right angles to the falx cerebri. It separates the cerebrum from the cerebellum. The third cranial nerve, which controls pupil size, travels through this area. It may be compressed as **intracranial pressure** rises or the brain is displaced due to swelling or hemorrhage. This will cause pupillary disturbances that may manifest on either the same or the opposite side as the problem. If the pressure is great enough, both pupils may dilate and fix.

Other anatomic points of interest within the skull are the cribriform plate and the foramen magnum. The **cribriform plate** is an irregular and bony plane at the base of the skull. It has surfaces against which the brain may abrade, lacerate, or contuse in severe deceleration. The *foramen magnum* is the largest opening in the skull. It is located at the base of the skull where it meets the spinal column. The foramen magnum is the point where the spinal cord exits the cranium.

The *cerebellum* is located directly under the tentorium. It lies posterior and inferior to the cerebrum. The cerebellum "fine tunes" motor control and allows the body to move smoothly from one position to another. Additionally, it is responsible for maintaining muscle tone.

The *pons* links the cerebellum, the cerebrum, and the upper portion of the spinal cord together. It is a bulb-shaped structure directly above the medulla oblongata. The pons acts as the communication interchange between the various components of the central nervous system and spinal cord.

The last nervous system structure still within the cranial vault is the *medulla oblongata*. It is recognizable as a bulge in the very top of the spinal cord. The medulla controls three basic functions—pulse rate, respiration, and blood pressure. Because of its location, just above the foramen magnum, a rise in intracranial pressure often affects this structure.

The Spinal Cord   CNS messages leave the medulla via the *spinal cord*, which is the body's main communication conduit. It carries commands to and from the brain, collecting or dispersing them through the peripheral nervous system. (See Figure 15-5.) The cord fills most of the spinal foramen of the vertebral column. It is at great risk for injury if any swelling, displacement, or constriction occurs.

Early in fetal development, the cord runs the entire length of the column. However, the skeletal system grows much faster than the specialized cells of the nervous system. By full maturity, the cord is effectively pulled up into the spinal column, ending at the 2nd-lumbar level by adulthood. During this growth, the spinal nerve roots are drawn into the lower spinal foramen. The area looks like the tail of the horse and is termed **cauda equina** (Latin for tail of the horse). This is the area into which a needle is introduced to withdraw cerebrospinal fluid for diagnostic purposes (called a spinal tap).

The peripheral nerves branch from the central nervous system in pairs between each vertebrae and between the skull and the atlas (C1). These peripheral nerves divide into somatic and autonomic tracts that innervate the body. The **autonomic nervous system** controls body organs not under conscious control, while the **somatic nervous system** controls skeletal muscles and dermatomes. **Dermatomes** are body regions corresponding to various nerve roots. (See Figure 15-6.) As the peripheral roots branch off the spine, they perceive sensation lower and lower on the body. The lower cervical and first thoracic branches control sensation and skeletal movement in the upper extremity. The thoracic branches govern sensation over the chest and back, while lumbar and sacral branches provide sensation for the lower extremities. Four locations are of special interest to us, because they represent levels of

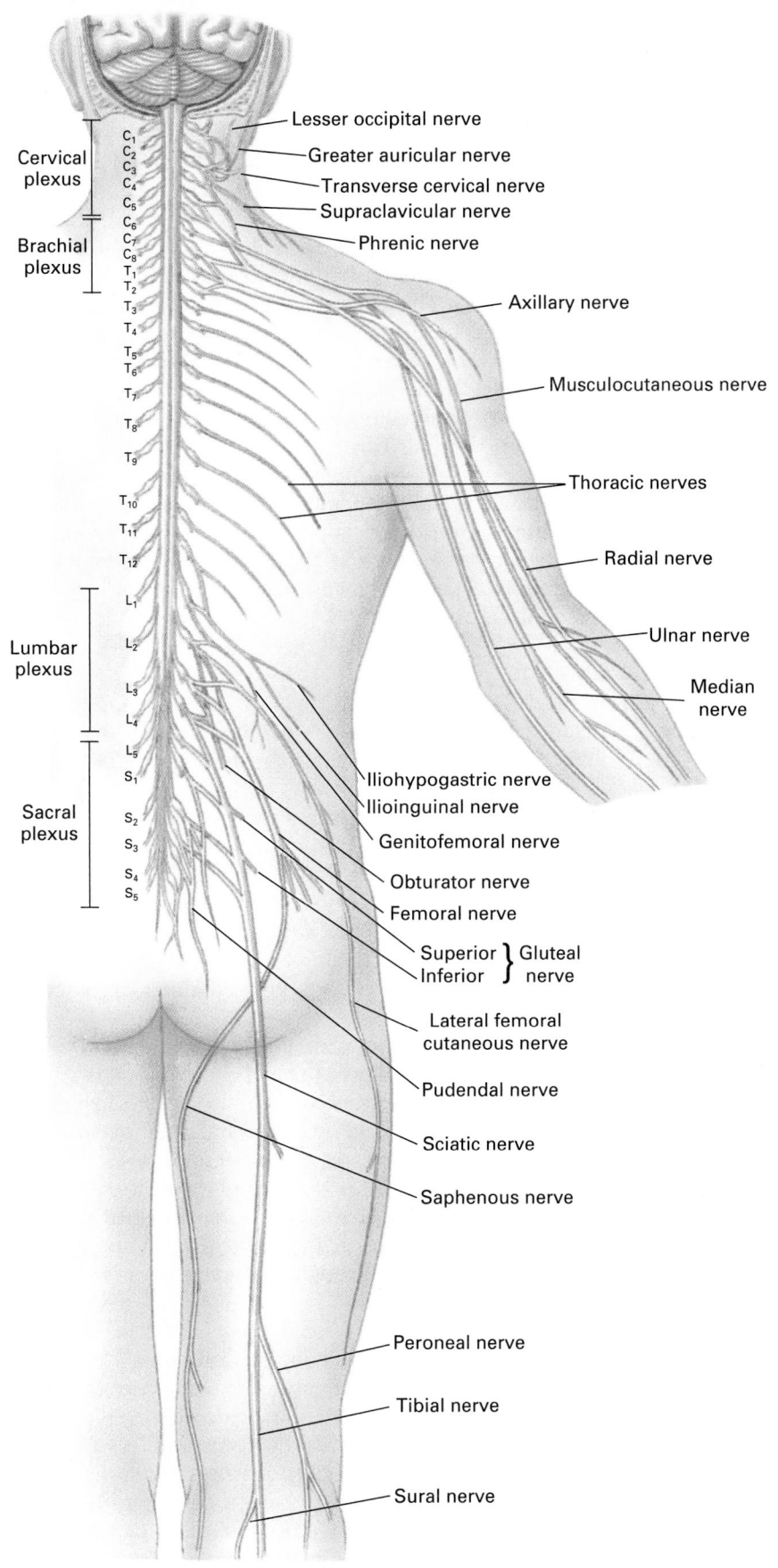

FIGURE 15-5 The spinal cord and its branches.

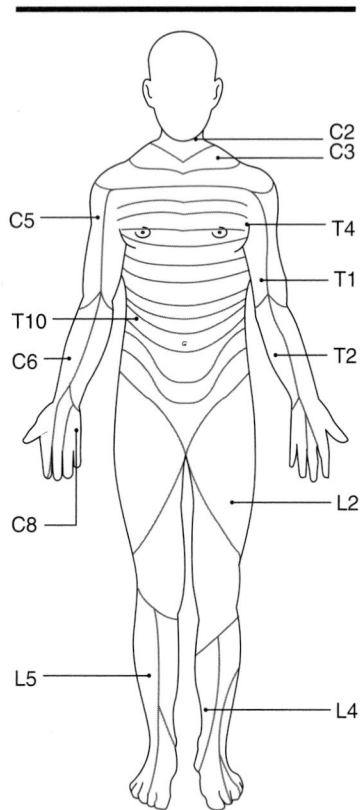

FIGURE 15-6 The dermatomes. Each dermatome corresponds to a spinal nerve.

■ **vitreous humor** clear watery fluid filling the posterior chamber of the eye. It is responsible for giving the eye its spherical shape.

■ **iris** pigmented portion of the eye. It is the muscular area that constricts or dilates to change the size of the pupil.

■ **lacrimal ducts** passageways carrying the lacrimal fluid (tears) from the lacrimal glands to the eye.

spinal cord control and are easy to locate. These locations include: the third cervical nerve, sensing the collar area; the fourth thoracic nerve, sensing the nipple line; the tenth thoracic nerve, sensing the umbilicus; and the first sacral nerve, sensing the soles of the feet.

CNS Circulation   Four major arterial vessels provide blood flow to the brain. The first two are the carotid arteries. These vessels ascend along the anterior surface of the neck and enter the cranium through its base. The two posterior vessels are the *vertebral arteries.* They ascend along and through the vertebral column. The carotid and vertebral arteries connect through the *circle of Willis* in the base of the brain. The circle of Willis is an arterial circle that assures good circulation to the body of the brain, even if one of the large feeder vessels is obstructed. Various arteries branch out from the circle of Willis and supply the substance of the brain itself. Venous drainage occurs initially through the dural sinuses. These ultimately drain into the internal jugular veins and then into the superior vena cava.

The spinal cord receives its blood supply from the *spinal arteries.* These vessels branch out from the vertebral arteries that travel the length of the vertebral column. The *anterior spinal artery* supplies the anterior two-thirds of the spinal cord, while the *posterior spinal artery* supplies the posterior one-third. The spinal veins follow a path similar to that of the spinal arteries and provide venous drainage of the cord.

Special Sense Organs

The head region includes vital sense organs subject to injury from kinetic impact. Two of the most important sense organs are the eye and the ear.

The Eye   The eyes provide much of the input that we use to interact with our environment. Although they are placed prominently on the face, the eyes are well-protected from trauma by a series of facial bones. The frontal bones project above the globe of the eye, while the nasal bones protect medially. The bone of the cheek, or zygoma, completes the physical protection both laterally and inferiorly. These bones collectively form the orbit or eye socket. The soft tissue of the eyelid and the eyelashes give additional protection to the critical ocular surface.

The eye is a spherical globe, filled with liquid. (See Figure 15-7.) Its major compartment (the posterior chamber) contains a gelatinous fluid called **vitreous humor.** Lining the compartment is a light- and color-sensing tissue known as the retina. The *lens* separates the posterior and anterior chamber. It is responsible for focusing light and images on the retina by the action of small muscles that change its thickness. A fluid similar to vitreous humor, called aqueous humor, fills the anterior chamber. The chamber also contains the **iris**—the colored portion of the eye that regulates the amount of light reaching the retina. Light enters the eye through the opening in the center of the iris called the *pupil.*

In examining the eye, you can easily identify several of its components such as the colored iris and the central black pupil. Bordering the iris is the *sclera*, the white and vascular area that forms the remaining, underlying surface of the exposed eye. The cornea, a very thin, clear, and delicate layer, covers both the pupil and iris. Continuous with the cornea and extending out to the interior surface of the eyelid is the *conjunctiva*—a delicate, smooth layer that slides over itself and the cornea when the eye closes or blinks.

When you look at a healthy eye, you will note that it is bathed in fluid. Produced by the lacrimal glands, this fluid flows through **lacrimal ducts** over the cornea. Because the cornea does not have blood vessels, the fluid pro-

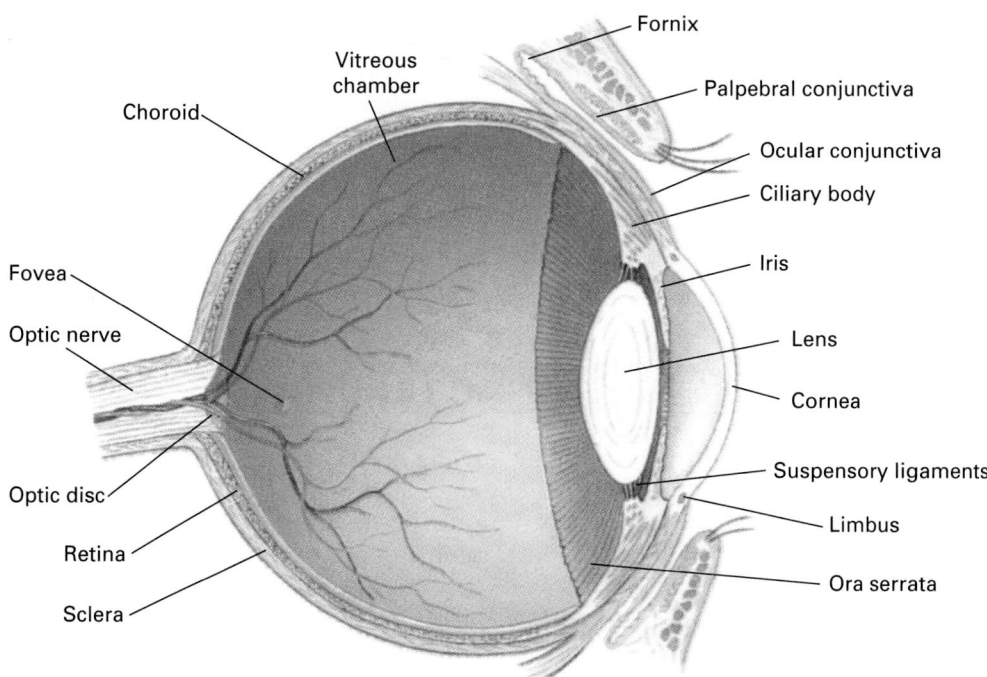

Fornix

Vitreous
chamber

Choroid

Palpebral conjunctiva

Ocular conjunctiva

Ciliary body

Iris

Fovea

Lens

Optic nerve

Cornea

Suspensory ligaments

Optic disc

Limbus

Retina

Ora serrata

Sclera

FIGURE 15-7 The human eye.

vides crucial lubrication, oxygen, and nutrients. If, for example, a contact lens is left in an unconscious patient, it may prevent this all-important fluid from traveling across the cornea, thus damaging the surface of the eye.

The last major elements in the eye are the cranial nerves. These nerves control the various small muscles located in the orbits, which in turn control the motion of the eye. These muscles allow the eye to rotate through a wide degree of motion.

The Ear   Another essential sensory organ is the ear. Its important structures are interior and exceptionally well protected from nearly all trauma. Only trauma involving great pressure differentials (e.g., blast and diving injuries) or basilar skull fracture are likely to damage this area. The ear provides us with two very useful functions—hearing and positional sense. Hearing occurs when sound waves cause the tympanic membrane (eardrum) to vibrate. The eardrum transmits the vibrations through three very small bones (the ossicles) to the **cochlea**, the organ of hearing. These vibrations stimulate the auditory nerve, which in turn transmits the signal to the brain.

The **semicircular canals** are responsible for position and motion sense. They are three hollow, fluid-filled rings set at different angles. When the head moves, fluid in these rings shifts. Small cells with hairlike fingers sense the motion and signal the brain to help maintain balance. This positional sense is present even when the eyes are closed. If injury or illness disturbs this center, excess signals are sent to the brain. Patients then experience a "spinning" feeling known as **vertigo**.

The Neck

The neck region is predominantly a soft-tissue area containing several structures susceptible to trauma. The spinal column is midline and posterior. Lateral to the spine are large muscle masses that strengthen and support the

■ **cochlea** snail-shaped structure within the inner ear containing the receptors for hearing.

■ **semicircular canals** the three rings of the inner ear. They sense the motion of the head and provide positional sense for the body.

■ **vertigo** loss of positional sensation and the perception that the horizon and all points of reference are moving.

spine and neck and permit a large range of motion for the head. Anterior to the spinal column is the *trachea*, the hollow tube supported by C-shaped cartilage. It shares its posterior surface with the smooth tissue of the *esophagus*. Superior to the trachea is the *larynx*, a cartilaginous structure consisting of the thyroid and cricoid cartilages. It is hollow like the trachea and houses the vocal cords, their supporting structures, and the epiglottis. The carotid arteries and the jugular veins are lateral to the trachea and the larynx. Both have internal and external divisions and carry large volumes of blood to or from the head and brain. The carotid arteries are high-pressure vessels that bleed profusely if lacerated. The jugular veins will also bleed profusely, although they generally carry much lower pressures.

HEAD, NECK, AND SPINAL TRAUMA

The head, neck, and spine are frequently the object of trauma because of their anatomical locations. The head may be the initial point of impact in auto accidents or falls, because it protrudes from the body. Because the head is associated with our individuality, it is also often the target of intentional blunt or penetrating injury. The neck and spine, because of its support of the head and body, may experience severe kinetic forces. Extension, flexion, compression, or lateral movement may lead to fracture, instability, and subsequent risk of spinal cord injury.

In considering trauma to the head, neck, and spine, it is best to segregate the following types of injury: superficial, internal (CNS), sensory organ, and neck injuries. Superficial injuries involve the scalp, underlying fascia, and skeletal structures. Internal injury includes brain and spinal cord trauma. Sense organ injury involves the eye and inner ear, while neck trauma may involve skeletal or soft tissues.

Superficial Injury

Superficial injuries take place in the protective structures of the brain and the spinal cord. These structures are often the first areas impacted by trauma.

Scalp Injuries
The scalp is an area frequently subjected to soft-tissue injury. Contusions, lacerations, avulsions, and significant hemorrhage are often obvious. They may manifest differently here than elsewhere on the body. This is because the scalp covers the unyielding bony tissue of the skull. Minor swelling or internal bleeding has but one way to expand—outward. A bump will be quite noticeable to your palpation or close inspection. Sometimes, however, this arrangement may confound assessment. In blunt trauma, the underlying fascia may tear, while the overlying skin remains intact. You may palpate a depression suggestive of depressed skull fracture where one does not exist. If a fracture does occur, internal bleeding and hematoma may fill the depression or result in a spongy or firm bump.

The scalp does not firmly attach to the skull from the frontal region to the occiput, nor does it firmly attach laterally. A glancing blow may cause a tearing and folding back of the scalp (an avulsion), thus exposing the skull. Although the injury may appear grotesque, it will generally heal well, unless there is gross contamination.

Bleeding from the scalp and facial areas can be profuse. An ample blood supply flows through this region to protect the brain from heat loss in cold weather. Because the scalp vessels are larger and not quite as muscular as other vessels, blood loss can be rapid and difficult to control. Severe and persistent bleeding from the scalp can contribute to shock.

Fractures   Fractures in the area of the head and neck can range from simple, minor breaks to breaks severe enough to cause life-endangering instability. Fractures of the cranium, facial region, and vertebral column are rarely of life-threatening proportions by themselves. It is the potential for central nervous system injury or airway threat that is your deep, overriding concern. Therefore, any potential fracture should receive your utmost consideration.

Skull Fractures.   Because of its spherical shape, the skull will not fracture, unless trauma is extreme. Such fractures may present as linear, depressed, comminuted, or basilar in nature. (See Figure 15-8.) Linear fractures are small cracks in the skull. In contrast, depressed fractures are actual inward displacements of the skull's surface. Comminuted fractures involve fragments of the skull that may penetrate the meninges and cause physical harm to the cerebrum or cerebellum underneath.

A common type of skull fracture involves the base of the skull. This area is permeated with *foramina* (openings) for various cranial nerves and blood vessels. It also has hollow or open structures such as the sinuses, the orbits of the eye, the nasal cavity, the external auditory canal, and the inner ear. These spaces weaken the skull and make the basilar area prone to fracture.

Signs of so-called basilar skull fractures vary with the location of injury. If the fracture involves the auditory canal and the lower lateral areas of the skull, hemorrhage may migrate to the mastoid (just posterior and slightly inferior to the ear). This will cause discoloration called **Battle's sign**. Another classic sign of basilar skull fracture is **bilateral periorbital ecchymosis**,

■ **Battle's sign** black-and-blue discoloration over the mastoid process (just behind the ear) that is characteristic of a basilar skull fracture.

■ **bilateral periorbital ecchymosis** black-and-blue discoloration of the area surrounding the eyes. It is usually associated with basilar skull fracture. (Also called raccoon eyes.)

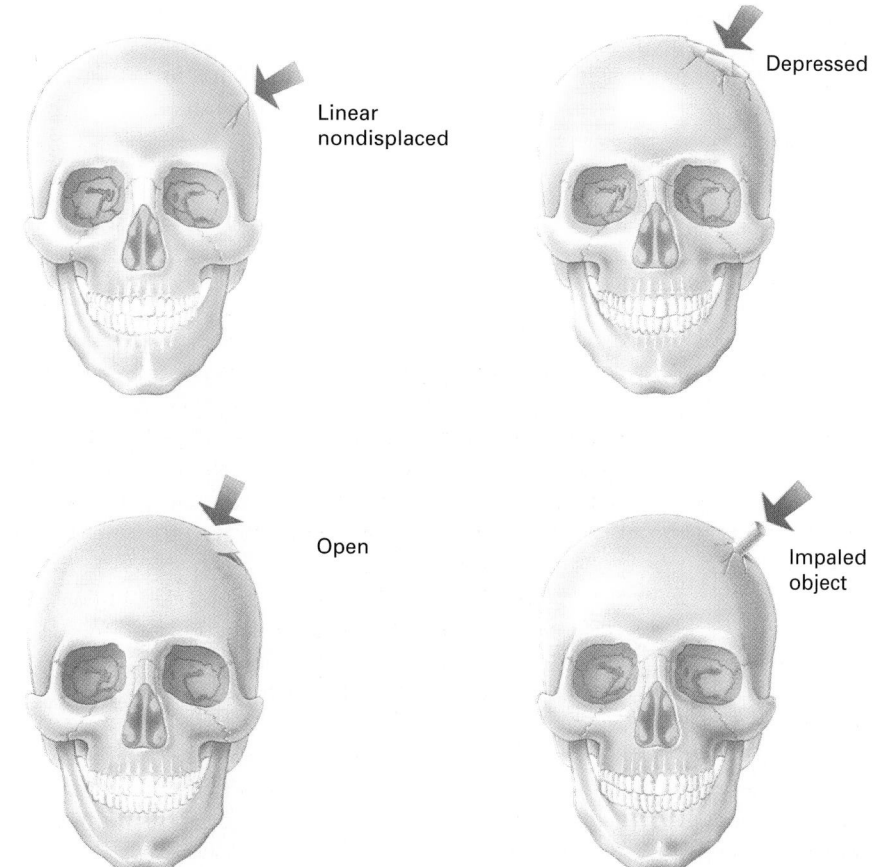

Linear
nondisplaced

Depressed

Open

Impaled
object

FIGURE 15-8   Various types of skull fractures.

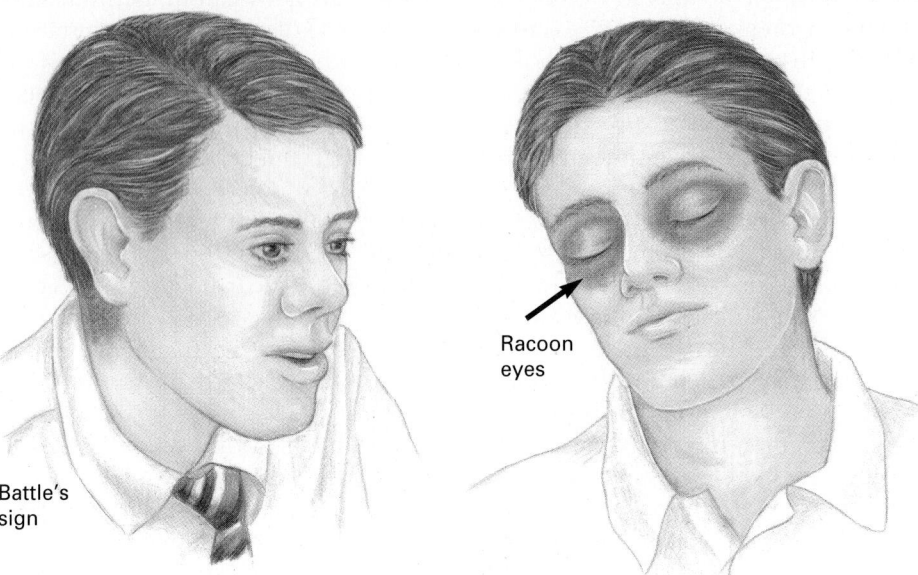

FIGURE 15-9 Battle's sign and raccoon eyes may indicate a basilar skull fracture.

Racoon eyes

Battle's sign

commonly called *raccoon eyes*. (See Figure 15-9.) It is a dramatic discoloration around the eyes, associated with orbital fractures and hemorrhage into the surrounding tissue. Remember that the discoloration of both Battle's sign and raccoon eyes may not appear during your care for the patient.

Basilar fractures can tear the dura and permit cerebrospinal fluid to seep through the nasal cavity or external auditory canal. (See Figure 15-10.) An open wound between the brain and the body's surface, and the subsequent loss of cerebrospinal fluid, is of concern. But the condition may also be beneficial. If intracranial pressure is increasing, loss of cerebrospinal fluid may help slow the rise. The central nervous system can regenerate the fluid at some later time.

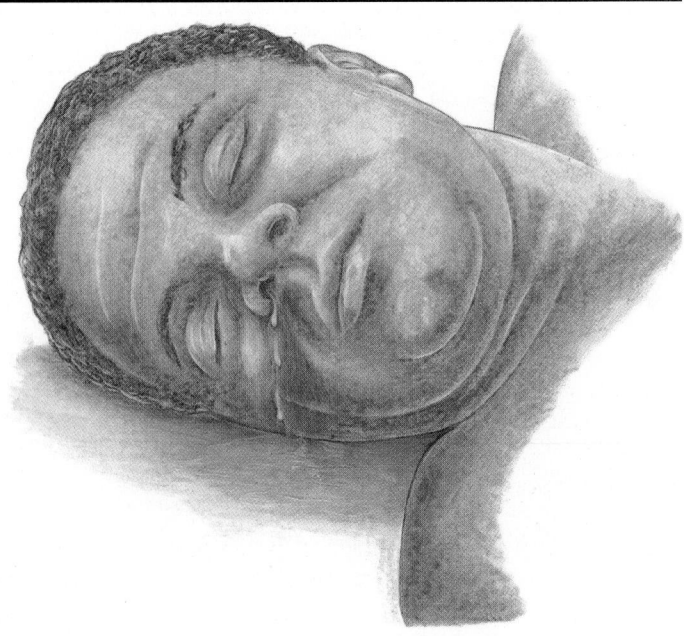

FIGURE 15-10 Drainage of blood or other fluid from the nose or ear may indicate a basilar skull fracture.

Spinal Column Injury. Abnormal motion, direct trauma, and compressional forces may cause spinal column injury. Movement beyond the normal range, including hyperextension, hyperflexion, or extreme lateral or rotational motion, may cause or contribute to injury. Falls against irregular surfaces or contact with moving objects such as a baseball bat or industrial machinery may also cause blunt injury. Projectiles, such as a bullet, may penetrate the soft tissue and directly damage the vertebral column. Compressional injury can also occur. Consider the forces as a diver impacts the bottom of a shallow pool head first. The body pushes against the head, compresses the neck, and subjects the cervical spine to tremendous forces (called **axial loading**). These forces may produce compressional fracture, intervertebral disc rupture, or both.

■ **axial loading** extreme compressional forces applied to the axis of the vertebral spine.

Spinal fracture is more common in the cervical and lumbar regions than elsewhere. The cervical spine has a high incidence of injury, because it supports the head and permits a wide range of motion. Its relationship with the head is like that of a column of dominoes balancing a 20-pound bowling ball. While the vertebral "dominoes" are held together with substantial ligaments, strong kinetic forces can cause injury. The lumbar region is frequently injured by either axial loading (as in a fall) or by tangential forces (as in a seatbelt injury). The thoracic region, on the other hand, is protected by the ribs, shoulder and back muscles, and the **scapula**. The pelvic ring and the musculature of the buttocks and lower back provide protection for the sacrum.

■ **scapula** large, flat, and irregular bone located in the posterior shoulder that articulates with the humerus.

With fracture, the ability of the column to protect the spinal cord is lost. The space between the cord's exterior and the interior of the spinal foramen is very small, especially in the cervical region. Any motion, both direct (as in trying to move the head) or indirect (as in trying to lift a heavy object), may displace the cervical vertebra and cause pressure, contusion, or laceration of the spinal cord.

Facial Injury. Fractures of the facial bones are usually less dangerous than those of the vertebrae. Most will be stable with minor complications. However, they do represent significant trauma and potentially serious complications. Fractures to this region may result from great forces and will often appear grotesque. They may involve the zygoma, maxilla (upper jaw), and mandible. Zygomatic fractures may entrap the muscles of the eye and limit its motion. **Maxillary** fractures may present with little more than pain, crepitation, moderate deformity, and limited instability of the upper-jaw area. Mandible fractures may present with deformity, pain, false motion, or limitation of the normal range of motion.

■ **maxillary** having to do with, or related to, the maxilla, or the bone of the upper jaw.

Severe trauma and crushing facial fractures may require aggressive airway support. For example, a suicide attempt that involves a shotgun placed under the jaw will create a blast that deflects away from the skull. The blast injures the mandible, hard palate, maxilla, and zygoma. The resultant damage destroys the rigid support of the nasal and oral cavities, thereby posing a serious threat to the airway. This injury may be life-threatening and difficult to manage.

Internal CNS Injury

Internal injuries to the central nervous system affect either the brain or spinal cord. Brain injuries generally relate to one of two distinct problems. The first set of problems, such as the concussion and the contusion, improve with time. The second set gets worse. This set includes intracranial, subdural, and epidural hemorrhages.

Brain Injury The scalp, skull, meninges, and cerebrospinal fluid protect the brain from strong acceleration or deceleration. To some degree, the brain floats in the cerebrospinal fluid much as you might do sitting in a bath tub.

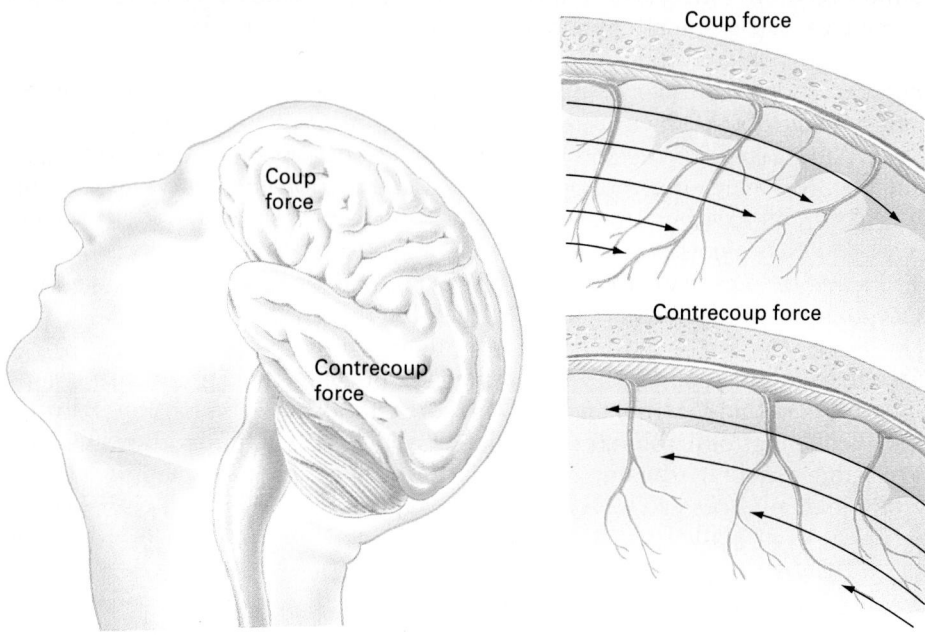

Coup force

Coup force

Contrecoup force

Contrecoup force

FIGURE 15-11 Coup and contrecoup movement of the brain.

■ **contrecoup** occurring on the opposite side; an injury to the brain opposite the site of impact.

When deceleration occurs, the brain "sloshes" forward, pushing the cerebrospinal fluid out of the way. Therefore, the brain gradually decelerates rather than stopping abruptly. Except for the most serious decelerations, this mechanism protects the contents of the skull very well. If the injury is too great, however, the brain will impact the interior of the skull, causing soft-tissue injuries such as contusions, lacerations, and hemorrhages. Extreme force may also cause the brain to "slosh" forward and then rebound, causing injury to the surface opposite the initial impact. This phenomenon is called **contrecoup** (pronounced kontra koo) injury. (See Figure 15-11.)

Keep in mind that the brainstem is the major point where the brain is tethered. In forceful acceleration or deceleration, the brain may tear or twist at this attachment. A wide variety of injuries may result, ranging from an interruption of normal brain function, to tissue damage, to actual hemorrhage.

A confounding problem with head trauma is that brain injury may occur simultaneously in several locations. The brain may impact the skull at the point of trauma, then "slosh" back and receive another injury, while a twisting motion injures the brain stem. In addition to being injured at several locations, the brain may be injured in different ways. It may suffer contusion, laceration, or internal hemorrhage. It may also be compressed by increasing pressure due to hemorrhage or edema.

■ **concussion** a transient period of unconsciousness. In most cases, the unconsciousness will be followed by a complete return of function.

Concussion/Contusion. The **concussion** is a transient loss of consciousness. If head trauma violently shakes the brain, it may disrupt its electrochemical function. Dysfunction is brief, usually abating in under three to five minutes. (In some cases, however, dysfunction can extend to as much as one hour.) Since the brain is not physically injured, complete recovery is expected. Concussion can occur simultaneously with other internal central nervous system injury.

■ **contusion** closed wound in which the skin is unbroken, although damage has occurred to the tissue beneath.

The **contusion** is a more significant jarring than concussion, with resultant cellular damage. Injured tissues may dysfunction and swell, beginning an increase in intracranial pressure and a decrease in cerebral perfusion. Localized injury to the brain may manifest by a characteristic dysfunction. An example is a patient whose personality changes after forehead trauma contuses the frontal lobe. Expect the level of consciousness and other physical signs to improve after a contusion or concussion.

Intracranial Hemorrhage. Hemorrhage can occur at several locations within the brain, each presenting with a different pathologic process. These injuries, from the deepest to the most superficial, are intracerebral, subdural, and epidural hemorrhage. In contrast to concussion and contusion, you should expect the intracranial hemorrhage patient to deteriorate after your arrival.

Intracerebral hemorrhage results from a ruptured blood vessel within the substance of the brain. Although blood loss is generally minimal, it is particularly damaging. Tissue edema results because blood, outside the blood vessels, irritates the nervous tissue. Intracerebral hemorrhage often presents much like a stroke with the manifestations occurring very quickly. The particular presentation relates to area of the brain involved. Normally, the signs and symptoms will progress with time.

■ **intracerebral hemorrhage** bleeding directly into the tissue of the brain.

Bleeding within the meninges, specifically beneath the dura and within the subarachnoid space, is called **subdural hematoma**. It occurs very slowly and is subtle in presentation, because blood loss is usually due to rupture of a small venous vessel. (See Figure 15-12.) Because the subdural hemorrhage is above the pia mater, it does not cause cerebral irritation as in the case of the intracerebral hemorrhage. The patient usually does not show overt signs and symptoms until hours or even days later. As a result, subdural hemorrhage is difficult to detect in the field.

■ **subdural hematoma** collection of blood directly beneath the dura mater.

✳ The subdural hematoma may not present with signs or symptoms for hours or even days after the injury.

Suspect subdural hemorrhage in an otherwise medical (non-trauma) patient who demonstrates neurologic signs and symptoms. A careful history may uncover a recent mechanism of injury that could cause this presentation. You will frequently encounter such cases with the elderly or with chronic alcoholics. Because the aging process and chronic alcoholism shrink the brain, both groups are prone to subdural hematoma. If you are called to treat a patient suspected of chronic alcohol use, investigate for recent head trauma. Also be alert for any signs suggestive of internal CNS injury.

Bleeding between the dura mater and the skull's interior surface is called **epidural hematoma**. (See Figure 15-13.) It usually involves arterial vessels,

■ **epidural hematoma** accumulation of blood between the dura mater and the cranium.

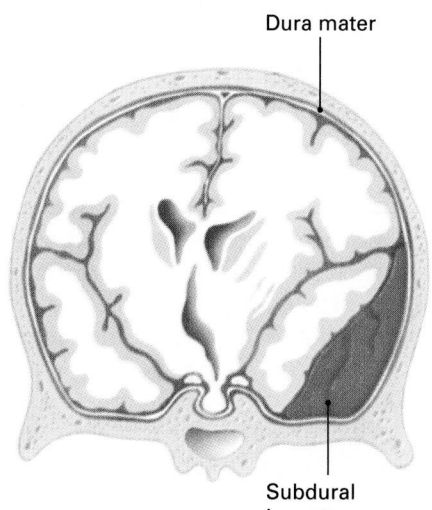

Dura mater

Subdural hematoma

FIGURE 15-12 Subdural hematoma.

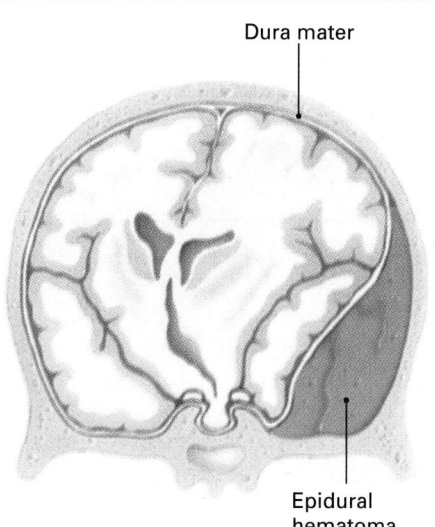

Dura mater

Epidural hematoma

FIGURE 15-13 Epidural hematoma.

often the middle meningeal artery. The condition progresses rapidly, while the patient moves quickly toward unconsciousness. Since the bleeding is from a relatively high-pressure vessel, intracranial pressure builds rapidly, compressing the cerebrum and increasing the pressure within the skull. The hemorrhage-induced intracranial pressure reduces oxygenated circulation to the nerve cells. Bleeding may be so extensive that it displaces the brain away from the injury site and pushes it toward the foramen magnum. Although the progression is both rapid and life threatening, immediate surgery can frequently reverse it.

The concussion, contusion, intracerebral hemorrhage, subdural hematoma, and epidural hematoma sometime occur in combination with one another. Occasionally the injury will cause the patient to sustain a concussion and epidural hematoma simultaneously. The concussion results in immediate unconsciousness, which lasts only minutes. The patient becomes conscious and alert, then exhibits a lowering of his or her level of consciousness. This interim period of consciousness, called a *lucid interval*, is frequently associated with the epidural hematoma.

Increasing Intracranial Pressure. Knowledge of the circulation of blood through brain tissue is critical in understanding the pathophysiology and significance of internal head injury. Since the cranium is a rigid container for the brain, any expansion in either the cerebrospinal fluid or in the vasculature must be matched by an equal reduction in the other. The most mobile volume within the skull is the vascular space. Should any swelling, bleeding, or fluid accumulation occur, it reduces the circulating blood volume and cerebral blood flow. With reduced cerebral blood flow, the brain becomes hypoxic and carbon dioxide concentrations rise. Hypercarbia dilates cerebral blood vessels and causes the systemic blood pressure to rise in an attempt to increase cerebral circulation. This reflex also increases the rate at which the intracranial pressure rises.

As the cycle of hypercarbia, increasing blood pressure, and increasing intracranial pressure continues, the pressure upon the brain displaces it away from the site of hematoma, hemorrhage, or edema and toward the foramen magnum. (See Figure 15-14.) This movement compresses the third cranial nerve, resulting in pupillary dilation. The movement also pushes the medulla oblongata into the foramen magnum, producing changes in the vital signs. The pulse rate slows; respirations become rapid, deep, or erratic; and blood pressure rises. This collective change in vital signs is called *Cushing's reflex*—a condition associated with increasing intracranial pressure. (See Figure 15-15.)

Pressure on the medulla oblongata may cause other neurologic signs and symptoms. The patient may vomit without nausea, and the level of consciousness will deteriorate. Since the medulla is an element of the **reticular activating system**, or system that causes consciousness, increased pressure leads to disorientation. Ultimately, the patient will become unconscious.

Spinal Cord Injury Any reason to suspect head injury is also a reason to suspect and treat the patient for a spinal fracture. Whenever the mechanism of injury includes events that could cause spinal cord trauma, treat the patient accordingly until proven otherwise. You can only gain that proof in the emergency department with X-ray and other diagnostic tests.

Injuries to the spinal column raise major concerns over injury to the spinal cord. The spinal cord almost fills the spinal foramen, especially in the cervical region. Displaced vertebrae or herniated intervertebral discs may impinge on the cord causing pressure, dysfunction, or cell death. Because the cells of the central nervous system have a difficult time repairing themselves, any injury may be permanent.

✱ Increasing intracranial pressure may cause slowing pulse rate, deep or erratic respirations, and an increasing blood pressure (Cushing's Reflex).

■ **reticular activating system** the system responsible for consciousness. A series of nervous tissues keeping the human system in a state of consciousness.

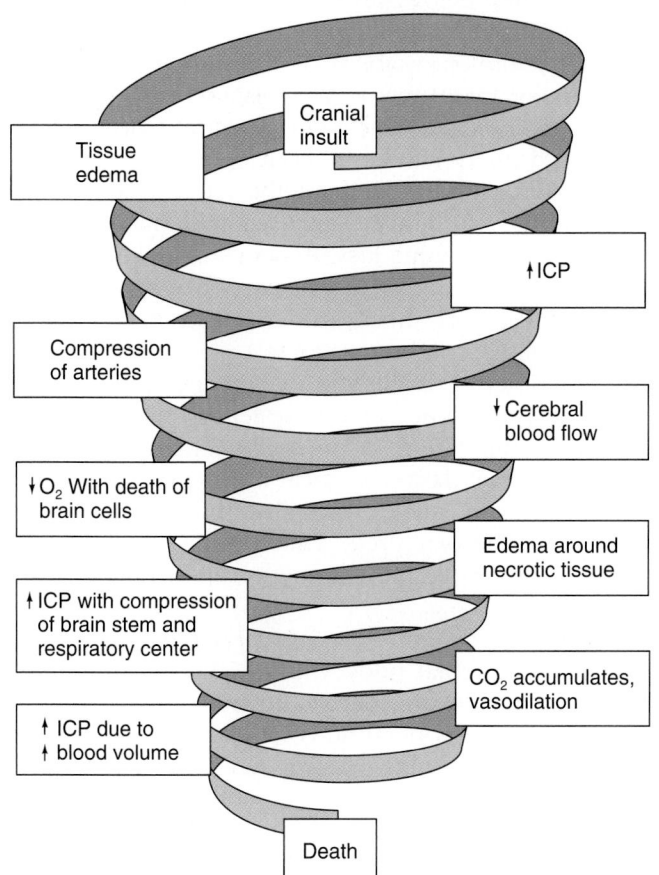

FIGURE 15-14 Pathway of deterioration following central nervous system insult.

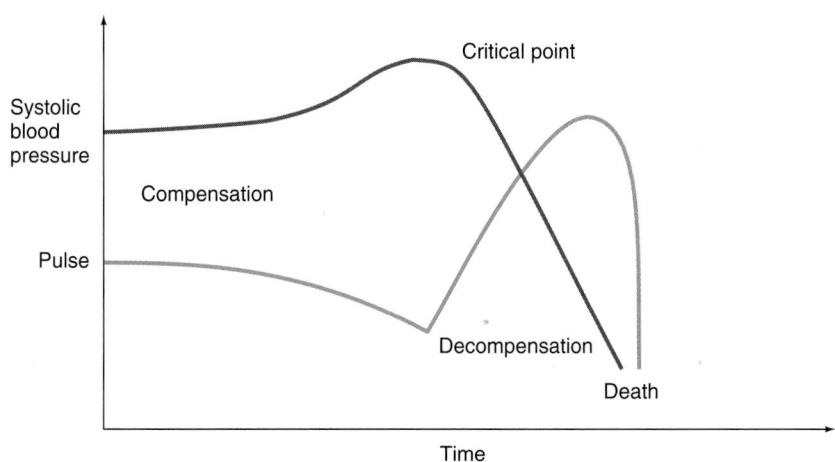

FIGURE 15-15 The response of systolic blood pressure and pulse during Cushing's Reflex.

The signs and symptoms of spinal cord injury may vary with the degree of damage and the general condition of the patient. At the injury site, they may range from pain, pain with motion, tenderness, point tenderness (tenderness at a specific location), to the complete absence of pain. More systemic signs may include bilateral paresthesia (a tingling or prickly sensation), anesthesia (absence of sensation), weakness, or paralysis. When a cord injury occurs, the patient often has normal sensation and muscle control down to the dermatome corresponding to the affected vertebra. Below this point, he or she experiences bilateral sensory and motor loss. However, the absence of this severe presentation does not rule out vertebral fracture or instability of the column. Nor does it rule out the potential for catastrophic injury should you mishandle the spine.

Central nervous system injury also affects activities under autonomic control. Blood vessels below the cord injury will be without nervous control and relax (dilate). In the shock patient, this will prevent the affected area from assisting with the normal response to shock. The vascular container will expand, thereby contributing to blood volume loss. In shock, the skin may be warm and dry, rather than cool and clammy, in the areas controlled by nerves below the cord injury. In the absence of shock, the area may be cooler or warmer and drier than skin that still has autonomic control.

There are several presentations characteristic of cervical spine injury. Cervical injury compromises the sympathetic nervous system so that it will no longer counter parasympathetic stimulation in the male. This results in a painful penile erection, called *priapism*. Lower cervical injury may also cause a patient to move the upper extremities into the so-called "hold-up" position. The muscles pulling the arms down are paralyzed, while those lifting them are intact. Any attempt by the patient to move the extremities will result in arms moving upward and into this position.

Vertebral injury may damage blood vessels, peripheral nerve roots, or the connective tissue surrounding the vertebral body without affecting the cord. Signs and symptoms may vary from localized pain to pain involved with attempted motion. Signs of individual peripheral nerve root damage, generally involving one or more discrete dermatomes or possibly limited to one side of the body, may also appear.

Forces that injure the spinal column are usually transmitted from somewhere else. The damage created by the transfer of energy may create more apparent injury in an area other than the spinal cord. For example, a bleeding head wound and/or a patient's complaint of headache may distract you from cervical compression fracture. Hence, you need to recognize the potential for spinal injury even if the patient has more dramatic signs and symptoms elsewhere.

Sense Organ Injury

Although injuries to the sense organs are neither as frequent nor as life-endangering as spinal fracture, they still present serious potential problems for the patient. Therefore, you must watch for the negative effects of trauma on the eye and ear.

Eye Injury As a rule, the orbit protects the eye from trauma. However, the anterior eye structures are extremely delicate, and the fluid within the chambers may not regenerate if lost. If significant penetrating injury occurs, especially if accompanied by loss of the aqueous or vitreous humor, the patient's sight may be threatened. Any object penetrating the eye will probably disturb the integrity of the anterior and/or posterior chambers. In addition to direct trauma, removal of an object may allow the fluids to leak from the chambers and further threaten the patient's vision.

Blunt trauma may result in several ocular presentations. Hemorrhage into the anterior chamber will pool and display a level of blood in front of the pupil and iris. This condition, called *hyphema*, is not emergent. Even so, it does require evaluation by an ophthalmologist. A less serious, but equally dramatic, eye injury is *conjunctival hemorrhage*. This condition results when a small vessel bursts, leaving the surface of the eye blood red. It will often clear without significant intervention or permanent vision impairment.

Two other, more serious ocular problems are central retinal artery occlusion and retinal detachment. *Acute retinal artery occlusion* is a vascular emergency in which an embolus (a traveling clot) blocks the blood supply to the eye. The patient complains of sudden and painless loss of vision in one eye. In *retinal detachment*, the retina separates from the posterior wall of the eye. The patient complains of a dark curtain obstructing part of the field of view. Both of these conditions are true emergencies that place the patient's future sight at risk.

Small foreign particles that land on the surface of the eye can also cause ocular emergencies. The object may embed in the interior of the lid and then drag across the cornea as the eye blinks. Corneal abrasions or lacerations result, often causing intense pain even after the object clears.

A *blowout fracture* is a fracture of the thin bones comprising the orbit of the eye. Most commonly, the inferior shelf fractures, involving the maxilla and/or zygoma. The patient often experiences significant swelling and pain in the maxillary sinus region. The fracture entraps the extraocular muscles, reducing the range of motion of the eye. Although these injuries are not life-threatening, they warrant evaluation by the emergency department staff.

Ear Injury   Injury rarely affects the middle and inner ear due to their location and the skeletal integrity that surrounds them. The tympanum (the ear drum) may rupture due to rapid pressure changes such as those experienced by the blast of an explosion or a SCUBA diving accident. Basilar skull fracture, which involves the auditory canal or the middle ear, may also damage the organs of hearing and positional sense. Damage to the internal ear may result in hearing loss, vertigo, or both.

Neck Injury

The neck is a critical area because it contains part of the upper airway and many major blood vessels. Damage could occur to the trachea, larynx, or esophagus. The internal and external carotid arteries or jugular veins might rupture or tear. Any of these conditions can seriously endanger the patient's life.

The trachea and larynx are the most anterior structures of the neck. Although they lay recessed from the face and chest, injury can still damage the integrity of the tracheal rings or larynx. Thus weakened, the airway may collapse on inspiration, leading to a severe respiratory problem. Penetrating wounds or tears to the trachea may force air into the neck during expiration. Through assessment, you may feel a crackling sensation (subcutaneous emphysema) or notice a gradual increase in the diameter of the neck. Both are signs of injury.

The carotid and jugular vessels are major circulatory system components found on both sides of the neck. Deep lacerations or other penetrating wounds to this area may result in severe bleeding. Carotid artery hemorrhage will be profuse, difficult to control, and may quickly lead to shock. The jugular veins, although rather low-pressure vessels, still carry large volumes of blood and will also bleed profusely. There is also a real concern for air aspiration. The jugular veins, at times, maintain a pressure less than atmospheric. An open wound may draw air into a vessel, affecting the heart or pulmonary circulation (pulmonary emboli).

✳ If a large neck wound exists, it may allow for aspiration of air into the venous system.

ASSESSMENT

Assessment of the trauma patient with possible head, neck, or spinal injury must be orderly and comprehensive. Do not simply direct your exam at expected injuries. You must organize and frequently practice the assessment process to uncover the most critical injuries rather than just the most obvious ones. Review the dispatch information, survey the scene, provide a quick primary assessment, and conduct a comprehensive secondary assessment. Also evaluate the vital signs, and obtain a patient history. These assessment elements are as crucial for the patient suffering a head, neck, and spine injury as they are for any other type of trauma or medical patient. However, if you identify problems involving the ABCs, diminished levels of consciousness, or developing shock, intervention and possible transport may precede the complete assessment.

Upon arrival at the scene, the first step in assessment is a rapid scene survey. During this survey, identify any mechanism of injury that could cause head, neck, or spine injury. Ask yourself: "What, if any, forces were great enough to cause significant brain and/or spinal cord injury?" Look specifically for the strength of impact and the kinetic energy involved. Is the windshield broken? Are there vehicle interior deformities? Was the fall from a height over 15 feet? Was trauma transmitted through or to the head or spinal column? If you can answer yes to any of these questions, then treat the patient as though head and spinal injuries exist. Both head and spinal injuries may be present without recognizable signs or symptoms. Hence, keep a high index of suspicion for these injuries whenever you respond to trauma.

Establish a baseline of central nervous system function early in your care, and follow it with frequent serial assessments. This will help identify whether the patient is improving, remaining stable, or deteriorating. Give careful attention to detail so you will notice the slightest change in level of consciousness, orientation, or other neurologic signs.

Primary Assessment

Perform the primary assessment and any interventions indicated by the findings. Central nervous system injury can easily account for problems with the ABCs. Therefore, their assessment and protection is of utmost significance. The D and E of the primary assessment also evaluate signs and symptoms that relate to CNS injuries. Performing a good primary assessment will quickly determine the extent of on-scene treatment required by the patient. (See Figure 15-16.) It will also determine if you will better serve the patient by providing rapid transport. Such a case arises, for example, with the epidural hematoma patient.

Airway　Assess the airway for the loss of airway control and the potential for vomiting. (See Figure 15-17 and Figure 15-18.) Unresponsive patients who have CNS injury may lose the gag reflex and normal mechanisms of airway protection. They may also vomit, sometimes without any prior nausea. It may be advisable to secure the airway with an endotracheal tube if you suspect a head injury.

Facial trauma may also endanger the airway. Assess the nasal and oral passages carefully, keeping alert for any potential airway threat. Watch for fluids, edema, or possibly airway collapse due to massive facial fractures. If the injury threatens the airway, protect it with a nasopharyngeal airway, oropharyngeal airway, or endotracheal tube, while observing cervical spine precautions. (See Chapter 11.) Employ advanced airway care procedures if the patient has a lowered level of consciousness or reduced or absent gag reflex.

Breathing　Your respiratory evaluation can reveal diagnostic signs suggestive of head injury. Determine the pattern of respiration early in the assessment. Identify any erratic, abnormally deep, or other unusual respiratory patterns. Central neurogenic hyperventilation (very deep and rapid), Cheyne-Stokes (cyclic increasing, decreasing, then apneic), Biot's (erratic and gasping), ataxic (irregular, forced, and gasping), or agonal (infrequent gasping) respira-

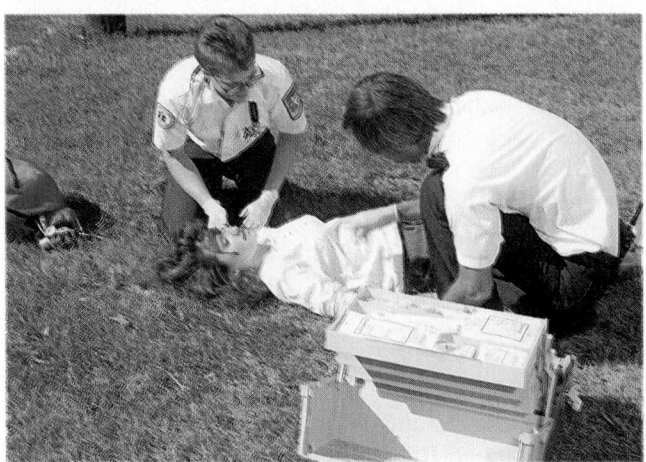

FIGURE 15-16 When treating a patient with a possible head injury, quickly assess the ABCs.

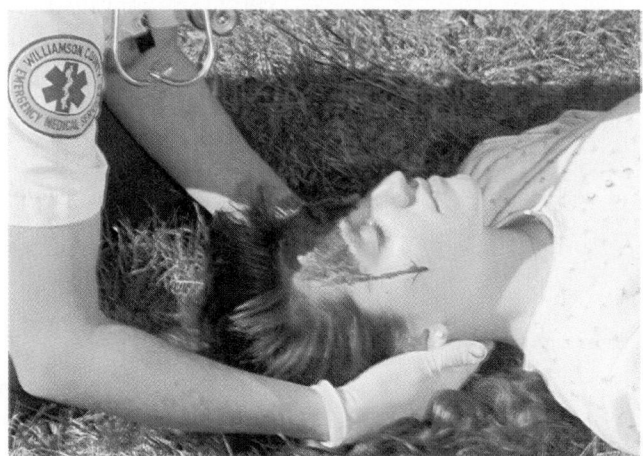

FIGURE 15-17 Manually immobilize the cervical spine. Use the modified jaw-thrust maneuver to open the airway if necessary.

Since neck may be injured, do not use normal method of opening airway . . .

Use modified jaw thrust

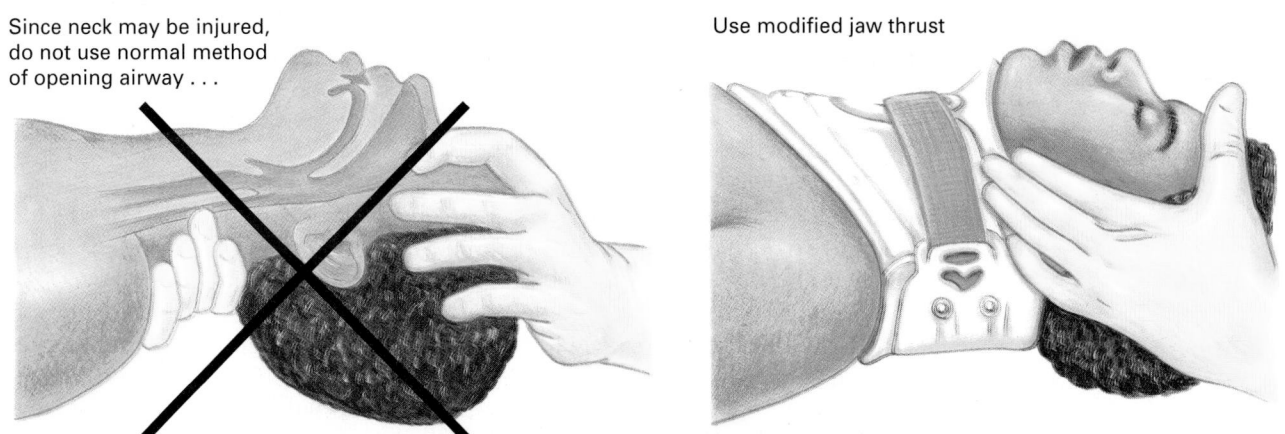

FIGURE 15-18 The modified jaw-thrust maneuver should be used in patients suspected of having a spinal injury.

tions may reflect brain stem injury and the need for rapid transport. Any indication of head injury requires hyperventilation using 100 percent oxygen.

Circulation Check the circulatory status during your primary assessment. The results may support the possibility of head injury and injury to, or pressure on, the medulla oblongata. If the pulse is slow and bounding, it may be a part of Cushing's reflex, especially if accompanied by a rapid and deep respiratory effort.

Disability The disability component of the primary assessment is important whenever you suspect central nervous injury. Critical elements of a rapid CNS assessment occur at this point during the primary patient evaluation. Establish the level of consciousness by assessing the patient's level of orientation or response to stimuli. To establish a CNS baseline, quickly check to see if the patient is oriented to time, place (or event), person, and one's own person. If the patient does not respond to questioning, look for a response to

✳ If head injury is suspected, the patient should be hyperventilated with high-flow oxygen.

✳ A baseline for the initial level of consciousness should be determined for comparison during serial assessments.

verbal or painful stimuli. Record the patient's best response, and compare it to subsequent evaluations to identify any deterioration or improvement. If the evaluation reveals any response lower than orientation to place (or the event), suspect CNS injury. Carefully monitor the patient for further deterioration, and prepare for rapid transport to the emergency department. If the patient appears fully oriented and if there are no other reasons to suspect head or spine injury, continue the secondary assessment and provide the necessary on-scene care.

Expose   During the expose stage of primary assessment, you will examine the head, neck, chest, and abdomen for early visible signs of developing life threat. At this time, focus on indications of central nervous system injury. Carefully investigate any sign of penetrating or blunt neck trauma. Be especially watchful for open wounds to the carotid arteries, jugular veins, the trachea, or esophagus. Watch the abdomen for "belly breathing," and note any difference in muscle tone or skin temperature between the upper and lower extremities and left and right sides.

At the conclusion of the primary assessment, review your findings. Determine if the patient may have an internal head injury. If so, plan for immediate transport. If you suspect spinal injury, carefully immobilize the patient and then transport. If you uncover neck injury, rule out an open vascular injury. If such an injury exists, seal it with an occlusive dressing, stop severe hemorrhage, and assure the airway remains patent. Then begin the secondary assessment, either while en route or at the scene.

The Secondary Assessment

The secondary assessment progress in relatively the same way for the head, neck, and spine patient as for other trauma patients. It should include a complete head-to-toe evaluation, vital signs, and a modest patient history. Any findings should support the "whole picture" of the incident. If any element of assessment does not agree with the suspected problem, re-evaluate the patient, mechanism of injury, and patient history. Also, periodically re-evaluate any finding of injury, dysfunction, or patient complaint to determine if any progression is occurring.

Head-to-Toe Assessment   The head-to-toe assessment begins with the head. Palpate and inspect the cranium over its entire surface. Carefully observe for any deformity, wound (whether open or closed), or fluid loss. Visualize the region behind the ear. Keep in mind that the characteristic discoloration of Battle's sign does not usually present in the prehospital setting. Assess the external auditory canal and nasal cavity for cerebrospinal fluid, blood, or both. Be careful to visualize and palpate the regions of the head without moving it or the spine. Check the facial region for soft-tissue injury or fracture. Palpate the frontal, zygomatic, nasal and maxillary bones as well as the mandible. Any swelling, crepitus, or instability will establish injury. Carefully palpate the orbital ridge and nasal region, since they are commonly involved in trauma. Any early signs of orbital swelling suggests a basilar skull fracture or blowout fracture.

Be careful in your estimation of the quantity and significance of blood loss involving the head. The tendency is to overestimate hemorrhage because the blood is very apparent and because the head is associated with our personal identity. But blood loss from the head alone rarely accounts for hypovolemic shock. If the signs and symptoms of shock exist, look elsewhere for a possible cause. An exception to this rule, however, occurs with children, where blood loss can be both significant in relative volume and a threat to life.

* Both head and spine injury may occur without recognizable signs and symptoms; therefore, you must maintain a high level of suspicion for these injuries.

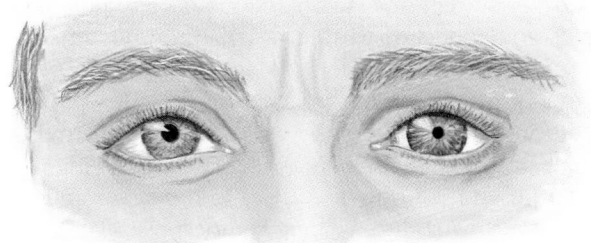

FIGURE 15-19 Anisocoria (unequal pupils) may indicate underlying CNS injury.

Give special attention to assessment of the eyes. (See Figure 15-19.) They are a direct window into the brain and can quickly and accurately tell the general condition of the central nervous system. The eye reflects the level of cerebral function and may identify some specific problems. If the pupil responds briskly to light-intensity changes, presume that the eye (and brain) are well perfused. If the pupil responds slowly, CNS depression is present, either due to the effects of drugs, hypoxia, or circulatory insufficiency. If the pupil is dilated and fixed, suspect severe CNS injury or hypoxia. If the pupillary signs are bilateral, presume the problem includes both hemispheres, while unilateral response reflects a problem on one side. (See Figure 15-20.) Examine the pupils for signs of trauma, impaled objects, and the presence of contact lenses. Specifically look for loss of aqueous or vitreous humor, foreign objects, or hyphema.

* The pupils are a direct window into the brain and can quickly and accurately tell the general condition of the central nervous system.

Re-examine the nasal and oral cavities to ensure that they remain unobstructed from tissue swelling or deformity. Assure that loose teeth, dentures, swollen tissue, or foreign objects do not threaten the airway. Check the maxilla and mandible for any crepitation or instability. Notice if the blood flowing from the nose, mouth, or ears demonstrates the target sign or "halo sign" (a dark circle surrounded by a lighter one) when dropped on a pillow or towel. This is suggestive of cerebral spinal fluid in the blood and basilar skull fracture. (See Figure 15-21.)

Palpate the neck over its entire surface—laterally, anteriorly, and posteriorly. Any tenderness, point tenderness, local warmth, or outright pain along the

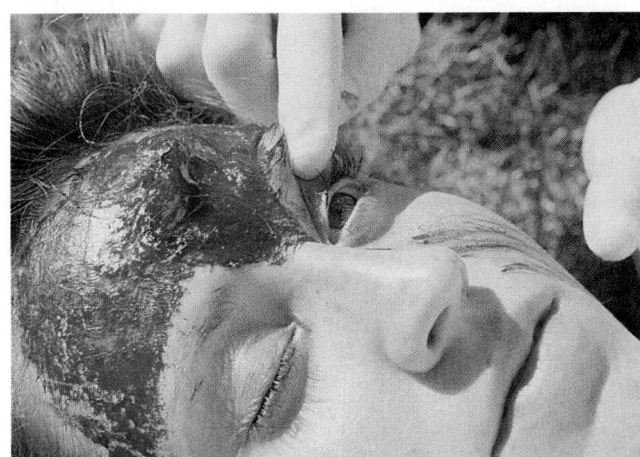

FIGURE 15-20 During the secondary assessment, be sure to inspect both eyes.

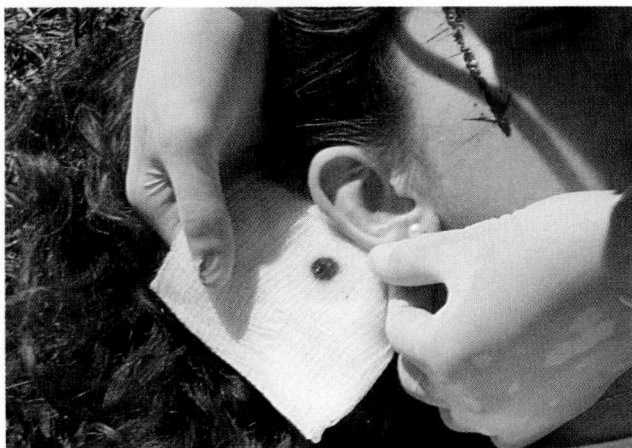

FIGURE 15-21 "Halo Test" to detect the presence of cerebrospinal fluid. If CSF is present, it will diffuse faster across a paper towel or sponge because it is thinner than blood.

vertebral column calls for immediate spinal immobilization. Blunt soft-tissue injury, as determined by swelling, tenderness, or subcutaneous emphysema laterally or anteriorly, should direct your concern to the vasculature and trachea traversing this region. Any open wound calls for hemorrhage control and protection against vascular aspiration of air. The neck assessment includes palpation of the trachea to ensure its integrity has not been lost. Any deformity, swelling, crepitus, or development of subcutaneous emphysema suggests injury.

* Any sizeable open neck wound should be sealed against the possibility of vascular aspiration of air.

Palpate the entire vertebral column during the head-to-toe assessment. Examine for specific signs and symptoms including pain, tenderness, deformity, and local warmth (suggesting early development of edema and injury).

Look for signs and symptoms of CNS injury during the remainder of the physical assessment. Any **flaccid** area, reduced sensation, weakness, or outright paralysis will direct your attention to head or spinal injury. Suspect temperature variation affecting a specific region, making it either cooler or warmer than the rest of the body, as being of CNS origin. Determine whether the loss of muscle tone or temperature variation is unilateral or bilateral and at what anatomic level the dysfunction begins.

■ **flaccid** relaxed, flabby, or without muscle tone.

Vital Signs   A reading of vital signs gives further indications of CNS injury. As you take the vitals, keep the following tips in mind.

❑ *Pulse.* Determine a baseline pulse rate during the primary assessment. If it is slow initially, or slows with subsequent evaluation, suspect head injury. Also note its strength. A slow pounding pulse is a sign of head injury.

❑ *Blood Pressure.* Blood pressure evaluation may support the probability of head injury. A high or rising blood pressure reflects an increase in intracranial pressure and is one element of Cushing's Triad (increasing blood pressure, slowing pulse rate, and erratic respiration). If serial blood pressure evaluation demonstrates an upward trend, suspect the presence of increasing intracranial pressure.

❑ *Respirations.* In head injury, respirations become erratic and deep. Suspect any unusual respiratory pattern in the unconscious patient to be of CNS origin.

Monitor the patient who is experiencing the effects of a head injury, or for that matter, any unconscious patient, for dysrhythmias. CNS injury can produce bradycardia due to brain stem pressure, tachycardia due to vagus nerve interruption, and general cardiac irritability secondary to hypoxia, hypercarbia, or other metabolic disturbance.

Glasgow Coma Scale   You can use the Glasgow Coma Scale to determine the patient's CNS status. It is an objective number that can be compared against later CNS assessment. You can also communicate this number to the emergency department physician. (See Table 15-1.) Determine the patient's best eye opening, motor, and verbal response. If the Glasgow Coma Score is below 12, consider immediate transport. A score of 7 or below reflects coma. (Three is the lowest score, while 15 is the highest.)

Patient History   Patient questioning is one of the key aspects of assessing head or spinal injuries. The elements of the chief complaint and past medical history can contribute greatly to the overall picture of what happened or may be happening. Questioning will allow you to monitor closely the level of consciousness and simultaneously determine the mechanism and symptoms of injury. Evaluate the chief complaint for any indication of CNS problem. Ask

TABLE 15-1 Glasgow Coma Scale

	Test	Patient's Response	Score
Eye Opening	Spontaneous speech	Opens eyes on own	4
		Opens eyes when asked in a loud voice	3
	Pain	Opens eyes when pinched	2
	Pain	Does not open eyes	1
Best Motor Response	Commands	Follows simple commands	6
	Pain	Pulls hand away when pinched	5
	Pain	Pulls a part of body away when pinched by an examiner	4
	Pain	Flexes body inappropriately to pain (decorticate posturing)	3
	Pain	Body becomes rigid in an extended position when pinched by an examiner (decerebrate posturing)	2
	Pain	No motor response to pain	1
Verbal Response (Talking)	Speech	Carries on a conversation correctly and tells examiner where he/she is, who he/she is, and the month and year	5
	Speech	Confused and disoriented	4
	Speech	Speech is clear but makes no sense	3
	Speech	Makes garbled sounds that examiner cannot understand	2
	Speech	Makes no sounds	1

- Assess the patient's score in each category, and total the scores of the three categories. A total score of 7 or less indicates coma.
- Assess the patient's score in each category frequently, and record each observation and the time it was made. Keep a parallel record of vital signs.

about any regional tingling sensations, numbness, weakness, or paralysis. Investigate any complaint of headache in detail to determine exactly where the patient feels the pain and how he or she perceives it. Although you may not use all this information to guide care, it may be very valuable to the emergency department staff.

Investigate any unusual symptoms mentioned by the patient. In the developing head injury, the patient may experience changes in vision, hearing, sensation, and motor control that may identify the location of the injury. As the problem progresses, the level of consciousness may decline, and the patient may be unable to relate this information to either you or the emergency department staff. For this reason, be sure to record the results of the neurologic assessment and patient questioning.

Attempt to elicit the immediate history of the event from the patient. He or she may be unaware of the circumstances preceding or immediately following the accident. Loss of memory preceding an event is called *retrograde amnesia*, while loss after it is called *antegrade amnesia*. Both are commonly found and may reflect the effects of emotional trauma rather than physiologic trauma.

Relatives and bystanders may also notice CNS changes in the patient. They may possess a history that precedes your arrival and may see a progression before you might recognize it. While casual observers may not be reliable, police or fire personnel are usually objective in noting the circumstances of an emergency. Be especially aware of personality changes in the patient (including bizarre behavior) and a changing level of consciousness.

MANAGEMENT

The management of the head, spine, and neck injury is a crucial part of total trauma care. You must ensure that your actions—or lack of actions—do not further harm the patient. Thus, do not leave the patient at the scene when assessment indicates rapid transport. Also do not fail to stabilize and care for the patient when on-scene care is appropriate. Proper actions include: rapid transport of the head injury patient with some interventions en route, complete spinal immobilization for the spinal injury patient, and special care for the patient with special sense organ injuries.

Immediate Spinal Immobilization

Immobilize the cervical spine immediately when you suspect injury either before or during the primary assessment. (See Figure 15-22.) If you are the team member stabilizing the head, approach the patient from the front or back. Support the head by grasping the mastoid and the angle of the mandible with the medial part of the palm of your hand. Gently bring the head to the neutral position, unless the patient feels pain or you feel resistance. Maintain manual stabilization with sufficient force to take the weight of the head off the spine and prevent its motion. This support prevents movement posteriorly, anteriorly, or laterally. It is crucial to maintain the spine in a neutral position during the entirety of your care—a task that is not as easy as it first seems.

Oxygen and Hyperventilation

If there is an indication that the patient might have sustained a head injury, administer 100 percent oxygen. If respirations are abnormal, then hyperventilate. Be cautious if you are ventilating a patient without the benefit of an

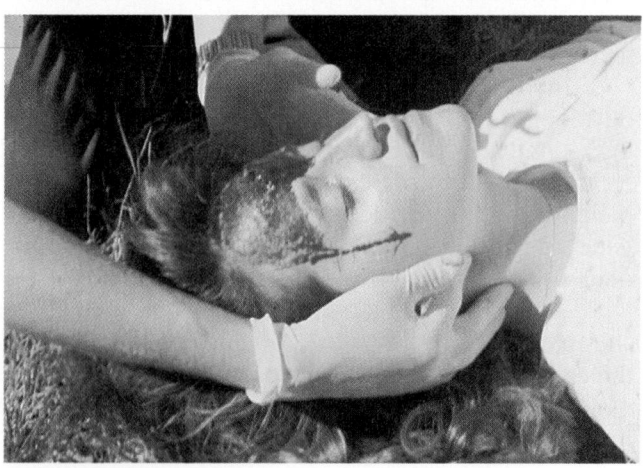

FIGURE 15-22 Maintain manual immobilization of the cervical spine while applying a rigid cervical collar.

endotracheal tube. Gastric distention and emesis may occur secondary to gastric insufflation. Hyperventilation and high-flow oxygen will reduce both the circulating carbon dioxide level and cerebral hypercarbia. They will also elevate the oxygen saturation of the blood and increase oxygen delivery to the brain. These effects will slow the development of the cerebral edema, the progression of intracranial pressure, and reduce the extent of injury.

Endotracheal Intubation

The airway is particularly susceptible to compromise in head injury. Protect it early in the unconscious patient, using the endotracheal tube with cervical precautions. Have one rescuer maintain the head position, while you attempt oral, nasal, or digital intubation. Although we discuss oral intubation in Chapter 11, it needs special modification for the spinal trauma patient. Here you should accomplish oral intubation without the normal flexion of the neck and extension of the head. One care provider should rigidly immobilize the head by holding stabilization, while you introduce the laryngoscope. Someone may apply downward pressure on the thyroid cartilage to aid in your visualization of the vocal cords. Oral intubation under these circumstances is at best difficult. This is especially true in the patient who still has muscle tone, lies supine on the floor or ground, and has vomitus and secretions in the airway.

✶ Oral intubation for the spinal injury patient must be accomplished without the normal flexion of the neck and extension of the head.

Two other useful airway techniques for spinal injury patients are nasal and digital intubation. Nasal intubation is a blind procedure you might use in a breathing patient. It allows the cervical spine to remain in the neutral position. Insert the endotracheal tube into the largest naris. Then direct it posteriorly, curving it toward the floor of the nasal cavity. Advance the tube the length of an oral airway (the distance between the earlobe and the corner of the mouth). At this point, slowly continue insertion, while you listen for the sounds of respiration. Gently manipulate the tube until the respiratory sounds are loudest, and then advance it during inspiration. With luck, the tube will enter the trachea and the airway will be secure. There are specially designed endotracheal tubes (the Endotrol) that have tips that you can direct. Such a tube will assist you in proper placement. Nasotracheal intubation is difficult, and determining proper placement is essential.

In digital intubation, you "walk" your index and second finger along the patient's tongue until you feel and lift the epiglottis. Stiffen the endotracheal tube with a stylet and insert it along your fingers and the epiglottis. During this procedure, it may be helpful for an assisting EMT or paramedic to place pressure on the thyroid cartilage to displace it slightly downward. This motion brings the tracheal opening more in line with the oral airway and increases the probability of proper tube placement. Gently advance the tube beyond your fingers and a few centimeters into the patient's trachea. Remember to protect your fingers with a bite block anytime they are placed in a patient's mouth.

Once placement of the tube appears to be correct, check it with auscultation of the axillary areas, bilaterally. Watch for symmetrical chest wall excursion. Also listen to the epigastric area for sounds of esophageal intubation. If you hear good breath sounds and no epigastric sounds, the tube is most likely in the trachea. Inflate the cuff, and hyperventilate the patient.

Attempts at endotracheal intubation can increase the parasympathetic (vagal) tone. This, in turn, may increase intracranial pressure and bradycardia or other cardiac dysrhythmias already present from the head injury. Therefore, assure that the intubation occurs rapidly. Then precede with hyperventilation, using 100 percent oxygen. Some EMS systems use pharmacological agents to reduce the vagal effects of intubation.

✶ Intubation in the head injury patient must be accomplished rapidly. It should be preceded and followed by patient hyperventilation.

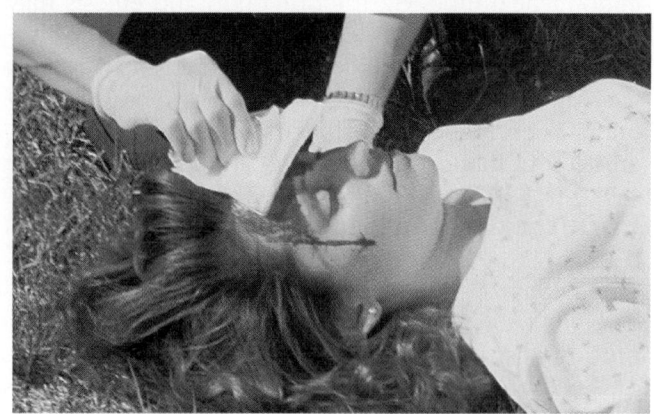

FIGURE 15-23 Control any bleeding.

Hemorrhage Control/Shock Care

Control any severe bleeding from the head, neck, or facial area with direct pressure. (See Figure 15-23.) If you suspect a depressed skull fracture, apply the pressure to the surrounding area. If hemorrhage originates from the neck or if there is an open injury to this area, seal the wound with an occlusive dressing. Keep the body at a 15-degree angle, with the head down (unless contraindicated). This position will ensure that pressure in the jugular veins remains positive. It also reduces the chance for air emboli.

Spinal injury may cause compromise of vascular control below the lesion. At best, this will keep the area from assisting with the compensatory mechanisms of shock (vasoconstriction) and, at worst, will contribute to hypovolemia. Apply and inflate the PASG if the signs of shock begin to appear. Use it cautiously if the patient is "belly breathing." Abdominal pressure may further compromise the diaphragm's efforts to move air. Consider initiating two large bore IVs with trauma tubing, running normal saline or lactated Ringer's solution, with pressure infusers ready. Observe respiration carefully for any signs of compromise from pulmonary edema, fluid overload, or from the PASG impinging on respiratory excursion.

Spinal Immobilization

A cervical collar will help to limit any cervical motion and is essential in the spinal immobilization procedure. (See Figure 15-24.) Select a rigid collar, properly sized for the patient. The collar should fit snugly and limit motion of the cervical spine, but it should not cause hyperextension. Apply it without moving the spine or causing patient discomfort. The sole purpose of the cervical collar is to aid immobilization. Never count on it for any stabilization of the injured area. Continue uninterrupted manual immobilization until you replace it with mechanical immobilization.

One of the most difficult movement tasks you will encounter in prehospital care is the rapid extrication of a potential spinal injury patient. You must move the patient quickly, yet any uncontrolled motion may permanently damage the spinal cord. Institute extreme care to keep the spine in alignment, while you move the patient to the waiting long spine board and stretcher. Use teamwork to keep the patient's nose, navel, and toes in the same plane without any flexion, extension, lateral motion, or rotation. (See Figure 15-25.) If sitting, as in a car, rotate the patient 90 degrees and carefully lower him or her to the board. Quickly secure the patient to the spineboard. Then move the patient to the ambulance, and transport with further care en route.

✳ When rapid extrication of the spine-injured patient is required, it must be accomplished with extreme care to keep the spine aligned.

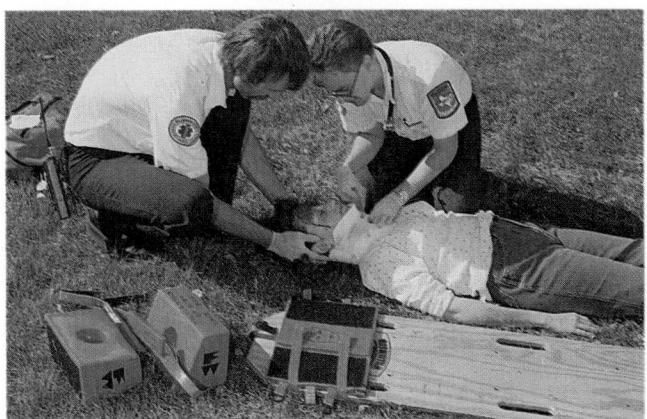

FIGURE 15-24 Apply a rigid cervical collar.

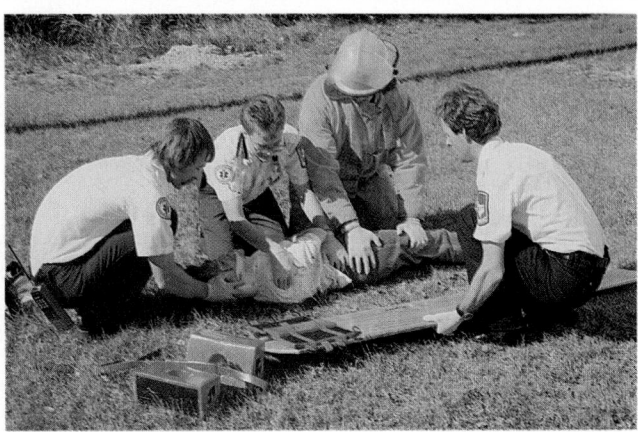

FIGURE 15-25 The patient should be moved as a unit, keeping the entire spine in alignment.

Use the short spineboard or vest-type immobilization for a seated patient if the situation is not so emergent. These devices provide a platform to which you can affix the shoulders, sacrum, and occiput to immobilize the patient's spine. You can then safely move the patient to the supine position and secure the patient, device, and long board together.

Prior to applying a movement device such as the vest or short spine board, evaluate the patient for motor and sensory function. Determine the level of neurologic function before applying mechanical immobilization. Serial assessment should continue during the application and patient transport to the hospital. If you note any change in the patient's signs or symptoms, determine the cause.

Maintain the neutral position during immobilization and movement. Place firm padding between the patient's occiput and the spine board or vest while the patient is sitting. If the patient is found supine or if you move the patient to this position through rapid extrication, approximate the padding size. Ensure that it does not cause extension of the neck, and be careful to place the padding behind the occiput rather than the neck.

Prevent the head from any lateral or turning motion by using a cervical immobilization device (CID). Select a commercial device or fabricate one from a blanket. It should place gentle but stabilizing pressure on the lateral aspects of the head and trap it firmly. You will then affix the CID to the spine board. (See Figures 15-26 and 15-27.) The head is further held in position with tape

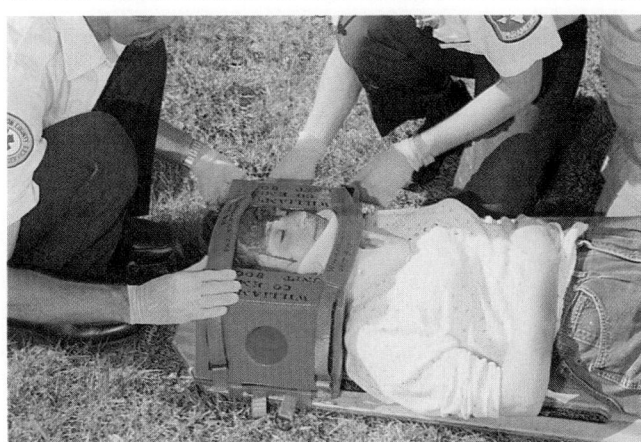

FIGURE 15-26 Stabilize the neck prior to transport.

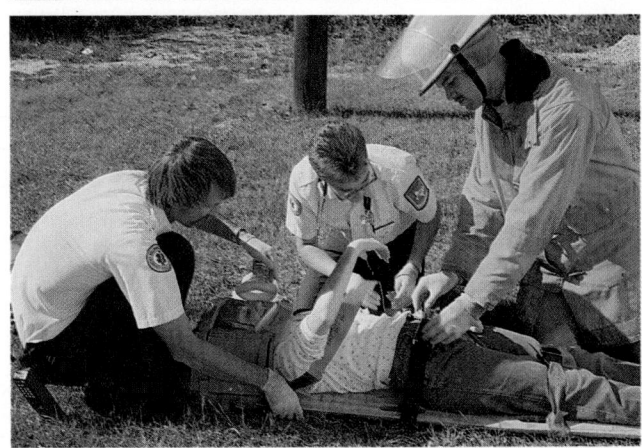

FIGURE 15-27 Secure the arms and legs.

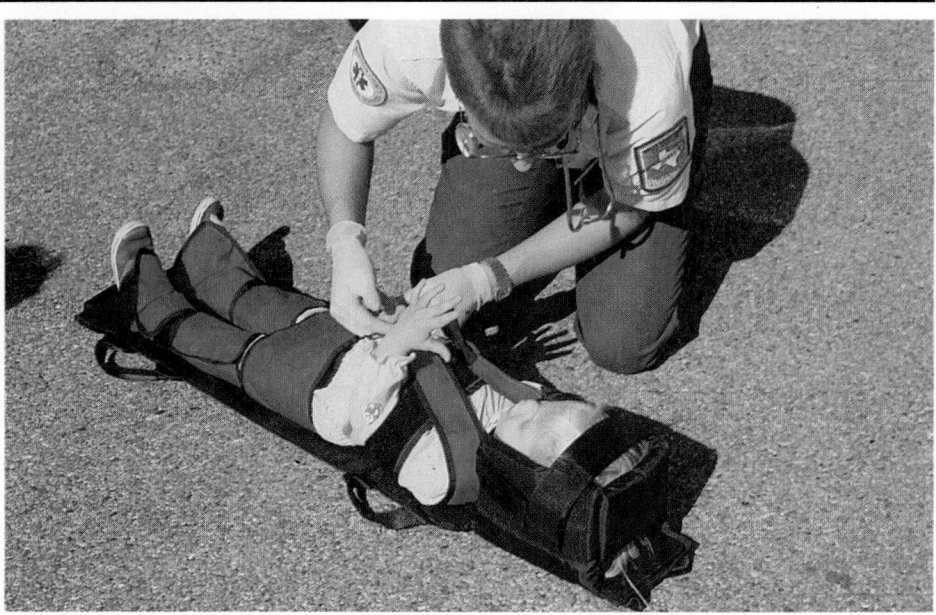

FIGURE 15-28 Pediatric immobilization devices are effective in immobilizing the spine of a child.

or velcro strapping, which crosses the forehead and the chin flange of the cervical collar. Ensure that the tape on the collar does not restrict breathing or flex the neck. (See Figure 15-28.)

If the patient is found standing and you suspect spine injury, immobilize him or her as found. (See Figures 15-29 to 15-31.) Place the long spine board behind the patient, and secure him or her carefully. First, secure the head, shoulders, pelvis, and extremities. Then lower the patient to the supine position and transport to the emergency department.

Watch the patient with spine injury for hypothermia. Loss of nervous control over the peripheral capillary beds reduces the body's ability to maintain core temperature and control heat loss. Keep the patient warm and reduce any heat loss except when the environment is extremely warm. Then, be careful to ensure that the patient does not overheat.

✳ Watch for and prevent hypothermia in the patient with central nervous system injury.

Wound Care

Once you address the greater concern for CNS injury, care for specific wounds to the head and neck. Impaled objects, whether penetrating the skull, the

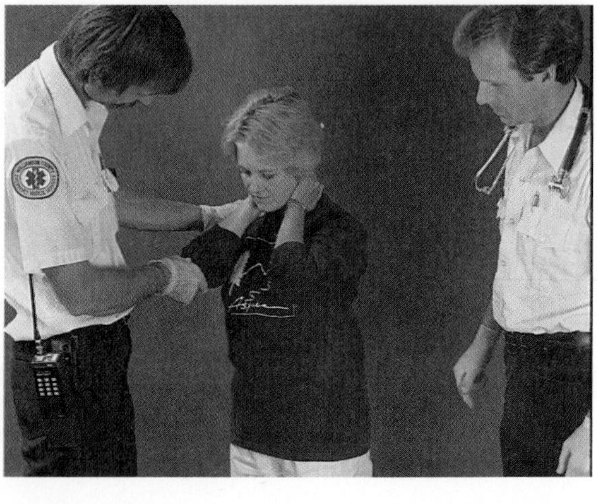

FIGURE 15-29 The standing patient who complains of neck pain following an injury should also receive spinal immobilization.

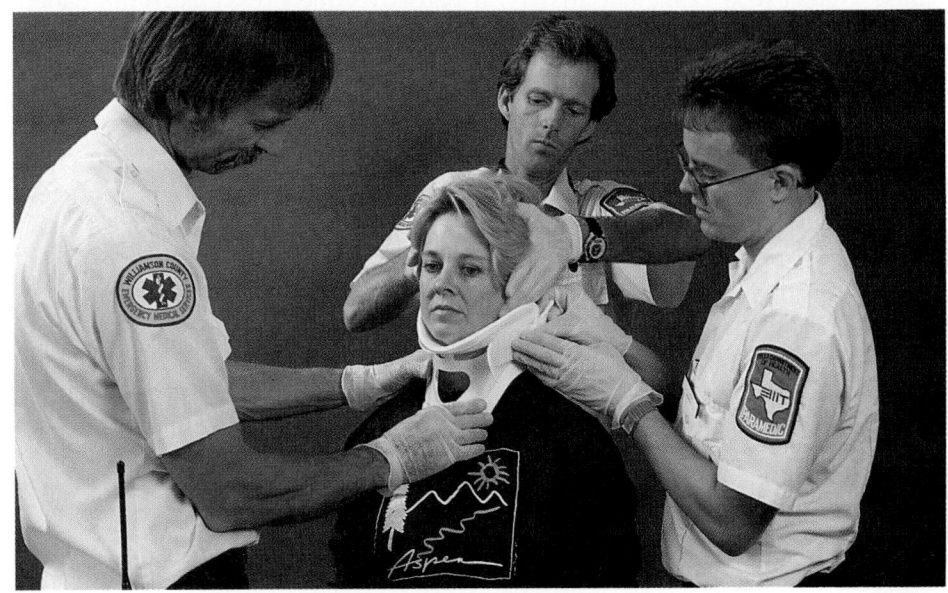

FIGURE 15-30 The cervical spine should be manually immobilized and a rigid cervical collar placed.

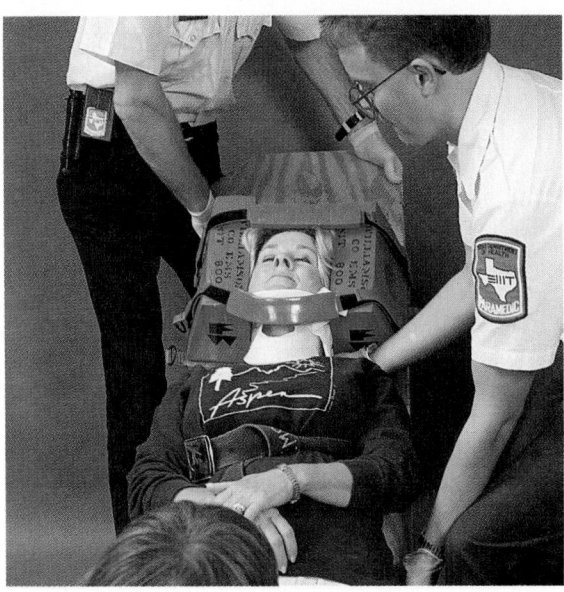

FIGURE 15-31 The long spine board can be applied while the patient remains standing.

neck, or the facial region, should be left in place. Protect them from further motion either by the object being bumped or from the forces of inertia during patient movement. The only exception to this rule is the object impaled in the cheek, threatening the airway. Safe removal is possible since the cheek contains no critical structures, and you can control bleeding.

In facial trauma, the nose may bleed profusely. If the hemorrhage appears to be anterior, tilt the head slightly back and have the patient squeeze the nose between his or her fingers. Clotting time is around 10 minutes, so the pressure should be held for at least that long. The patient may require nasal packing at the emergency department to control posterior nasal bleeding. If the patient swallows a large amount of blood, be watchful for vomiting.

In eye injuries, you will protect the eye and gently transport the patient. Keep impaled objects from jostling by using a cup style dressing. Cover both eyes to reduce the sympathetic motion of the injured eye. Eye injuries can cause a great deal of patient anxiety. If you cover the eyes, talk to the patient during your care and alert him or her of any planned movement, such as transport to the ambulance, before it occurs. In the case of an unconscious or semiconscious patient, tie the hands to keep him or her from touching the wound. Leave the patient with an eye injury in a supine position, if possible.

Drug Therapy

Once you have cared for the patient's emergent needs, you may receive orders from medical control for certain pharmacological interventions. These may include oxygen, furosemide (Lasix), methylprednisolone (Solu-Medrol), and diazepam (Valium). It is essential that you consult with the system medical director regarding the indications, dosage, and protocols for use of any drug mentioned in this text.

✱ It is essential that you consult with the system medical director regarding the indications, dosage, and protocols for use of any drug mentioned in this text.

Oxygen   Oxygen is the first-line drug used in the care of the patient with suspected head injury, cerebral edema, intracerebral hemorrhage, epidural hematoma, and subdural hematoma. Coupled with the use of hyperventilation, it has the potential to limit cerebral edema and ensure that the brain remains as well oxygenated as possible. Hyperventilation also reduces the level of carbon dioxide in the blood, further reducing the potential harm caused by injury to the brain.

Administer oxygen by partial or nonbreather mask at high flow in the patient who is conscious and breathing adequately. Monitor the administration with pulse oximetry, keeping the saturation in the high 90s. In the patient who is unconscious and not breathing well, ventilate at 24 full breaths per minute using the bag-valve device connected to a reservoir with an oxygen flow of 15 liters per minute. If possible, secure the airway with an endotracheal tube to assure optimal ventilation, oxygenation, and carbon dioxide removal.

Furosemide   You may also be called upon to use a second diuretic, furosemide (Lasix), for the head injury. It is a potent diuretic frequently administered during congestive heart failure and pulmonary edema. It may also be of benefit in treating the syndrome of increasing intracranial pressure. Lasix causes some vasodilation as well as rapid diuresis. These two effects reduce the cardiovascular volume and blood pressure, hence reducing the progression of cerebral edema. The drop in systemic blood pressure may cause the cerebral blood flow to slow, increasing hypoxia and hypercarbia.

Lasix often comes in a preloaded syringe and is given in an IV bolus of 20–80 mg. Administer the medication very slowly, over 1 to 2 minutes. It is generally contraindicated in the pregnant female, as it may cause some fetal abnormalities.

Methylprednisolone (Solu-Medrol)   Methylprednisolone (Solu-Medrol) is indicated in patients with suspected spinal cord injury. It is a steroid that minimizes swelling of the spinal cord, thereby reducing the extent of injury. Methylprednisolone is an anti-inflammatory drug.

Administer Methylprednisolone in an initial bolus of 30 mg/kg. Deliver it very slowly over a 15-minute period. Establish a maintenance infusion 45 minutes later, administering 5.4 mg/kg/hr. Administer methylprednisolone via intravenous route only. There are no contraindications or significant precautions to be observed in the use of this drug in the emergency setting.

Diazepam   Diazepam (Valium) is another anticonvulsant and anti-anxiety agent useful in treating the head injury patient. It is the first-line drug in the control of major motor seizures. Do not mix valium with other drugs, and remember that it is a relatively short-acting drug.

The standard dosage is between 2–15 mg IV bolus. Administer it very slowly, no more than 5 mg per minute. Use a large vein to reduce venous irritation. If the patient is seizing, you may administer the drug intramuscularly and titrate it to effect. Watch the patient carefully, and give a follow-up dose of Valium if its effects begin to subside. It is essential that you consult with the system medical director regarding the indications, dosage, and protocols for use of any drug mentioned within this text.

SUMMARY

Head, neck, and spine injuries are severe and significant injuries frequently encountered in prehospital care. They often present with signs and symptoms unreflective of their real significance. They may progress quietly and rapidly, resulting in patient demise. Ensure that your assessment and care of the patient with a head, neck, or spine injury anticipates problems rather than awaits the development of signs and symptoms. Ventilate the possible head injury patient at 20 to 25 breaths per minute with 100 percent oxygen. Protect the airway with endotracheal intubation if the gag reflex is diminished or absent. Provide the spine injury patient with immediate and continued immobilization from scene arrival until you relinquish patient responsibility to the emergency department staff. Neck injuries also deserve special care. Penetrating injury should increase suspicion for vascular or respiratory injury, including airway compromise or air emboli. Seal any open wound to the neck with an occlusive dressing, and control any significant blood loss. Better patient care and reduced morbidity and mortality will result from your aggressive focus on the head, neck, and spine injury patient.

FURTHER READING

American College of Surgeons, Committee on Trauma. *Advanced Trauma Life Support Course: Student Manual*. American College of Surgeons, 1984.

Butman, A.M., and J.L. Paturas. *Pre-Hospital Trauma Life Support*. Akron, OH: Emergency Training, 1990.

Campbell, J.E. *Basic Trauma Life Support*, 2nd ed. Englewood Cliffs, NJ: Prentice-Hall, Inc., 1988.

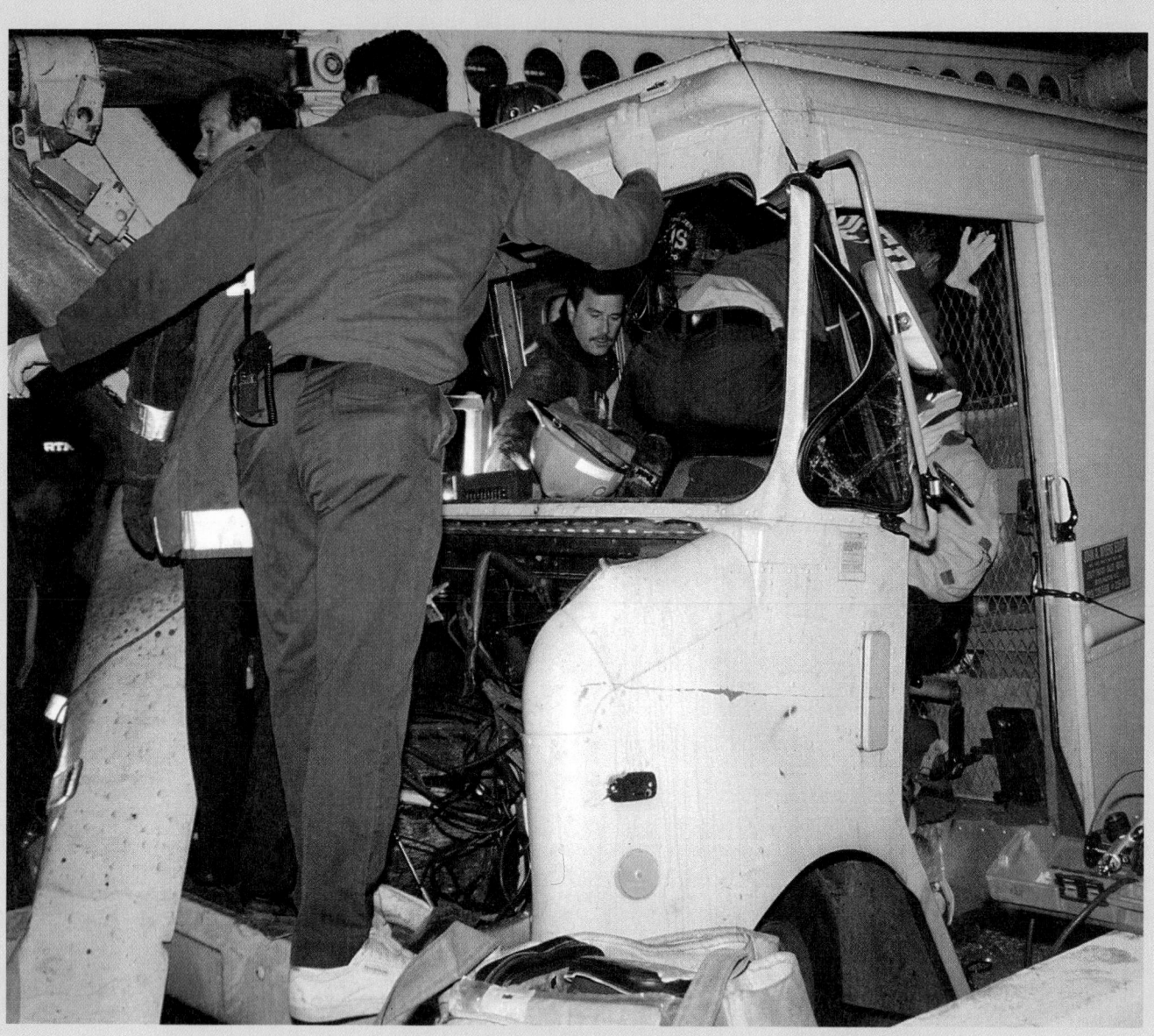

16

BODY CAVITY TRAUMA

Objectives for Chapter 16

After reading this chapter, you should be able to:

1. Describe the incidence, mortality, and morbidity of body cavity injury in the trauma patient. (See p. 470.)

2. Locate and explain the function of the organs and major structures found within the thorax and abdomen. (See pp. 471–473.)

3. Explain the process of respiration, including the function of the bellows system, the pleura, and the airway. (See pp. 471–473.)

4. Identify various injuries associated with chest and abdominal trauma. (See pp. 476–482.)

5. Describe the signs and symptoms most commonly found in cases of chest and abdominal trauma, noting the causes and/or effects of each condition. (See pp. 476–482.)

6. Describe how the elements of primary assessment relate to chest and abdominal injury. (See pp. 482–485.)

7. Describe a complete secondary assessment of the chest and abdomen, including the following tasks. (See below pages.)

- Inspection and examination (pp. 485-488)
- Vital signs (p. 488)
- Patient history (p. 489)

8. Identify, order, and describe the care steps for chest and abdominal penetrating and blunt trauma. (See pp. 489–496.)

Medic Rescue 3 responds to a small tavern downtown where a patient has been shot during an argument. Upon arrival, the paramedics find several police officers securing the scene. Officers have the suspected assailant in handcuffs. One officer says: "You'll find the victim inside the bar. He was shot once in the chest with a .357 magnum."

Paramedics spot the patient on the floor, sitting up against the wall. He's holding a blood-stained towel in place. Paramedics quickly learn that the 24-year-old male has some minor bleeding from the left upper chest. Assessment reveals the patient to be conscious, alert, and somewhat agitated. He seems to have some trouble speaking in complete sentences and is slightly ashen in color. The patient's airway is clear, but he is laboring for each breath. Paramedics determine the respiratory rate is 36 and breaths are shallow. Pulses (both central and distal) are strong but rapid. The chest has one small entrance wound, with a spray of burnt gunpowder around it. A small stream of blood seeps from the wound with no visible gurgling or bubbles. One paramedic evaluates the posterior chest to find a larger, more jagged wound losing little blood with no signs of air exchange. The rest of the primary assessment reveals no other signs of injury.

Paramedics seal the wounds with occlusive dressings and apply high-flow oxygen. The patient's color improves, although he is having more difficulty moving air. They apply pulse oximetry and obtain a reading of 92 percent. The blood pressure is 100 by palpation (environmental noise is too loud to get a good reading). Although background noise makes it difficult to hear lung sounds, they appear diminished on the left. The team notices that the patient now is returning to the earlier ashen color. They also observe that his jugular veins are becoming more prominent. The trachea looks to be midline. The patient strains with each respiration, and his level of consciousness diminishes.

Paramedics load the patient onto the stretcher and transfer him to the ambulance. En route to the hospital, they give a report to medical command. They receive orders to infuse lactated Ringer's solution rapidly and to repeat the breath sounds. The breath sounds are now severely diminished on the left and the trachea seems displaced to the right.

Medical control orders needle decompression of the left chest. One paramedic removes the occlusive dressings, with no change in the patient's condition. The paramedic then inserts a large bore needle in the intercostal space and a gush of air exits. The crew now reapply the dressings, taping only three sides. They slit a sterile glove finger and secure it to the needle hub. The patient's respirations improve. So does his level of consciousness and oxygen saturation reading.

At the emergency department, the staff places a chest tube and applies suction. They fully evaluate the patient and take him to the ICU to observe for a few days. He recovers completely.

INTRODUCTION

The body cavity includes the thorax, abdomen, and pelvic cavity. Trauma to this part of the body can directly involve the respiratory, cardiovascular, digestive, or urinary systems. Depending upon the type of trauma, multiple systems may be involved. In the case of vehicular accidents, trauma to the body cavity is the second-highest cause of death. Other forms of trauma can also result in life-threatening injuries.

To combat mortality from body cavity trauma, you need to understand the basic anatomy, physiology, and pathophysiology of organs and structures found within this area. With this knowledge, you can provide efficient and appropriate assessment and management of body cavity injuries.

✱ Always suspect chest or abdominal cavity injury in the patient with multiple injuries.

ANATOMY AND PHYSIOLOGY

Trauma assessment rests upon knowing the location and function of each organ within the body cavity. Forces directed at a specific area of the body cavity will most likely affect the organs within that area. Therefore, if you know the direction and strength of these forces, you can anticipate the specific organ or organs involved and the potential degree of injury.

To orient yourself to the body cavity, think of it as one large space, extending from above the clavicles downward into the pelvis. This space is divided into two smaller cavities by the *diaphragm*, a strong sheet of muscle that actively participates in respiration. The upper cavity is the *thorax*. The thorax contains the lungs and the **mediastinum**, a central region that houses the heart, trachea, esophagus, major blood vessels, and several nerve pathways. The lower *abdominal cavity* is subdivided into three cavities: the abdomen, the retroperitoneal space, and the pelvic cavity.

■ **mediastinum** central cavity within the thorax containing the heart, great vessels, trachea, and esophagus.

The Thorax

The thorax acts as both a container and a dynamic component of the respiratory process. (See Figure 16-1.) It houses the major functional parts of the respiratory and circulatory systems. It also changes volume very dramatically to accommodate respiration (the bellows system).

The thorax is composed of skeletal and soft tissue. It is made up of twelve C-shaped rib pairs, articulating directly with the vertebral column posteriorly. Through cartilage attachments, the upper six ribs directly join with the sternum anteriorly, while the next four attach indirectly. Because the last two ribs do not attach anteriorly, they can move through a modest range of motion.

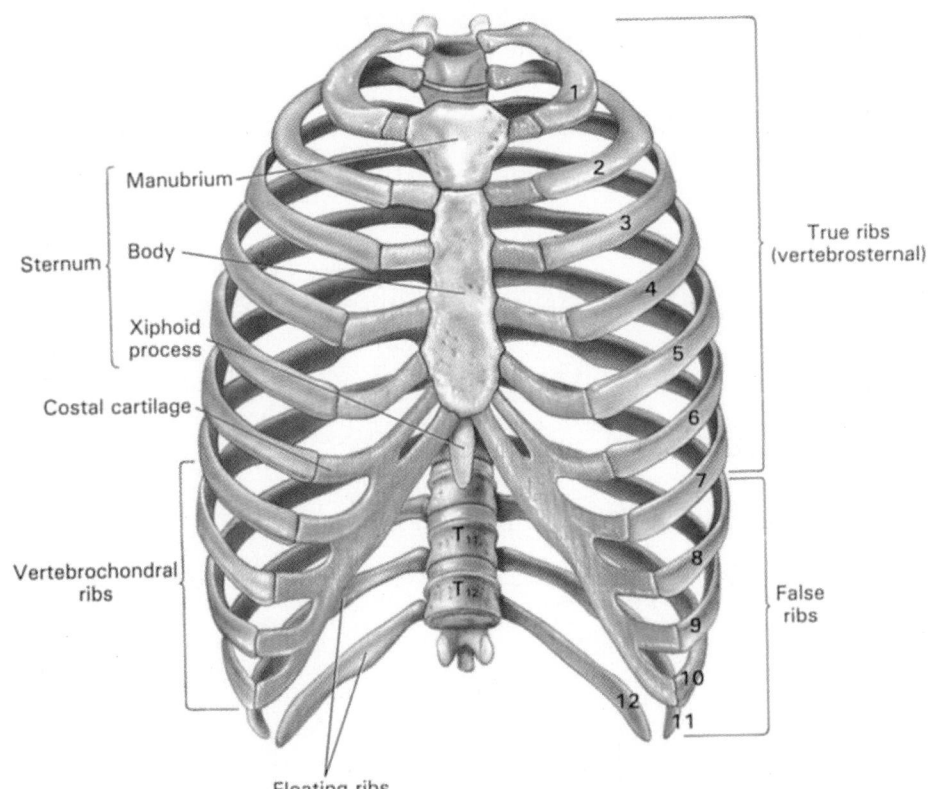

FIGURE 16-1   The thorax.

Thoracic Cage

The framework of the shoulder covers the upper thorax. (See Figure 16-2.) Sitting over the upper rib anteriorly, each clavicle articulates with the sternum medially and the humerus and scapula distally. The scapula overrides the upper four ribs posteriorly. Both the musculature and the structure of the shoulder girdle protect the upper thorax from the effects of trauma extremely well.

The ribs, which form the rigid structure of the thorax, lie at a downward orientation from posterior to anterior. They lift to a more horizontal position by contraction of the **sternocleidomastoid** and **intercostal muscles**. The sternocleidomastoid muscles raise the sternum and the anterior ribs, while the intercostal muscles bring the ribs closer together and help lift the lower ribs. The result of this motion is an increase in the anterior-posterior dimension of the chest. Simultaneously, the diaphragm contracts, thus displacing the abdominal contents downward and increasing the superior-inferior dimension of the thorax.

Expansion of the thorax outward and movement of the diaphragm downward dramatically increases the total volume of the chest. This volume increase causes the pressure within to fall. Air from the outside rushes in to equalize the pressure and *inspiration* occurs. When the muscles of respiration relax, the ribs settle, the diaphragm rises, and the volume of the chest decreases. This volume decrease causes pressure within to rise. As air rushes out, *expiration* occurs.

Mediastinum

The central region of the chest is the *mediastinum*. It is bordered laterally by the lungs, inferiorly by the diaphragm, and superiorly by the neck and shoulders. It houses several structures essential to body function. These include the *trachea, vena cava, aorta,* and *esophagus.* Each structure is a major conduit for the respiratory, venous, arterial, and digestive systems respectively. The heart, the principal organ of the cardiovascular system, is also located within the mediastinum.

The heart is a hollow, muscular pump that powers the entire cardiovascular system. (See Chapter 21.) The cardiac septum divides the heart into right

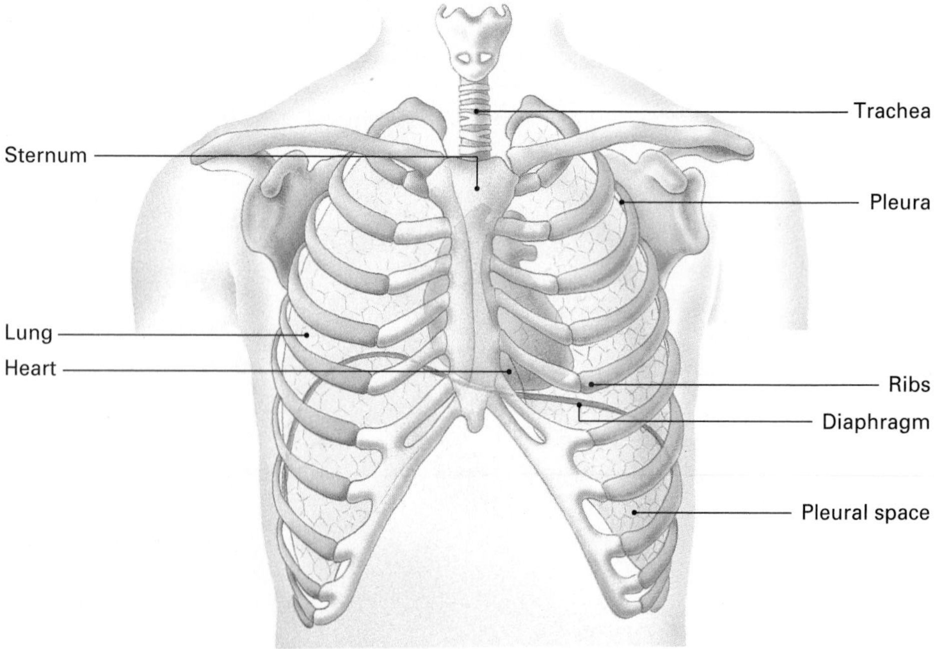

■ **sternocleidomastoid** muscle of the lateral neck and anterior thorax attaching at the mastoid, clavicle, and sternum. It serves as an accessory muscle of respiration and lifts the sternum and anterior chest during deep respiration.

■ **intercostal muscles** muscles between the ribs that serve to expand the chest.

FIGURE 16-2 The organs of the thorax.

and left sides. The tricuspid and mitral valves further divide the heart into upper and lower chambers (the atria and ventricles). The heart walls are made up of very special muscle tissue (cardiac muscle), which provides a constant and rhythmic pumping action. Coronary arteries, found on the exterior of the heart muscle, supply the heart with oxygenated blood.

Surrounding the heart is a strong, thin sac called the **pericardium.** A small amount of fluid lays between the pericardium and the outer-most cardiac tissue, the *endocardium*. Like the pleura of the lungs, the pericardium does not stretch. If filled with fluid, the pericardium may inhibit cardiac filling.

The arch of the aorta and the *ligamentum arteriosum* suspend the heart centrally in the chest. The aorta attaches to the base of the heart and is firmly stabilized against the thoracic spine, posteriorly. To some degree, the innominate and subclavian arteries immobilize the aorta as they branch from the arch. The *ligamentum arteriosum* also helps maintain the position of the heart and the curve of the aorta.

The lungs fill the chest cavity on either side of the mediastinum. They occupy between 6–8 liters of space, with the right lung slightly larger than the left. The left lung is smaller because of the heart's position in the mediastinum. Each lung has regions called *lobes*—the right lung has three lobes, while the left lung has two.

Pleura   The *pleura* ensures that the lungs expand and contract along with the inside of the thorax. It is a double layer of smooth and delicate tissue lining the interior of the thorax (**parietal pleura**) and the exterior of the lungs (**visceral pleura**). Between these two layers is a potential space containing a small amount of pleural fluid to lubricate and hold the two layers together. The force securing the lungs, to the thorax resembles that which holds two pieces of glass together when water gets between them. Unless you allow air to enter, the two "panes" (or the lungs and thorax) remain firmly together.

Alveoli   The **alveolus** is a hollow, grape-shaped chamber where oxygen and carbon dioxide exchange takes place. There are about 300 million of these hollow spaces in the respiratory system, with a combined surface area half that of a basketball court. This surface allows an efficient and effective exchange of carbon dioxide and oxygen. The alveoli also give the lungs their spongy compliance, volume, and light weight. The alveoli are flexible and elastic. With each breath, they vary their diameter and change their volume to accommodate the chest motion. Under normal circumstances, air will enter the airway and travel into the alveoli during inspiration.

The Bellows System   The bellows system is responsible for the movement of air in and out of the alveoli. The following elements of the bellows system must be functional for normal respiration to occur.

❏ Skeletal muscles, which change the volume of the thorax.
❏ Pleura, which causes the chest walls and lungs to move together.
❏ Alveoli, which respond to changes in thoracic volume.
❏ Airway, which permits air to travel in and out with each breath.

These elements must work together to bring oxygen in and remove carbon dioxide from the alveoli.

The changing **intrathoracic** pressure is also responsible for some hemodynamic effects. The reduction of this pressure during inspiration assists venous return to the heart, while the increasing pressure during expiration helps move arterial blood out of the thorax.

■ **pericardium** two-layered sac surrounding the heart.

■ **parietal pleura** fine fibrous sheath covering the interior of the thorax.

■ **visceral pleura** fine lining covering the lungs. With the parietal pleura, it forms the seal holding the lungs to the interior of the thoracic cage.

■ **alveolus** one of the millions of microscopic chambers within the lung. It is the location where the gasses of respiration are exchanged. (pl. alveoli)

■ **intrathoracic** within the thoracic cavity.

The Abdomen

The diaphragm is a dynamic organ that forms the upper border of the abdomen. It is a dome-shaped muscle that attaches to the lower border of the rib cage and moves up and down with each breath. The uppermost point of its travel during a deep expiration is somewhere just below the nipple line. The lower point of travel is a few inches below the xiphoid. Thus, any penetrating or blunt trauma to this region may involve organs of the abdomen, thorax, or both.

Abdominal Cavity   The lower ribs and lumbar spine, as well as the muscles of the lower back, form the posterior boundary of the abdomen. Laterally, it is bound by the flank muscles and anteriorly by the abdominal muscles. Its inferior border is the pelvis. Three regions further subdivide the abdomen: the abdominal space, the retroperitoneal space, and the pelvic cavity. The **retroperitoneal** space contains the kidneys, aorta, vena cava, and part of the duodenum and pancreas. Its organs lack the protective covering of the peritoneum, hence the name. The *pelvic cavity* contains the organs within the pelvis: the bladder, rectum, and, in the female, the **genitalia**. The *abdominal* cavity houses the remaining organs, all of which are covered by peritoneum.

For assessment purposes, we divide the abdomen into four quadrants by drawing an imaginary set of lines through the umbilicus, one superior to inferior and the other left to right. The *right-upper quadrant* contains the liver, right kidney, gall bladder, duodenum, and part of the pancreas. The *left-upper quadrant* includes the stomach, left kidney, spleen, and most of the pancreas. The *left-lower quadrant* houses the sigmoid colon, while the *right-lower quadrant* contains the appendix. All quadrants hold some of the small bowel, although the lower quadrants have the largest portion. The large bowel begins in the right lower quadrant and travels upward, across, and downward through all the remaining quadrants.

Alimentary Canal   The *alimentary* canal is a continuous tube that begins with the esophagus and ends at the rectum. Its first component, the esophagus, empties into the stomach. Here hydrochloric acid and **enzymes** mix and churn with the food. When the mixture, called *chyme*, reaches a semi-liquid consistency, the lower end of the stomach allows it to travel into the **duodenum**. In this area, pancreatic juices and bile assist with the digestive breakdown. The material continues its motion through the canal via **peristalsis**, a wavelike muscular motion of the bowel. The next two segments of the small bowel, the **jejunum** and the **ileum** absorb most, if not all, of the nutrients.

The digested food next enters the large bowel at the *ileocecal valve*, a one-way structure in the right-lower quadrant. The large bowel contains bacteria that break down the remaining material and release the water within it. The large bowel absorbs the water and other fluids, returning them to the liver and then the circulatory system. As the digested and relatively dehydrated material ends its travel through the alimentary canal, it moves to the *rectum*, a holding area. The anus is the sphincter muscle that retains the material until the body is ready to release it.

Accessory Organs   Besides the alimentary canal, there are accessory organs that assist in digestion. These include the liver, gall bladder, and pancreas. The *liver* occupies the area below and under the rib cage in the right-upper quadrant and, to a smaller extent, the left-upper quadrant. A large and vascular organ, it detoxifies the blood coming from the digestive field. It also stores body energy reserves, produces plasma proteins, and performs many other functions. Beneath and behind the liver is the *gall bladder*, a storehouse

■ **retroperitoneal** behind the layers of the peritoneum. The organs within this space include the kidneys, spleen, and part of the pancreas.

■ **genitalia** reproductive organs of either the male or the female.

■ **enzyme** biochemical catalyst that speeds chemical reactions. The enzyme itself does not normally change during the process.

■ **duodenum** first part of the small bowel. About 10 inches in length, it receives the secretions of the liver and the pancreas.

■ **peristalsis** wavelike muscular motion of the esophagus and bowel that moves food through the digestive system.

■ **jejunum** second portion of the small bowel. It is approximately 8 feet in length and is located between the duodenum and ileum.

■ **ileum** third and longest portion of the small bowel. It is approximately 12 feet in length and extends from the jejunum to the ileo-cecal valve.

for **bile**. Bile is a product of the liver and helps in the digestion of fats. The gall bladder will constrict in response to digestive material passing from the stomach (especially fats) and excrete bile, through the bile duct, into the duodenum.

The *pancreas* also excretes digestive juices through the common bile duct into the duodenum. Because they are very caustic, pancreatic juices efficiently assist with the breakdown of food in the small bowel. The pancreas also produces **insulin**, the hormone necessary to move glucose across the cell membrane for use in metabolism. The pancreas is found in both upper quadrants, with most of its mass in the left.

Another occupant of the left-upper abdominal quadrant is the *spleen*. This large vascular organ helps protect the body against invasion of foreign organisms. Not only does the spleen help produce white blood cells, it also houses the system that gives us immunity from disease.

The kidneys lay behind and beneath the spleen on the left, and behind the liver on the right. These organs filter blood and draw water and waste products from it. The kidneys concentrate waste and preserve the water/salt balance of the human system. Urine, their product, travels through the ureters to the urinary bladder.

The abdomen also contains the abdominal aorta and vena cava. They are large vessels traveling along the posterior wall, next to the spinal column. Major branches from both vessels supply blood to, or receive blood from, the organs of the abdomen. They continue inferiorly to provide circulation to the pelvis and lower extremities.

Peritoneum   The **peritoneum** is a delicate tissue covering both the organs (except those in the retroperitoneal space) and the interior of the abdominal cavity. Fluid within the peritoneum allows smooth motion between the various internal organs. The peritoneal space is a sensitive and relatively sterile area. Therefore, blood, other body fluid, or fecal material can easily inflame this space.

Two specialized and important tissues of the abdominal cavity are the **mesentery** and the **omentum**. The mesentery is a double fold of peritoneum extending from the posterior wall of the abdomen to the small bowel. It provides the small bowel with circulation and innervation. It also keeps the bowel from becoming entangled during the process of digestion. Like the mesentery, the omentum is a double layer of peritoneum. It suspends downward from the duodenum and the stomach and hangs in front of the abdominal organs. After a person's youth, it becomes covered with fatty tissue and insulates the anterior abdomen from trauma and temperature extremes. The peritoneum covers the anterior abdominal organs but not the kidneys, aorta, vena cava, and parts of the duodenum and pancreas.

The Pelvic Cavity

The pelvic cavity contains the bladder, rectum and, in the female, the reproductive organs. This cavity also houses the iliac artery and vein, supplying and returning blood from the lower extremities. The pelvic cavity is the space from the opening of the pelvis (the pelvic inlet) to the pelvic floor. It is generally well-protected from trauma.

BODY CAVITY INJURIES

Injuries of the chest, abdomen, and pelvic cavity pose a serious threat to life due to blood loss, respiratory embarrassment, and compromise of critical organ function. They deserve serious evaluation and immediate consideration when they are subjected to trauma. To this end, you need to understand what

■ **bile** a yellow to green viscous fluid secreted by the liver and stored in the gall bladder. It is secreted into the small bowel, aids in digestion of fats, and gives the stool its normal coloration.

■ **insulin** pancreatic hormone needed to transport simple sugars from the interstitial spaces into the cells.

■ **peritoneum** fine fibrous tissue surrounding the interior of most of the abdominal cavity and covering most of the small bowel and some of the abdominal organs.

■ **mesentery** double fold of peritoneum that supports the major portion of the small bowel, suspending it from the posterior abdominal wall.

■ **omentum** sheet of peritoneum and fat tissue, covering and protecting the anterior surface of the interior abdomen.

✱ Chest injuries account for one out of four trauma deaths in this country.

internal injuries can occur, how they endanger body function, and the consequences that may follow.

Chest Injuries

There are two types of chest injuries: those that compromise the bellows system and the movement of air and those that injure the internal structures. An injury can render the bellow system ineffective in three ways.

❑ Pain can restrict chest excursion.
❑ Air can enter the pleural space and prevent adequate air exchange.
❑ The chest wall can fail to move in unison.

Internal injuries can contuse or lacerate lung or mediastinal tissue, including the great vessels, trachea, esophagus, or the heart.

Rib Fractures   Simple rib fracture can affect the efficiency of respiration. The fracture of a rib is very painful and will cause the patient to limit chest excursion with each breath. This limits tidal volume and dramatically reduces the alveolar air (the air delivered to the alveoli for oxygen and carbon dioxide exchange). Additionally, your patient will not breathe deeply since such chest motion causes extreme pain. Shallow breathing results in alveolar collapse and the natural reflex to correct this, sighing, is suppressed by the pain. This alveolar collapse, called **atelectasis**, results in less efficient respiration and over the long term may lead to pneumonia or other respiratory infection.

Pulmonary Contusion   During trauma, compression of the chest may contuse the lungs as it would any other body tissue. Pulmonary tissue will swell and edema develops, much like tissue anywhere else in the body. Pulmonary contusion reduces lung compliance and increases respiratory effort. It also interferes with the diffusion of carbon dioxide, increasing $PaCO_2$ and decreasing the blood's pH.

Flail Chest   Severe trauma may fracture several ribs. If three or more ribs fracture in multiple locations, the chest area may become unstable. (See Figure 16-3.) In this injury, called *flail chest*, the segment moves due to intrathoracic pressures rather than by muscular control. As the patient inspires, the intact chest wall moves outward, and the intrathoracic pressure falls. The reduced intrathoracic pressure draws the unstable, or flail segment, inward. As the chest relaxes and moves inward during expiration, the intrathoracic pressure increases and causes the flail segment to move outward. The motion of the flail segment is opposite to the rest of the chest and is called *paradoxical*. (See Figure 16-4.) It results in severe respiratory compromise because the air from beneath the segment travels to and from the good lung tissue instead of in and out of the airway. This paradoxical motion limits the useful air exchange from beneath the area of injury and reduces the efficiency of the remaining bellows system.

Traumatic Asphyxia   Another extreme condition often associated with severe rib injury is **traumatic asphyxia**. This condition involves some mechanism that holds or pushes the chest wall inward. This may occur either by the nature of the rib fractures or by a compressional force trapping the patient such as the auto seat and the steering wheel. The compression severely limits chest **excursion** and results in hypoventilation. It also may tamponade intrathoracic hemorrhage and cause a backflow and back up of venous blood,

■ **atelectasis** collapse of the alveoli of the lung.

■ **traumatic asphyxia** compression of the chest due to a crush injury. It limits chest excursion yet tamponades hemorrhage.

■ **excursion** extent of movement of a body part such as the chest during respiration.

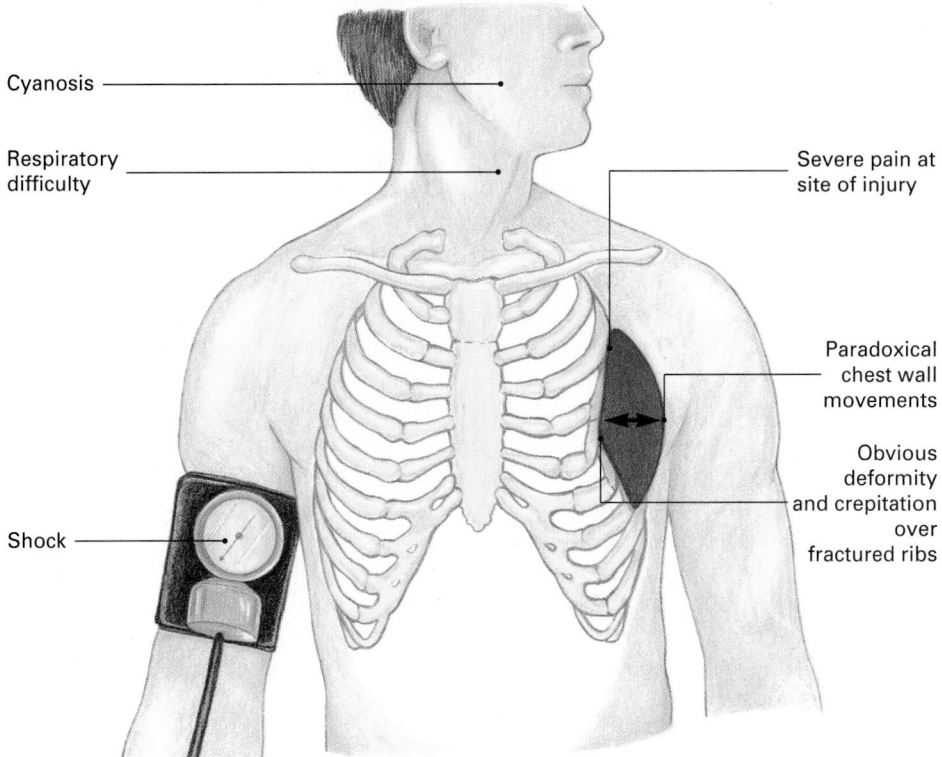

Cyanosis

Respiratory difficulty

Severe pain at site of injury

Paradoxical chest wall movements

Obvious deformity and crepitation over fractured ribs

Shock

FIGURE 16-3 Flail chest.

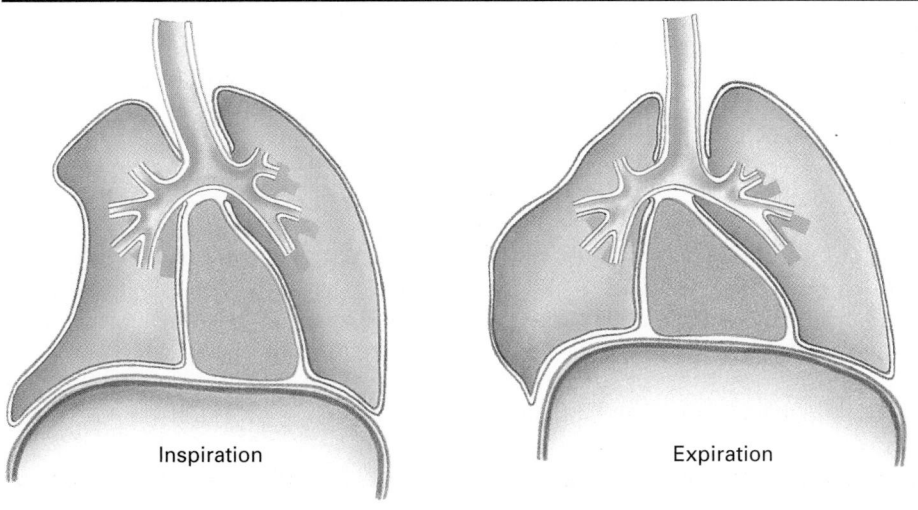

Inspiration

Expiration

FIGURE 16-4 Paradoxical movement of the chest wall seen in flail chest.

especially within the neck and the head. The classical presentation of traumatic asphyxia includes bloodshot eyes, bulging blue tongue, distended neck veins, and a cyanotic upper body. The prognosis is grave. While release of the chest pressure may help the patient to breathe, it may also lead to rapid hypovolemia, shock, and death.

Pneumothorax   The bellows system may also fail because of loss of pleural seal integrity. If an internal or external wound allows air, blood, or fluid to enter the area between the pleural tissues, the potential space becomes an actual space. Expansion of the pleural space reduces the effective

* Hypoxia is the most important concern in chest trauma.

lung expansion and compromises respiration. If the pleural space expands because of air from an interior wound, it is called a *closed pneumothorax*. If the wound is external, it is called an *open pneumothorax*. The opening may be the result of a torn bronchus, bronchiole, or alveolus. It can be caused by penetrating or blunt trauma, COPD, or congenital defect. The larger the tear and the structure involved, the more rapid the progression of the pneumothorax. In small tears, pneumothorax may self-seal, and the body will gradually reabsorb the air. If the tear involves larger airways, the pneumothorax may be progressive. Penetrating trauma (open pneumothorax) will usually require a rather large hole to allow the exchange or passage of air. Such trauma normally results in gurgling or frothy blood at the wound site.

Compression of a hyperinflated chest during an auto accident may precipitate a pneumothorax. As the driver sees the impending impact, he or she takes a deep gasp of air and holds it. During the crash, the chest impacts the steering wheel or dashboard and compresses the hyperinflated thorax against the closed glottis. The alveoli and bronchioles rupture like a sealed paper bag between two hands clapping. This phenomenon, called the *paper bag syndrome*, results in a closed pneumothorax.

Be cautious in using intermittent positive pressure ventilation (IPPV), because it may induce or worsen a pneumothorax in the chest trauma patient. Positive pressure may rupture lung tissue already damaged or weakened by the injury. It may also push air past a wound that would not otherwise allow air to enter the pleura.

Tension Pneumothorax   If a wound permits air to enter the pleural space, it may also act as a one-way valve, producing a condition called **tension pneumothorax**. Tension pneumothorax is a progressive pneumothorax that enlarges, builds in pressure, and begins to infringe upon the function of the opposite lung and the circulatory system. (See Figure 16-5.) The valve allows air to enter the pleural space during inspiration. As the patient brethes out, the valve closes and air cannot exit. The problem progresses and pressure within the thorax grows. This condition will:

❑ Increase the effort of respiration.
❑ Push the mediastinum against the unaffected lung.
❑ Retard venous return to the heart.
❑ Reduce the heart's ability to fill.
❑ Possibly kink the vena cava where it travels through the diaphragm.

The overall effect upon the patient is extreme dyspnea and, eventually, acute circulatory compromise.

Movement of the mediastinum away from the affected side may cause the trachea to shift from midline. It is a late sign, present only after there has been a significant shifting of the mediastinum. Therefore, tracheal deviation is not a good sign to guide care. Instead, look for severe dyspnea, unilaterally absent or severely diminished breath sounds, subcutaneous emphysema, and signs and symptoms of shock without any other apparent cause.

The pleural space may also fill with fluid, most commonly blood (*hemothorax*). The accumulation will normally be slow and result in minimal respiratory embarrassment during the time the patient is in the prehospital setting. If the hemothorax involves a large vessel, blood loss may be severe and hypovolemia will be the primary patient problem. Remember that each lung occupies about 3 to 4 liters of space. Any rapid blood loss capable of causing respiratory compromise will probably result in hypovolemic shock. A mixed presentation of pneumothorax and hemothorax together is also common. (See Figure 16-6.)

■ **tension pneumothorax** buildup of air under pressure within the thorax. By compressing the lung, it severely reduces the effectiveness of respiration.

✳ Tension pneumothorax requires immediate decompression, if permitted by local protocols.

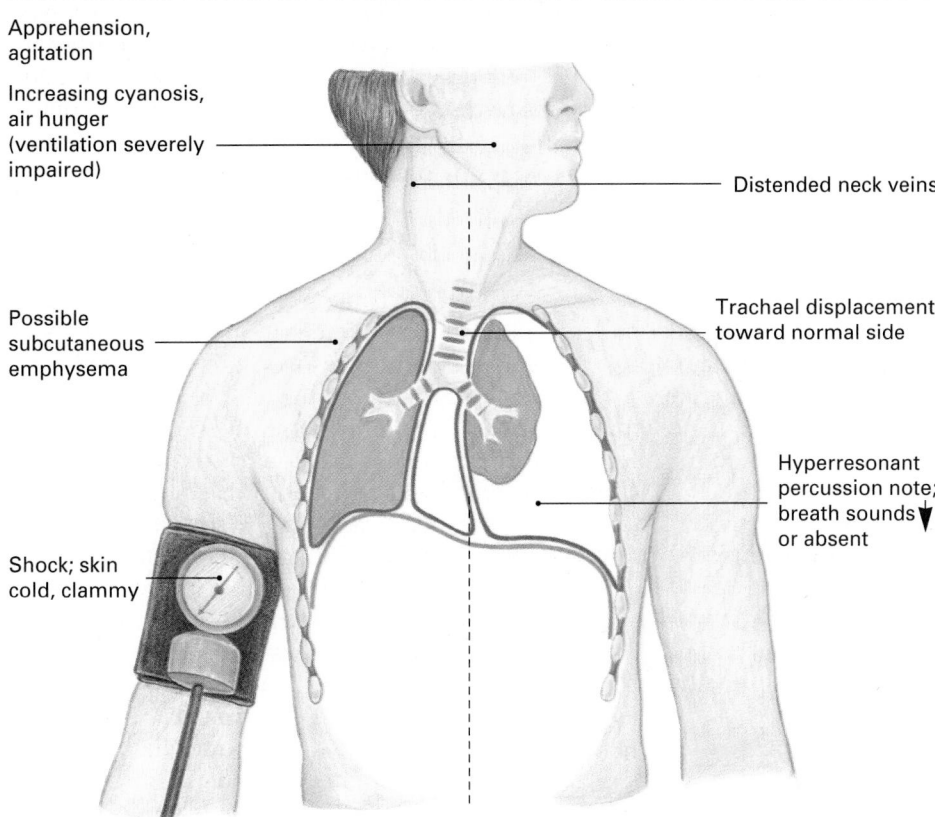

Apprehension, agitation

Increasing cyanosis, air hunger (ventilation severely impaired)

Possible subcutaneous emphysema

Shock; skin cold, clammy

Distended neck veins

Trachael displacement toward normal side

Hyperresonant percussion note; breath sounds ▼ or absent

FIGURE 16-5 Physical findings of tension pneumothorax.

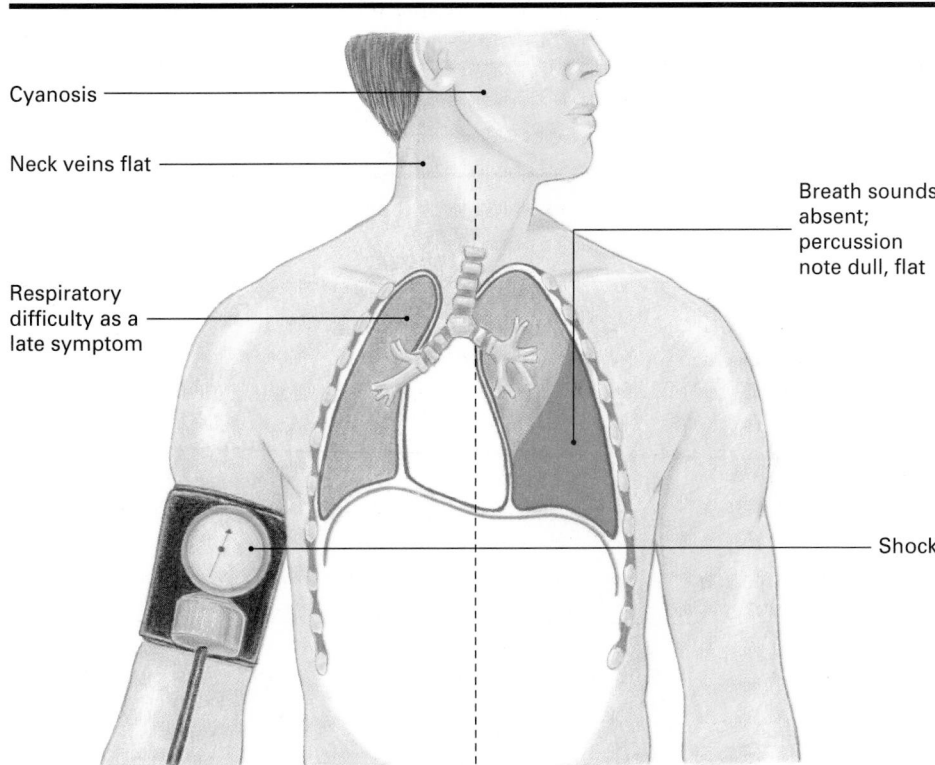

Cyanosis

Neck veins flat

Respiratory difficulty as a late symptom

Breath sounds absent; percussion note dull, flat

Shock

FIGURE 16-6 Physical findings of massive hemothorax.

Cardiac Injury

Decelerating trauma can affect structures within the mediastinum, including the heart and great vessels. Kinetic forces can contuse the heart, injuring the myocardium. This injury often has a better prognosis than myocardial infarction, even though it presents similarly. The myocardial contusion patient may display acute signs and symptoms, including life-threatening dysrhythmias while in your care. (Dysrhythmia recognition and care will be discussed in Chapter 21.)

Pericardial tamponade can occur secondary to either blunt or penetrating trauma. A coronary artery may tear, allowing blood to enter the pericardial space. As the sac fills with blood, it progressively restricts the passive filling of the heart. Cardiac output then drops quickly and without warning. In this injury, the compensatory mechanisms for shock cause systemic vasoconstriction in order to maintain blood pressure. The patient's systolic pressure will remain relatively normal, while the diastolic pressure rises. This narrowing of the pulse pressure is characteristic of tamponade, as are distending jugular veins and distant heart sounds. (See Figure 16-7.) If the syndrome continues, pericardial tamponade will eventually stop blood flow through the heart, resulting in cardiopulmonary arrest. This condition is unresponsive to CPR, defibrillation, and drug therapy.

Injuries to Other Structures in the Mediastinum

The aorta, the largest artery in the body, connects to the heart at its base. If sudden deceleration occurs, especially if it is lateral, the heart may twist on the aorta. This movement can cause the layers of the vessel to tear apart, causing a ballooning of the wall known as an *aneurysm*. Blood flows into and expands the defect. In the process, it often impinges the left subclavian artery and diminishes circulation to the left upper extremity. The patient may complain of a tearing sensation in the central chest or back and numbness or tingling in the left upper extremity. The patient may also exhibit a diminished or absent pulse. The defect may rupture with rapid hemorrhage into the mediastinum. A very high percentage of the patients who suffer a traumatic aortic aneurysm do not survive.

Other injuries of the mediastinal contents include: rupture of the esophagus or trachea and laceration to the inferior or superior vena cava. A tracheal tear may allow free air into the mediastinum, especially if the patient coughs

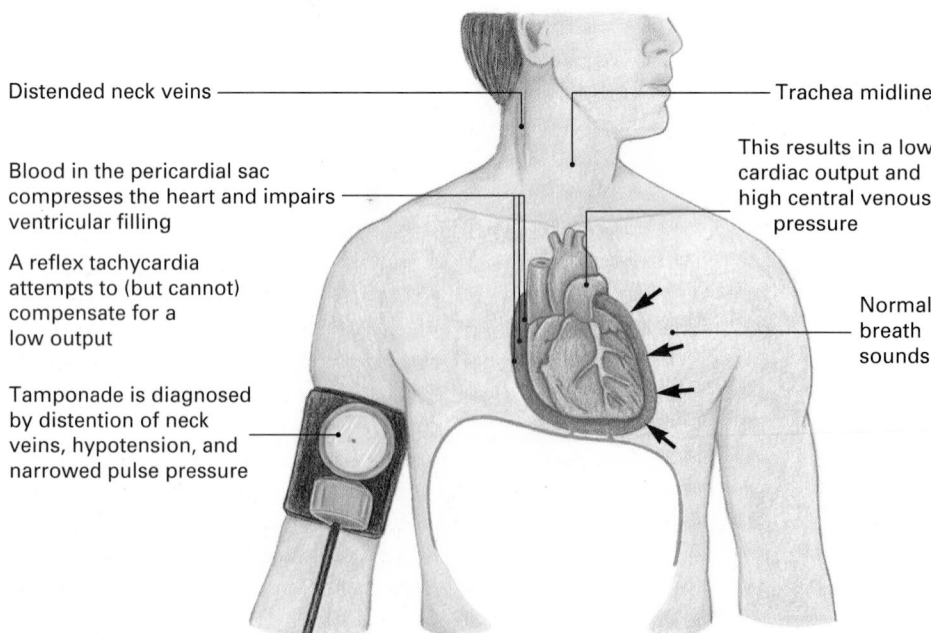

FIGURE 16-7 Physical findings of cardiac tamponade.

or is placed on IPPV. Esophageal injury may allow gastric or other foreign materials into the mediastinum. While these injuries may cause only minor problems in the field setting, they may eventually result in patient demise from infection. Vena cava damage, whether superior or inferior, may account for rapid, extensive, shock-inducing hemorrhage. Penetrating trauma most frequently causes these injuries.

Severe blunt abdominal trauma has been known to rupture the diaphragm and force abdominal contents into the thoracic cavity. This injury reduces the dynamics of the respiratory system and frequently makes the abdomen appear hollow or empty.

Abdominal Injury

Life-threatening injury to the abdomen presents with less obvious signs and symptoms than other trauma. Assessment of this area is more difficult because the abdominal container is soft and pliable. Also, the effects of hemorrhage or abdominal organ dysfunction are often delayed. Thus, it is very difficult to predict the nature and the extent of injury.

Penetrating Trauma　Penetrating trauma to the abdomen may cause severe injury. With high-speed projectiles, such as bullets, the injury is dependent upon the energy expended by the projectile and the particular organ involved. The liver, kidneys, and spleen are very susceptible to injury from the cavitational wave, while the small and large bowels are not. It is also important to note that you cannot determine the depth of a wound, its pathway, or the organs and tissues affected from an entrance wound alone.

Evisceration　Evisceration is a rupture or laceration of the abdominal wall that allows abdominal contents to escape through the opening. The small bowel is the most common protruding viscera. As the bowel protrudes, it may obstruct the wound. At the same time, however, pressure from the protrusion may occlude the bowel's blood supply. The atmosphere may also expose the bowel to drying. Finally, as the bowel exits and reenters the wound, the pathogens in the atmosphere and on bodily surfaces may contaminate it. Any of these conditions pose significant threats to bowel survival.

Blunt Trauma　Blunt trauma is responsible for several types of injuries within the abdomen. Solid organs may contuse, lacerate, or fracture. Hollow organs may rupture, and abdominal vasculature may tear. Hemorrhage, organ dysfunction, irritation, or destruction of the abdominal lining and organs may also occur with these injuries.

Solid-Organ Injury. During deceleration or acceleration, the posterior abdominal wall and the anterior abdominal surface may trap and compress the solid abdominal organs. Tissues are compressed, resulting in swelling, hemorrhage, and, possibly, organ failure. If the forces of injury are severe enough, they may cause the solid organs to fracture. Frequently, the organ's peritoneal envelope contains the hemorrhage, and may rupture with time. Although the result may be delayed, rapid exsanguination can follow.

Hollow-Organ Injury. Deceleration may also compress hollow organs. If kinetic forces are great enough, the organ may rupture and spill its contents into the abdominal cavity. The large bowel contains bacteria and other pathogens that, if spilled, cause severe infection. The gall bladder, stomach, and small bowel contain caustic fluids that will chemically damage the abdominal contents if released into the peritoneal space.

Other Trauma-Related Injuries. Traumatic jarring or deceleration of abdominal organs may also cause them to tear at their sites of attachment. Blood vessels often tear where they branch from the abdominal aorta or vena cava or at the organ they supply. Injuries involving the blood supply to any abdominal organ can result in rapid and extensive blood loss and organ dysfunction. Ligamentous detachment can also lead to abdominal organ trauma. When the various organs within the cavity decelerate, ligaments and other connective tissue may restrain them.

The *ligamentum teres* suspends the liver. In deceleration, the ligament may slice the liver as cheese is sliced by a wire cutter. The laceration is severe, often resulting in rapid hemorrhage.

The design of the pelvic cavity protects its internal structures. Even so, some injuries may still occur. In rapid deceleration, the full bladder may rupture when the seat belt slows the body and expresses great force along the top of the pelvic ring. A similar injury may occur to a full sigmoid colon or rectum. The spilling of abdominal contents or blood into the peritoneal space will generally present in one of two ways.

- ❏ Spillage of blood, urine, small bowel contents, and gastric or other digestive fluids (bile or pancreatic juices) are very irritating. These substances will inflame the peritoneum within 12 hours.
- ❏ Spillage of the highly infectious contents of the large bowel will inflame more slowly (about 12–24 hours).

The first indication of either of the above evolving injuries may be *rebound tenderness.*

Genitalia Injury

Injury to the female genitalia most commonly results from direct trauma to the area. Child molestation and rape are common causes. (See Chapter 31.) The mechanism of injury normally involves forceful placement of objects into the vaginal canal. Tearing of the internal genitalia presents with moderate to severe internal and/or external bleeding.

The external male genitalia suffer injury more frequently. The penis and testicles are well supplied with nerves and a blood vessel. Injury can be very painful. Laceration can cause significant blood loss, while blunt trauma may lead to a sizable hematoma.

ASSESSMENT

During assessment of the trauma patient, you will direct your attention to the chest and abdomen several times. (See Figure 16-8.) Careful evaluation of the mechanism of injury will either suggest or rule out the probability of body cavity injury. The primary survey will quickly identify any life threats that call for immediate care. The physical exam may call your attention to more subtle signs of injury, while questioning may permit the patient to relate symptoms, indicative of thoracic or abdominal injury. Your assessment must be complete and thorough enough to identify any injury and specific enough to determine proper care. If you overlook any evidence, further injury or mistreatment may result.

Mechanism of Injury

The mechanism of injury may be the first and most obvious indication that a chest or abdominal injury exists. The gross nature of the incident may reveal

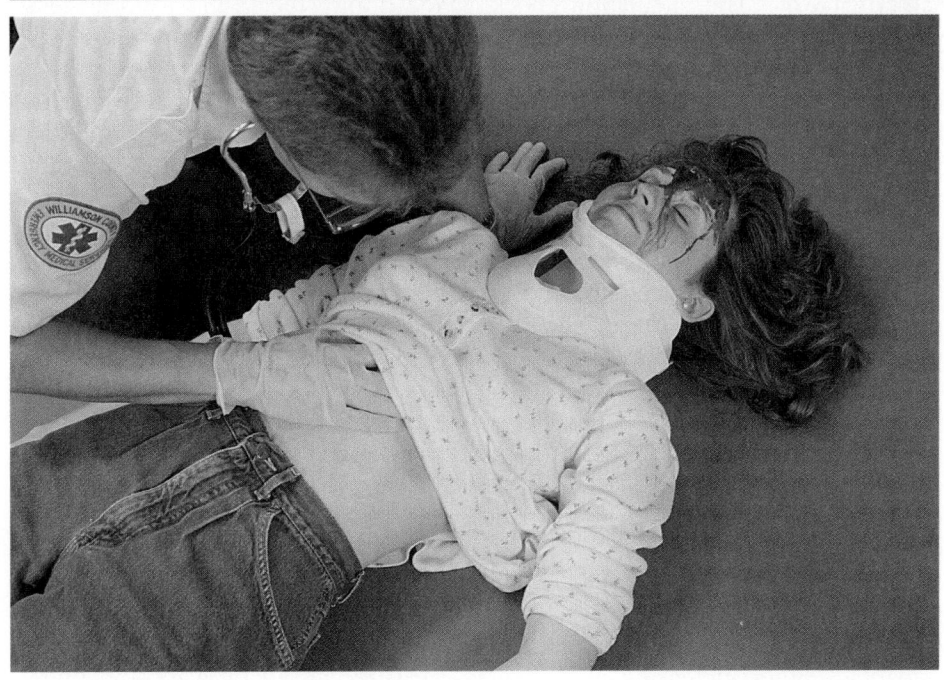

FIGURE 16-8 The chest and abdomen must be inspected for injury.

the direction, strength, and point of contact of the insult. Examine the auto damage (or other traumatic events). Then mentally relive the events that may have occurred in the passenger compartment. Try to picture the patient's impact against the interior. Observe any steering wheel or dash deformity. Determine if a seatbelt or air bag restrained the patient. If so, speculate on what effect it may have had upon the impact.

Primary Assessment

With any thoracic or abdominal trauma, you should suspect cervical spine injury. Only after immobilizing the head and neck should you begin the A-B-C-D-E of primary assessment. Your initial survey will reveal the potential for, and the effects of, body cavity trauma.

✳ Assume that a spinal injury also exists in any patient with body cavity trauma.

Airway and Breathing Evaluation of the airway may suggest chest injury. But the real evaluation of respiratory system function begins with the assessment of breathing. Remember to *look*, *listen*, and *feel* as you evaluate respiratory effectiveness and search for signs of chest trauma.

"Look" for equal, smooth, and symmetrical excursion of the chest. It should rise and settle gently in a rhythmic manner. Inspiration should be slightly shorter in duration than expiration. If the respiratory effort varies from normal patterns, suspect chest injury.

"Listen" to identify problems deep within the chest as well as the more common sounds of upper airway restriction. Wheezes or gurgling may reflect pulmonary edema, blood in the respiratory tract, or lower airway narrowing.

"Feel" air traveling through the airway. The movement of air may not reflect the nature and extent of chest or abdominal injury, but it may at least show that the patient is breathing. Keep in mind that normal respiration is extremely quiet and unobtrusive. At the trauma scene, it can be hard to distinguish normal breathing from apnea unless you look, listen, and feel very carefully. Chest wall movement may occur despite a complete airway obstruction. It is essential to confirm air movement even when the chest is moving.

Circulation   The circulation check, made during the primary assessment, plays a key role in body cavity evaluation. Indications of hypovolemic shock—rapid and weak pulse, cool clammy skin, poor capillary refill, and a diminishing level of consciousness—may mean an internal blood loss within the chest or abdominal cavity. If these signs and symptoms are present and if you are unable to locate an external site of hemorrhage, suspect bleeding within the body cavity.

Disability   Assessment for disability (including level of consciousness) may also heighten the suspicion of chest or abdominal injury. If the patient displays restlessness, anxiety, or central nervous system depression, suspect respiratory or circulatory compromise of body cavity origin.

Expose and Examine   As assessment continues, expose the head, neck, chest, and abdomen. Be careful to protect the patient from the environment and from embarrassment of being viewed by bystanders. It is often best to cover a patient with a sheet or blanket to limit the vision of onlookers. Such a cover will also maintain body temperature and protect the patient from adverse weather.

Neck.   The neck examination may reveal jugular venous distention (JVD), secondary to either increasing intrathoracic pressure caused by a tension pneumothorax or a venous backflow resulting from pericardial tamponade, traumatic asphyxia, or heart failure (myocardial contusion). Remember that you may find JVD in the normotensive supine patient. It is a significant finding only in a patient who is otherwise hypovolemic or whose upper torso is elevated higher than 45 degrees.

The neck exam may also reveal tracheal displacement. A shift to the contralateral side may suggest tension pneumothorax. A shift to the ipsilateral side may point to an airway obstruction. Should the trachea be tugging toward one side with each inspiration, it may suggest **hemothorax** or simple (nontension) pneumothorax. Finally, the neck exam may identify subcutaneous emphysema. This finding often occurs with tension pneumothorax. Increased pressure within the thorax "pushes" air into the soft tissues, causing a crackling sensation during palpation. The air will frequently migrate upward to the neck and head.

Chest.   Examine the chest carefully for signs of external trauma. Note any contusions, abrasions, lacerations, or any penetrating wounds. Because assessment occurs so quickly after the injury, recognition of some of these signs may be difficult, if not impossible. Watch the chest's motion to determine if it is moving normally. Look for any paradoxical movement, any area that is moving less than the rest of the chest, or any retraction between the ribs, at the sternal notch or above the clavicles. Note any deformity in the thoracic cage, even if it appears to be stable and supporting normal respiration.

If you note respiratory distress, you may wish to auscultate the chest quickly to determine the effectiveness of the respiratory effort. Place the diaphragm of the stethoscope in each axilla, just above the nipple line. This location contains the least soft tissue between the skin and the lung tissue. It also lets you listen to the sounds in the distant reaches of the lung fields. If you hear normal respiratory sounds, presume that good air exchange is occurring. The sounds should be equal bilaterally. If not, you should suspect an injury or obstruction.

Abdomen.   Quickly observe and palpate the abdomen for signs of injury. Evaluate any discoloration, abrasion, laceration, evisceration, penetrating wound, or impaled object for the internal injury it may represent. Note if the

■ **hemothorax** blood within the pleural cavity.

abdomen (or any quadrant) is rigid or tender, exhibits rebound tenderness, or contains an unusual or pulsing mass. If so, you should suspect internal hemorrhage and perform further assessment later. Observe the abdomen for any signs of abnormal movement. Strong pulsation may reflect abdominal aortic aneurysm. Exaggerated abdominal wall movement with respiration may indicate lower cervical spine injury.

Evaluating the Primary Survey   With each step of the primary survey, you should identify and immediately care for any threat to life. Administer oxygen to any patient with respiratory distress or potential for shock. Protect the airway if the patient is otherwise unable to protect it. Assist respirations by bag masking the patient if he or she is unable to move adequate air due to nervous or bellows system failure. Seal any opening in the chest with an occlusive dressing, and limit the motion of any flail segment. If signs point to a developing tension pneumothorax, consider pleural decompression. Finally, if the potential for shock exists or if any signs of shock appear, treat the patient aggressively with fluid resuscitation and PASG application.

Always suspect hemorrhagic body cavity injury in any patient who suffers from the severe forces of trauma. Assess carefully for any sign or symptom forewarning of hypovolemia. After completing the primary assessment, decide whether to transport immediately or remain at the scene. If the patient has or had an altered level of consciousness or signs of respiratory or circulatory embarrassment, transport without delay. When in doubt, you should transport.

Secondary Assessment

The secondary assessment gives you the chance to examine suspected injuries determined either from the mechanism of injury or the results of the primary assessment. Even when a serious injury might call for immediate transport, completely evaluate the chest and abdomen as soon as practical. If the patient's condition does not require immediate transport, continue the head-to-toe assessment, with special emphasis on the body cavity. Reassess the head and neck and then observe, palpate, and auscultate the entire chest. Assessment should be complete and all-inclusive. Use no single sign, but several in combination, to confirm the existence of a certain injury. Perform the entire chest assessment and use all the results to identify what may be going on within. A frequent short-fall of many field care providers is to find one or two signs of a particular injury and then focus on the suspected problem. However various chest injuries, as well as many abdominal ones, present with similar signs and symptoms. If assessment is not comprehensive, you may miss the true injury.

Chest Assessment   Assess the chest completely and comprehensively. As with the primary survey, begin by observing the breathing.

Inspection.   Observe the excursion and rhythmic motion of the chest. Determine the rate of respiration and the approximate tidal volume. Multiply the two values to determine the minute volume and the relative effectiveness of the respiratory effort. Use pulse oximetry to determine if respirations are effective. (See Figure 16-9.) Maintain an oxygen saturation (SPO_2) above 94 percent when possible. If the saturation drops much below 91 percent, employ aggressive respiratory care.

Evaluate the chest carefully for discoloration or local swelling. Any developing erythema, ecchymosis, or deformity will become more visible with time. Periodic assessment ensures that the effects of delayed development do

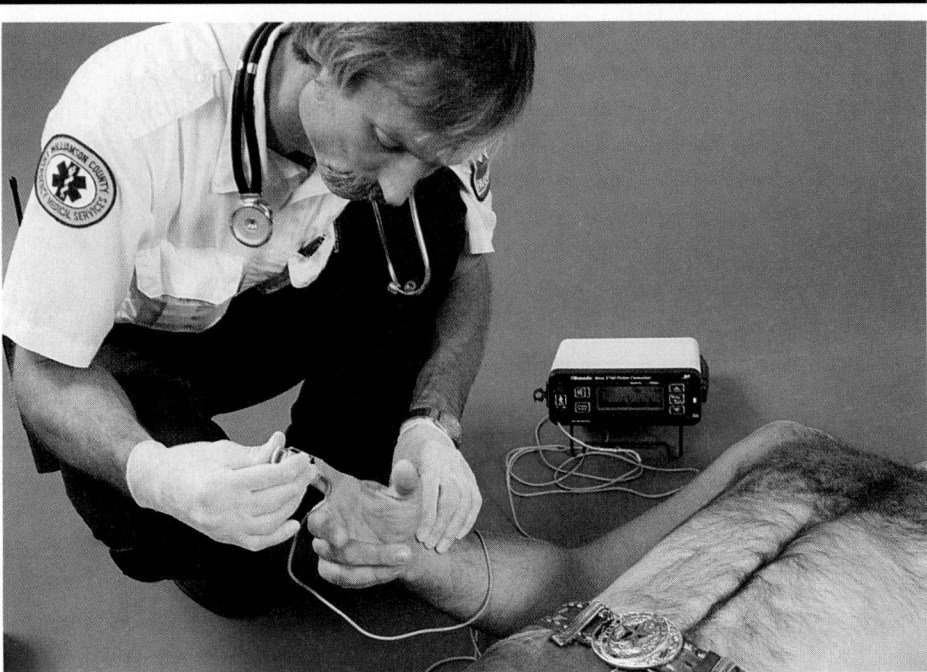

FIGURE 16-9 Pulse oximetry is effective in determining the status of oxygenation.

not go unnoticed. Direct special attention at the ribs and sternum, since the forces of trauma often trap the soft tissues between the offending object and these bony structures. If there is a penetrating wound, look for an exit wound, especially if a rifle, shotgun, or handgun was used. Examine the wound or wounds closely for air movement or frothy blood, both indicative of an open pneumothorax (sucking chest wound).

Look for other signs of respiratory distress outside the thoracic region. Any use of accessory muscles to assist the respiratory effort, such as the sterno-cleidomastoids or abdominal muscles, suggest respiratory problems. Anxiety, restlessness (especially in the presence of shock), or reduced level of consciousness hint of a possible respiratory problem. Systemic discoloration (cyanotic or ashen skin) may also be due to respiratory insufficiency.

Palpation. Palpate the entire chest. Gently localize any crepitation, subcutaneous emphysema, or deformity, and note it for the record. Place your hands on the lower borders of the patient's chest, and evaluate the motion associated with each breath. This will allow you to count respirations easily and to determine rate, regularity, and symmetry of chest excursion. If a rib fracture exists, gentle compression of the lateral chest inward should elicit pain or crepitus. (See Figure 16-10.)

Auscultation. Auscultation should evaluate the complete thorax. Listen to the anterior and posterior chest at the lung bases, apices, and axillae and at the suprasternal notch. Lung sounds should be faint, but without rales or rhonchi. Sounds should also be equal in all regions. Be especially alert to the development of fine rales in the lower fields. These may be an early sign of pulmonary edema, which is frequently associated with lung contusion. Should lung sounds be unequal, search for the cause. Identify the presence of pneumothorax, tension pneumothorax, hemothorax, localized pulmonary edema, or bronchial obstruction.

Also listen to the heart sounds. If they are displaced from the normal position, which is just left of the sternum, a tension pneumothorax may be

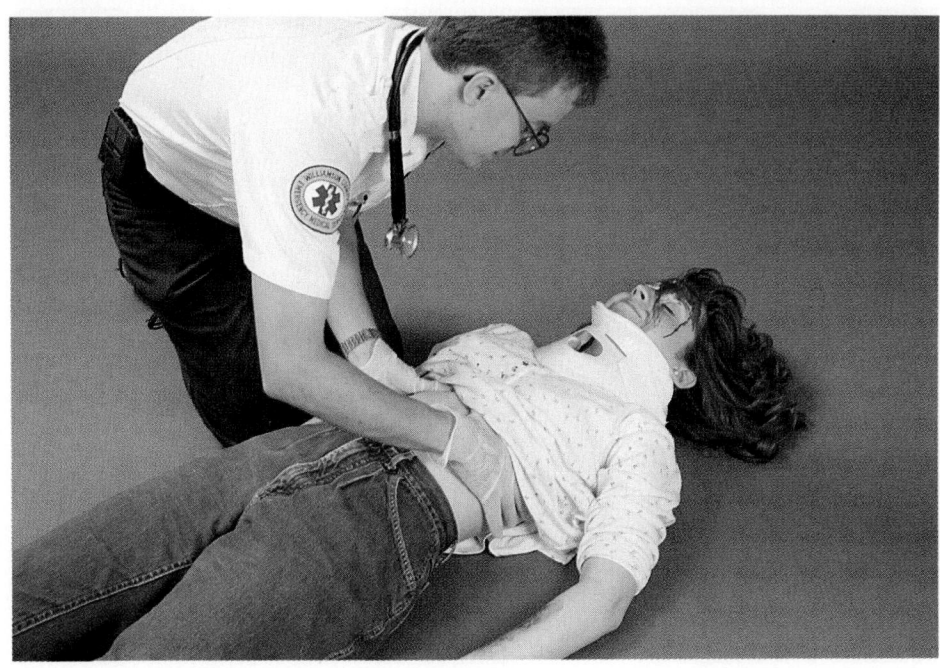

FIGURE 16-10 Palpate the chest, noting any crepitus or subcutaneous emphysema.

developing. If the heart sounds are distant and/or muffled, pericardial tamponade may be the cause. If a gallop (S_3) is heard, it may signal congestive heart failure secondary to myocardial contusion.

Percussion. Percuss the chest to assist in the confirmation of a particular injury. If chest resonance is dull, it may reflect accumulation of fluid, most likely blood, in the thorax. If the vibration is hyperresonant, there may be air under pressure within, a sign of tension pneumothorax. Check one side against the other (anterior against posterior and superior against inferior) to determine if inequality exists. Localize the absence or reduced resonance. Then determine whether it is bilateral or regional.

Abdominal Assessment The abdominal assessment should also include careful and complete observation and palpation. Remember, the abdominal area lacks the bony protection of the chest. Therefore, patients with abdominal injury may not present with overt signs and symptoms.

Inspection. Carefully remove the patient's remaining clothing so you can visualize the abdomen in its entirety. Look for any signs of discoloration or deformity as well as any sites of pulsation. (See Figure 16-11.) These signs develop over time and serial assessment may be the only way to ensure that you do not miss them.

The mechanism of injury, as well as any associated signs and symptoms, helps determine the potential for injury. It is also important to remember that the signs and symptoms of underlying problems in the abdomen progress more slowly and inconspicuously than those of chest injury. Spilling of bowel contents or blood into the peritoneal space may not manifest with pain until hours after the injury.

Palpation. Evaluate each quadrant by pushing lightly with fingers of one hand over those of the other hand. Feel for guarding, tenderness, pulsation, or masses. Release the pressure quickly, and note any discomfort (rebound ten-

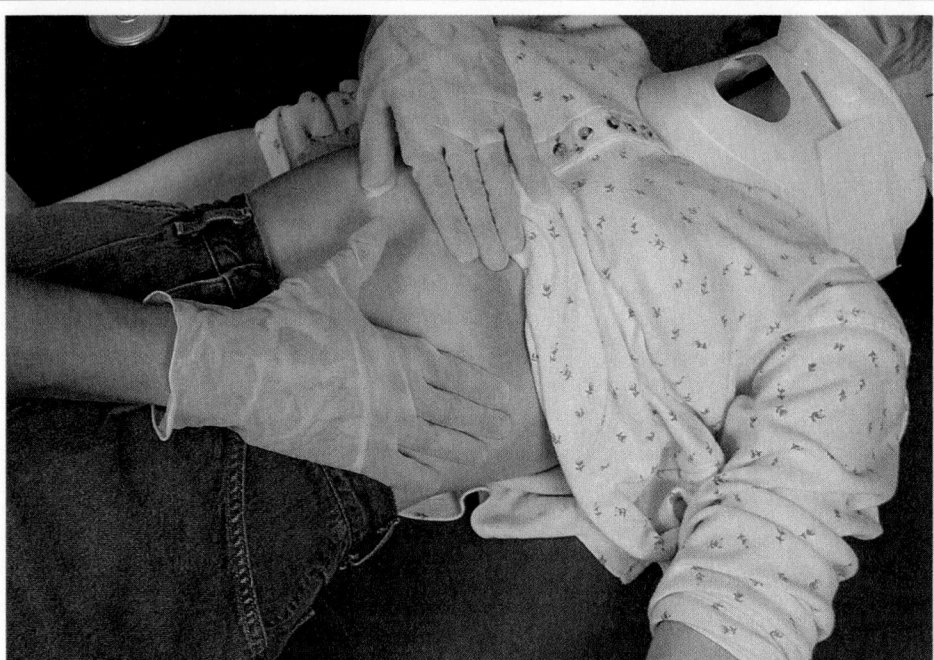

FIGURE 16-11 Note any contusions possibly indicative of serious, underlying injury.

derness). Relate any findings to the organs that lie beneath. Evaluate any other signs and symptoms in search of potential injury. Palpate the flanks and lower back. Ensure that no pain is felt on touch and that no deformities, swelling, or local warmth or coolness exist.

Vital Signs   Determination of an abdominal injury often rests less upon frank abdominal signs than upon elimination of injury and blood loss elsewhere. Therefore, careful evaluation of the rest of the patient and accurate vital signs are essential to assessment of abdominal and chest injuries.

To develop accurate vital signs, establish a baseline pulse, respiratory rate and character, and blood pressure. Then carefully monitor these signs over time to determine any trends.

Pulse. You evaluated the pulse briefly during the primary assessment. Now, carefully reassess it for signs of developing shock. A rapid thready pulse in an anxious or CNS-depressed patient may be the only early indication of chest or abdominal hemorrhage.

Blood Pressure. Blood pressure can be helpful in assessing the patient with chest or abdominal injury. The hypotension associated with shock, although a late sign, should direct attention to the source of blood loss (possibly into the body cavity). A narrowing pulse pressure (the difference between the systolic and diastolic pressure) may be a sign of pericardial tamponade. If the pulse is stronger during inspiration (*pulsus paradoxus*), it may be even more specific of tamponade. Note that pulse strength normally increases with expiration.

✳ Note that pulse strength normally increases with expiration.

Respirations. A complete evaluation of the patient's breathing may give you more information about chest trauma. Determine the exact rate and depth of respiration. Time the respirations for at least 30 seconds. Assess for regularity of breathing, and ask if the respiratory effort in any way affects any chest pain the patient feels.

Patient History   You begin developing a history as soon as you start assessment. As you evaluate the patient for symptoms of injury, note any complaint of pain, tenderness, or abnormal feeling. Palpate carefully, and elicit patient feedback. More painful, but less significant, injury elsewhere often distracts the patient. Explain to him or her that you will address the major complaint shortly, but first you must complete a thorough exam.

Thoracic Symptoms.   As you progress into the survey, focus on questions related to the thoracic area. Ask specifically if the breathing is getting easier or harder. In traumatic chest compression, the alveoli may collapse (atelectasis) and the patient may complain that "I had the wind knocked out of me." The patient will find it difficult to move air at first. As the alveoli reexpand, respiration will become less and less difficult. On the other hand, the patient may complain that it takes more and more effort to breathe. The lungs become stiff and edematous after a pulmonary contusion. Thus, the effort needed to move air becomes greater. Increased respiratory effort may also reflect an increasing pneumothorax, hemothorax, tension pneumothorax, or other progressing chest injury.

Abdominal Symptoms.   Abdominal symptoms can be very useful in determining the nature of any internal injury. Identify the exact location and type of pain experienced by the patient. Record the description carefully in the patient's own words. Determine specifically if the pain is sharp, dull, tearing, constant, periodic, or throbbing. Identify the onset and progression of any abdominal or chest pain. Did the pain begin immediately after the injury or was it delayed? If so, for how long? Is the pain growing worse, remaining the same, or getting better since the onset? Is there any position, movement, or activity that makes it either better or worse?

Document any findings and then attempt to determine whether they reflect a specific organ or multiple-organ injury. Summarize and prioritize these findings. Decide what structures within the thorax, abdomen, and pelvis may be injured. Then place the injuries in order of significance for the patient's overall condition. This will help you to identify the priorities for care.

MANAGEMENT

As patient management begins, stabilize the spine, secure the airway, and support breathing as required by the results of the primary assessment. Any significant trauma to the chest signifies vertebral injury until proven otherwise. Intubate any patient who is unable to protect the airway. All trauma patients, and especially patients with body cavity injury, should receive high-flow oxygen. If necessary, provide positive pressure ventilation, while being cautious of the injuries it may induce in the thoracic trauma patient. If the patient exhibits any early signs of shock, begin PASG application and fluid resuscitation. Start two large-bore IVs peripherally, while other members of your team prepare, apply, and inflate the PASG. Assist the infusion by using pressure infusion bags (or BP cuffs). If the abdomen shows signs of internal hemorrhage, consider inflating the abdominal compartment of the PASG, not only for its hemodynamic effect, but also for potential hemorrhage control. (Inflate the abdominal compartment only after or with inflation of the leg compartments.)

Transport immediately if the patient presents with any uncorrectable breathing or airway problem, any signs or symptoms of central nervous system depression, or any signs of developing shock. Additionally, if the mechanism of injury suggests a threat to life, transport and provide care en route.

Once you address the primary care priorities, the specific steps of body cavity injury care can begin.

Thoracic Trauma Care

Soft-Tissue Injury Care   Soft-tissue injuries of the chest are important because of the potential for injury beneath. Superficial contusions, abrasions, and minor lacerations can be cared for after the patient is completely stable. The only exception is the open chest wound. If a wound penetrates the thorax (see Figure 16-12), seal it as if it were a sucking chest wound (open pneumothorax). Cover the wound with an occlusive dressing such as petroleum gauze, a defibrillator pad, or the inside of a trauma dressing wrapper. Secure three sides with tape so any excessive intrathoracic pressure will escape, thus preventing tension pneumothorax. (See Figure 16-13.)

If you suspect any internal chest injury, place the patient on the injured side, unless otherwise contraindicated. Monitor him or her closely for tension pneumothorax or other dyspnea-inducing problems. Placing the patient on the injured side allows gravity to assist the inflation of the unaffected lung. The weight of the injured or affected lung and the mediastinum will pull downward. This ensures that the unaffected lung fully inflates with each breath.

Pain Medication   Some situations may call for the administration of pain medication. The following are two commonly prescribed drugs.

Nitronox. Within some EMS systems, protocol may suggest the use of Nitronox. This is an analgesic that may help manage the patient's pain, permitting him or her to take deeper breaths. Nitronox is a mixture of 50 percent oxygen and 50 percent nitrous oxide. The patient self-administers it through a mask arrangement. This protects a patient from receiving too much drug, thereby preventing central nervous system depression. Nitronox is a short-acting agent whose effects will subside within 2–5 minutes. Nitrous oxide has proven safe in the field setting, and you should consider it when approved by medical control.

Nitronox does have a few side effects that affect its administration in trauma. Some patients will experience nausea and possibly vomiting. Anticipate this and be prepared for it. Nitrous oxide also may increase

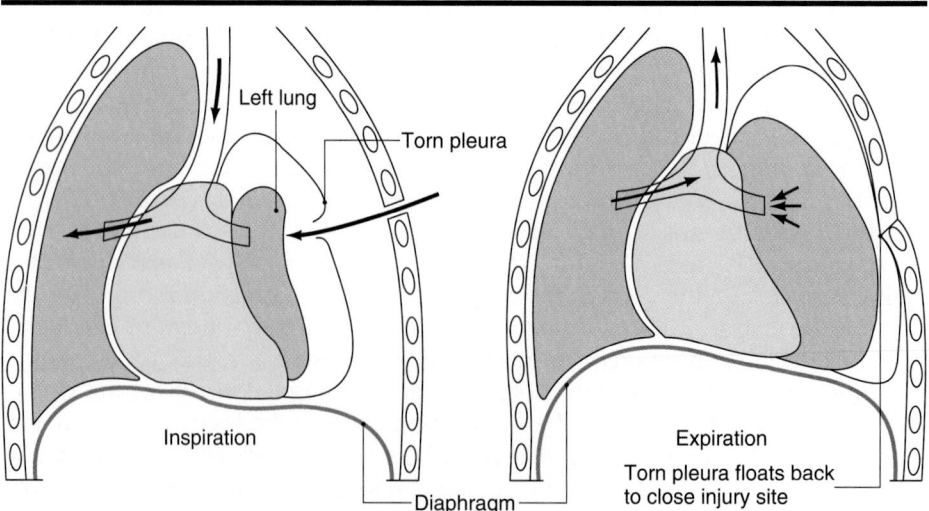

FIGURE 16-12 Sucking chest wound.

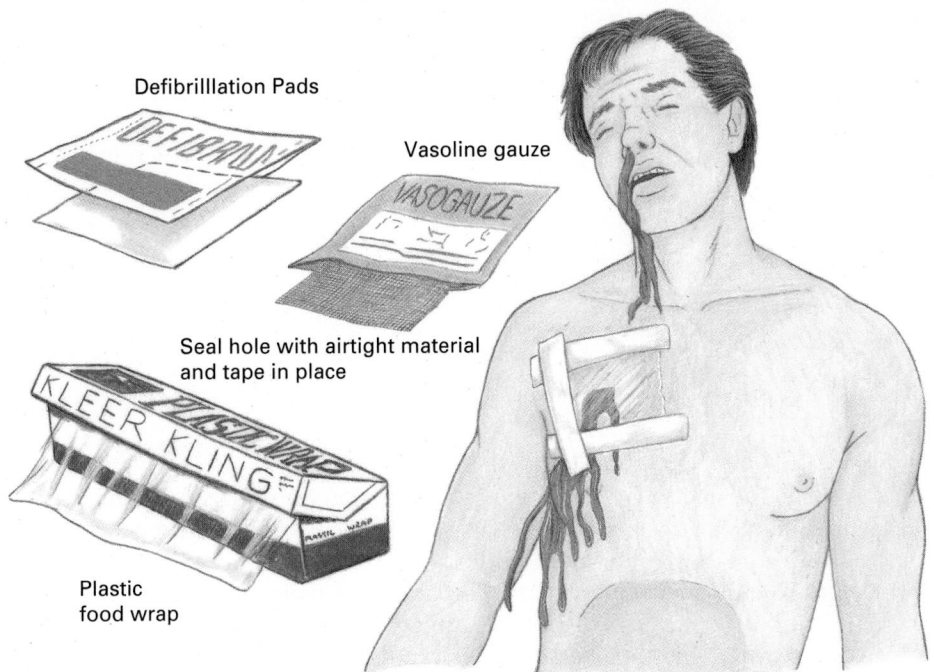

FIGURE 16-13 Prehospital treatment of a sucking chest wound should include the placement of an occlusive dressing secured on three sides.

intracranial pressure. Thus limit its use with the head injury patient. Finally, nitrous oxide will move, by diffusion, to air spaces in the body. These may include gas bubbles in an obstructed bowel or the air pocket in a pneumothorax. Exclude possible pneumothorax before you consider Nitronox for a chest injury patient.

Morphine Sulfate. You may also consider morphine sulfate for the chest injury patient. It may be an effective agent in reducing the pain of rib fracture and helping the patient breathe more deeply. However, morphine is also a respiratory depressant. It may reduce your patient's drive to breathe and lead to hypoventilation. Do not use morphine sulfate in patients with possible abdominal injury. It may mask the signs and symptoms of that injury, making it all but impossible for the emergency department staff to determine the source of the problem.

Flail Chest Care   Extensive rib fractures may result in paradoxical chest wall motion and need special care. Flail chest severely compromises respiration as air moves from under the flail segment into the unaffected lung regions and then back again. It is essential that you stop the paradoxical motion and this ineffective air exchange. Apply gentle pressure, as with a bulky trauma pad or pillow, to inhibit the outward excursion of the segment. (See Figure 16-14.)

Use positive pressure ventilation to assist breathing for the patient. This will reverse the operation of the bellows system and help negate the motion of the flail segment. The positive pressure you create by squeezing the device or the bag valve mask forces air into the chest and pushes both the normal chest wall and the flail segment outward. Passive exhalation permits both the flail segment and the normal chest wall to move inward. This external-powered respiration gets the flail segment and the normal chest wall working in

✳ Nitronox should not be used in cases of pneumothorax or in instances where bowel obstruction is possible.

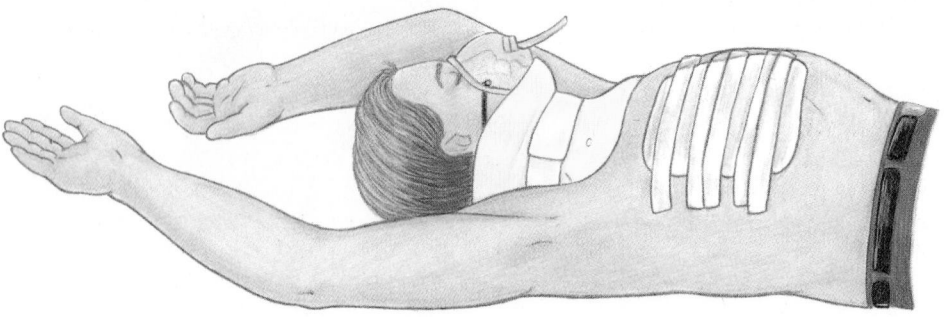

FIGURE 16-14 Flail chest should be treated with oxygen and gentle splinting of the flail segment with a pillow or a pad.

Tape pad in place, extending tape to both sides of chest

unison again. The conscious patient with spontaneous breathing may resist your attempts to assist respirations. This will usually abate once you accomplish effective air exchange and diminish the pain associated with respiration. It is helpful if the patient can signal when he or she feels the need for a breath.

Be careful in the use of positive pressure ventilation for any significant chest trauma as it may exacerbate injury to the pulmonary tissues, possibly beneath the flail segment. The bag-valve device may increase the incidence of associated pneumothorax and tension pneumothorax. It is rare that you will be called upon to use the demand valve to assist the chest trauma patient. Its high-pressure inspiration significantly increases the incidence of simple and tension pneumothorax.

Traumatic Asphyxia Care   The final trauma-induced chest wall defect is *traumatic asphyxia*. Prepare to transport any patient with this problem to the hospital rapidly. Administer aggressive care during extrication and while en route. Anticipate the rapid development of hypovolemia as you release the chest compression. Remember that the pressure compressing the chest and limiting respiration may also tamponade hemorrhage. Once you release compression, the patient may bleed internally and exsanguinate. Initiate two IV access lines with large-bore catheters and trauma tubing. Prepare to run two 1000 mL bags of either normal saline or lactated Ringer's solution with pressure infusion. Prepare, apply, and be ready to inflate the PASG. Provide 100 percent oxygen by nonrebreather or bag-valve-mask and be ready to intubate the patient if unconsciousness ensues. Be prepared for this patient to deteriorate rapidly to trauma arrest.

Sodium Bicarbonate. Medical control may order sodium bicarbonate for potential acidosis caused by traumatic asphyxia. Prolonged hypoxia followed by the release of chest compression may cause acidotic blood to return to the central circulation. Bicarbonate will counteract this problem by buffering the shift of the blood's pH. It will bind to the free hydrogen ions and form water and carbon dioxide, thus bringing the acidity of the blood more toward normal. Use it only when the hypoxia has been present for more than 10 minutes. Administer it via IV bolus at a dosage of 1 mEq per kilogram of body weight during or shortly after the decompression of the patient's chest.

Use great care in administering this drug as it will place a high concentration of sodium ions in the vascular space, thus increasing the risk for systemic and pulmonary edema. (Edema is more of a concern in the overhydrated or CHF patient than in one suffering from hypovolemia.) The alkalizing effects of bicarbonate may also reduce the effectiveness of the catecholamines you may use in cardiac arrest or protracted hypotension. Guide any administration of sodium bicarbonate by protocol and medical control.

Tension Pneumothorax Care   If you suspect a closed pneumothorax or have sealed an open pneumothorax, frequently evaluate the patient for the signs and symptoms of tension pneumothorax. Look specifically for any tracheal displacement, unequal breath sounds, jugular vein distention, or unusual response to percussion. Be especially alert for any increasing dyspnea or drop in the patient's level of consciousness or level of orientation.

Tension pneumothorax is a serious, life-threatening insult to the respiratory and cardiovascular system. If it is present, relieve the pressure quickly by needle decompression, when protocol permits. There are two field approaches to pleura decompression. The first is the midclavicular approach. Approximate the second or third intercostal space at the midclavicular line. Locate the middle of the clavicle on the affected side and move the fingers down to the first or second intercostal space. The second site is the midaxillary line at or around the fifth intercostal space. Locate the intersection of the midaxillary and nipple line, and palpate the nearest intercostal groove.

At either location, insert a large bore (10–14 gauge) over-the-needle catheter just above the lower rib at a 90-degree angle. Advance the needle until you hear the sound of escaping air. (See Figure 16-15.) At this point, advance the catheter and remove the needle. Secure the hub of the catheter with tape and cover it with a finger of a rubber glove. Tie or tape the glove finger securely around the hub. Cut the finger tip to allow air to escape and not reenter. (See Figure 16-16.)

Once you relieve the tension pneumothorax, monitor the patient frequently for redevelopment of the emergency. The catheter may become blocked or kinked, allowing the chest to repressurize. It may be necessary to decompress the chest by inserting another needle close to the original site.

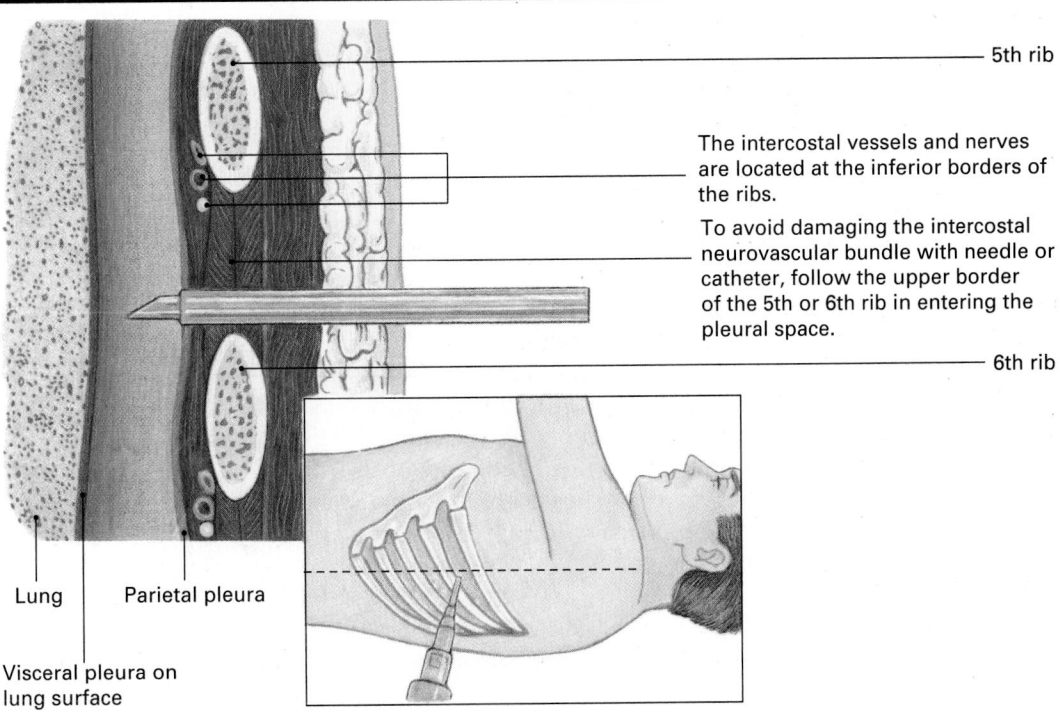

5th rib

The intercostal vessels and nerves are located at the inferior borders of the ribs.

To avoid damaging the intercostal neurovascular bundle with needle or catheter, follow the upper border of the 5th or 6th rib in entering the pleural space.

6th rib

Lung   Parietal pleura

Visceral pleura on lung surface

FIGURE 16-15   Needle decompression of a tension pneumothorax.

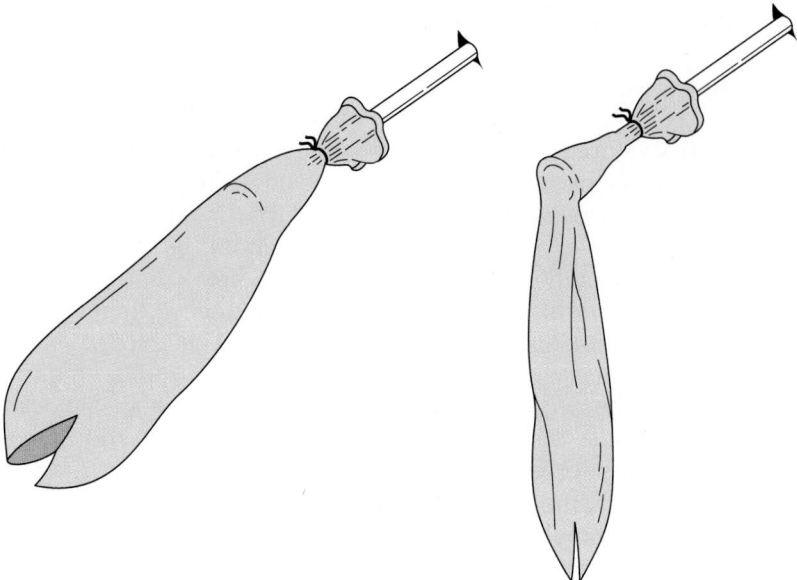

FIGURE 16-16 One-way valve constructed out of the finger of a latex glove.

Cardiac Contusion Care   Treat the cardiac contusion patient as aggressively as you would the patient with myocardial infarction. Implement cardiac protocols (to be discussed in Chapter 21) as appropriate, including oxygen, lidocaine, bretylium, procainamide, and atropine.

Pericardial Tamponade Care   Pericardial tamponade is a dire emergency rarely correctable in the field setting. The procedure to relieve the pressure within the pericardial sac (pericardiocentesis) is extremely difficult under the best of conditions and carries extreme hazards for the patient. (See Figure 16-17.) In the process, the care provider inserts a large bore spinal needle into the pericardial sac and aspirates the blood that restricts cardiac filling. However, if the needle penetrates the myocardium, the resulting hole may permit a rapid redevelopment of the injury. Unless you have specific training and are permitted to attempt this procedure by protocol, package the patient and transport immediately.

Traumatic Aortic Aneurysm Care   Any patient you suspect of suffering traumatic aortic aneurysm should receive rapid and gentle transport to definitive care. Bouncing, sudden movement, or an increase in blood pressure, such as that caused by anxiety, may cause the injury to progress or rupture. Although you must maintain good perfusion, treat shock conservatively. Obtain any blood pressure measurement using the right, upper extremity or one of the lower extremities. An attempt to obtain a blood pressure through use of the left, upper extremity may cause additional back pressure on the aneurysm, thus increasing the likelihood of its rupture. The patient should receive two large bore IV sites with 1,000 milliliter solution bags readied for infusion. If the aneurysm should rupture, the patient will need very rapid fluid resuscitation.

Impaled Object Care   If an object is found to be impaled in the chest, immobilize it as you find it. Cover the entry wound with an occlusive dressing and a bulky dressing. Completely stabilize the object so patient transport will not cause the object to move or dislodge. If the object is very large or

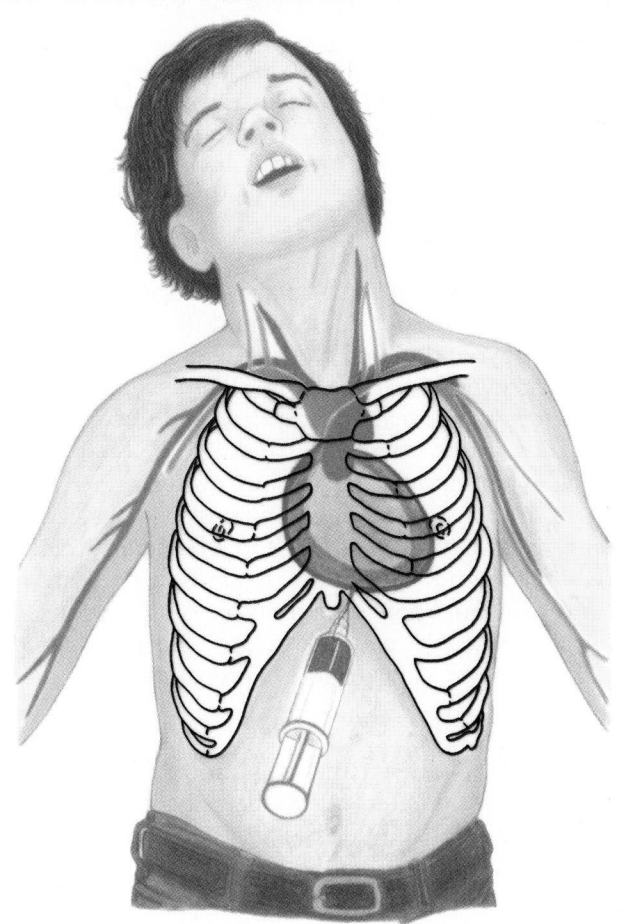

FIGURE 16-17 Technique for pericardiocentesis.

unwieldy, attempt to cut it. Fully immobilize the object prior to and during efforts to shorten it. Remove the object only if it interferes with attempts to perform CPR in the cardiopulmonary arrest patient. Its removal may increase internal bleeding and further contribute to hypovolemia.

Abdominal Trauma Care

Direct care of the patient with suspected abdominal trauma in anticipation of internal hemorrhage and the need for rapid surgery. Immediately transport the patient with any significant signs, symptoms, or mechanism of injury that suggests internal bleeding. While en route to the emergency department, insert two large bore catheters and start IV fluids. Apply the PASG and be ready for inflation. Evaluate vital signs frequently, along with other signs possibly indicating the early development of shock. These signs include capillary refill, blood pressure, skin color, patient anxiety or restlessness, and pulse rate and strength.

* The primary consideration in the management of the abdominal trauma patient is to determine that an abdominal injury exists. The exact injury is less important than developing a reasonable suspicion of trauma.

In the presence of any significant sign or symptom of shock, it is imperative to provide aggressive fluid replacement to the abdominal trauma patient. Rapid blood loss can result from various sources and leave the patient with irreversible shock if you do not treat early. The crystalloid solutions you use in the field will only remain in the vascular space for a short period. Thus, for every milliliter of blood lost, you must infuse three milliliters of IV fluid. If the patient has lost 500 mL of blood preceding your arrival, he or she needs 1,500 mL of fluids immediately and three times the blood volume lost during each minute thereafter.

If you delay care until the signs and symptoms of shock are obviously apparent, it may be necessary to infuse more fluid than possible in the field setting. The patient should receive aggressive fluid resuscitation en route to the hospital and blood replacement once there. After you have taken emergency measures aimed at preventing or treating shock, you can begin care for the specific abdominal injuries.

Penetrating Abdominal Injury Care   Cover penetrating wounds of the abdominal cavity, as you would with any open wound. If it appears that the bowel is protruding, cover the wound with a wet sterile dressing and then an occlusive dressing. The occlusive dressing ensures that the tissues will remain moist. It will also provide a barrier against evaporation and contamination. If an object remains impaled in the abdomen, carefully immobilize it in place. Restrain the hands of a patient with either an evisceration or an impaled object to prevent them from manipulating the wound.

If you find a penetrating wound caused by a rifle or handgun, examine the patient for an exit wound. If found, dress both wounds with occlusive dressing as a measure to prevent an open pneumothorax. If a projectile expends all its energy within the patient, it may not emerge. Realize that you cannot anticipate the complete pathway of damage. So prepare to treat internal and severe hemorrhage.

Blunt Abdominal Injury Care   Care for the blunt abdominal injury is basically supportive. Unless otherwise required, place the patient in the most comfortable position, usually on the side, and flex the legs. Then transport the patient to a trauma center as rapidly and as smoothly as possible. Jarring may increase both the patient's discomfort and the rate of hemorrhage.

SUMMARY

Injury to the body cavity and the structures within is a frequent cause of serious injury and patient death. In response to this type of trauma, provide aggressive assessment, care, and transport. Evaluate the mechanism of injury, and determine various indices of suspicion for specific chest and abdominal injury. Through the primary survey, look for immediate life threats and correct them as found. If there is any reason to suspect serious internal injury, perform only a quick primary assessment and transport the patient immediately. Otherwise, provide more intensive field assessment and care. Assess the chest and abdomen carefully during the physical assessment, looking for the subtle signs of injury. Evaluate the patient's history and symptoms as well as the vital signs to continue your search for body cavity injury. Ensure that your focus remains on total patient care.

Injury to the chest and abdomen account for a very high percentage of trauma deaths. Therefore, you should have a high index of suspicion for injury to this region and prepare for aggressive intervention. Such an approach will give emergency medical service its best opportunity to reduce patient mortality and morbidity.

FURTHER READING

American College of Surgeons, Committee on Trauma. *Advanced Trauma Life Support Course: Student Manual.* American College of Surgeons, 1989.

Bledsoe, B.E. *Atlas of Paramedic Skills.* Englewood Cliffs, NJ: Prentice-Hall, Inc., 1987.

Butman, A.M., and J.L. Paturas. *Pre-Hospital Trauma Life Support.* Akron, OH: Emergency Training, 1986.

Campbell, J.E. *Basic Trauma Life Support,* 2d. ed., Englewood Cliffs, NJ: Prentice-Hall, Inc., 1988.

Hardaway, R.M. *Shock—The Reversible Stage of Dying.* Littleton, MA: PSG Publishing Company, Inc., 1988.

Jastremski, M.S., M. Dumas, and L. Penalver. *Emergency Procedures.* Philadelphia, PA: W. B. Saunders Company, 1992.

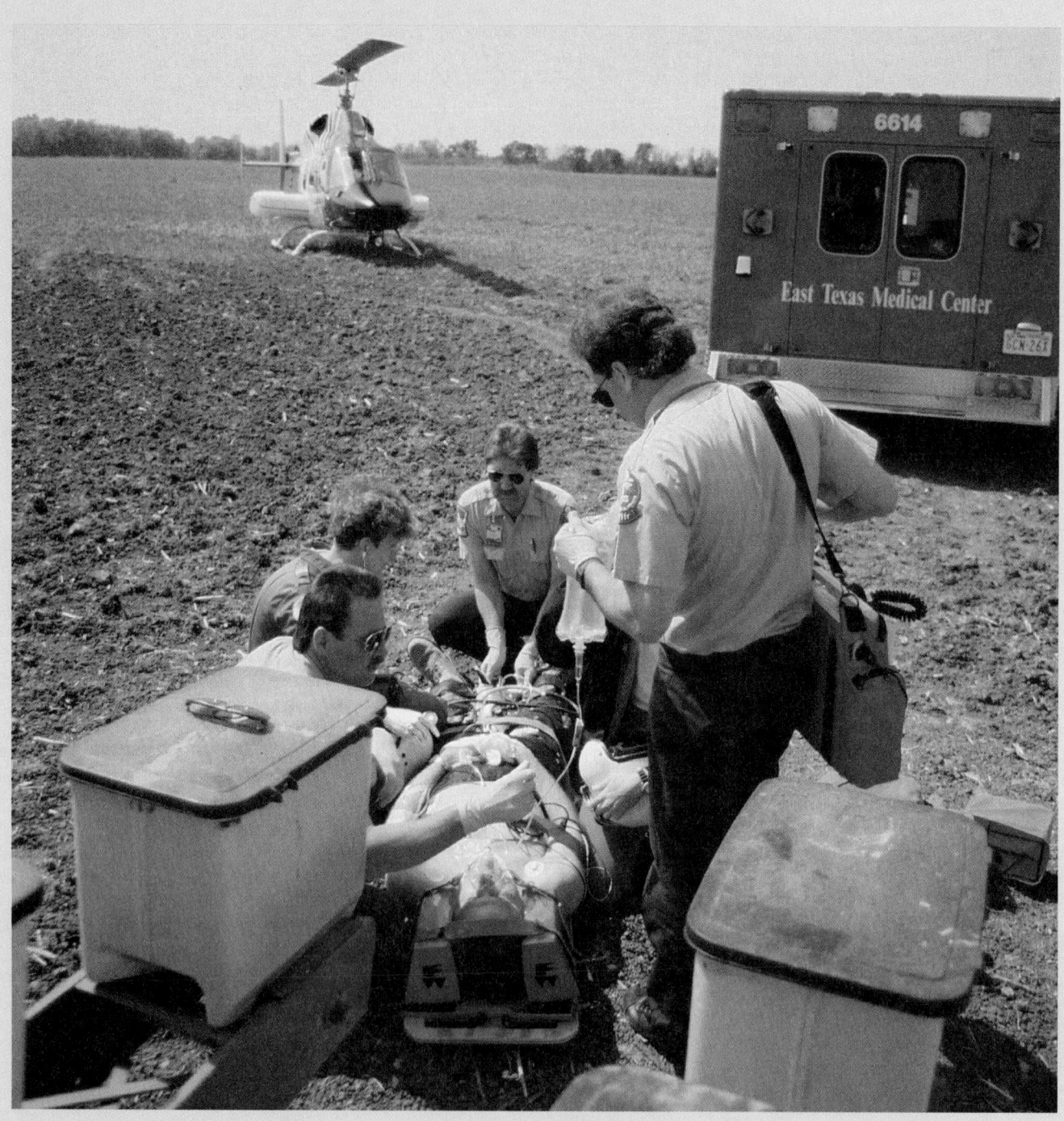

17

MUSCULOSKELETAL INJURIES

Objectives for Chapter 17

After reading this chapter, you should be able to:

1. Identify the bones of the extremities, and describe their general structure. (See p. 504.)

2. Describe the structure, attachment, and general action of the muscles of the extremities. (See pp. 505–506.)

3. Compare and contrast strains, sprains, subluxations, dislocations, and fractures. (See pp. 506–510.)

4. List the signs and symptoms normally associated with musculoskeletal injury, and describe their relative importance to the patient assessment process. (See pp. 513–515.)

5. Order and describe the steps of assessment for trauma patients as they apply to various extremity injuries. (See pp. 513–515)

6. Describe the signs and symptoms of circulatory or nervous loss to a distal extremity, and identify the steps taken to correct this deficit. (See pp. 515–517.)

7. Explain fracture or dislocation immobilization techniques for the following locations: pelvis, hip, femur, knee, tibia and fibula, ankle, foot, shoulder, humerus, elbow, radius and ulna, wrist, hand, and finger. (See pp. 517–519.)

The dispatch center sends Unit 93 to a local nursing home to pick up a patient who has fallen out of bed. Upon arrival, the paramedics find the patient lying on a hallway floor. The 85-year-old female resident explains that she fell while walking to the recreation hall. She denies vertigo or any other symptoms either now or prior to the fall. Physical assessment by the paramedics determines that her pain is limited to the thigh area. The patient also explains that she felt a snap as her hip gave way and she fell. Further physical assessment reveals an angulated left thigh, crepitation, and instability beyond the hip joint. The attending nurse states that Mrs. Jones rarely complains and has had few medical problems. Her medications include an oral hypoglycemic agent or a diuretic.

Evaluation of vital signs reveals a blood pressure of 110/90, a pulse of 90, and respirations of normal depth and at a rate of 22. The elderly patient's hands and unaffected leg are moist and cool, while the leg with the injury is very cold. During palpation of the distal pulse, the senior paramedic finds it to be diminished when compared to the right leg. She places the patient on moderate-flow oxygen and notices that oximetry shows a saturation of 96 percent.

Next, paramedics gently move the patient to a spineboard via an orthopedic stretcher. Once in the ambulance, they start an intravenous line, hang normal saline, and set it to run at a "to-keep-open" rate. A dextrose stick indicates the patient's glucose to be 120 mg/dl. Paramedics transport her uneventfully to the emergency department. Here X-rays confirm a hip fracture. Due to her age, the patient spends several weeks in the hospital and then several months ambulating in the nursing home.

INTRODUCTION

Musculoskeletal injuries occur second only to soft-tissue injuries. They usually result from direct or transmitted kinetic forces. However, they may occasionally be caused by penetrating insult. While most musculoskeletal injuries do not require more than basic care, you must apply these basic skills properly to ensure that no harm occurs during care and transport.

Assessment and care of musculoskeletal injuries for the unstable patient differs from that of the stable patient. You will provide unstable patients with immediate transport, directing your care at emergent life support. Management will not include the detailed and time-consuming splinting process. However, you still must consider possible musculoskeletal injuries when choosing movement and packaging techniques for unstable patients.

You will provide the stable patient with an isolated long bone injury, or who is moderately injured, with complete assessment and immobilization of any injured area. Assess any injury carefully to ensure that circulation, motor control, and sensation remain intact during immobilization and transport. Affix the injury site in a physiologic position to allow the greatest comfort, adequate circulation, and efficient immobilization. Stabilize adjacent joints to prevent motion from being transmitted to, or through, the injury site. If you meet these objectives, you will ensure that your patients receive optimal stabilization of their suspected injuries.

To respond properly to musculoskeletal emergencies, you must maintain and build upon the knowledge and skills of the Basic EMT. In addition to these basic skills, you will need a deeper understanding of the structure and function of the musculoskeletal system, knowledge of the process and progression of injury, and a complete grasp of the assessment and care modalities that these injuries require.

ANATOMY AND PHYSIOLOGY

The musculoskeletal system is a complex system of levers and fulcrums that provide motion and support for the body. It consists of two distinct subsystems: the *skeleton* and the *muscles*. The skeleton is the superstructure of the human body, while the muscles supply the power of motion to the superstructure and various organs.

The Skeleton

A total of 206 bones comprise the skeleton. (See Figure 17-1.) As the body's living framework, the skeleton provides many functions. Also, like other systems, it has many components that enable motion.

Purpose   Besides acting as the body's structural form, the skeleton serves several other important purposes. First, the skeleton protects the vital organs. Second, it allows us to move about efficiently against the forces of gravity. Third, the skeleton stores many salts and other materials needed for metabolism. Finally, it is responsible for producing the red blood cells used to transport oxygen.

Although the skeleton is not often thought of as alive, it is exactly that. Its cells are alive and living in a matrix of protein fibers and salt deposits. These living cells are constantly changing the structure and dynamics of the human frame.

A continuous supply of blood brings the bones oxygen and nutrients and removes carbon dioxide and waste products. As with any body tissue, if the blood supply is damaged or lost, bone tissue will become ischemic and die. The bone will not show evidence of this degeneration during emergency care. However, the effects may be devastating afterwards.

General Structure   Numerous bones make up the framework of the body. They are divided into two major subdivisions: the axial and the appendicular skeletons. The *axial skeleton* consists of the skull, the vertebral column, and the thorax. The components of this subdivision have been discussed in Chapters 15 and 16. The *appendicular skeleton* consists of the shoulder girdle and bones of the upper extremity and the pelvis and bones of the lower extremity.

Extremity Long Bones. The extremity long bones are similar in design and structure. Both upper and lower extremities affix to the axial skeleton and **articulate** with joints supported by several bones. Each has a single long bone proximally and paired bones distally. The terminal member (the hand or the foot) is made up of numerous bones with differing purposes, yet parallel design.

■ **articulate** to join together and permit motion.

The long bones in both the upper and lower extremities also consist of three regions, differing in anatomy and purpose. (See Figure 17-2.) The **diaphysis** is the long narrow cylinder or shaft of the bone. The articular and widened end is the **epiphysis**. Between the two is the **metaphysis**, which transitions from the hollow support member to the articular end. Below are descriptions of the main components of the long bones.

■ **diaphysis** hollow shaft of the long bones.

■ **epiphysis** ends of the long bone, including the epiphyseal, or growth plate, and support structures underlying the joint.

❑ *The Diaphysis.* The diaphysis is the central portion of the long bone. It consists of dense, compact bone. However, the actual weight-bearing portion of the shaft is a very thin and light hollow tube. Its interior is filled with *yellow bone marrow* that stores fat in a semi-liquid form. The fat is a readily available energy source that the body can quickly and easily use.

■ **metaphysis** growth zone of the bone, active during the development stages of youth. It is located between the epiphysis and the diaphysis.

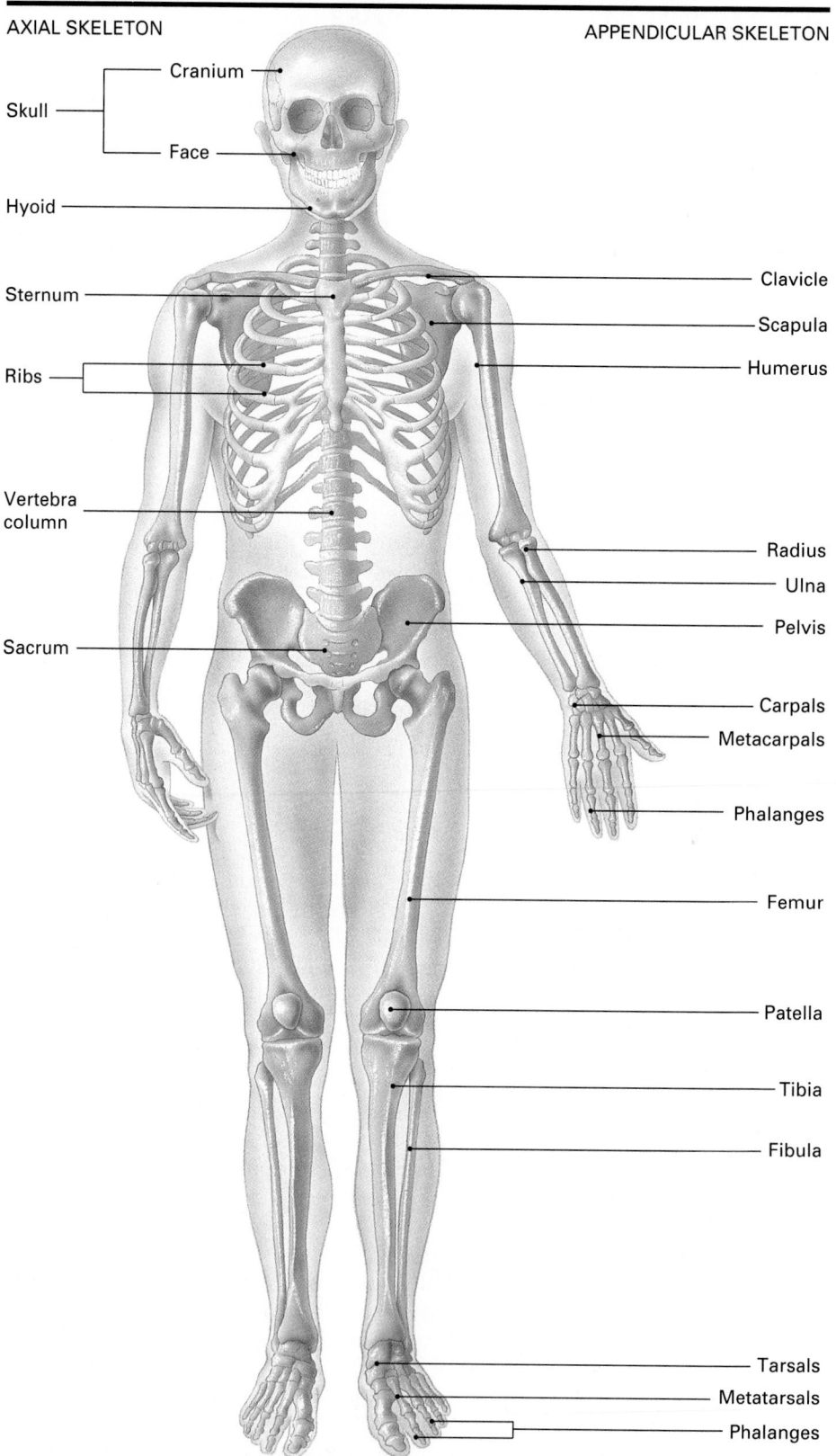

FIGURE 17-1   The human skeleton.

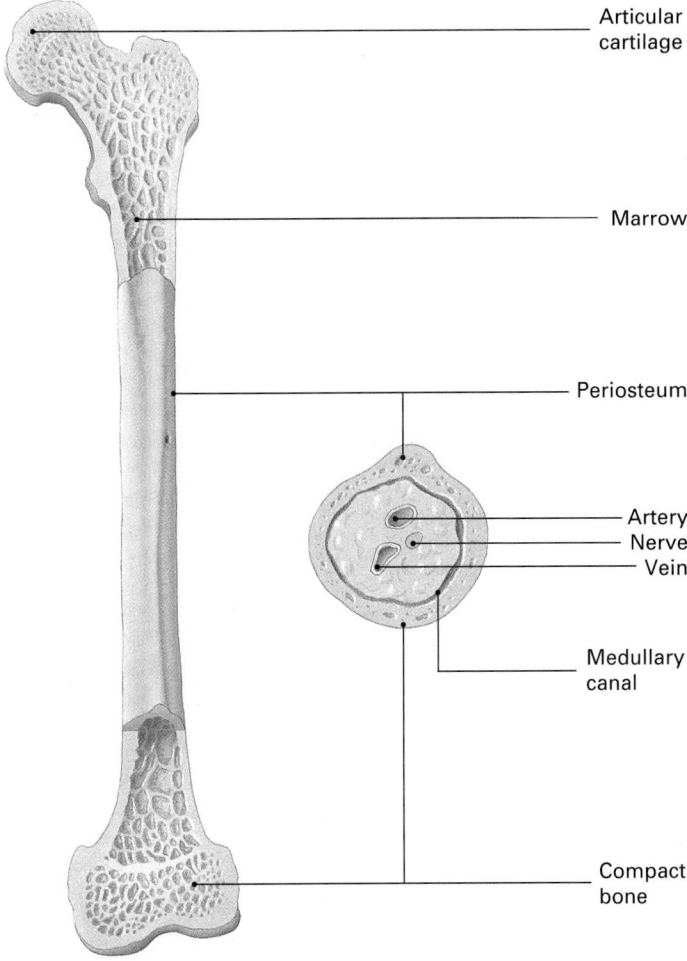

Articular cartilage

Marrow

Periosteum

Artery
Nerve
Vein

Medullary canal

Compact bone

FIGURE 17-2 The internal anatomy of a long bone.

❑ *The Periosteum.* The exterior of the diaphysis is covered with a tough membrane called the **periosteum**. Vascular and innervated, it initiates the repair cycle when the bone fractures. Blood vessels and nerves penetrate both the periosteum and compact bone by traveling through small passages called **haversian canals**. These canals allow the essential blood to pass into the interior and circulate to the bone ends.

❑ *The Epiphysis.* Toward the epiphysis, the bone structure changes dramatically. The hard, compact bone of the shaft changes into a network of fibers and strands. This network serves to spread the stress and pressure of support over a larger surface. The tissue in cross-section resembles a rigid bony sponge (**cancellous bone**). Covering this network of fibers is a thin layer of compact bone supporting the articular surface. *Red bone marrow* fills the chambers of the cancellous bone of the larger long bones and is responsible for the manufacture of erythrocytes.

❑ *The Metaphysis.* The *metaphysis* is an intermediate region between the epiphysis and diaphysis. It expands the dense, thin, and solid hollow tube of the diaphysis into the cancellous honeycomb of the epiphysis.

Cartilage. A layer of connective tissue, called **cartilage** covers the epiphyseal surface. It is a smooth, strong, and flexible material that functions as the

■ **periosteum** tough, hard covering of bone.

■ **haversian canals** small perforations of the long bones through which the blood vessels and nerves travel into the bone itself.

■ **cancellous bone** spongy bone tissue found at the distal and proximal ends of the long bones.

■ **cartilage** connective tissue providing the articular surfaces of the skeletal system.

actual surface of articulation between bones. The cartilage allows for very easy movement between the ends of adjacent bones such as the femur and tibia. This tissue also absorbs some of the impact associated with walking, running, or any jarring activity.

Joints and Ligaments. The bones are held together by a relatively sophisticated structure, the *joint*. **Ligaments**, which are connective tissue bands, hold the joints together. They stretch and permit joint motion, while holding the bone ends firmly in place. The ends of the ligaments attach to the joint end of each of the associated bones. Ligaments surround the articular region and cross it at many oblique angles. This arrangement ensures that the joint is held strongly together yet is flexible enough to move through the designed range of motion.

The ligaments surrounding a joint form what is known as the **synovial** capsule. This chamber holds a small amount of fluid to lubricate the articular surfaces. This oily, viscous fluid assists joint motion by reducing friction.

Upper Extremity

Each upper extremity consists of the shoulder girdle, arm, forearm, and hand. The shoulder is composed of the clavicle and scapula, which sit high on the thoracic cage. The scapula is an irregularly-shaped bone located posteriorly and buried within the musculature of the upper back. It provides the glenoid depression, or *fossa*. This shallow socket holds the humerus. The scapula moves freely over the posterior thorax, providing some of the shoulder's large range of motion. The upper-back musculature effectively protects the scapula from fracture in all but the most direct and severe trauma.

The clavicle is anterior to the scapula and is not as well protected. It holds the scapula and shoulder joint at a fixed distance from the sternum. The clavicle frequently fractures. It is, in fact, the most commonly fractured bone of the human body.

The humerus is the single bone of the proximal upper extremity. (This region is properly referred to as the arm.) It is secured against the shallow glenoid fossa of the shoulder joint proximally. The humerus articulates with the radius and ulna at the elbow.

The radius and ulna form the forearm. They move in conjunction with the humerus and with each other. This articulation provides the ability to rotate the distal forearm to the palm up (**supination**) or palm down (**pronation**) position. It simultaneously allows for folding of the elbow. The radius is on the thumb side of the forearm.

The radius and ulna articulate with the carpal bones of the wrist. They, in turn, articulate with the metacarpals of the palm of the hand. The metacarpals articulate with the phalanges of the fingers. Each finger consists of three phalanges: the proximal, the middle, and the distal. The thumb has only two: the proximal and distal.

Lower Extremity

Each lower extremity is comprised of the pelvis, thigh, leg, and foot. The pelvis supports and allows much of the motion of the lower extremity. A pair of fused bones and the sacrum compose the pelvis. The pubis, ilium, and iliac join collectively, making up the innominates. The two innominates, together with the sacrum, form the pelvic ring. This rigid ring is very strong and provides the basis for movement of the lower extremities and support when standing. The actual articular surface for the femur is the *acetabulum*. It is a hollow depression in the lateral pelvis into which the head of the femur fits.

The femur is the largest and strongest of the long bones. During the normal stress of walking, it often withstands pressure up to 1,200 pounds per square inch along its diaphysis. With such strength, a fracture of the femur must involve tremendous force. Therefore, it probably will cause other related soft-tissue, vascular, or nervous injury.

The femur is not a straight long bone. At its superior end, where the head meets the acetabulum, the femur makes an almost 90-degree turn. The head is supported by the neck, a narrow shaft, at almost a right angle to the upper-most aspect of the widened femoral shaft. This configuration permits the wide range of motion found in the joint and accounts for the femur's great strength.

Meeting the femur distally is the tibia. It pairs with the fibula, a smaller, much more delicate bone. The tibia is the only bone of the lower leg that articulates with the femur. Since the fibula does not, its only function is to add control to the placement and motion of the foot during walking or other ambulation.

Both the tibia and fibula join the talus and calcaneus to form the ankle. The tibia forms the medial malleolus (protuberance of the ankle), while the fibula forms the lateral malleolus. In turn, the talus articulates with the tarsals. The tarsals, in turn, articulate with the metatarsals. Both articulate with the pha-langes of the foot, in a parallel configuration to the bones of the wrist and hand.

The Muscular System

More than 600 muscle groups make up the muscular system. As you might expect, a large number of EMS calls involve injuries to this extensive system.

Purpose The muscles of the body can be divided into three main types. Of these, the most specialized is the myocardium—a very specific and unique tissue. The myocardium is the muscle of the heart. It contracts rhythmically on its own, emitting an electrical impulse in the process. In this way, it provides the lifelong rhythmic contraction and pumping function of the heart. (The par-ticular properties of the myocardium are discussed in Chapter 21.)

The second type of muscle is *smooth muscle*. These muscles are not under conscious control. We find them within the vascular system, the bronchioles, the bowel, and in many other organs. The autonomic nervous system controls them. Smooth muscle contracts to reduce (or relaxes to expand) the diameter of the lumen of the blood vessels, the bronchioles, or the digestive tract.

The remaining type of muscle tissue is *skeletal muscle*. Skeletal muscles are muscles over which we have conscious control. The skeletal muscles are associated with mobility of the extremities and the body in general. The largest component of the muscular system, they are the muscles most com-monly traumatized.

Structure The skeletal muscles lie beneath the protective layer of the skin and subcutaneous fat. Like other tissues, they have an ample supply of blood vessels and nerves. Individual muscle fibers layer together to form a muscle body, such as the triceps.

Skeletal muscles attach to the bones at a minimum of two locations. These attachments are called the origin and the insertion, depending upon how the bones move with contraction. The point of attachment that remains stationary is the **origin**, while the point that moves is the **insertion**.

Tendons are specialized connective tissue bands that accomplish the insertion and, in some cases, the origin. These very fibrous ribbons, actually a part of the muscle, are extremely strong and will not stretch. They are so strong that in some instances they will break an area of bone loose rather than tear. The Achilles tendon demonstrates the strength of this particular tis-sue. It can be felt as the band posterior to the malleoli of the ankle. This ten-don is the muscle-controlled cord that allows us to lift the entire body weight and stand on our toes. Muscles usually pair, one on each side of a joint. This

■ **origin** attachment of a muscle to the bone that does not move (or experiences the least movement) when the muscle contracts.

■ **insertion** attachment of a muscle to the bone that moves when the muscle contracts.

■ **tendon** band of connective tissue that attaches muscle to bone

configuration is essential because the muscle is only able to shorten with force. One muscle mass will move the extremity in one direction by contraction, while the opposing mass stretches. The opposing mass can then contract, stretching the opposite muscle and moving the extremity in the opposite direction. This arrangement causes the straightening of the limb (called *extension*) and then the bending at the joint (called *flexion*).

By adding more individual muscles to a joint, with different origins and insertions, the body can control a wide variety of motion. The shoulder demonstrates this relationship. The shoulder muscles permit the humerus various degrees of motion. These include moving the extremity away from the body (**abduction**) or toward the body (**adduction**), as well as rotating the humerus at the elbow through about 60 degrees or circling the entire extremity through a 180-degree arch.

The forearm demonstrates the sophistication of the muscle-tendon relationship. As the anterior muscles controlling the fingers contract, you can feel them tensing in the forearm, while the fingers flex. You can visualize and palpate the movement of the tendons in the distal forearm and wrist as the fingers flex and extend. It is easy to appreciate the damage a deep transverse laceration can cause to the underlying connective tissue and muscle control of distal skeletal structures.

The muscle tissue is responsible not only for the body's ability to move about, but also for the production of heat energy. A chemical reaction between oxygen and simple sugars produces the energy of motion. Heat, water, and carbon dioxide are created as by-products of this reaction. The body then excretes water in the urine, expires carbon dioxide through respiration, and dissipates heat through radiation or convection. The body must constantly meet the requirements of muscle tissue for oxygen, nutrients, and elimination of their waste products.

The blood vessels and major nerve pathways travel deep within the muscle masses and along the long bones. This orientation minimizes the effects of most trauma. A fracture or dislocation of the bone, however, may injure these structures.

PATHOPHYSIOLOGY

The various injury processes that may occur to the muscular and skeletal systems are easy to identify. Blunt trauma may contuse muscles, or muscles may strain when excessive force or fatigue overexerts the fibers. Various joints may injure because of extreme stress, as in a sprain. Or they become displaced partially or completely, as in subluxation or dislocation. The long bones themselves can disrupt through various types of fractures.

Muscular Injury

Muscular injury is common and may present painfully. Injuries may include contusions, strain, sprain, cramp, and spasm. None of these should contribute significantly to hypovolemia, with the exception of a severe contusion and accompanying internal hemorrhage.

Contusion Blunt trauma frequently causes contusion. As with all contusions, small blood vessels rupture, causing dull pain, leakage of blood into the interstitial spaces, and the classical discoloration. The injury may allow pooling of blood beneath tissue layers and a resultant hematoma. Infrequently, large volumes of blood may accumulate and contribute to hypovolemia. This

■ **abduction** movement of a body part or extremity away from the midline.

■ **adduction** movement of a body part or extremity toward the midline.

✳ Muscular injuries rarely contribute significantly to hypovolemia, with the exception of a severe contusion accompanied by internal hemorrhage.

may occur when the injury involves large vessels in the major muscle masses of the thigh, buttocks, calf, or arm.

Strain   A strain is an overstretching of the muscle and presents as pain. Extreme energy stretches the muscle mass beyond its normal limits of motion. The result is damage to fibers without internal bleeding or discoloration. Patients normally report pain when attempting to use the specific muscle affected.

Muscle Cramp   Muscle cramping is not really an injury, but an "angina" of the tissue. Muscle pain results when circulation fails to supply the muscle mass with oxygen or fails to remove the waste products of metabolism. The pain begins during or immediately after vigorous exercise or after the limb has been left in an unusual position for a period of time. Changing position may reduce or eliminate the pain. Once rest allows circulation to restore the metabolic balance, the pain usually subsides.

Muscle Spasm   Muscle spasm causes pain similar to that of the muscle cramp as the muscle mass contracts firmly. A spasm may feel much like the deformity of a fracture to palpation. As with the cramp, the spasm will subside uneventfully with restored circulation.

Penetrating Muscle Injury   Muscle injury may also occur with open wounds. Deep lacerations may penetrate the skin and subcutaneous tissues, thus affecting the muscle mass, tendons, and ligaments. Massive wounds that involve a large percentage of a muscle, or wounds that affect the tendons, may reduce the strength of the distal limb or render muscular control ineffective. As the tendons are cut, the muscle will retract them into the soft tissue. The opposing muscle will contract, moving the limb and also pulling the distal tendon away from the injury. Such injuries often call for surgical intervention to identify and rejoin the damaged connective bands.

Joint Injury

Joint injuries include the sprain, the subluxation, and the dislocation. The following sections detail the mechanics behind each of these injuries.

Sprain   The sprain is a tearing of the connective tissue of the joint capsule, specifically a ligament or ligaments. This injury causes exquisite pain at the site followed shortly by inflammation and swelling. Ecchymotic discoloration will occur over time, but not usually during the prehospital period. The ligaments have torn under tremendous tension. Therefore, the joint is exceedingly weakened. Continued use may cause complete joint failure.

Subluxation   A **subluxation** (partial dislocation) occurs when the joint stressfully separates, stretching the ligaments. It differs from the sprain in that it more significantly reduces the integrity of the joint. In a subluxation, the articular surfaces are not held together tightly since there is more ligament damage. The site is painful; the range of motion is limited; and the joint is unstable. Hyperflexion, hyperextension, or lateral rotation beyond the normal range of motion are commonly responsible for this injury. Extreme force pulling along the axis of the limb may also cause this injury. Swelling and pain will normally accompany this injury.

■ **subluxation** incomplete dislocation of a joint. The surfaces remain in contact, while the joint is somewhat deformed.

Dislocation   **Dislocation** is a frank displacement of the bone ends from the joint. The joint fixes in an abnormal position, with noticeable deformity of the joint area. It will be painful and swollen. There is danger that the injury is entrap-

■ **dislocation** displacement of a bone or other structure from its normal anatomical location.

ping, compressing, or tearing blood vessels and nerves. Dislocation occurs when the joint moves beyond its normal range of motion with great force. The very nature of the injury means that it has associated ligament damage and may also involve injury to the capsule and trauma to the articular cartilage.

Fractures

■ **fracture** disruption of the bone tissue. Types of fractures include: comminuted, greenstick, impacted, linear, oblique, spiral, and reverse.

The most dramatic of skeletal injuries is the **fracture**. As a break in the continuity of the bone, it may involve not only skeletal tissue but blood vessels, nerves, and other tissues within and surrounding the bone. If the fracture damages internal blood vessels or nerves, it may limit the degree of repair possible and the post-accident use of the limb. You will deal with many types of fractures. These most commonly include open, closed, impacted, hairline, and greenstick fractures. (See Figure 17-3.)

Closed Fracture   The *closed fracture* does not have an associated open wound. The prognosis for a closed fracture is generally better than for the open fracture. (See Figure 17-4.)

Open Fracture   An *open fracture* is any fracture with an associated open wound. The wound communicates with the fracture site and provides a route for infectious materials to enter. Injury may occur when a penetrating object, such as a bullet, enters the body and then fractures the bone. It may also result when the bone breaks and pushes through the skin.

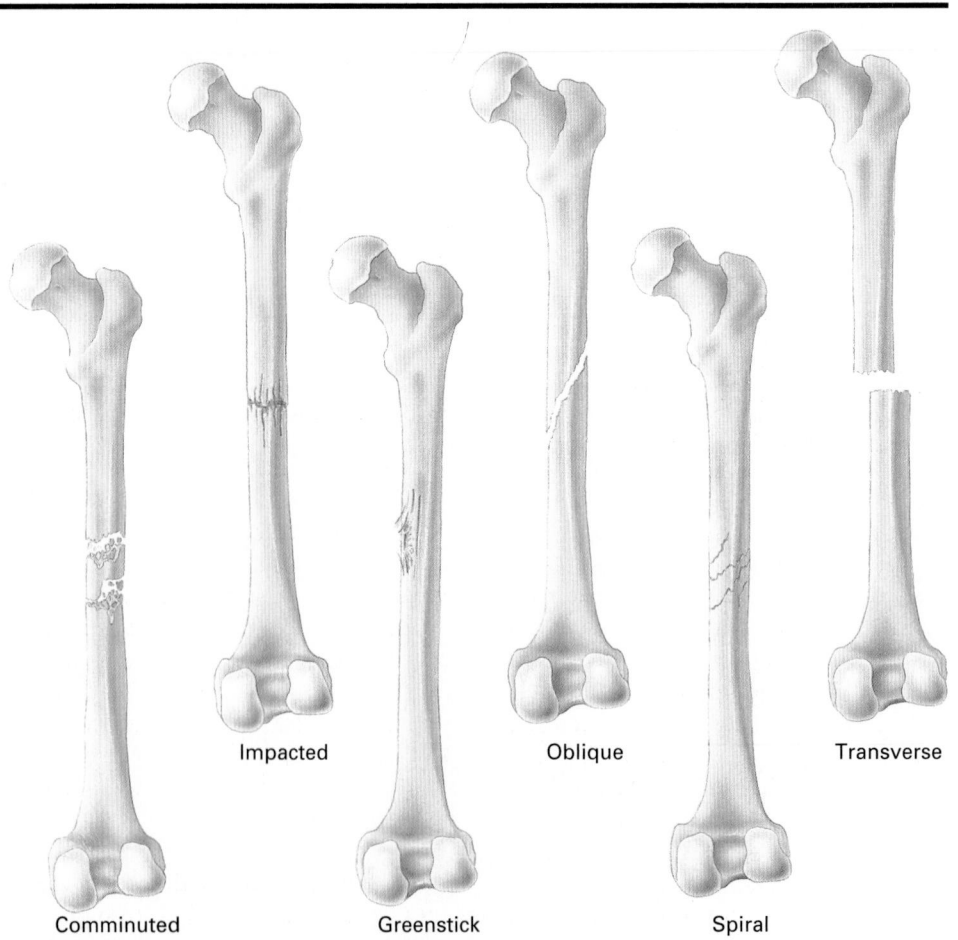

Impacted   Oblique   Transverse

FIGURE 17-3 Types of fractures.   Comminuted   Greenstick   Spiral

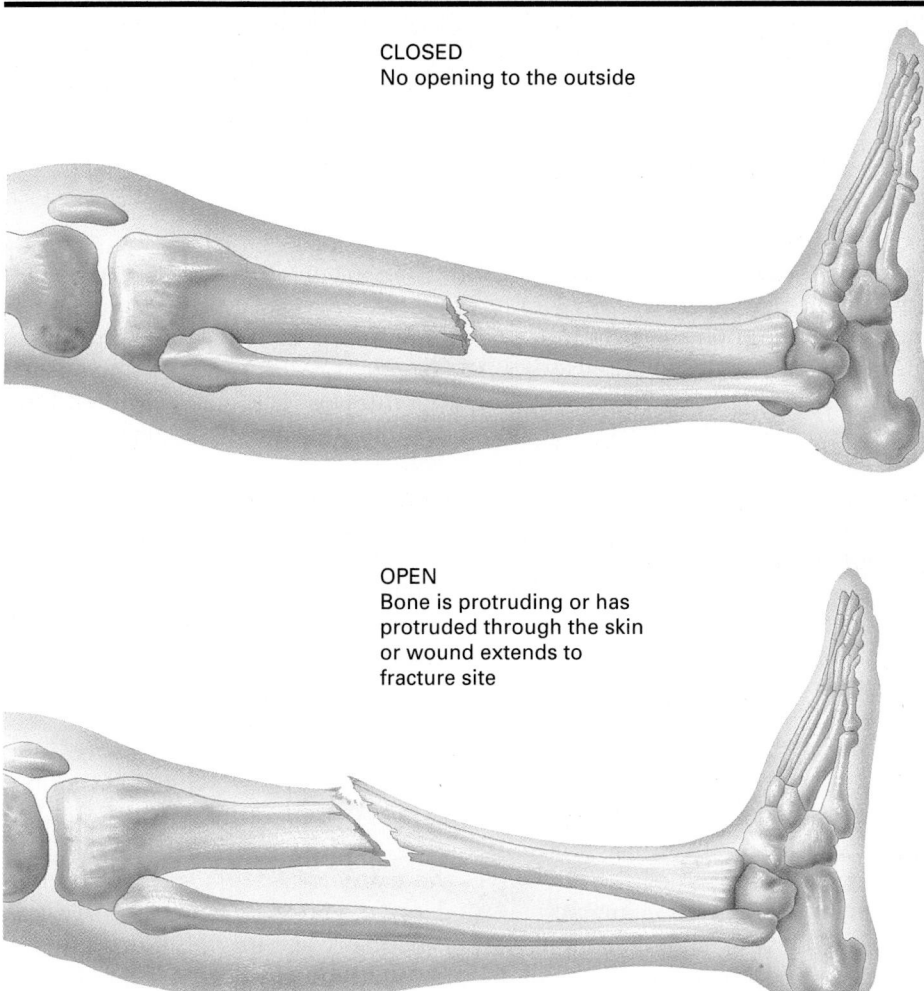

CLOSED
No opening to the outside

OPEN
Bone is protruding or has
protruded through the skin
or wound extends to
fracture site

FIGURE 17-4 Classification of fractures.

Hairline and Impacted Fractures   Two types of fractures that remain in-line and stay relatively stable are the hairline and the impacted fractures. The *hairline fracture* is a small crack in the bone that does not cause the bone ends to displace. The *impacted fracture* occurs when the ends of the broken bone compress together, providing the fracture with some stability. In either fracture, the only evidence of a problem may be the mechanism of injury and pain. The patient may use the limb normally. But it is noticeably weak and may, with stress, collapse post-accident. The only way to rule out such an injury is with an X-ray in the emergency department.

Greenstick Fractures   The *greenstick fracture* is a partial break, disrupting only one side of the long bone. It most frequently affects pediatric patients because their bone structure is less mature and more flexible than that of adults. While incomplete as a fracture, it is significant because of the partial nature of the break. During the natural repair, the injured side experiences growth, while the other does not. The probable result will be a bone that increases angulation as it heals. Occasionally, the emergency department staff will break the bone completely to ensure proper repair.

Fractures in the Geriatric Patient   Skeletal injuries for the other end of the age spectrum, the geriatric patient, are quite different. The strength of the skeletal system diminishes with advancing age. Bones may degenerate to a point where they fracture easily or spontaneously. The patient frequently describes "feeling a snap" before falling. The injury process is relatively atraumatic. Thus, the patient feels less uncomfortable than someone suffering an equivalent break because of trauma.

General Musculoskeletal Considerations

If we examine the skeletal structure and the musculature together, we can better anticipate the potential effects of trauma. It is important to note that long bones are smallest through the diaphysis and largest at the epiphyseal area, or joint. On the other hand, the diameter of the extremity is greatest surrounding the midshaft due to the placement of the skeletal muscles. This anatomical relationship is significant when looking at the potential for nervous or vascular injury.

Since there is a limited amount of soft tissue surrounding a joint, joint fractures, dislocations, and, to a lesser degree, subluxations and sprains may cause severe problems beyond the direct injury. Any swelling, deformity, or displacement may compromise the nerve and vascular supply to the distal extremity. Fractures near a joint may actually sever blood vessels or nerves. Dislocation may trap and compress these structures between the two displaced bone ends. The chance of blood vessel and nerve damage is much greater for injuries of the joint than for fractures of the long bone shaft.

The circulation supplying the epiphyseal area of a long bone enters the bone through the diaphysis. If a fracture close to the epiphysis displaces the bone ends, it may compromise this circulatory supply, with devastating results. The distal end of the bone may die without adequate circulation. This may destroy the joint and its function.

Once injury occurs, the stability of the extremity is reduced. Any further movement can increase pain, soft-tissue damage, and the possibility of vascular or nerve involvement. Manipulation of the injury site may also increase the likelihood of introducing bone fragments or fat emboli into the venous system. Even slight manipulation can cause internal trauma. When, for example, the femur fractures, the bone ends are about the size of a broken broom handle. If, during extrication, splinting, and patient movement, they flail about within the soft tissue, the internal damage may be more severe than that which initially occurred with the fracture.

Another complication associated with long bone fracture is muscle spasm induced by the pain of injury. In a long bone fracture, pain causes the opposing muscles to contract. This forces the broken bone ends to override the fracture site. The result, in the case of the femur, is two broom-handle-sized bones being driven into the muscles of the thigh. It is easy to appreciate the damage and pain resulting from an unstabilized fracture.

Specific Musculoskeletal Considerations

Certain long bone injuries deserve of special attention. They may present management problems or necessitate immediate care and transport due to significant blood loss or threat to the limb.

Lower Extremities   The lower extremities may suffer a number of types of fractures or dislocations. (See Figure 17-5.) The following sections discuss the most frequent sites of injury.

Pelvic Fractures. Pelvic fractures most commonly occur across the iliac crests or through the pelvic ring. Either fracture requires a great deal of force, although the pelvic ring fracture is generally much more severe. The injury

* The chance of blood vessel and nerve damage is much greater for injuries of the joint than for fractures of the long bone shaft.

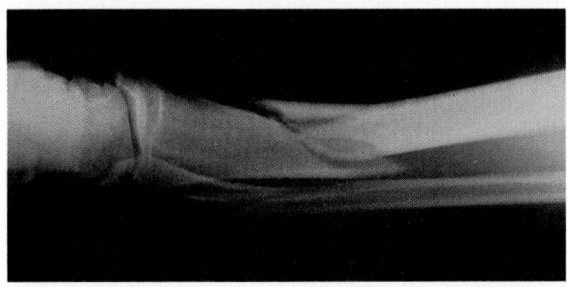

FIGURE 17-5 Radiograph of comminuted fracture of the left tibia and fibula secondary to an automobile/pedestrian accident.

✱ Pelvic fractures are frequently associated with severe hemorrhage, often in excess of 2 liters.

usually affects two sites because of the circular anatomy of the pelvis. The ring fracture usually involves the vasculature that runs along its interior and then to the lower extremities. Pelvic fractures frequently cause severe internal hemorrhage, often in excess of 2 liters. They may also result in the loss of circulation to one or both lower extremities.

Hip Dislocation. The hip joint may dislocate in two ways. The anterior dislocation displaces the femoral head anteriorly. The patient's foot and knee rotate laterally. There may be a noticeable prominence in the inguinal area, reflecting the head of the dislocated femur. The posterior dislocation displaces the head of the femur into the buttocks. The patient will generally flex the knee and rotate the leg and foot internally.

Femur Fractures. Fractures of the femur in the proximity of the hip may be difficult to differentiate from the anterior dislocation. While you may expect the broken leg to be slightly shorter than the unbroken one, the difference may be slight and unnoticeable if the legs are not straight and parallel. Fractures involving the femur, either midshaft or otherwise, may affect the surrounding vasculature or significant soft tissue. The bleeding that follows can be extensive. Fractures of the femur, the pelvis and, to a limited degree, the humerus can involve significant blood loss, possibly contributing to, or inducing, hypovolemia.

Knee Dislocation/Fracture. Knee dislocations will normally present with the knee at an angle and firmly fixed in position. The dislocation carries a high incidence of vascular and nervous injury because of the proximity of blood vessels and nerves to the injury site. Dislocation may also occur in combination with the fracture, since the energy needed to cause one is commonly sufficient to cause the other. Dislocations of the patella are more common than those of the knee. But, to the untrained examiner, it may be difficult to distinguish one dislocation from the other. Patellar dislocations carry a lower incidence of vascular injury than do knee dislocations.

Treat any fracture within three inches of a joint, especially the knee, the elbow, or the ankle, similar to the treatment for a dislocation. Immobilize the joint as found.

Lower-Leg Fractures. Fractures of the lower-leg bones, the tibia and the fibula, can occur separately or together. Direct trauma suffered during an auto or athletic accident frequently causes these injuries. The tibia will most commonly fracture, since it is the anterior bone and is responsible for weight bearing. If the fibula is intact, the extremity may not angulate, but it will not be able to bear weight. If only the fibula is broken, the limb may be rather stable.

Foot/Ankle Fractures. Foot and ankle fractures most often result from crush injuries or structural fatigue. The injuries are reasonably stable, even though

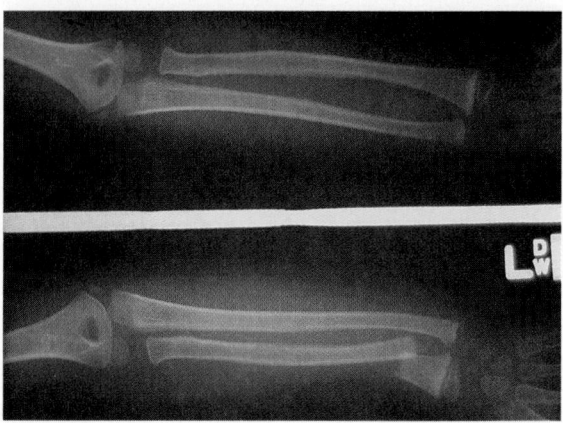

FIGURE 17-6 Radiograph of fractured left radius in a child. Right forearm is included for comparison.

the extremity cannot bear weight. With any injury to this area, be concerned about the status of distal circulation and nervous status.

Upper Extremities   A number of sites in the upper extremities seem prone to fractures or dislocations. (See Figure 17-6.) The following sections describe some common upper-extremity injuries.

Shoulder Dislocation.   Shoulder dislocation may occur anteriorly, posteriorly, or inferiorly. The posterior dislocation presents with a hollow shoulder, the limb angled forward, the elbow internally rotated, and the arm away from the chest. The anterior displacement presents with a prominent shoulder and with the arm close to the chest as well as forward of the anterior axillary line. The inferior displacement locks the patient's extremity above the head.

Humerus Fracture.   Fracture may occur along the entire length of the humerus. Here the injury is particularly hard to stabilize because of the structure and mobility of the shoulder joint. The axillary artery runs through the axilla, making it difficult to apply any mechanical traction to the limb. Humerus fracture also presents a potential hazard for circulatory compromise.

Elbow Fracture.   Fractures in and around the elbow are particularly dangerous, especially in children. The soft-tissue depth is minimal, and the skeletal diameter is large. Any fracture has a good probability of blood vessel or nerve involvement. Such damage may result in the eventual loss of function distal to the injury.

Forearm Fracture.   The forearm may fracture anywhere along its length and may involve the radius, ulna, or both. Commonly fractures will occur at the distal end of the radius, breaking it just above the articular surface. Known as *Colle's fracture*, it may present with the wrist turned up at an unusual angle. As with most joint fractures, the major concern is for distal circulation and innervation.

Hand and Wrist Fractures.   Hand and wrist fractures are commonly associated with direct trauma. They present with very noticeable deformity and significant pain. These fractures are of serious concern to the patient. Since the hand and wrist bones are small, any fracture is in the close proximity of a joint. Exercise concern for vascular and nervous involvement.

Effects of Fractures and Dislocations   Fractures and dislocations affect living tissue that requires a constant and rich supply of oxygenated blood. While the central nervous system, the heart, and the kidneys will dysfunction more rapidly and more acutely than the skeletal system, the long bones may degenerate over time and leave the limb unable to carry out its intended function. Musculoskeletal injuries are of relatively low priority in the seriously injured patient. Yet their proper care is important to the patient's overall well being and recovery.

ASSESSMENT

Evaluation of the fracture, dislocation, or muscular injury occurs late in the assessment process. These injuries infrequently threaten life or seriously contribute to the development of shock. On the other hand, they occur often in patients who present without other serious injury. In most circumstances, the fracture and dislocation will receive complete assessment and stabilization.

Primary Assessment

It is imperative that you begin trauma assessment with the A-B-C-D-Es of the primary assessment. You then follow it with the head-to-toe examination, vital signs, and evaluation of the patient history. In all cases, you will defer musculoskeletal injury assessment and care until you can rule out the potential for life threat. Consider and evaluate the patient for the risk of cervical-spine injury. This may not be easy, since primary kinetic forces resulting in musculoskeletal injury may also be strong enough to cause injury to the spine.

* Muscular injury assessment and care must be deferred until the potential for life threat is ruled out.

Assess the **A**irway, **B**reathing, and **C**irculation as adequate, or correct any problem immediately. If you cannot achieve this in the field, transport the patient immediately and give care focusing on the A-B-Cs en route. Identify any alteration in mental status or central nervous system depression before continuing with the assessment. Assess the head, neck, chest, and abdomen for signs of serious trauma. Then complete the entire primary assessment.

While skeletal injury does not often account for life-threatening hemorrhage, fracture of the pelvis or bilateral femur fractures may induce hypovolemia. If the mechanism of injury suggests either of these fractures, observe and palpate the pelvis and femurs early. If you find evidence of injury, apply the PASG and inflate all compartments to a pressure immobilizing the pelvis and the lower extremities. Remember that femur fractures can account for blood loss in excess of 1,500 mL each, while the pelvis may account for more than 2,000 mL. Consider any patients with these injuries as candidates for immediate transport.

* Patients with pelvic or femur fractures should be considered for immediate transport.

Secondary Assessment

After you have ruled out potential life threat and attended to any serious problems, you may begin secondary assessment. The process may occur at the scene or en route to the hospital. The head-to-toe exam will help you to reevaluate the head, neck, chest, and abdomen in more depth than in the initial assessment. Be sure to examine for the signs and symptoms of internal or external injury or hemorrhage.

Lower-Extremity Assessment   Once the assessment reaches the pelvis, evaluation of the major musculoskeletal areas begins. Assess the pelvis by applying gentle pressure to the iliac crests in a posterior direction, then medially. Next, apply posterior pressure to the symphysis pubis. If there is any crepitus, pain, or instability, stabilize the patient for a possible fractured pelvis.

Observe and palpate the extremities carefully for signs and symptoms of fracture, dislocation, or other injury. Expose and visualize the extremity before you palpate it. Remove any restrictive clothing or cut it away carefully, whichever is most effective. In doing so, avoid manipulation of a potential

* Any unusual limb placement, asymmetry, or limb length inequality should arouse suspicion of musculoskeletal injury.

injury site. View the area entirely to locate any deformity, discoloration, or other signs of injury. Any unusual limb placement, asymmetry, or limb length inequality should arouse suspicion of musculoskeletal injury. Question the patient about pain, inability to move, or pain when attempting motion. Your assessment must be gentle, yet complete.

If you identify no specific injury, palpate the extremity for instability, deformity, crepitation, false motion, or any regions of unusual warmth or coolness. Palpate the entire lateral and medial surface, then the anterior and posterior surface. Record any abnormal signs. As the assessment arrives at the foot, carefully examine the distal circulation. (See Figure 17-7.) Assess pulses for presence and then compare bilaterally. Test the skin for blanching, capillary refill, and warmth. Observe the skin for discoloration, noting any erythema, ecchymosis, or other abnormal hue. Approximate the level at which any deficit begins and note any relation to long bone injury.

Evaluate sensation and muscle strength distal to the injury. Check tactile (touch) response by stroking the bottom of the foot with the blunt end of a bandage scissors or other similar instrument. Ask the patient to describe the feeling. If the patient is responsive and if there is no indication that the limb is injured, ask the patient to push down with the balls of both feet against your hands. Then ask the patient to pull upward with the top of the feet, again against your hands. If any unilateral weakness or pain is felt, note it in the record and look for the cause.

Upper-Extremity Assessment Assess the upper extremity in a similar way. (See Figure 17-8.) Expose, observe, and then palpate it. Determine tactile response by using the back of the patient's hand. Test muscular strength by having the patient squeeze two of your fingers. Identify any deficit, and attempt to locate the cause. Evaluate the upper extremity before using it for blood pressure determination.

When the assessment for an extremity suggests injury, treat the limb as though a fracture or dislocation exists. The only way to rule out a fracture is X-ray examination. Nothing more than slight discomfort will result from treating a soft-tissue or muscular injury as a fracture. Failure to immobilize an injury properly, however, may further damage soft, skeletal, connective, vascular, or nervous tissue.

Reassess and record the distal pulse, skin temperature, and capillary refill times during splint application, patient packaging, and transport. You should give special attention to the distal pulse and sensation before, during, and after any splinting as well as periodically during transport and patient care. Any limb manipulation caused by these activities, or swelling of the affected limb, may produce an obstruction of an artery or compression of a nerve. If you do not detect the compromise, the result may be prolongation of the healing process or loss of the limb.

If possible, find the exact site of injury and determine if it involves the joint area or long bone shaft. Make a visual image of the wound in your mind. This will enable you to describe it in the record and to the receiving physician. The splinting device (e.g., the PASG for a femur fracture) may hide the site from view, leaving the attending physician unable to determine what exists within. A good narrative description of the wound may delay the need to remove the splint to view the injury.

One complication of musculoskeletal injury to the extremities is *compartment syndrome*. This condition results from bleeding into a closed space surrounded by membranes that will not stretch. The hemorrhage then compresses the blood vessels and nerves. Suspect compartment syndrome in any patient with an extremity injury who has lost the pulse or function in the hand or foot. Compartment syndrome most often occurs in the forearm or the leg.

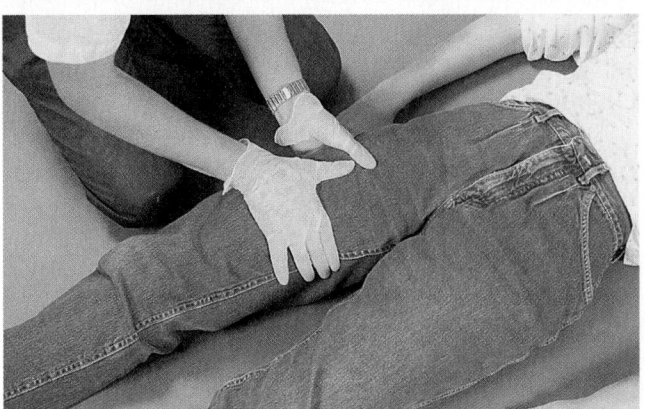

FIGURE 17-7 Assessment of the lower extremity.

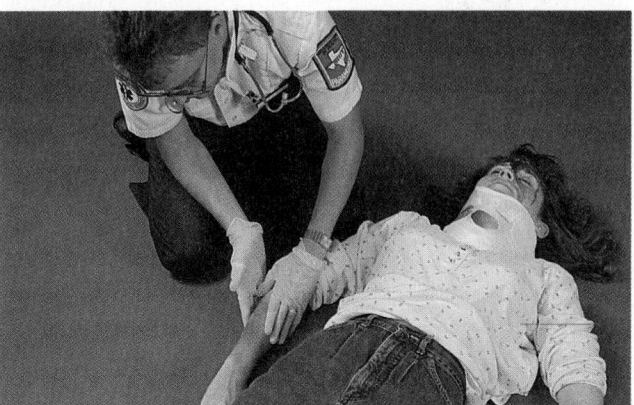

FIGURE 17-8 Assessment of the upper extremity.

Patient History During the physical exam, question the patient about the symptoms of injury. Determine the nature and location of pain and tenderness or dysfunction. Assure your verbal investigation is detailed and complete. Your description of the fracture or dislocation event may also be helpful. The patient may state that he or she felt the bone "snap" or the joint "pop out." Determine if the bone snapped, thus causing the fall or vice versa. Evaluate the patient for the amount of pain and discomfort he or she experienced with the injury. The elderly patient may present with a fractured hip and limited pain, usually related to a degenerative disease and secondary fracture. Such a presentation may suggest a less aggressive approach to care that focuses upon patient comfort rather than upon traction splinting and shock care.

Determine the mechanism of injury from the patient's explanation and observation of the environment. It is helpful for you mentally to relive the incident and determine what injury or injuries may have occurred. If you suspect any injury, your assessment should either rule it out or treat the patient as though the injury exists.

As you conclude the trauma assessment, identify all injuries found, prioritize them, and establish the order of care. The moments taken to sort out what is wrong with the patient and to plan care steps will increase efficiency, reduce on-scene time, and ensure that the patient receives the proper care at the right time.

✱ At the conclusion of the trauma assessment, identify all injuries found, prioritize them, and establish the order of care.

MANAGEMENT

Some patients with musculoskeletal injuries require immediate transportation, while many others will receive on-scene care. The care for these two types of patients differs greatly. In seriously injured patients, you can neither assess nor care for fractures as precisely as you may desire. Other priorities are more important. In contrast, patients with limited and isolated injuries must receive detailed splinting and packaging to ensure that no further harm occurs.

Immediate Transport

Once you make the decision to transport an unstable or potentially unstable patient, you must consider long bone and muscle injury. It is neither practical nor appropriate to splint each fracture while the patient exsanguinates from internal hemorrhage. You must, however, rapidly extricate the patient, using techniques of immobilization and movement to protect the body as a whole, including potential fractures.

✱ It is neither practical nor appropriate to splint each fracture while the patient exsanguinates from internal hemorrhage.

Using axial traction for movement causes the extremities to align. This technique moves the patient gently by applying the "pull" to the shoulders while stabilizing the head. As movement occurs, the travel of the patient causes the upper extremities to align against the body and the lower extremities to align together. Continuing movement will keep the limbs in position and limit their flailing about. While this procedure is certainly not ideal, it minimizes further trauma to the musculoskeletal system when rapid transport is the first priority.

If the use of axial traction is inappropriate, select other techniques that minimize limb movement. For example, during removal from the auto or other accident scene, secure the upper extremities to the body and the legs to each other.

Securing the patient to the long spineboard will immobilize his or her extremities. You can adequately accomplish patient packaging by securing the head with a cervical immobilization device. Cross the shoulders and chest with straps, encircling the pelvis (and hands), legs, and feet. If you move the patient as a unit, you will minimally displace any fracture or dislocation during transport.

On-Scene Care

✱ If immediate transport is not required and if the patient is stable, the long bone and muscular injuries can be cared for according to the priorities established during the secondary assessment.

If you do not need to transport the patient immediately, you can treat long bone and muscular injuries individually and according to the priorities you established during the secondary assessment. Fractures of the pelvis, femur, and humerus generally take priority over other musculoskeletal injuries. Fractures or dislocations involving circulatory or nervous deficit should also be given a high priority.

General Considerations Proper assessment of suspected fractures and dislocations usually involve frequent serial evaluation of the distal circulatory and nervous functions before, during, and after splinting. Determine the presence of the pulse, and compare its strength and rate with that of the opposite limb. Monitor distal temperature carefully and time capillary refill. Any deviation from baseline findings should be reason to check the splint for tightness and possible circumferential constriction.

The adage "immobilize the adjacent joints" is appropriate for both fractures and dislocations. Whichever splint and splinting process you choose must effectively immobilize the proximal and distal joint to prevent any transmitted motion. Transmitted motion can occur in many ways. The flexion/extension motion of the normal joint is one way. Rotational and lateral motions also occur, especially once injury damages the joint structure. The elbow demonstrates this well. In an elbow injury, if the palm of the hand rotates from supine to prone, the radius and ulna move at the injury site. This motion can induce further pain, if not further injury. You can eliminate this motion only if you effectively immobilize the joints proximal and distal to the injury.

Fractures, dislocations, and connective tissue injury may be very difficult to differentiate from one another. If any question exists, err on the side of over-immobilization. Limb stabilization will rarely harm a patient, while failure to stabilize may allow significant soft-tissue injury to occur.

Limb Positioning The best position for splinting an extremity is the neutral position. This provides the least tension on the ligaments and tendons of the limb. You can approximate the neutral position by leaving the various joints half-way between full extension and full flexion. While this position is physiologically ideal, it is sometimes difficult to obtain in the field.

A situation deserving special consideration is the hand injury. The hand's articulations are sophisticated and essential to human function. Therefore, care of such an injury is critical. Bring the injured hand to the neutral position (also called the position of function) to ensure that you maintain patient comfort and that the limb receives no further damage. Obtain this position by placing the hand as if it were holding a softball. You may accomplish this position comfortably by surrounding a roll of roller bandage with a trauma dressing and placing it in the patient's palm.

Shaft fractures are not as easy to immobilize as they might first seem. The major long bones are embedded within large muscle masses, such as the hamstring and the quadriceps of the thigh or the biceps and the triceps of the arm. These muscles make it difficult to splint the bone ends in any position other than aligned. If you attempt to immobilize a fracture in an angulated position, the splint may be ineffective.

Align a fracture gently and carefully. Explain to the patient what is about to happen. Tell him or her that alignment will hurt, but the pain will be less after the procedure. There will also be less pain during movement to the ambulance and travel to the hospital. Stabilize the proximal limb as found, while the distal limb is brought into alignment. Accomplish this with gentle traction. Once you align the limb, bring it immediately to its final position for transport. Assess the distal circulation and nervous function. If there is any noticeable resistance during the alignment process, discontinue it. Assess the pulse and nervous function immediately. If present, splint the limb. If either the pulse or innervation is compromised, gently manipulate the limb before splinting it. If initial attempts do not restore the pulse or sensation, immobilize the limb and transport the patient quickly.

While alignment is an uncomfortable process, it is necessary if splinting is to be effective. The splints you will most commonly use for fractures are the air splint, the PASG, and the traction splint. By their nature, they force alignment of the limb. The structure of the padded board splint and fracture straps also require the same aligned limb for proper immobilization. The ladder and vacuum splints can conform to the limb angle without alignment. However, the ladder splint has limited ability to immobilize firmly.

Once you position the limb acceptably, immobilize it completely. One team member holds the limb in position and monitors the distal pulse, as you apply the splint. Use gentle traction to align the extremity and continue it until you firmly secure the limb to the device. The splint should maintain both limb immobilization and gentle traction during the entire prehospital period. At the conclusion of the splinting process, carefully reassess the pulse and sensation.

Fractures within three inches of the joint or dislocations are splinted very differently than midshaft fractures. You should splint joint injuries in the position found, because of the danger of vascular or nervous injury that may result from manipulation of such fractures. Also, the initial position is easier to splint. The exception is a patient with no circulation distal to the injury. In this case, gently move the limb, while palpating for the return of a distal pulse. If you do not regain the pulse with a minimum of movement, splint the limb and transport the patient without delay.

Many areas of the extremities call for special techniques of immobilization. It is essential to look at each injury separately and identify any special considerations of care.

Lower-Extremity Management   Stabilize the pelvis and control hemorrhage. It is a standard practice to apply the PASG for pelvic fractures, because of the potential for severe blood loss and the difficulty in immobilizing the broken pelvic ring. Inflate the PASG until it affixes the pelvis and hip joint. Start two large-bore IVs, and hang two 1,000 mL bags of lactated Ringer's solution or normal saline. Use trauma tubing and pressure infusion sets for rapid infusion. The lines need only run at a to-keep-open rate until the early signs of shock develop. Consider this patient a candidate for rapid transport.

* If distal pulses or innervation are compromised due to a skeletal injury, gently manipulate the limb to achieve its return and then splint.

* Fractures or dislocations in the vicinity of a joint should generally be splinted in the position found.

Immobilize fractures and dislocations of the hip in the position found. You may use the long spineboard to splint the patient entirely and accommodate the injury. Use pillows, blankets, and other padding to maintain the initial position and ensure patient comfort.

Femur fractures can originate from two sources: severe trauma and degenerative disease. Patients with disease-induced fractures present with a clouded history of trauma and relative patient comfort. Care for the patient, as with the hip fracture patient, by immobilizing him or her as found and then by gentle transport.

The patient with a femur fracture resulting from trauma will be in extreme discomfort. Often, you will find him or her writhing in pain. For this patient, distal traction will best reduce the pain and muscle spasm. The traction splint is the best avenue for care of the hemodynamically stable patient with an isolated femur fracture. If the early signs of shock are present, or if the history reflects that the patient has sustained enough trauma to induce shock, the PASG may be a better choice. Use only the amount of traction necessary to align or stabilize the limb and no more. Limited traction will begin a cycle of reduced pain, muscle relaxation, and limb lengthening. If you use mechanical traction (e.g., the traction splint), monitor and readjust the splint to ensure a constant gentle pull on the limb.

Immobilize fractures or dislocations of the knee as you find them. The common presentation is with the knee at an angle of 90 degrees, or slightly greater. Leave the limb in this position unless distal pulses are lost. Place padded board splints lateral and medial to the fracture to immobilize the injury effectively. Anterior and posterior ladder splints or the vacuum splint will also accomplish fixation. Care for ankle and foot injuries with either the full-leg air, vacuum, or pillow splint. Each device will immobilize the injury. However, the pillow and vacuum splints will better conform to the position of the patient's extremity.

After you splint the limb, it is beneficial to secure it to the uninjured leg. This will afford some protection against uncontrolled movement. It may also reassure the patient that he or she still has some control over the extremity.

Upper-Extremity Management   Immobilize shoulder injuries, like all joint injuries, as found, unless the pulse or feeling distal to the injury is absent. Immobilize the anterior and posterior dislocation as found with a sling and swath and, if needed, place a pillow under the arm and forearm. Any inferior dislocation (with the upper extremity fixed above the head) calls for ingenuity by you. Immobilize the extended arm in that position. Tie a long, padded splint with cravats to the torso, shoulder girdle, arm, and forearm to serve this purpose. Move the patient to the long spineboard, and affix the splint and patient to the spineboard.

Splint humeral fractures with the elbow either fixed or extended. If flexed, allow the patient to sit and do not include the elbow in the arm sling. Then swath the extremity. If the extremity is extended, secure it with a padded board splint along the medial aspect of the limb. Then secure the arm and splint against the supine body. Ensure that you do not push the splint into the axilla. Such pressure may impinge the axillary artery and reduce circulation to the extremity.

Splint the elbow with a single padded board or ladder splint. Either way, sling and swathe with the wrist slightly above the elbow in the sitting or supine patient. This position will increase venous return and reduce the swelling and pain.

You can effectively immobilize musculoskeletal injuries of the forearm, wrist, hand or fingers with a padded board or air splint. Place a roll of bandage material or some similar object in the patient's hand to maintain the position of function. Then secure the extremity to the padded board or inflate the splint. It is necessary that the distal extremity be accessible to determine adequacy of perfusion and sensation. Place the wrist above the elbow to assist venous return and reduce distal swelling.

Pain frequently accompanies the fracture, dislocation, or other musculoskeletal injury. If a patient with these injuries does not have respiratory or cardiovascular compromise, you may provide pain relief to increase comfort and reduce anxiety. Nitronox is the drug of choice, because it is self-administered and has a short half-life. Also consider morphine sulfate. Titrate its administration to pain relief, and halt it immediately if any respiratory depression or hypotension develops. You may need to administer naloxone (Narcan) if the patient's respiratory depression or hypotension becomes severe. In all cases, consult with medical control.

The trauma patient needs psychological as well as physiological support. Too often we concentrate all efforts on the patient's injuries, forgetting the emotional impact of the incident and the emergency care. You can be very effective in treating the patient's emotional response to trauma. It is important to remember that patients are not frequently exposed to injury. They do not know what effects the injury will have on their life, nor what to expect from medical care in the prehospital, emergency department, or the in-hospital setting. A concerned attitude, frequent and compassionate communication, and a professional demeanor will go far to calm and reassure patients. Simple attention to the patient may make his or her experience with prehospital emergency medical service one he or she will remember positively.

✱ Do not concentrate all efforts on the patient's injuries and neglect the emotional impact of the incident and the emergency care.

SUMMARY

It is rare that musculoskeletal injury threatens the life of the patient. General care of the injuries presented in this chapter take second priority to the many other life-threatening injuries accompanying trauma. However, once the patient is stable and ruled out as a candidate for rapid transport, you can then assess and care for fractures, dislocations, strains, and sprains.

Provide your patient with a careful and detailed assessment. Look for any pain, pain on motion, instability, false motion, or other signs or symptoms of injury. Be especially watchful of associated vascular or nervous injury by carefully assessing the distal extremity. If you suspect a fracture or dislocation, splint the joint area as found. Gently align the midshaft region, unless you experience resistance. Frequently assess distal feeling and pulses (or capillary refill) before, during, and after your splint application. Be sure musculoskeletal care is an integrated part of your total trauma patient care.

FURTHER READING

American College of Surgeons, Committee on Trauma. *Advanced Trauma Life Support Course: Student Manual.* American College of Surgeons, 1989.

Butman, A.M., and J.L. Paturas. *Pre-Hospital Trauma Life Support.* Akron, OH: Emergency Training, 1986.

Campbell, J.E. *Basic Trauma Life Support,* 2nd ed. Englewood Cliffs, NJ: Prentice-Hall, Inc., 1988.

DoCarmo, P.B. *Basic EMT Skills and Equipment: Technique and Pitfalls.* St. Louis, MO: C.V. Mosby Co., 1988.

Grant, H.D., R.H. Murray, and J.D. Bergeron. *Emergency Care.* 5th ed. Englewood Cliffs, NJ: Prentice-Hall, Inc., 1990.

Phillips, C. *Basic Life Support Skills Manual,* 2nd ed. Englewood Cliffs, NJ: Prentice-Hall, Inc., 1986.

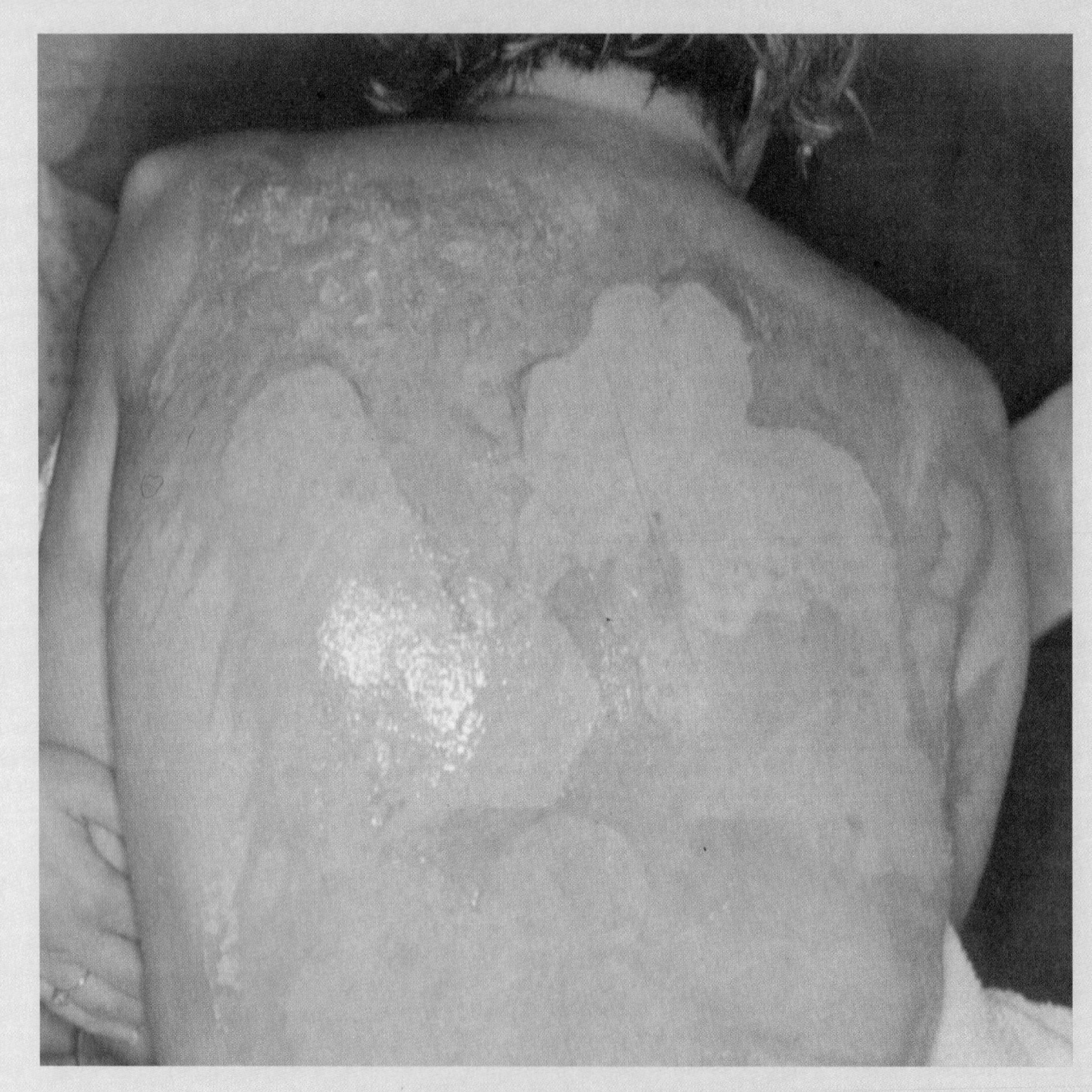

18

SOFT-TISSUE TRAUMA AND BURNS

Objectives for Chapter 18

After reading this chapter, you should be able to:

1. Describe the structure and function of skin. (See pp. 522–525.)

2. Identify the characteristics of a contusion, abrasion, laceration, incision, avulsion, and amputation. (See pp. 525–528.)

3. Name the four types of burns. (See pp. 529–533.)

4. Explain the precautions to take when approaching a possible radiological incident, including the effect of time, distance, and shielding upon exposure. (See p. 531.)

5. Discuss the common causes of inhalation injuries. (See pp. 532–533.)

6. Explain the three degrees of thermal burns as well as the depth and effects that these burns have on the human body. (See pp. 533–534.)

7. Identify the two methods of approximating the burn surface area, and apply them to several burn patient descriptions. (See pp. 535–536.)

8. Describe difficulties in assessing and caring for soft-tissue injuries. (See pp. 538–551.)

9. List the anatomical areas that, when burned, will increase the overall severity of the burn. (See pp. 541–542.)

10. List the advantages and the disadvantages of each of the following methods of bleeding control. (See below pages.)

- Direct pressure (p. 544)
- Elevation (p. 544)
- Pressure point (p. 544)
- Tourniquet (pp. 544–545)

11. Identify the circumstances in which each of the above techniques, or a combination, might be best. (See p. 544.)

12. List and explain the care steps for chemical burns, noting the special considerations given to lime and phenol burns. (See pp. 548–550.)

The paramedics of Fire Rescue respond with trucks 23 and 56 to a working structural fire. Upon arrival, they find two fire units already deployed, with firefighters engaging a wood frame home fully engulfed in flames. As paramedics position their vehicle, the south wall of the structure collapses on a firefighter. Within minutes, other firefighters extinguish the burning wall and free the victim.

Paramedics proceed to help. Upon removal of the firefighter's turnout gear, they expose relatively painless, dark, discolored burns to his posterior thorax, lower back, and the left upper extremity circumferentially. They also find angulation, false motion, and pain in the right forearm. Respirations appear adequate, although the patient is coughing up sooty sputum and is slightly hoarse. The firefighter is conscious, alert, and without much pain, despite the very severe burns. His airway seems clear, except for the hoarseness. Vital signs reveal normal breathing in terms of volume and rate and a strong, regular pulse at a rate of about 100. Distal pulses are also strong and capillary refill is timed at two seconds. The patient is fully conscious and oriented and is joking about the incident.

The rescue crew now take some initial care steps. They cut away all the clothing, including a still-smoldering belt. They then cover the burn site with a dry, sterile sheet and start an IV line, running normal saline at a wide-open rate. They apply oxygen through a nonrebreathing mask and observe an oximetry reading of 97 percent. The paramedics quickly load the patient into the ambulance and begin rapid transport. They take a quick blood pressure (120/88) and respirations (26 and shallow), noting that the patient is now experiencing some breathing effort.

While one of the paramedics is splinting the right limb, the patient begins to cough deeply and to experience severe dyspnea. The dyspnea progresses, and the level of consciousness drops. Oxygen saturation falls to 86 percent. One of the paramedics begins to bag-valve-mask with supplemental oxygen, while her partner prepares the intubation equipment.

Medical control orders the crew to intubate. They make an attempt during transport. The airway is edematous, and visualization of the vocal cords is difficult. Paramedics withdraw the tube when auscultation of breath sounds, failure to obtain chest rise, and a dropping oxygen saturation indicate esophagal placement. They hyperventilate the patient and attempt another intubation. They are again unsuccessful.

As they withdraw the tube, the ambulance arrives at the emergency department. The physician places a large-bore catheter in the cricothyroid membrane and attempts transtracheal jet insufflation. The technique is successful. After an emergency tracheostomy, the firefighter begins spontaneous respirations and maintains a strong pulse. But his level of consciousness does not improve. The hospital staff transfer him to the burn unit for definitive care.

INTRODUCTION

The skin is one of the largest, most important, and least appreciated organs of the human body. Covering the entire body, it protects us from fluid loss and bacterial invasion. It also provides a massive surface for sensation and a natural radiator to dissipate excess body heat. With all these responsibilities, the skin still remains durable, flexible, and very able to repair itself.

Known collectively as the **integumentary system**, the skin is the first tissue of the human body to experience the effects of trauma. Because skin covers the entire body surface, any penetrating injury or the kinetic forces of blunt injury must pass through it before impacting on other vital organs. This transmission of energy often manifests with signs observable only by careful examination of the skin. Therefore, the skin is of great significance in both primary and secondary patient assessment.

■ **integumentary system** skin, consisting of the epidermis and dermis.

OVERVIEW OF SOFT-TISSUE INJURIES

Trauma to the skin may present as abrasions, hematomas, lacerations, punctures, avulsions, and amputations. Although such injuries infrequently cause threat to life, they may endanger blood vessels, nerves, connective tissue, and other important internal structures. Uncontrolled blood loss may lead to hypovolemia and shock, while the wound may provide a pathway for infection. Care for these injuries is easy to provide, although several objectives must be met.

Burns are a specific subset of soft-tissue injury with a pathologic process all their own. While the term "burn" suggests combustion, the actual burn process is much different. The human body is predominantly water and will not support combustion. Instead, it changes chemically, evaporating the water and denaturing the proteins that make up cell membranes. The result can be widespread damage to the integumentary system.

Inhalation injury often accompanies burn injury. The products of combustion can cause severe respiratory burns from either thermal or chemical interaction with the airway tissue. Carbon monoxide may also "poison" the patient by reducing the ability of red blood cells to carry oxygen. It is in fact the most common source of poisoning in the United States.

Chemicals may also cause burns. Chemicals can affect the body tissue at a molecular level in much the same way as the thermal burns. The insult may not cause the rapid evaporation of fluid, although it will destroy the cell's membranes. The resulting injury will affect the patient in a way similar to that of the thermal burn.

You must have a good understanding of the structure and function of the integumentary system as well as the pathologic processes that affect it. This understanding will ensure that you can optimally assess and care for the patient who sustains either a wound or burn injury.

ANATOMY AND PHYSIOLOGY OF THE SKIN

The skin is an "envelope" that contains the human body. As you will remember from Chapter 12, "The Pathophysiology of Shock," the body is composed of about 60 percent water. Yet it survives in an atmosphere with a relatively low external humidity. The body also survives in an environment filled with microorganisms that would raise havoc within the body if they could freely enter and grow. Because of the skin, the body maintains its water and wards off many microorganisms.

Layers of Skin

The skin is comprised of three layers of tissue: the epidermis, the dermis, and the subcutaneous tissue. (See Figure 18-1.) Together they form the body's outermost shell.

The Epidermis The first and outermost layer is the **epidermis**. It is a layer of dying and dead cells being pushed outward by new cells growing from beneath. As these cells reach the surface, they abrade away with everyday activity. The constant movement outward provides a barrier that is difficult for bacteria and other pathogens to penetrate.

Glands beneath the epidermis secrete an oil called **sebum**. This oil lubricates the epidermis and assists in making it watertight. It also coats the outer layers and makes the epidermis pliable. In addition, sebum provides a barrier to the flow of water or other fluids either in or out of the skin.

■ **epidermis** outermost layer of the skin comprised of dead or dying cells.

■ **sebum** fatty secretion of the sebaceous gland. It helps keep the skin pliable and waterproof.

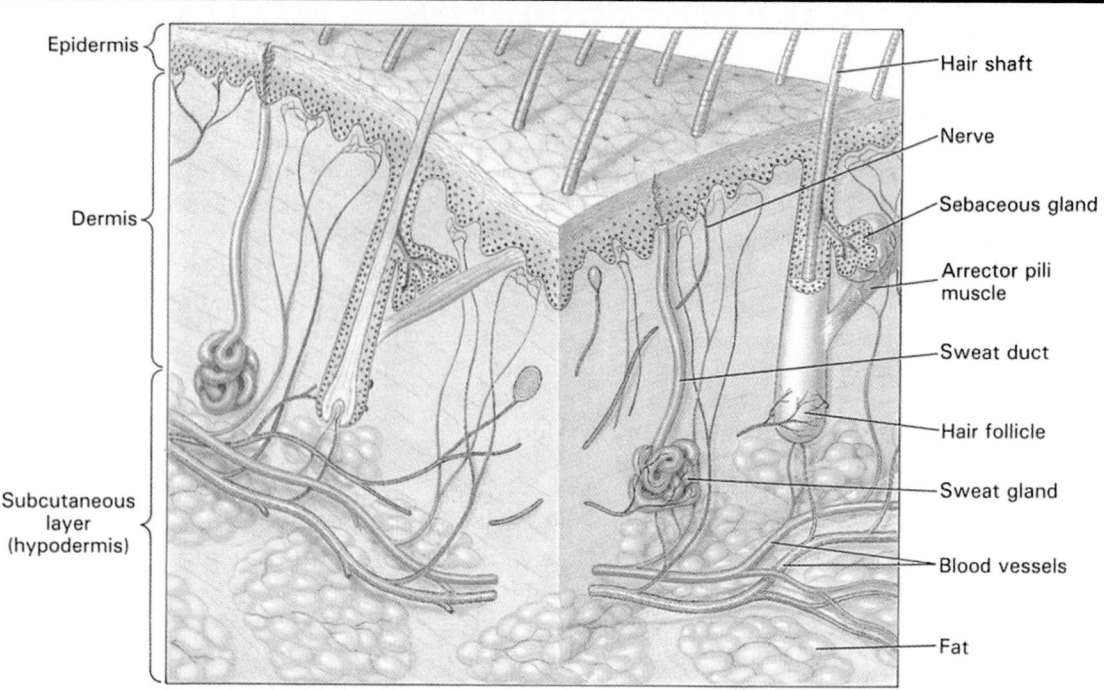

Epidermis
Dermis
Subcutaneous
layer
(hypodermis)

Hair shaft
Nerve
Sebaceous gland
Arrector pili
muscle
Sweat duct
Hair follicle
Sweat gland
Blood vessels
Fat

FIGURE 18-1 Anatomy of the skin.

dermis true skin, also called the corium. It is the layer of tissue producing the epidermis and housing the structures, blood vessels, and nerves normally associated with the skin.

sebaceous glands glands within the dermis secreting sebum.

tunica intima interior layer of the blood vessels. It is smooth and provides for the free flow of blood.

tunica media the middle, muscular layer of the blood vessels. It controls the vessel lumen size.

tunica adventitia outer fibrous layer of the blood vessels. It maintains their maximum size.

The Dermis   Directly below the epidermis is the tissue layer called the **dermis**. It consists of many different structures, including blood vessels, glands, and nerve endings. It is here that **sebaceous glands** produce sebum and secrete it into hair follicles. Sudoriferous glands in the dermis also secrete sweat to the surface of the skin. As the water in sweat evaporates, passing air carries the vapor and associated heat energy away with it. The change of a fluid to a vapor (evaporation) is an efficient method of cooling. This process allows us to maintain a normal body temperature even in ambient temperatures of greater than 100 degrees (as long as evaporation is possible).

The Subcutaneous Tissue   Additional regulation of body temperature occurs as warm blood from the body's core travels through the peripheral circulation. Vessels direct blood either to the dermal surface or to beneath the *subcutaneous tissue*. Subcutaneous tissue, which is composed of adipose (fat) and connective tissues, serves as a strata of insulation. The shunting of blood into the deeper areas allows the skin's temperature to drop. This slows the movement of heat to the environment and conserves heat energy. If the warm core blood is brought to the surface, skin temperature rises. Accordingly, the temperature difference between the body surface and the environment increases, as does the rate of heat exchange. This causes body cooling.

Blood Vessels

Blood is an important medium traveling through the skin. It is a fluid consisting of water, electrolytes, proteins, and cells. Blood travels through arteries, arterioles, veins, venules, and capillaries. Any soft-tissue wound or burn can affect the flow of blood through these vessels. Therefore, it is important for you to have an understanding of their basic structure.

The arteries, arterioles, veins, and venules are made up of three layers: the **tunica intima**, the **tunica media**, and the **tunica adventitia**. The intima is the interior, smooth lining. It allows for the free flow of blood and prevents absorption of the blood's nutrients and oxygen as well as waste products such as carbon dioxide. The media is the muscular part of the tube. It allows the central nervous system to control the vessel's internal diameter, or **lumen**. The size of the lumen determines how much flow will pass to a particular organ or extremity. Muscle fibers of the tunica media are found in two orientations. Most are wrapped around the vessel circumferentially and cause lumen constriction when they contract. Others run lengthwise, with their function not well understood. The outer layer of the vessel is the adventitia. It consists of connective tissue defining the maximum lumen when the muscles relax.

■ **lumen** opening, or space, within a needle, artery, vein, or other hollow vessel.

The final blood vessel is the capillary. Its wall is only one cell thick. It therefore allows the easy transfer of oxygen, carbon dioxide, nutrients, and waste products between the cardiovascular system, the interstitial spaces, and the body cells.

Functions of the Skin

The skin varies in thickness from almost a centimeter on the heel of the foot to microscopic dimensions on the surface of the eye. Extremely flexible, the skin ordinarily regenerates itself. This durable, thin organ provides a number of valuable functions.

❏ The skin protects the human body from many dangers found in the environment, such as pathogens.
❏ The skin functions as an organ of sensation, perceiving temperature, pressure (touch), and pain.
❏ The skin contains vital fluids and aids in temperature regulation through secretion of sweat and shunting of blood.
❏ The skin provides a barrier against infection and insulation from trauma.

Although many people often take the skin for granted, soft-tissue injury can subject a patient to severe blood and fluid loss, infection, hypothermia, and other injuries. Therefore, as a paramedic, you need to become familiar with the pathophysiology of wounds and burns to the skin.

PATHOPHYSIOLOGY OF SOFT-TISSUE INJURY

Soft tissues can be injured through two very different mechanisms. One is trauma and the other is burns. Trauma is a violent transfer of energy that produces either an open or closed wound on the skin. Burns induce a denaturing of the cell membrane through contact with heat, electricity, chemicals, or radiation. An understanding of these two injury mechanisms will help you to better apply the assessment and management process.

Wounds

Wounds are soft-tissue injuries affecting the epidermis, dermis, and subcutaneous tissues. They can be either blunt or penetrating. Common wounds include contusions, abrasions, lacerations, incisions, punctures, avulsions, and amputations. Each wound is different and deserves special consideration.

■ **contusion** closed wound in which the skin is unbroken, although damage has occurred to the immediate tissue beneath.

Contusions   **Contusions** are blunt, non-penetrating injuries that crush and damage small blood vessels. Blood is drawn to the inflamed tissue, caus-

■ **erythema** general reddening of the skin due to dilation of the superficial capillaries.

■ **ecchymosis** blue-black discoloration of the skin due to leakage of blood into the tissues.

■ **hematoma** collection of blood beneath the skin or trapped within a body compartment.

■ **abrasion** scraping or abrading away of the superficial layers of the skin. An open soft-tissue injury.

■ **laceration** open wound, normally a tear with jagged borders.

■ **incision** very smooth or surgical laceration, frequently caused by a knife, scalpel, razor blade, or piece of glass.

ing a reddening called **erythema**. Blood also leaks into the surrounding interstitial spaces through damaged vessels. As the free blood loses its oxygen, it becomes dark red and then blue, resulting in **ecchymosis**. Since ecchymosis is a delayed sign in wound progression, you will need to evaluate trauma patients carefully and serially.

Contusions are more pronounced in areas where the offending agent and skeletal structures (such as the ribs or the skull) trap the skin. Occasionally, a chest injury will display an erythematous or ecchymotic outline of the ribs and sternum, reflecting the impact with the auto dashboard or other blunt object. Early evidence of the injury may be difficult to identify. But as time passes, it will become more and more evident.

Soft-tissue bleeding can occur within the tissue and at times be quite significant. When the injury involves a larger vessel, most commonly an artery, the blood can actually separate tissue and pool in a pocket called a **hematoma**. These injuries are very visible in cases of head trauma because of the unyielding skull underneath. Although less pronounced in other areas, hematomas can contain significant hemorrhage. Severe hematomas to either the thigh, leg, or arm may contribute significantly to hypovolemia. The thigh, for example, has been known to contain over a liter of fluid before swelling becomes apparent.

Abrasions   **Abrasions** are typically the most minor of injuries that penetrate the epidermis and violate the protective envelope of the skin. They involve an abrasive action that removes layers of the epidermis and the upper reaches of the dermis. Bleeding is usually limited because the injury involves only superficial capillaries. If the injury compromises a large surface of the epidermis, it carries the danger of secondary infection.

Lacerations   A **laceration** is an open wound penetrating more deeply into the dermis than the abrasion. A laceration tends to involve a smaller surface area, being limited to the immediate tissue surrounding the penetration. It endangers the deeper and more significant vasculature: arteries, arterioles, venules, and veins, as well as nerves, tendons, ligaments, and perhaps some underlying organs. Because of the potential for involvement of other structures, you will need to evaluate the laceration site carefully. (See Figure 18-2.) As with the abrasion, the injury breaks the protective barrier and provides a pathway for infection.

Incisions   An **incision** is a surgically smooth laceration. Often caused by a sharp instrument such as a knife, straight razor, or piece of glass, this wound tends to bleed freely. In all other ways, it is a laceration.

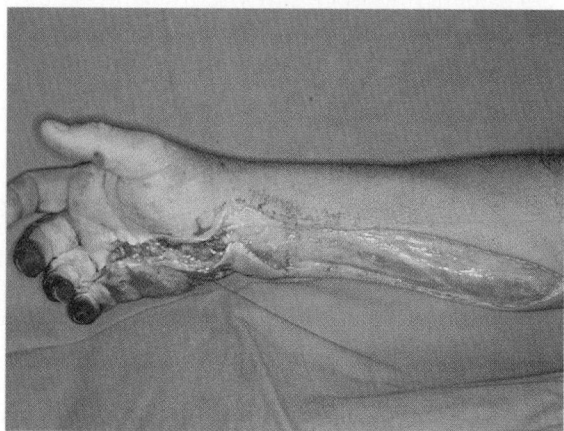

FIGURE 18-2 Severe hand injury resulting from contact with a high-pressure grease gun. The initial injury appeared very minor. (Courtesy of Scott and White Hospital and Clinic)

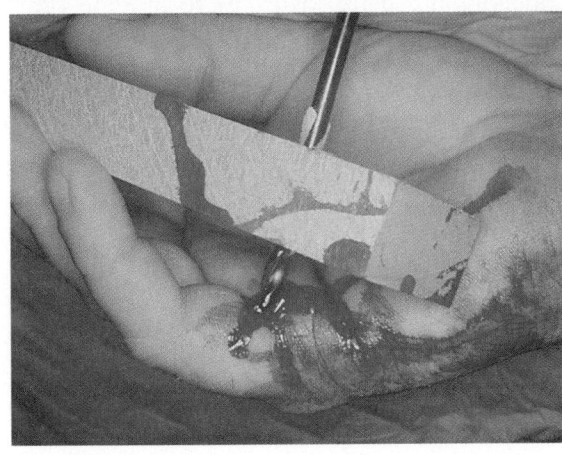

FIGURE 18-3 Penetrating injury with retained foreign body. (Courtesy of Scott and White Hospital and Clinic)

Punctures A second special type of laceration is the **puncture**. It involves a small entrance wound with damage into the interior of the body. (See Figure 18-3.) The wound will normally seal itself and present in a way unreflective of the extent of injury. Besides the depth of damage, the puncture carries the danger of infection. The penetrating object introduces bacteria and other pathogens into the wound, thus opening the way to serious infection. Low oxygen levels in deep wounds compound the problem because of the more favorable environment for bacterial growth.

■ **puncture** specific soft-tissue injury involving a deep, narrow wound to the skin and underlying organs. It carries an increased danger of infection.

Avulsions **Avulsion** occurs when a flap of skin, although torn or cut, is not completely loose. Avulsion is frequently seen with blunt trauma to the skull where the scalp is torn and folds back. It may also occur with animal bites and machinery accidents. (See Figure 18-4.) Its seriousness depends upon the area involved, the condition of the circulation to (and distal to) the injury site, and the degree of contamination.

A special type of avulsion is the degloving injury. The mechanism of injury tears the skin off the underlying muscle, blood vessels, and bone. It is a particularly gruesome injury, occurring occasionally with farm and industrial machinery. The device traps the skin as the skeletal tissue underneath pulls away with great force. The wound exposes a large area of tissue and is often severely contaminated. The injury carries with it a poor prognosis. If, how-

■ **avulsion** forceful tearing away or separation of body tissue. The avulsion may be partial or complete.

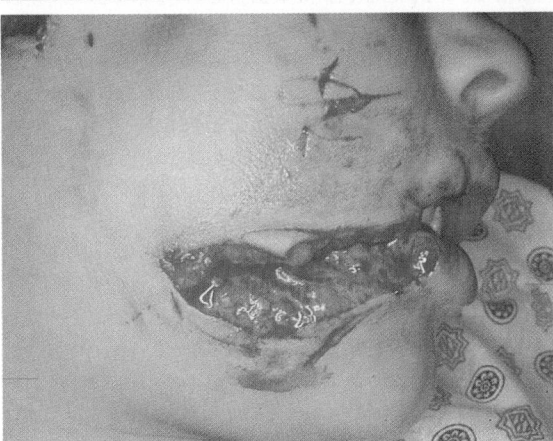

FIGURE 18-4 Avulsion in a young child resulting from a dog bite. (Courtesy of Scott and White Hospital and Clinic)

ever, the vasculature and the innervation remain intact, there may be some hope for use of the extremity or the digit.

A variation of the degloving process is the ring injury. As a person jumps or falls, the ring is caught, pulling the skin of the finger against the weight of the victim. The force may tear the upper layers of tissue away from the phalanges, exposing the tendons, nerves, and blood vessels. Although the ring injury involves a smaller area, it is otherwise similar to the degloving injury.

■ **amputation** severance, removal, or detachment, either partial or complete, of a body part.

Amputations   The partial or complete severance of a digit or limb is an **amputation**. It often results in the complete loss of the limb at the site of severance. The surgeon may reattach the amputated part or use the skin for grafting, as he or she repairs the remaining limb. If this skin is unavailable, the surgeon may have to cut the bone and musculature back further to close the wound. This will reduce the length of the limb as well as its future usefulness.

Hemorrhage

Soft-tissue injuries frequently cause blood loss, ranging from inconsequential to life threatening. The loss can be arterial, venous, or capillary. Bleeding can be easy or almost impossible to control. Hemorrhage is usually dark red in venous injury, red in capillary injury, and bright red in arterial injury. The rate of hemorrhage also progresses from oozing capillary to flowing venous to pulsing arterial bleeding. In practice, it may be hard to differentiate between the origins of hemorrhage. However, it is important for you to determine the rate and quantity of blood loss. This information will help you decide upon the most effective means of stopping the blood flow.

Elements in the blood may assist in the control of blood loss through the clotting process. Plasma and the platelets release proteins at the site of disturbed flow and injury to the blood vessel. They form a matrix of fibers and capture the red blood cells, occluding flow. This clotting mechanism takes about ten minutes in the normal, healthy adult. It is more rapid if the injury involves a small blood vessel; it is less rapid if the vessel is a large artery or vein.

Often the nature of the vessel injury may be more important than the size or type of vessel. If a moderately-sized vein or artery is cut cleanly, the muscles in its wall will contract. This retracts the severed vessel into the tissue. As the muscle is drawn back from the wound, it thickens and restricts the lumen. This tamponades flow, reduces the rate of loss, and assists the clotting mechanisms. Therefore, clean lacerations and amputations generally do not bleed profusely. If the vessel is not severed cleanly but is laid open instead, the muscle contraction will open the wound, thereby increasing blood loss. Such an injury accompanies laceration that either parallels or involves a large blood vessel.

Another type of injury that may result in heavy, difficult-to-control bleeding is the crushing wound. It is a combination of lacerations and contusions that present with generalized bleeding from the wound. Because the injury does not cleanly sever the vessels, they bleed without the natural control of retraction. The actual bleeding source is difficult to locate and control.

Burns

Burns, as you have read, result from the disruption of proteins in the cell membranes. It is important that you learn to determine the cause, degree, and extent of burn. This information will help you accurately report the condition to medical control—an essential step in the care of a severely burned patient.

Types of Burns   Soft-tissue burns occur secondary to thermal (heat), electrical, chemical, or radiation insult to the body. While the result of the burn mechanism is much the same, the process of damage differs. The following sections describe each of these four types of burns.

Thermal Burns.   The thermal burn actually causes damage by increasing the rate at which the molecules within an object move and collide with each other. The measure of the energy of this motion is *temperature*. At a temperature greater than absolute zero, the molecules of any object move about. As the temperature of the object increases, the speed of the molecules and the incidence of collision with other molecules also increases. This changing internal energy causes many substances, such as steel, to expand with increasing temperature. Heat energy may also cause chemical changes. As temperature increases, substances such as gasoline may combine with oxygen. The nature of matter may change as well. Water, for example, may change into ice or steam. An egg becomes hard as the proteins break down in a hot frying pan.

Such changes also take place in the burn patient. As molecular speed increases, the cell components, especially membranes and proteins, begin to break down just like the egg in a frying pan. The result of exposure to extreme heat is progressive injury and cell death.

The extent of burn injury relates to the amount of heat energy transferred to the patient's skin. That energy in turn depends upon three components of the burning agent: its temperature, the concentration of heat energy it possesses, and the length of contact time. Obviously, the greater the temperature of an agent, the greater the potential for damage.

It is also important to consider the amount of heat energy possessed by the object or substance. A blast of heated air from an oven at 350 degrees is much less damaging than hot cooking oil at the same temperature. Also, momentary contact with hot oil would result in less damage than if it is poured into one's shoe.

The burn is a progressive process. Thus, the greater the heat energy transmitted by the burn process to the body, the deeper the wound. Initially, the burn damages the epidermis by the increase in temperature. As the contact with the substance continues, the heat energy penetrates further and deeper into the body tissue. It may involve the epidermis, dermis, subcutaneous, muscular, skeletal, and other internal tissue.

Electrical Burns.   The power of electricity results from a flow of electrons from a point of high concentration to one of low concentration. The difference between the two concentrations is called the *voltage*. The rate of flow, or the current, is known as the *amperage*. A third variable is *resistance*. The copper of electrical wire allows free flow of electrons and has very little resistance. Tungsten (the filament in a light bulb) is moderately resistant and will heat, glow, and emit light as you apply more and more current.

The human body, like tungsten, is relatively resistant to the flow of electricity. If you subject the human body to a voltage differential, it will allow the current to pass. As it does, it creates heat energy. For small voltages, the energy is of little consequence. But if the voltage or current is high, it can cause profound damage. The longer the duration of contact, the greater the potential for injury.

Thermal injury due to electrical current occurs as energy travels from the point of contact to the point of exit. (See Figure 18-5.) At both these points, the concentration of electricity is great, as is the degree of damage you might expect. The smaller the area of contact, the greater the concentration of current flow and the greater the injury. Between the entrance and exit points, the

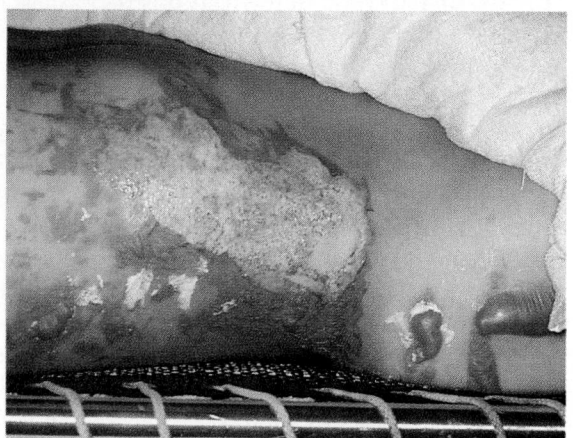

FIGURE 18-5 Exit wound from electrocution injury. Patient is a male who came into contact with 72,000-volt power lines. (Courtesy of Scott and White Hospital and Clinic)

energy spreads out over a larger cross-sectional area and generally causes less injury. Electric current may follow blood vessels and nerves since they offer less resistance than muscle and bone. This may lead to serious injury deep within the involved limbs.

Electrical contact may also disrupt control of muscle tissue. Muscles are controlled by complicated electrochemical reactions that can be severely disrupted by the passage of current, especially alternating current. If the current continues for a period of time, it may immobilize the muscles of respiration. The result is prolonged respiratory arrest, anoxia, hypoxemia, and eventually death. The electrical current may also disrupt the heart's electrical system, causing ventricular fibrillation accompanied by ineffective pumping action.

At times, electrical energy may cause flash burns secondary to the heat of current passing through adjacent air or by the ignition of clothing or other combustibles. Air is very resistant to the passage of electrical current. If the current is strong enough and the space is small, the electricity will arc, producing tremendous heat. If the patient's skin is close by, the heat may severely burn or vaporize tissue. Additionally, the heat may ignite articles of clothing and result in the more common thermal burn.

Chemical Burns. Chemical burns denature the biochemical makeup of the cell membrane and destroy the cell. Such injury is not transmitted through the tissue as is the thermal injury. A chemical burn must destroy the tissue before chemically burning any deeper. This generally limits the "burn" process unless very strong chemicals are involved. Chemical burns may be caused by agents too numerous to mention. They are most commonly either strong acids or bases (alkali).

Radiation Injury. The earth has been bombarded with nuclear radiation since before recorded time. It is a daily, natural phenomenon. The danger becomes apparent with exposure to synthetic sources that greatly increase the intensity of radiation. Industry and medicine use radioactive materials for diagnostic testing and for energy production. The risk of injury occurs from accidents associated with improper handling, either in the on-site environment or during transport.

Nuclear radiation causes damage through a process known as **ionization**. A radioactive energy particle travels into a substance and changes an internal atom. In the human body, the affected cell either repairs the damage, dies, or goes on to produce damaged cells (cancer). The cells most sensitive to radiation injury are *erythrocytes*, cells responsible for erythrocyte production (marrow), cells lining the intestinal tract, and cells involved in human reproduction.

■ **ionization** the process of changing a substance into separate charged particles (ions).

We commonly encounter three types of radiation. These include:

❑ *Alpha Radiation.* The nucleus of an atom releases **alpha radiation** in the form of a neutron. It is a very weak energy source and travels only inches through the air. Paper or clothing will easily stop alpha radiation. It also will not penetrate the epidermis of the skin. It is really only a hazard if the patient inhales or ingests contaminated material.

❑ *Beta Radiation.* The second radiological particle is **beta radiation**. Its energy is greater than that of alpha radiation. It will travel 6–10 feet through air or will penetrate a few layers of clothing. Beta particles will invade the first few millimeters of skin, thus creating the potential for external as well as internal contamination.

❑ *Gamma Radiation.* **Gamma radiation**, also known as X-rays, is the most powerful ionizing radiation. It has the ability to travel through the entire body or ionize any atom within. Gamma radiation evokes the greatest concern for external exposure. It is the most dangerous and most feared type of radiation because it is difficult to protect against.

■ **alpha radiation** lowest level of nuclear radiation. A weak source of energy, it is stopped by clothing or the first layers of skin.

■ **beta radiation** medium-strength radiation stopped with light clothing or the uppermost layers of skin.

■ **gamma radiation** powerful electromagnetic radiation emitted by radioactive substances. It is stronger than alpha and beta radiation.

Exposure to radiation and the effects of ionization can occur through two mechanisms. A strong radioactive source, composed of an unstable material such as uranium, may expose the unshielded person to ionizing radiation. The second mechanism of exposure is contamination by dust, debris, or fluids that contain very small particles of radioactive material. The contaminant gives off weaker levels of radiation. However, close proximity to the body and longer contact time may produce greater exposure and contamination. Note that most substances, including human tissue, will not give off radiation. The patient alone is not the danger in the radiological incident. Any danger comes from a radioactive source such as the contaminated material on the patient.

Three aspects of radiation exposure are of importance to you. They include: duration of exposure; the distance from the source; and the shielding between you, the patient, and the source. Knowledge of these three factors can limit your exposure and potential for injury.

❑ *Duration.* Radiation exposure is an accumulative danger. The longer you or the patient remain exposed to the source, the greater the potential for injury.

❑ *Distance.* Radiation strength reduces quickly as you travel farther from the source. It is similar to the intensity of light from a light bulb. At a few feet, we can easily read by it, while at a few hundred feet the light barely casts a shadow. Mathematically, the relationship is inverse and squared. As we double our distance from the source, its strength drops to one fourth. As we triple the distance, its strength diminishes to one ninth, and so on.

❑ *Shielding.* The more material between you and the source, the less you will experience radioactive exposure. With alpha and beta radiation, shielding is very easy and reasonably effective. With gamma sources, you need dense objects such as earth, concrete, metal, and lead to provide any real protection.

It is very difficult to determine the onset of radiological exposure. Radiation is invisible and cannot be felt. It does not present with any immediate side effects, unless the exposure is extremely high. Instead, the results of an exposure may present serious medical problems years after the incident.

The injuries and side effects of exposure relate to the dose and occur in either the acute or delayed time parameters. Acute symptoms include nausea, vomiting, and malaise. If the dose is extremely high, it may lead to severe illness and death. In some cases, burns may evolve, especially if a limb receives very high doses of beta or gamma radiation. Moderate or prolonged exposure to radiation may produce long-term and delayed problems. Infertility is a potential injury, since the cells producing the egg and sperm are very susceptible to ionization damage. Cancer is another delayed and severe side effect. It may occur years or even decades after an incident.

✱ Inhalation injury may be associated with burns, especially if the injury occurred in an enclosed space.

Inhalation Injury   The burn environment frequently causes inhalation injury. This is especially true if the injury occurs in a closed space or when the patient is unconscious. A patient who is unconscious or entrapped in a smoke-filled area will eventually breathe in the gases, heated air, flame, or steam. The result is sustained airway and respiratory injury.

You can expect to find the following inhalation conditions in a burn environment. Keep them in mind as you survey the scene and take the necessary protective measures.

Toxic Inhalation.   Modern residential and commercial construction uses synthetic resins and plastics that release toxic gases when they burn. They can form such toxic compounds as potassium cyanide and hydrogen sulfide. If a patient inhales these gases, they will react with the lung tissue, causing internal chemical burns or an actual systemic poisoning. The signs and symptoms of these injuries may not display until an hour or two after inhalation.

Airway Thermal Burn.   Another, though less frequent, injury is the airway thermal burn. Very moist mucosa lines the airway and insulates it very well against heat damage. It takes great thermal energy to evaporate the fluid and injure the cells. Hot air or flame inspiration rarely has enough heat energy to cause significant thermal airway burns.

An occasional cause of thermal airway burn is super-heated steam. Steam is created under great pressure and heats to well above 212°F. A common hazard to firefighters, it develops when a stream of water strikes a hot spot and vaporizes explosively. The blast may dislodge the firefighter's self-contained breathing apparatus, and he or she may inhale the super-heated steam. It contains enough energy to severely burn the upper airway. It also may damage the lower respiratory tract, although this happens infrequently.

With any thermal or smoke-related chemical burn injury to the respiratory tract, there is the danger of airway restriction, severe dyspnea, and possible respiratory arrest. The airway is a narrow tube, lined with extremely vascular tissue. If damaged, it will swell rapidly, seriously reducing the size of the airway lumen. (See Figure 18-6.) The patient may present with a minor

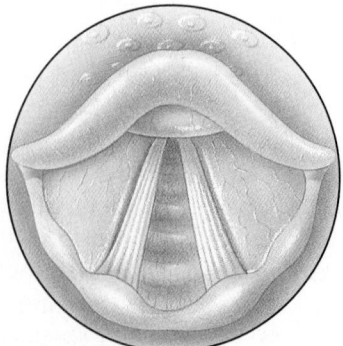 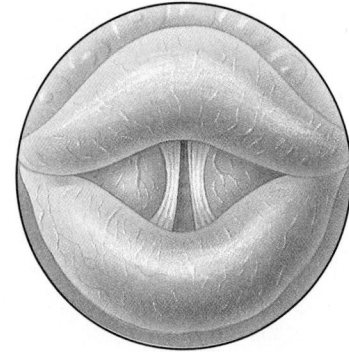

FIGURE 18-6   Laryngeal edema from inhalation injury.

hoarseness, followed precipitously by dyspnea. The injury may be so extensive as to induce complete respiratory obstruction and arrest.

Carbon Monoxide Poisoning. An additional concern associated with the burn environment is carbon monoxide poisoning. Suspect it in any patient who has been within an enclosed space during combustion. Poisoning occurs because the hemoglobin of the blood has a much greater affinity for carbon monoxide than for the essential oxygen. If your patient inhales it, even in the smallest quantities, carbon monoxide will displace oxygen. The result is hypoxemia. Although difficult to detect, hypoxemia will subtly embarrass the patient's oxygen delivery to vital organs. If associated with airway burns, it will further compound the respiratory compromise.

✳ Carbon monoxide poisoning is a frequent hazard that should be suspected in any patient who was in an enclosed space during combustion.

Degree of Burn   After you determine the source of the burn and any associated inhalation injury, you need to assess the burn's severity. Burns are normally classified by degrees. (See Figure 18-7.) The *first-degree burn* involves only the upper layers of the epidermis and dermis. It is an irritation of the living cells in this region and results in some pain, minor edema, and erythema. It will normally heal without complication. (See Figure 18-8.)

The *second-degree burn* penetrates slightly deeper and produces blisters. Heat energy travels into the dermis, involving more of the tissue and resulting in greater destruction. The second-degree burn is similar to the first in that it is reddened, painful, and edematous. (See Figure 18-9.) You can differentiate it from the first-degree burn only after blisters form. First- and

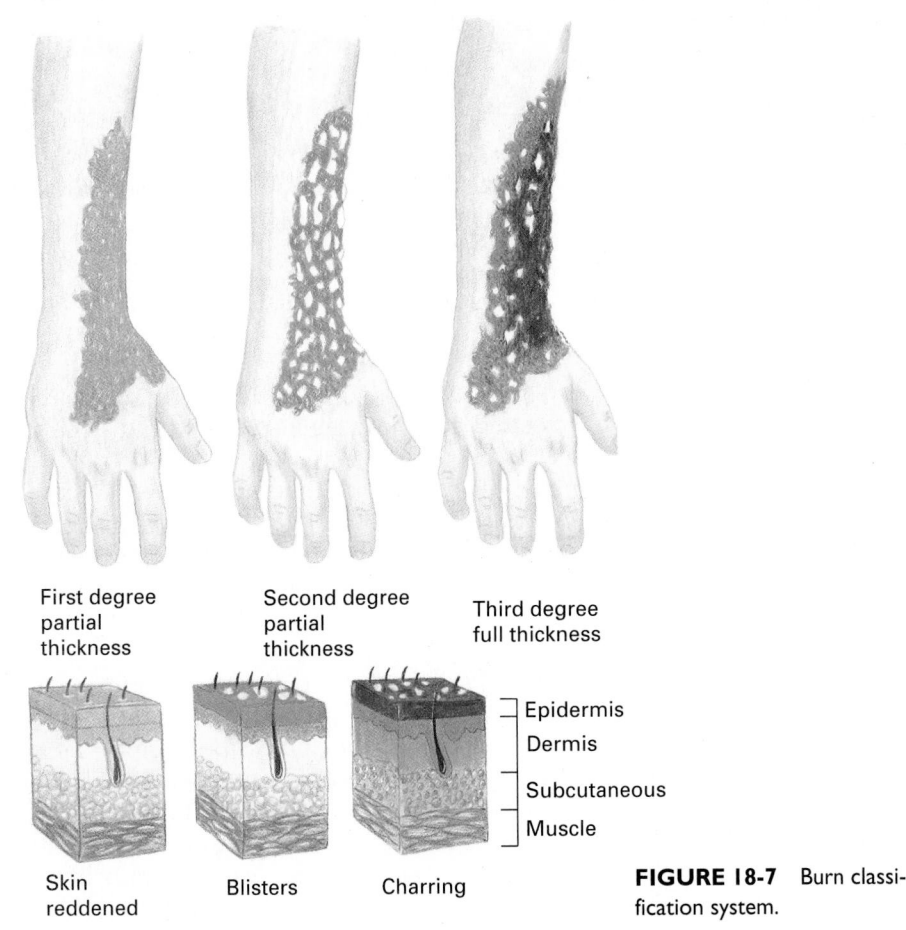

First degree
partial
thickness

Second degree
partial
thickness

Third degree
full thickness

Epidermis
Dermis
Subcutaneous
Muscle

Skin
reddened

Blisters

Charring

FIGURE 18-7   Burn classification system.

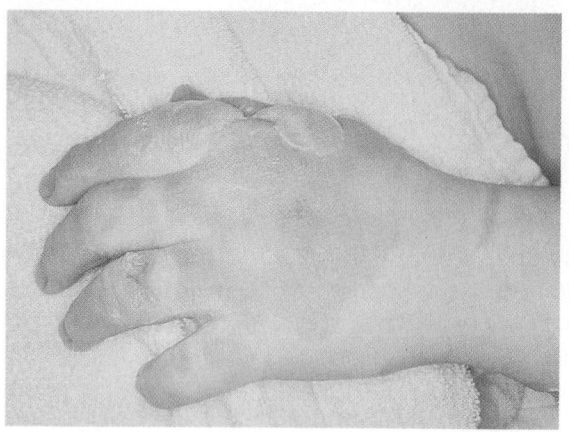

FIGURE 18-8 Burn injury of the hand with primarily first- and second-degree burns. (Courtesy of Scott and White Hospital and Clinic)

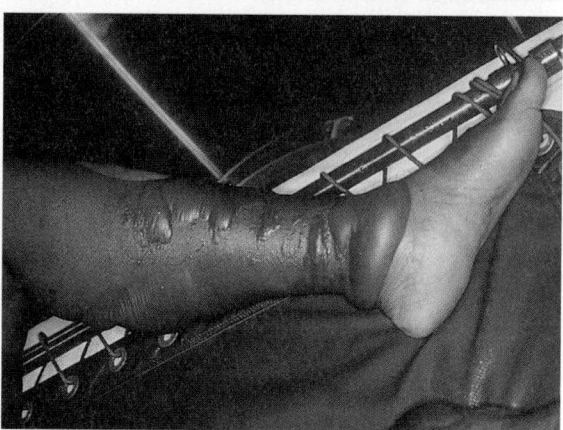

FIGURE 18-9 Second-degree burns are characterized by the formation of fluid-filled blisters. (Courtesy of Scott and White Hospital and Clinic)

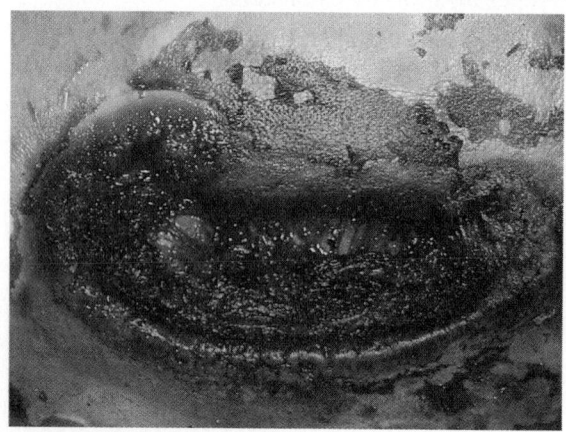

FIGURE 18-10 Third-degree burn. (Courtesy of Scott and White Hospital and Clinic)

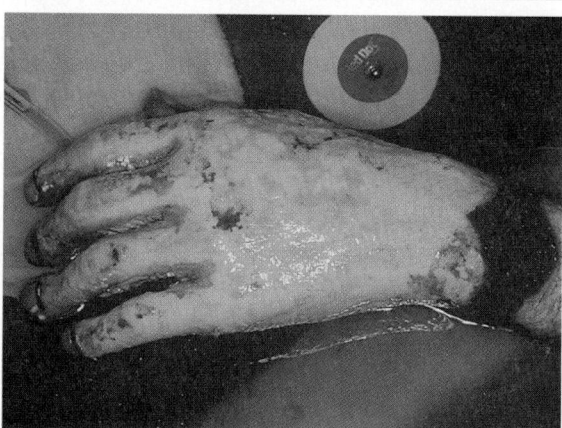

FIGURE 18-11 Third-degree burns result in complete loss of the skin. (Courtesy of Scott and White Hospital and Clinic)

second-degree burns are also referred to as partial-thickness burns. This is because the dermis is still intact and complete regeneration of the skin is very likely.

A special and common type of partial-thickness burn is the sunburn. Ultraviolet radiation causes the burn rather than the normal thermal process. The radiation penetrates only superficially and damages the uppermost layers of the dermis. Although it may present as the classical first- or second-degree injury, it will be limited in its damage when you compare it to the thermal second-degree burn.

Third-degree burns, or full-thickness burns, penetrate the entire dermis. These burns destroy the tissue's regenerative properties and the peripheral nerve endings. (See Figure 18-10.) The injury is painless because of the nerve destruction. The burn will take on various discolorations due to the nature of the burning agent and the damaged, dying, or dead tissue. Third-degree burns may involve injury to blood vessels, nerves, muscle tissue, bone, or internal organs. Because the burn destroys the entire dermis, healing is difficult unless the wound is small or skin grafting is possible. (See Figure 18-11.)

Extent of Burn Surface Area   Prehospital care providers use one of two methods to estimate burn surface area. In the field setting, we most commonly use the *rule of nines* to make gross estimations. Less frequently, we use the *palmar surface* (based upon the size of the patient's hand) to assess smaller wounds more accurately.

Rule of Nines.   The rule of nines identifies eleven topographical regions of the body, each of which occupies approximately 9 percent of body surface area. (See Figure 18-12.) These regions include the entire head and neck, the front of the chest, the front of the abdomen, the posterior chest, the lower back (the posterior abdomen), the anterior surface of each lower extremity, the posterior surface of each lower extremity, and each upper extremity. The remaining 1 percent of surface area is assigned to the genitalia.

Since the anatomy of the infant and the child differs significantly from that of the adult, we modify the rule of nines for them. We divide the head and neck area into the anterior and posterior surface and award 9 percent for each. We reduce the surface area of each lower extremity by 4 1/2 percent to ensure the total body surface area remains at 100 percent. This is at best a gross approximation of the area burned. Health care workers regard it as such.

Palmar Surface.   An alternative system for burn approximation uses the surface of the patient's hand to approximate the affected body area. The palm of one hand represents about 1 percent of the body surface area, whether the patient is an adult, a child, or an infant. If you can visualize the palmar surface area and apply it to the burn area mentally, then you can obtain an estimate of the total skin surface affected.

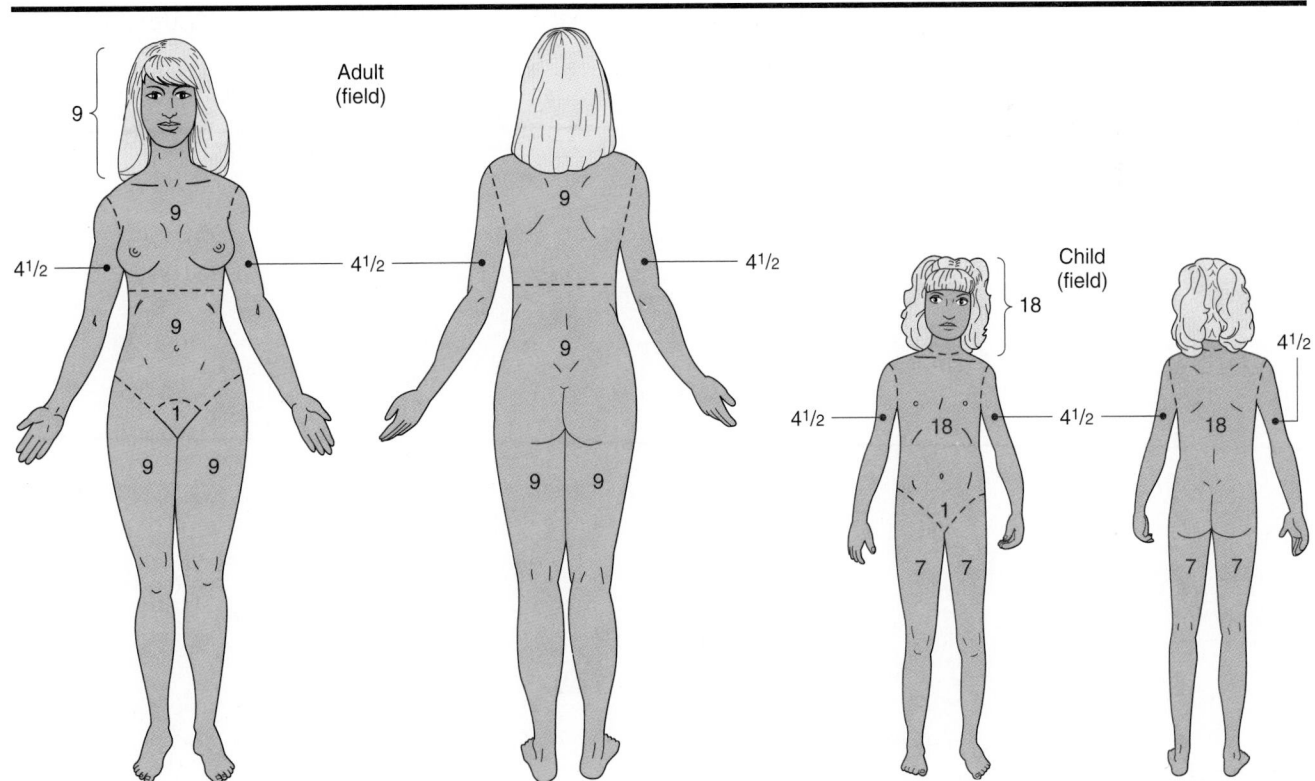

FIGURE 18-12   The rule of nines.

The system is easier to use for the local burns, while the rule of nines is simpler and more appropriate for larger burns. Many other burn approximation routines exist that are both more specific to age and, in general, more accurate. However, they are more complicated and time consuming to use. Both the rule of nines and the palmar surface method provide reasonable approximations of burn surface area if you apply them properly in the field.

Systemic Complications   Burns cause several systemic complications. These include hypothermia, hypovolemia, and the formation of an eschar.

Hypothermia. A burn may disrupt the body's ability to regulate core temperature. The destruction of tissue reduces or eliminates the ability of the skin to contain the fluid within. The burn process releases plasma and other tissue, which seep into the wound. There they evaporate and rapidly remove heat energy. If the burn is extensive, the uncontrolled loss of body heat may induce hypothermia.

Hypovolemia. Hypovolemia also may complicate the severe burn. The inability of damaged blood vessels to contain plasma will cause a shift of proteins and fluid into the burn tissue. Loss of plasma protein will reduce the blood's ability, via osmosis, to draw fluids from the uninjured tissues. This in turn will reduce the body's natural response to fluid loss and may produce a profound hypovolemia. (See Figure 18-13.) Although this is a serious complication of the extensive burn, it takes hours to develop. Modern aggressive fluid resuscitation can counteract this aspect of the burn process.

Eschar. The denaturing of the skin further complicates the injury in the third-degree thermal burn. As the burn destroys the dermal cells, they become hard and leathery, producing what is known as an **eschar**. The skin as a whole tightens over the wound site, restricting the flow of blood and increasing the pressure of any edema beneath. If the burn is **circumferential**, the

■ **eschar** hard, leathery product of deep third-degree burn. It consists of dead and denatured skin.

■ **circumferential** encircling or going around the complete exterior.

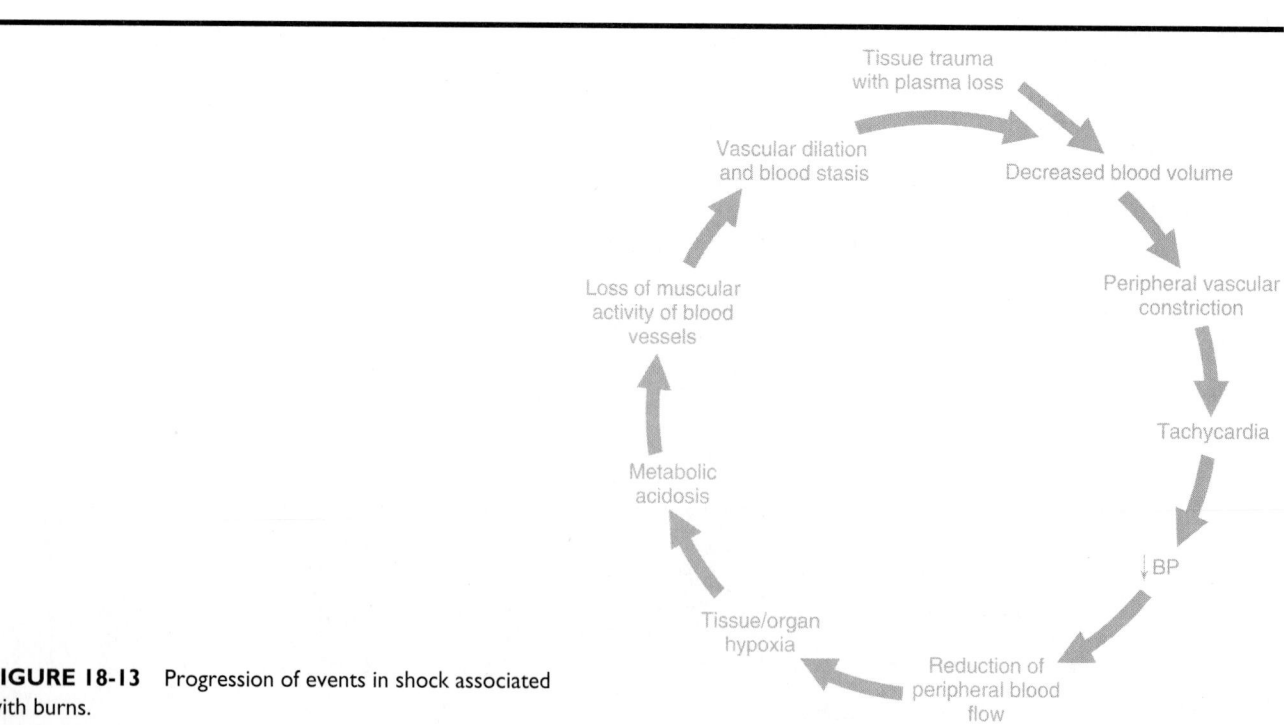

FIGURE 18-13   Progression of events in shock associated with burns.

constriction may be severe enough to occlude all blood flow into the distal extremity. In the case of the thoracic burn, it may drastically reduce chest excursion and respiratory tidal volume. (See Figure 18-14.)

Special Considerations   Although infection is the most persistent killer of burn victims, it does not directly concern you in the field setting. Pathogens invade the wound shortly after the burn occurs and up until the wound heals. Their hazard to life occurs as they grow to massive numbers, a process taking days or weeks to develop.

Special factors that more immediately affect your field decisions involve the patient's overall health and age. The geriatric, pediatric, ill, or trauma patient has greater difficulty handling the burn injury than does the healthy individual. The pediatric patient suffers from a high surface area to body weight ratio, which means the fluid reserves for the burn are low. Geriatric patients have reduced mechanisms for fluid retention, lower fluid reserves, and are more apt to have underlying disease. Ill patients are already using body energy to fight their disease. With the burn, these patients now have two

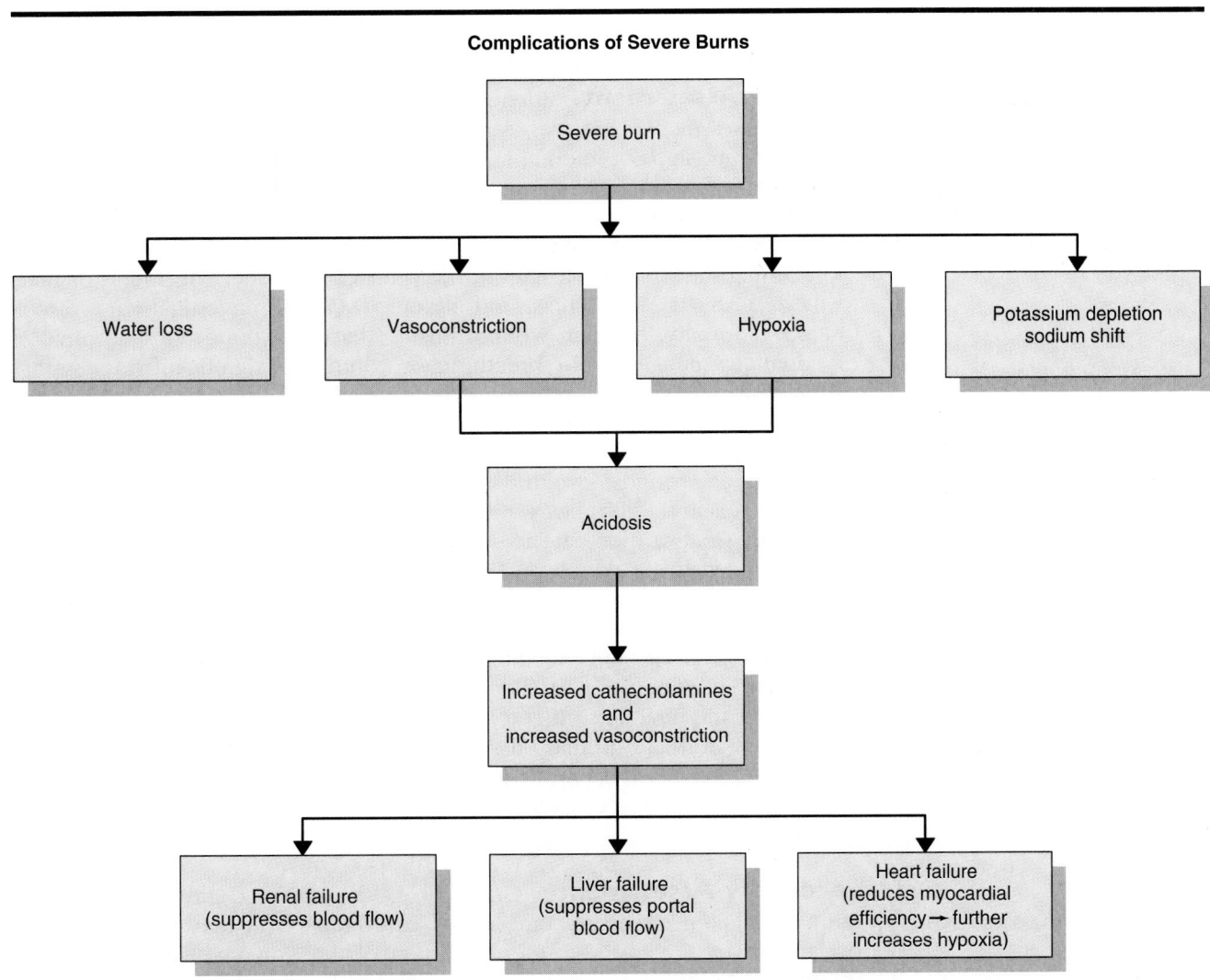

FIGURE 18-14 Complications of severe burns.

medical stresses to combat. Burn fluid loss also compounds the blood loss of trauma patients. They, too, must recover from two injuries.

ASSESSMENT OF SOFT-TISSUE INJURY

Evaluation of the skin tells more about the condition of the body than any other aspect of patient assessment. Not only is the skin the first body organ to experience the effects of trauma, it is the first and often the only organ to display them. Therefore, assessment of the skin, and the associated wounds and burns, must be deliberate, careful, and complete.

While the soft-tissue injury process varies, assessment is simple and well structured. Apply it carefully and completely to ensure that you establish the nature and extent of each injury. This will help you to place soft-tissue injuries in the appropriate priority for care.

Wounds

Assessment of patients with soft-tissue wounds follows the same general progression as other assessments. First, you survey the scene, ruling out potential hazards. Next, you perform a quick primary assessment. Then you complete each element of the secondary assessment: the head-to-toe survey, vital signs, and patient history.

Primary Assessment   Identification of wounds forms a key part of the primary assessment. However, remember that wounds are often the only or most apparent signs of internal injury. Severe and life-threatening hemorrhage may also accompany soft-tissue injuries. In either case, the evaluation of wounds begins after you assess and secure the ABC's and quickly determine the patient's general neurologic status.

During the "Expose" aspect of the primary assessment, examine wounds to the face, head, neck, chest, and abdomen. Quickly investigate any discoloration, deformity, or open wound. Ensure that the wound does not involve or endanger the airway or breathing or contribute significantly to hypovolemia. Focus immediate care upon controlling severe blood loss or the more serious injuries that the soft-tissue trauma may suggest.

Scan the entire body for external bleeding. If the mechanism of injury suggests open wounds, sweep the body areas hidden from sight with gloved hands. This action will quickly rule out otherwise unseen, rapid, and pooling blood loss. Control moderate to severe hemorrhage immediately. The control does not need to be definitive, but it should stop any continuing significant blood loss. When more time can be spent, properly dress and bandage the wound.

Quickly survey the bleeding wound to determine the type of hemorrhage: arterial, venous, or capillary. Approximate and compare the volume of loss against the time since the accident. The result will be the rate of loss. At the conclusion of the primary assessment, make the decision either to transport immediately or remain at the scene and provide complete care. Consider the rate and volume of any blood loss and any uncontrollable bleeding in this decision.

Secondary Assessment   Once you have completed the primary assessment and taken necessary emergency care steps, you may begin the secondary survey. The head-to-toe evaluation of the skin involves observation, inquiry, and palpation. It must follow a planned and comprehensive process, although the actual order is not critical.

* Wound assessment must be comprehensive to ensure that the extent of each injury is known so that care can be appropriately prioritized.

Observe. Begin wound assessment by observing a particular body region. Identify any discoloration, deformity, or frank wounds. Determine if any discoloration is local, distal, or systemic. Contusions, blood-vessel injuries, dislocations, and fractures may cause local discoloration, including erythema or ecchymosis. Distal discoloration may reflect the pale, cyanotic, or ashen color of a limb distal to the point of circulation loss. You may find systemic discoloration such as a pale, ashen, or gray hue in all limbs, suggesting hypovolemia and shock.

Inspect any wound in detail. Visualize to determine its depth, and evaluate the potential for damage to underlying bones, muscle, or body organs. If possible, identify the offending agent, and determine the amount of force transmitted to the interior. Your assessment should also determine the nature and quantity of any wound contamination and the depth of its introduction. Observe the wound in such a way that you can describe it to the attending physician after you dress and bandage the injury. This information will help the emergency department staff to prioritize patient injuries. It will also help with the documentation in the run report.

✱ The wound should be observed in such a way that it can later be described to the attending physician.

Inquire. Question the patient about the mechanism of injury, any pain or pain on movement, and the loss of function or sensation specific to an area. Additionally, attempt to determine what happened and the exact nature of any pain or sensory or motor loss. Question the patient about signs or symptoms before touching an area.

Palpate. Finally, palpate the entire body surface. Attempt to locate any deformity, asymmetry, temperature variation, unexpected masses, and localized loss of skin or muscle tone. Also note any tenderness or loss of sensation. (Employ universal precautions during palpation.)

Prioritize soft-tissue wounds to identify the order of care to follow. The few moments taken to sort out injuries and to plan the management process will save time in the field. This will also ensure that you provide early care for injuries with the highest priority.

Thermal Burns

Like the assessment of wounds, the assessment of thermal burns follows established procedures for performing the primary and secondary surveys. However, because of the inherent environmental danger involved in a thermal burn incident, you must first conduct a full scene survey.

Scene Survey Rescuer and patient safety depend upon a complete and thorough survey of the scene. Stop the burning process so it no longer threatens you or the patient. Extinguish any overt flame and quickly survey the patient for other sources that may continue the burn process. Assure that the patient's environment is free from the danger of structural collapse, contamination, electricity, and any other hazards.

Include a quick check of the patient's posterior surface. Burn patients may be an actual source of hazard to you and to themselves. Leather articles will smolder for hours and continue to induce thermal injury. Specifically look at any shoes, belts, or watchbands. Watches, rings, and other jewelry may also hold and transmit heat. Be careful as you check these items. They may be hot enough to burn you.

✱ Look for and extinguish smoldering shoes, belts, or watchbands early in the assessment of burn patients.

Except in the very local burn, view the patient's entire body surface. Remove any clothing that was or could have been involved in the burn. If any of the clothing within the wound resists removal, cut around it as necessary.

Once the scene is safe and the patient's clothing is not burning, examine the burn mechanism. Is there any possibility that the patient was unconscious during the fire or trapped within the building? If so, place a special emphasis upon airway assessment and management. Watch for any signs of airway restriction, and be alert to the possibility of carbon monoxide poisoning.

Primary Assessment   Start your primary survey by ruling out any danger of associated trauma or the possibility of spine injury. Otherwise, protect the patient from further cervical injury.

Next, assure the airway is patent. If not, protect it. Give the burn patient special consideration under this priority. Look for the signs of any thermal or inhalation injury during the initial airway exam. Carefully visualize the nasal hairs to ensure they have not been singed. Examine any sputum and the areas around the mouth and nose for carbonaceous residue or any other evidence of inhalation. Airway sounds reflecting irritation or mucosal damage, such as hoarseness or coughing, should alert you to the potential for airway injury and progressive restriction to follow. Consider a patient with any signs of respiratory involvement as a potential acute emergency, and provide immediate transport and care.

Institute high-flow oxygen, and ready the equipment for endotracheal intubation. Burn patients may progress rapidly from mild dyspnea to total respiratory arrest. While the intubation of a respiratory burn patient may be difficult in the field, there are distinct advantages to performing it early. The edema is progressive and will gradually reduce the airway lumen. If intubation waits until the patient arrives at the emergency department, the airway may be so edematous that it is difficult if not impossible to intubate.

If you elect (and medical control approves) field intubation for the burn patient, perform it quickly and carefully. The airway is already narrowing, and the normal trauma associated with intubation could make matters worse. The technique will also be complicated if the patient is conscious and fights the process. Under these circumstances, you may find nasotracheal intubation useful. Also consider oral intubation, using a topical lidocaine spray. In either case, select the crew members with the most experience to attempt this procedure. This will ensure that it is completed quickly.

As with all intubation, it is best to maintain an airway using the largest endotracheal tube possible. Have several smaller than normal-sized tubes ready, since the edema may limit the available size of the airway. Select the largest one that you think may easily pass through the cords.

The remainder of the primary assessment progresses as with any trauma patient. Establish the patient's level of consciousness or responsiveness. As you "Expose" and examine the patient, look for any circumferential burns of the head, neck, chest, extremity, or abdomen. The signs and symptoms of the severe burn will usually not affect the patient within the prehospital environment. The pain may actually be paradoxical to the severity of the burn. Less severe first- and second-degree burns are very uncomfortable, while extensive third-degree burns are often almost without pain.

The other classical and deadly problems associated with extensive soft-tissue burn will not develop until well after you have concluded prehospital care. Hypovolemia is frequently delayed because the fluid loss is gradual and progressive. Infection, the greatest cause of patient mortality, occurs days and often weeks after post-burn.

Rapidly transport any patient with third-degree burns over a large portion of the body. Patients with associated injury to the face, joints, hands, or feet are also candidates for immediate transport. Other cases include patients sustaining an inhalation of smoke, steam, or flame, or any geriatric, pediatric, ill, or trauma patient.

✱ In severe airway burns, if intubation waits until the patient arrives at the emergency department, the airway may be so edematous that it may be difficult or impossible to intubate once there.

Secondary Assessment The head-to-toe examination and the rest of the secondary assessment continues at the scene only if you can rule out significant and life-threatening burns. Otherwise, institute such assessment during transport. It is essential that you accurately approximate the depth and extent of the burn area. This will guide you in providing care. It will also help emergency department personnel to prepare for patient arrival.

✱ The head-to-toe examination should continue at the scene only if significant and life-threatening burns can be ruled out.

Apply the rule of nines to determine the total body surface area (BSA) burned. Add 9 percent if the burn involves an entire "rule of nines" region. If it only involves a portion, add that proportion of 9 percent. For example, if 1/3 of the upper extremity is burned, the surface area approximation is 3 percent (1/3 of 9 percent = 3 percent).

The depth of a burn injury is also an important consideration. Identify areas of painful sensation as *partial-thickness burns*. Consider those that present with limited or absent pain as probable *full-thickness burns*. This differentiation is difficult because partial-thickness injury and pain commonly surrounds the third-degree burn. (See Table 18-1.)

The third consideration in determining the severity of a burn is the area affected. The face, hands, feet, joints, genitalia, and circumferential burns deserve particular consideration. Each present with special problems to patients and their recovery. You have already assessed the face for burns to eliminate respiratory involvement. But this area also needs special consideration for aesthetic reasons. Facial damage and scarring may be more debilitating than any joint or limb burn. Carefully assess and give a high priority to these injuries, even if you do rule out respiratory involvement.

Consider burns involving the feet or the hands as serious. These areas are critical for much of the patient's daily activities. Serious burns and the associated scar tissue make thermal foot injury very debilitating. Assess these areas and communicate the degree and specific burn area to the receiving physician. Joints carry a similar danger. Scar tissue will replace the skin, with joint flexibility and mobility suffering. Give any burn appearing as full thickness and involving the hands, feet, or joints a higher priority than a burn of equal surface area and depth elsewhere.

TABLE 18-1 Characteristics of Various Depths of Burns			
	First Degree	**Second Degree**	**Third Degree**
Cause	Sun or minor flash	Hot liquids, flashes, or flame	Chemicals, electricity, flame, hot metals
Skin color	Red	Mottled red	Pearly white and/or charred, translucent, and parchment-like
Skin	Dry with no surface blister	Blisters with weeping	Dry with thrombosed blood vessels
Sensation	Painful	Painful	Anesthetic
Healing	3–6 days	2–4 weeks, depending on depth	Requires skin grafting

TABLE 18-2 Injuries that Benefit from Burn Center Care

A. Second-degree burn greater than 15 percent of body surface area (BSA)
B. Third-degree burn greater than 5 percent BSA
C. Significant face, feet, hands, perineal burns
D. High-voltage electrical injury
E. Inhalation injury
F. Chemical burns causing progressive tissue destruction
G. Associated significant injuries

Source: American Burn Association.

Also pay particular attention to burns surrounding an extremity, the thorax, the abdomen, or the neck. Due to the nature of a third-degree burn, the area underneath may be drastically compressed as an eschar forms. Constriction may hinder respirations, restrict distal blood flow, or cause hypoxia of the tissues beneath. Carefully assess any burn encircling a part of the body for distal circulation or other signs of vascular embarrassment.

Finally, assign a higher priority to any burn affecting pediatric, geriatric, ill, or otherwise injured patients. The serious burn causes great stress on these patients. Massive fluid and heat loss as well as infection challenge the human system. Consider the burn more serious when accompanied by any other patient problem. Once the depth, extent, and other contributing factors to burn severity have been determined, categorize the patient as either minor, moderate, or severely burned. The following criteria can be used as a guide.

1. Minor
   - Sunburns
   - Limited partial-thickness burn
2. Moderate
   - Partial-thickness burn over 15 percent BSA
   - Limited full-thickness burn
3. Severe
   - Partial-thickness burn over 30 percent BSA
   - Full-thickness burn over 5 percent BSA
   - Inhalation injury

Any involvement of a critical area, such as hands, feet, joints, face, or genitalia represent an increase in one level of severity. The same holds true for pediatric, geriatric, other trauma, or acute medical patients. Any signs or symptoms of respiratory involvement identifies the patient as a severe emergency. Such patients require immediate transport to a Burn Center, if possible. (See Table 18-2.)

Chemical Injuries

In dealing with the chemical burn, be sure the incident does not contaminate anyone else. Make certain that the source is isolated and no longer a danger to the patient or others. Remove any clothing that you suspect may be contaminated, and isolate it from accidental contact. Save it and then dispose of it properly.

✱ In dealing with the chemical burn, it is of the utmost concern that no one else is contaminated.

Personal protection is a priority. Always wear gloves, though you should never presume they protect you from the agent. Take appropriate protective action against airborne dust or toxic fumes, both for you and the patient. Identify the type of agent, its exact chemical name, the length of contact time, and the precise patient areas affected. Rule out contact with phenol, sodium, or dry lime. Examine any wound carefully to establish the depth, extent, and nature of the injury. Identify and enter in your report any first-aid given prior to your arrival.

Electrical Injuries

Be certain that the power has been shut off before you approach the scene. Until it is, do not allow anyone to approach the patient or the proximity of the electrical source. Handling of live wires is a dangerous activity under the best of conditions, even for specially trained personnel. Do not attempt it unless you are specially trained, equipped, and authorized.

* Until the power is off, no one should be allowed to approach the patient or the proximity of the electrical source.

Once the scene is secure, assess the patient and prepare him or her for transport. Search for both an entrance and an exit wound. Look specifically for possible points of contact with both the ground and the electrical source. In some circumstances, multiple entrance and exit wounds will be present. As with thermal burns, look for smoldering shoes, belts, or other items of clothing. They may continue the burning process well after the current is shut off. Also, it is necessary to monitor the patient for possible cardiac disturbances. Assure that emergency department personnel examine any patient who has sustained a significant electrical shock. The damage caused by the current may be internal and not apparent to you or your patient during assessment. Consider this patient a high priority for immediate transport.

Radiation Exposure

The potential radiation incident must be a concern during the dispatch and response phase of the emergency call. Because radiation is neither seen nor felt, it can endanger EMS personnel unless you take the proper precautions. If you suspect radiation exposure, approach the scene very carefully. If the incident has occurred at a power generator plant or in an industrial or a medical facility, seek out persons knowledgeable in the hazardous substance being used. Also ensure that the scene is secure and protect bystanders, rescuers, and patients from exposure.

* Because radiation can be neither seen nor felt, it can endanger EMS personnel unless proper precautions are taken.

If patients are close to an unremovable source, have them brought to you. If patients have been contaminated, disrobe and wash them with soap and water, then rinse the contaminated area thoroughly before your assessment begins. It is necessary to document carefully the circumstances of exposure. If possible, identify the source. Determine the patient's proximity to the source during exposure as well as the length of exposure. The actual assessment will be quite simple and reveal minimal signs or symptoms of injury. Only extreme exposure will result in the classical presentation of nausea, vomiting, and malaise. Burns are extremely rare, although they may occur if the exposure was intense and long-term. Even though the patient seems well, the consequences of high-dose radiation exposure can be devastating.

MANAGEMENT OF SOFT-TISSUE INJURY

Once you have completed assessment of the soft-tissue injury, you can take certain management steps, either in the field or en route to the hospital. Blood loss control, prevention of shock, and decontamination of affected areas take priority. The following sections describe some of the most important care steps.

* The management of wounds is a late priority in the care of the trauma patient, unless extensive bleeding is noted.

Wounds

Unless you note extensive bleeding, the management of wounds by dressing and bandaging is a late priority in the care of the trauma patient. Apply the appropriate objectives of wound care after you appropriately care for higher-priority injuries.

Objectives of Bandaging   The objectives of bandaging are simple, straightforward, and essential to quality emergency care. They include hemorrhage control, sterility (or in the field, a degree of cleanliness), and immobilization. Any wound dressing and bandaging must employ and accomplish these objectives.

Hemorrhage Control. Occasionally, bleeding from a soft-tissue injury can be difficult to control. If the bleeding continues despite initial use of direct pressure, examine the wound to determine the exact site of blood loss. Then apply direct pressure to that point. Too often hemorrhage continues because the bandaging technique distributes the pressure over the entire wound site rather than focusing upon the bleeding source. The pressure causing the hemorrhage is no greater than the patient's systolic blood pressure. Digital pressure can easily compress the vessel and hence should halt any blood loss. It may be necessary to maintain digital pressure for the duration of your care.

Elevation assists in controlling hemorrhage, although it is generally not as effective as direct pressure. Elevation may also benefit the wound by reducing extremity arterial pressure and increasing venous return. Both minimize potential edema and help maintain optimal circulation to the affected area. The use of pressure points may assist with bleeding control and the clotting process. Locate the pulse point immediately proximal to the wound and apply firm pressure. Maintain the pressure for at least 10 minutes, if not for all of your prehospital time.

A combination of techniques for hemorrhage control may be effective when bleeding is resistant to direct pressure. Direct pressure, elevation, and pressure points together will halt all but the most difficult bleeding. An exception to the effectiveness of normal blood loss techniques may occur with the severe crush injury. (See Figure 18-15.) In a crush injury, several blood vessels tear, making it difficult to pinpoint the bleeding. Even if you can find the source, it is hard to apply direct pressure. In such cases, the use of the tourniquet may be useful. The tourniquet is generally the last choice for controlling

* A combination of techniques for hemorrhage control may be effective when bleeding is resistant to direct pressure.

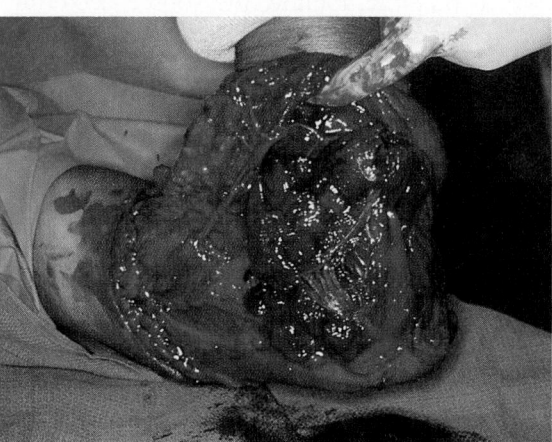

FIGURE 18-15   Crush injury to the elbow. This wound should be both dressed and splinted. (Courtesy of Scott and White Hospital and Clinic)

hemorrhage. If you properly apply it, it will stop the flow of blood; however, it has serious risks. Keep the following precautions in mind whenever you consider the use of a tourniquet.

1. If the pressure is insufficient, the tourniquet will halt venous return. However, it will not affect arterial flow. The result is an increase in the rate and the volume of blood loss.
2. When the tourniquet is applied properly, the entire limb distal to the device is without circulation. Hypoxia may permanently damage the tissue beyond the tourniquet.
3. When you restore the circulation, the blood returning to the central circulation is highly hypoxic and acidic.

Do not use the tourniquet unless you cannot control severe bleeding by any other means. Apply it in a way that does not injure the tissue beneath. During prehospital care, a readily-available and effective tourniquet may be a sphygmomanometer (regular for the upper extremity and thigh for the lower). Inflate it to 20–30 mmHg above the patient's systolic blood pressure and beyond the pressure where the patient's hemorrhage ceases. Once you apply it, leave the tourniquet in place until the patient arrives at the emergency department. Monitor the cuff pressure during transport to ensure that it does not lose pressure. Alert the hospital staff to your use of the tourniquet during transport as well as upon arrival.

✱ Once applied, the tourniquet should be left in place until the patient arrives at the emergency department.

Sterility. Once you halt the severe bleeding, keep the wound as sterile as possible. Field conditions may limit this to keeping the wound as clean as is *reasonably* possible. Under normal conditions, you need not cleanse the wound. But, if grossly contaminated, irrigate it with normal saline or lactated Ringer's solution. You may also carefully remove larger particles—glass, debris, and so forth—if you can accomplish this swiftly and without inducing further harm.

Try to make the dressing appear as neat as time and the environment allow. The neat appearance will calm and reassure the patient, while the cleanliness reduces contamination and, hopefully, post-trauma infection.

Immobilization. The last bandaging objective is immobilization. Fixation of the wound site will help with the natural clotting mechanisms and reduce the patient's discomfort. Maintaining gentle pressure with the bandage may offer the patient some comfort and reduces swelling. Immobilize the limb to the body or to a rigid surface such as a padded board or ladder splint. Do not use elastic bandaging material. Rapid edema occurring immediately after an injury will cause increasing pressure to the tissue underneath the elastic. This pressure may reduce or halt circulation.

Frequently monitor any limb that you bandage circumferentially to ensure that the distal pulse remains strong. If you cannot locate the distal pulse, monitor capillary refill, skin color, and temperature. If signs or symptoms suggest that the distal circulation is compromised, check, and possibly loosen, the bandage. Any circumferential pressure around a limb retards the venous return of blood from the extremity. This increases the edema and pain of the injury, while reducing the circulation through the extremity.

Special Wound Care
Treat painful contusions or those with the potential for large debilitating edema with cold and moderate-pressure bandages. Do not use ice. Ice will cool beyond therapeutic value and possibly cause tissue freezing and further harm. In caring for any soft-tissue injury, you are

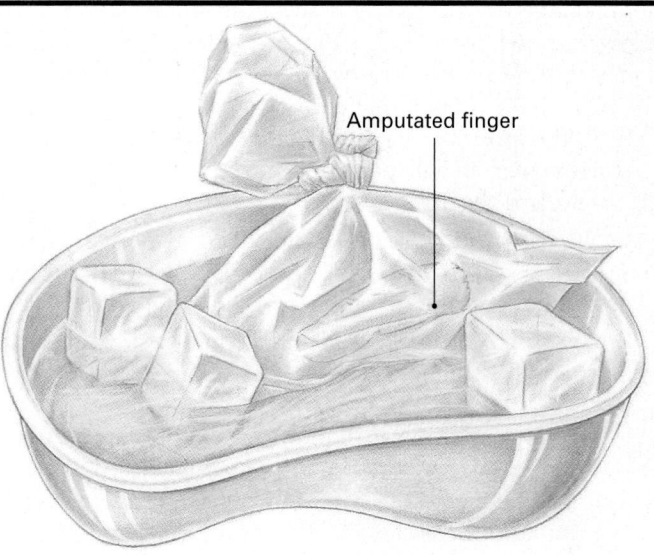

FIGURE 18-16 Amputated parts should be put in a dry bag, sealed, and placed in cool water that contains a few ice cubes.

responsible for describing the wound in detail to the emergency department staff. This will avoid the need for them to remove the dressing and evaluate the wound until they can care for other more serious injuries. If the description of the wound is inaccurate, patient care and your credibility will suffer.

✱ Current recommendation for managing separated body parts includes dry cooling and rapid transport.

Current recommendations for managing separated body parts includes dry cooling and rapid transport. Place the amputated part in a plastic bag, and keep it cool by cold water immersion. (See Figure 18-16.) The water in which the bag and body part sits may have a few ice cubes in it, but avoid direct contact between the ice and the injured part. Transport any avulsed or amputated part to the hospital receiving the patient. (See Figures 18-17 through 18-20.) Even if the part cannot be totally reattached, the skin may be used to cover the limb end. Except in very special circumstances, do not wait to find the part. Transport the patient and any found body tissue immediately. Do not delay patient transport while looking for a body part. (See Figures 18-21 through 18-23.)

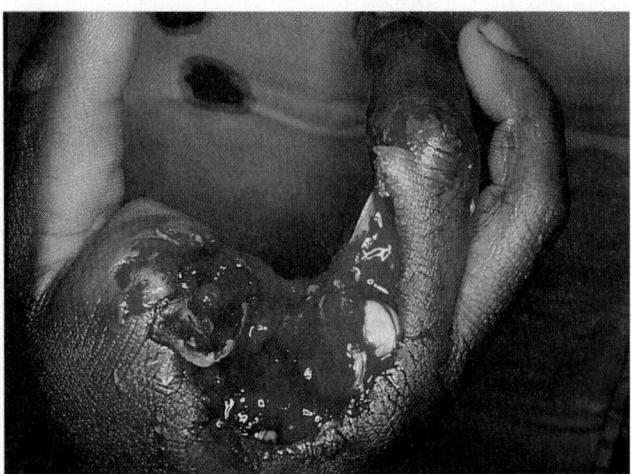

FIGURE 18-17 Amputation of the index and long fingers of the right hand. (Courtesy of Scott and White Hospital and Clinic)

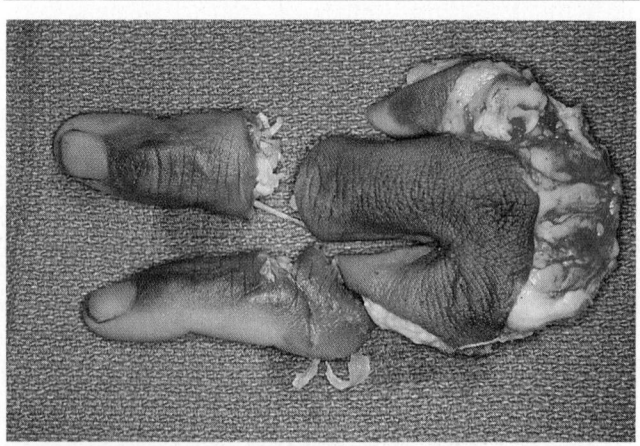

FIGURE 18-18 The amputated parts should be transported with the patient to the hospital. Even if replantation cannot be performed, the skin, blood vessels, and bone can be used in the repair. (Courtesy of Scott and White Hospital and Clinic)

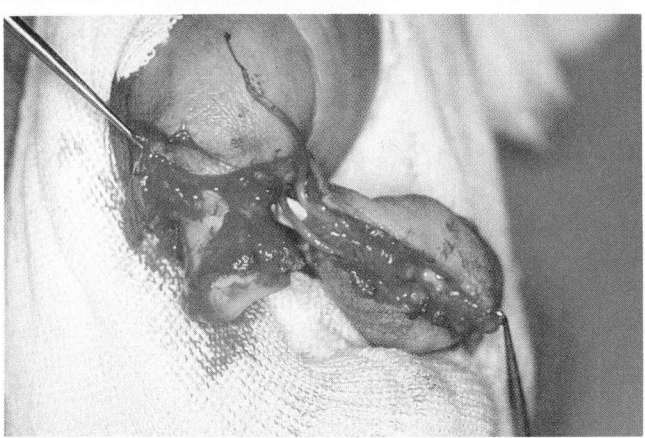

FIGURE 18-19 Near amputation of the thumb of the right hand. (Courtesy of Scott and White Hospital and Clinic)

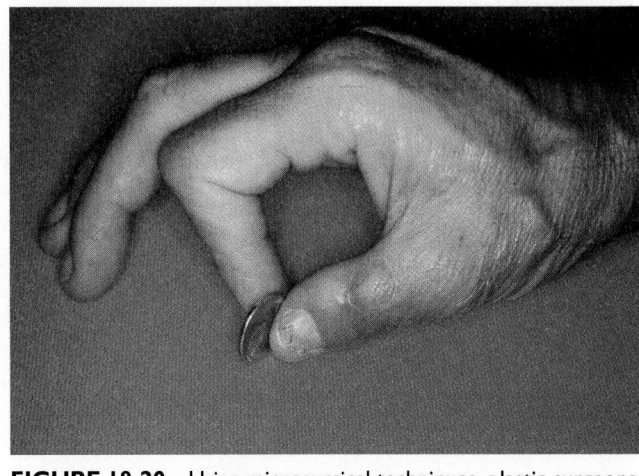

FIGURE 18-20 Using microsurgical techniques, plastic surgeons replanted the thumb, with good function preserved. (Courtesy of Scott and White Hospital and Clinic)

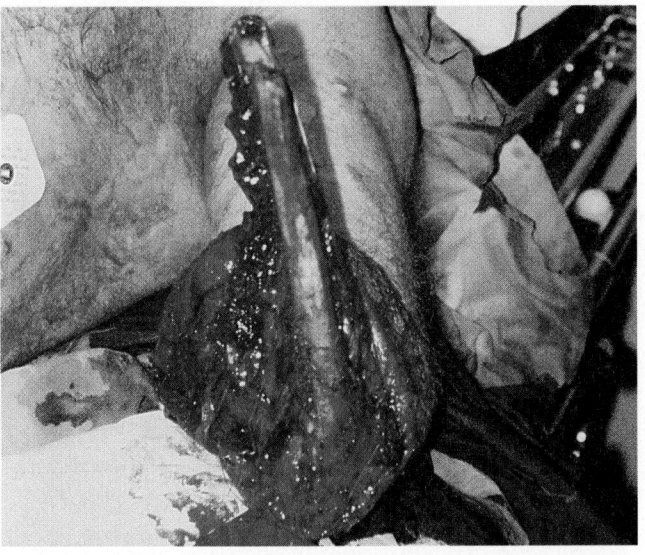

FIGURE 18-21 Complete amputation of the distal forearm and hand, from an agricultural injury. (Courtesy of Kenneth Phillips, D.O.)

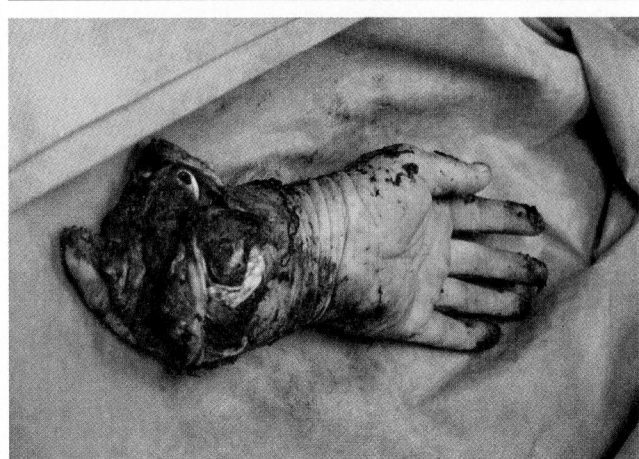

FIGURE 18-22 Paramedics located the amputated hand and transported it to the hospital with the patient. (Courtesy of Kenneth Phillips, D.O.)

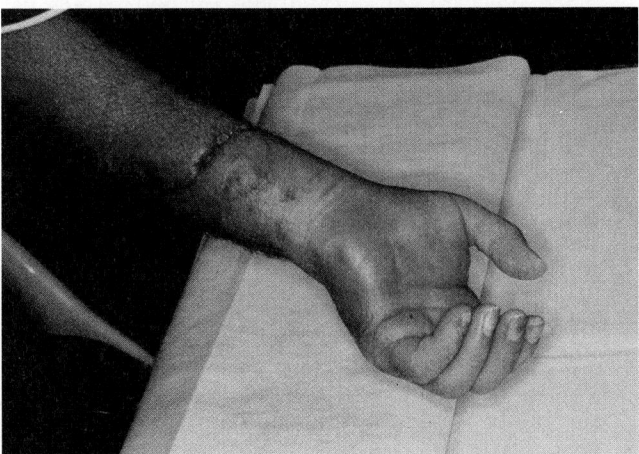

FIGURE 18-23 The hand was replanted using microsurgical techniques. Success of the replant is highly dependent upon care provided in the field by paramedics. (Courtesy of David Zehr, M.D.)

Burns

Treatment of burns varies with the cause. In all cases, however, management depends upon the extent and depth of exposure.

Thermal or Electrical Burns   Management of thermal or electrical burns may be divided into two categories: local and minor burns and moderate to severe burns. The following sections describe some of the actions that may be taken in each of these cases.

Local and Minor Burns. Use local cooling to treat minor soft-tissue burns that involve only a small proportion of the body surface area at a partial thickness. Care for only those burns that involve less than 10 percent of the BSA in this way. Cooling of larger surface areas might subject the patient to hypothermia. Cold, or cool water immersion, has some effect in reducing pain and may limit the depth of the burning process. It will only be effective if used immediately in the post-burn period.

It is also important to remove any article of clothing or jewelry that might possibly act to contain edema. As the injury site accumulates body fluid, it will increase in size. If the swelling encounters any constriction, it increases tissue pressure and may tourniquet the vasculature. The result may be loss of pulse and circulation distal to the burn.

Moderate to Severe Burns. Use dry, sterile dressings to treat partial-thickness burns over 30 percent of the body or full-thickness burns over 5 percent of the BSA. They will keep air movement past the sensitive first- and second-degree burn to a minimum. Sterile dressings will also provide padding against minor bumping. In the third-degree burn, they will provide a barrier to possible contamination.

Establish intravenous routes in any patient with moderate to severe burns. Introduce two large-bore catheters and hang 1000 mL bags of either normal saline or lactated Ringer's solution. Current fluid resuscitation formulas recommend 4 mL of fluid for every kilogram of patient weight multiplied by the percentage of body surface area burned. The patient will need half this fluid in the first eight hours of care. This particular fluid resuscitation protocol is known as the *Parkland formula* and is most applicable to prehospital care.

If the wound size is great, medical control may ask you to administer aggressive fluid therapy during prehospital care. If all the normal IV access sites are burned, you may place the catheter through the burned tissue. Be careful with insertion. The skin may be leathery, yet the tissue underneath is very delicate.

Chemical Burns   Decontaminate the patient who has come in contact with any chemical capable of tissue damage early in the assessment/care process. Stop the damage by irrigating the site with large volumes of cool water. (See Figure 18-24.) Water will not only rinse away the offending material, it will dilute any water soluble agents. The cooling effect of the water also reduces the heat and the rate of chemical reaction and, ultimately, its effects upon the skin. If the contamination is widespread, douse the patient with large volumes of water. Use a garden hose or low-pressure water from a fire truck. Assure that the water is cool, not cold.

Once the patient has been rinsed for a few minutes, remove the clothing. Take care that the rescuers do not become contaminated. If the agent is dangerous, save all clothing and contain all the rinse water for proper disposal at a later time.

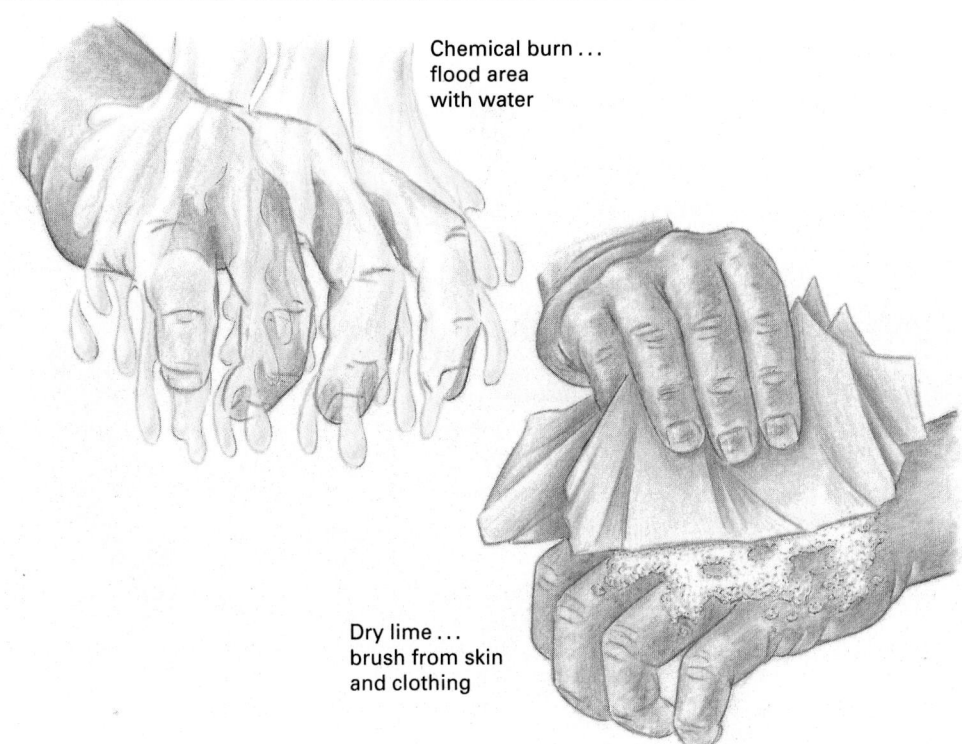

Chemical burn ...
flood area
with water

Dry lime ...
brush from skin
and clothing

FIGURE 18-24 Chemical burns should be flushed with large quantities of water. Dry lime should be first brushed away before applying water.

Next, scrub the wound with a mild soap and a gentle brush. Scrub rigorously enough to remove any remaining corrosive. However, be careful not to cause further soft-tissue damage. After scrubbing, gently irrigate the wound with a constant flow of water. While the pain and the burning process may appear to subside, it is important to continue the irrigation until the patient arrives at the emergency department. If practical, transport the corrosive container or a sample with the patient.

DO NOT USE ANY ANTIDOTE OR A NEUTRALIZING AGENT. Neutralizing agents often react violently with the agent they neutralize. They may ultimately increase the heat of the reaction and induce thermal burns. In some cases, the antidote or neutralizing agent is more damaging to the skin than the contaminant.

✱ Do not use any antidote or any neutralizing agent on chemical burns.

Irrigate chemical splashes that involve the eye with large volumes of water. (See Figure 18-25.) Alkali burns are especially damaging and call for you to flush the eye for at least 15 minutes. Irrigate acid burns for at least 5 minutes. Flush splashes of an unknown agent for up to 20 minutes. However, do not delay transport while irrigating.

Some substances either do not dissolve in water or may react violently with it. Treat substances such as phenol, dry lime, and sodium differently.

❏ *Phenol.* Phenol is a gelatinous caustic used in industry as a powerful cleaner. It is very difficult to remove since it is sticky and insoluble in water. Alcohol, which will dissolve it, is frequently available where phenol is used. Use the alcohol to remove the phenol and follow it with large volumes of water.

❏ *Dry Lime.* Dry lime is a strong corrosive that reacts with water. It produces heat and subsequent chemical and thermal injury. Brush dry lime off gently, but as completely as possible. Then rinse the contaminated

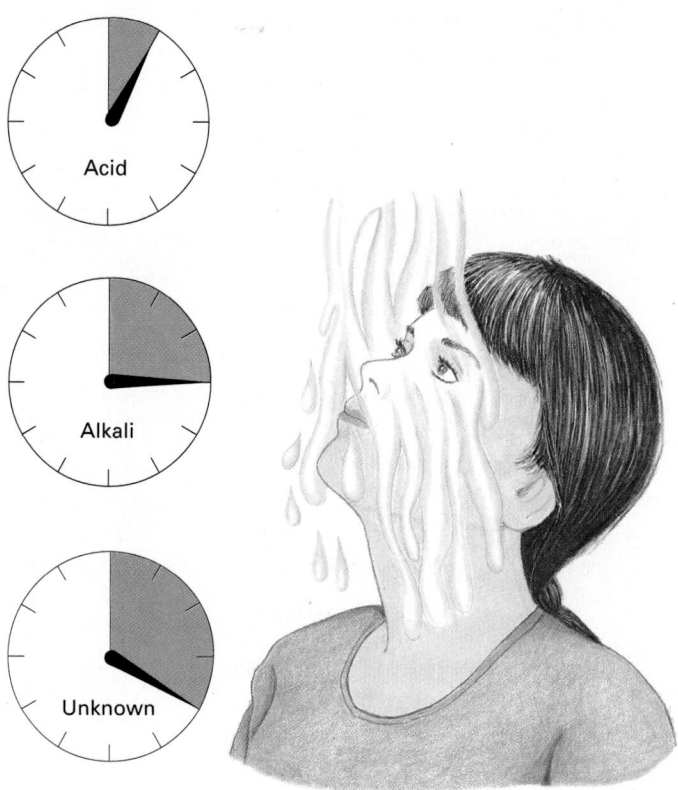

FIGURE 18-25 Treatment for chemical burns to the face and eye is copious, prolonged irrigation with water.

area with large volumes of cool to cold water. While the water will react with the lime, it will also cool the area and remove any loose substance. In using water, the lime may react with it rather than with the water of the body's soft tissues.

❑ *Sodium.* Sodium is an unstable metal that reacts destructively with many substances, including human tissue. It will react vigorously with water, creating extreme heat, explosive hydrogen gas, and possible ignition. It is normally stored under oil since it will react with oxygen in the air. If a patient has been contaminated with sodium, decontaminate gently and quickly by gentle brushing. Then cover the wound with oil used to store the substance.

Radiation Exposure   In radiation rescue, assure that professionals in the field isolate the source, contain it, and test the scene for safety. If this is impossible, move the patient to a remote site where you can give care without danger either to you or the patient. Plan the removal well, using as much shielding as possible. Keep exposure times to a minimum.

If patient removal is chosen, use the oldest rescuers as the evacuation team. This approach is prudent because the effects of radiation exposure become evident many years after it occurs. If older rescuers are used, it will be more likely that they are past the reproductive years and will have fewer years of life left if and when a problem does surface. This concern is especially important for pregnant females and young adults of both sexes. Radiation damages the reproductive system very easily.

If the exposure is due to contamination either by liquid or dust, rinse the patient with copious amounts of water. Carefully disrobe the patient, then scrub and rinse again. As with chemical contamination, save all clothing and water used for decontamination so that these materials may be disposed of safely. Perform decontamination before moving the patient to the ambulance. If possible, use persons knowledgeable in the radiation techniques and who possess appropriate protective gear.

Once decontaminated, treat the radiation patient as any other patient. Because the human body alone cannot be a source of ionizing radiation, this patient poses no threat to you or your crew. However, any contaminated material on the patient, or any contamination transferred to you, will provide a source of radiation exposure.

SUMMARY

Soft-tissue injury may compromise the skin—the protective envelope that protects and contains the human body. Any trauma must penetrate it to harm the interior organs and threaten life. Any damage to the skin may interfere with its ability to contain water within the body and to prevent damaging agents from entering. For these reasons, assessment and care of soft-tissue injuries are important.

Assess wounds carefully since they may be the only overt signs of serious internal injury. Realize that discoloration and swelling take time and may not be as apparent in the field as when you present the patient at the emergency department. Look carefully for the early signs of these wounds and use the mechanism of injury to locate potential sites of trauma. Employ the objectives of bandaging when caring for soft-tissue injury. Control hemorrhage, immobilize the injury site, and keep the wound as clean as possible.

Assess the burn to determine its depth and the body surface area it involves. Be sensitive to any respiratory, joint, hand, foot, or circumferential regions affected by the burn. Give special consideration to the pediatric, geriatric, ill, or injured patient who is also burned. Determine the overall severity from these factors and, if the condition warrants, institute aggressive care. Anticipate airway compromise and fluid loss. Secure the airway very early in prehospital care. Initiate IV access, and begin fluid administration.

Chemical, radiation, or electrical burns require special care and assessment. Chemical burns need rapid and effective decontamination. Radiation burns call for extreme care in removing the patient from the source and in providing decontamination and supportive aid. An electrical burn requires careful assessment to determine the area and depth of burn involvement as well as wound site dressing and cardiac monitoring.

While soft-tissue injuries often are not a high priority, they do represent a high incidence of patient injury and are significant to the overall assessment and care of the trauma victim.

FURTHER READING

American College of Surgeons, Committee on Trauma. *Advanced Trauma Life Support Course: Student Manual.* American College of Surgeons, 1989.

Butman, A.M., and J.L. Paturas, *Pre-Hospital Trauma Life Support.* Akron, OH: Emergency Training, 1990.

Campbell, J.E. *Basic Trauma Life Support*, 2nd ed. Englewood Cliffs, NJ: Prentice-Hall, Inc., 1988.

Grant, H.D., R.H. Murray, and J.D. Bergeron, *Emergency Care*, 5th ed., Englewood Cliffs, NJ: Prentice-Hall, Inc., 1990.

Lodge, D.W., and H.D. Grant, *Handbook of Emergency Care Procedures.* Englewood Cliffs, NJ: Prentice-Hall, Inc., 1989.

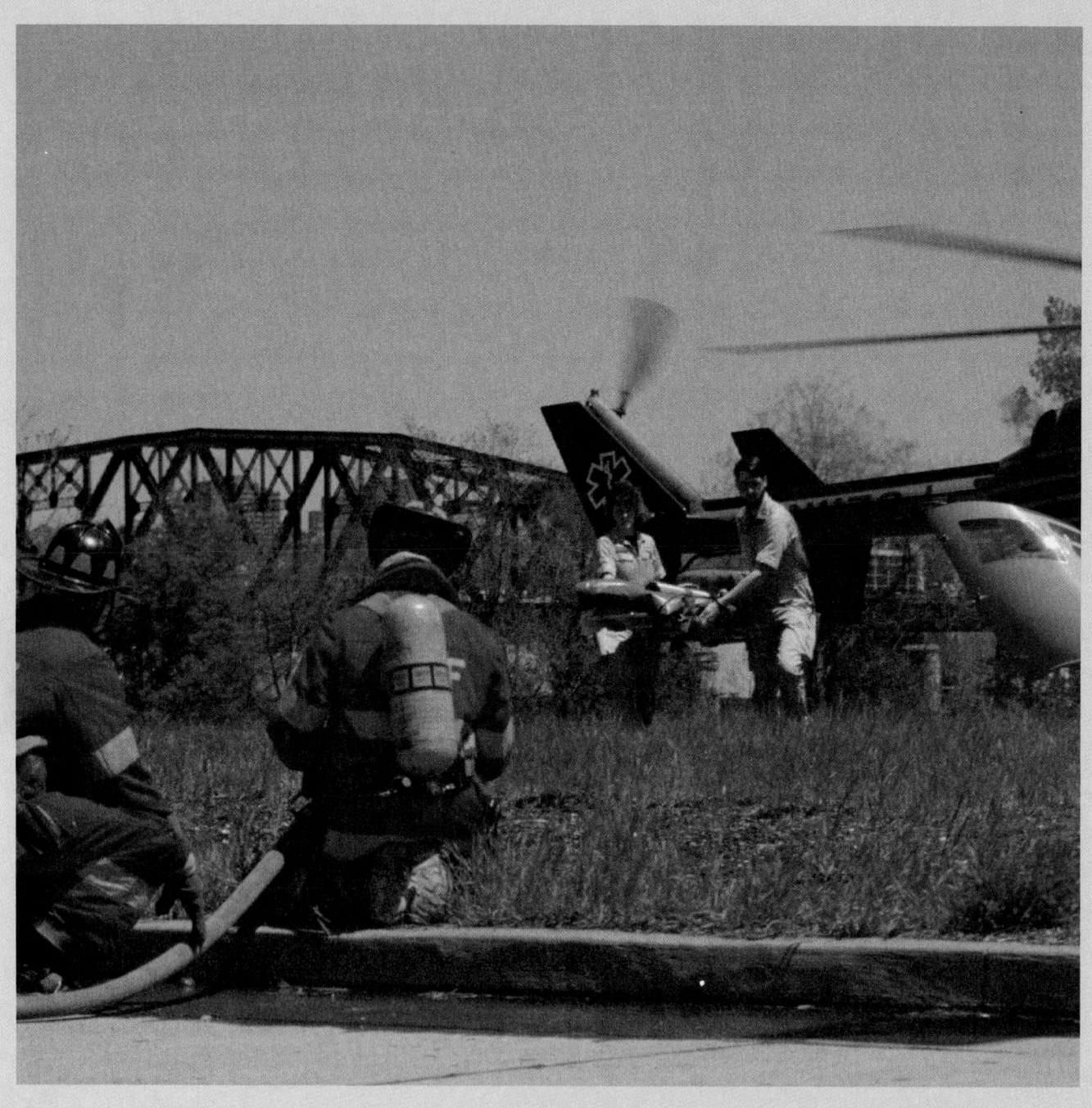

19

SHOCK TRAUMA RESUSCITATION

Objectives for Chapter 19

After reading this chapter, you should be able to:

1. Identify the importance of rapid recognition and treatment of shock in trauma patients. (See p. 554.)

2. Compare and contrast compensated, decompensated, and irreversible shock. (See pp. 557–559.)

3. List mechanisms that compensate for blood loss, and describe how they provide this function. (See pp. 557–558.)

4. Identify signs and symptoms of hypovolemic shock, and explain why they occur. (See pp. 557–559.)

5. List findings related to hypovolemic shock for each element of the primary assessment. (See pp. 560–562.)

6. Identify and explain the various steps taken in the care of patients with differing degrees of blood loss. (See pp. 563–567.)

7. Explain benefits of, and indications and contraindications for, using the pneumatic antishock garment (PASG). (See pp. 565–566.)

8. Explain how catheter length and diameter and fluid pressure affect the rate of intravenous infusion. (See pp. 566–567.)

9. List signs and symptoms of circulatory overload in a patient receiving rapid crystalloid infusion. (See p. 567.)

10. Describe the preparation of a patient for air medical transport. (See p. 567.)

11. Identify the benefits of helicopter use, and list the criteria for establishing a landing zone. (See pp. 568–570.)

An outlying basic life support unit calls for Metro-Rescue 9, an advanced life support (ALS) unit. The victim of a farm accident lies trapped under a tractor, bleeding profusely. While en route, Rescue 9 calls dispatch to alert the Life Flight helicopter.

Upon arrival, the crew of Rescue 9 sees a young male with his leg pinned beneath an overturned tractor and the adjoining ground soaked with blood. The patient is pale with cool, moist skin. The ALS crew finds him conscious but anxious and somewhat combative. The patient is unsure of what happened. He is breathing with shallow breaths, has a weak radial pulse of 120, and 3-second capillary refill. Primary assessment reveals no injuries, except those found on the trapped limb. Blood pressure is 90 by palpation, respirations are 22 and shallow, oxygen saturation is 92 percent, and the level of consciousness continues to diminish. Extrication is expected in 3 minutes. Rescue 9 asks dispatch to send Life Flight to the scene.

The on-scene paramedic contacts medical control, relays patient information, and obtains permission for two IVs. Lines are started with large-bore catheters and trauma tubing. One 1000 mL bag of normal saline and one of lactated Ringer's are hung, both running wide open. Oxygen is applied via non-rebreather mask, while the pneumatic antishock garment (PASG) is readied on a long spine board.

Removal of the tractor reveals a crush wound to the right thigh. The ALS crew locates the source of hemorrhage, and they apply direct digital pressure. Bleeding slows and pressure dressings replace digital pressure. The crew then moves the patient to the long spine board, where they apply and inflate the PASG. Next, they quickly load him into the ambulance to await the helicopter.

A second set of vital signs reveals respirations at 26 with very shallow breaths, a carotid pulse of 136, and oxygen saturation at 86 percent. The patient responds to verbal stimuli. When Life Flight arrives, the on-scene paramedic gives an abbreviated report, and the patient is quickly moved to the helicopter. In flight, pressure IV infusers are applied and inflated to 300 mm Hg. The two bags empty and are replaced with a second lactated Ringer's solution running slowly and one unit of O negative blood.

Twelve minutes later, they arrive at the trauma center. There has been some improvement in respiration, a lowering pulse rate, and oxygen saturation has risen to 90 percent. At the emergency department, blood is drawn, typed, and crossmatched. Meanwhile, a second unit of O negative blood is administered. Physician assessment and X-ray reveal no femur fracture. The ED team takes the young man to surgery where the surgeon repairs the femoral artery. Three days later, Rescue 9 receives a call from the patient's parents thanking the crew. Their son is doing fine and will be coming home this weekend.

INTRODUCTION

Trauma presents a key challenge in prehospital care. It is the third leading cause of death in the United States, claiming some 140,000 lives each year. Unlike progressive diseases such as heart attack, stroke, or cancer, trauma strikes suddenly and unexpectedly. It often strikes people at the prime of their lives and ranks as the most common cause of death among people under age 34. Extensive treatment of trauma—surgery, intensive care, and in-hospital recovery—makes it a costly medical condition. Rehabilitation may take years and disability may continue for a victim's lifetime. As a result, your actions at a traumatic incident carry great responsibility. Your efforts may reduce morbidity and/or limit disability.

TRAUMA MANAGEMENT

Trauma spurred the start of prehospital care in the mid-1960s. Since then, however, it has been overshadowed by an emphasis on cardiac and medical emergency response. Recent programs such as Advanced Trauma Life Support (ATLS) for physicians and Basic Trauma Life Support (BTLS) and Prehospital Trauma Life

Support (PHTLS) for prehospital providers have refocused our attention on trauma management. Today, aggressive trauma care is the object of much study. It now receives a strong emphasis in training and is an important element of paramedic response.

Because of the seriousness of trauma, your actions must be well planned and efficient in dealing with a patient who may be in shock. You will begin by evaluating the accident scene for mechanism of injury and by establishing an index of suspicion. You will then focus on the "A, B, C, D, and E" of primary assessment. That is, you will concentrate on the systems and anatomical areas where the greatest life threat exists—**A**irway; **B**reathing; **C**irculation; **D**isability (nervous or skeletal system injury); **E**xposure of injury to the head, neck, chest, abdomen, and pelvis.

After you have established the mechanism of injury and completed the primary assessment, the results are measured against trauma triage criteria. If a patient displays any of the physical findings, or if the accident analysis reveals any of the listed mechanisms of injury, the patient should receive aggressive care during rapid transport to the trauma center. This shock/trauma resuscitation gives you the best opportunity to impact the chances for patient survival.

The steps below outline the process of information gathering and the care most appropriate for the trauma patient. (Each of these steps will be taken up on pages 00–00.)

1. Review of the dispatch information
2. Survey of the scene
3. Primary assessment
   - Shock/trauma resuscitation
4. Secondary assessment
   - Head-to-toe exam
   - Vital signs
   - Patient history
5. Management
6. Transportation

The first three steps should occur in order. If the primary assessment reveals no life threat, and if the patient does not meet trauma triage criteria, the process continues and scene care is indicated. Elements of the secondary assessment—head-to-toe exam, vital signs, and patient history—will be provided and may occur simultaneously or in any order. Patient injuries will be prioritized and managed at the scene in order of seriousness. Packaging and transport to the closest facility will follow. However, any trauma patient must be frequently evaluated for any findings that suggest shock/trauma resuscitation and rapid transport to a trauma center.

If the existence, or even threat, of shock is recognized, treat the patient aggressively. Rapid transport coupled with invasive and non-invasive procedures can combat hypovolemia and support the body's compensatory mechanisms. Modalities of care include the PASG, advanced airway techniques, oxygen-supplemented positive pressure ventilation, and rapid intravenous infusion. These procedures, followed by the trauma center's sophisticated interventions, will improve the shock patient's prognosis.

In order to anticipate, recognize, or treat shock, you must first understand the causes and manifestations of shock. Unlike heart attack and other medical emergencies, trauma affects several body organs and systems at once. In addition to the physical injury, internal and/or external blood loss will often affect the cardiovascular system and begin the shock syndrome. This syndrome consists of a

* Because of the seriousness of trauma, your actions must be well planned and efficient in dealing with a patient who may be in shock.

* Any trauma patient must be frequently evaluated for any findings that suggest shock/trauma resuscitation and rapid transport to a trauma center.

series of compensatory actions and resultant signs and symptoms. An appreciation of shock and these responses begins with an understanding of the relevant anatomy and physiology.

ANATOMY AND PHYSIOLOGY OF THE CARDIOVASCULAR SYSTEM

The cardiovascular system maintains the human body by providing transportation of nutrients and waste products, distribution of heat and body fluids, destruction of pathogens, and self-repair of damaged blood vessels. Hemorrhage and shock disrupt many of these functions. As a result, shock then puts body organs, and ultimately the entire organism, at risk for anoxic death. This is why an understanding of the cardiovascular system helps us prevent and/or lessen shock.

The cardiovascular system is made up of blood, blood vessels, and the heart, with each element playing an important role in normal body function. Blood, the substance most commonly lost in trauma, circulates throughout the body. It carries nutrients (including oxygen) to the body cells and removes waste products (including carbon dioxide). Blood vessels (which lose fluid in trauma) make up the container and help direct blood flow to and from vital organs. The heart pumps blood through the vessels and powers the entire system. The heart, vessels, and blood work together to ensure all cells receive a supply of nutrients and are relieved of their waste products.

Blood consists of two major components: red blood cells, called erythrocytes, and fluid, called plasma. Erythrocytes contain hemoglobin, an iron compound that carries oxygen from the lungs to body cells. **Plasma** is a fluid that suspends the erythrocytes and carries them and other blood components to the far reaches of the body. These two elements make up an essential fluid accounting for 7 percent of the body weight, or about 5 to 6 liters in the normal 75 Kg. (165 lbs.) person.

Blood fills the vessels—arteries, arterioles, capillaries, venules, and veins—to form a dynamic elastic container. Muscle fibers surround these vessels in order to change the lumen and, in concert, the container size. Vessels either constrict or dilate to compensate for fluid loss or retention. This effect is most noticeable in the venous system since it holds about 60 percent of blood volume and maintains a rather low pressure.

Arterioles have the ability to affect blood pressure and direct blood flow from the heart to various organs. They can open and close with a valve-like function and can vary their lumen by as much as a factor of five. If a majority of arteries dilate, resistance to blood flow (peripheral resistance) drops as does blood pressure. If they constrict, blood pressure rises. Thus, through the control of arterioles, the central nervous system can regulate blood pressure. Arterioles also play an important role in directing blood flow to body organs. If arterioles leading to a particular organ dilate, the organ receives more blood. If pre-organ arterioles constrict, blood flow is reduced. Together, these actions allow regulation of organ blood flow while maintaining a stable blood pressure.

Arterioles and venules work together to help control body fluid balance among vascular and interstitial spaces. Through their action, the cardiovascular system can either draw fluid from, or pass fluid to, these areas and body cells. If pre-capillary arterioles dilate and post-capillary venules constrict, blood is pushed into the capillary bed and fluid moves out of the vascular compartment. If pre-capillary arterioles constrict and venules dilate, blood flows from the capillary bed and fluid flows into the vascular space. This control allows the body to regulate fluid placement and to use body cells and spaces as a fluid reservoir.

■ **plasma** the fluid portion of the blood consisting of serum and protein substances in solution.

The heart is a two-sided, double-action pump generating the major force and pressure of the cardiovascular system. It ejects its contents into the arterial circulation. This outflow, in combination with vessel valve function, creates arterial pressure and directs blood flow to desired body tissues.

The heart's pumping efficiency depends on several factors. It must receive blood from venous vessels (**preload**) and have a moderate resistance to pump against (**afterload**). If the ventricles are forcefully filled through good venous return and atrial contraction, the walls of the heart stretch. This action increases the volume and force of the ejected blood.

The vascular system retains plasma through a complicated system of biochemical equilibrium. Protein and electrolyte concentrations are different in each of the vascular, interstitial, and intracellular spaces. However, they exert equal osmotic pressures. The system achieves a balance, and this balance continues even when intake and output of fluid are unequal.

Fluid loss from the vascular container may be caused by various mechanisms, including burns, diarrhea, reduced fluid intake, granulating wounds, sweating due to fever or environmental extremes, or hemorrhage. This chapter principally addresses blood loss through hemorrhage, whether it be external or internal.

■ **preload** the volume of blood delivered to the atria prior to ventricular diastole.

■ **afterload** the pressure or resistance against which the heart must pump.

PATHOPHYSIOLOGY

Shock is the transition between normal body function and balance (called homeostasis) and death. Up to a point, the body's response to any hemorrhage is efficient and well designed. This response is termed **compensated shock**. After the body can no longer compensate, the compensatory mechanisms fail. Circulation soon fails as well, and the patient moves quickly toward death. **Decompensated shock** is the second stage of this process. The final stage occurs when body cells and organs are so damaged from anoxia that even if oxygenated circulation is restored they will die. This is **irreversible shock** and may occur during the late stages of compensated shock or shortly after decompensated shock. Our objective in prehospital care is to recognize compensated shock early, treat it aggressively, and prevent it from becoming decompensated and, ultimately, irreversible shock. (See Chapter 12.)

Compensated Shock

The human system adjusts to varying levels of fluid intake and loss. A healthy young individual can drink a few liters at one sitting without experiencing fluid overload. He or she can also lose a large fluid volume sweating on a hot day, again without experiencing adverse effects. In either case, the body uses mechanisms that respond to fluid fluctuations and allow unimpeded body function. The body responds in a similar way to the loss of blood—so long as the loss is minor and relatively uncomplicated.

As blood flows from a wound, initial fluid adjustment mechanisms activate. Veins respond first since they hold about 60 percent of the circulating blood volume and are able to reduce their capacity significantly. By constricting their walls, they compensate for blood loss of about 1 to 2 units (0.5 to 1 L). This mechanism permits blood donation or minor hemorrhage without major systemic consequences. If blood loss is slowed, or stops, the body will draw fluid from interstitial areas and body cells to replenish lost volume. Arterioles constrict and venules dilate. Interstitial and cell fluid is drawn into the circulation and assists in filling the vascular container. Since the body is over 60 percent water, there is a tremendous reservoir to draw from (about 40 L). While this mechanism is not as rapid as venous constriction, it is reasonably quick and may return several liters to active circulation.

■ **compensated shock** a hemodynamic insult to the body in which the body responds effectively. Signs and symptoms are limited, and the human system functions normally.

■ **decompensated shock** a continuing hemodynamic insult to the body in which the compensatory mechanisms break down. The signs and symptoms become very pronounced, and the patient moves rapidly toward death.

■ **irreversible shock** the final stage of shock in which the organs and cells are so damaged that recovery is impossible.

✱ Our objective in prehospital care is to recognize compensated shock early, treat it aggressively, and prevent it from becoming decompensated and, ultimately, irreversible shock.

The addition of body fluid helps to fill the vascular container and to maintain circulation. But it also dilutes the remaining blood. Erythrocytes, lost through hemorrhage, are not readily replaced. As a result, the blood is not able to carry as much oxygen. Clotting factors are also diluted, and the body begins to loose its ability to control hemorrhage. Because this process reduces the overall efficiency of the cardiovascular system, the body starts to show the early signs and symptoms of shock. The greater and more rapid the hemorrhage, the more severe the problem becomes.

Eventually, veins become maximally constricted and fluid replacement can no longer keep pace with the loss. Blood return to the heart slows, preload diminishes, ventricular filling is not complete, and cardiac output drops. Blood pressure drops as does the body's ability to direct blood flow. The body, through baroreceptors in the neck, recognizes the drop and employs several reflex actions. Catecholamines—epinephrine and norepinephrine—are released into the blood stream, causing arterioles to constrict and the heart rate to increase. Blood is shunted away from non-vital tissues, to the heart, brain, and skeletal muscles. These actions help maintain blood pressure and the body's control of circulation.

These compensatory actions cause some of the classic signs of shock. One of the first apparent signs is anxiety and restlessness. This agitated state results from catecholamine release and the beginnings of decreased cerebral perfusion. Other signs develop as preload and cardiac output begin to drop. To compensate, the pulse rate increases, yielding a weak, rapid pulse. In fact, the pulse may be diminished or absent in the distal extremities. Yet other signs emerge as the central nervous system calls for the arterioles to constrict, especially to non-vital organs like the skin. Shunting of blood away from the skin results in cooling and stagnation of blood flow. This in turn causes the moist, clammy feeling associated with shock. The reduction in red blood cells near the skin's surface makes the patient look pale. As remaining blood cells lose their oxygen, the patient becomes ashen or cyanotic.

As the progression of shock becomes more severe, even circulation to critical organs becomes inadequate. There may be a subtle and progressively lowering level of consciousness, indicated by decreased orientation to time, place (or event), person, and one's own person.

In a hypoxic state like severe shock, the muscles of respiration work less efficiently and move less air. Increasing levels of carbon dioxide cause an increasing respiratory rate. The result is a more rapid, shallow, and less effective respiratory pattern: the respirations normally associated with shock states.

Eyes are yet another area where early signs of shock may be manifested. The eyes are a window into the brain and accurately reflect the status of cerebral perfusion. In shock, they may give the first hint that problems exist. The sparkle and rate of pupillary response are dependent upon good circulation. Dull and lack-luster eyes or diminished pupillary response reflect reduced circulatory effectiveness.

Decompensated Shock

If the blood loss continues, the body's compensatory mechanisms will eventually breakdown. Reduction of container size and shunting of blood to vital organs and other mechanisms will no longer assure adequate cardiac preload. As cardiac output and arterial blood pressure drop, blood flow to critical organs ceases. The patient soon becomes completely unconscious. Vital signs disappear and death rapidly ensues. This is decompensated shock.

Decompensated shock may occur very quickly or may be delayed, depending upon the rate of blood loss and overall patient condition. As the body compensates for blood loss, vessels constrict and limit blood flow to some tissues, including blood vessels. As time passes, these blood vessels tire and relax, trigger-

✳ One of the first apparent signs of shock is anxiety and restlessness.

ing decompensation. In the otherwise healthy individual, this event occurs about one hour into the shock syndrome and is the basis for the Golden Hour concept.

If blood loss is very rapid, compensatory mechanisms may not have time to be effective. In the elderly, the very young, and those with pre-existing conditions, compensatory mechanisms may not respond as vigorously. As a result, they will not tolerate hemorrhage and shock effectively.

✱ Decompensated shock occurs about one hour into the shock syndrome and is the basis for the Golden Hour concept.

Irreversible Shock

While the body struggles to survive under the stress of compensation, several negative conditions develop. The low-flow state and poor oxygen-carrying capacity of the blood leave much of the body hypoxic. As body cells are deprived of oxygen, they use an inefficient, anaerobic biochemical process to survive. In doing so, they produce lactic acid and accumulate other waste products. These contaminants build up in noncritical body organs and compound the existing hypoxia.

As the muscles of vessel walls become exhausted and relax, their lumens dilate, enlarging the vascular container beyond its pre-shock state. Immediate return of all the lost blood would not fill the vascular space. Even if the vascular system could be filled, the hypoxic heart would have trouble maintaining a normal stroke volume, strength of contraction, blood pressure, and, ultimately, circulation. Because of hypoxia, the arterioles lose their ability to constrict, support blood pressure, and direct circulation. The pulmonary muscles become exhausted from working in an acidic and hypoxic environment. Finally, the entire human system falls subject to poor circulation, oxygenation, and the build up of waste products. It becomes impossible to reverse the effects of shock once irreversible shock takes hold.

ASSESSMENT

Assessment of the trauma patient must search for early indications of shock rather than to wait for the classic signs and symptoms. (See Figure 19-1.) The body is able to adjust well to fluid loss with few overt signs. Should assessment overlook these

✱ Assessment of the trauma patient must search for the early indications of shock rather than to wait for the classic signs and symptoms.

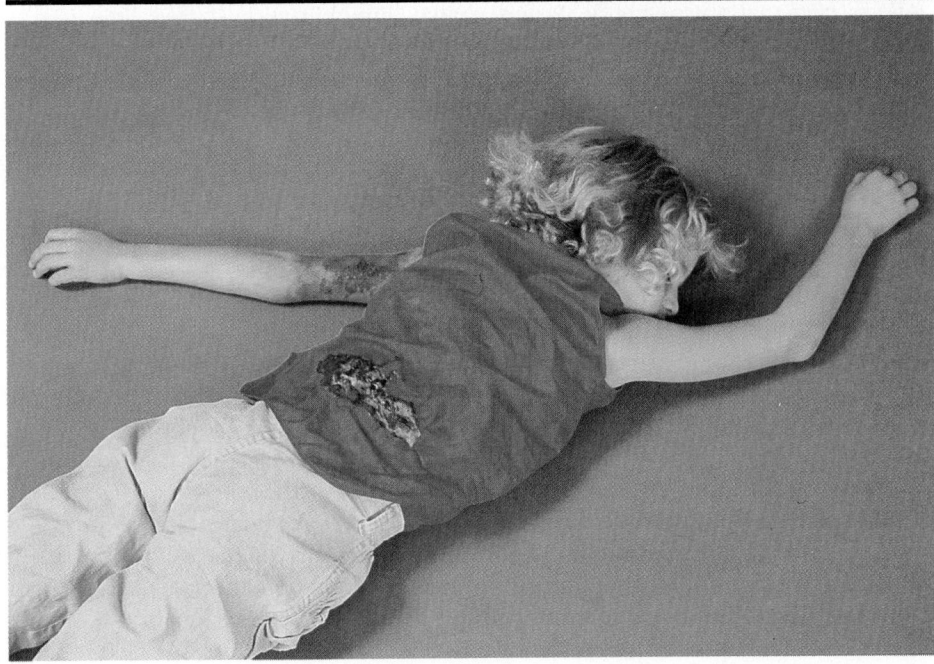

FIGURE 19-1 The victim of serious injury requires prompt and careful evaluation by the paramedic.

early signs, the condition will deteriorate until the more obvious signs of circulatory insufficiency emerge. Delayed recognition slows trauma intervention and impedes potential for survival. You must apply deliberate anticipation and examination to discover the early signs and symptoms of shock, thus ensuring the best opportunity for patient survival. Evaluate your patient early, carefully, and frequently from the time of on-scene arrival until delivery to the emergency department.

Review of Dispatch Information

Trauma assessment begins with review of the dispatch information while you are en route to the scene. Use this information to plan assessment and the major steps of trauma management. Identify the general nature of the call, its location, number of injured persons, and other data to determine your scene approach and patient care. Also search out equipment you may need, and assure that it is handy and in operational order. In trauma, you have no more than 10 minutes to provide assessment and scene care. Pre-planning will help you move quickly and efficiently toward this goal.

Survey of the Scene

Upon arrival, quickly survey the scene to exclude hazards, identify the mechanism of injury (and related indices of suspicion), and locate all patients. Analysis of the mechanism of injury may provide the most revealing aspect of trauma patient assessment. It indicates what injuries may have happened even before patient signs and symptoms yield clues. If the force, direction, and location of impact suggest substantial internal injury, treat the patient for such injury. Treatment should occur even if vital signs and assessment do not support the suspicion. Head, chest, and abdominal injuries are notorious for silently causing shock and death.

Primary Assessment

Once at the patient's side, your first task is primary assessment. (See Figure 19-2.)

C-Spine   Stabilize the cervical spine unless blunt trauma can be ruled out. Kinetic forces fracturing any long bone, rib, or the skull suggest enough trauma to fracture the vertebral column. Likewise, any large contusion or soft-tissue injury reflects potential spinal injury. Proper spinal immobilization carries little risk of patient injury; the same cannot be said of an injured, unstabilized spine. One of your crew should be assigned to stabilize the head manually while the primary assessment continues. Manual stabilization should be released only after it has been replaced by a cervical collar and mechanical stabilization such as fixation to a long spine board and then a cervical immobilization device.

Airway   The airway needs rapid assessment to ensure it remains patent. Examine for any fluids (vomitus, blood, etc.), obstruction, or signs of trauma. Apply suction as necessary, remove any obstructions, and intubate if there is a threat to the airway from tissue swelling. If the patient is unconscious, protect the airway with positioning, nasopharyngeal airway placement, or endotracheal intubation, as necessary. Once you choose a management technique, continue the assessment while crew members ready equipment, prepare the patient, and start the procedure.

Breathing   Evaluate breathing to determine approximate rate, depth, and minute volume. If the patient has experienced significant trauma, give supplemental high-flow oxygen. If respiratory volume is not within normal limits, assist respirations with a bag-valve-mask and supplemental oxygen. Ready any equipment and employ procedures while assessment continues.

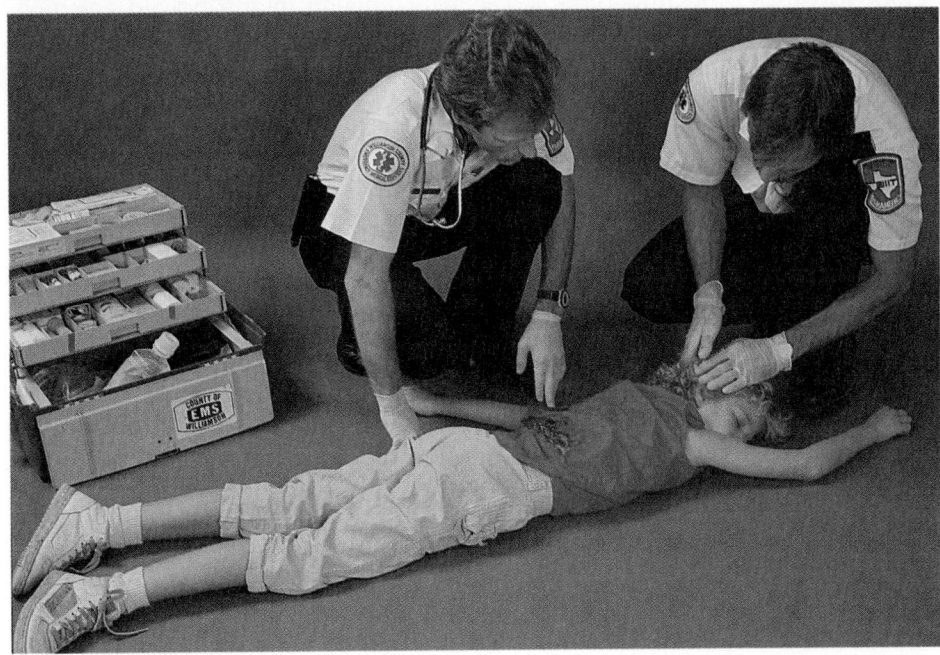

FIGURE 19-2 The first step in assessment of the shock trauma patient is completion of the primary survey.

Circulation Check circulation by evaluating pulse and peripheral perfusion. Determine if the pulse rate is slow, normal, or fast, (determine the exact rate later). Then check the pulse strength. Is it weak, normal, or strong? Compare carotid and radial pulse strength to determine if any difference exists. Finally, evaluate blanching of the peripheral skin to determine capillary refill time. After depressing a nailbed, color should return in under two seconds. If more than three seconds elapse, there is reduced peripheral perfusion. Should any sign point to developing hypovolemia, target the patient for PASG application, and two large bore IVs, hung with two 1,000 mL bags of solution, trauma tubing, and pressure infusers. (See Figure 19-3.)

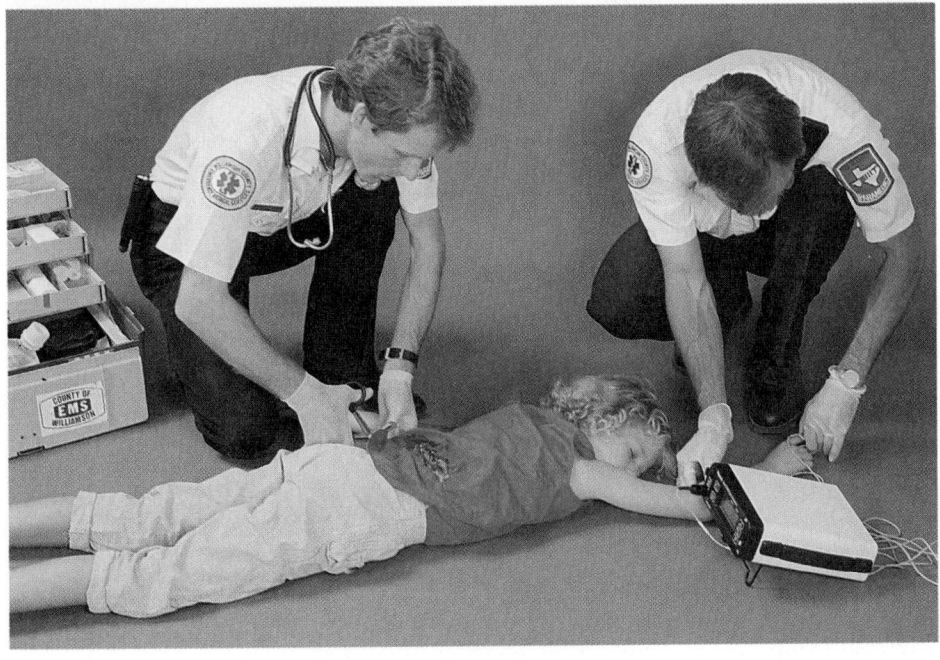

FIGURE 19-3 The paramedic should use every tool and skill available to assist the shock trauma patient.

Disability By this time, you should have enough information to determine roughly the level of consciousness. Categorize the patient's status using the following AVPU system:

A = Alert and oriented
V = Responsive to verbal stimuli
P = Responsive to painful stimuli
U = Completely unresponsive

If the patient is responsive, ask him or her to move all four limbs. This will quickly locate any extremity injury or identify neurologic deficit. If the patient can move all extremities without noticeable pain, you can proceed with the assessment while presuming that no serious extremity injuries exist.

Expose As the primary assessment comes to a close, expose the patient for visual evaluation of the head, neck, chest, abdomen, and pelvis. (See Figure 19-4.) You should observe for the following conditions:

❑ *Wounds:* Contusions, abrasions, lacerations
❑ *Deformities:* Hematomas, subcutaneous emphysema, abnormal angulation or positioning
❑ *Abnormal Motion:* Paradoxical respiration, use of accessory breathing muscles, sternal retraction, or abdominal pulsation

Scan the body for signs of external hemorrhage, sweep hidden areas with the hands, and control any moderate to severe hemorrhage as it is found. Visualize the major body areas to rule out serious hemorrhage, remove clothing as needed, and assess entrapped areas as extrication exposes them. (See Figure 19-4.)

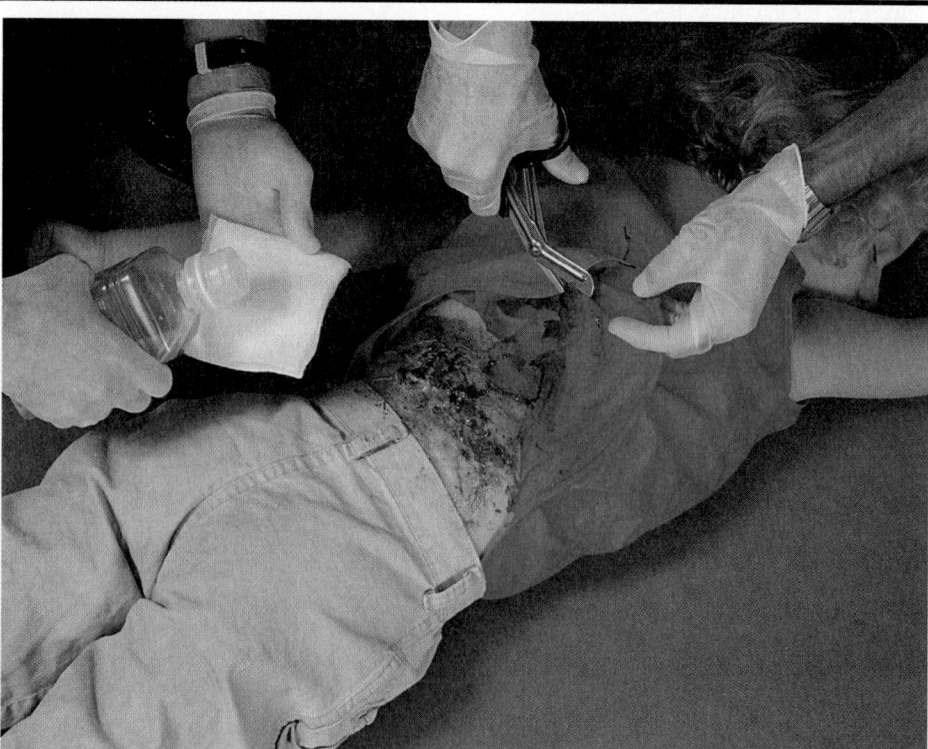

FIGURE 19-4 Exposure and initial treatment should be rapidly completed.

Decision to Transport

At completion of the primary survey, you have all the information needed to select immediate transport or on-scene treatment. While emphasis in this chapter is on rapid transport with care en route, you will best serve the majority of patients by providing scene care. These patients need the reduced risk of injury aggravation that results from splinting, bandaging, and careful packaging of the patient. If the patient is not a candidate for rapid transport, assessment continues. This will include a head-to-toe exam, determination of vital signs, and a complete patient history (not necessarily in that order).

Certain injuries and patient conditions by themselves merit rapid transport and aggressive care. (See Figure 19-5.) Institute aggressive care and rapid transport to a trauma center if the patient meets any of the criteria in Table 19-1. Repeat the primary assessment any time the patient receives significant intervention, a few minutes have passed, or a change is noted in the patient's presentation. Serial primary assessments will help identify signs or symptoms of

✳ Repeat the primary assessment any time the patient receives significant intervention, a few minutes have passed, or a change is noted in the patient's presentation.

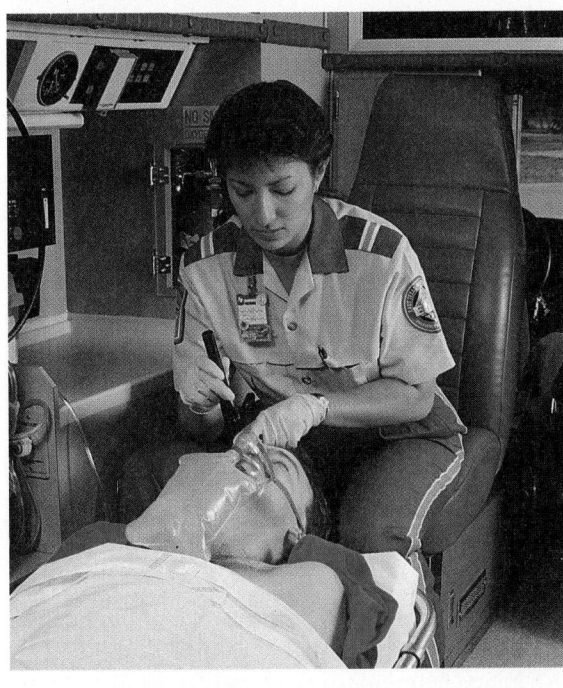

FIGURE 19-5 If shock is present, the patient should be transported immediately with stabilization attempted en route.

TABLE 19-1 Conditions for Rapid Transport	
Mechanism of Injury	**Physical Findings**
Fall greater than 20 feet	Pulse greater than 120 or less than 50
Death of a car occupant	Systolic blood pressure less than 90
Struck by a vehicle traveling over 20 MPH	Respiratory rate < 10 or > 29
Ejected from the vehicle	Glasgow Coma Scale less than 13
Severe vehicle deformity	Penetrating trauma (except extremities)
Rollover with signs of impact	Greater than 2 proximal long bone fractures
	Flail chest
	Burns to greater than 15 percent of B. S. A.
	Burns to face or airway

TABLE 19-2
The Trauma Score

Respiratory Rate (per minute):	Score:
10–29	4
above 29	3
6–9	2
1–5	1
none	0

Respiratory Expansion:	Score:
Normal:	1
Retraction:	0

Blood Pressure (systolic):	Score:
above 89	4
76–89	3
50–75	2
0–49	1
no pulse	0

Capillary Return:	Score:
Normal:	2
Delayed:	1
None:	0

Glasgow Coma Scale:	
13–15	= 5
9–12	= 4
6–8	= 3
4–5	= 2
below 4	= 0

✻ Suspect shock in any patient who displays signs and symptoms of compensation, who has a mechanism of injury that could produce shock, or who has sustained a series of injuries that may induce it.

developing shock, thus alerting you to gradual patient deterioration. Only when transport is underway and the skills of shock care have been applied does a complete physical evaluation of the trauma patient begin. In severely unstable patients, you may never have enough time to assess the patient completely.

Trauma Score

The Trauma Score (see Table 19-2) is a numeric value assigned to a patient based upon assessment. It consists of five components, including the results of the Glasgow Coma Scale. (See Chapter 15.)

The Trauma Score ranges from 0 to 16 points. Research has found patients with scores of 12 or above do relatively well while scores below 10 indicate a poor prognosis. Aggressive intervention has the greatest effect in patients who score between 4 and 12. The Trauma Score provides an objective number describing the seriousness of the patient's condition. It can be used to report the patient's condition to the hospital physician, thus allowing him or her to plan for care upon arrival. Medical control may also use the score to determine the need for advanced life support or for purposes of research and quality improvement.

SHOCK/TRAUMA RESUSCITATION

You should suspect shock in any patient who displays signs and symptoms of compensation, who has a mechanism of injury that could produce shock, or who has sustained a series of injuries that may induce it. If you suspect shock, you should plan shock management well and execute it aggressively. Remember, the human body can compensate for only a limited time and blood loss. The effectiveness of prehospital care and eventual patient survival may depend more upon the time between accident and arrival at the emergency department than upon your skills and abilities as a paramedic.

Correction of Critical Life Threats

Shock/trauma resuscitation occurs simultaneously with the ABCs of the primary assessment. Critical threats to life are immediately corrected as the assessment continues.

Airway Airway is of first concern. If endangered by fluid, swelling, or collapse, secure it with an endotracheal tube. If the patient is unable to protect the airway, intubate. In potential cervical spine injury, immobilize the head firmly in the neutral position and attempt nasotracheal intubation (ideally with a directable tipped tube). If the technique seems ineffective or time consuming, attempt digital placement of the tube.

After properly placing the tube, tape it firmly in place and note the depth of insertion. Endotracheal tubes often become displaced during extrication and patient movement. The use of end-expiratory CO_2 detectors may help verify proper tube placement and removal of CO_2 during the respiratory exchange.

Breathing Once the airway is secure, ventilate if respirations are too fast, too slow, or do not move an adequate volume of air. Apply the bag-valve-mask to the endotracheal tube or tight-sealing mask. Ventilations should be full and at a rate of 20 to 25 breaths per minute. Provide the patient with supplemental oxygen at 15 L per minute via the bag-valve-mask and reservoir. Remember, hypovolemic patients may have erythrocytes and hemoglobin in short supply. Therefore, use high-flow oxygen and positive pressure ventilation to assure that the patient is well oxygenated.

If pulse oximetry is available, gauge ventilation to keep the SpO_2 as high as possible. Any SaO_2 less than 90 percent is cause for concern and immediate attention. In low hemoglobin states, such as shock, pulse oximetry may give a high reading that could mislead you. The hematocrit and available hemoglobin may actually be very low due to a loss of blood and dilution of the remaining blood by interstitial fluids and fluids from your resuscitation. The oxygen-carrying ability of the blood may be so reduced that even oxygen at a saturation of 100 percent cannot adequately supply the body cells.

Circulation Control any moderate to severe hemorrhage. Accomplish this immediately with digital pressure applied directly to the source of hemorrhage. Maintain pressure until control is assumed by a dressing and bandage. If direct pressure is ineffective, try direct pressure and elevation. If that is ineffective, then try direct pressure, elevation, and pressure points. An effective bandage-dressing combination is a roller dressing and a sphygmomanometer. Place the roller dressing at the site of hemorrhage, apply the cuff and inflate slowly until bleeding stops. Use this technique only as a rapid emergency approach under dire circumstances. If time permits, replace hemorrhage control with a more standard dressing and bandage combination. Use a tourniquet, only as a last resort.

In amputations, hemorrhage is often easy to control. Severed blood vessels retract into the limb stump, thicken, and occlude bleeding. This usually occurs during the first 10 minutes after an accident. On the other hand, crushing injuries may bleed severely from multiple locations, and bleeding can be almost impossible to stop. Such injuries may require a tourniquet to arrest hemorrhage.

Application of the PASG

Consider the pneumatic antishock garment (PASG) to control blood loss and to help the body compensate for shock. Currently, its method of action and degree of benefit are being questioned; however, it is well established as being able to control lower extremity hemorrhage and to increase peripheral vascular resistance. The increase in vascular resistance will help maintain the blood pressure in states of shock.

The PASG begins **autotransfusion** around 250 mL of blood. While this falls well below what experts previously thought, the PASG still provides a significant contribution to the hypovolemic patient. The process that autotransfuses the blood also reduces the vascular container size, thus doubling the effect.

■ **autotransfusion** a process that causes the displacement of the patient's blood from one region to another.

The only current contraindications to the application of the trousers are pulmonary edema and penetrating chest trauma. Pulmonary edema is infrequently associated with hypovolemic shock, but anticipate it with severe chest injury or underlying heart disease. Auscultate for breath sounds while applying and inflating the PASG, and check frequently thereafter. If rales or rhonchi appear, stop the inflation. Use of PASG in gunshot wounds, stab wounds, or other penetrating trauma has been shown to be of little value and may increase patient mortality.

Relative PASG contraindications include late pregnancy and impaled objects protruding from the abdomen (or lower extremities). In such cases, apply the device and inflate the unaffected compartments only. Head injury is also a relative contraindication as the garment may increase intracranial pressure. This contraindication only applies when the patient's systolic blood pressure is above 100 mm/Hg, which is not normally associated with hypovolemic shock.

Apply the garment and initially inflate to pressure of at least 40 mm/Hg. Most autotransfusion occurs around 40 mm/Hg, while higher pressures increase peripheral resistance. Guide the inflation by patient response—skin color, level of consciousness, pulse rate, and general appearance. Evaluate blood pressure periodically, keeping in mind that it is only a relative measure of circulatory status and somewhat time consuming.

Do not deflate the PASG in the field for any reason. It will reduce circulating blood volume and peripheral resistance rapidly. Such an insult to an already hypovolemic patient may have catastrophic results. Several associated deaths have already resulted from such deflations.

Fluid Therapy

✳ Fluid therapy should be initiated either quickly (well under 1 minute) at the scene or while en route to the hospital.

Fluid therapy begins very early in shock patient care. It should be initiated either quickly (well under 1 minute) at the scene or while en route to the hospital. In trauma patients, fluid therapy is an emergency procedure, not an elective one. As a paramedic, you must be proficient at this skill through frequent practice. The following strategies will help guide you in the administration of fluids.

Strategies
A pre-packaged trauma IV kit often speeds the procedure. It should contain packaged large bore catheters, tape, trauma tubing, prep pads, bacteriostatic ointment, a 1,000 mL bag of crystalloid solution, and a commercial pressure infuser. This packaging ensures that set-up is easy, rapid, and complete.

✳ The most ideal locations for IVs in the trauma patient are the antecubital fossa and the external jugular veins.

In administering fluids rapidly to a trauma patient, the venipuncture site is very important. In medical patients a distal vein is ideal; however, the trauma patient requires a vein large enough to pass a large bore catheter and peripheral enough so as not to require a long catheter. The most ideal locations are the antecubital fossa and the external jugular veins. Both locations provide good access to large veins and lay rather close to the surface. Often, an IV will be easier to initiate after PASG application because of increased venous pressure.

Central lines are not recommended in cases of trauma for a number of reasons. First, they are placed in deep veins, thus requiring longer catheters. Second, central lines often obstruct other aggressive resuscitation techniques. Third, they take much more time to complete. As a result, you will find it much easier and less time consuming to obtain two or three peripheral lines than one central line.

Another important factor to consider in shock/trauma resuscitation is catheter size and length. Fluid flow is a factor of catheter diameter to a power of four (Poiseuille's law). By doubling the internal diameter of the catheter, the fluid will flow sixteen times faster. Hence, it is essential to pass the largest catheter into the vein that is as reasonably possible. Additionally, shorter catheters reduce the resistance to fluid flow. For this reason, a larger central line catheter (which must be reasonably long) may not infuse fluid as quickly as a shorter and smaller peripheral one.

■ **Seldinger technique** a technique for guiding a larger catheter into a vein previously entered with a small catheter, using a wire dilator.

Placement of a large bore catheter can be difficult in a normotensive patient, much less one in shock. A procedure that facilitates IV insertion is the **Seldinger technique**. It involves normal peripheral venipuncture, using a moderately sized over-the-needle catheter. Once the catheter is in place and the needle is withdrawn, a guide wire is passed through it. The catheter is then withdrawn, and a dilator and number 8 or 9 French catheter are threaded along the wire guide into the vein. The wire and dilator are removed leaving the large catheter in place. The technique is simple, quite effective, and allows the passage of a large catheter into a relatively small peripheral vein.

Restrictions on fluid flow may also be caused by fluid administration sets. The smaller the diameter and the longer the set, the slower the fluid will flow. Administration sets for trauma use should be short in length and large in diameter. Trauma IV tubing is now available and suggested for advanced life support units. Blood tubing has high-flow characteristics as well as the added benefit that the tubing can be used by emergency department staff to administer blood.

The last consideration regarding flow is the pressure used. One can easily demonstrate the effect of pressure on fluid flow through an IV administration set by simply raising the fluid bag. The drip rate and flow out of the needle will increase. Gravity may not create enough pressure for trauma patients who need large volumes of solution quickly. Use of a thigh blood pressure cuff or a commercially available pressure infusion device may be necessary. Pressures of 200 to 300 mm/Hg will double the rate of fluid delivery.

Precautions   Benefits to rapid fluid infusion must be weighed against patient concerns. Rapid infusion in a patient who does not need it or in one who has underlying heart problems may precipitate pulmonary edema and congestive heart failure. Monitor breath sounds, respiratory effort, and blood pressure carefully. Slow or stop the IVs at the first sign of circulatory overload: dyspnea, rales, rhonchi, or dropping oxygen saturation.

The standard of care for a patient who has lost or is losing a large volume of blood is two large-bore IV sites. Connect them to trauma tubing running from one 1,000 mL bag of normal saline and one of lactated Ringer's solution. Lactated Ringer's solution is most ideal for fluid resuscitation, yet normal saline is compatible with whole blood administration. Apply pressure infusion devices and inflate to 200 to 300 mm Hg of pressure. Provide frequent serial vital signs and patient assessments, placing a special focus on breath sounds, rate and quality of pulse, and the patient's level of consciousness.

There are limits to the effectiveness of crystalloid infusions. First, three liters of crystalloid expand the vascular volume by only 1 liter. This is because much of the fluid leaks from the capillaries into the interstitial and cellular spaces. Second, the infusing fluid is also not a complete replacement for blood. It does not contain either the hemoglobin needed to carry oxygen to the body cells or the clotting factors. Infusing more than three liters of crystalloid may severely dilute the blood so it does not carry enough hemoglobin and will not clot effectively. For these reasons, field crystalloid infusion is limited to 3 liters.

Entrapment, and other special circumstances, may cause you to be on scene for more than 10 minutes. Establish communication with the trauma center. While starting the IVs, consider drawing a tube of blood and sending it to the hospital with a supervisor or the police. This allows the emergency department to type and crossmatch blood prior to patient arrival. Under dire circumstances, suggest bringing blood and the emergency physician to the scene.

AIR MEDICAL TRANSPORT

In recent years, the helicopter has become widely available to ALS systems throughout the country. Helicopters transport patients rapidly (about 140 mph), bypassing traffic and flying directly to the nearest trauma center. Since trauma care is often a race against time, air medical service provides a welcome, life-saving addition to the prehospital care system.

The helicopter should be used when it will significantly reduce transport time for severely injured trauma patients. In making this decision, consider the normal activation and warm-up time (3 to 5 minutes) and the flight time to the scene. It is counterproductive to wait 15 minutes at the scene for a helicopter when it will reduce transport time by 10 minutes. On the other hand, if the helicopter arrives during a prolonged extrication or during rush hour, the time savings may be well worth it. As a general rule, if transport by ground will exceed 30 minutes, use of the helicopter may be indicated.

Coordination of helicopter response should be assigned to someone other than the paramedic in-charge. Your responsibilities should be directed toward the assessment and care of the patient. In preparation for flight, assure that the patient's airway is secure. Also, establish a good IV, immobilize the patient's spine, and complete a thorough assessment. The flight crew will want these critical procedures completed before loading the patient because of the small working environment within the helicopter. (See Figure 19-6.) It will also be essential to provide the flight crew with a full patient report.

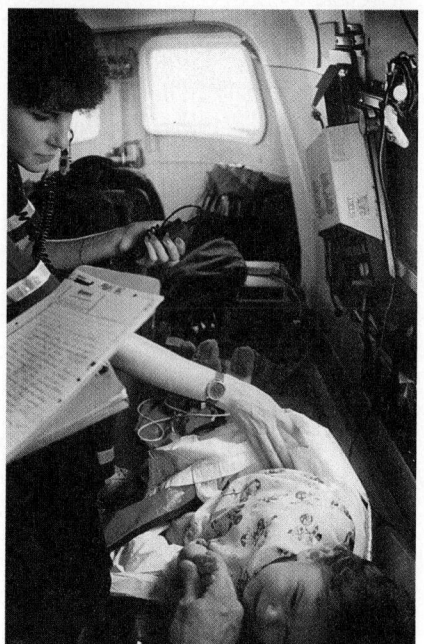

FIGURE 19-6 The work space in the helicopter is small so complete crucial procedures before loading the patient.

The landing area at the scene of the accident should be established by someone knowledgeable with the criteria for helicopter landing zones. The landing zone should be as level as possible and clear of dust, debris, and snow. Prop wash—the powerful blast of air that occurs with landing—can blow debris into the medical care site, on to bystanders, or possibly into the rotors. Dust and snow may turn into clouds that obscure or blind the pilot's vision. (See Figure 19-7.)

A landing zone should be a minimum of 60 × 60 feet for small helicopters, 75 × 75 feet for medium ones, and 120 × 120 feet for large ones. It should be free of wires, trees, and other obstructions that may impede landing or interfere with patient loading. If you observe obstructions or other possible hazards, direct

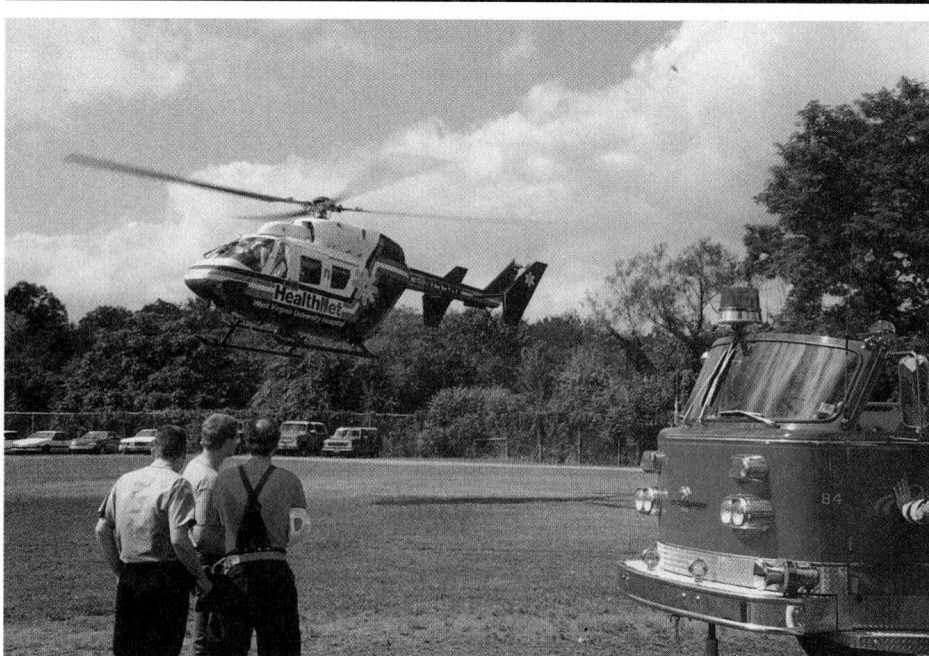

FIGURE 19-7 Assure the helicopter landing zone is free of debris, utility lines, and other hazards.

someone to radio the information to the incoming pilot. Wires and poles that are visible from the ground may be invisible to the pilot and flight crew.

In daylight, firmly anchored traffic cones will mark the corners of the landing zone. At night, the landing zone should be illuminated by lights pointed at the zone surface. Do not direct lights into the air or at the helicopter. They may blind the pilot and make a safe landing difficult. Be especially watchful of camera crews looking for a good shot of the helicopter landing. Flares should not be used since they may be blown with the prop wash, igniting leaves, debris, or spilled fuel.

Once the helicopter lands, it should be approached from the front and only under the direction of the flight crew. Frequently, the crew will approach the patient while the rotors are still turning (a hot off-load). If the patient is properly prepared for transport and a well-organized patient report is ready, the crew may load the patient while the rotors continue to turn (a hot load). If you are asked to help load the patient, stay close to the flight crew. Follow their instructions carefully, and avoid the area of the tail rotor. It spins at speeds in excess of 2,000 rpm and is almost invisible. After you have loaded the patient, move forward away from the helicopter, staying in clear view of the pilot.

SUMMARY

The critical trauma patient needs rapid assessment and aggressive care to obtain the best chance for survival. Use the dispatch information and scene survey to plan assessment and care. Provide a rapid and complete primary assessment, and correct any problems as they are found. Determine the need for rapid transport or on-scene care. If the patient is displaying the signs and symptoms of shock, treat aggressively with PASG application and inflation, rapid infusion of fluids, and immediate transport to the trauma center.

In responding to the trauma emergency, keep to the priorities of emergency care. They include:

A = Airway and cervical spine
B = Breathing
C = Circulation
D = Disability
E = Expose and correct any severe hemorrhage or any life threat detected by the primary survey

If you keep to these priorities, the trauma patient will have the best possible chance to survive the syndrome called shock.

FURTHER READING

American College of Surgeons, Committee on Trauma. *Advanced Resources for Optimal Care of the Injured Patient*. American College of Surgeons, 1990.

American College of Surgeons, Committee on Trauma. *Advanced Trauma Life Support Course: Student Manual*. American College of Surgeons, 1989.

Baxt, William G. *Trauma, The First Hour*. 1st ed. Englewood Cliffs, NJ: Prentice-Hall, Inc., 1985.

Butman, Alexander M. and James L. Paturas. *Pre-Hospital Trauma Life Support*. Akron, OH: Emergency Training, 1990.

Campbell, John E. *Basic Trauma Life Support*. 2nd ed. Englewood Cliffs, NJ: Prentice-Hall, Inc., 1988.

Hardaway, Robert M. *Shock: The Reversible Stage of Dying*. 1st ed. Littleton, MA: PSG Publishing Company, Inc., 1988.

Jastremski, Michael S., Marc Dumas and Lisa Penalver. *Emergency Procedures*. 1st ed. Philadelphia, PA: E. B. Saunders Company, 1992.

Macdonald, Steven C., Alexander Butman, Marvin A. Wayne and Norman McSwain. *Using Anti-Shock Trousers: A Guide for the EMT*. 1st ed. Akron, OH: Emergency Training, 1982.

Maull, Kimball, Jackie Kirby, and Dennis Rowe. *Trauma Update for the EMT*. 1st ed. Englewood Cliffs, NJ: Prentice-Hall, Inc., 1992.

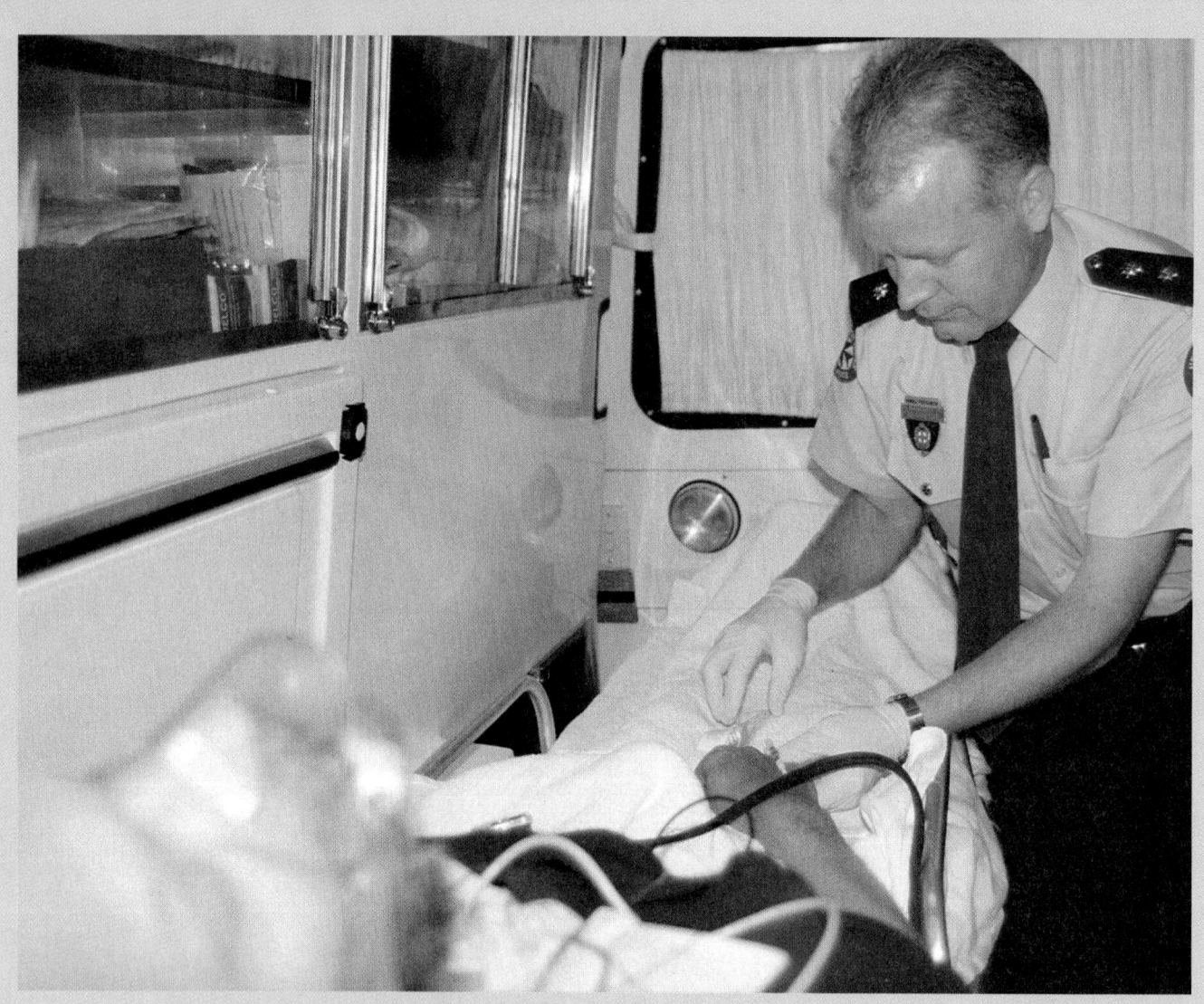

20

RESPIRATORY EMERGENCIES

Objectives for Chapter 20

After reading this chapter, you should be able to:

1. Identify the historical factors to elicit when evaluating the respiratory system. (See p. 575.)

2. Identify specific observations and physical findings to evaluate in the patient with a respiratory complaint. (See pp. 576–580.)

3. Describe the techniques of inspection, auscultation, and palpation of the chest. (See pp. 576–579.)

4. Define the following terms. (See below pages.)

- snoring (p. 578)
- stridor (p. 578)
- wheezing (p. 578)
- rhonchi (p. 578)
- rales (p. 579)
- friction rub (p. 579)

5. Review the basic principles of respiratory management. (See pp. 581–599.)

6. Describe the difference between the normal respiratory drive and the respiratory drive of the patient with chronic obstructive pulmonary disease (COPD). (See pp. 583–586.)

7. Review the pharmacology, action, dosage, side effects, contraindications, and routes of administration of the following drugs. (See below pages.)

- epinephrine (p. 589)
- albuterol (p. 590)
- isoetharine (p. 590)
- metaproterenol (p. 591)
- terbutaline (p. 591)
- methylprednisolone (p. 593)
- aminophylline (p. 594)

8. Discuss the pathophysiology, assessment, and management of the following conditions. (See below pages.)

- emphysema (pp. 583–589)
- chronic bronchitis (pp. 585–586)
- asthma (pp. 586–594)
- pneumonia (pp. 594–597)
- toxic inhalation (pp. 595–597)
- pulmonary embolism (p. 597)
- hyperventilation syndrome (pp. 597–598)
- central nervous system dysfunctions (pp. 598–599)

Central 9-1-1 dispatches Ellis County EMS to a "medical emergency" in a rural part of the county. The response time is approximately 12 minutes. Upon arrival at the rural farm house, the paramedics are met by an EMT-Basic from the local volunteer fire department. She reports they have a 55-year-old white male with difficulty breathing. The First Responder states that oxygen is already being administered. The paramedics grab the drug box, monitor/defibrillator, airway kit, and stretcher. They then enter the small farmhouse.

Paramedics find the patient seated at the kitchen table, obviously short of breath. They quickly perform a primary assessment. The airway is clear, the patient is moving air, and has a strong pulse. Paramedics replace the nasal cannula positioned by the First Responder with a venturi mask that delivers an FiO_2 of 35 percent.

The paramedics then complete the secondary assessment. The patient has diminished breath sounds, occasional rhonchi, and is using the accessory muscles of respiration. There is a hint of cyanosis around the mouth. Paramedics learn that several years ago, doctors at the V.A. hospital diagnosed the patient as having emphysema. Over the last 24 hours, the patient has had progressive dyspnea and didn't sleep at all the previous night. Vital signs reveal a blood pressure of 140/78 mm/Hg, a pulse of 96, and a respiratory rate of 28. The monitor shows a sinus rhythm. Pulse oximetry reveals an SpO_2 of 90 percent, while receiving supplemental oxygen. The patient is mentally alert. He is currently taking theophylline and amoxicillin. He still smokes a pack of cigarettes per day and has a 30 pack/year history.

The patient wants to be transported to the V.A. hospital. The paramedics contact medical control and provide the patient report. The medical control physician approves transport to the V.A. hospital as it is only 5 miles farther than the nearest hospital. The transport time will be approximately 40 minutes.

The medical control physician orders the placement of an IV of D5W at a "to keep open" rate. In addition, he orders a nebulizer treatment with 0.5 milliliters of albuterol (Ventolin) placed in 3 milliliters of normal saline. Because of the long transport time, he also orders the administration of 125 milligrams of methylprednisolone (Solu-Medrol) by IV drip over 20 minutes. Halfway through the nebulizer treatment, the patient shows marked improvement. His respiratory rate slows to 20, and his SpO_2 increases to 94 percent. Transport to the hospital is uneventful. He remains in the hospital 2 days and is discharged home.

INTRODUCTION

The respiratory system is a vital body system responsible for providing oxygen to the tissues as well as removing the metabolic waste product carbon dioxide. Oxygen is required for the conversion of essential nutrients into energy and must be constantly available to all body tissues.

Respiratory emergencies are among some of the most common EMS emergencies. As a paramedic, you must promptly recognize and treat respiratory problems appropriately. This chapter will discuss pathophysiology, patient assessment, and management of some of the most frequently encountered respiratory emergencies.

REVIEW OF RESPIRATORY ANATOMY AND PHYSIOLOGY

The anatomy and physiology of the respiratory system was presented in detail in Chapter 11. As mentioned in that chapter, the airway is divided anatomically into the *upper airway* and the *lower airway*. (See Figure 20-1.) The upper airway is responsible for warming and humidifying incoming air. It is also very effective in air purification.

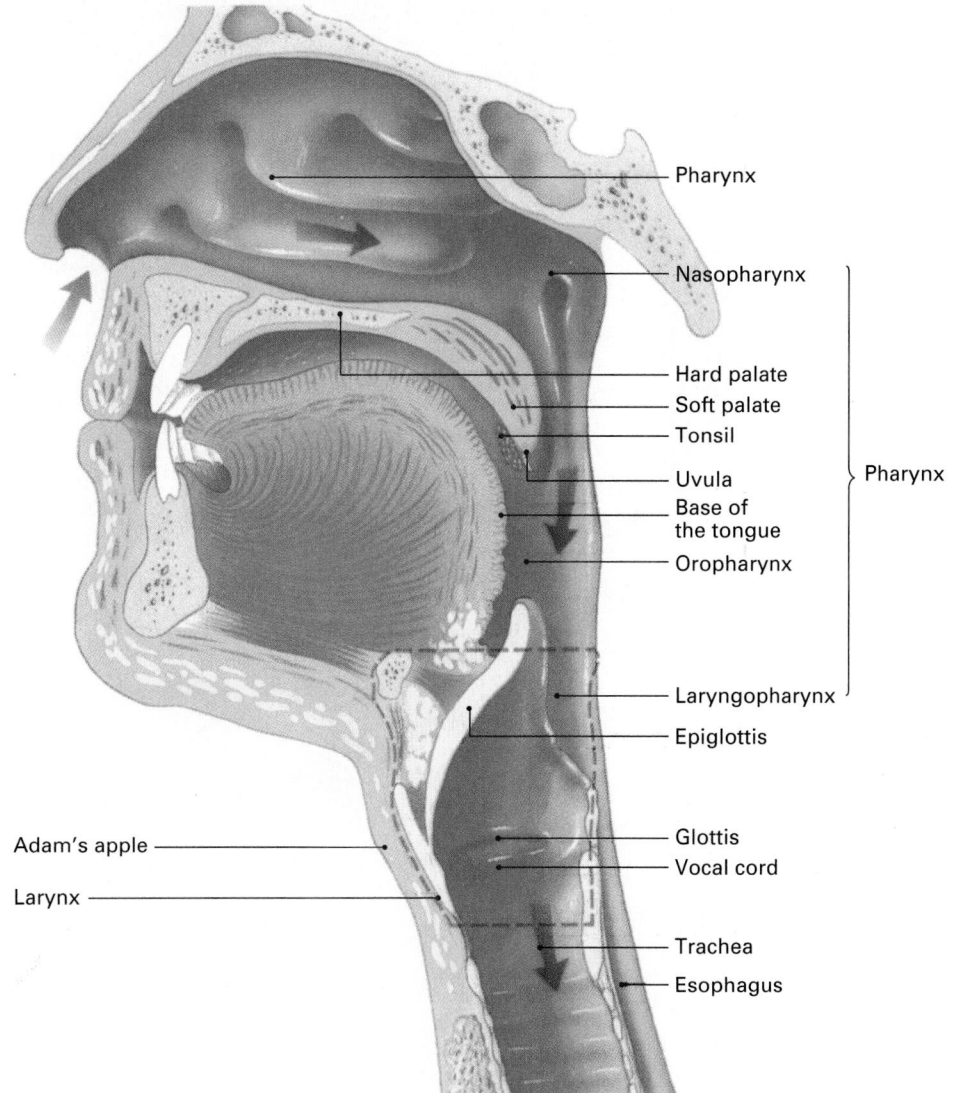

Pharynx

Nasopharynx

Hard palate

Soft palate

Tonsil

Uvula

Base of
the tongue

Oropharynx

Pharynx

Laryngopharynx

Epiglottis

Adam's apple

Glottis

Vocal cord

Larynx

Trachea

Esophagus

FIGURE 20-1 Anatomy of the upper airway.

Air enters the upper airway through the mouth and nose. During inspiration, air exits the upper airway and passes through the larynx into the trachea. At the *carina*, the trachea divides into the right and the left mainstem *bronchi*. The right mainstem bronchus is almost straight, whereas the left mainstem bronchus angles more acutely to the left. (See Figure 20-2.) The mainstem bronchi then divide into the secondary bronchi. These secondary bronchi ultimately divide into the *bronchioles*, or the small airways. The bronchioles contain smooth muscle that can contract, thus reducing the diameter of the airway. After approximately 22 divisions, the bronchioles become *respiratory bronchioles*. They contain only muscular connective tissue and have a limited ability for gas exchange. The respiratory bronchioles then divide into the *alveolar ducts*. These terminate in the *alveolar sacs*.

Most of the gas exchange takes place in the alveoli, although limited gas exchange may occur in the alveolar ducts and respiratory bronchioles. (See Figure 20-3.) The alveoli are kept open because of the presence of an important chemical called *surfactant*, which tends to decrease the surface tension of the alveoli.

The lungs are covered by connective tissue called *pleura*. Unattached to the lung, except at the hilum (the point at which the bronchi enter the lungs),

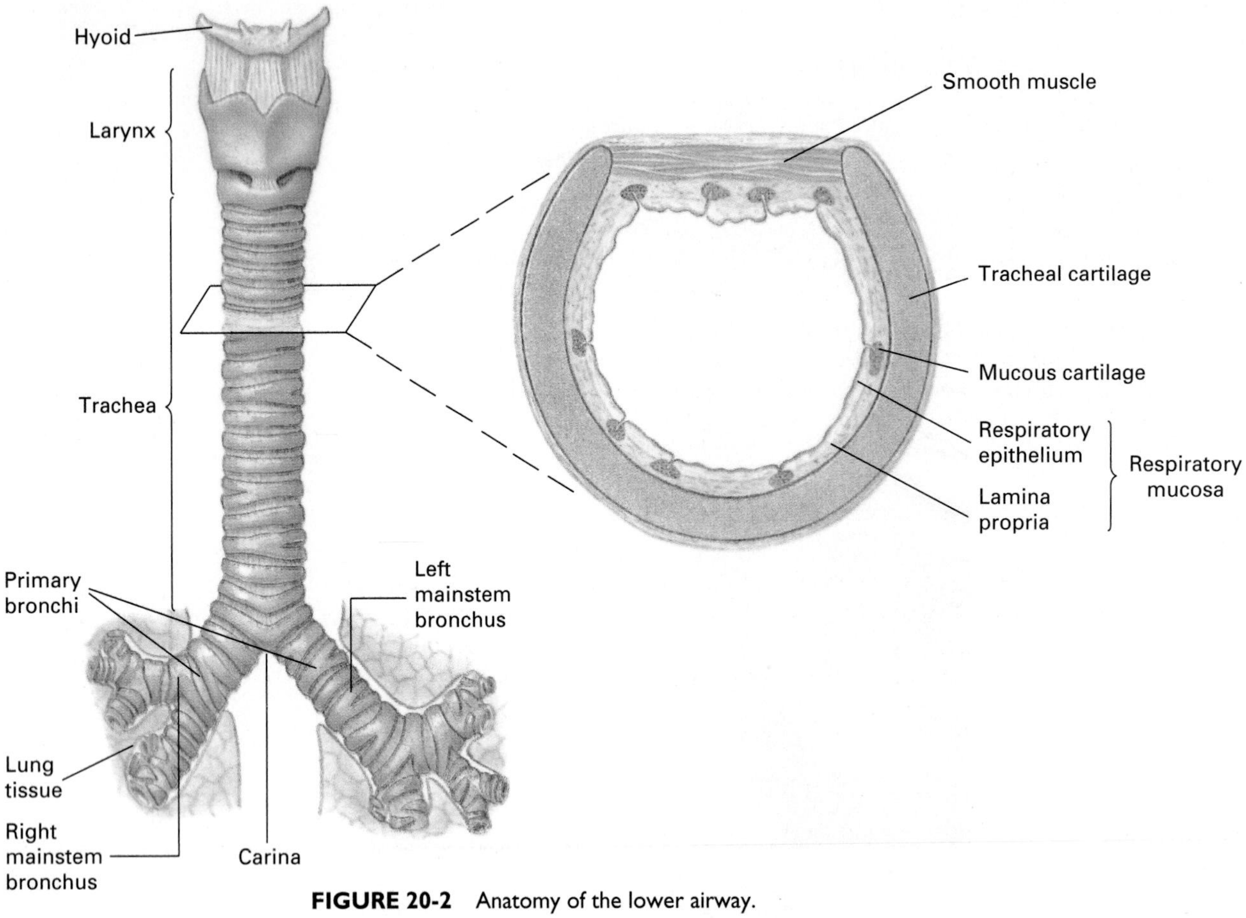

Hyoid

Larynx

Trachea

Smooth muscle

Tracheal cartilage

Mucous cartilage

Respiratory
epithelium

Lamina
propria

Respiratory
mucosa

Primary
bronchi

Left
mainstem
bronchus

Lung
tissue

Right
mainstem
bronchus

Carina

FIGURE 20-2 Anatomy of the lower airway.

the pleura consists of two layers. The *visceral pleura* covers the lungs and does not contain nerve fibers. In contrast, the *parietal pleura* lines the thoracic cavity and contains nerve fibers. A small amount of *pleural fluid* usually can be found in the pleural space, a potential space between the two layers of pleura.

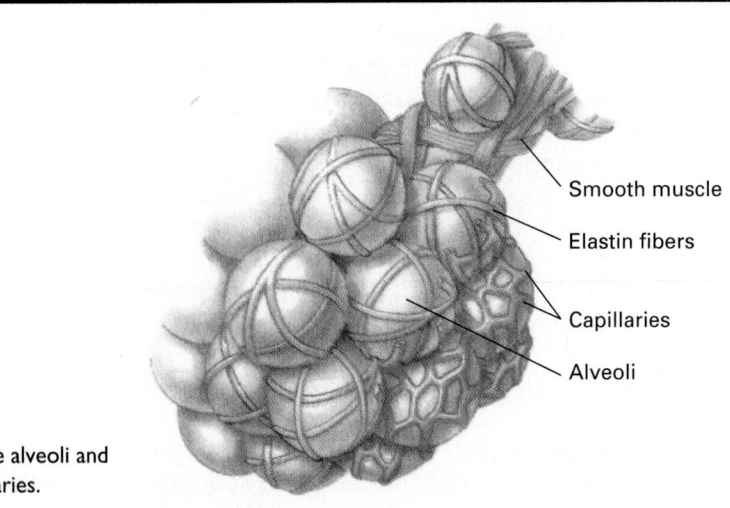

Smooth muscle

Elastin fibers

Capillaries

Alveoli

FIGURE 20-3 The alveoli and the pulmonary capillaries.

Blood supply to the lungs is through two systems: the pulmonary arteries and veins and the bronchial arteries and veins. The *pulmonary arteries* transport deoxygenated blood from the heart and present it to the lungs for oxygenation. The *pulmonary veins* then transport the oxygenated blood from the lungs back to the heart. The lung tissue itself receives little of its blood supply from the pulmonary arteries and veins. Instead, *bronchial arteries* that branch from the aorta provide most of the blood supply. *Bronchial veins* return blood from the lungs to the superior vena cava.

This entire system provides for respiration—the exchange of gases between a living organism and its environment. *Pulmonary respiration* occurs in the lungs when the respiratory gases are exchanged between the alveoli and the red blood cells in the pulmonary capillaries through the capillary membranes. *Cellular respiration*, on the other hand, occurs in the peripheral capillaries. It involves the exchange of the respiratory gases between the red blood cells and the various tissues.

ASSESSMENT OF THE RESPIRATORY SYSTEM

Assessment of the respiratory system is a vital aspect of prehospital care. You must quickly assess the airway and ventilation status during the primary survey. If the secondary survey reveals that the respiratory system appears to be involved in the patient's problem, focus on this aspect of the assessment.

History

The history and physical exam should be directed at problem areas as determined by the patient's chief complaint or primary problem. If the chief complaint is "shortness of breath," or **dyspnea**, ask the following questions. (The answers to these or similar questions will provide you with a pertinent patient history.)

■ **dyspnea** difficult or labored breathing.

❑ How long has the dyspnea been present?
❑ Was the onset gradual or abrupt?
❑ Is the dyspnea better or worse by position? Is there associated orthopnea (dyspnea while lying supine)?
❑ Has the patient been coughing?
  • If so, is the cough productive?
  • What is the character and color of the sputum?
  • Is there any **hemoptysis**?

■ **hemoptysis** expectoration of blood from the respiratory tree.

❑ Is there any pain associated with the dyspnea?
  • If so, what is the location of the pain?
  • Was the onset of pain sudden or slow?
  • What was the duration of the pain?
❑ Does the pain radiate to any area?
❑ Does the pain increase with respiration?
❑ What is the patient's past medical history?
❑ What current medications is the patient taking? (Pay particular attention to oxygen therapy, oral bronchodilators, corticosteroids, and antibiotics.)
❑ Does the patient have any allergies?

Physical Examination

Physical examination of the respiratory system should follow the standard steps of patient assessment. They are inspection, palpation, percussion, and auscultation.

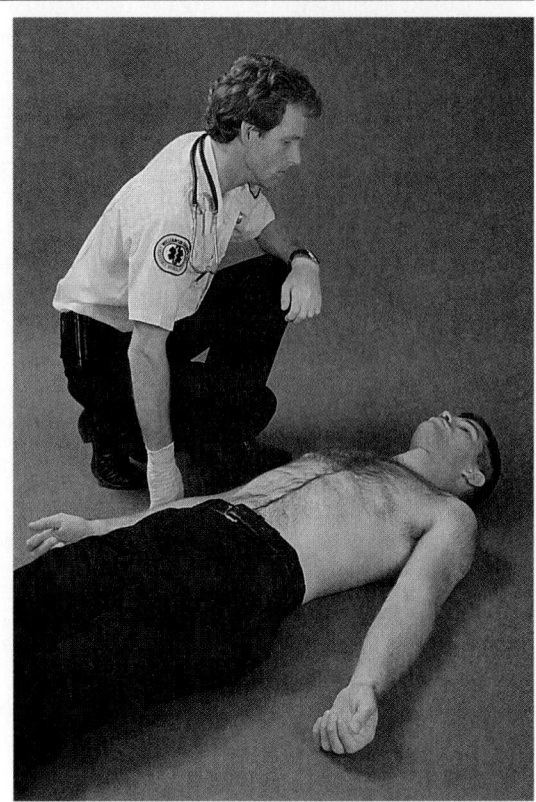

FIGURE 20-4 The first step in evaluating the respiratory emergency is to check the ABCs.

Primary Survey   As in other emergencies, conduct a primary assessment, ensuring a patent airway. (See Figure 20-4.) If the airway is compromised, quickly institute basic airway management techniques. When assessing the airway, keep the following principles in mind.

❑ Noisy breathing nearly always means partial airway obstruction.
❑ Obstructed breathing is not always noisy.
❑ The brain can survive only a few minutes in **asphyxia**.
❑ Artificial respiration is useless if the airway is blocked.
❑ A patient's airway is useless if the patient is apneic.
❑ If you note airway obstruction, do not waste time looking for help or equipment.

■ **asphyxia** a decrease in the amount of oxygen and an increase in the amount of carbon dioxide as a result of some interference with respiration.

Once you have secured a patent airway, ensure that the patient has adequate ventilation and circulation.

Secondary Survey   Begin your secondary survey by looking for any of the following conditions.

■ **hypoxia** state in which insufficient oxygen is available to meet the oxygen requirements of the cells.

❑ Anxiety, discomfort, or stress—these may possibly indicate **hypoxia**.
❑ Difficulty in speaking due to dyspnea.
❑ Distraction from questioning due to the symptoms present.
❑ Alert verbal response versus confusion.
❑ Position of the patient.
❑ Obesity, which can result in hypoventilation.

Following observation, the vital signs should be determined, including the rate and depth of the respiratory pattern. Determine if any abnormal respiratory patterns are present. A patient will occasionally exhibit *pulsus paradoxus*, a drop in the systolic blood pressure of 10 Torr or more with each respiratory cycle. Pulsus paradoxus is associated with **chronic obstructive pulmonary disease (COPD)** and cardiac tamponade. As a rule, you should not take the time to look for pulsus paradoxus.

During the secondary survey, turn your attention to the respiratory system. Inspection should be completed after first looking for signs of respiratory distress. Obvious signs include:

❏ **Nasal flaring**
❏ Intercostal muscle retraction
❏ Use of the accessory respiratory muscles
❏ **Cyanosis**
❏ Pursed lips
❏ **Tracheal tugging**

Next, the anterior-posterior dimensions and general shape of the chest should be inspected. (See Figure 20-5.) An increased anterior-posterior diameter is suggestive of chronic obstructive pulmonary disease. The chest should be inspected for symmetrical movement. Any asymmetry may be suggestive of trauma. A paradoxical movement is suggestive of flail chest. Note any chest scars, lesions, wounds, or deformities.

Following inspection, palpate the chest, both front and back, for any abnormalities. (See Figure 20-6.) Note any tenderness, crepitus, subcutaneous emphysema, or air leakage. Palpate the anterior chest first, then the posterior.

■ **chronic obstructive pulmonary disease (COPD)** characterized by a decreased ability of the lungs to perform the function of ventilation.

■ **nasal flaring** excessive widening of the nares with respiration.

■ **cyanosis** bluish discoloration of the skin due to an increase in reduced hemoglobin in the blood. The condition is directly related to poor ventilation.

■ **tracheal tugging** retraction of the tissues of the neck due to airway obstruction or dyspnea.

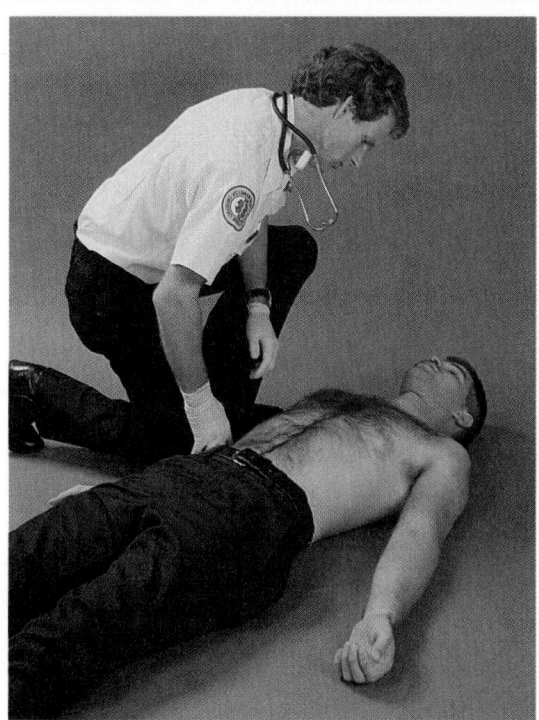

FIGURE 20-5   Inspection of the chest.

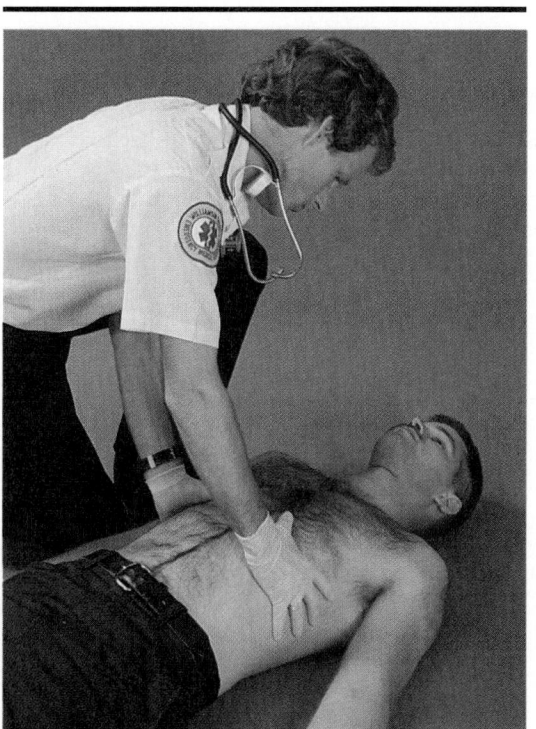

FIGURE 20-6   The chest should be palpated.

Inspect your gloved hands for blood each time they are removed from behind the patient's chest. In some instances, it may be appropriate to evaluate the patient's **tactile fremitus**, the vibration felt in the chest during speaking. When evaluating tactile fremitus, compare one side of the chest with the other. Simultaneously, palpate the trachea for tracheal deviation suggestive of a tension pneumothorax. (See Chapter 16.)

Following palpation, and if indicated, quickly percuss the chest. Limit percussion to suspected cases of pneumothorax and pulmonary edema. (See Figure 20-7.) A hollow sound on percussion is often indicative of pneumothorax or emphysema. In contrast, a dull sound is indicative of pulmonary edema, hemothorax, or pneumonia.

Finally, auscultate the chest. Begin by listening to the patient without a stethoscope and from a distance. Note any loud stridor, wheezing, or cough. If possible, the patient should be in the sitting position and the chest auscultated in a symmetrical pattern. (See Figure 20-8.) When the patient cannot sit up, auscultate the anterior and lateral parts of the chest. Each area should be auscultated for one respiratory cycle. While the patient breathes in and out deeply with the mouth open, note any abnormal breath sounds and their location. (See Figure 20-9.)

Many terms are used to describe abnormal breath sounds. The following are some of the more common terms.

❑ *Snoring.* Occurs when the upper airway is partially obstructed, usually by the tongue.
❑ *Stridor.* Harsh, high-pitched sound heard on inspiration and characteristic of an upper airway obstruction such as croup.
❑ *Wheezing.* Whistling sound due to narrowing of the airways by edema, bronchoconstriction, or foreign materials.
❑ *Rhonchi.* Rattling sounds in the larger airways associated with excessive mucus or other material.

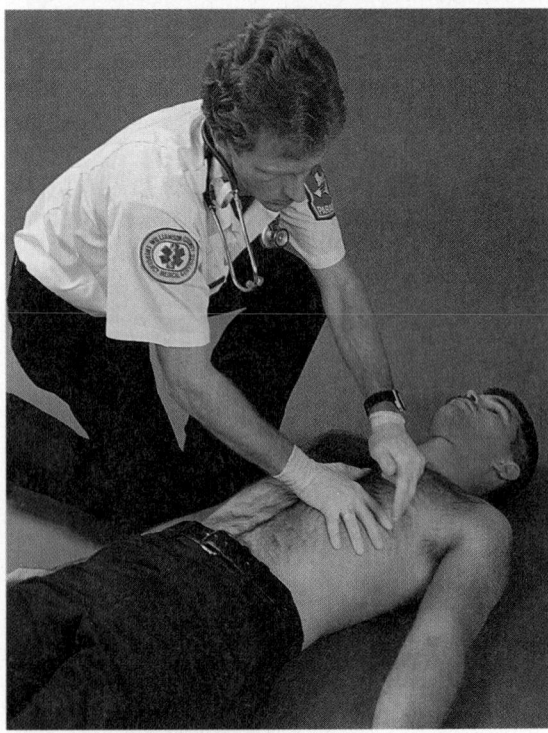

FIGURE 20-7 If indicated, the chest should be percussed.

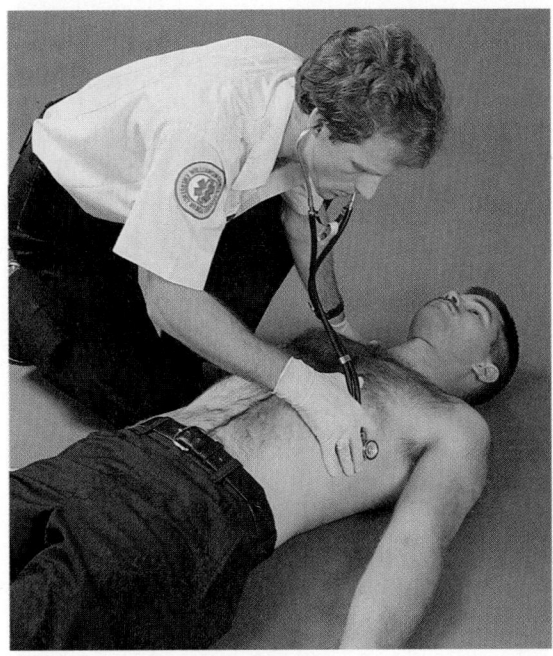

FIGURE 20-8 The chest should be auscultated.

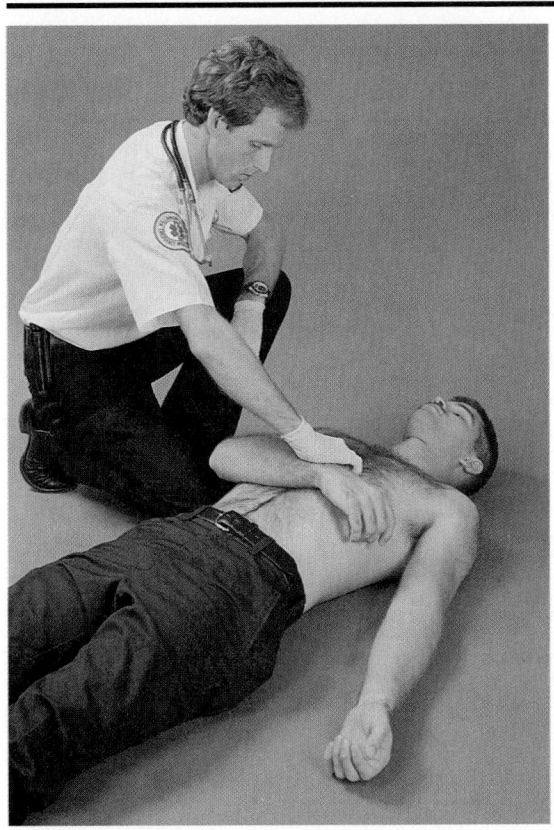

FIGURE 20-9 The respiratory rate should be counted. It is often helpful to take the pulse of patients when counting respirations. The patient will think that you are taking the pulse and will not consciously modify his or her respiratory rate.

❑ *Rales.* Fine, moist crackling sounds associated with fluid in the smaller airways.

❑ *Friction Rub.* Occurs when the pleura become inflamed, as in pleurisy; sounds like dried pieces of leather rubbing together.

Pulse Oximetry

Pulse oximetry offers a rapid and accurate means for assessing oxygen saturation. The device can be quickly applied to a finger. The pulse rate and oxygen saturation can be continuously recorded. Use of the pulse oximeter, if available, is encouraged for any patient complaining of dyspnea or respiratory problems. (See Figures 20-10 through 20-13.) For additional discussion of pulse oximetry, see Chapter 11.

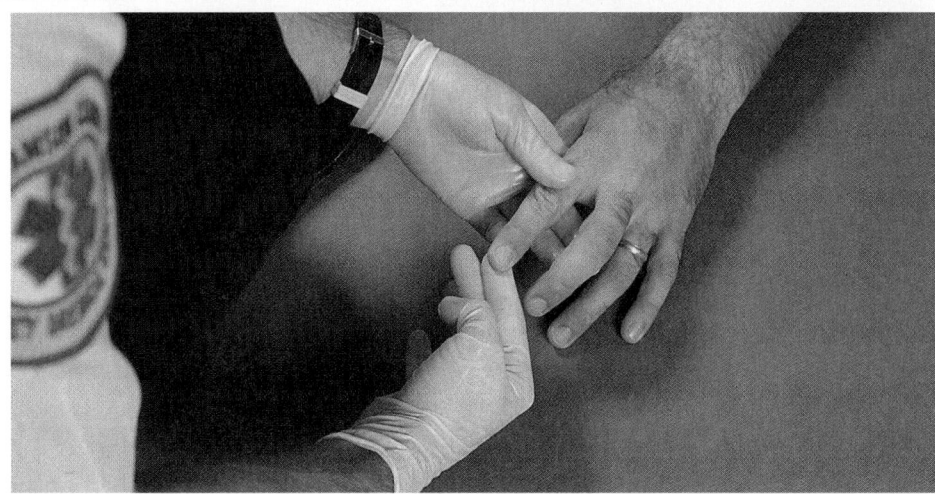

FIGURE 20-10 Prior to placing the oximeter probe, the fingers should be inspected. Any clubbing may indicate chronic respiratory or cardiac disease.

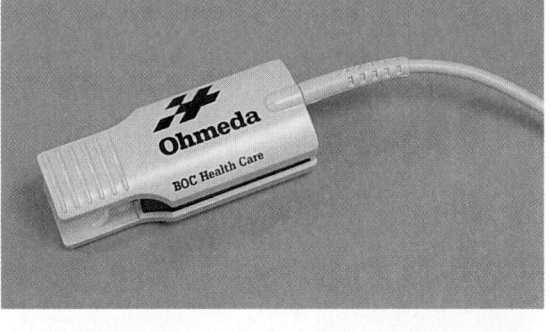

FIGURE 20-11 Sensing unit for pulse oximetry. This device transmits light through a vascular bed, such as in the finger, and can determine the oxygen saturation of red blood cells.

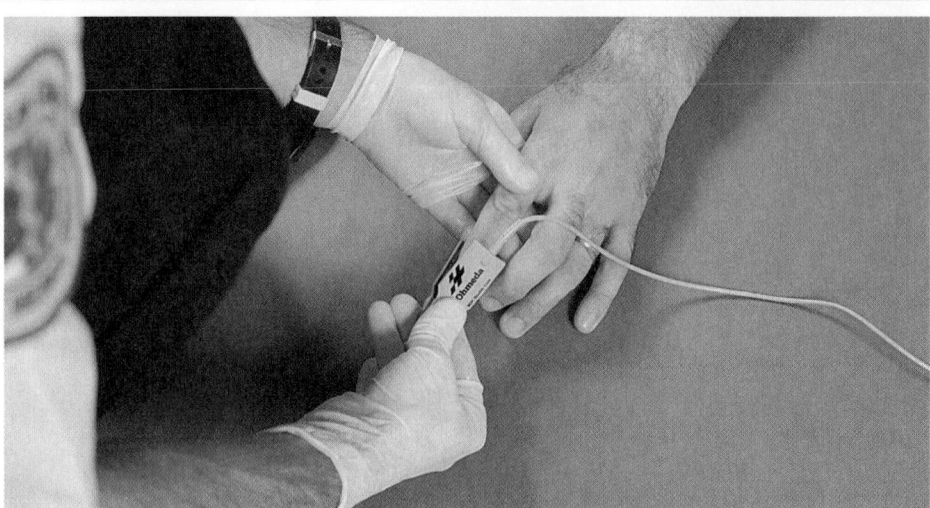

FIGURE 20-12 To use the pulse oximeter, it is only necessary to turn the device on and attach the sensor to a finger.

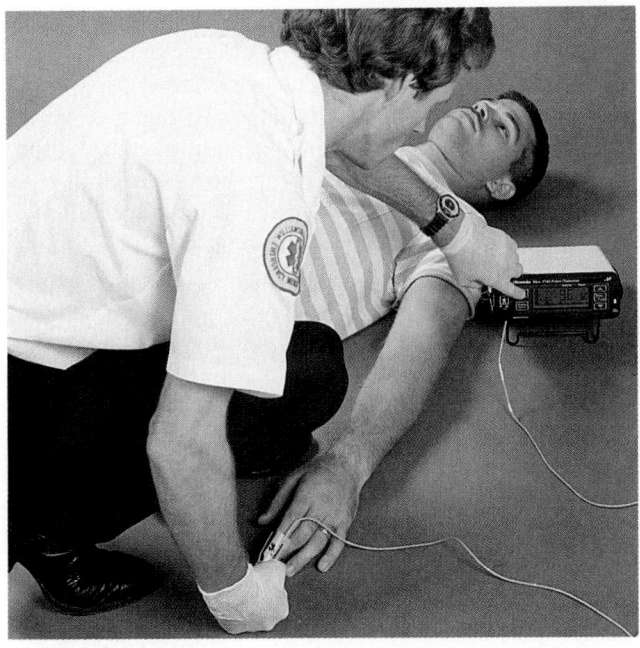

FIGURE 20-13 The desired graphic mode on the oximeter should be selected. The oxygen saturation and pulse rate can be continuously monitored.

PATHOPHYSIOLOGY AND MANAGEMENT OF RESPIRATORY DISORDERS

The following sections will address the pathophysiology and management of the more common respiratory disorders encountered in prehospital care. The discussion begins with a look at some general principles that can and should be applied to ALL respiratory emergencies.

Management Principles of Respiratory Emergencies

In cases of acute respiratory insufficiency, several principles should guide your actions in the prehospital setting. These include:

❑ The airway always receives first priority. In trauma victims who may have associated cervical spine injuries, protect and maintain the airway without extending the neck.

❑ Any patient with respiratory distress should receive oxygen.

❑ Any patient whose illness or injury suggests the possibility of hypoxia should receive oxygen.

❑ If there is a question whether oxygen should be given, as in chronic obstructive pulmonary disease, administer it. *Oxygen should never be withheld from a patient suspected of suffering hypoxia.*

✳ In any respiratory emergency, the first priority is to open and maintain the airway.

✳ Do not deprive the COPD patient of oxygen.

Keep these precautions in mind as you read through the descriptions of pathophysiology, assessment, and management of respiratory disorders frequently encountered in the field.

Upper-Airway Obstruction

The most common cause of upper-airway obstruction is the relaxed tongue. In an unconscious patient in the supine position, the tongue can fall into the back of the throat and obstruct the upper airway. Additionally, the upper airway can become obstructed by such common materials as food, dentures, or other foreign bodies. A typical example of upper-airway obstruction is the "cafe coronary," which tends to occur in middle-aged or elderly patients who wear dentures. These people often are unable to sense how well they have chewed their food. Thus, they accidentally inhale a large piece of food, often meat, that obstructs their airway. Concurrent alcohol consumption is often implicated in the "cafe coronary." The upper airway can be obstructed in a variety of ways such as facial or neck trauma, upper-airway burns, and allergic reactions. It can also become blocked by swelling of the epiglottis or subglottic area because of epiglottitis or croup.

Assessment Assessment of the patient with an upper-airway obstruction varies, depending upon the cause of the obstruction and the history of the event. The unresponsive patient should be evaluated for snoring respirations, possibly indicating tongue or denture obstruction. If confronted by a patient suffering a "cafe coronary," determine whether the victim can speak. Speech indicates that, at present, the obstruction is incomplete. If the victim is unresponsive and has been eating, strongly suspect a food bolus lodged in the trachea. If a burn is present or suspected, assume laryngeal edema until proven otherwise.

Patients who may be having an allergic reaction to food will often report an itching sensation in the palate followed by a "lump" in the throat. The situation may progress to hoarseness, inspiratory stridor, and complete obstruction. Pay particular attention to the presence of urticaria (hives). Intercostal muscle retraction and use of the strap muscles of the neck for breathing suggest attempts to ventilate against a partially closed airway.

* An obstructed airway requires immediate intervention.

Management Management of the obstructed airway is based on the nature of the obstruction. Blockage by the tongue can be corrected by opening the airway, using either the head-tilt/chin-lift, jaw-thrust, or modified jaw-thrust maneuver. The airway can be maintained by employing either a nasopharyngeal or oropharyngeal airway. If possible, remove obstructing foreign bodies using the following basic airway maneuvers.

Conscious Adult Patient. In an adult patient who is conscious, take the following steps.

1. Determine if there is a complete obstruction or poor air exchange. Ask the patient: "Are you choking?" "Can you speak?" If the patient can speak, he or she should be asked to produce a forceful cough to expel the foreign body.
2. If the patient has complete obstruction or poor air exchange, provide up to five abdominal thrusts in rapid succession. If the thrusts prove unsuccessful, repeat until the obstruction is relieved or the patient becomes unconscious. In children or very obese or pregnant patients, use chest thrusts in lieu of abdominal thrusts.

Unconscious Adult Patient. If the patient is unconscious or loses consciousness, take the following steps.

1. Use the jaw-thrust, chin lift, or modified jaw-thrust maneuver in an attempt to open the airway.
2. Pinch the patient's nostrils and attempt to give two ventilations. If the attempts to ventilate fail, the head should be repositioned and the attempt repeated. If this fails . . .
3. Straddle the patient and administer up to five abdominal thrusts in quick succession. If this fails . . .

4. Try the tongue-jaw lift and, if the foreign body is seen, attempt finger sweeps. If successful, ventilation should be resumed. If unsuccessful . . .

5. Continue the abdominal thrusts and finger sweeps, while preparing the laryngoscope and the Magill forceps. The airway should be visualized with the laryngoscope. If the foreign body can be seen, it should be grasped with the Magill forceps and removed. Once removed, ventilations should begin as well as the supplemental administration of oxygen.

In cases of airway obstruction caused by laryngeal edema, establish the airway by the head-tilt, jaw-thrust, or triple airway maneuver. Supplemental oxygen should then be administered. Next, start an IV with a crystalloid solution and administer epinephrine. The patient should then receive diphenhydramine (Benadryl). Transtracheal ventilation may be required if the patient does not respond to the treatments described.

Obstructive Lung Disease

Obstructive lung disease is widespread in our society. The most common obstructive lung diseases encountered in prehospital care are emphysema, chronic bronchitis, and asthma. This section will discuss each of these disease processes, detailing the pathophysiology, assessment, and treatment.

Emphysema   *Emphysema* results from destruction of the alveolar walls distal to the terminal bronchioles. It is more common in men than women. The major factor contributing to emphysema in our society is cigarette smoking. Continued exposure to noxious substances, such as cigarette smoke, results in the gradual destruction of the walls of the alveoli. This process decreases the alveolar membrane surface area, thus lessening the area available for gas exchange. The loss of membrane results in an increased ratio of air to lung tissue in the lung. Additionally, the number of pulmonary capillaries in the lung is decreased, thus increasing resistance to pulmonary blood flow. This condition ultimately causes pulmonary hypertension, which in turn may lead to right heart failure, **cor pulmonale**, and death. (See Figure 20-14.)

■ **cor pulmonale** hypertrophy of the right ventricle resulting from disorders of the lung.

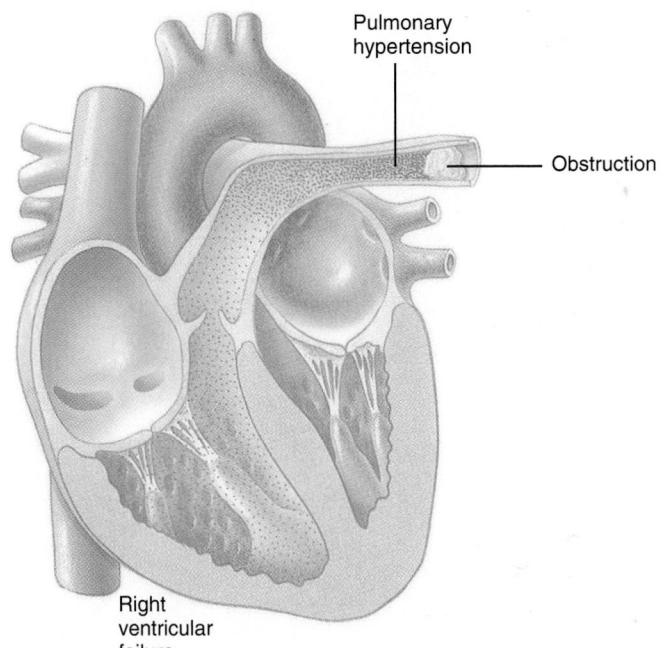

Pulmonary hypertension

Obstruction

Right ventricular failure

FIGURE 20-14 Chronic obstructive pulmonary disease of long standing can cause pulmonary hypertension, which in turn may lead to cor pulmonale.

Emphysema also causes weakening of the walls of the small bronchioles. When the walls of the alveoli and small bronchioles are destroyed, the lungs lose their capacity to recoil and air becomes trapped in the lungs. Thus, residual volume increases, while vital capacity remains relatively normal. As the disease progresses, the PaO_2 further decreases, which may lead to increased red blood cell production and polycythemia (an abnormally high hematocrit). The $PaCO_2$ also increases and becomes chronically elevated, forcing the body to depend upon hypoxic drive to control respirations.

Patients with emphysema are more susceptible to acute respiratory infections, such as pneumonia, and to cardiac dysrhythmias. Chronic emphysema patients ultimately become dependent on bronchodilators, corticosteroids, and, in the final stages, supplemental oxygen.

Assessment. The patient with emphysema may report a history of recent weight loss, increased dyspnea on exertion, and progressive limitation of physical activity. (See Figure 20-15.) Unlike chronic bronchitis, discussed in subsequent sections, emphysema is rarely associated with a cough, except in the morning. The patient should be questioned about cigarette and tobacco usage. This is generally reported in pack/years. The patient should be asked the number of cigarette packs (20 cigarettes/pack) smoked per day and the number of years he or she has smoked. The number of packs smoked per day should be multiplied by the number of years smoked. For example, a man who has smoked 2 packs per day for 15 years would have a 30 pack/year smoking history. Medical problems related to smoking, such as emphysema, chronic bronchitis, and lung cancer, usually begin after a patient surpasses a 20 pack/year history, although this can vary significantly.

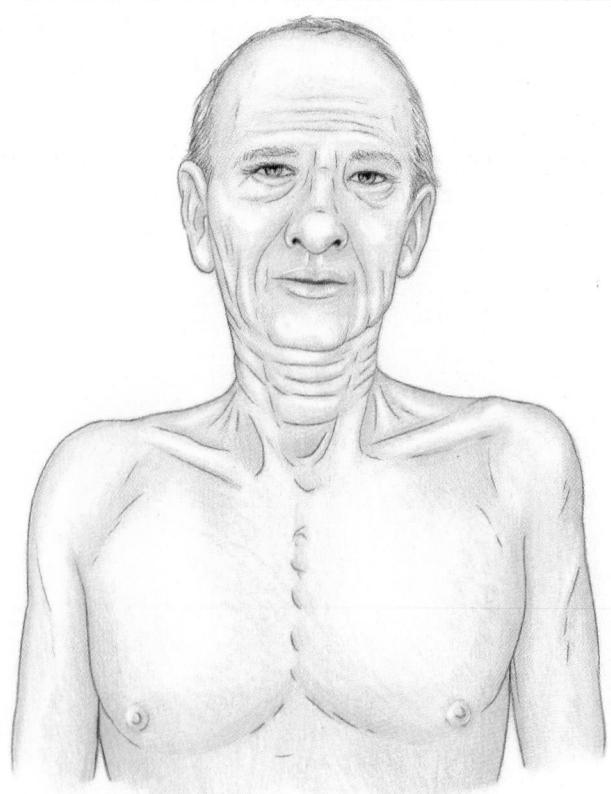

FIGURE 20-15 Typical appearance of patient with emphysema. There are well-developed accessory muscles and suprasternal retraction.

Physical exam of the emphysema patient usually reveals a barrel chest evidenced by an increase in the anterior/posterior chest diameter. You may also note decreased chest excursion with a prolonged expiratory phase and a rapid resting respiratory rate. Patients with emphysema are often thin since they must use a significant amount of their caloric intake for respiration. They tend to be pink in color due to **polycythemia** and are referred to as "pink puffers." Emphysema patients often have hypertrophy of the accessory respiratory muscles. The patient will often involuntarily purse his or her lips to create increased airway pressure. Clubbing of the fingers is common. Breath sounds are usually diminished. Wheezes and rhonchi may or may not be present. The patient may exhibit signs of right heart failure as evidenced by jugular venous distention, peripheral edema, and hepatic congestion.

■ **polycythemia** an excess of red blood cells.

Management. Although emphysema differs in the disease process from chronic bronchitis, the two respiratory disorders share several of the symptoms and the pathophysiology. As a result, you will treat the two disorders in a similar manner. The discussion of management of emphysema will be taken up with chronic bronchitis. (See next section.)

Chronic Bronchitis Chronic bronchitis results from an increase in the number of the mucous-secreting cells in the respiratory tree. It is characterized by the production of a large quantity of sputum. This often occurs after prolonged exposure to cigarette smoke. Unlike emphysema, the alveoli are not severely affected and diffusion remains normal. Gas exchange is decreased because there is lowered alveolar ventilation, which ultimately results in hypoxia and hypercarbia. (See Figure 20-16.) Hypoxia may increase red blood cell production, which in turn leads to polycythemia (as occurs in emphysema). Increased $PaCO_2$ levels may lead to irritability, decreased intellectual abilities, headaches, and personality changes. Physiologically, an increased $PaCO_2$ causes pulmonary vasoconstriction, resulting in pulmonary hypertension and, eventually, cor pulmonale. Unlike emphysema, the vital capacity is decreased, while the residual volume is normal or decreased.

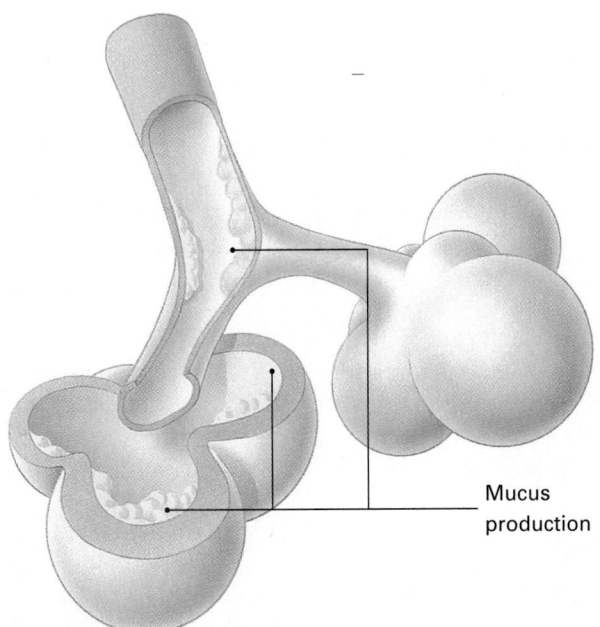

Mucus production

FIGURE 20-16 Chronic mucous production and plugging of the airways occur in chronic bronchitis.

Assessment. The patient with chronic bronchitis often will have a history of heavy cigarette smoking. There may also be a history of frequent respiratory infections. In addition, these patients usually produce considerable quantities of sputum daily.

Patients with chronic bronchitis tend to be overweight and can be cyanotic. Because of this, they are often referred to as "blue bloaters." This can be contrasted with the "pink puffer" image of emphysema patients described above. Auscultation of the thorax often will reveal rhonchi due to occlusion of the larger airways with mucous plugs. The patient may also exhibit signs and symptoms of right heart failure such as jugular venous distention, ankle edema, and hepatic congestion.

Management. The primary goal in the emergency management of the patient with either emphysema or chronic bronchitis is to relieve hypoxia and reverse any bronchoconstriction that may be present. However, many of these patients are dependent upon hypoxic respiratory drive. As a result, the supplemental administration of oxygen may decrease respiratory drive and inhibit ventilation. You must continually monitor the patient and be prepared to assist ventilations if signs of respiratory depression develop.

The first step in treating a patient suffering an exacerbation of emphysema or chronic bronchitis is to establish an airway. Then the patient may be placed in a seated or semi-seated position to assist the accessory respiratory muscles. Administer supplemental oxygen at low flow rate, generally less than 2 liters per minute. Alternately, you may use a venturi mask at a low concentration (24–35 percent). A nasal cannula can often be used, but you must constantly monitor the respiratory rate and depth. If hypoxia or respiratory failure is evident, then the concentration of delivered oxygen should be increased. An intravenous line should be established with lactated Ringers or normal saline at a "to keep open" (TKO) rate. Then, if ordered by the medical control physician, administer a bronchodilator medication such as albuterol or metaproterenol through a small volume nebulizer or particle inhaler (Rotohaler).

Asthma

✱ Asthma is a chronic inflammatory disease.

Asthma is a common respiratory illness that affects many persons. During a time when deaths from other respiratory diseases are steadily declining, deaths from asthma have significantly increased during the last decade. Most of the increased asthma deaths have occurred in patients who are 45 years of age or older. In addition, the death rate for black asthmatics has been twice as high as their white counterparts. Approximately 50 percent of patients who die from asthma do so before reaching the hospital. Thus, EMS personnel are frequently called upon to treat patients suffering an asthma attack. Prompt recognition, followed by appropriate treatment, can significantly improve the patient's condition and enhance their chances of survival.

Pathophysiology   Asthma is a chronic inflammatory disorder of the airways. In susceptible individuals, this inflammation causes symptoms usually associated with widespread but variable airflow obstruction. In addition to airflow obstruction, the airway becomes hyperresponsive. The airflow obstruction and hyperresponsiveness are often reversible with treatment. The conditions may also reverse spontaneously.

Asthma may be induced by one of many different factors. These items, commonly referred to as "triggers" or "inducers," vary from one individual to the next. In allergic individuals, environmental allergens are a major cause of inflammation. These may occur both indoors and outdoors. In addition to allergens, asthma may be triggered by cold air, exercise, foods, irritants, and certain medications. Often, a specific trigger cannot be identified.

Within minutes of exposure to the offending trigger, a two-phase reaction occurs. The first phase of the reaction is characterized by the release of chemical mediators such as *histamine*. These mediators cause contraction of the bronchial smooth muscle and leakage of fluid from peribronchial capillaries. This results in both bronchoconstriction and bronchial edema. These two factors can significantly decrease expiratory airflow causing the typical "asthma attack." Often, the asthma attack will resolve spontaneously in 1–2 hours or may be aborted by the use of inhaled bronchodilator medications such as albuterol. However, within 6–8 hours after exposure to the trigger, a second reaction occurs. This late phase is characterized by inflammation of the bronchioles as cells of the immune system (eosinophils, neutrophils, and lymphocytes) invade the mucosa of the respiratory tract. This leads to additional edema and swelling of the bronchioles and a further decrease in expiratory airflow.

The second phase reaction will not typically respond to inhaled beta-agonist drugs such as epinephrine or albuterol. Instead, anti-inflammatory agents such as corticosteroids are often required. It is important to point out that the severe inflammatory changes seen in an acute asthma attack do not develop over a few hours or even a few days. The inflammation will often begin several days or several weeks before the onset of the actual asthma attack.

Assessment   The most common presenting symptoms of asthma are dyspnea and wheezing. Wheezing results from turbulent airflow through the inflamed and narrowed bronchioles. Many asthmatics will present with a persistent cough. This is primarily due to hyperresponsiveness of the airway. It is important to point out that many asthmatics do not wheeze. Their initial presentation may be a frequent and persistent cough. As asthma severity increases, the patient may exhibit hyperinflation of the chest due to trapping of air in the alveoli. In addition, **tachypnea** will occur. The patient may start to use accessory muscles to aid respiration.

✳ Not all wheezing is asthma.

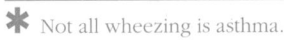
■ **tachypnea** rapid respiration.

Symptoms of a severe asthma attack include speech dyspnea (the inability to complete a phrase or sentence without having to stop to breathe), pulsus paradoxus (a drop of systolic blood pressure of 10 mmHg or more with inspiration), tachycardia, and decreased oxygen saturation on pulse oximetry. As hypoxia develops the patient may become agitated and anxious.

Primary Survey.   Begin the initial prehospital assessment of the asthmatic by completing the primary survey. After you have ruled out immediate threats to the airway, breathing, or circulation, turn your attention to the secondary assessment.

Secondary Survey.   During the secondary survey, try to obtain a brief patient history. Most asthmatics will report that they suffer from asthma. In addition, the patient's home medications may assist in confirming a history of asthma. Common asthma medications include inhaled beta-agonists (albuterol, metaproterenol), inhaled corticosteroids (betamethasone, beclomethasone), inhaled cromolyn sodium, and inhaled anticholinergics (ipratropium bromide). Often the patient will be taking oral bronchodilators such as theophylline or may be taking oral corticosteroids (prednisone). Determine when symptoms started and what the patient has taken in an attempt to abort the attack. Also, find out whether the patient is allergic to any medications. Question the patient about hospitalizations for asthma. If the patient has been hospitalized, ask whether the patient has ever required intubation and mechanical ventilation. A prior history of a patient requiring mechanical ventilation places the patient into a high-risk category until proven otherwise.

After you obtain the pertinent history, perform a brief physical examination. Place particular emphasis on the chest and neck. Examination of the chest should begin with inspection. Note any increase in the diameter of the chest that may indicate air trapping. Also, note the use of accessory muscles, including retraction of the intercostal muscles or use of the strap muscles of the neck. Following inspection, palpate the chest, noting any deformity, crepitus, or asymmetry. Next, auscultate the posterior chest. Note any abnormal breath sounds such as wheezing or rhonchi. Listen to the symmetry of breath sounds. Unilateral wheezing may indicate an aspirated foreign body or a pneumothorax.

Accurate vital signs should be obtained. One of the most important vital signs is the respiratory rate. An increase in the respiratory rate is one of the earliest symptoms of a respiratory problem. Many EMS personnel inaccurately measure the respiratory rate. The easiest method is to simply place your fingers on the patient's radial artery as if you were measuring the pulse rate. This will make the patient think you are obtaining the pulse rate, and he or she will not alter their breathing pattern. The respiratory rate should be measured for at least 30 seconds. At the same time, note any alterations in the respiratory pattern. Pulse oximetry is an excellent adjunct to respiratory assessment. It will provide you with data regarding the oxygen saturation status (SpO_2) as well as an audible measure of the pulse rate.

Most EMS systems should be able to measure the Peak Expiratory Flow Rate (PEFR). (See Figures 20-17 and Table 20-1.) The PEFR measures the airflow rate during a maximum exhalation and is a reliable indicator of airflow. The PEFR, measured in liters per minute, can be used to measure asthma severity and to monitor the patient's response to therapy. The more severe the asthma attack, the lower will be the PEFR.

The PEFR is obtained using a Wright Meter, which is fairly inexpensive and easy to use. A disposable mouth piece is placed into the meter. The patient is instructed to make a maximum inhalation and then make a maximal exhalation into the meter. This should be repeated twice, with the highest reading recorded as the patient's PEFR.

Management   Treatment of asthma is designed to correct hypoxia, reverse any bronchospasm, and treat the inflammatory changes associated with the disease. Oxygen should be administered at a high concentration (100 percent). Intravenous access should be established and the patient placed on an

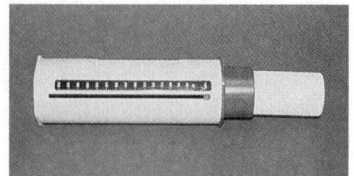

FIGURE 20-17 Wright Meter for determining Peak Expiratory Flow Rate (PEFR).

✳ In addition to oxygen, ß agonists are the mainstay of emergent asthma therapy.

TABLE 20-1 Spirometry and Peak Flow Values for Adults			
SEVERITY	FEV1 (Liters)	FEV1/FVC (%)	PEAK FLOW (Liters/Min.)
Normal	4.0–6.0	80–90	550–650 (Males) 400–500 (Females)
Mild	3.0	70	300–400
Moderate	1.6	50	200–300
Severe	0.6	40	100

ECG monitor. Initial treatment should be directed at reversing any bronchospasm present. The most commonly used drugs are the inhaled beta-agonist preparations such as albuterol (Ventolin, Proventil). (See Tables 20-2 through 20-6.) These can be easily administered with a small volume, oxygen-powered nebulizer. (See Procedure 20-1.) The patient's response to these medications should be monitored by improvement in PEFR, pulse oximetry readings, or both.

In addition to inhaled beta-agonists, early administration of corticosteroids should be considered. (See Table 20-7.) While the inhaled beta-agonists will help with bronchoconstriction, they will do little for the underlying inflammation, which is the principal problem. If you anticipate a long transport time, medical control may request the administration of methylprednisolone or a similar corticosteroid. It is important to point out that the beneficial effects of corticosteroid administration will probably not be detected until 6–8 hours following administration.

If symptoms are severe and do not improve with administration of the inhaled beta-agonists, the intravenous administration of aminophylline may be indicated. If the patient is not currently taking a theophylline preparation, administer a loading dose of 5–6 mg/kg of aminophylline over 20–30 minutes. (See Table 20-8.) This should be followed by a maintenance infusion of 0.8–1.0 mg/kg/hr. Remember that both the inhaled beta agonists and aminophylline may increase heart rates and/or cause tremors, nausea, and vomiting.

TABLE 20-2 Epinephrine 1:1,000	
Class:	Sympathomimetic
Actions:	Bronchodilation
Indications:	Bronchial asthma
	Exacerbation of chronic obstructive pulmonary disease (COPD)
	Allergic reactions
Contraindications:	Patients with underlying cardiovascular disease
	Hypertension
	Pregnancy
	Patients with tachyarrhythmias
Precautions:	Should be protected from light
	Blood pressure, pulse, and EKG must be constantly monitored.
Side effects:	Palpitations, tachycardia
	Anxiousness
	Headache
	Tremor
Dosage:	0.3–0.5 mg
Route:	Subcutaneously
Pediatric Dosage:	0.01 mg/kg up to 0.3 mg

TABLE 20-3 Albuterol (Proventil) (Ventolin)

Class:	Sympathomimetic (β_2 selective)
Action:	Bronchodilation
Indications:	Asthma Reversible bronchospasm associated with COPD
Contraindications:	Known hypersensitivity to the drug Symptomatic tachycardia
Precautions:	Blood pressure, pulse, and ECG should be monitored. Use caution in patients with known heart disease.
Side Effects:	Palpitations, anxiety, headache, dizziness, and sweating
Dosage:	*Metered Dose Inhaler* 1–2 sprays (90 µg per spray) *Small Volume Nebulizer* 0.5 ml (2.5 mg) in 2.5 ml normal saline over 5–15 minutes *Rotohaler* One 200 µg Rotocap® should be placed in the inhaler and breathed by the patient.
Route:	Inhalation
Pediatric Dosage	0.15 mg (0.03 ml)/kg in 2.5 ml normal saline

TABLE 20-4 Isoetharine (Bronkosol)

Class:	Sympathomimetic (β_2 selective)
Actions:	Bronchodilation Increases heart rate
Indications:	Asthma Reversible bronchospasm associated with chronic bronchitis and emphysema
Contraindications:	Patients with history of hypersensitivity to the drug
Precautions:	Blood pressure, pulse, and EKG must be constantly monitored
Side Effects:	Palpitations, tachycardia Anxiety, tremors Headache
Dosage:	*Hand nebulizer* 4 inhalations *Small Volume Nebulizer* 0.5 ml (1:3 with saline)

TABLE 20-5 Metaproterenol (Alupent)

Class:	Sympathomimetic (β_2 selective)
Actions:	Bronchodilation Increases heart rate
Indications:	Bronchial asthma Reversible bronchospasm associated with chronic bronchitis and emphysema
Contraindications:	Patients with cardiac dysrhythmias or significant tachycardia
Precautions:	Blood pressure, pulse, and EKG must be constantly monitored. Occasional nausea and vomiting reported
Side Effects:	Palpitations, anxiety, headache, nausea, vomiting, dizziness, and tremor
Dosage	*Metered Dose Inhaler* 2–3 inhalations; can be repeated in 3–4 hours if required *Small Volume Nebulizer* 0.2–0.3 ml diluted in 2–3 ml normal saline administered over 5–15 minutes
Route:	Inhalation only
Pediatric Dosage:	0.05–0.3 ml in 4 ml normal saline

TABLE 20-6 Terbutaline (Brethine)

Class:	Sympathomimetic
Action:	Bronchodilator Increases heart rate
Indications:	Bronchial asthma Reversible bronchospasm associated with COPD
Contraindications:	Patients with known hypersensitivity to the drug
Precautions:	Blood pressure, pulse, and ECG must be constantly monitored
Side Effects:	Palpitations, tachycardia, PVCs Anxiety, tremor, headache
Dosage:	*Metered Dose Inhaler* 2 puffs, 1 minute apart *Subcutaneous Injection* 0.25 mg; may be repeated in 15–30 minutes
Route:	Inhalation Subcutaneous injection
Pediatric Dosage:	0.01 mg/kg subcutaneously

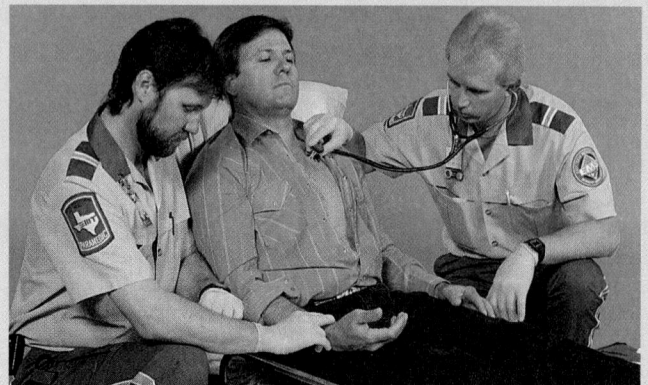

20-1A. Complete the primary assessment.

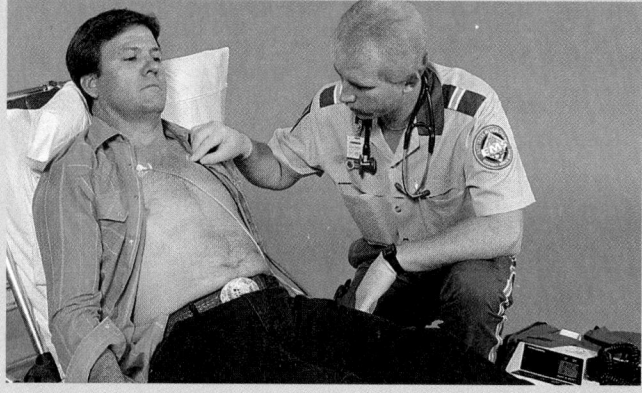

20-1B. Auscultate the chest.

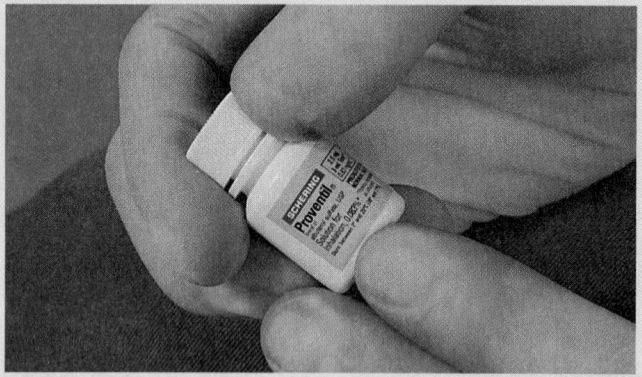

20-1C. Select the desired medication.

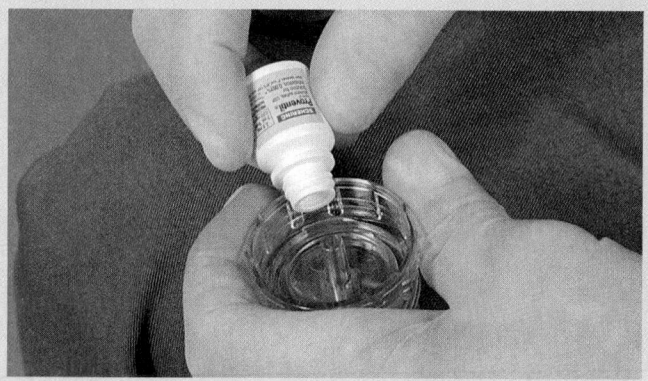

20-1D. Add medication to the nebulizer.

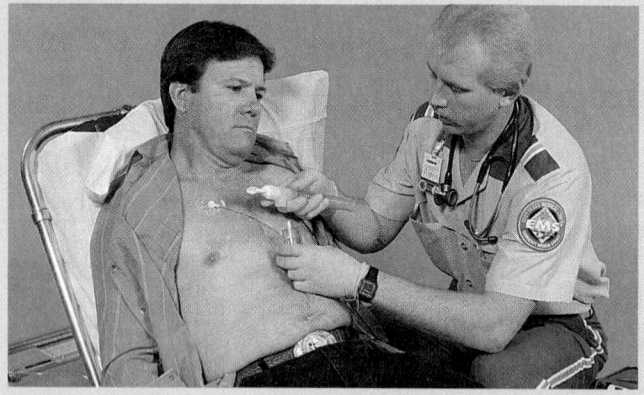

20-1E. Determine pre-treatment pulse rate.

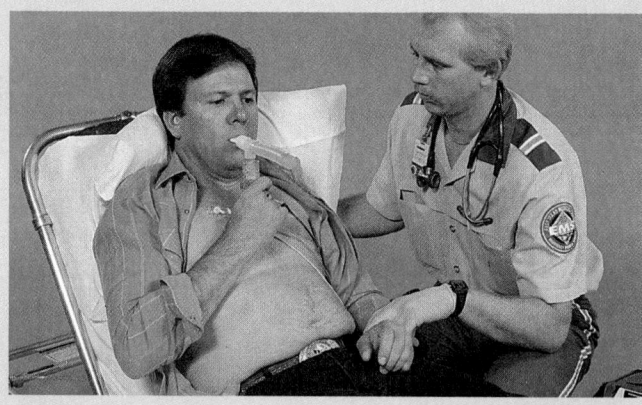

20-1F. Administer the medication.

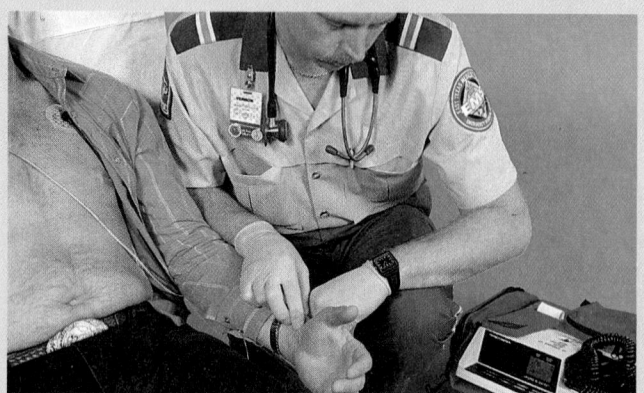

20-1G. Determine post-treatment pulse rate.

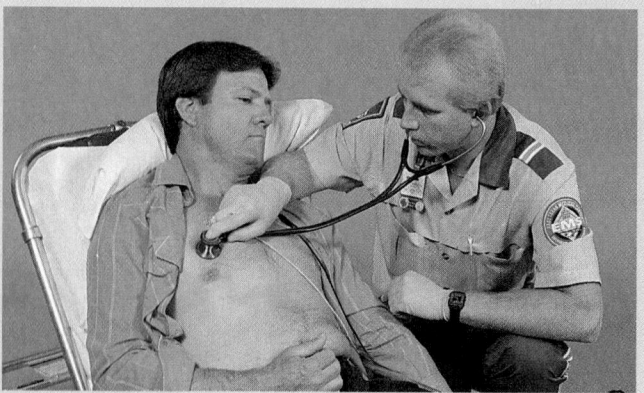

20-1H. Reassess breath sounds.

TABLE 20-7　Methylprednisolone (Solu-Medrol)

Class:	Steroid
Actions:	Anti-inflammatory Suppresses immune response (especially in allergic reactions)
Indications:	Severe anaphylaxis Possibly effective as an adjunctive agent in the management of spinal cord injury
Contraindications:	None in the emergency setting
Precautions:	Must be reconstituted and used promptly Onset of action may be 2–6 hours and thus should not be expected to be of use in the critical first hour following an anaphylactic reaction.
Side Effects:	GI bleeding Prolonged wound healing Suppression of natural steroids
Dosage	125–250 mg
Routes:	IV IM
Pediatric Dosage:	30 µg/kg

Many patients will wait before summoning EMS. The longer the time interval from the onset of the asthma attack until treatment, the less likely it will be that bronchodilator medications will work. Often, after a prolonged asthma attack, the patient may become fatigued. A fatigued patient can quickly develop respiratory failure and subsequently require intubation and mechanical ventilation. Always be prepared to provide airway and respiratory support for the asthmatic.

Special Cases　While most cases of asthma conform to the preceding descriptions, you may run into several special cases in the field. Asthma conditions that require special concern include status asthmaticus and asthmatic attacks in children.

Status Asthmaticus. *Status asthmaticus* is defined as a severe, prolonged asthma attack that cannot be broken by repeated doses of epinephrine. It is a serious medical emergency that requires prompt recognition, treatment, and transport. The patient suffering status asthmaticus frequently will have a greatly distended chest from continued air trapping. Breath sounds, and often wheezing, may be absent. The patient is usually exhausted, severely acidotic, and dehydrated. The management of status asthmaticus is basically the same as for asthma. You should recognize that respiratory arrest is imminent and be prepared for endotracheal intubation. Transport should be immediate, with aggressive treatment continued en route.

TABLE 20-8 Aminophylline

Class:	Xanthine bronchodilator
Actions:	Smooth muscle relaxant Causes bronchodilation Mild diuretic properties Increases heart rate
Indications:	Bronchial asthma Reversible bronchospasm associated with chronic bronchitis and emphysema Congestive heart failure
Contraindications:	Patients with history of hypersensitivity to the drug Hypotension
Precautions:	Monitor for arrhythmias Monitor blood pressure Do not administer to patients on chronic theophylline preparations until the theophylline blood level has been determined.
Side Effects:	Convulsions, tremor, anxiety, dizziness Vomiting Palpitations, PVCs, tachycardia
Dosages:	*Method 1* 250–500 mg in 90 or 80 ml of D5W respectively infused over 20–30 minutes (approximately 5–10 mg/kg/hr) *Method 2* 250–500 mg (5–7 mg/kg) in 20 ml of D5W infused over 20–30 minutes
Route:	Slow IV Infusion
Pediatric Dosage:	5–6 mg/kg loading dose to be infused over 20–30 minutes; maximum dose not to exceed 12 mg/kg per 24 hours.

Asthma in Children. Asthma in children is common. The pathophysiology and treatment are essentially the same as in adults, with altered medication dosages. Several additional medications are used in the treatment of childhood asthma. Asthma in children is discussed in greater detail in Chapter 30.

Pneumonia

Pneumonia is an infection of the lungs and a common medical problem, especially in the aged and those infected with the Human Immunodeficiency Virus (HIV). In fact, pneumonia is one of the leading causes of deaths in both groups of patients.

Pathophysiology   Pneumonia is a common respiratory disease caused when an infectious agent invades the lung. Bacterial and viral pneumonias are the most frequent, although fungal and other forms of pneumonia do exist. The infection begins in a part of the lung and often spreads to nearby alveoli. It may ultimately involve the entire lung.

Assessment   The patient with pneumonia will generally appear ill. He or she may report a recent history of fever and chills. These chills are commonly described as "bed shaking." There is usually a generalized weakness and **malaise**. The patient will tend to complain of a deep, productive cough and may be able to expel yellow sputum, often streaked with blood. Many cases involve associated chest pain. Therefore, pneumonia should be considered in any patient who presents complaining of chest pain, especially if accompanied by fever and/or chills. In pneumonias involving the lower lobes, patients may complain of nothing more than upper-abdominal pain.

■ **malaise** discomfort or uneasiness often associated with disease.

Physical examination will commonly reveal fever, tachycardia, and a cough. Respiratory distress may be present. Auscultation of the chest may reveal wheezes, rhonchi, or rales. There usually is decreased air movement in consolidated (filled with infection) areas. Percussion of the chest may reveal dullness over the consolidated areas.

Management   Pneumonia is generally diagnosed on the basis of physical examination, X-ray, and laboratory cultures. Therefore, diagnosis in the field is unlikely. The primary treatment is antibiotics to which the causative organism is susceptible. In the field, however, antibiotics are not indicated and treatment is purely supportive. Place the patient in a comfortable position, and administer supplemental oxygen. The medical control physician may sometimes order a breathing treatment with a beta agonist. Because some bronchospasm is often associated with pneumonia, these drugs will afford the patient some symptomatic relief.

Toxic Inhalation

Inhalation of toxic substances into the respiratory tract can cause pain, inflammation, or destruction of pulmonary tissues. Significant inhalations can affect the alveoli's ability to exchange oxygen, thus resulting in hypoxemia.

Pathophysiology   The possibility of inhalation of products toxic to the respiratory system should be considered in any dyspneic patient. Causes of toxic inhalation include superheated air, toxic products of combustion, chemical irritants, and inhalation of steam. Each of these agents can result in upper airway obstruction due to edema and laryngospasm. In such cases, bronchospasm and lower-airway edema may additionally appear. In severe inhalations, disruption of the alveolar/capillary membranes may result in life-threatening pulmonary edema.

Assessment   When assessing the patient with possible toxic inhalation exposure, determine the nature of the inhalant or the combusted material. Several products can result in the formation of corrosive acids or alkalis that irritate and damage the airway. These include:

- ❑ Ammonia (ammonium hydroxide)
- ❑ Nitrogen oxide (nitric acid)
- ❑ Sulfur dioxide (sulphurous acid)
- ❑ Sulfur trioxide (sulfuric acid)

It is also crucial to determine the duration of the exposure, whether the patient was in an enclosed area at the time of the exposure, or if he or she experienced a loss of consciousness. Loss of consciousness may mean that the airway became vulnerable due to loss of the airway protective mechanisms.

During physical examination, pay particular attention to the face, mouth, and throat. Note any burns or particulate matter. Next, auscultate the chest for the presence of any wheezes or rales. Wheezing may indicate bronchospasm, while rales may suggest pulmonary edema.

Management   After the safety of rescue personnel has been assured, remove the patient from the hazardous environment. Next, establish and maintain an airway. Remember that the airway is often irritable and attempts at endotracheal intubation may result in laryngospasm, completely obstructing the airway. Laryngeal edema, as evidenced by hoarseness, brassy cough, and stridor, is ominous and may require prompt endotracheal intubation. Humidified oxygen at high concentration should be administered. As a precaution, start an IV of a crystalloid solution to provide rapid venous access. Transport should be prompt.

✳ The paramedic's first concern in any toxic inhalation situation is personal safety.

Carbon Monoxide Inhalation

Carbon monoxide exposure is potentially life-threatening because of its affect on hemoglobin. Carbon monoxide can be encountered in industrial sites, such as mines and factories. In addition, it is a particular hazard for fire-fighters and rescue personnel.

Pathophysiology   Carbon monoxide is an odorless, tasteless, colorless gas produced from the incomplete burning of fossil fuels. It is present in the environment in various concentrations primarily because of automotive exhaust emissions. Most poisonings occur from automobiles and home-heating devices used in poorly ventilated areas. Carbon monoxide is often used in suicide attempts.

Carbon monoxide easily binds to the hemoglobin molecule. It has an affinity for hemoglobin 200 times that of oxygen. Once bound, receptor sites on the hemoglobin can no longer transport oxygen to the peripheral tissues. The result is hypoxia at the cellular level and, ultimately, metabolic acidosis.

Assessment   When confronted by a patient suffering possible carbon-monoxide poisoning, determine the source of exposure, its length, and the location. Less time is required to develop a significant exposure in a closed space compared to one in an area that is fairly well ventilated.

Signs and symptoms of carbon-monoxide poisoning include headache, irritability, errors in judgment, vomiting, chest pain, confusion, agitation, loss of coordination, loss of consciousness, and even seizures. On physical examination, the skin may be cyanotic or it may be bright cherry red (a very late finding). There may be other signs of hypoxia such as peripheral cyanosis or confusion.

✳ The patient suffering carbon-monoxide poisoning should initially receive the highest possible concentration of oxygen.

Management   Upon detection of carbon-monoxide poisoning, remove the patient from the site of exposure. The airway should be assured and maintained. Administer supplemental oxygen at the highest possible concentration. If respiratory depression is noted, respirations should be assisted. If shock is present, it should be treated. Prompt transport is essential.

Hyperbaric oxygen therapy may be used in the treatment of severe carbon-monoxide poisoning. Many EMS systems have protocols established whereby patients suffering carbon-monoxide poisoning are transported to hospitals with hyperbaric oxygen therapy facilities. Hyperbaric oxygen increases the PaO_2, thus promoting increased oxygen uptake on parts of the hemoglobin molecule not yet bound by carbon monoxide.

Pulmonary Embolism

A pulmonary embolism is a blood clot (or some other particle) that lodges in a pulmonary artery, effectively blocking blood flow through that vessel. This condition is potentially life-threatening because it can significantly decrease pulmonary blood flow, thus leading to hypoxemia.

Pathophysiology   Sources of pulmonary emboli include air embolism, such as can occur during the placement of a central line; fat embolism, such as can occur following a fracture; amniotic fluid embolism; and blood clots. Factors predisposing a patient to blood clots include prolonged immobilization, thrombophlebitis, use of certain medications, and atrial fibrillation.

When a pulmonary embolism occurs, the blocked blood flow through the affected artery causes the right heart to pump against increased resistance. This results in an increase in pulmonary capillary pressure. The area of the lung supplied by the occluded pulmonary vessel can no longer effectively function in gas exchange, although it is still ventilated.

Assessment   Signs and symptoms of a patient suffering a pulmonary embolism will vary, depending upon the size and location of the obstruction. The patient suffering acute pulmonary embolism may report a sudden onset of severe unexplained dyspnea, which may or may not be associated with chest pain. There may be a recent history of immobilization such as hip fracture, surgery, or debilitating illness.

The physical examination may reveal labored breathing, tachypnea, and tachycardia. In massive pulmonary emboli, there may be signs of right heart failure such as jugular venous distention and, in some cases, falling blood pressure.

Management   The patient suffering suspected pulmonary embolism should have an airway established and maintained. Assist ventilations as required. Administer supplemental oxygen at the highest possible concentration. Establish an IV of lactated Ringer's or normal saline at a "to keep open" rate. Transport the patient as quickly as possible.

The diagnosis of pulmonary embolism is often difficult and requires a high index of suspicion. Treatment in the hospital setting may include the use of various medications in an attempt to dissolve the clot.

Hyperventilation Syndrome

Hyperventilation syndrome is characterized by rapid breathing, chest pains, numbness, and other symptoms usually associated with anxiety or a situational reaction. However, many serious medical problems can cause hyperventilation. To avoid improper treatment, consider hyperventilation indicative of a serious medical problem until proven otherwise.

Pathophysiology   Hyperventilation syndrome frequently occurs in anxious patients. The patient often senses that he or she cannot "catch his or her breath." The patient will then begin to breathe rapidly. Hyperventilation in a purely anxious patient results in the excess elimination of CO_2, causing a respiratory alkalosis.

Assessment   With a hyperventilating patient, you may elicit a history of fatigue, nervousness, dizziness, chest pain, and numbness and tingling around the mouth, hands, and feet. The physical examination will reveal an anxious patient with tachypnea and tachycardia. Spasm of the fingers and feet—the so-called carpopedal spasm—may also be present. If the patient has a history of seizure disorder, the hyperventilation episode may precipitate a seizure.

Management   The primary treatment for hyperventilation syndrome is reassurance. Mechanisms that will assist in increasing the PCO_2, such as breath holding or breathing into a paper bag, are discouraged in prehospital care. It is important to exclude other medical causes before determining that a patient is hyperventilating. Do not withhold oxygen.

The hyperventilating patient can often present a dilemma for prehospital personnel. Although anxiety is the most common cause of hyperventilation, other more serious diseases can present in exactly the same manner. For example, pulmonary embolism or acute myocardial infarction can exhibit symptoms similar to hyperventilation syndrome. Hyperventilating patients require oxygen. Allowing them to rebreathe into a paper bag can be deadly. Many EMS systems permit paramedics to use rebreathing techniques only on physician order.

Central Nervous System Dysfunction

Central nervous system dysfunction, with the exception of drug overdose and massive stroke, are a relatively rare cause of respiratory emergencies. However, always consider the possibility of central nervous system dysfunction in any dyspneic patient.

Pathophysiology   Central nervous system dysfunction can be a causative factor in respiratory depression and arrest. Causes include head trauma, stroke, brain tumors, and various drugs. Several medications, such as narcotics and barbiturates, make the respiratory centers in the brain less responsive to increases in $PaCO_2$. These agents also depress areas of the brain responsible for initiating respirations.

Management   If central nervous system dysfunction is suspected, establish and maintain an airway. If respiratory depression is noted or if respirations are absent, initiate mechanical ventilation. Administer supplemental oxygen, and establish an IV of 5 percent dextrose in water at a "to keep open" rate. Specific therapy should be directed at the underlying problem, if it is known.

Dysfunction of the Spinal Cord, Nerves, or Respiratory Muscles

Several disease processes can affect the spinal cord, nerves, and/or respiratory muscles. Dysfunction of these structures can lead to hypoventilation and progressive hypoxemia.

Pathophysiology   Several disease processes can interfere with respiratory function. These include spinal cord trauma, polio, and myasthenia gravis. Certain tumors can also impinge on the spinal cord, depressing respiratory function. These disorders result in an inability of the respiratory muscles to contract normally, thus causing hypoventilation. Tidal and minute volume are decreased.

Management   Management of spinal cord and respiratory muscle dysfunction is purely supportive. Establish an airway, and provide ventilatory support. If myasthenia gravis is present and if transport time is long, the physician may request the administration of one of several agents effective in treating such patients.

SUMMARY

Respiratory emergencies are commonly encountered in prehospital care. Recognition and treatment must be prompt. The primary treatment is to correct hypoxia. Necessary steps include establishing and maintaining the airway, assisting ventilations as required, and administering supplemental oxygen. Appropriate pharmacological agents may be subsequently ordered by the medical control physician.

FURTHER READING

Guyton, A. C. *Textbook of Medical Physiology. 8th ed.* Philadelphia, PA: W.B. Saunders Company, 1991.

National Heart, Lung, and Blood Institute. *International Consensus Report on Diagnosis and Management of Asthma.* U.S. Department of Health and Human Services, Bethesda, MD, 1992.

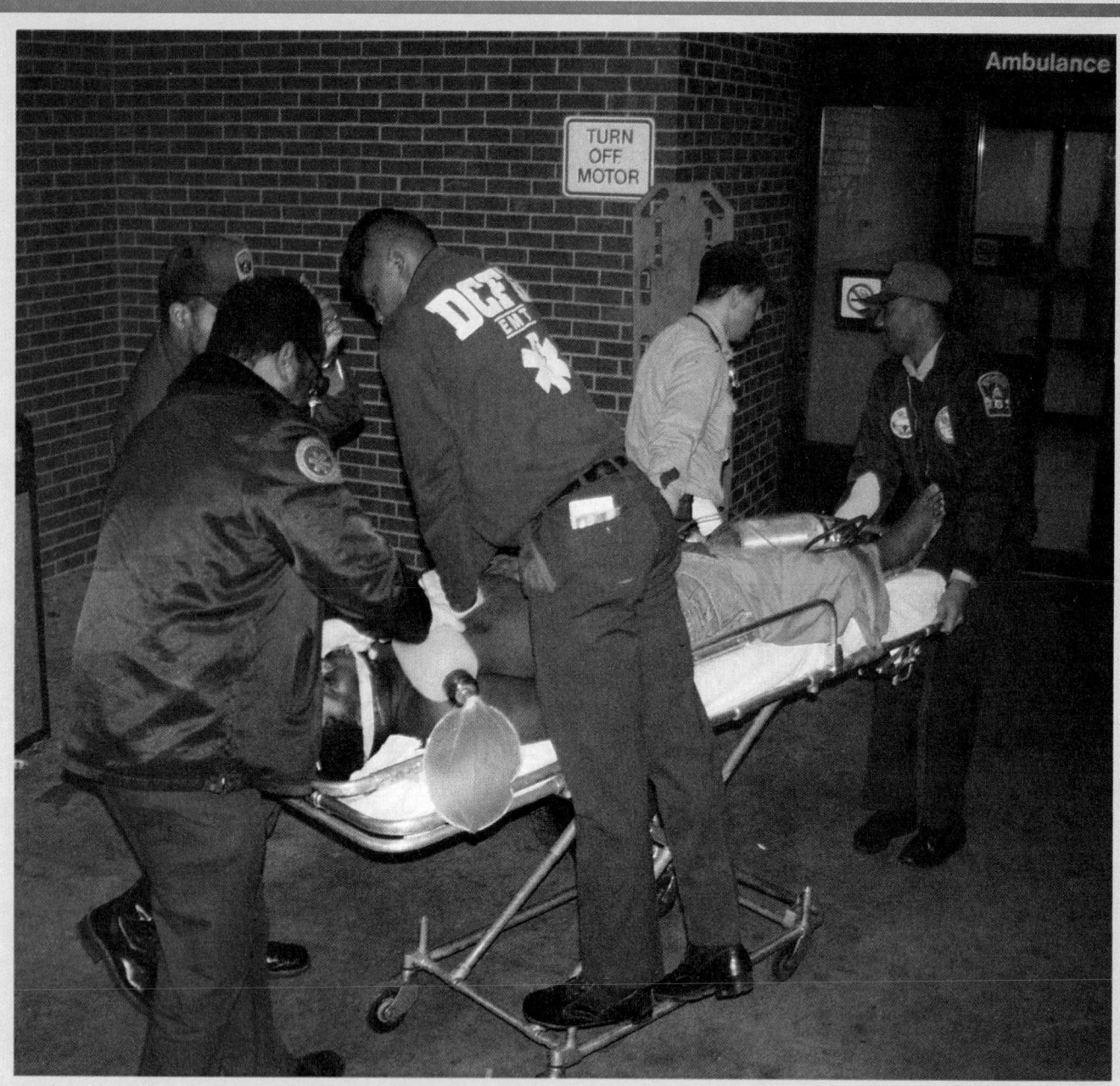

21

CARDIOVASCULAR EMERGENCIES

Objectives for Chapter 21

After reading this chapter, you should be able to:

1. Describe the size, shape, location, and orientation of the heart. (See p. 603.)
2. Describe the normal anatomy of the heart and peripheral circulatory system. (See pp. 603–609.)
3. Name and describe the location of the cardiac valves. (See pp. 604–606.)
4. Describe the anatomy of the coronary arteries and veins. (See pp. 606–607.)
5. Describe the differences between the structural and functional aspects of the arterial and venous systems. (See pp. 607–609.)
6. Describe the structure and function of capillaries. (See p. 608.)
7. Describe the course of blood flow through the heart and lungs. (See pp. 604–609.)
8. Describe the cardiac cycle. (See pp. 609–610.)
9. Define the following terms. (See below pages.)
   - stroke volume (p. 609)
   - afterload (p. 610)
   - preload (p. 609)
   - cardiac output (p. 610)
   - Starling's Law (p. 609)
10. Describe the innervation of the heart. (See pp. 610-612.)
11. Name major electrolytes that affect cardiac function. (See p. 612.)
12. Describe the electrical properties of the heart. (See pp. 612–616.)
13. Describe the normal sequence of electrical conduction through the heart. (See p. 615.)
14. Describe cardiac depolarization and repolarization. (See pp. 613–614.)
15. Name three areas of the heart with pacemaking capabilities, and list the intrinsic rates of each. (See p. 616.)
16. Describe the basic concepts of ECG monitoring. (See pp. 616–619)
17. Describe the grids and markings on ECG paper. (See p. 619)
18. Define the following terms or phrases. (See below pages.)
    - isoelectric line (p. 619)
    - U wave (p. 620)
    - P wave (p. 619)
    - P-R interval (p. 620)
    - QRS complex (p. 619)
    - QRS duration (p. 620)
    - T wave (p. 620)
    - ST segment (p. 620)
19. Define refractory period, and describe the difference between the relative refractory period and the absolute refractory period. (See p. 625.)
20. Explain which information can and cannot be obtained from the rhythm strip analysis. (See p. 618.)
21. Name twelve causes of dysrhythmias. (See pp. 627.)
22. Describe the etiology, ECG findings, clinical significance, and treatment for common dysrhythmias. (See pp. 6027–683.)
23. Name common chief complaints of cardiac patients. (See p. 683)
24. Describe appropriate history and physical assessment goals for cardiac patients. (See pp. 683–688.)
25. Describe the pathophysiology of atherosclerosis. (See pp. 688–689.)
26. List major risk factors for atherosclerosis. (See p. 689.)
27. Describe the pathophysiology, signs, symptoms, and management of the following patient problems. (See below pages.)
    - angina pectoris (pp. 689–690)
    - acute MI (pp. 690–694)
    - left ventricular failure (pp. 694–697)
    - pulmonary edema (pp. 694–697)
    - right ventricular failure (pp. 697–699)
    - cardiogenic shock (pp. 699–701)
    - cardiac arrest (pp. 701–704)
    - pulseless electrical activity (PEA) (pp. 703–704)
    - abdominal aortic aneurysm (pp. 705–706)
    - dissecting aortic aneurysm (pp. 706–707)
    - acute arterial occlusion (p. 707)
    - acute pulmonary embolus (p. 707)
    - deep venous thrombosis (p. 708)
    - varicose veins (p. 708)
    - peripheral arterial atherosclerotic disease (p. 708)
    - hypertensive emergency (p. 709)
28. Describe some common drugs used in cardiovascular emergencies. (See pp. 710–712.)
29. Describe the indications for and the use of the following techniques. (See below pages.)
    - ECG monitoring (pp. 712–715)
    - precordial thump (p. 715)
    - defibrillation (pp. 715–717)
    - cardioversion (p. 717)
    - carotid sinus massage (pp. 717–721)
    - transcutaneous cardiac pacing (p. 721)

As the crew of Paramedic Unit 428 sits down to dinner, a car speeds into the station's driveway. A frantic woman runs around the parked ambulance yelling, "Help, Help!" The paramedics rush to assist her. When the woman sees them coming, she cries: "My husband is sick!" She then points to the car.

Upon approaching the car, the paramedics find an elderly man in the front seat. He is unresponsive and pulseless. While one paramedic pulls the patient from the car and begins CPR, the other paramedic retrieves equipment from the ambulance. One of the EMTs calls the fire department for assistance.

When paramedics question the wife, they learn that the 65-year-old patient developed chest pain approximately 30 minutes ago. As the couple drove to the hospital, the man became nauseated. Approximately a block from the EMS station, he went into cardiac arrest.

Paramedics immediately apply "quick-look" paddles to the patient's chest. The ECG reveals ventricular fibrillation. The paramedic charges the defibrillator and delivers a 200 joule shock. The ECG remains unchanged. A second 300 joule shock is delivered. The ECG is still unchanged. A third shock is delivered at 360 joules, with the same result.

The engine company arrives within 2 minutes. With the crew's help, CPR is continued, an IV started, an endotracheal tube placed, and the patient ventilated with 100 percent oxygen. One of the paramedics administers 1 mg of epinephrine intravenously. Another delivers a fourth shock at 360 joules. This converts the patient to an idioventricular rhythm, which subsequently improves to a sinus tachycardia with a pulse. The patient's blood pressure is 110 by palpation. The ECG shows a few PVCs developing. The paramedics now administer 100 mg of lidocaine and begin a lidocaine drip at 2 milligrams per minute.

Paramedics rapidly transport the patient to the hospital. He never regains spontaneous respirations in the ambulance. However, at the hospital the patient is placed on a ventilator in the CCU. Cardiac enzyme studies and a 12-lead ECG confirm the presence of an anterior wall myocardial infarction. The patient slowly improves and is weaned from the ventilator. He subsequently undergoes cardiac rehabilitation. The attending physician discharges him on three different medications.

INTRODUCTION

Cardiovascular disease is a major cause of death and disability in the United States. It has been shown that many patients suffering cardiovascular emergencies, especially heart attacks, die within the first hour after the onset of symptoms. Yet prompt, definitive intervention, especially early defibrillation, has proven effective in preventing many of these deaths. It was such facts that led to the development of emergency medical service, as we know it today.

This chapter will thoroughly discuss advanced prehospital care of cardiovascular emergencies. First, we will review the pertinent anatomy and physiology. Then we will examine ECG monitoring, patient assessment, and recognition and treatment of cardiovascular disorders.

■ **cardiovascular disease** disease affecting the heart, peripheral blood vessels, or both.

✱ Cardiovascular disease is the number one cause of death in the United States.

ANATOMY AND PHYSIOLOGY

The *cardiovascular system* includes two components—the heart and the peripheral blood vessels. Prehospital personnel must thoroughly understand the anatomy and physiology of each.

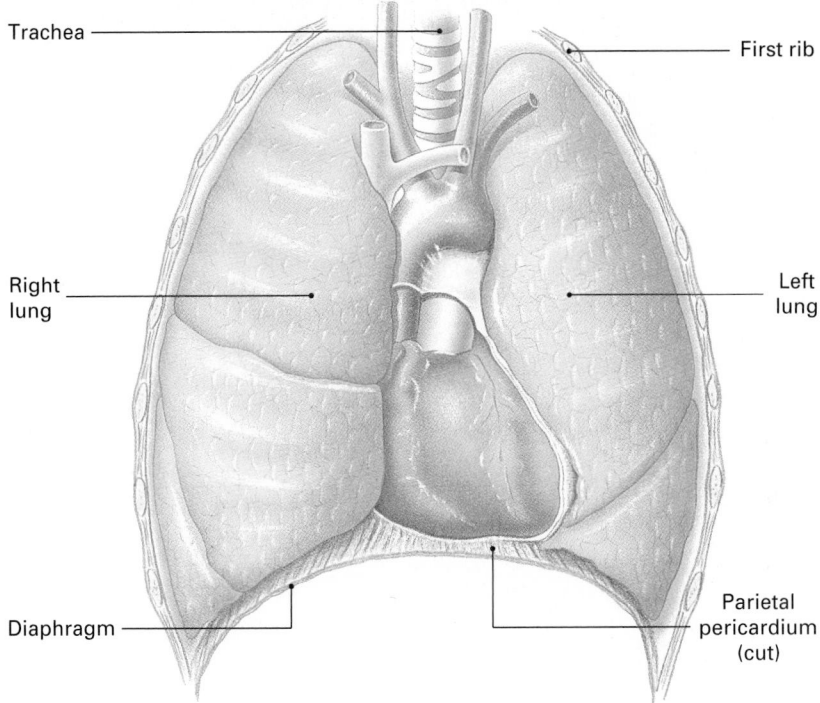

Trachea

First rib

Right lung

Left lung

Diaphragm

Parietal pericardium (cut)

FIGURE 21-1 Location of the heart within the chest.

Anatomy of the Heart

The *heart* is a four-chambered muscular organ, approximately the size of a closed fist. It is located in the center of the chest in the mediastinum. (See Figure 21-1.) Approximately two-thirds of its mass is located to the left of the midline, with the remainder located to the right. It lies anterior to the spinal column and posterior to the sternum. The lower border of the heart, which forms a blunt point, is called the *apex*. The apex is positioned immediately above the diaphragm to the left of the midline. The top portion of the heart, referred to as the *base*, is located at approximately the level of the second rib. The great vessels enter the heart through the base.

Tissue Layers   The heart consists of several readily identifiable layers. (See Figure 21-2.) Surrounding the heart is a protective sac called the *pericardium*. The pericardium consists of two layers: the *visceral pericardium* and the *parietal pericardium*. The visceral pericardium is the layer in contact with the heart muscle itself. The parietal pericardium is the outer, fibrous layer. Situated between these two layers is *pericardial fluid*, which acts as a lubricant during cardiac contraction. Generally, only a scant amount of pericardial fluid is present. However, during certain disease states, and with certain injuries, the pericardial sac becomes filled with blood or fluid. This condition can adversely affect cardiac output.

The outermost lining of the heart, the *epicardium*, is **contiguous** with the visceral pericardium. The thick middle layer of heart wall, containing the bulk of the muscle mass, is the *myocardium*. The innermost layer, which lines the chambers, is the *endocardium*.

The myocardial muscle cells are unique. They physically resemble skeletal muscle, but they have electrical properties like smooth muscle. Within the myocardial cells are specialized structures that promote the rapid spread of the myocardial electrical impulse from one muscle cell to another.

■ **contiguous** in contact or closely related.

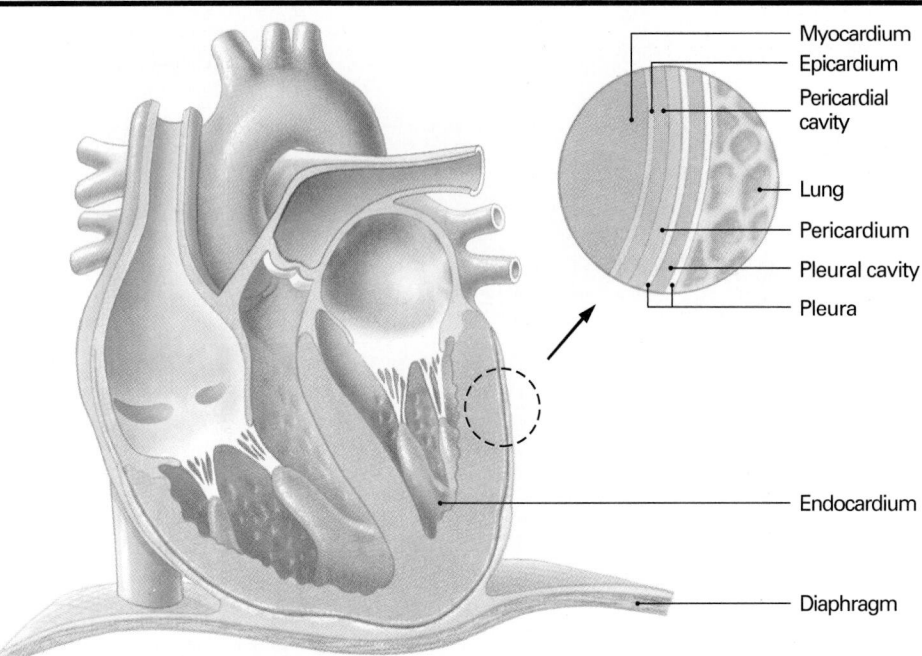

Myocardium
Epicardium
Pericardial cavity
Lung
Pericardium
Pleural cavity
Pleura
Endocardium
Diaphragm

FIGURE 21-2 Layers of the heart.

Chambers The heart contains four chambers. (See Figure 21-3.) The two superior chambers, which receive incoming blood, are called *atria*. The larger, inferior chambers are called the *ventricles*. The right and left atria are separated by the *interatrial septum*. The ventricles are separated by the *interventricular septum*. Both septa contain fibrous connective tissue as well as contractile muscle. The walls of the atria are much thinner than those of the ventricles and do not contribute significantly to the heart's pumping action.

The right atrium receives blood from the periphery of the body via the superior and inferior vena cavae. (See Figure 21-4.) The left atrium receives incoming oxygenated blood from the lungs via the pulmonary veins. The ventricles receive blood from the atria and in turn pump the blood out of the heart. The right ventricle receives blood from the right atrium and pumps it to the lungs through the pulmonary arteries. Because the pulmonary circulation does not offer a great deal of resistance, the right side of the heart is a low-pressure pump. As a result, the *myocardial muscle mass*, or thickness, is significantly less on the right than on the left.

The left ventricle receives blood from the left atrium and pumps it out of the heart into the aorta. Because of the high level of resistance present in the peripheral circulation, the left side of the heart is a high-pressure pump.

Valves The heart contains two sets of valves. (See Figure 21-5.) Both sets are made of endocardial as well as connective tissue. The *atrioventricular (AV) valves* are those between the atria and the ventricles. The valve separating the right atrium from the right ventricle is the *tricuspid valve*. The tricuspid valve contains three distinct leaflets. The *mitral valve* separates the left atrium from the left ventricle and contains only two leaflets. The valve leaflets are connected to specialized muscles in the ventricles called *papillary muscles*. When relaxed, these muscles open the valves and allow blood to flow between the two chambers. Specialized fibers called *chordae tendonae* connect the leaflets to the papillary muscles. These fibers prevent the valves from prolapsing into the atria during ventricular contraction.

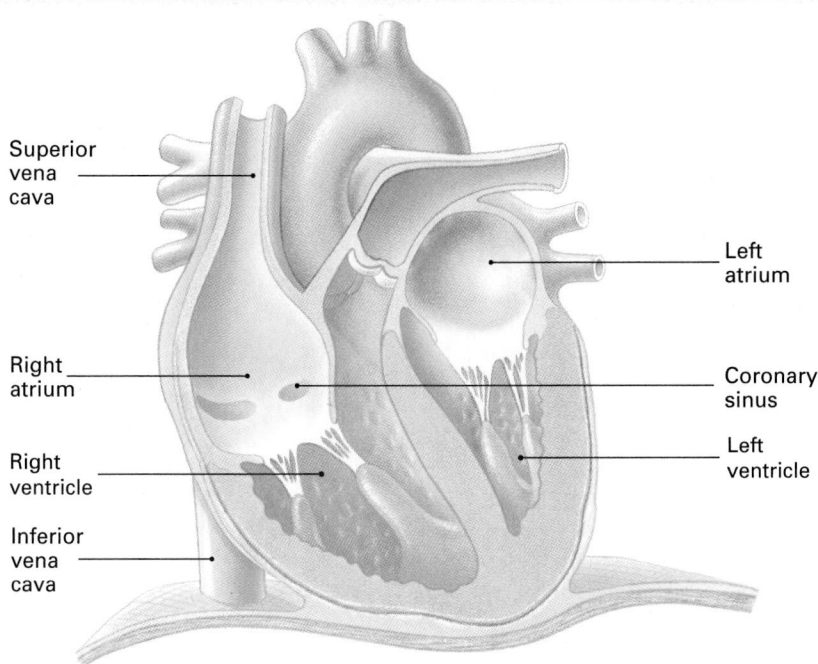

Superior
vena
cava

Left
atrium

Right
atrium

Coronary
sinus

Right
ventricle

Left
ventricle

Inferior
vena
cava

FIGURE 21-3 The chambers of the heart.

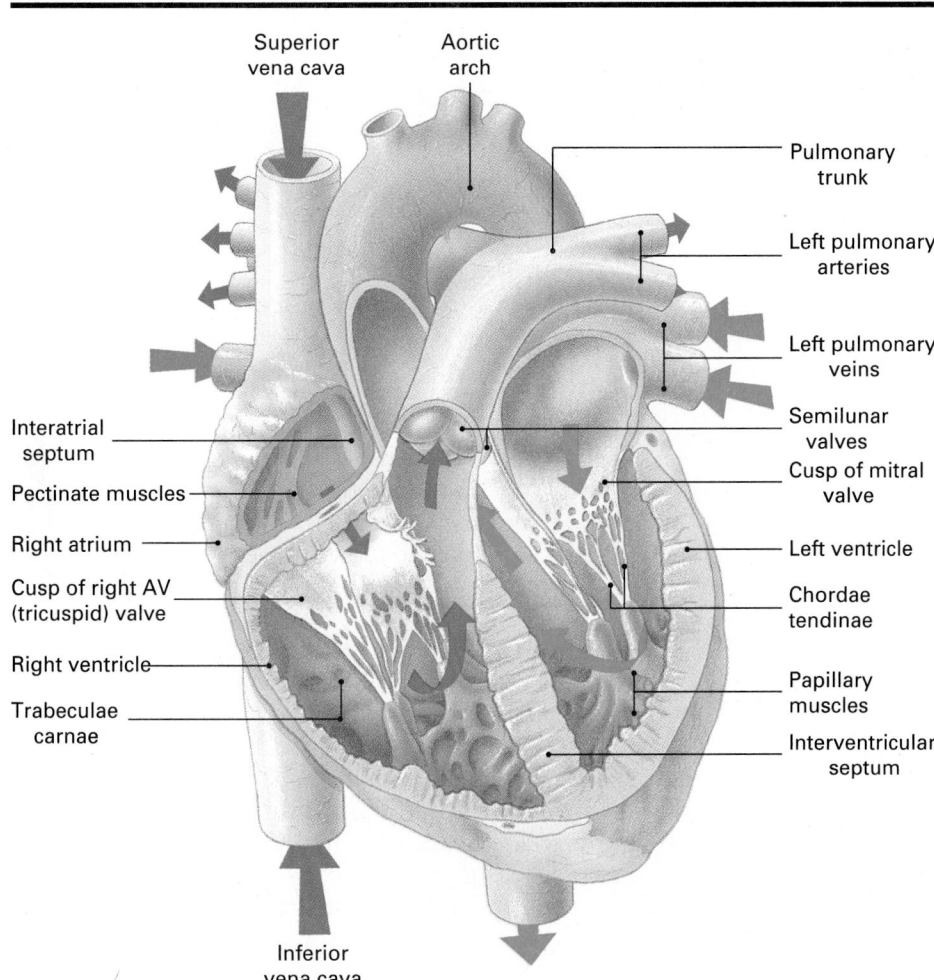

Superior
vena cava

Aortic
arch

Pulmonary
trunk

Left pulmonary
arteries

Left pulmonary
veins

Semilunar
valves

Interatrial
septum

Cusp of mitral
valve

Pectinate muscles

Right atrium

Left ventricle

Cusp of right AV
(tricuspid) valve

Chordae
tendinae

Right ventricle

Papillary
muscles

Trabeculae
carnae

Interventricular
septum

Inferior
vena cava

FIGURE 21-4 Blood flow
through the heart.

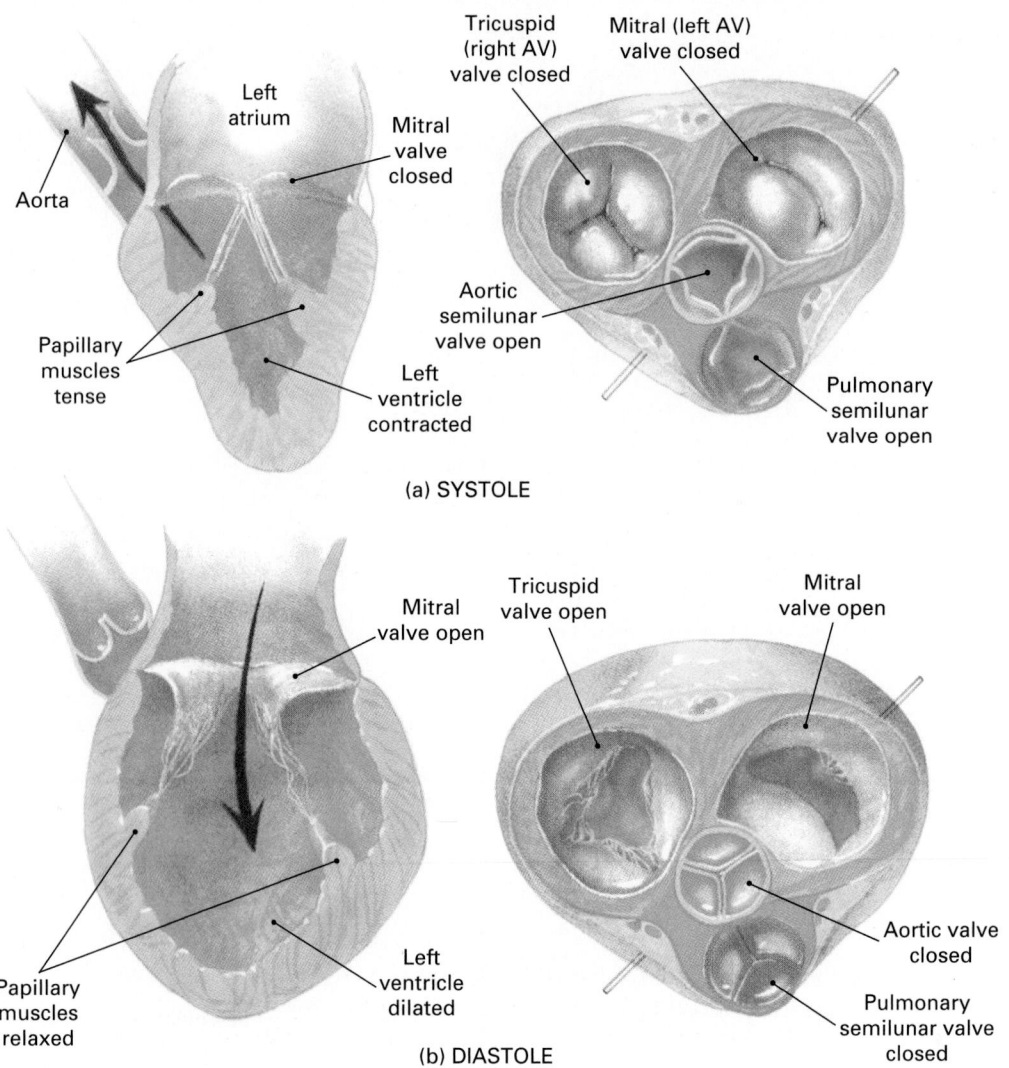

FIGURE 21-5 The valves of the heart.

The *semilunar valves* are located between the ventricles and the arteries into which they empty. The *pulmonic valve* is between the right ventricle and the pulmonary artery. The *aortic valve* is between the left ventricle and the aorta. These valves prevent the backflow of blood into the ventricles during diastole.

Vessels The *great vessels* are the largest blood vessels in the body. They are attached to the base of the heart and transport blood both to and from the heart. Deoxygenated blood enters the heart through the *vena cava*. The *superior vena cava* receives blood from the head and upper extremities, and the *inferior vena cava* receives blood from areas below the heart. Deoxygenated blood continues through the right side of the heart until it is emptied into the *pulmonary artery*, which transports it to the lungs for oxygenation. Oxygenated blood then returns to the heart, from the lungs, via the four *pulmonary veins*. The pulmonary veins deliver blood to the left atrium. Oxygenated blood ultimately leaves the heart via the aorta.

The heart is richly supplied with blood vessels, which transport nutrients and oxygen to the cardiac muscle and electrical conductive system. (See

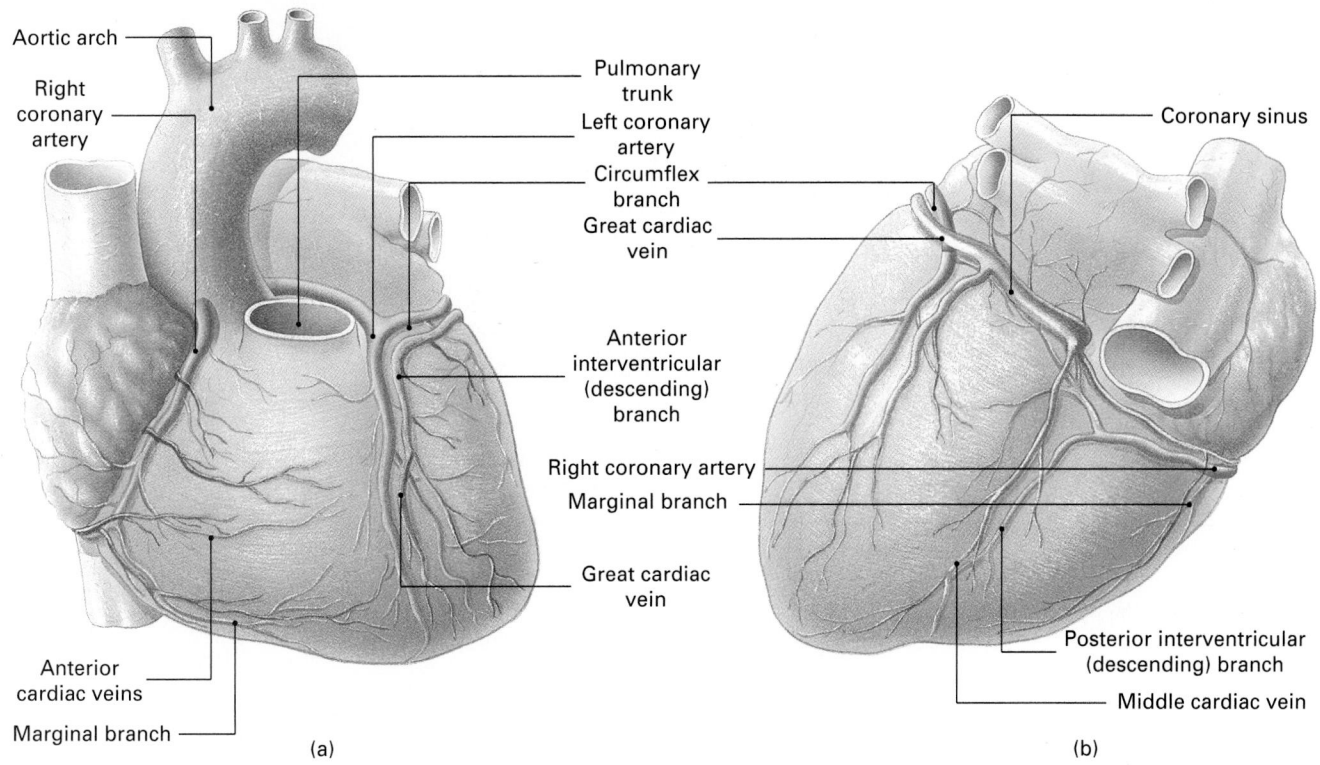

FIGURE 21-6 The coronary circulation: (a) anterior; (b) posterior.

Figure 21-6.) These vessels, referred to as the *coronary arteries*, originate in the aorta just above the leaflets of the aortic valve. The main coronary arteries lie on the surface of the heart. Blood is supplied to the myocardial muscle mass through small penetrating arterioles. The *left coronary artery* supplies the left ventricle, the interventricular septum, and part of the right ventricle. The two major branches of the left coronary artery are the *anterior descending artery* and the *circumflex artery*. The *right coronary artery* supplies a portion of the right atrium and ventricle and part of the conduction system. The two major branches of the right coronary artery are the *posterior descending artery* and the *marginal artery*.

The many **anastomoses** between the various branches of the coronary arteries allow for the development of collateral circulation. *Collateral circulation* is a protective mechanism that allows for an alternate path of blood flow in the event of vascular occlusion. The coronary vessels receive blood during diastole as the aortic valve leaflets cover the arterial openings during systole.

■ **anastomosis** a communication between two or more vessels.

Deoxygenated blood is removed from the heart through the *coronary veins*. The major vein draining the left ventricle is the *coronary sinus*. The coronary veins roughly correspond to the coronary arteries and drain into the right atrium.

Anatomy of Peripheral Circulation

The *peripheral circulation* transports oxygenated blood from the heart to the tissues and subsequently transports deoxygenated blood back to the heart. Oxygenated blood leaves the heart via the arterial system, while deoxygenated blood returns to the heart via the venous system.

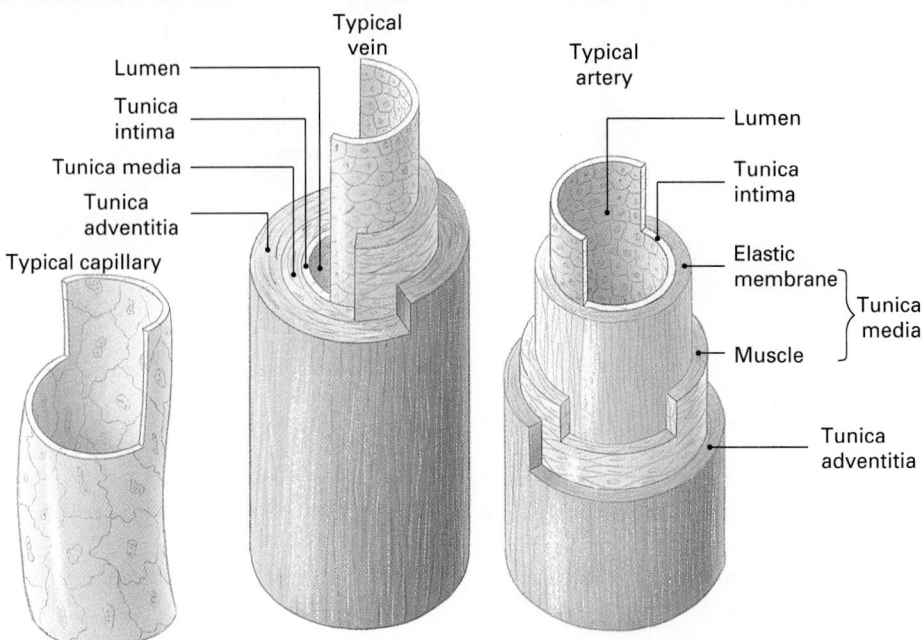

Lumen
Tunica intima
Tunica media
Tunica adventitia
Typical capillary
Typical vein
Typical artery
Lumen
Tunica intima
Elastic membrane
Muscle
} Tunica media
Tunica adventitia

FIGURE 21-7 The layers of the peripheral arteries.

The vessels of the peripheral circulation are made up of several layers. (See Figure 21-7.) The innermost lining of the blood vessels, the *tunica intima*, is a single cell layer thick. The middle layer, the *tunica media*, consists of elastic fibers and muscle. This layer gives blood vessels their strength and recoil, which results from the difference in pressure inside and outside the vessel. The tunica media is much thicker in arteries than in veins. The outermost lining is a fibrous tissue covering called the *tunica adventitia*. It provides the vessel with strength to withstand the pressures generated by the contraction of the heart. The *lumen* of a vessel is the cavity inside it. The diameter of vessels varies significantly.

The amount of blood a vessel can transport is directly related to its diameter. The larger the diameter, the greater the blood flow. In fact, blood flow increases in direct proportion to the fourth power of the radius of the vessel. For example, a vessel with a relative radius of 1 would transport 1 mL per minute of blood at a pressure difference of 100 mmHg. If the vessel radius was increased to 4, keeping the pressure difference constant, the flow would increase to 256 mL (4^4) per minute. This relationship is represented by **Poiseuille's Law**, which states that the blood flow through a vessel is directly proportional to the fourth power of the vessel's radius.

Arterial System

The *arterial system*, which carries blood from the heart, functions under high pressure. The larger arterial vessels are called *arteries*. The arteries eventually branch into smaller structures called arterioles. The *arterioles*, the smallest branches of the arterial tree, control blood flow to various organs by their degree of resistance. The arterioles continue to divide until they become *capillaries*, which are the points of connection between the arterial and venous systems. The walls of the capillaries are a single cell layer thick, which allows for exchange of gases, fluids, and nutrients between the vascular system and the tissues.

Venous System

The *venous system* transports blood back to the heart from the peripheral tissues. It functions under low pressure. Blood flow is aided by the action of surrounding muscles and by the presence of one-way

■ **Poiseuille's Law** a law of physiology stating that blood flow through a vessel is directly proportional to the radius of the vessel to the fourth power.

valves within the veins. Blood enters the venous system through the capillaries. The capillaries drain into the *venules*. The venules drain into the *veins*, which ultimately drain into the vena cava, which returns blood to the heart.

Physiology of Circulation

It is important for you to understand the pathway of normal blood flow through the heart. The superior and inferior vena cava return blood from the body to the right atrium. The blood then leaves the right atrium, through the tricuspid valve, and enters the right ventricle. The right ventricle contracts, forcing blood through the pulmonary valve into the pulmonary arteries. The blood is transported, through the pulmonary arteries, to the lungs. The pulmonary arteries then divide, until they terminate as the pulmonary capillaries. In the pulmonary capillaries, the blood takes in oxygen and gives off carbon dioxide.

Oxygenated blood then leaves the pulmonary capillaries and enters the pulmonary veins, which ultimately deliver the blood to the left atrium. Blood leaves the left atrium through the mitral valve and enters the left ventricle. The left ventricle then contracts, forcing blood through the aortic valve and into the aorta. From the aorta, blood is supplied to the coronary arteries and peripheral circulation.

Although the heart is functionally divided into the right and left sides, it acts as a unit. For example, the right and left atria contract at the same time, filling both ventricles to their maximum capacities. Subsequently, both ventricles contract at the same time, ejecting blood into both the pulmonary and systemic circulations. The pressure of the contraction causes the tricuspid and mitral valves to close and the aortic and pulmonic valves to open at the same time.

The period from the end of one heart contraction until the end of the next one is referred to as the **cardiac cycle**. The first phase of the cardiac cycle, known as **diastole**, is the phase at which ventricular filling begins. This is the relaxation phase. Diastole is much longer than **systole**, the contraction phase (0.52 second compared to 0.28 second). During diastole, most cardiac filling occurs, and the coronary arteries are filled. As the heart rate increases, the length of diastole decreases. So does the length of systole, although to a lesser degree. Systole, also referred to as *ventricular contraction*, is the phase during which blood is ejected from the heart.

The amount of blood ejected from the left and right ventricles is exactly the same. However, the resistance against which each ventricle must pump is different. The right ventricle pumps only against the resistance of the pulmonary system and is thus a low-pressure system. The left ventricle must pump against the entire systemic circulation and is a high-pressure system.

The amount of blood ejected from each ventricle during one contraction is called the **stroke volume**. (See Figure 21-8.) The average stroke volume varies between 60–100 mL, with the average being 70 mL. This capacity can increase significantly in a healthy heart. The stroke volume is a reflection of three factors: preload, cardiac contractility, and afterload. Each ventricle can pump out only what it receives from the venous system. The ventricles fill during diastole. The pressure in the ventricle at the end of diastole is referred to as **preload**, or *end-diastolic volume*. Preload influences the force of the next contraction, which is based on **Starling's Law of the Heart**. This law states that the more the myocardial muscle is stretched, up to a limit, the greater its force of contraction will be. In other words, the greater the volume of blood filling the chamber, the more forceful the cardiac contraction. Therefore, the greater the venous return, the greater the preload and the greater the stroke volume.

■ **cardiac cycle** the period of time from the end of one cardiac contraction to the end of the next.

■ **diastole** the period of time when the myocardium is relaxed and cardiac filling and coronary perfusion occur.

■ **systole** the period of the cardiac cycle when the myocardium is contracting.

■ **stroke volume** the amount of blood ejected by the heart in one cardiac contraction.

■ **preload** the pressure within the ventricles at the end of diastole; commonly called the end-diastolic volume.

■ **Starling's Law of the Heart** law of physiology stating that the more the myocardium is stretched, up to a certain amount, the more forceful the subsequent contraction will be.

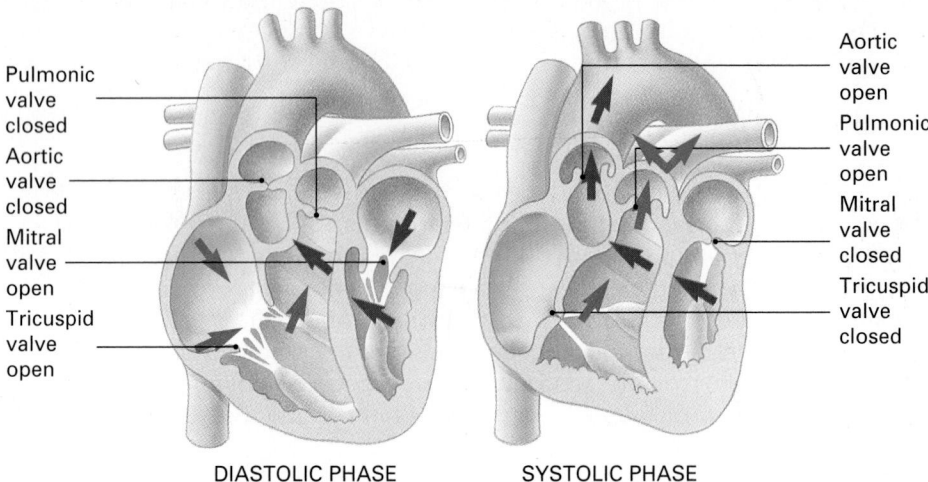

Pulmonic
valve
closed
Aortic
valve
closed
Mitral
valve
open
Tricuspid
valve
open

Aortic
valve
open
Pulmonic
valve
open
Mitral
valve
closed
Tricuspid
valve
closed

DIASTOLIC PHASE   SYSTOLIC PHASE

FIGURE 21-8 Relation of blood flow to cardiac contraction.

■ **afterload** the resistance against which the heart must pump.

■ **cardiac output** the amount of blood pumped by the heart in one minute.

In addition, the pressure against which the ventricle must pump also affects stroke volume. The greater the resistance, the less the stroke volume. The resistance against which the ventricle must contract is called the **afterload**. An increase in peripheral vascular resistance will decrease stroke volume. Conversely, a decrease in peripheral vascular resistance, up to a point, will increase stroke volume.

Cardiac output is also related to stroke volume. **Cardiac output** can be defined as the volume of blood pumped by the heart in one minute. It is a function of stroke volume and heart rate, as shown in the below formula.

Stroke Volume (mL) × Heart Rate (bpm) = Cardiac Output (mL/min)

The normal heart rate is 60–100 beats per minute, and the average stroke volume is 70 mL. Thus an average cardiac output is about 5 L per minute, as shown below.

Stroke Volume × Heart Rate = Cardiac Output

(70 mL) × (70 bpm) = (4900 mL/min)

Blood pressure is directly related to cardiac output and peripheral resistance. The following formula shows this relationship.

Blood Pressure = Cardiac Output × Systemic Vascular Resistance

In other words, if the peripheral resistance is kept constant and cardiac output is increased, blood pressure will increase. Conversely, if peripheral resistance is kept constant and cardiac output decreases, blood pressure will fall. Because of the body's compensatory mechanisms, these changes generally occur only in very sick patients. For example, if cardiac output falls, as can occur after myocardial infarction, the baroreceptors detect this change and increase peripheral vascular resistance to maintain blood pressure. In addition, the heart is stimulated to increase its rate, contractile state, or both to help correct the deficit in cardiac output.

Nervous Control of the Heart

The heart is regulated by both the sympathetic and parasympathetic components of the autonomic nervous system. (See Figure 21-9.) The sympathetic nervous system innervates the heart through the *cardiac plexus*. The sympa-

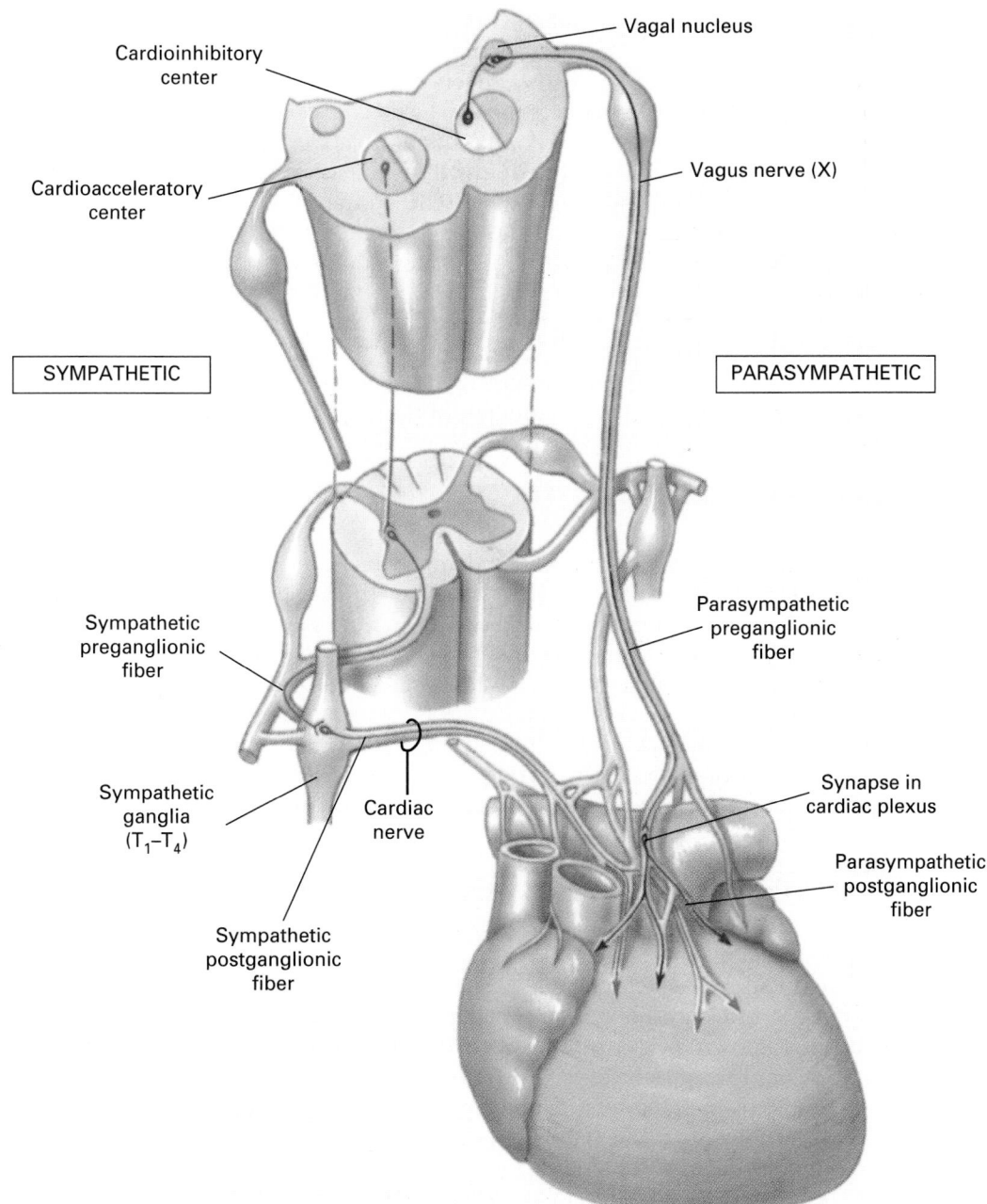

FIGURE 21-9   Nervous control of the heart.

thetic nerves arise from the thoracic and lumbar regions of the spinal cord. These nerves leave the spinal cord and form the sympathetic chain, which runs alongside the spinal column. The cardiac plexus arises from ganglia in the sympathetic chain and innervates both the atria and ventricles. The chemical neurotransmitter for the sympathetic nervous system, and thus for the cardiac plexus, is *norepinephrine*. Release of norepinephrine causes an increase in heart rate and cardiac contractile force, primarily through its actions on beta receptors.

Parasympathetic control of the heart occurs through the *vagus nerve*, or the tenth cranial nerve. The vagus nerve descends from the brain to innervate the heart and other organs. Vagal nerve fibers primarily innervate the atria, although some fibers innervate the upper portion of the ventricles. The neurotransmitter for the parasympathetic nervous system, and thus the vagus nerve, is *acetylcholine*. Release of acetylcholine slows the heart rate and slows atrioventricular condition. Several maneuvers can cause stimulation of the vagus nerve. These include Valsalva (straining against a closed glottis), pressure on the carotid sinus, and distention of the urinary bladder.

The two cardiac control systems, the sympathetic and parasympathetic, are in direct opposition to one another. The normal state is a balance between the two. In stressful situations, the sympathetic system becomes dominant. However, parasympathetic control dominates during sleep.

The term **chronotropy** refers to heart rate. A drug or agent that is a *positive chronotropic agent* is one that increases heart rate. Conversely, a *negative chronotropic agent* decreases heart rate. The term **inotropy** refers to the strength of a muscular contraction of the heart. Thus, a *positive inotropic agent* is one that increases the strength of the cardiac contraction, and a *negative inotropic agent* is one that decreases it.

Role of Electrolytes

Cardiac function, both electrical and mechanical, is strongly influenced by electrolyte imbalances. Electrolytes that affect cardiac function include sodium (Na^+), calcium (Ca^{++}), and potassium (K^+). Sodium plays a major role in depolarization of the myocardium. Calcium plays a role in myocardial depolarization and myocardial contraction. Hypercalcemia can result in increased contractility, whereas hypocalcemia has been associated with decreased myocardial contractility and increased electrical irritability. Potassium plays a major role in repolarization. Hyperkalemia results in decreased automaticity and conduction, whereas hypokalemia causes increased irritability.

Electrophysiology

The heart is composed of three types of cardiac muscle: atrial muscle, ventricular muscle, and specialized excitatory and conductive muscle fibers. The atrial and ventricular fibers contract in the same way as does skeletal muscle. However, there is a major difference. Within the cardiac muscle fibers are special structures known as the **intercalated discs**. (See Figure 21-10.) These discs connect cardiac muscle fibers and conduct electrical impulses quickly from one muscle fiber to the next. The intercalated discs conduct electrical impulses 400 times faster than the standard cell membrane. This special feature allows cardiac muscle cells to function together in a **syncytium**. That is, when one cell becomes excited, the action potential spreads rapidly across the entire group of cells, resulting in a coordinated contraction.

Within the heart are two syncytia—the atrial syncytium and the ventricular syncytium. The *atrial syncytium* contracts in a superior-to-inferior direction, so that blood is expressed from the atria to the ventricles. The *ventricular syncytium*, on the other hand, contracts in an inferior-to-superior direction, expelling blood from the ventricles into the aorta and pulmonary arteries. The two syncytia are separated from one another by the fibrous structure that supports the valves and physically separates the atria from the ventricles. The only way an impulse can be conducted from the atria to the ventricles is through the *atrioventricular (AV) bundle*. Cardiac muscle functions according to an "all or none" principle. That is, if a single muscle fiber becomes depolarized, the action potential will spread through the whole syncytium. Stimulation of an atrial fiber will cause complete depolarization of the atria, and stimulation of a ventricular fiber will cause complete depolarization of the ventricles.

■ **chronotropy** pertaining to heart rate.

■ **inotropy** pertaining to cardiac contractile force.

■ **intercalated discs** specialized band of tissue inserted between myocardial cells that increase the rate in which the action potential is spread from cell to cell.

■ **syncytium** group of cardiac muscle cells that physiologically function as a unit.

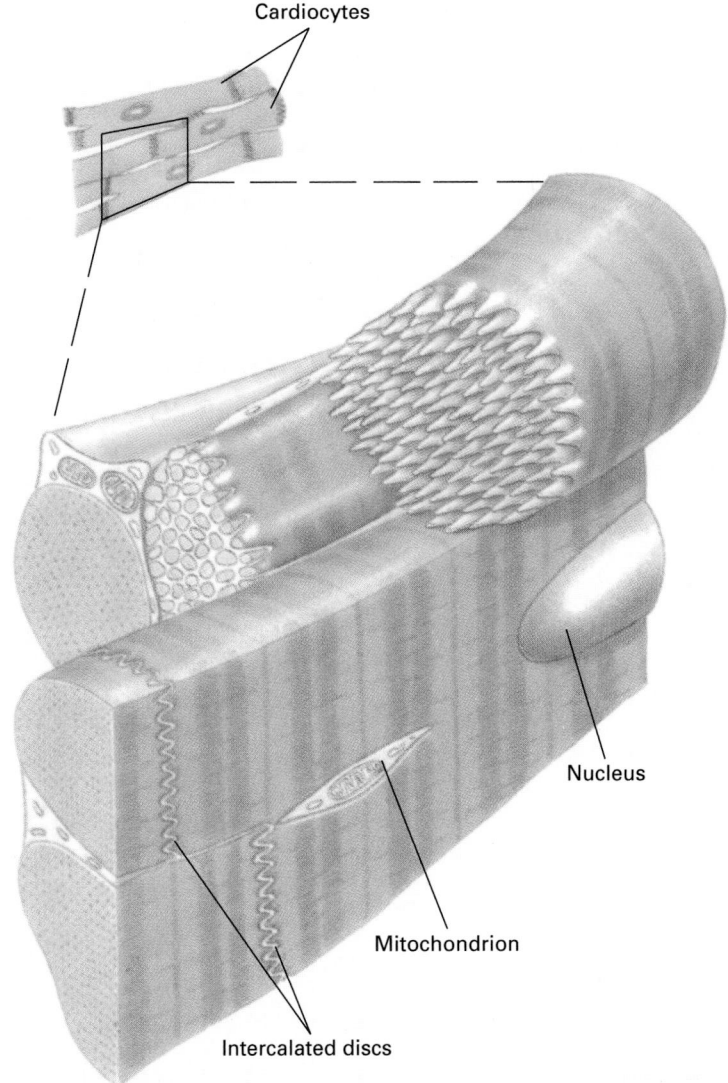

Cardiocytes

Nucleus

Mitochondrion

Intercalated discs

FIGURE 21-10 Microscopic appearance of cardiac muscle. The intercalated discs speed transmission of the electrical potential quickly from one cell to the next.

Cardiac Depolarization The concept of *cardiac depolarization* is essential to the interpretation of electrocardiograms (ECGs). Normally, there is an ionic difference on the two sides of a cell membrane. Sodium (Na$^+$) is actively pumped out of the cell membrane by the sodium-potassium pump. This causes more negatively charged anions to remain inside the cell than positively charged cations, which results in a difference in voltage across the cell membrane. Thus the inside of the cell is more negatively charged than the outside. This difference, referred to as the **resting potential**, can be measured experimentally by placing one probe inside the cell and another outside the cell and determining the difference in millivolts. In the resting myocardial cell, the difference is approximately -90 mV. (See Figure 21-11.)

When the myocardial cell is stimulated, the membrane surrounding the cell changes instantaneously to allow sodium ions to rush into the cell, bringing their positive charge. This charge is so strong that it causes the normal negative resting potential to disappear completely. In fact, it causes the inside of the cell to become positively charged at approximately +20 mV as compared to the outside. This influx of sodium and change of membrane polarity is referred to as the **action potential**. After the influx of sodium, there is a slower influx of calcium ions (Ca^{++}) through the calcium channels, which

■ **resting potential** the normal electrical state of cardiac cells.

■ **action potential** the stimulation of myocardial cells, as evidenced by a change in the membrane electrical charge, that subsequently spreads across the myocardium.

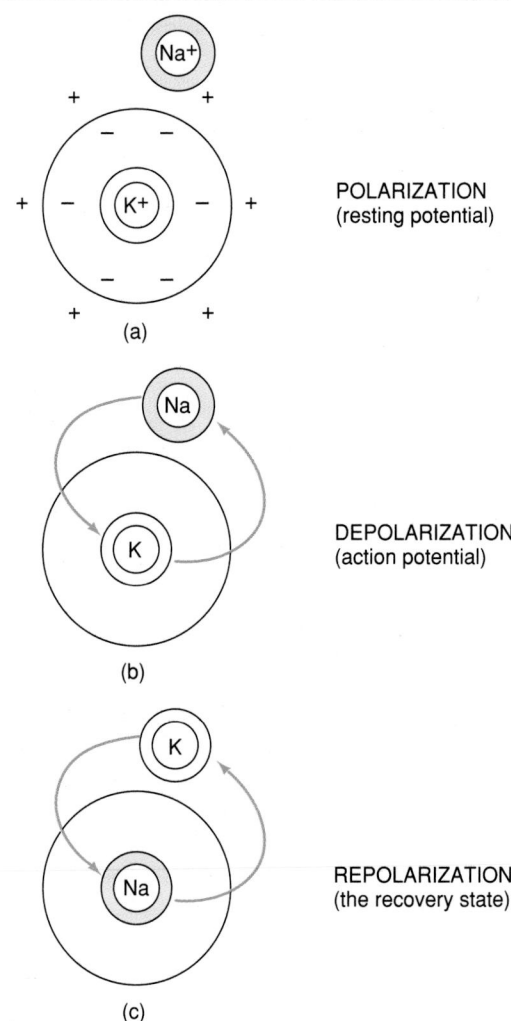

POLARIZATION
(resting potential)

(a)

DEPOLARIZATION
(action potential)

(b)

REPOLARIZATION
(the recovery state)

(c)

FIGURE 21-11 Schematic of ion shifts during depolarization and repolarization.

causes the inside of the cell to become even more positive. Once depolarization occurs in a muscle fiber, it is transmitted throughout the entire syncytium, via the intercalated discs, until the entire muscle mass is depolarized. Contraction of the muscle follows depolarization.

The cell membrane remains permeable to sodium for only a fraction of a second. Thereafter, sodium influx stops, and potassium escapes from inside the cell. This causes a change in the charge inside the cell back to a negative value. In addition, sodium is actively pumped outside the cell, allowing the cell to return to its normal resting state. This return to the resting state is called **repolarization**.

■ **repolarization** the return of a muscle cell to its pre-excitation resting state.

Cardiac Conductive System The description above applies generally to cardiac muscle in both the atrial and ventricular syncytia. However, another type of cardiac muscle fiber, known as the conductive fibers, has not yet been discussed. The *conductive fibers* of the heart are specialized muscle cells designed to transmit the depolarization potential rapidly through the heart. They transmit the impulse much more quickly than it could be transmitted through regular myocardial cells.

The conductive system stimulates the ventricles to depolarize in the proper direction. As mentioned earlier, the atria contract in a superior-to-inferior direction, and the ventricles contract in an inferior-to-superior direction.

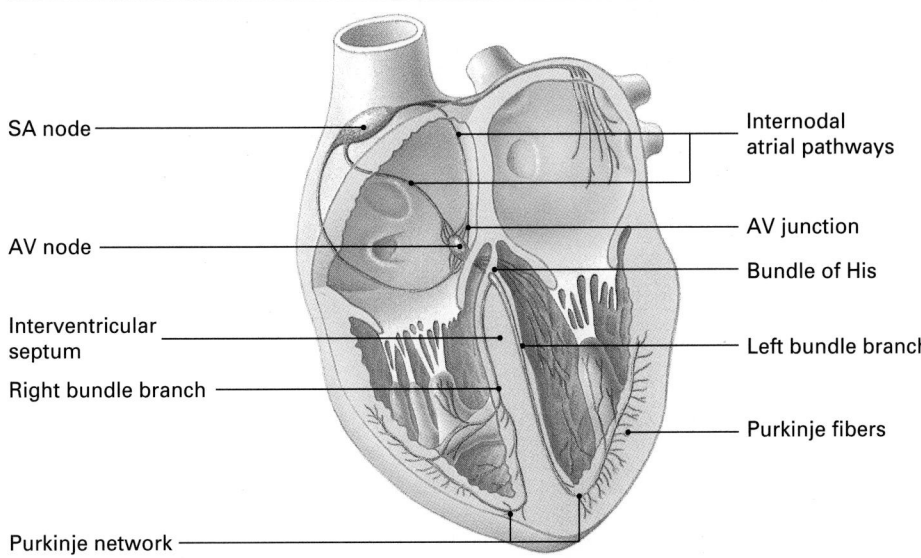

FIGURE 21-12 The cardiac conductive system.

This allows blood to flow in the proper direction. If the depolarization impulse originated in the atria and was allowed to spread passively to the ventricles, then ventricular depolarization would occur in a superior-to-inferior direction and would be ineffective. Therefore, the purpose of the conduction system is to initiate an impulse, spread it through the atria, transmit it quickly to the apex of the heart, and there stimulate the ventricles to depolarize in an inferior-to-superior direction. (See Figure 21-12.)

The cells of the cardiac conductive system have several important properties. First, they have *excitability*. That is, they can respond to an electrical stimulus, like all other myocardial cells. Second, they have *conductivity*. They can propagate the electrical impulse from one cell to another. Finally, they have the unique property of *self-excitation*. That is, an individual conductive cell is capable of self-depolarization without an impulse from an outside source. This property, shared by all cells of the conductive system, is called **automaticity**. Generally, the cell in the cardiac conductive system with the fastest rate of discharge, or automaticity, becomes the pacemaker of the heart. As a rule, the highest cell in the conductive system has the fastest rate of automaticity. Normally, this cell is in the *sinoatrial (SA) node*, which is located high in the right atrium. However, if a cell of the conductive system fails to discharge and depolarize, the cell with the next fastest rate then becomes the pacemaker.

Knowledge of the anatomy of the cardiac conductive system is essential to understanding ECG readings. The SA node, located high in the right atrium, is connected to the AV node by the *internodal pathways*. The internodal pathways conduct the depolarization impulse to the atrial muscle mass and, through the atria, to the AV junction. The impulse is slowed at the AV junction to allow time for ventricular filling. Then, as the impulse passes through the AV junction, it enters the AV node. The AV node is connected to the AV fibers, which conduct the impulse from the atria to the ventricles. The AV fibers then become the *bundle of His*, which transmits the impulse through the interventricular septum.

The bundle of His subsequently divides into the right and left bundle branches. The *right bundle branch* delivers the impulse to the apex of the right ventricle, where it is spread across the myocardium by the *Purkinje system*. At the same time, the impulse is carried into the *left bundle branch*. The left bundle branch divides into the *anterior and posterior fascicles*, which ulti-

■ **automaticity** the capability of self-depolarization. Refers to the pacemaker cells of the heart.

mately terminate into the Purkinje system. At the same time that the impulse is transmitted to the right ventricle, the Purkinje system spreads it across the mass of the myocardium. Repolarization predominantly occurs in the opposite direction.

Each component of the conductive system has its own intrinsic rate of self-excitation. These include:

$$SA\ node\ =\ 60\text{--}100\ \text{beats per minute}$$

$$AV\ node\ =\ 40\text{--}60\ \text{beats per minute}$$

$$Purkinje\ system\ =\ 20\text{--}40\ \text{beats per minute}$$

RECOGNITION OF DYSRHYTHMIAS

✱ A paramedic must be capable of interpreting all rhythm strips, relying only on medical control when a question arises about interpretation.

As a paramedic, one of your most important skills will be to obtain and interpret ECG rhythm strips. Subsequent treatment received by your patient will be based upon a rapid, accurate interpretation.

Introduction to ECG Monitoring

Interpretation of ECGs is a fundamental paramedic skill. Although most EMS systems have the capability of telemetry, so that the ECG reading can be verified by the medical control physician, the paramedic is still the person who must interpret the tracing.

This section will address ECG monitoring as well as recognition and interpretation of dysrhythmias. This text presents basic information. ECG interpretation is a skill that can be mastered only through classroom instruction and repeated practice.

■ **electrocardiogram (ECG)** the graphic recording of the heart's electrical activity. It may be displayed either on paper or on an oscilloscope.

The Electrocardiogram   The **electrocardiogram (ECG)** is a graphic record of the electrical activity of the heart. It tells you nothing whatsoever about the heart's pumping ability. The heart is the largest generator of electrical energy in the body. The body acts as a giant conductor of electricity, and its electrical activity can be sensed by electrodes placed on the skin. These electrodes detect the total amount of electrical activity occurring within the heart at a given time.

The ECG machine records the positive and negative electrical impulses from the heart over time. Positive impulses are recorded as upward deflections on the paper, and negative impulses as downward deflections. The absence of any electrical impulse results in the recording of an *isoelectric line*, which is a flat line.

The electrical impulses present on the skin surface are a very low voltage. These impulses are amplified by the ECG machine and recorded on ECG graph paper or on an oscilloscope.

ECG Leads   You can obtain many views of the heart's electrical activity by monitoring the voltage change through various electrodes placed on the body surface. Each pair of electrodes is referred to as a *lead*. In the hospital, 12 leads are normally used. As a rule, only 3 leads are generally utilized in the field. (One lead is adequate for detecting life-threatening dysrhythmias.) However, with the advent of thrombolytic therapy and computer interpretation, 12-lead ECGs are becoming more commonplace in the field. Limited discussion of the 12-lead ECG will be presented later in this chapter.

There are three types of ECG leads: bipolar leads, augmented leads, and precordial leads. A *bipolar lead*, the kind most frequently used, has one positive electrode and one negative electrode. On a bipolar lead, any electrical impulse within the body moving toward the positive electrode will cause a positive deflection on the ECG paper. Any electrical impulse moving toward the negative electrode will cause a negative deflection. The absence of a positive or negative deflection means either that there is no electrical impulse or that the impulse is moving perpendicular to the lead. Leads I, II, and III, commonly called *limb leads*, are bipolar leads. These are the most frequently used leads in the field.

The electrodes of the three bipolar leads are placed in the following areas of the body.

Lead	Positive Electrode	Negative Electrode
I	left arm	right arm
II	left leg	right arm
III	left leg	left arm

These three leads form a triangle around the heart, referred to as *Einthoven's triangle*. (See Figure 21-13.) The direction from the negative to the positive electrode is referred to as the axis of the lead. Each lead is designed to look at a different axis of the heart. Lead I forms the top of Einthoven's triangle and is said to have an axis of 0°. Lead II forms the right side of the tri-

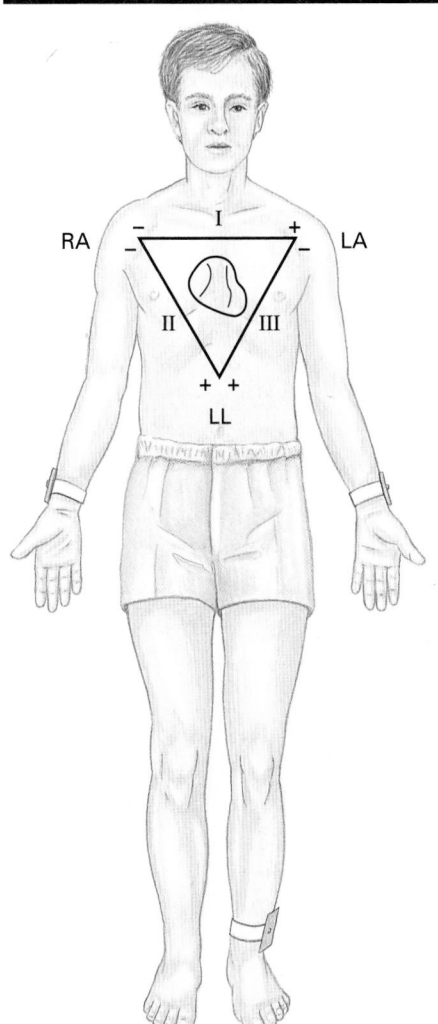

FIGURE 21-13 Einthoven's triangle as formed by Leads I, II, and III.

angle and has an axis of 60°, while Lead III forms the left side of the triangle and has an axis of 120°.

The bipolar leads provide only three views of the heart. Because additional views are sometimes useful, *augmented*, or *unipolar leads*, were developed. These leads evaluate different axes than the bipolar leads, but they utilize the same set of electrodes. They do this by electronically combining the negative electrodes of two of the bipolar leads to obtain an axis that is in between. The augmented leads are designated aVR, aVL, and aVF.

The six leads described so far can be obtained by using three standard electrodes. In addition, the *precordial leads* can be placed across the surface of the chest to measure electrical cardiac activity in a horizontal axis. These leads are helpful in viewing the left ventricle and septum. The precordial leads are designated V1 through V6.

Routine ECG Monitoring   Only one lead is generally used in routine monitoring, whether in the ambulance, emergency department, or coronary care unit. The most common monitoring leads are Lead II or the *modified chest lead 1 (MCL$_1$)*. (See Figure 21-14.) Lead II is most frequently used because most of the heart's electrical current flows toward the positive axis of Lead II. This gives the best view of the ECG waves. MCL$_1$ is a special monitoring lead that is selectively used in some systems. It is useful in determining the origin site of abnormal complexes such as premature beats. However, to avoid confusion, Lead II will be used as the monitor lead throughout this text.

Considerable information can be obtained from a single monitoring lead. Data include:

❏ The rate of the heartbeat.
❏ The regularity of the heartbeat.
❏ The length of time it takes to conduct the impulse through the various parts of the heart.

The following information CANNOT be obtained from a single lead.

❏ The presence or location of an infarct.
❏ Axis deviation or chamber enlargement.
❏ Right-to-left differences in conduction or impulse formation.
❏ The quality or presence of pumping action.

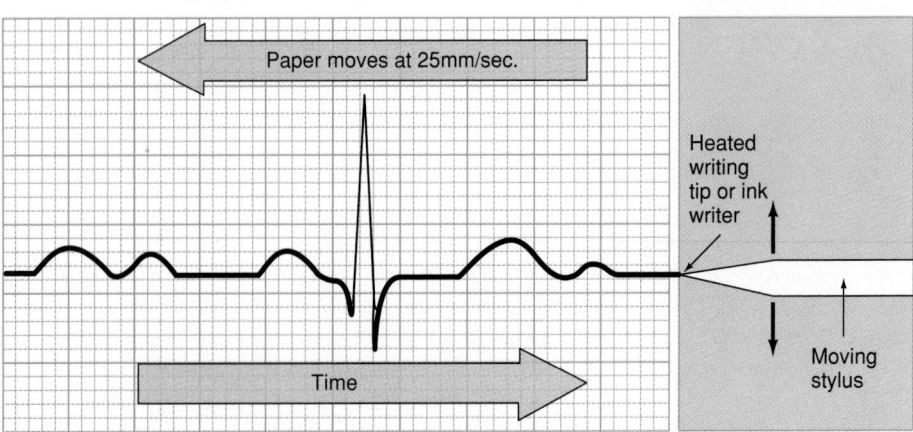

FIGURE 21-14   Recording of the ECG.

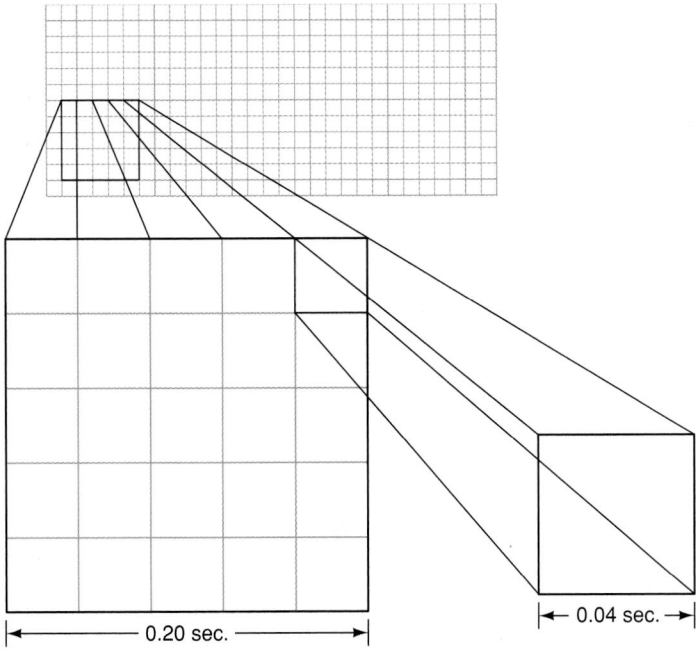

FIGURE 21-15   The ECG paper and markings.

|←——— 0.20 sec. ———→| |← 0.04 sec. →|

ECG Graph Paper   The ECG graph paper is standardized to allow comparative analysis of ECG patterns. (See Figure 21-15.) The paper moves across the stylus at a standard speed of 25mm/sec. The amplitude of the ECG deflection is also standardized. When properly calibrated, the ECG stylus should deflect two large boxes when 1 mV of voltage is present. Most machines have calibration buttons, and a calibration curve should be placed at the beginning of the first ECG strip. Many machines do this automatically when they are first turned on.

The horizontal axis represents time, while the vertical axis represents voltage. The ECG paper is divided into small and large boxes. There are five small boxes in a large box. The following relationships apply to the horizontal axis.

$$1 \text{ small box} = 0.04 \text{ sec}$$
$$1 \text{ large box} = 0.20 \text{ sec} (0.04 \text{ sec} \times 5 = 0.20 \text{ sec})$$

These increments are used to measure the duration of the ECG complexes and time intervals. The vertical axis reflects the voltage amplitude in millivolts. Two large boxes equal 1 mV.

In addition to the grid, ECG paper has time interval markings at the top. These marks are placed at 3-second intervals. Each 3-second interval contains 15 large boxes (0.2 sec × 15 boxes = 3 sec). The time markings are used to calculate heart rate.

Relationship of the ECG to Electrical Events in the Heart   The ECG tracing has specific components that reflect electrical changes in the heart. (See Figure 21-16.) The first component of the ECG, corresponding to depolarization of the atria, is called the *P wave*. On Lead II, it is a positive, rounded wave that precedes the QRS complex. The *QRS complex* reflects ventricular depolarization. The *Q wave* is the first negative deflection after the P wave. The *R wave* is the first positive deflection after the P wave, and the *S wave* is the first negative deflection after the R wave. All three waves are not always present, and the shape of the QRS complex can vary from individual to individual.

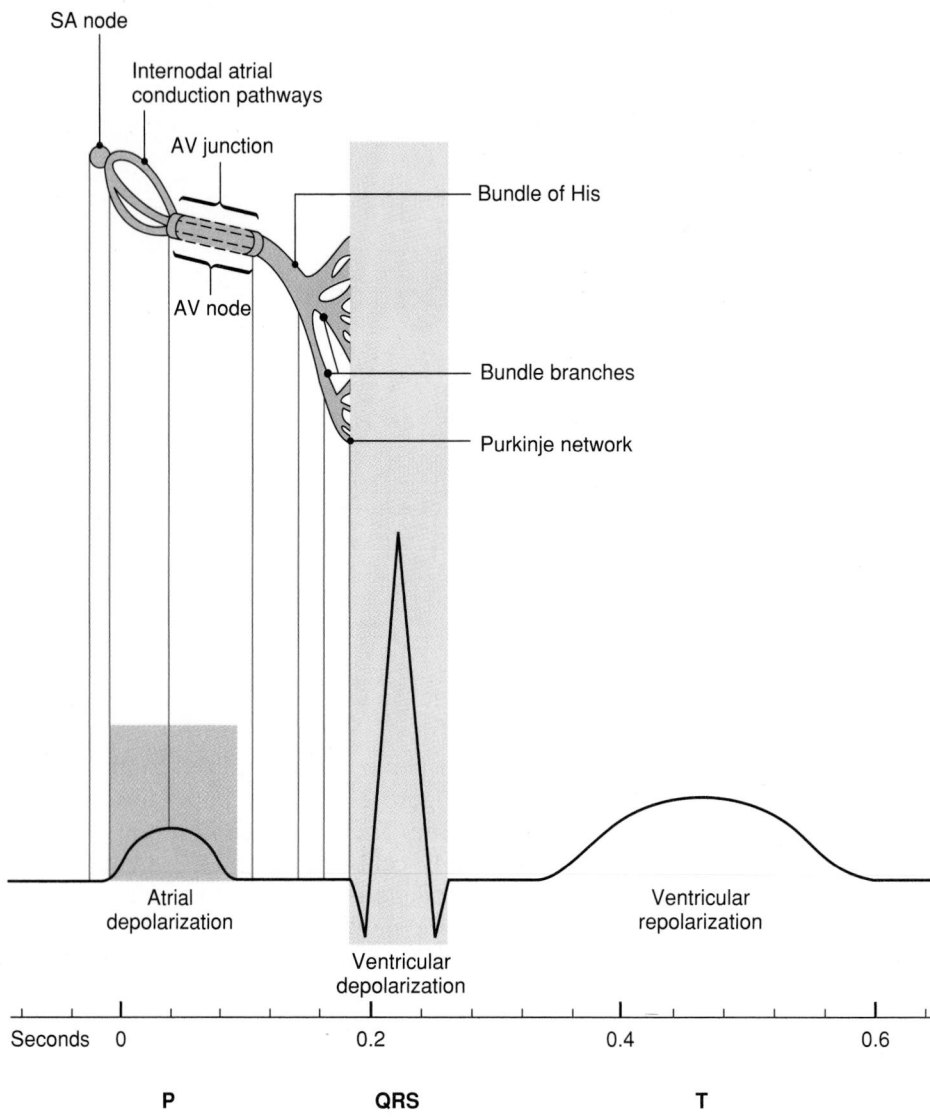

SA node

Internodal atrial
conduction pathways

AV junction

AV node

Bundle of His

Bundle branches

Purkinje network

Atrial
depolarization

Ventricular
depolarization

Ventricular
repolarization

Seconds   0   0.2   0.4   0.6

P   QRS   T

FIGURE 21-16   Relationship of the ECG to electrical activities in the heart.

The next wave, which is normally positive in Lead II, is the *T wave*. The T wave is rounded and usually moves in the same direction as the QRS complex. The T wave reflects repolarization of the ventricles. Occasionally, a *U wave* can be seen. This follows the T wave and is usually positive. The U wave may be associated with electrolyte abnormalities, or it may be a normal finding.

In addition to the wave forms described above, the ECG tracing reflects important time intervals. The distance from the beginning of the P wave to the beginning of the QRS complex is called the *P-R interval*. This represents the time necessary for the impulse to be transmitted from the atria to the ventricles. The *QRS duration* is the interval from the first deflection to the last deflection of the QRS complex. It represents the time interval necessary for ventricular depolarization. The *S-T segment* is the distance from the S wave to the beginning of the T wave. Usually this is an isoelectric line; however, it may be elevated or depressed in certain disease states such as ischemia. (See Figures 21-17 to 21-24.)

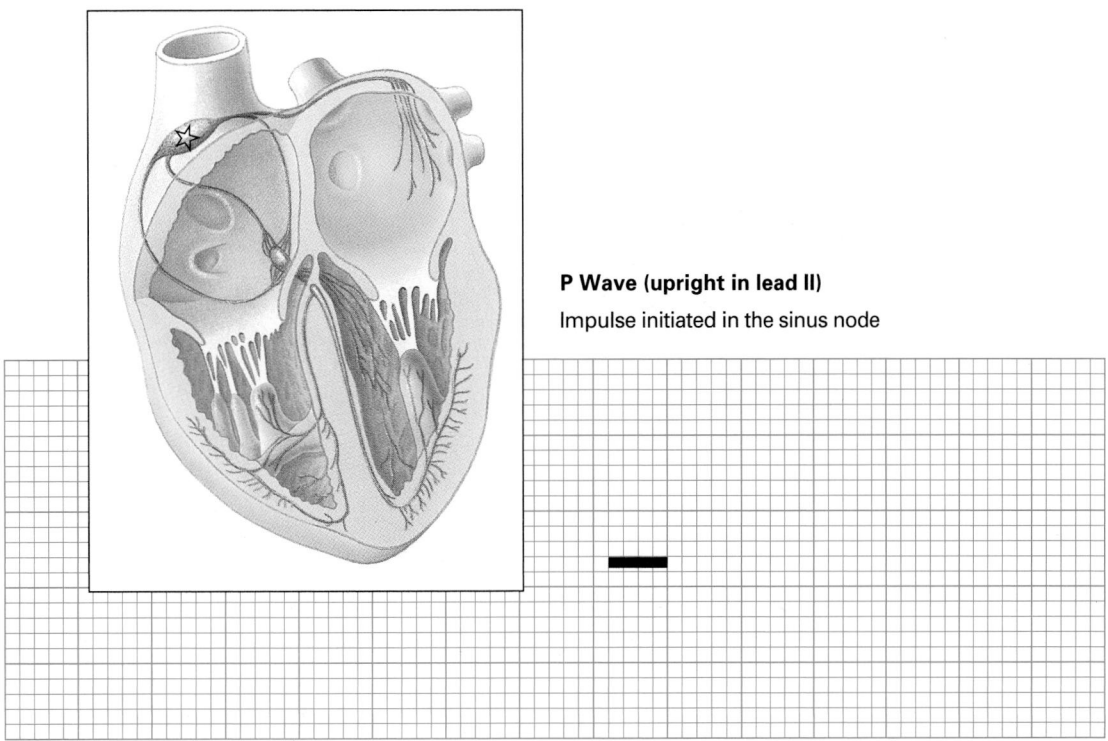

P Wave (upright in lead II)

Impulse initiated in the sinus node

FIGURE 21-17   Impulse initiation in the SA node.

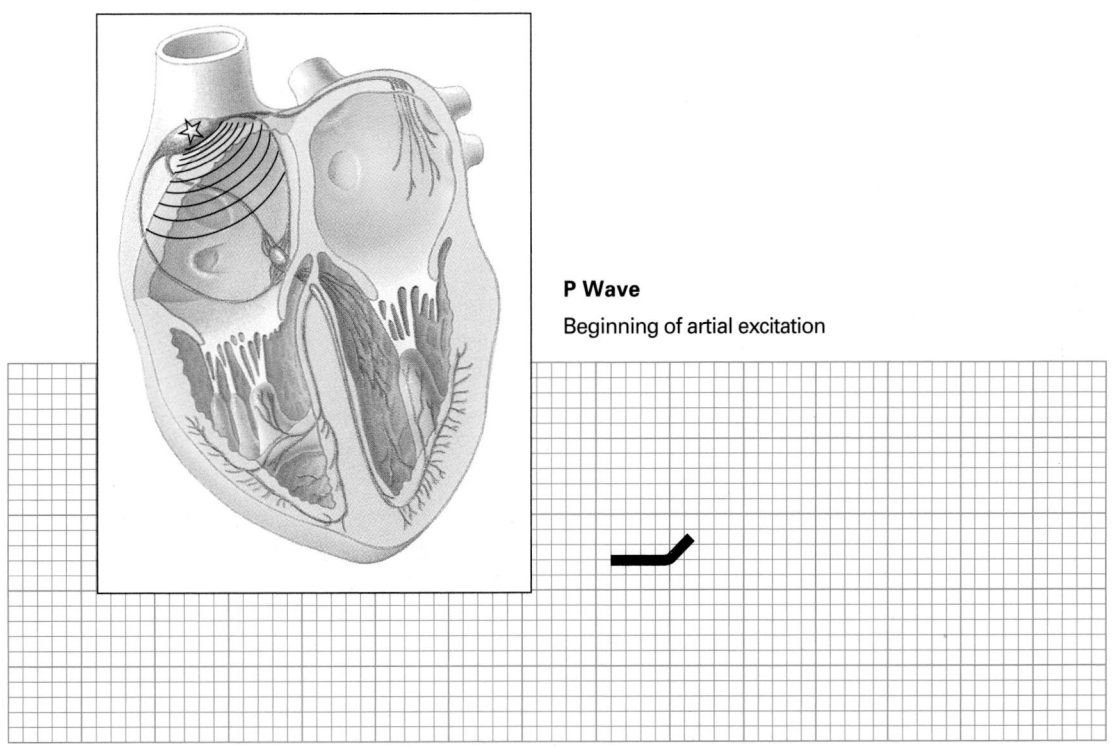

P Wave

Beginning of artial excitation

FIGURE 21-18   Beginning of atrial excitation.

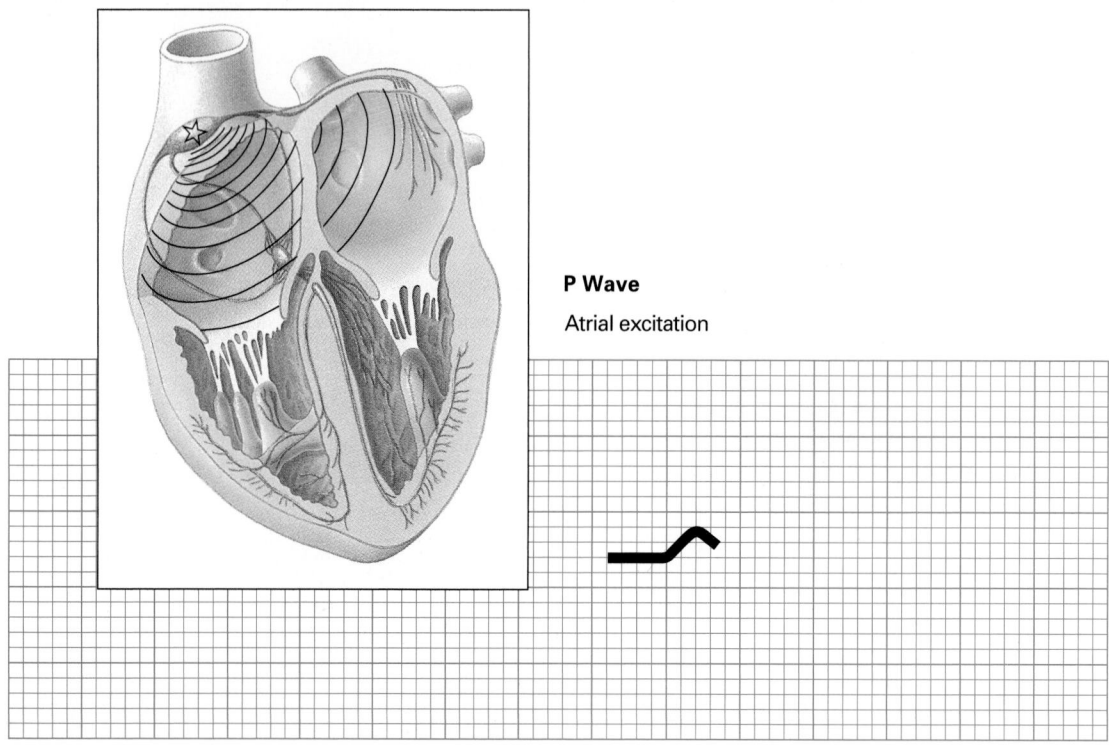

P Wave

Atrial excitation

FIGURE 21-19 Atrial excitation.

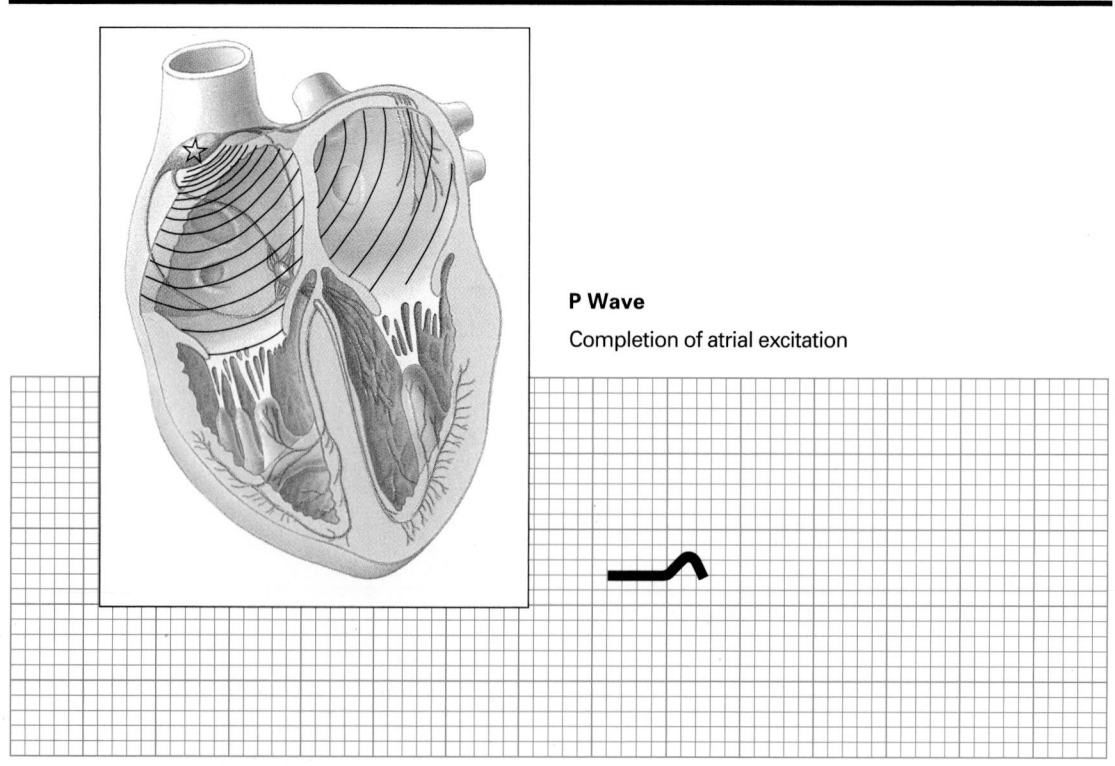

P Wave

Completion of atrial excitation

FIGURE 21-20 Completion of atrial excitation.

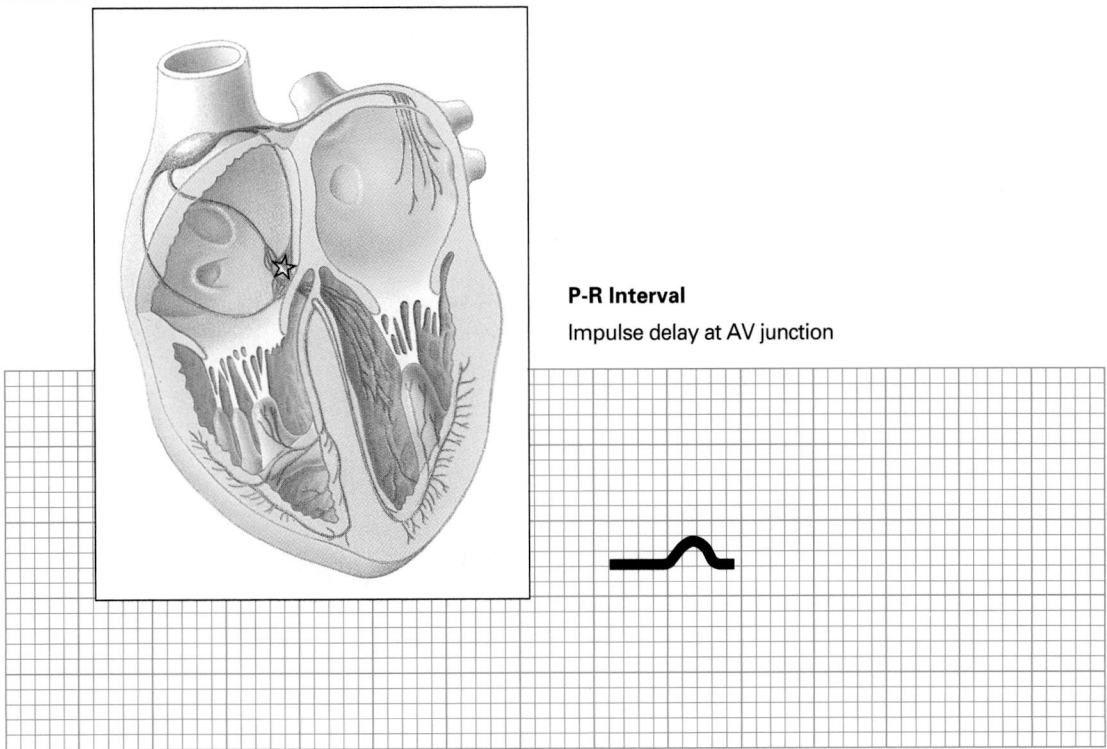

P-R Interval

Impulse delay at AV junction

FIGURE 21-21 Impulse delay at the AV junction.

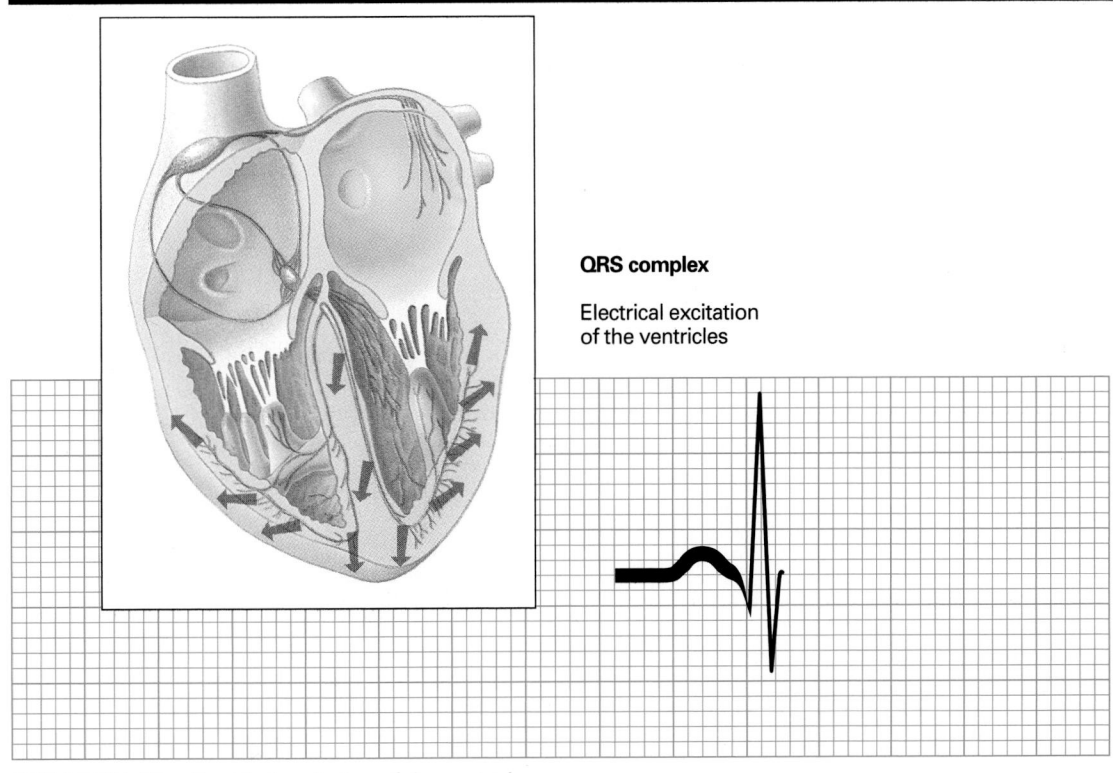

QRS complex

Electrical excitation
of the ventricles

FIGURE 21-22 Electrical excitation of the ventricles.

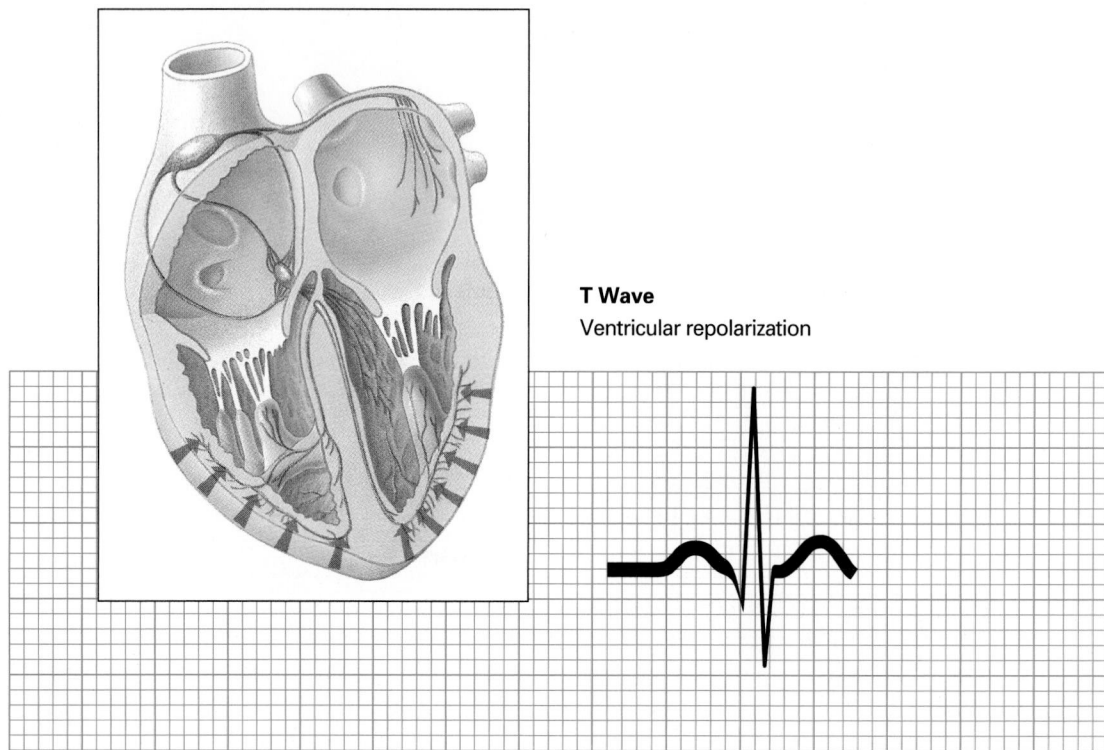

T Wave
Ventricular repolarization

FIGURE 21-23 Ventricular repolarization.

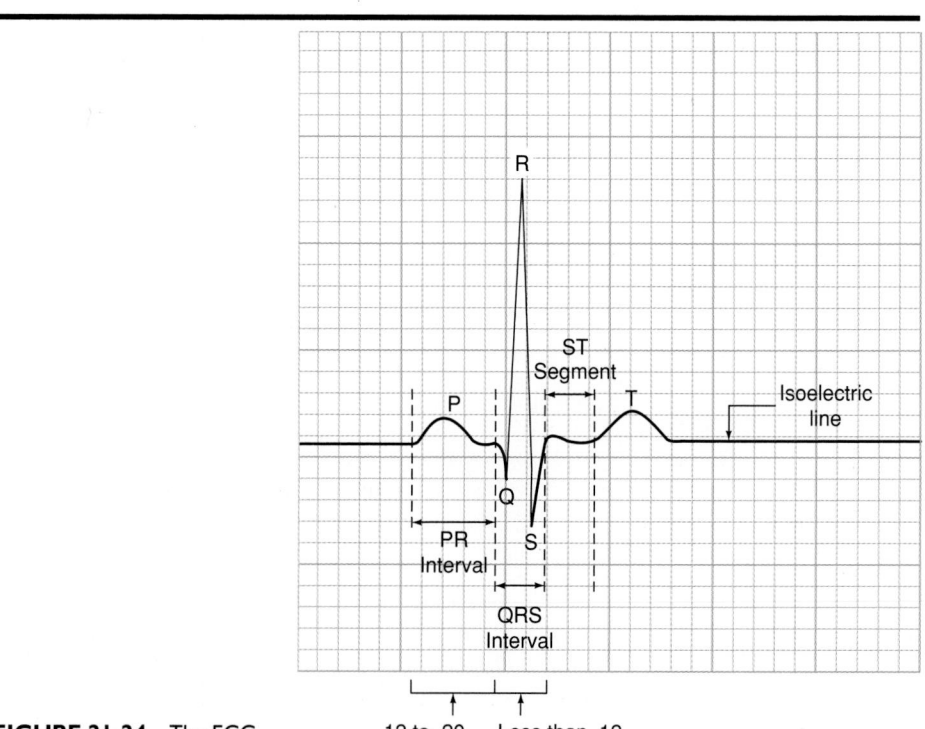

FIGURE 21-24 The ECG.

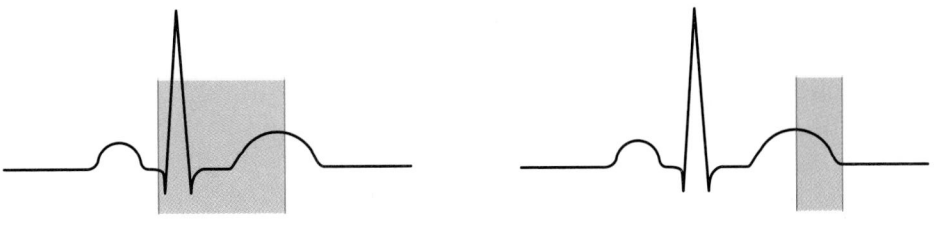

Absolute Refractory Period

Relative Refractory Period

FIGURE 21-25 Refractory periods of the cardiac cycle.

Because of the all-or-none nature of myocardial depolarization, there is a time interval when the heart cannot be restimulated to depolarize. This **refractory period** is a period of time when the myocardial cells have not yet repolarized and cannot be stimulated again. (See Figure 21-25.) There are two aspects of the refractory period—the absolute refractory period and the relative refractory period. The **absolute refractory period** is the time when stimulation will not produce any depolarization whatsoever. This usually lasts from the beginning of the QRS complex to the apex of the T wave. The **relative refractory period** is a period when a sufficiently strong stimulus may produce depolarization. This usually corresponds to the down slope of the T wave.

As mentioned, the autonomic nervous system and the cardiac conductive system are closely interrelated. The vagus nerve provides parasympathetic (cholinergic) control to the SA node and, to a lesser degree, to the AV node. The cardiac plexus innervates the atria and the ventricle and provides sympathetic (adrenergic) control.

Artifacts are deflections on the ECG produced by factors other than the heart's electrical activity. Common causes of artifacts include:

❏ Muscle tremors
❏ Shivering
❏ Patient movement
❏ Loose electrodes
❏ 60 hertz interference
❏ Machine malfunction

■ **refractory period** the period of time when myocardial cells have not yet completely repolarized and cannot be stimulated again.

■ **absolute refractory period** the period of the cardiac cycle when stimulation will not produce any depolarization whatever.

■ **relative refractory period** the period of the cardiac cycle when a sufficiently strong stimulus may produce depolarization.

Interpretation of Rhythm Strips

The key to interpretation of rhythm strips is a logical, systematic approach to each strip. Attempting to "eyeball" the strip in a nonanalytical way often leads to an incorrect interpretation. The analytical approach to rhythm strip interpretation should include the following basic criteria.

1. Always use a consistent analytical approach.
2. Memorize the rules for each dysrhythmia.
3. Analyze a given rhythm strip according to a specific format.
4. Compare your analysis to the rules for each dysrhythmia.
5. Identify the dysrhythmia based upon similarity to established rules.

✳ The key to interpretation of rhythm strips is to approach each in a logical, systematic manner.

Basic Steps   There are several standard formats for ECG analysis. The format presented here includes the following items.

1. Rate
2. Rhythm
3. P waves
4. P-R interval
5. QRS complexes

Step 1: Analyze the Rate.   The first step in ECG strip interpretation is to analyze the heart rate. Usually this means ventricular rate. However, if the atrial and ventricular rates are different, you must calculate both.

The normal heart rate is 60–100 beats per minute. A heart rate greater than 100 beats per minute is a **tachycardia**. A heart rate less than 60 beats per minute is a **bradycardia**.

The rate can be calculated in any of the following ways.

❑ *Six-Second Method.* The heart rate can be calculated by counting the number of complexes within a 6-second interval. Mark off a 6-second interval by noting two 3-second marks at the top of the ECG paper. Then multiply the number of complexes within the 6-second strip by 10, which will give the heart rate per minute.

❑ *Heart Rate Calculator Rulers.* Commercially available heart rate calculator rulers allow you to determine heart rate rapidly. Always use them according to the accompanying directions.

❑ *R-R Interval.* The R-R interval is related directly to heart rate. The R-R interval method is accurate only if the heart rhythm is regular. It can be calculated in the following ways:

1. Measure the duration between R waves in seconds. Divide this number into 60, giving the heart rate per minute.

    Example: 60 ÷ 0.65 second = 92 (heart rate)

2. Count the number of large squares within an R-R interval, and divide the number of squares into 300.

    Example: 300 ÷ 3.5 large boxes = 86 (heart rate)

3. Count the number of small squares within an R-R interval, and divide the number of squares into 1,500.

    Example: 1,500 ÷ 29 small boxes = 52 (heart rate)

❑ *Triplicate Method.* Another method, also useful only with regular rhythms, is to locate an R wave that falls on a dark line bordering a large box on the graph paper. Then assign numbers corresponding to the heart rate to the next six dark lines to the right. The order is: 300, 150, 100, 75, 60, and 50. The number corresponding to the dark line closest to the peak of the next R wave is a rough estimate of the heart rate.

Step 2: Analyze the Rhythm.   The next step is to analyze the rhythm. First, measure the R-R interval across the strip. Normally, the R-R rhythm is fairly regular. Some minimal variation, associated with respirations, should be expected. If the rhythm is irregular, note if it fits one of the following patterns.

❑ Occasionally irregular (only one or two R-R intervals on the strip are irregular)

❑ Regularly irregular (patterned irregularity or group beating)

❑ Irregularly irregular (no relationship between R-R intervals)

■ **tachycardia** a heart rate greater than 100 beats per minute.

■ **bradycardia** a heart rate less than 60 beats per minute.

Step 3: Analyze the P Waves. The P waves reflect atrial depolarization. Normally, the atria depolarize away from the SA node and toward the ventricles. In Lead II, this is seen as a positive, rounded P wave. When analyzing the P waves, ask yourself the following questions.

- ❑ Are P waves present?
- ❑ Are the P waves regular?
- ❑ Is there one P wave for each QRS complex?
- ❑ Are the P waves upright or inverted (compared to the QRS complex)?
- ❑ Do all the P waves look alike?

Step 4: Analyze the P-R Interval. The P-R interval represents the time necessary for atrial depolarization and conduction of the impulse up to the AV node. The normal P-R interval is 0.12–0.20 sec (3–5 small boxes). Any deviation is an abnormal finding. The P-R interval should be consistent across the strip.

Step 5: Analyze the QRS Complex. The QRS complex represents ventricular depolarization. When evaluating the QRS complex, ask yourself the following questions.

- ❑ Do all of the QRS complexes look alike?
- ❑ What is the QRS duration?

The QRS duration is usually 0.04–0.12 sec. Anything longer than 0.12 sec (3 small boxes) is abnormal.

Analysis of a Normal Sinus Rhythm On a normal ECG, the heart rate is between 60 and 100 beats per minute. The rhythm is regular (both P-P and R-R). The P waves are normal in shape, upright, and appear only before each QRS complex. The P-R interval lasts 0.12–0.20 sec and is constant. The QRS complex has a normal morphology, and its duration is less than 0.12 sec. All of these factors indicate a normal sinus rhythm.

Introduction to Dysrhythmias

Any deviation from the heart's normal electrical rhythm is a **dysrhythmia.** (Absence of cardiac electric activity is called **arrhythmia.**) The causes of dysrhythmias include:

- ❑ Myocardial ischemia, necrosis, or infarction
- ❑ Autonomic nervous system imbalance
- ❑ Distention of the chambers of the heart (especially in the atria, secondary to congestive heart failure)
- ❑ Blood gas abnormalities, including hypoxia and abnormal pH
- ❑ Electrolyte imbalances (Ca^{++}, K^+, Mg^{++})
- ❑ Trauma to the myocardium (cardiac contusion)
- ❑ Drug effects and drug toxicity
- ❑ Electrocution
- ❑ Hypothermia
- ❑ CNS damage
- ❑ Idiopathic events
- ❑ Normal occurrences

■ **dysrhythmia** any deviation from the normal electrical rhythm of the heart.

■ **arrhythmia** the absence of cardiac electrical activity; often used interchangeably with dysrhythmia.

Dysrhythmias that occur in the healthy heart are of little significance. NO MATTER WHAT THE ETIOLOGY OR TYPE OF DYSRHYTHMIA, THE PATIENT AND HIS OR HER SYMPTOMS ARE TREATED, NOT THE DYSRHYTHMIA.

Mechanism of Impulse Formation   Several physiologic mechanisms can result in cardiac dysrhythmias. The depolarization impulse is normally transmitted through the conductive system and the myocardium. When the impulse is conducted normally, it is said to be conducted *antegrade*. However, in certain dysrhythmias, the depolarization impulse is conducted backwards. Backward conduction is said to be *retrograde*.

Ectopic Foci.   One cause of dysrhythmias is *enhanced automaticity*. This condition results when heart cells other than the pacemaker cells automatically depolarize, producing a contraction. Depolarizations that occur from cells other than the normal pacemakers are referred to as **ectopic beats**. Premature ventricular contractions and premature atrial contractions are examples of ectopic beats. The ectopic beat can be intermittent or sustained.

■ **ectopic beats** cardiac depolarization resulting from depolarization of cells in the heart that are not a part of the heart's normal pacemaker.

Reentry.   The phenomenon of *reentry* may be responsible for isolated premature beats, or *tachydysrhythmias*. Reentry occurs when two branches of a conduction pathway are altered by ischemia or other disease processes. Conduction is slowed in one branch, while the other has a unidirectional block. The depolarization wave is conducted slowly, in an antegrade fashion, through the branch with ischemia. It is blocked in the branch with a unidirectional block. After the depolarization wave is conducted through the slowed branch, it enters the branch with the unidirectional block and is conducted retrograde back to the origin of the branch. By this time, the tissue is no longer refractory, and stimulation again occurs. This can result in the development of rapid rhythms, such as paroxysmal supraventricular tachycardia or atrial fibrillation.

Classification of Dysrhythmias   Dysrhythmias can be classified in any number of ways. Examples of classification methods include:

- ❏ Changes in automaticity versus disturbances in conduction
- ❏ Major versus minor dysrhythmias
- ❏ Life-threatening versus non-life-threatening dysrhythmias
- ❏ Site of origin

This text classifies dysrhythmias by site of origin. The approach is closely related to basic physiology, so it is easy to understand. The dysrhythmias addressed in this section include the following categories.

Dysrhythmias Originating in the SA Node
- ❏ Sinus bradycardia
- ❏ Sinus tachycardia
- ❏ Sinus dysrhythmia
- ❏ Sinus arrest

Dysrhythmias Originating in the Atria
- ❏ Wandering pacemaker
- ❏ Premature atrial contractions
- ❏ Paroxysmal supraventricular tachycardia
- ❏ Atrial flutter
- ❏ Atrial fibrillation

Dysrhythmias Originating in the AV Junction

- ❏ Premature junctional contractions
- ❏ Junctional escape complexes and rhythm
- ❏ Accelerated junctional rhythm
- ❏ Paroxysmal junctional tachycardia

Dysrhythmias Originating in the Ventricles

- ❏ Ventricular escape complexes and rhythm
- ❏ Premature ventricular complexes
- ❏ Ventricular tachycardia
- ❏ Ventricular fibrillation
- ❏ Asystole
- ❏ Artificial pacemaker rhythm

Dysrhythmias Resulting From Disorders of Conduction

- ❏ AV blocks
  - First-degree AV block
  - Second-degree AV block (Mobitz I), or *Wenkebach phenomenon*
  - Second-degree AV block (Mobitz II)
  - Third-degree AV block
- ❏ Disturbances of ventricular conduction
- ❏ Pre-excitation syndrome

DYSRHYTHMIAS ORIGINATING IN THE SA NODE

Dysrhythmias originating in the SA node most often result from changes in autonomic tone. However, disease can exist in the SA node itself. Dysrhythmias that originate in the SA node include:

❑ Sinus bradycardia
❑ Sinus tachycardia
❑ Sinus dysrhythmia
❑ Sinus arrest

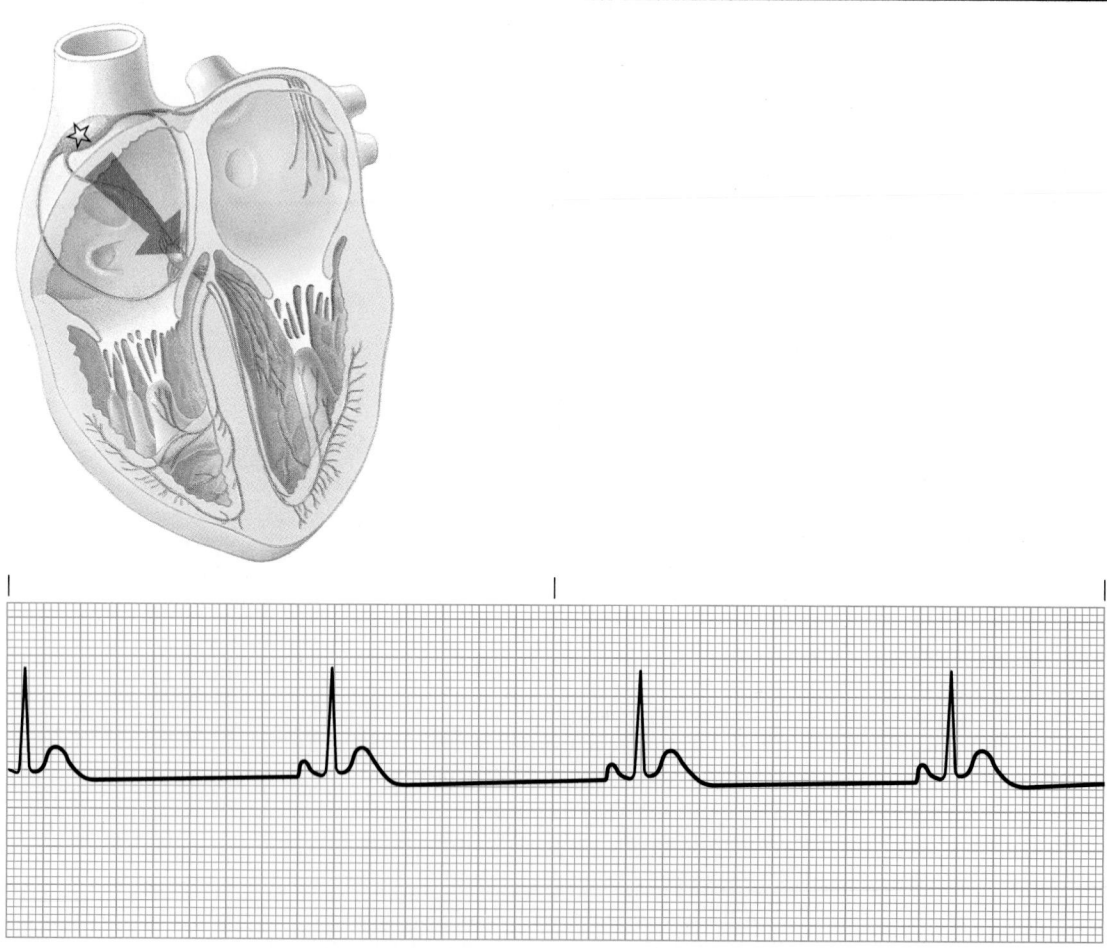

FIGURE 21-26 Sinus bradycardia.

Several ECG features are common to all dysrhythmias that originate in the SA node. These include:

❑ Upright P waves in Lead II
❑ Similar appearance in all P waves
❑ Normal P-R interval
❑ Normal QRS complex duration

Sinus Bradycardia

Description: *Sinus bradycardia* results from slowing of the SA node.

Etiology: Sinus bradycardia may result from any of the following conditions.

❑ Increased parasympathetic (vagal) tone
❑ Intrinsic disease of the SA node
❑ Drug effects (digitalis, propranolol, quinidine)

Sinus bradycardia is a normal finding in healthy, well-conditioned persons.

Rules of Interpretation/Lead II Monitoring (See Figure 21-26.)
    Rate: Less than 60
    Rhythm: Regular
    Pacemaker Site: SA node
    P Waves: Upright and normal in morphology
    P-R Interval: 0.12–0.20 sec and constant (normal)
    QRS Complex: 0.04–0.12 sec (normal)

Clinical Significance: The decreased heart rate can result in decreased cardiac output, hypotension, angina, or CNS symptoms. This is especially true for rates less than 50 beats per minute. Because of the slow heart rate, atrial ectopic or ventricular ectopic rhythms may occur.

Treatment: Treatment is unnecessary unless hypotension or ventricular irritability is present. If treatment is required, administer a 0.5 mg bolus of atropine sulfate. This can be repeated every 3–5 minutes until a satisfactory rate has been obtained or 0.04 mg/kg of the drug has been given. If atropine fails, consider transcutaneous cardiac pacing (TCP), if available. Isoproterenol is rarely required.

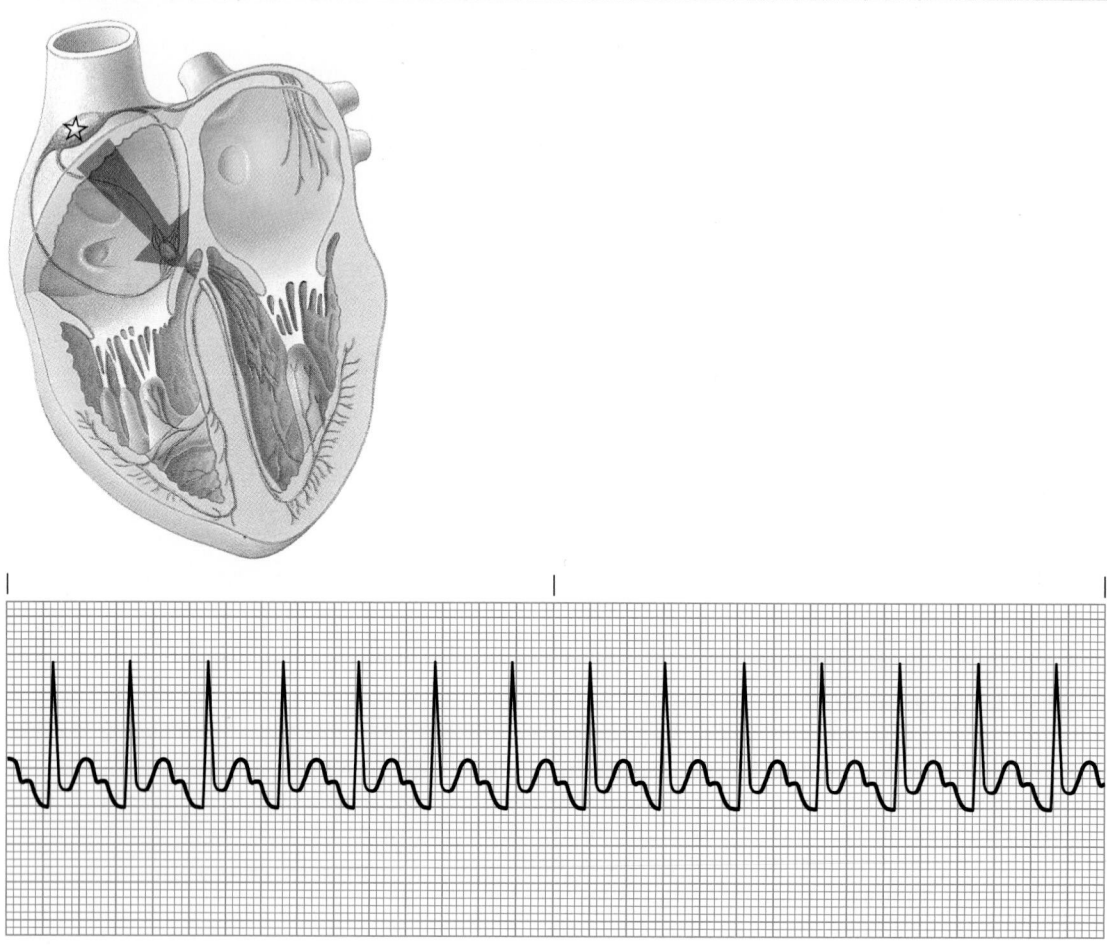

FIGURE 21-27 Sinus tachycardia.

Sinus Tachycardia

Description: *Sinus tachycardia* results from an increase in the rate of SA node discharge.

Etiology: Sinus tachycardia may result from any of the following conditions.

- ❏ Exercise
- ❏ Fever
- ❏ Anxiety
- ❏ Hypovolemia
- ❏ Anemia
- ❏ Pump failure
- ❏ Increased sympathetic tone

Rules of Interpretation/Lead II Monitoring (See Figure 21-27.)
    Rate: Greater than 100
    Rhythm: Regular
    Pacemaker Site: SA node
    P Waves: Upright and normal in morphology
    P-R Interval: 0.12–0.20 sec and constant (normal)
    QRS Complex: 0.04–0.12 sec (normal)

Clinical Significance: Sinus tachycardia is often a benign process. In some cases, it is a compensatory mechanism for decreased stroke volume. If the rate is greater than 140 beats per minute, cardiac output may fall because ventricular filling time is inadequate. Very rapid heart rates increase myocardial oxygen demand and can precipitate ischemia or infarct in diseased hearts. Prolonged sinus tachycardia accompanying acute MI is often an ominous finding suggestive of cardiogenic shock.

Treatment: Treatment is directed at the underlying cause. Hypovolemia or other causes should be corrected.

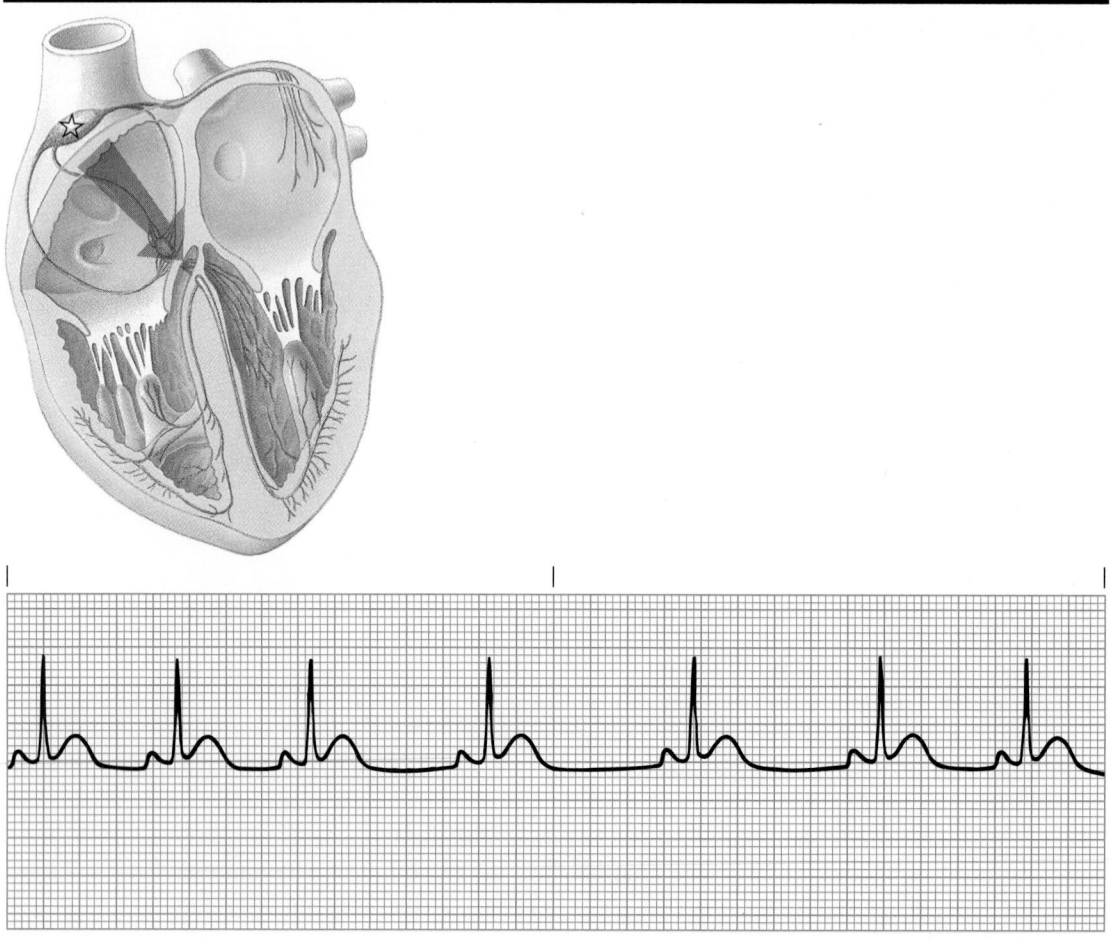

FIGURE 21-28 Sinus dysrhythmia.

Sinus Dysrhythmia

Description: *Sinus dysrhythmia* often results from a phasic variation of the R-R interval.

Etiology: Sinus dysrhythmia is often a normal finding and is sometimes related to the respiratory cycle and changes in intrathoracic pressure. Pathologically, sinus dysrhythmia can be caused by enhanced vagal tone.

Rules of Interpretation/Lead II Monitoring (See Figure 21-28.)
> *Rate:* 60–100 (varies with respirations)
> *Rhythm:* Irregular
> *Pacemaker Site:* SA node
> *P Waves:* Upright and normal in morphology
> *P-R Interval:* 0.12–0.20 sec
> *QRS Complex:* 0.04–0.12 sec

Clinical Significance: Sinus dysrhythmia is a normal variant, particularly in the young and the aged.

Treatment: Typically, none required.

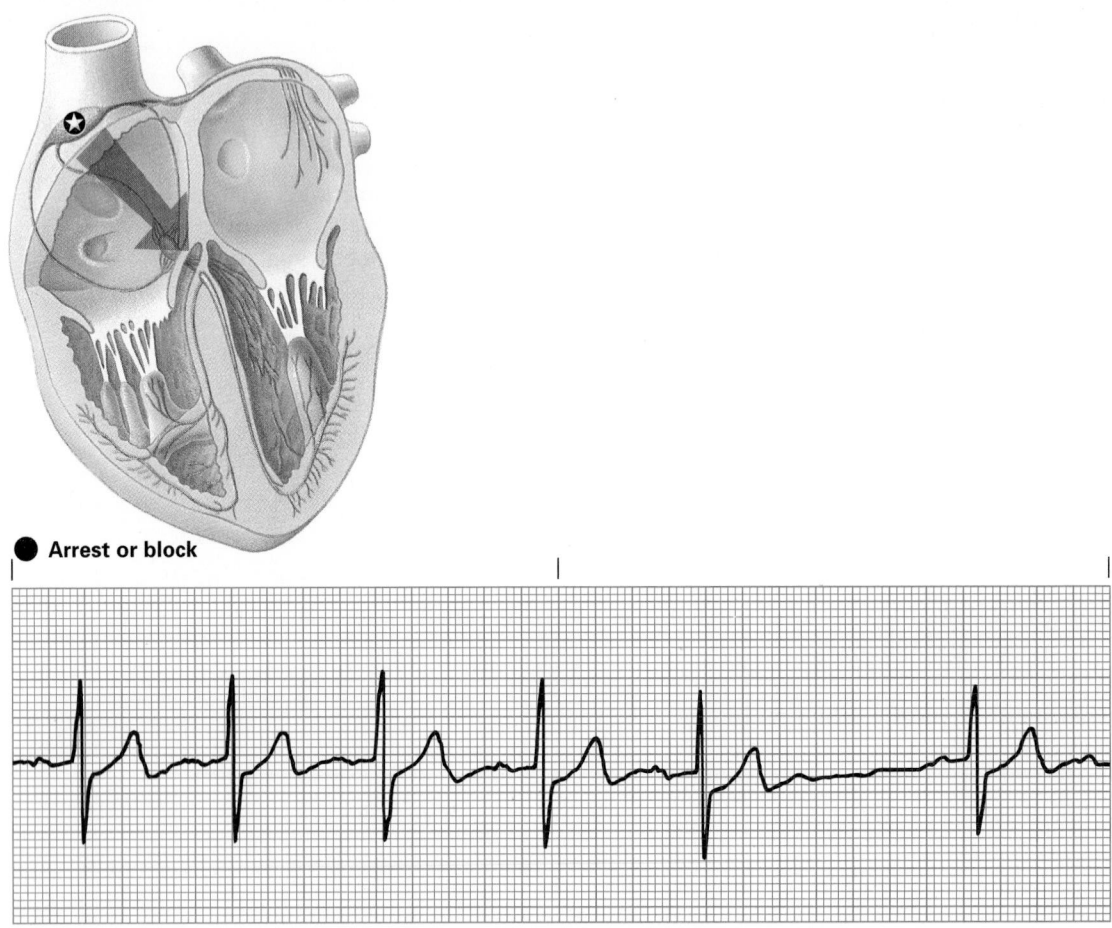

Arrest or block

FIGURE 21-29 Sinus arrest.

Sinus Arrest

Description: *Sinus arrest* is an episode of failure of the sinus node to discharge, resulting in short periods of cardiac standstill. This standstill can persist until pacemaker cells lower in the conductive system discharge (escape beats) or until the sinus node resumes discharge.

Etiology: Sinus arrest can result from any of the following conditions.

❑ Ischemia of the SA node
❑ Digitalis toxicity
❑ Excessive vagal tone
❑ Degenerative fibrotic disease

Rules of Interpretation/Lead II Monitoring (See Figure 21-29.)
   Rate: Normal to slow depending on the frequency and duration of the arrest
   Rhythm: Irregular
   Pacemaker Site: SA node
   P Waves: Upright and normal in morphology
   P-R Interval: 0.12–0.20 sec and constant
   QRS Complex: 0.04–0.12 sec

Clinical Significance: Frequent or prolonged episodes may compromise cardiac output, resulting in syncope and other problems. There is always the danger of complete cessation of SA node activity. Usually, an escape rhythm develops. However, cardiac standstill can occasionally result.

Treatment: If the patient is asymptomatic, then observation is all that is required. If the patient is extremely bradycardic or symptomatic, administer a 0.5 mg bolus of atropine sulfate. This can be repeated every 3–5 minutes until a satisfactory rate has been obtained or 0.04 mg/kg of the drug has been administered. If atropine fails, consider transcutaneous cardiac pacing (TCP), if available. Isoproterenol is rarely required.

DYSRHYTHMIAS ORIGINATING IN THE ATRIA

Dysrhythmias can originate outside the SA node in the tissue of the atria or in the internodal pathways. Ischemia, hypoxia, atrial dilation, and other factors can cause atrial dysrhythmias. Dysrhythmias originating in the atria include:

❑ Wandering pacemaker
❑ Premature atrial contractions
❑ Paroxysmal supraventricular tachycardia
❑ Atrial flutter
❑ Atrial fibrillation

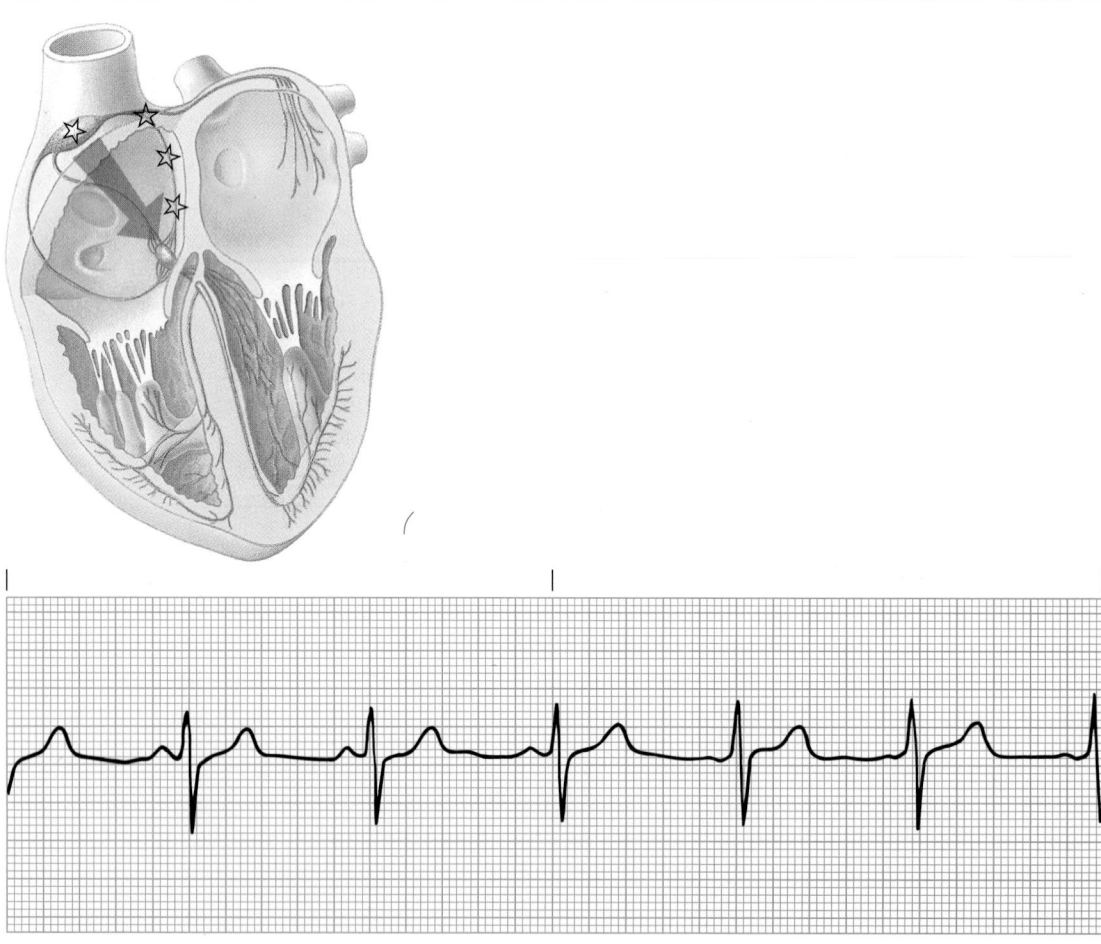

FIGURE 21-30 Wandering pacemaker.

Several ECG features are common to all dysrhythmias that originate in the atria. These include:

❑ P waves differ in appearance from sinus P waves
❑ The P-R interval may be normal, shortened, or prolonged
❑ Normal QRS complex duration

Wandering Pacemaker

Description: *Wandering pacemaker*, often called wandering atrial pacemaker, is the passive transfer of pacemaker sites from the sinus node to other latent pacemaker sites in the atria and AV junction. Often, more than one pacemaker site will be present, causing variation in R-R interval and P wave morphology.

Etiology: Wandering atrial pacemaker can result from any of the following conditions.

❑ A variant of sinus dysrhythmia
❑ A normal phenomenon in the very young or the aged
❑ Ischemic heart disease
❑ Atrial dilation

Rules of Interpretation/Lead II Monitoring (See Figure 21-30.)
   Rate: Usually normal
   Rhythm: Slightly irregular
   Pacemaker Site: Varies between the SA node, atrial tissue, and the AV junction
   P Waves: Morphology changes from beat to beat; P waves may disappear entirely.
   P-R Interval: Varies. May be less than 0.12 sec, normal, or greater than 0.20 sec.
   QRS Complex: 0.04–0.12 sec

Clinical Significance: Wandering pacemaker usually has no detrimental effects. Occasionally, it can be a precursor of other atrial dysrhythmias, such as atrial fibrillation. It sometimes indicates digitalis toxicity.

Treatment: If the patient is asymptomatic, observation is all that is required.

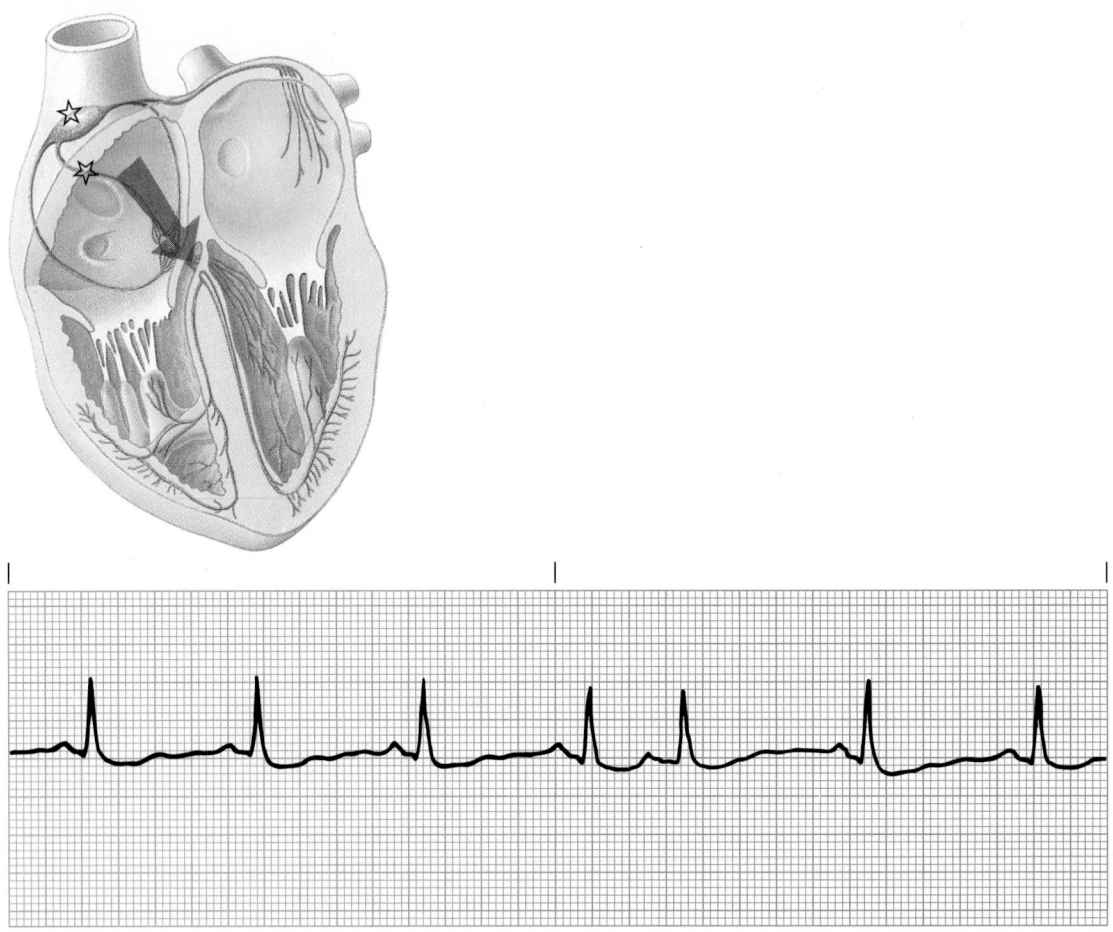

FIGURE 21-31 Premature atrial contractions.

Premature Atrial Contractions

Description: *Premature atrial contractions (PAC)* result from a single electrical impulse originating in the atria outside the SA node, which in turn causes a premature depolarization of the heart before the next expected sinus beat. Because it results in depolarization of the atrial syncytium, this impulse also depolarizes the SA node, interrupting the normal cadence. This creates a **noncompensatory pause** in the underlying rhythm.

Etiology: A premature atrial contraction can result from any of the following conditions.

❑ Use of caffeine, tobacco, or alcohol
❑ Sympathomimetic drugs
❑ Ischemic heart disease
❑ Hypoxia
❑ Digitalis toxicity
❑ No apparent cause

Rules of Interpretation/Lead II Monitoring (See Figure 21-31.)

Rate: Depends on the underlying rhythm

Rhythm: Depends on the underlying rhythm; usually regular except for the PAC

Pacemaker Site: Ectopic focus in the atrium

P Waves: The P wave of the PAC differs from the P wave of the underlying rhythm. It occurs earlier than the next expected P wave and may be hidden in the preceding T wave.

P-R Interval: Usually normal; however, can vary with the location of the ectopic focus. Ectopic foci near the SA node will have a P-R interval of 0.12 sec or greater, whereas ectopic foci near the AV node will have a P-R interval of 0.12 sec or less.

QRS Complex: Normal, 0.04–0.12 sec. However, it may be greater than 0.12 sec if the PAC is abnormally conducted through partially refractory ventricles. In some cases, the ventricles are in the refractory period and will not depolarize in response to the PAC. In these cases, the QRS complex is absent.

Clinical Significance: Isolated PACs are of minimal significance. Frequent PACs may indicate organic heart disease and may be forerunners of other atrial dysrhythmias.

Treatment: If the patient is asymptomatic, observation is all that is required in the field.

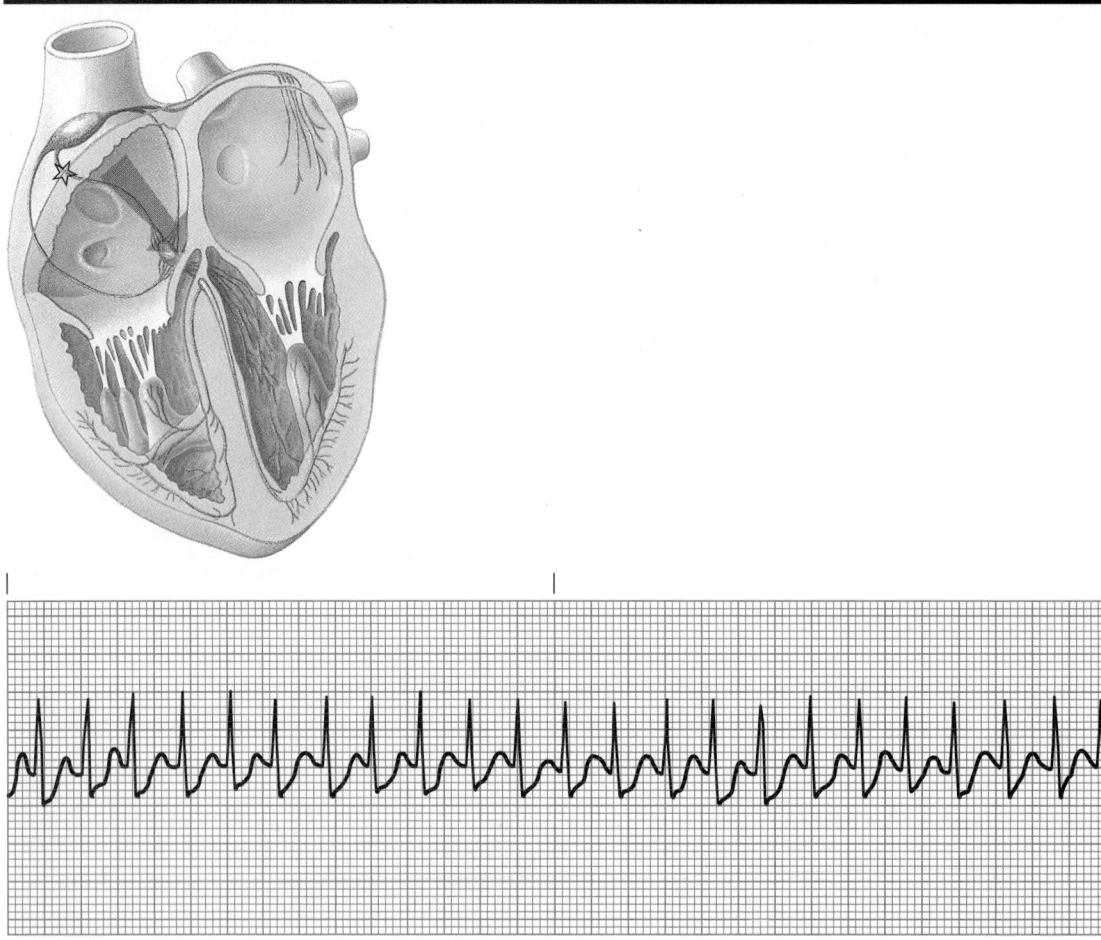

FIGURE 21-32   Paroxysmal supraventricular tachycardia.

Paroxysmal Supraventricular Tachycardia

Description: *Paroxysmal supraventricular tachycardia (PSVT)* occurs when rapid atrial depolarization overrides the SA node. It often occurs in paroxysm with sudden onset, may last minutes to hours, and terminates abruptly. It may be caused by increased automaticity of a single atrial focus or by reentry phenomenon at the AV node.

Etiology: Paroxysmal supraventricular tachycardia may occur at any age and often is not associated with underlying heart disease. It may be precipitated by stress, overexertion, smoking, or ingestion of caffeine. However, it is frequently associated with underlying atherosclerotic cardiovascular disease and rheumatic heart disease. PSVT is rare in patients with myocardial infarction. It can occur with accessory pathway conduction, such as Wolff-Parkinson-White syndrome.

Rules of Interpretation/Lead II Monitoring (See Figure 21-32.)
   Rate: 150–250 per minute
   Rhythm: Characteristically regular, except at onset and termination
   Pacemaker Site: In the atria, outside the SA node
   P Waves: The atrial P waves differ slightly from sinus P waves. The P wave is often buried in the preceding T wave. The P wave may be impossible to see, especially if the rate is rapid. Turning up the speed of the graph paper or oscilloscope to 50 mm/sec spreads out the complex and can aid in the identification of P waves.
   P-R Interval: Usually normal. However, it can vary with the location of the ectopic pacemaker. Ectopic pacemakers near the SA node will have P-R intervals close to 0.12 sec, whereas ectopic pacemakers near the AV node will have P-R intervals of 0.12 sec or less.
   QRS Complex: Normal; 0.04–0.12 sec

Clinical Significance: Young patients with good cardiac reserves may tolerate PSVT well for short periods of time. Patients often sense PSVT as palpitations. However, rapid rates can cause a marked reduction in cardiac output because of inadequate ventricular filling time. Coronary artery perfusion can also be compromised, since the diastolic phase of the cardiac cycle is reduced. PSVT can precipitate angina, hypotension, or congestive heart failure.

(continued)

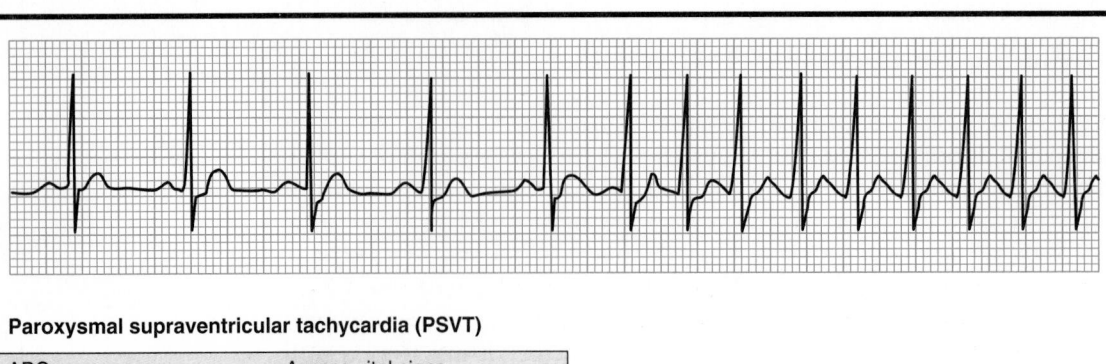

Paroxysmal supraventricular tachycardia (PSVT)

• Assess ABCs   • Assess vital signs • Secure airway   • Review history • Administer oxygen   • Perform physical examination • Start IV   • Order 12-lead ECG • Attach monitor, pulse oximeter, and   • Order portable chest   automatic sphygmomanometer   roentgenogram

If ventricular rate > 150 beats/ min
- Prepare for immediate cardioversion
- May give brief trial of medications based on arrhythmia
- Immediate cardioversion is seldom needed for heart rates < 150 beats/ min

Unstable, with serious signs or symptoms* — Yes →

No or borderline

Atrial fibrillation
Atrial flutter†

Consider use of
- *Diltiazem*
- β-*Blockers*
- *Verapamil*
- *Digoxin*
- *Procainamide*
- *Quinidine*
- *Anticoagulants*

Paroxysmal supraventricular tachycardia (PSVT)

Vagal maneuvers†

- *Adenosine* 6 mg, rapid IV push over 1–3s

  1-2 min

- *Adenosine* 12 mg, rapid IV push over 1—3s (may repeat once in 1–2 min)

Complex width ?

Narrow / Width‡

Blood pressure?

Normal or elevated / Low or unstable

- *Verapamil* 2.5–5 mg IV

  15-30 min

- *Verapamil* 5–10 mg IV

Consider
- *Digoxin*
- β-*Blockers*
- *Diltiazem*

Wide-complex tachycardia of uncertain type

- *Lidocaine* 1–1.5 mg/ kg IV push

  Every 15–30 min

- *Lidocaine* 0.5–0.75 mg/ kg IV push, maximum total 3 mg/ kg

- *Adenosine* 6 mg, rapid IV push over 1–3s

  1–2 min

- *Adenosine* 12 mg, rapid IV push over 1–3s (may repeat once in 1–2 min)

Ventricular tachycardia (VT)

- *Lidocaine* 1–1.5 mg/ kg IV push

  Every 5–10 min

- *Lidocaine* 0.5–0.75 mg/ kg IV push, maximum total 3 mg/ kg

- *Procainamide* 20–30 mg/ min, maximum total 17 mg/ kg

- *Bretylium* 5–10 mg/ kg over 8–10 min, maximum total 30 mg/ kg over 24 hours

---

- *Lidocaine* 1–1.5 mg/ kg IV push

- *Procainamide* 20–30 mg/ min, maximum total 17 mg/ kg

Synchronized cardioversion

---

* Unstable condition must be related to the tachycardia. Signs and symptoms may include chest pain, shortness of breath, decreased level of consciousness, low blood pressure (BP), shock, pulmonary congestion, congestive heart failure, acute myocardial infarction.
† Carotid sinus pressure is contraindicated in patients with carotid bruits; avoid ice water immersion in patients with ischemic heart disease.
‡ If the wide-complex tachycardia is known with certainty to be PSVT and BP is normal/ elevated, sequence can include *verapamil*.

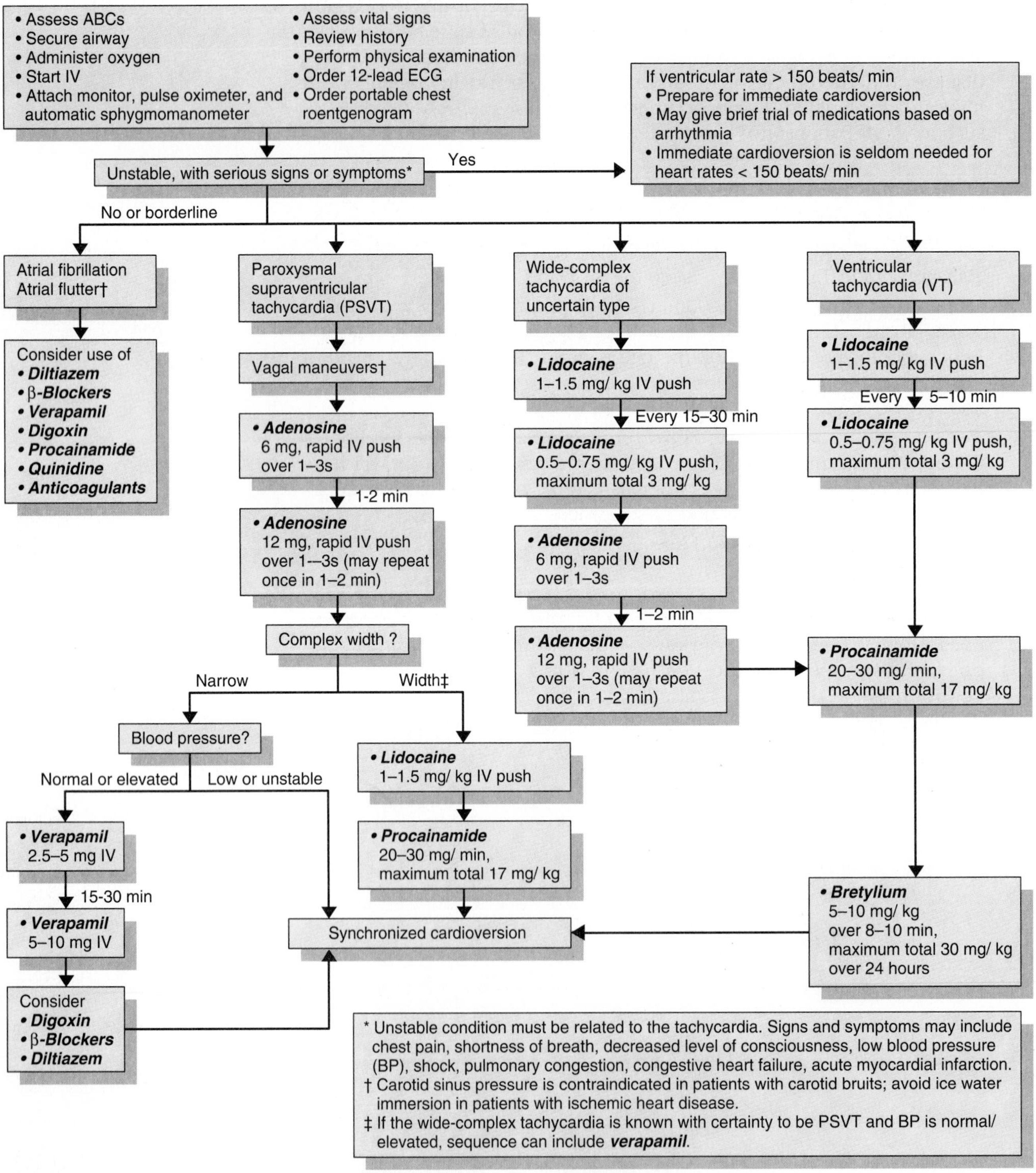

FIGURE 21-33 Recommended treatment of paroxysmal supraventricular tachycardia.

Paroxysmal Supraventricular Tachycardia (continued)

Treatment: If the patient is not tolerating the rapid heart rate, as evidenced by hemodynamic instability, attempt the following techniques in the order in which they are given. (See Figure 21-33.)

1. *Vagal Maneuvers.* Ask the patient to perform a Valsalva maneuver. This is a forced expiration against a closed glottis, or the act of "bearing down" as if to move the bowels. This results in vagal stimulation, which may slow the heart. If this is unsuccessful, attempt carotid artery massage, if the patient is eligible. Do not attempt this in patients with carotid **bruits** or known cerebrovascular or carotid artery disease.

   ■ **bruit** the sound of turbulent blood flow through a vessel; usually associated with atherosclerotic disease.

2. *Pharmacological Therapy.* Adenosine (Adenocard) is relatively safe and highly effective in terminating PSVT. This is especially true if the etiology of the dysrhythmia is reentry. Administer 6 mg of adenosine by rapid IV bolus over 1–3 sec through the medication port closest to the patient's heart or central circulation. If the patient does not convert after 1–2 minutes, administer a second bolus of 12 mg over 1–3 sec in the medication port closest to the patient's heart or central circulation. If this fails, and the patient has a normal blood pressure, medical control may request the administration of verapamil. Verapamil is contraindicated in patients with a history of bradycardia, hypotension, or congestive heart failure. It should not be used with intravenous beta blockers. It should be used with caution in patients on chronic beta blocker therapy. Hypotension that occurs following verapamil administration can often be reversed with 0.5–1.0 gm of calcium chloride administered intravenously.

3. *Electrical Therapy.* If the ventricular rate is greater than 150 beats per minute, or if the patient is hemodynamically unstable, synchronized cardioversion should be utilized. If time allows, sedate the patient with 5–10 mg of diazepam IV. Apply synchronized DC countershock of 100 joules. If this is unsuccessful, repeat the countershock at increased energy as ordered by the medical control physician. DC countershock is contraindicated if digitalis toxicity is suspected as the cause of the PSVT.

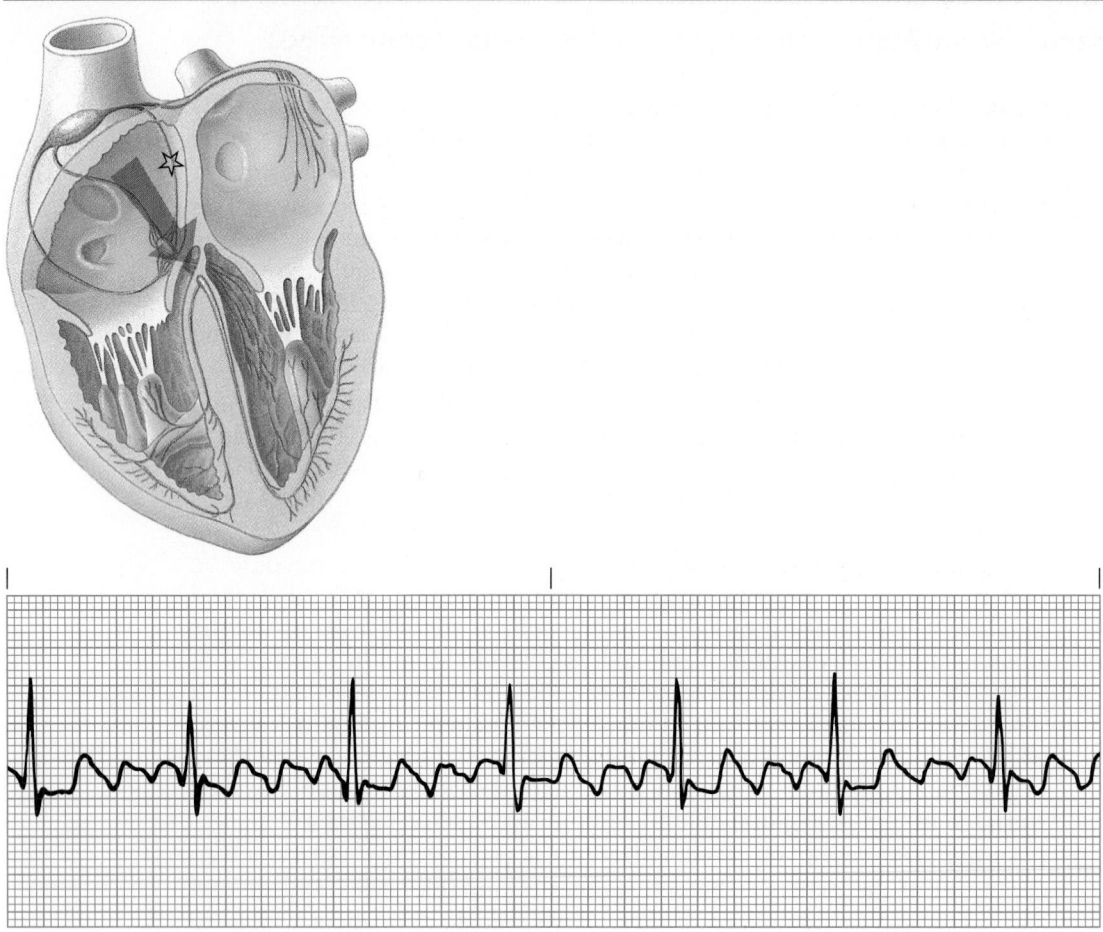

FIGURE 21-34 Atrial flutter.

Atrial Flutter

Description: *Atrial flutter* results from a rapid atrial reentry circuit and an AV node that physiologically cannot conduct all impulses through to the ventricles. The AV junction may allow impulses in a 1:1 (rare), 2:1, 3:1, or 4:1 ratio or greater, resulting in a discrepancy between atrial and ventricular rates. The AV block may be consistent or variable.

Etiology: Atrial flutter may occur in normal hearts, but it is usually associated with organic disease. It rarely occurs as the direct result of an MI. Atrial dilation, which occurs with congestive heart failure, is a cause.

Rules of Interpretation/Lead II Monitoring (See Figure 21-34.)

Rate: Atrial rate is 250–350 per minute. Ventricular rate varies with the ratio of AV conduction.

Rhythm: Atrial rhythm is regular. Ventricular rhythm is usually regular, but can be irregular if the block is variable.

Pacemaker Site: Sites in the atria outside the SA node

P Waves: Flutter (F) waves are present, resembling a sawtooth or picket-fence pattern. This pattern is often difficult to identify in a 2:1 flutter. However, if the ventricular rate is greater than 150, 2:1 flutter should be suspected.

P-R Interval: The P-R interval is usually constant but may vary.

QRS Complex: Normal, 0.04–0.12 sec

Clinical Significance: Atrial flutter with normal ventricular rates is generally well tolerated. Rapid ventricular rates may compromise cardiac output and result in symptoms. Atrial flutter often occurs in conjunction with atrial fibrillation and is referred to as "atrial fib-flutter."

Treatment: Treatment is indicated only for rapid ventricular rates with hemodynamic compromise. (See Figure 21-36 on page 650.)

1. *Electrical Therapy.* Immediate cardioversion is indicated in unstable patients. Unstable patients are those with heart rates greater than 150 with associated chest pain, dyspnea, a decreased level of consciousness, or hypotension. If time allows, sedate the patient with 5–10 mg of diazepam IV. Then apply synchronized DC countershock of 100 joules. If this is unsuccessful, repeat the countershock at increased energy as ordered by the medical control physician.

2. *Pharmacological Therapy.* Pharmacological therapy is utilized occasionally in patients with atrial flutter who are stable. This is especially true in cases where the rapid heart rate is causing congestive heart failure. Several medications are available to slow the ventricular rate. The most frequently used drug is diltiazem (Cardizem). In addition, verapamil, digoxin, beta blockers, procainamide, and quinidine can be used. Consult medical control or refer to local protocols concerning pharmacological therapy of atrial flutter.

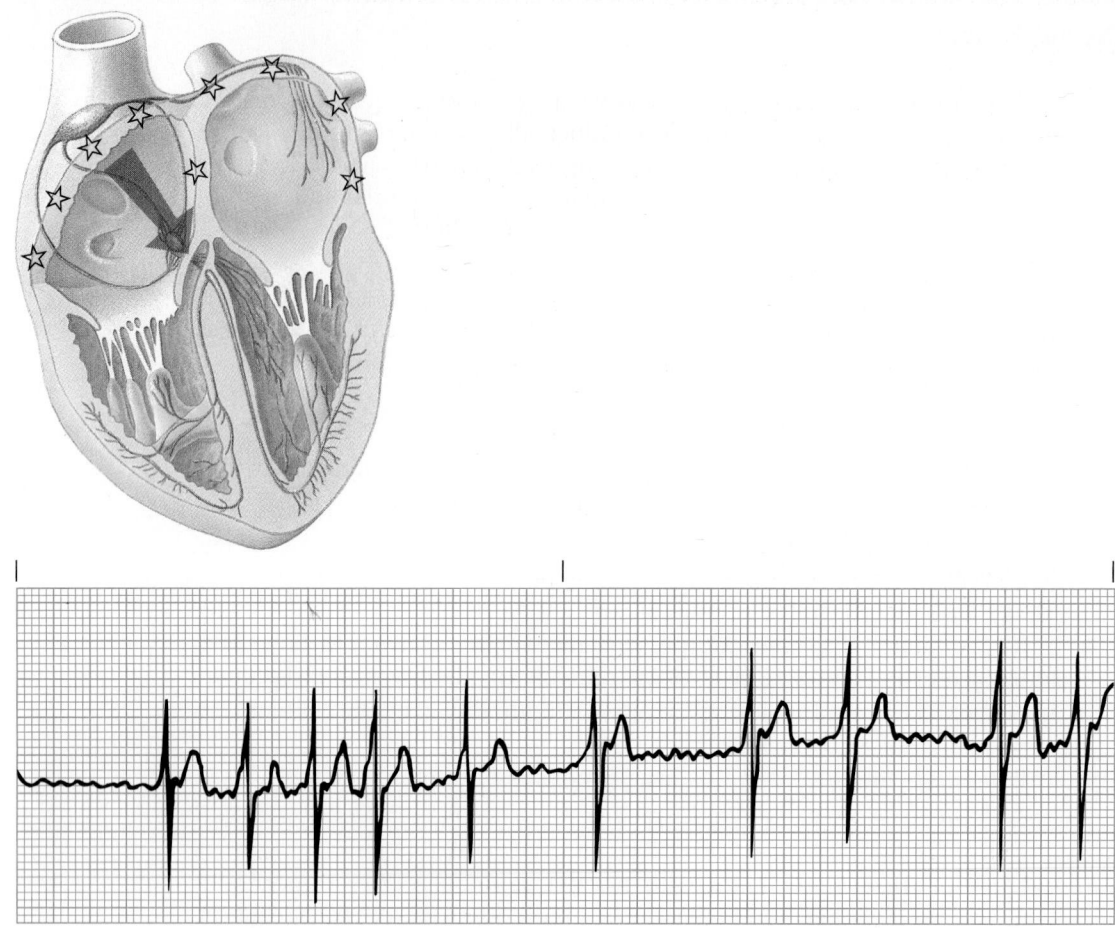

FIGURE 21-35 Atrial fibrillation.

Atrial Fibrillation

Description: *Atrial fibrillation* is a dysrhythmia that results from multiple areas of reentry within the atria or from multiple ectopic foci bombarding an AV node that physiologically cannot handle all of the incoming impulses. AV conduction is random and highly variable.

Etiology: Atrial fibrillation may be chronic and is often associated with underlying heart disease such as rheumatic heart disease, atherosclerotic heart disease, or congestive heart failure. Atrial dilation occurs with congestive heart failure and is often the cause of atrial fibrillation.

Rules of Interpretation/Lead II Monitoring (See Figure 21-35.)

Rate: Atrial rate is 350–750 per minute (cannot be counted). Ventricular rate varies greatly depending on conduction through the AV node.

Rhythm: Irregularly irregular.

Pacemaker Site: Numerous ectopic foci in the atria

P Waves: No discernible P waves are present. Fibrillation (f) waves are present, indicating chaotic atrial activity.

P-R Interval: None

QRS Complex: Normal, 0.04–0.12 sec

Clinical Significance: In atrial fibrillation, the atria fail to contract and the so-called "*atrial kick*" is lost, thus reducing cardiac output by 20–25 percent. There is frequently a *pulse deficit* (a difference between the apical and peripheral pulse rates). If the rate of ventricular response is normal, as often occurs in patients on digitalis, the rhythm is usually well tolerated. If the ventricular rate is less than 60, cardiac output can fall. Digitalis toxicity should be suspected in patients with atrial fibrillation with a ventricular rate of less than 60. If the ventricular response is rapid, coupled by the loss of "atrial kick," cardiovascular decompensation may occur, resulting in hypotension, angina, infarct, congestive heart failure, or shock.

(continued)

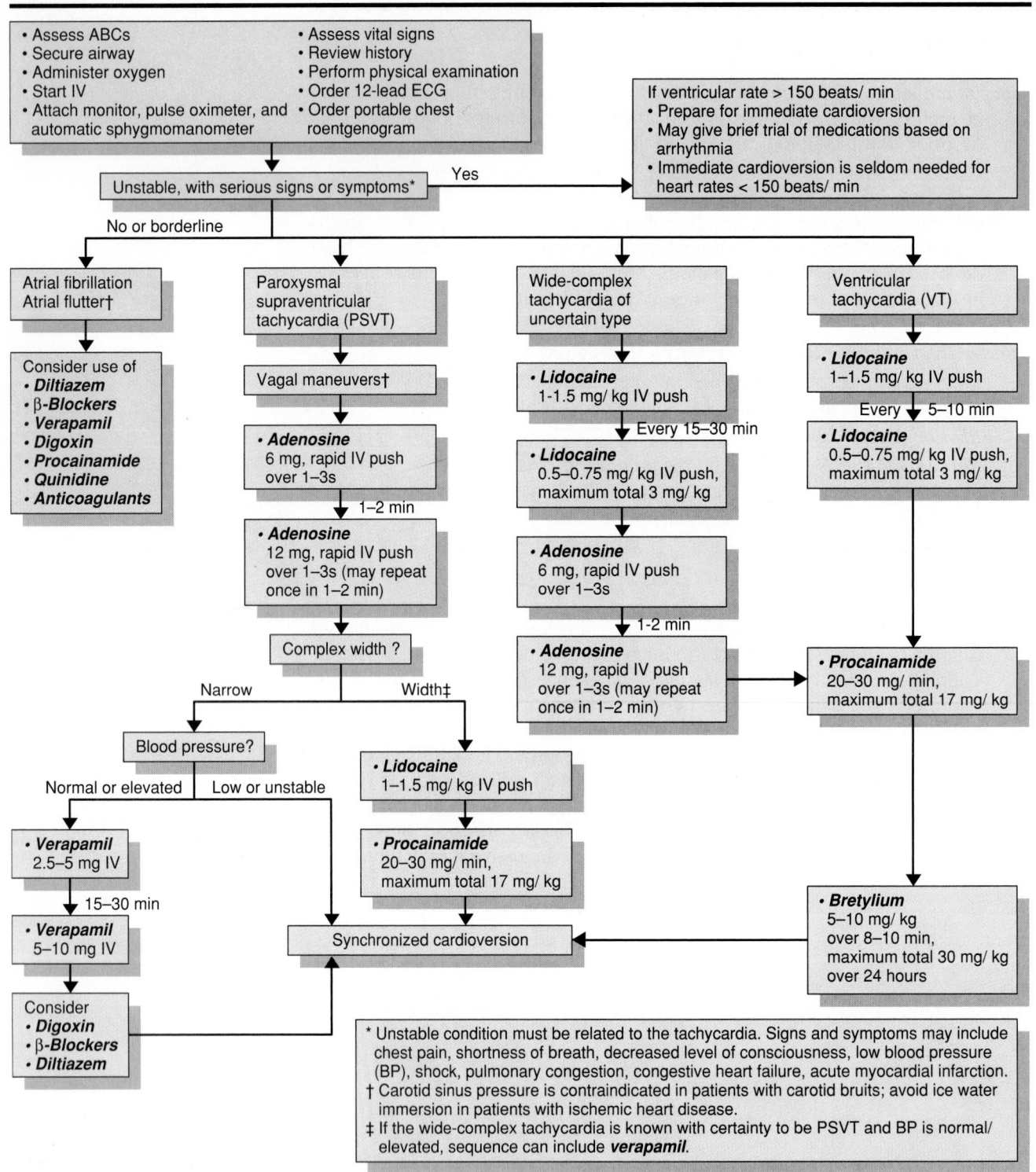

FIGURE 21-36 Recommended treatment of atrial fibrillation and atrial flutter.

Atrial Fibrillation (continued)

Treatment: Treatment is indicated only for rapid ventricular rates with hemo-dynamic compromise. (See Figure 21-36.)

1. *Electrical Therapy.* Immediate cardioversion is indicated in unstable patients. Unstable patients are those with heart rates greater than 150 with associated chest pain, dyspnea, a decreased level of consciousness, or hypotension. If time allows, sedate the patient with 5–10 mg of diazepam IV. Then apply synchronized DC countershock of 100 joules. If this is unsuccessful, repeat the countershock at increased energy as ordered by the medical control physician.

2. *Pharmacological Therapy.* Pharmacological therapy is utilized occasion-ally in patients with atrial fibrillation who are stable. This is especially true in cases where the rapid heart rate is causing congestive heart fail-ure. Several medications are available to slow the ventricular rate. The most frequently used drug is diltiazem (Cardizem). In addition, verap-amil, digoxin, beta blockers, procainamide, and quinidine can be used. Consult medical control or refer to local protocols concerning pharmaco-logical therapy of atrial fibrillation.

DYSRHYTHMIAS ORIGINATING IN THE AV JUNCTION

Dysrhythmias can originate within the AV node and the AV junction. The location of the pacemaker site will dictate the morphology of the P wave. Ischemia, hypoxia, and other factors have been identified as causes. Dysrhythmias originating in the AV junction include:

- ❑ Premature junctional contractions
- ❑ Junctional escape complexes and rhythm
- ❑ Accelerated junctional rhythm
- ❑ Paroxysmal junctional tachycardia

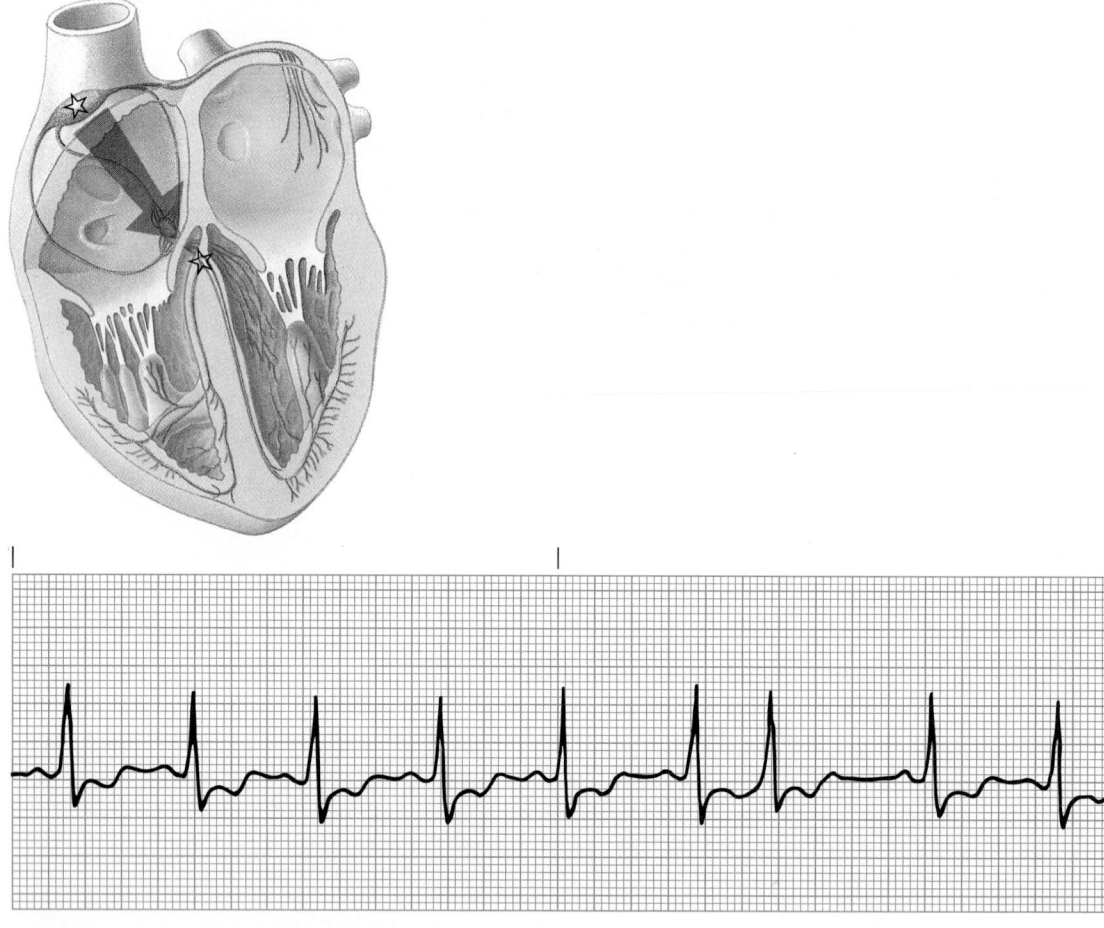

FIGURE 21-37 Premature junctional contractions.

Several ECG features are common to all dysrhythmias that originate in the AV junction. These include:

❑ Inverted P waves in Lead II as a result of retrograde depolarization of the atria. The relationship of the P wave to QRS depolarization is dependent on the relative timing of atrial and ventricular depolarization. The P wave can occur before the QRS complex, if the atria depolarize first; after the QRS, if the ventricles depolarize first; or during the QRS, if the atria and ventricles depolarize simultaneously. Depolarization of the atria during ventricular depolarization masks the P wave. Some atrial complexes that originate near the AV junction can result in negative P waves as well.

❑ P-R interval of less than 0.12 sec.

❑ Normal QRS complex duration.

Premature Junctional Contractions

Description: *Premature junctional contractions (PJCs)* result from a single electrical impulse originating in the AV node that occurs before the next expected sinus beat. A PJC can result in either a compensatory pause or noncompensatory pause, depending on whether the SA node is depolarized. A noncompensatory pause occurs if the SA node is depolarized by the premature beat, and the normal cadence of the heart is interrupted. A **compensatory pause** occurs only if the SA node discharges before the premature impulse reaches it.

■ **compensatory pause** the pause following an ectopic beat where the SA node is unaffected and the cadence of the heart is uninterrupted.

Etiology: A premature junctional contraction can result from any of the following conditions.

❑ Use of caffeine, tobacco, or alcohol

❑ Sympathomimetic drugs

❑ Ischemic heart disease

❑ Hypoxia

❑ Digitalis toxicity

❑ No apparent cause

Rules of Interpretation/Lead II Monitoring (See Figure 21-37.)

Rate: Depends on the underlying rhythm

Rhythm: Depends on the underlying rhythm, usually regular except for the PJC

Pacemaker Site: Ectopic focus in the AV junction

P Waves: Inverted; may appear before or after the QRS complex. P waves can be masked by the QRS complex or be absent.

P-R Interval: If the P wave occurs before the QRS complex, the P-R interval will be less than 0.12 sec. If the P wave occurs after the QRS complex, then technically it is an R-P interval.

QRS Complex: Normal; 0.04–0.12 sec. However, it can be greater than 0.12 sec if the PJC is abnormally conducted through partially refractory ventricles.

Clinical Significance: Isolated PJCs are of minimal significance. Frequent PJCs indicate organic heart disease and may be precursors to other junctional dysrhythmias.

Treatment: If the patient is asymptomatic, observation is all that is required in the field.

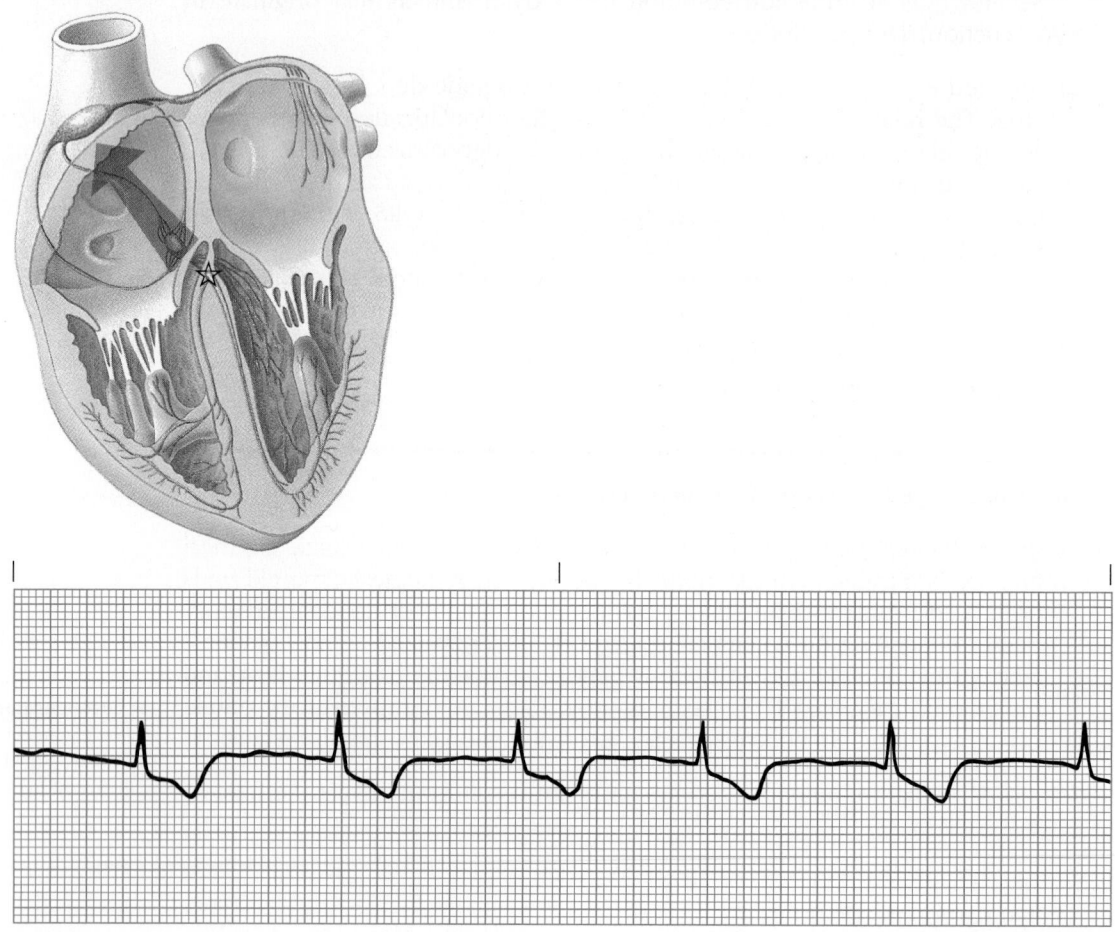

FIGURE 21-38 Junctional escape complex and rhythm.

Junctional Rhythm

Description: A *junctional escape beat,* or *junctional escape rhythm,* is a dysrhythmia that results when the rate of the primary pacemaker, usually the SA node, becomes less than that of the AV node. The AV node then becomes the pacemaker. The AV node usually discharges at its intrinsic rate of 40–60 beats per minute. This is a safety mechanism that prevents cardiac standstill.

Etiology: Junctional escape rhythm has several etiologies. These include increased vagal tone, which can result in SA node slowing; pathological slow SA node discharge; or heart block.

Rules of Interpretation/Lead II Monitoring (See Figure 21-38.)

 Rate: 40–60 per minute

 Rhythm: Irregular in single junctional escape complex; regular in junctional escape rhythm

 Pacemaker Site: AV junction

 P Waves: Inverted; may appear before or after the QRS complex. The P waves can be masked by the QRS or be absent.

 P-R Interval: If the P wave occurs before the QRS complex, P-R interval will be less than 0.12 sec. If the P wave occurs after the QRS complex, technically it is an R-P interval.

 QRS Complex: Normal; 0.04–0.12 sec. However, it may be greater than 0.12 sec.

Clinical Significance: The slow heart rate can decrease cardiac output, possibly precipitating angina and other problems. If the rate is fairly rapid, the rhythm can be well tolerated.

Treatment: If the patient is asymptomatic, observation is all that is required in the field. Treatment is unnecessary unless hypotension or ventricular irritability is present. If treatment is required, administer a 0.5 mg bolus of atropine sulfate. This can be repeated every 3–5 minutes until a satisfactory rate has been obtained or a total of 0.04 mg/kg of the drug has been given. If atropine fails, consider transcutaneous cardiac pacing (TCP), if available. Isoproterenol is rarely required.

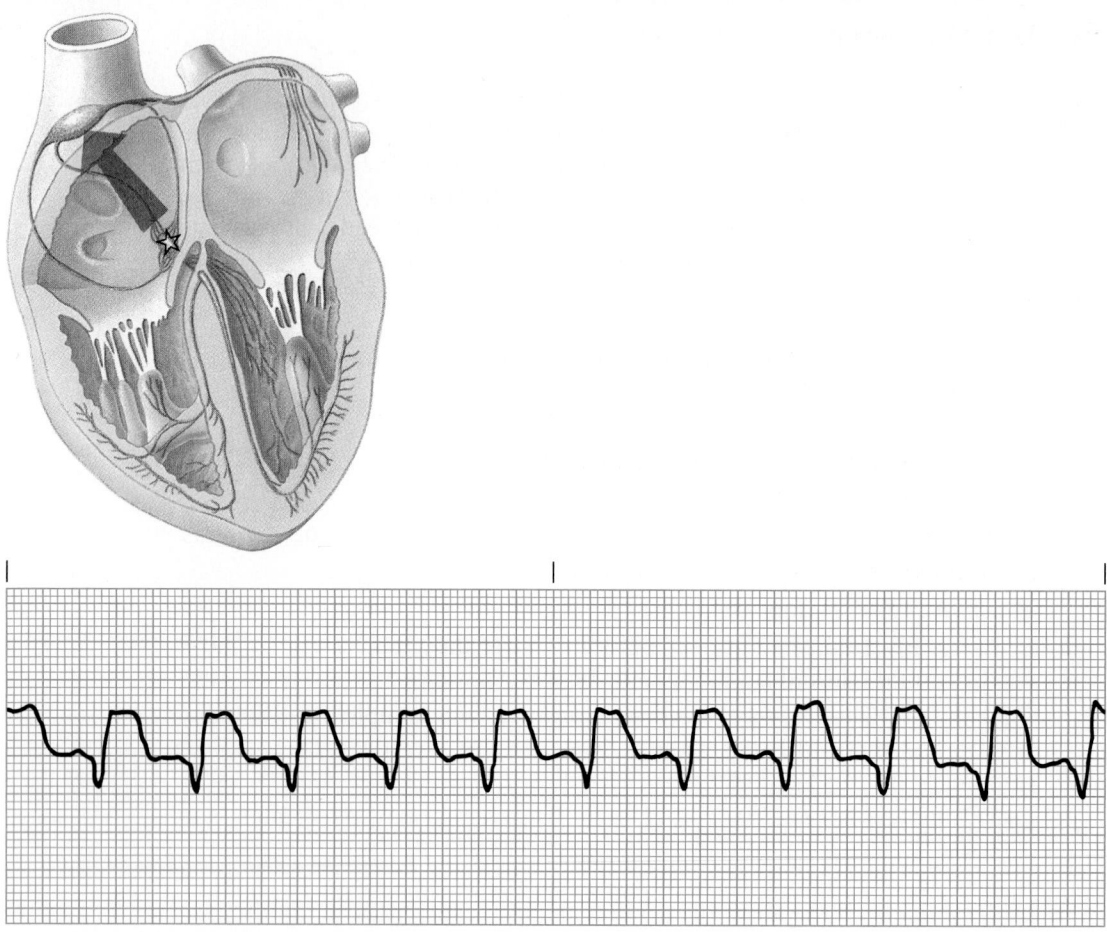

FIGURE 21-39 Accelerated junctional rhythm.

Accelerated Junctional Rhythm

Description: An *accelerated junctional rhythm* is one that results from increased automaticity in the AV junction, causing the AV junction to discharge faster than its intrinsic rate. If it is fast enough, the AV node can override the SA node. Technically, the rate associated with an accelerated junctional rhythm is not a tachycardia. However, when compared to the intrinsic rate of the AV junctional tissue (40–60 beats per minute), it is considered accelerated.

Etiology: Accelerated junctional rhythms often result from ischemia of the AV junction.

Rules of Interpretation/Lead II Monitoring (See Figure 21-39.)

> *Rate*: 60–100 per minute
>
> *Rhythm*: Regular
>
> *Pacemaker Site*: AV junction
>
> *P Waves*: Inverted; may appear before or after the QRS complex. P waves may be masked by the QRS or be absent.
>
> *P-R Interval*: If the P wave occurs before the QRS complex, the P-R interval will be less than 0.12 sec. If it occurs after the QRS, technically it is an R-P interval.
>
> *QRS Complex*: Normal; 0.04–0.12 sec

Clinical Significance: An accelerated junctional rhythm is usually well tolerated. However, since ischemia is often the etiology, the patient should be monitored for other dysrhythmias.

Treatment: Prehospital treatment is generally unnecessary.

Paroxysmal Junctional Tachycardia

Description: *Paroxysmal junctional tachycardia (PJT)* develops when rapid AV junctional depolarization overrides the SA node. It often occurs in paroxysms with sudden onset, may last minutes to hours, and terminates abruptly. It may be caused by increased automaticity of a single AV nodal focus or by a reentry phenomenon at the AV node. Paroxysmal junctional tachycardia is often more appropriately called *paroxysmal supraventricular tachycardia (PSVT)*, since it may be indistinguishable from paroxysmal atrial tachycardia due to the rapid rate.

Etiology: Paroxysmal junctional tachycardia may occur at any age and may not be associated with underlying heart disease. It may be precipitated by stress, overexertion, smoking, or ingestion of caffeine. However, it is frequently associated with underlying ASHD and rheumatic heart disease. PJT rarely occurs with myocardial infarction. It can occur with accessory pathway conduction, as in Wolff-Parkinson-White syndrome.

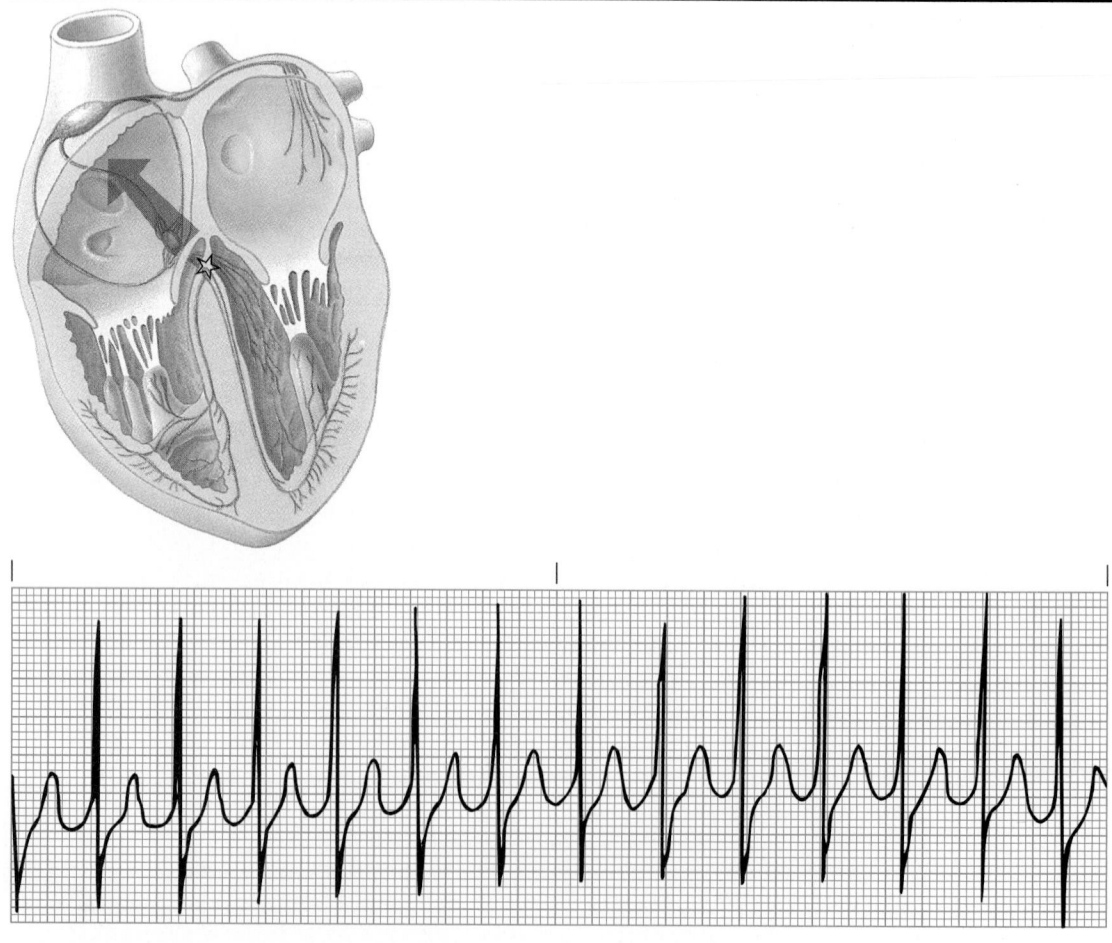

FIGURE 21-40 Paroxysmal junctional tachycardia.

Rules of Interpretation/Lead II Monitoring (See Figure 21-40.)

Rate: 100–180 per minute

Rhythm: Characteristically regular, except at onset and termination of paroxysms

Pacemaker Site: AV junction

P Waves: If present, P waves are inverted. They can occur before, during, or after the QRS complex. Turning up the speed of the graph paper or oscilloscope to 50 mm/sec spreads out the complex and aids in the identification of P waves.

P-R Interval: If the P wave occurs before the QRS complex, the P-R interval will be less than 0.12 sec. If it occurs after the QRS complex, technically it is an R-P interval.

QRS Complex: Normal; 0.04–0.12 sec

Clinical Significance: PJT may be well tolerated for a short period of time in young patients with good cardiac reserve. The patient will often sense it as palpitations. However, rapid rates can cause a marked reduction in cardiac output because of inadequate ventricular filling time. Coronary artery perfusion can also be compromised, since the diastolic phase of the cardiac cycle is reduced. PJT can precipitate angina, hypotension, or congestive heart failure.

Treatment: If the patient is not tolerating the rapid heart rate, as evidenced by hemodynamic instability, attempt the following techniques in the order in which they are given.

1. *Vagal Maneuvers*. Ask the patient to perform a Valsalva maneuver. This is a forced expiration against a closed glottis, or the act of "bearing down" as if to move the bowels. This results in vagal stimulation, which may slow the heart. If this is unsuccessful, attempt carotid artery massage if the patient is eligible. Do not attempt this in patients with carotid bruits or known cerebrovascular or carotid artery disease.

2. *Pharmacological Therapy*. Adenosine (Adenocard) is relatively safe and highly effective in terminating PJT. This is especially true if the etiology of the dysrhythmia is reentry. Administer 6 mg of adenosine by rapid IV bolus over 1–3 seconds through the medication port closest to the patient's heart or central circulation. If the patient does not convert after 1–2 minutes, administer a second bolus of 12 mg over 1–3 seconds in the medication port closest to the patient's heart or central circulation. If this fails, and the patient has a normal blood pressure, medical control may request the administration of verapamil. Verapamil is contraindicated in patients with history of bradycardia, hypotension, or congestive heart failure. It should not be used with intravenous beta blockers. It should be used with caution in patients on chronic beta blocker therapy. Hypotension that occurs following verapamil administration can often be reversed with 0.5–1.0 gm of calcium chloride administered intravenously.

3. *Electrical Therapy*. If the ventricular rate is greater than 150 beats per minute, or the patient is hemodynamically unstable, synchronized cardioversion should be utilized. If time allows, sedate the patient with 5–10 mg of diazepam IV. Apply synchronized DC countershock of 100 joules. If this is unsuccessful, repeat the countershock at increased energy as ordered by the medical control physician. DC countershock is contraindicated if digitalis toxicity is suspected as the cause of the PJT.

DYSRHYTHMIAS ORIGINATING IN THE VENTRICLES

Dysrhythmias can originate within the ventricles. The location of the pacemaker site will dictate the morphology of the QRS complex. Many factors, including ischemia, hypoxia, and medications, have been identified as causes. Dysrhythmias originating in the ventricles include:

- ❑ Ventricular escape complexes and rhythms
- ❑ Premature ventricular contraction
- ❑ Ventricular tachycardia
- ❑ Ventricular fibrillation
- ❑ Asystole
- ❑ Artificial pacemaker rhythm

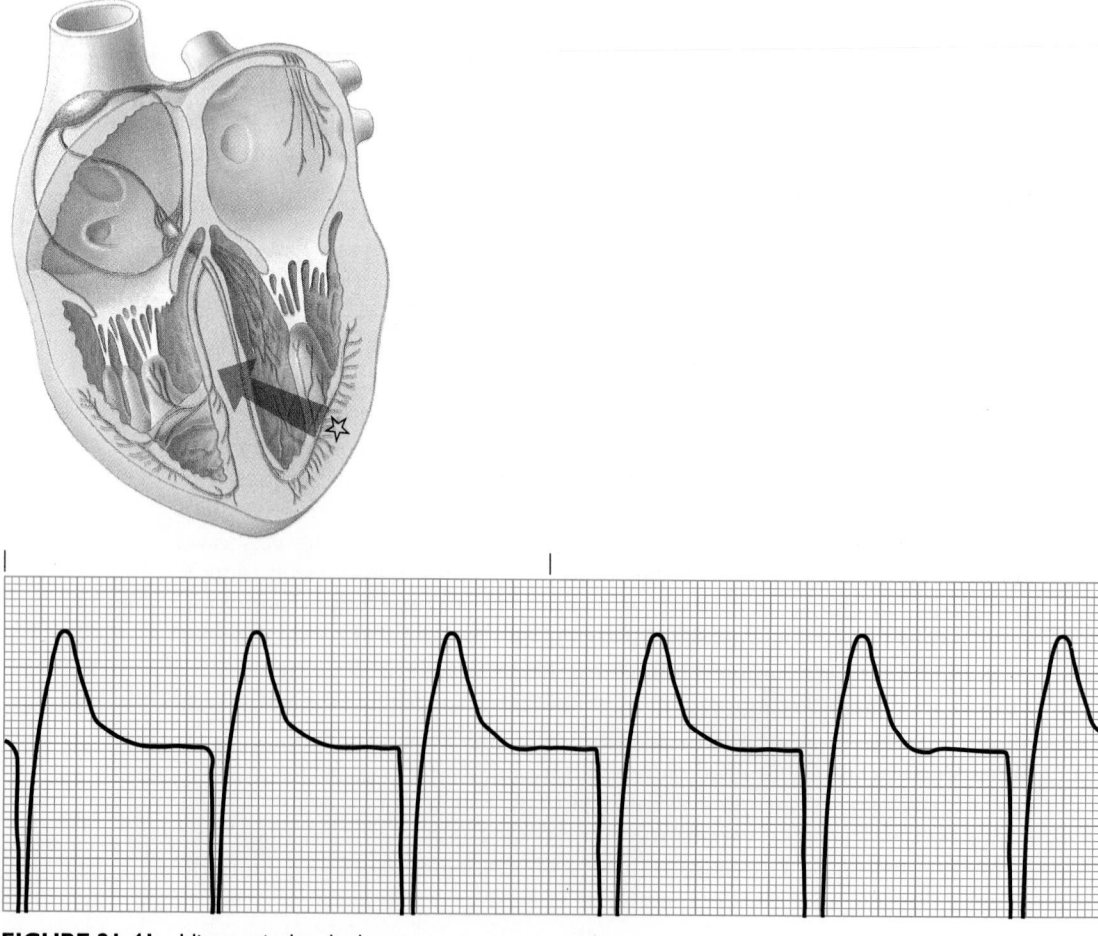

FIGURE 21-41 Idioventricular rhythm.

ECG features common to all dysrhythmias that originate in the ventricles include:

❏ QRS complexes of 0.12 sec or greater
❏ Absent P waves

Ventricular Escape Complexes and Rhythms (Idioventricular Rhythm)

Description: A ventricular escape beat, or *ventricular escape rhythm*, is a dysrhythmia that results when either impulses from higher pacemakers fail to reach the ventricles or the rate of discharge of higher pacemakers becomes less than that of the ventricles (normally 15–45 beats per minute). Ventricular escape rhythms serve as safety mechanisms to prevent cardiac standstill.

Etiology: Ventricular escape complexes and ventricular rhythms have several etiologies. These include slowing of supraventricular pacemaker sites or high-degree AV block. They are frequently the first organized rhythms seen following successful defibrillation.

Rules of Interpretation/Lead II Monitoring (See Figure 21-41.)
   Rate: 15–40 per minute (occasionally less)
   Rhythm: The rhythm is irregular in a single ventricular escape complex. Ventricular escape rhythms are usually regular unless the pacemaker site is low in the ventricular conductive system. Such placement makes regularity unreliable.
   Pacemaker Site: Ventricle
   P Waves: None
   P-R Interval: None
   QRS Complex: Greater than 0.12 sec and bizarre in morphology

Clinical Significance: The slow heart rate can significantly decrease cardiac output, possibly to life-threatening levels. The ventricular escape rhythm is a safety mechanism and should not be suppressed. Escape rhythms can be perfusing or nonperfusing and must be treated accordingly.

Treatment: If the escape rhythm is perfusing, the object of treatment is to increase the heart rate. Administer a 0.5 mg bolus of atropine sulfate. Repeat this every 3–5 minutes until a satisfactory rate has been obtained or 0.04 mg/kg of the drug has been given. If atropine fails, consider transcutaneous cardiac pacing (TCP), if available. Isoproterenol is rarely required. Lidocaine is contraindicated until the heart rate is corrected. If the rhythm is nonperfusing, follow the Pulseless Electrical Activity (PEA) protocol. This includes airway stabilization and CPR. Place an IV line, and administer 1 mg of epinephrine 1:10,000 IV. However, treatment should be directed at correcting the primary problem (hypovolemia, hypoxia, cardiac tamponade, acidosis, etc.). A fluid challenge should be considered.

Premature Ventricular Contractions

Description: A *premature ventricular contraction (PVC)* is a single ectopic impulse, arising from an irritable focus in either ventricle, that occurs earlier than the next expected beat. It may result from increased automaticity in the ectopic cell or a reentry mechanism. The altered sequence of ventricular depolarization results in a wide and bizarre QRS complex. In addition, the altered sequence of ventricular depolarization can cause the T wave to occur in the opposite direction to the QRS complex.

A PVC does not usually depolarize the SA node and interrupt its rhythm. That is, the normal cadence of the heart is not interrupted. The pause following the PVC is fully *compensatory*. Occasionally, a PVC falls between two sinus beats without interrupting the rhythm. This is called an **interpolated beat**.

■ **interpolated beat** a PVC that falls between two sinus beats without effectively interrupting this rhythm.

If more than one PVC occurs, each one can be classified as unifocal or multifocal. The morphology of the PVC depends on the location of the ectopic pacemaker. Two PVCs of different morphologies imply two pacemaker sites (multifocal). PVCs with the same morphology are considered unifocal. If the coupling interval (the distance between the preceding beat and the PVC) is constant, the PVCs are most likely unifocal.

PVCs often occur in patterns of group beating. These include:

❑ *Bigeminy.* Every other beat is a PVC.
❑ *Trigeminy.* Every third beat is a PVC.

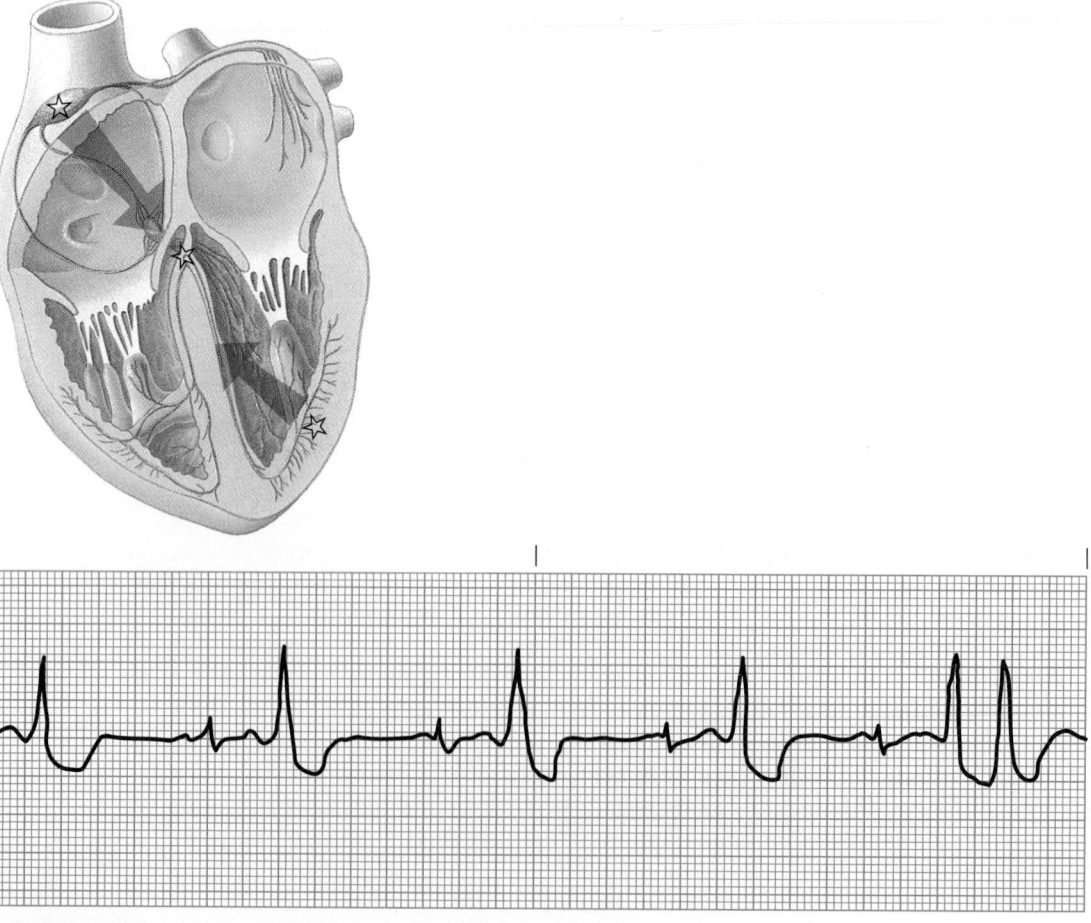

FIGURE 21-42 Premature ventricular contractions.

❑ *Quadrigeminy*. Every fourth beat is a PVC.

These terms can be applied to PACs and PJCs as well.

Repetitive PVCs are two PVCs together without a normal complex in between. These can occur in groups of two (couplets) or groups of three (triplets). More than three PVCs in a row are often considered to be ventricular tachycardia.

PVCs can trigger lethal dysrhythmias, such as ventricular fibrillation, if they fall within the relative refractory period (the so-called R on T phenomenon). PVCs are often classified by their relationship to the previous normal complex.

Etiologies: Etiologies for PVCs include:

❑ Myocardial ischemia
❑ Hypoxia
❑ Acid-base disturbances
❑ Electrolyte imbalances
❑ Increased sympathetic tone
❑ Idiopathic causes
❑ Normal variant

Rules of Interpretation/Lead II Monitoring (See Figure 21-42.)

Rate: Depends on underlying rhythm and rate of PVCs

Rhythm: Interrupts regularity of underlying rhythm; occasionally irregular

Pacemaker Site: Ventricle

P Waves: None; however, a normal sinus P wave (interpolated P wave) can sometimes be seen before a PVC.

P-R Interval: None

QRS Complex: Greater than 0.12 sec and bizarre in morphology

Clinical Significance: Patients often sense PVCs as "skipped beats." In a patient without heart disease, PVCs may be of no significance. In patients with myocardial ischemia, PVCs may indicate ventricular irritability and may trigger lethal ventricular dysrhythmias. PVCs are often classified as malignant or benign. Malignant PVCs have one of the following traits.

❑ More than 6 PVCs per minute
❑ R on T phenomenon
❑ Couplets or runs of ventricular tachycardia
❑ Multifocal
❑ Associated with chest pain

With PVCs, the ventricles often do not fill adequately, and there is often no pulse associated with them. If PVCs are frequent, then cardiac output may fall.

Treatment: If the patient has no history of cardiac disease and no symptoms, and if the PVCs are nonmalignant, no treatment is required. If the patient has a prior history of heart disease or symptoms, or if the PVCs are malignant, administer oxygen and place an IV line. Administer lidocaine at a dose of 1.0–1.5 mg/kg of body weight. Give an additional lidocaine bolus of 0.5–0.75 mg/kg every 5–10 minutes, if necessary, until a total of 3.0 mg/kg of the drug has been given. If the PVCs are effectively suppressed, start a lidocaine drip beginning at a rate of 2–4 mg/min. The dose of lidocaine should be reduced in patients with decreased cardiac output (i.e., CHF, shock), patients who are age 70 or greater, or patients who have hepatic dysfunction. These patients should receive a normal bolus dose first, followed by half the normal infusion. If the patient is allergic to lidocaine, or if a maximum dose of lidocaine (3 mg/kg) has been given, procainamide or bretylium should be considered.

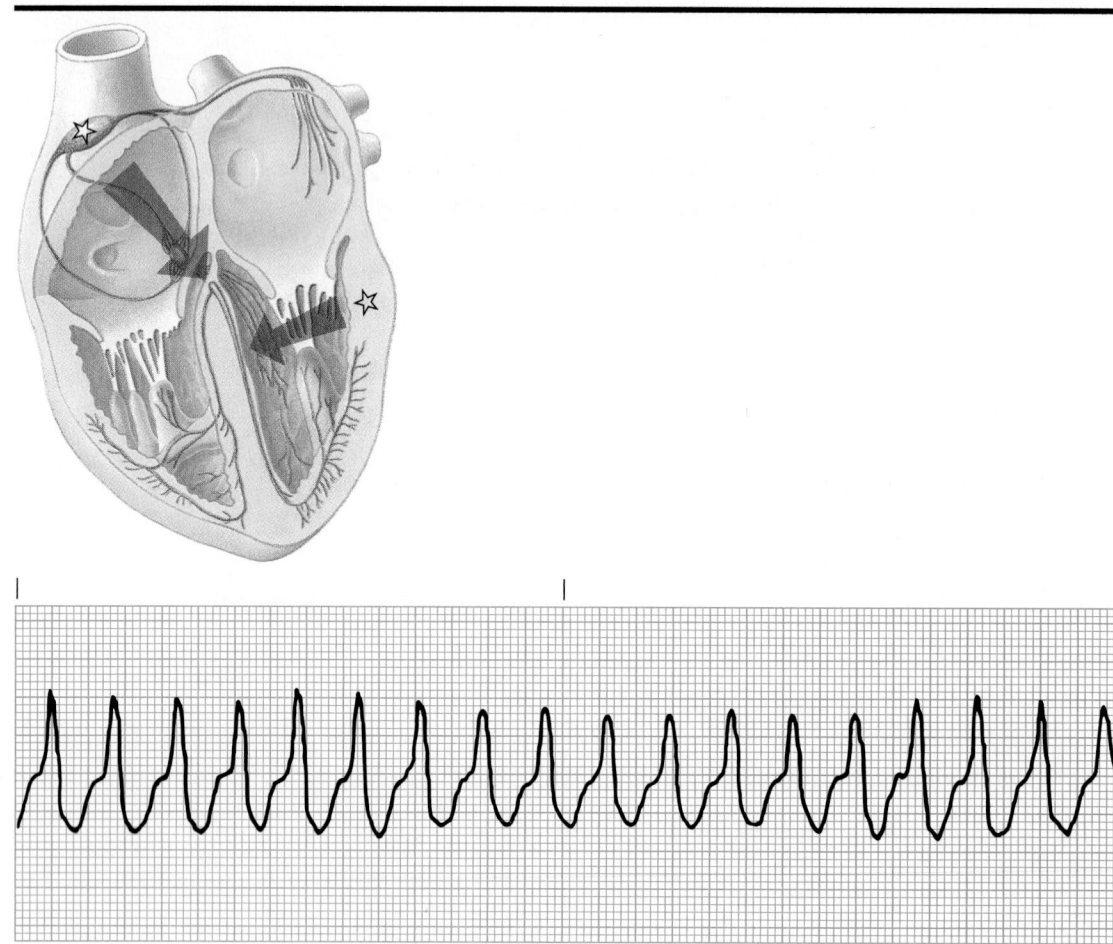

FIGURE 21-43 Ventricular tachycardia.

Ventricular Tachycardia

Description: *Ventricular tachycardia* is a rhythm that consists of three or more ventricular complexes in succession at a rate of 100 beats per minute or more. This rhythm overrides the normal pacemaker of the heart, and the atria and ventricles are asynchronous. Sinus P waves may occasionally be seen, dissociated from the QRS complexes.

Etiology: Several etiologies have been identified for ventricular tachycardia. As with PVCs, these include:

- ❏ Myocardial ischemia
- ❏ Hypoxia
- ❏ Acid-base disturbances
- ❏ Electrolyte imbalances
- ❏ Increased sympathetic tone
- ❏ Idiopathic causes

Rules of Interpretation/Lead II Monitoring (See Figure 21-43.)

Rate: 100–250 (approximately)

Rhythm: Usually regular; can be slightly irregular

Pacemaker Site: Ventricle

P Waves: If present, not associated with the QRS complexes

P-R Interval: None

QRS Complex: Greater than 0.12 sec and bizarre in morphology

Clinical Significance: Ventricular tachycardia usually results in poor stroke volume. This, coupled with the rapid ventricular rate, may severely compromise cardiac output and coronary artery perfusion. Ventricular tachycardia may be either perfusing or nonperfusing, and this dictates the type of treatment. Ventricular tachycardia may eventually deteriorate into ventricular fibrillation.

(continued)

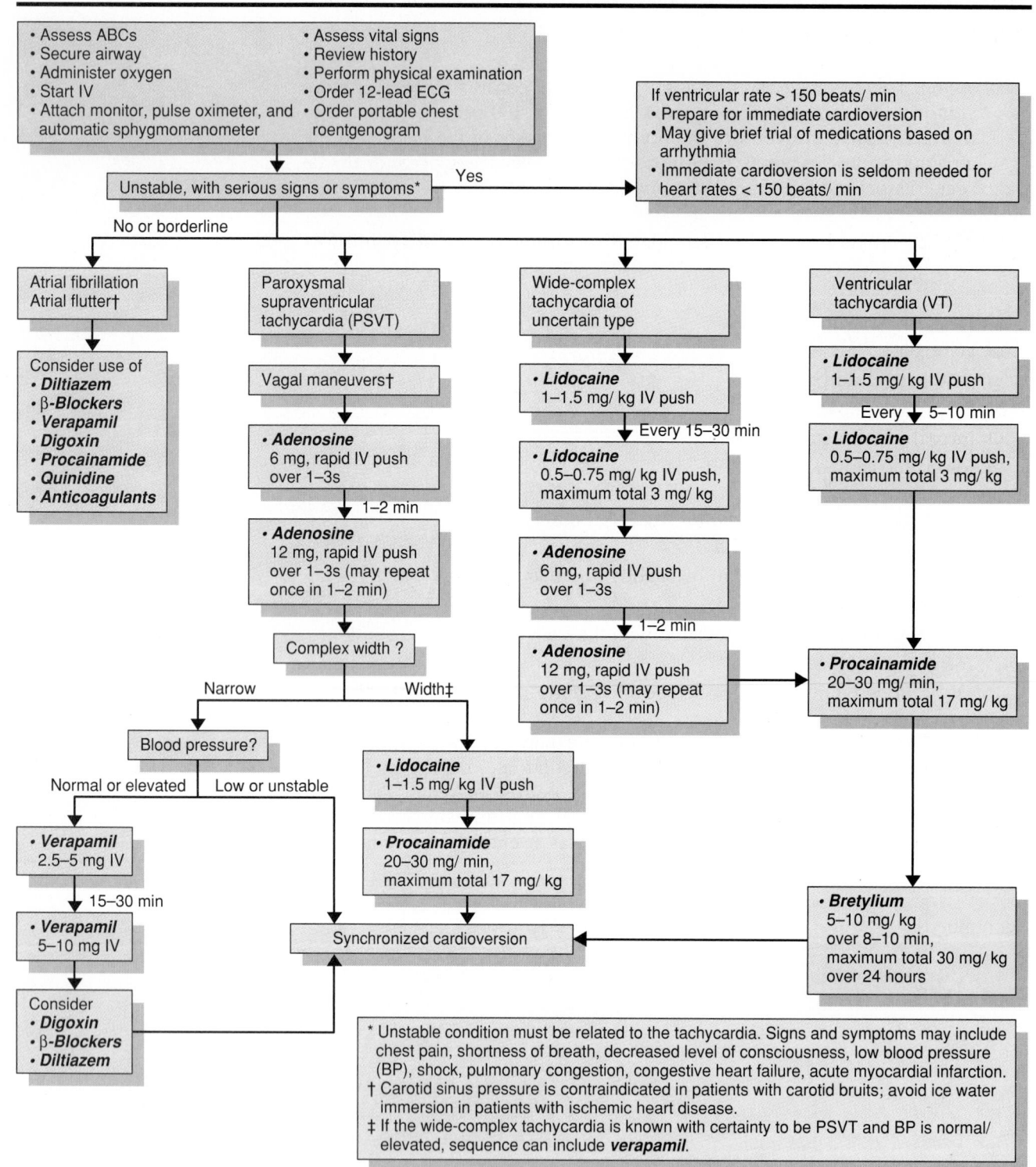

Assess ABCs
- Assess ABCs
- Secure airway
- Administer oxygen
- Start IV
- Attach monitor, pulse oximeter, and automatic sphygmomanometer

- Assess vital signs
- Review history
- Perform physical examination
- Order 12-lead ECG
- Order portable chest roentgenogram

If ventricular rate > 150 beats/ min
- Prepare for immediate cardioversion
- May give brief trial of medications based on arrhythmia
- Immediate cardioversion is seldom needed for heart rates < 150 beats/ min

Unstable, with serious signs or symptoms* — Yes

No or borderline

Atrial fibrillation Atrial flutter†

Consider use of
- *Diltiazem*
- β-*Blockers*
- *Verapamil*
- *Digoxin*
- *Procainamide*
- *Quinidine*
- *Anticoagulants*

Paroxysmal supraventricular tachycardia (PSVT)

Vagal maneuvers†

- *Adenosine*
  6 mg, rapid IV push over 1–3s

  1–2 min

- *Adenosine*
  12 mg, rapid IV push over 1–3s (may repeat once in 1–2 min)

Complex width ?

Narrow   Width‡

Blood pressure?

Normal or elevated   Low or unstable

- *Verapamil*
  2.5–5 mg IV

  15–30 min

- *Verapamil*
  5–10 mg IV

Consider
- *Digoxin*
- β-*Blockers*
- *Diltiazem*

Wide-complex tachycardia of uncertain type

- *Lidocaine*
  1–1.5 mg/ kg IV push

  Every 15–30 min

- *Lidocaine*
  0.5–0.75 mg/ kg IV push, maximum total 3 mg/ kg

- *Adenosine*
  6 mg, rapid IV push over 1–3s

  1–2 min

- *Adenosine*
  12 mg, rapid IV push over 1–3s (may repeat once in 1–2 min)

- *Lidocaine*
  1–1.5 mg/ kg IV push

- *Procainamide*
  20–30 mg/ min, maximum total 17 mg/ kg

Synchronized cardioversion

Ventricular tachycardia (VT)

- *Lidocaine*
  1–1.5 mg/ kg IV push

  Every 5–10 min

- *Lidocaine*
  0.5–0.75 mg/ kg IV push, maximum total 3 mg/ kg

- *Procainamide*
  20–30 mg/ min, maximum total 17 mg/ kg

- *Bretylium*
  5–10 mg/ kg over 8–10 min, maximum total 30 mg/ kg over 24 hours

* Unstable condition must be related to the tachycardia. Signs and symptoms may include chest pain, shortness of breath, decreased level of consciousness, low blood pressure (BP), shock, pulmonary congestion, congestive heart failure, acute myocardial infarction.
† Carotid sinus pressure is contraindicated in patients with carotid bruits; avoid ice water immersion in patients with ischemic heart disease.
‡ If the wide-complex tachycardia is known with certainty to be PSVT and BP is normal/ elevated, sequence can include *verapamil*.

FIGURE 21-44 Recommended treatment of ventricular tachycardia with pulse.

Ventricular Tachycardia (continued)

Treatment: If the patient is perfusing, as evidenced by the presence of a pulse, administer oxygen and place an IV line. Administer lidocaine at a dose of 1–1.5 mg/kg body weight intravenously. Administer additional doses of 0.5–0.75 mg/kg, until a total of 3.0 mg/kg has been administered. If this treatment is unsuccessful, attempt to administer procainamide at 20–30 mg/minute to a maximum of 17 mg/kg. If procainamide fails, 5–10 mg/kg of bretylium may be administered over 8–10 minutes to a maximum dose of 30 mg/kg. Use synchronized cardioversion if the patient becomes unstable, as evidenced by chest pain, dyspnea, or systolic blood pressure of less than 90 mm/kg.

If the patient's condition is unstable, as evidenced by an altered level of consciousness or falling blood pressure, then cardioversion should be the initial treatment after placement of an IV line and oxygen administration. If time allows, sedate the patient first. The treatment plan is illustrated in the protocol.

If the patient is nonperfusing, follow the protocol for ventricular fibrillation. (See Figure 21-44.)

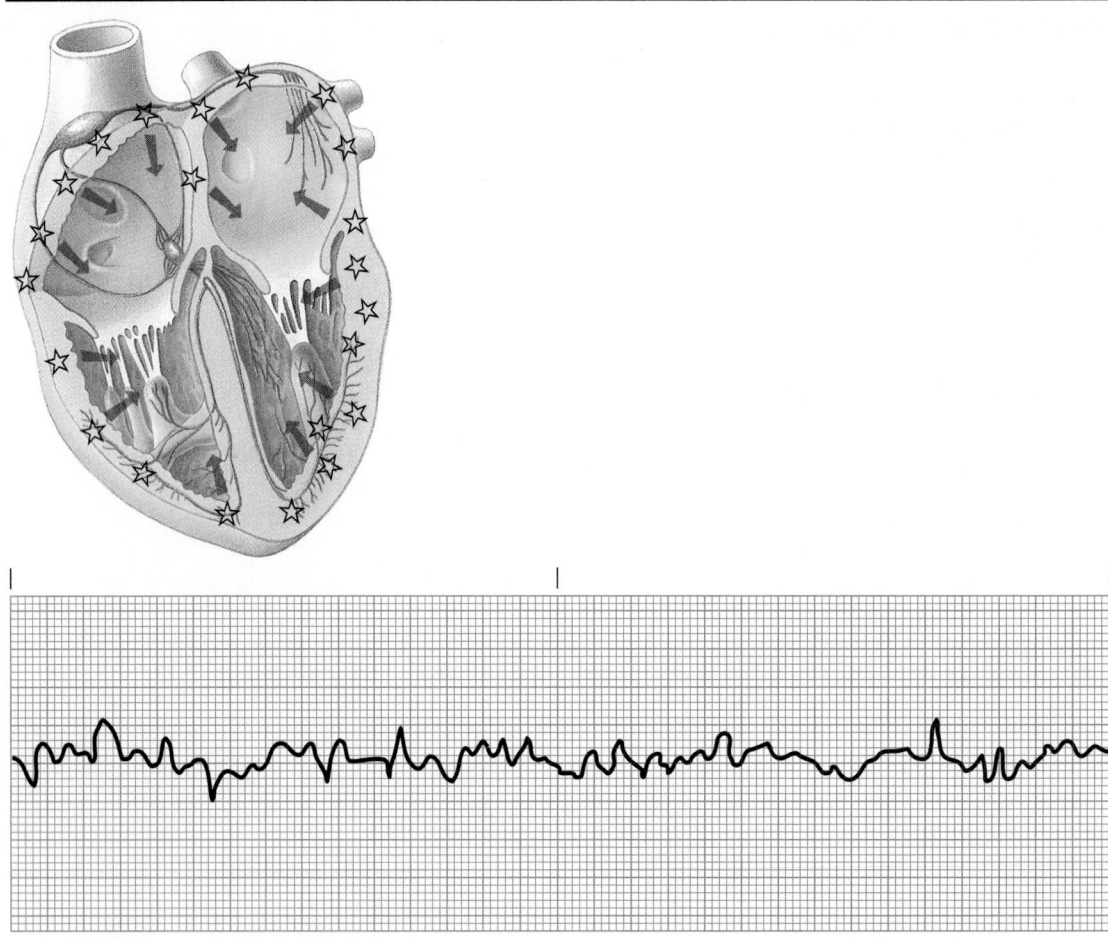

FIGURE 21-45 Ventricular fibrillation.

Ventricular Fibrillation

Description: Ventricular fibrillation is a chaotic ventricular rhythm usually resulting from the presence of many reentry circuits within the ventricles. There is no ventricular depolarization or contraction.

Etiology: A wide variety of causes have been associated with ventricular fibrillation. Most cases result from advanced coronary artery disease.

Rules of Interpretation/Lead II Monitoring (See Figure 21-45.)
    Rate: No organized rhythm
    Rhythm: No organized rhythm
    Pacemaker Site: Numerous ectopic foci throughout the ventricles
    P Waves: Usually absent
    P-R Interval: Absent
    QRS Complex: Absent

Clinical Significance: Ventricular fibrillation is a lethal dysrhythmia. There is no cardiac output or organized electrical pattern, thus resulting in cardiac arrest.

Treatment: Ventricular fibrillation and nonperfusing ventricular tachycardia are treated identically. Initiate CPR. Follow this with DC countershock at 200 joules. If this is unsuccessful, repeat at 200–300 joules. If this is still unsuccessful, repeat at 360 joules. Subsequently, control the airway and establish an IV line. Epinephrine 1:10,000 is the drug of first choice. This can be administered every 3–5 minutes as required. If unsuccessful, consider lidocaine, bretylium, or possibly sodium bicarbonate. (See Figure 21-64 on page 702.)

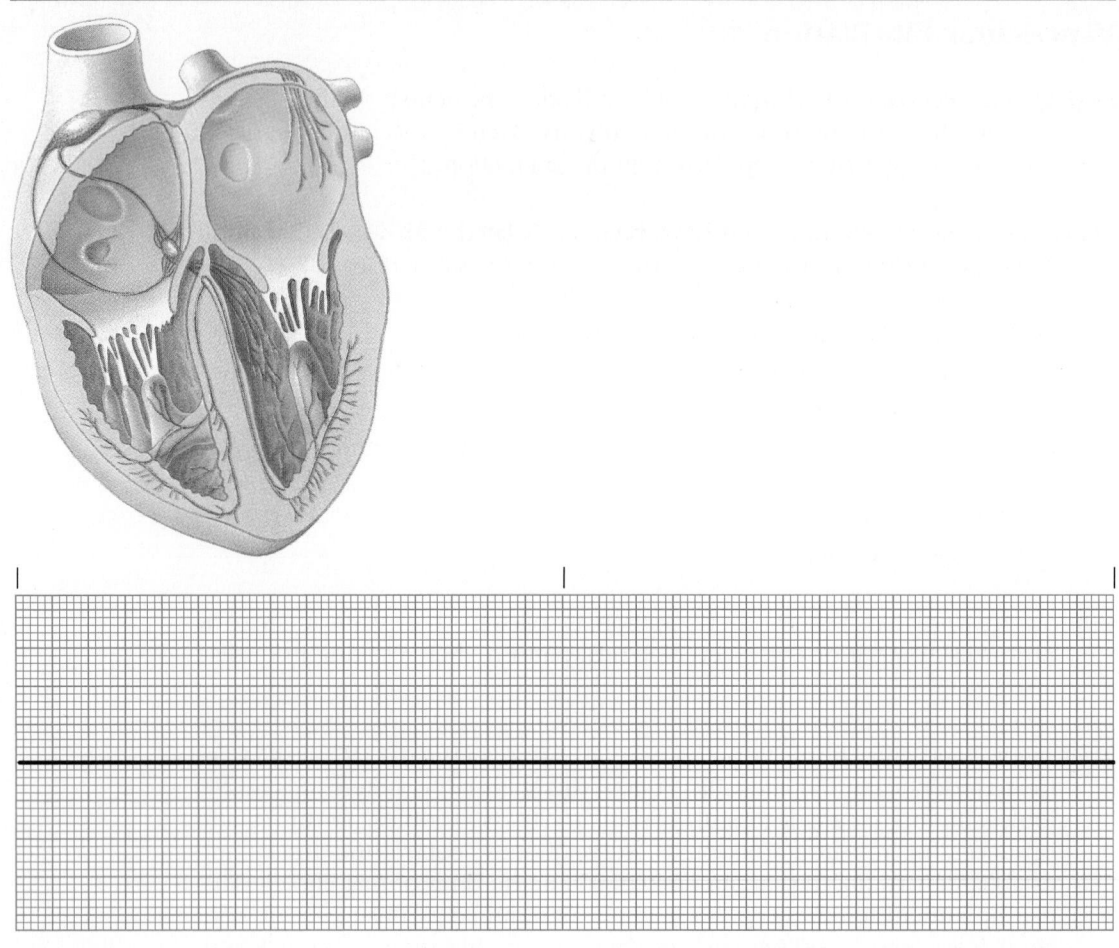

FIGURE 21-46 Asystole.

Asystole (Cardiac Standstill)

Description: *Asystole* is the absence of all cardiac electrical activity.

Etiology: Asystole may be the primary event in cardiac arrest. It is usually associated with massive myocardial infarction, ischemia, and necrosis. Asystole is often the end result of ventricular fibrillation. Asystole results from cases of heart block, in which no escape pacemaker takes over.

Rules of Interpretation/Lead II Monitoring (See Figure 21-46.)
    Rate: No electrical activity
    Rhythm: No electrical activity
    Pacemaker Site: No electrical activity
    P Waves: Absent
    P-R Interval: Absent
    QRS Complex: Absent

Clinical Significance: Asystole results in cardiac arrest. The prognosis for resuscitation is very poor.

Treatment: Asystole is treated with CPR, airway management, oxygenation, and medications. If there is any doubt about the underlying rhythm, attempt defibrillation. Medications include epinephrine, atropine, and, in certain situations, sodium bicarbonate. (See Figure 21-65 on page 703.)

Artificial Pacemaker Rhythm

Description: An *artificial pacemaker rhythm* is a rhythm generated by regular electrical stimulation of the heart through an electrode implanted in the heart and connected to a power source. The pacemaker lead may be implanted in any of several locations in the heart, although it is most often placed in the right ventricle or in both chambers (dual-chambered pacemaker.)

Pacemakers that fire continuously at a preset rate are called *fixed-rate pacemakers.* This firing occurs regardless of the electrical activity of the heart. *Demand pacemakers* contain a sensing device and fire only when the natural rate of the heart drops below the rate set for the pacemaker. In these cases, the pacemaker acts as an escape rhythm.

The ventricular pacemaker stimulates only the right ventricle, resulting in a rhythm that resembles an idioventricular rhythm. Dual-chambered pacemakers, commonly called *AV sequential pacemakers,* stimulate the atria first and then the ventricles. These are most beneficial for patients with marginal cardiac output who need the extra atrial "kick" to maintain cardiac output.

Pacemakers are usually inserted into patients with chronic high-grade

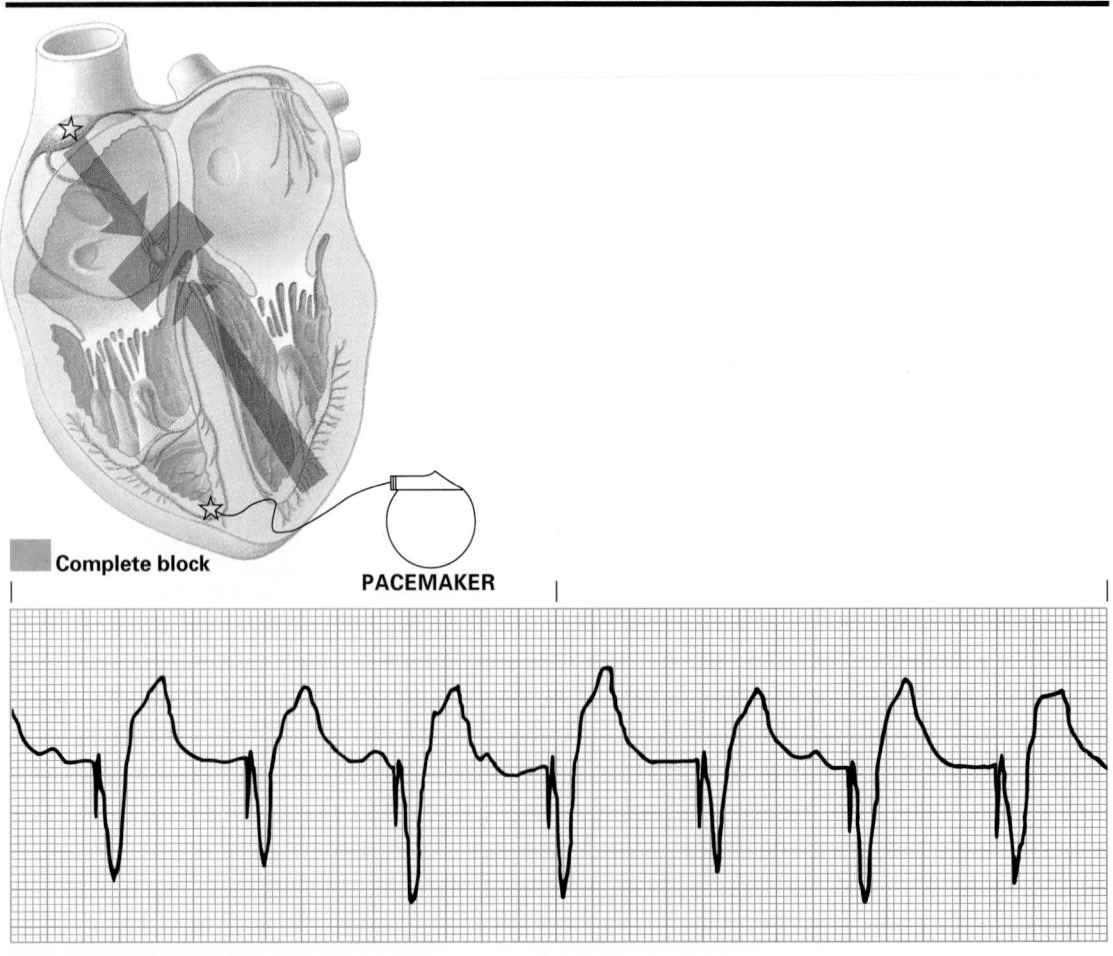

Complete block   PACEMAKER

FIGURE 21-47 Artificial pacemaker rhythm.

heart block, sick sinus syndrome, or who have had episodes of severe symptomatic bradycardia.

Rules of Interpretation/Lead II Monitoring (See Figure 21-47.)

Rate: Varies with the preset rate of the pacemaker

Rhythm: Regular if pacing constantly; irregular if pacing on demand

Pacemaker Site: Depends on electrode placement

P Waves: None produced by ventricular pacemakers. Sinus P waves may be seen but are unrelated to the paced QRS complexes. Dual-chambered pacemakers produce a P wave behind each atrial spike. A pacemaker spike is an upward or downward deflection from the baseline, which is an artifact created each time the pacemaker fires. The *pacemaker spike* tells you only that the pacemaker is firing. It reveals nothing about ventricular depolarization.

P-R Interval: If present, varies

QRS Complex: The QRS complexes associated with pacemaker rhythms are usually longer than 0.12 sec and bizarre in morphology. They often resemble ventricular escape rhythms. Each pacemaker spike should be followed by a QRS complex. If this occurs, the pacemaker is said to be "capturing." In patients with demand pacemakers, some of the patient's own QRS complexes may be seen. A pacemaker spike should not be associated with these complexes.

Problems with Pacemakers: Problems, although rare, can arise from pacemakers. One cause is battery failure. Most pacemaker batteries have relatively long lives and can be checked by the cardiologist. Batteries are usually changed before problems arise. However, if a battery fails, no pacing will occur and the patient's underlying rhythm, which may be bradycardic or asystolic, may return.

Occasionally, a pacemaker can "run away." This condition, rarely seen with new pacemakers, results in a rapid rate of discharge. Run-away pacemaker usually occurs when the battery runs low. Newer models gradually increase their rate as their batteries run low.

Demand pacemakers can fail to shut down when the patient's heart rate exceeds the limit set for the device. Thus the pacemaker competes with the patient's own natural pacemaker. Occasionally, a paced beat can fall in the vulnerable period, precipitating ventricular fibrillation.

Finally, pacemakers can fail to capture. This can occur when the leads become displaced or the battery fails. In such cases, pacemaker spikes are usually present but are not followed by P waves or QRS complexes. Bradycardia often results.

Considerations for Management: Always examine any unconscious patient for a pacemaker. Battery packs are usually palpable under the skin, often in the shoulder or axillary region. Bradydysrhythmias, asystole, and ventricular fibrillation resulting from pacemaker failure are treated as in any other patient. Ventricular irritability may be treated with lidocaine without fear of suppressing ventricular response to the pacemaker. Patients with pacemakers can be defibrillated as usual, but do not discharge paddles directly over the battery pack. External cardiac pacing, if available, can be used until definitive care is available. Patients with pacemaker failure should be promptly transported without prolonged field stabilization. Definitive care consists of battery replacement or temporary pacemaker insertion.

DYSRHYTHMIAS THAT ARE DISORDERS OF CONDUCTION

Several dysrhythmias result from improper conduction through the heart. The three general categories of conductive disorders include:

- ❏ Atrioventricular blocks
- ❏ Disturbances of ventricular conduction
- ❏ Pre-excitation syndromes

The dysrhythmias that will be discussed under this heading include:

- ❏ AV blocks
  - First-degree AV block
  - Second-degree AV block (Mobitz I)
  - Second-degree AV block (Mobitz II)
  - Third-degree AV block
- ❏ Disturbances of ventricular conduction
- ❏ Pre-excitation syndromes
  - Wolff-Parkinson-White syndrome

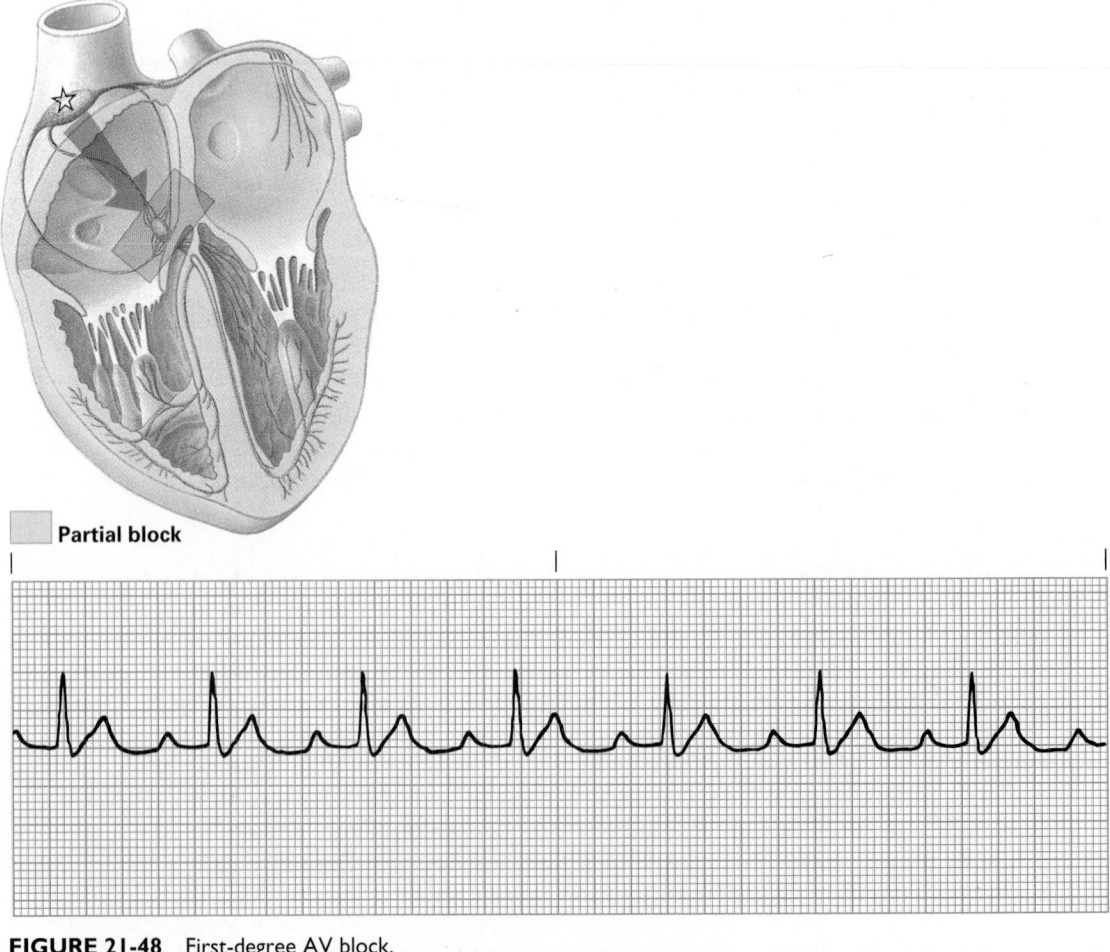

■ Partial block

FIGURE 21-48 First-degree AV block.

AV Blocks

An *AV block* is the delay or interruption of impulses between the atria and the ventricles. These dysrhythmias can be caused by pathology of the AV junctional tissue or by a physiological block, such as occurs with atrial fibrillation or flutter. Causes include AV junctional ischemia, AV junctional necrosis, degenerative disease of the conductive system, and drug toxicity (particularly from the use of digitalis).

AV blocks can be classified according to the site or degree of the block. Blocks may occur at the following sites.

❏ At the level of the AV node
❏ At the level of the bundle of His
❏ Below the bifurcation of the bundle of His

The following discussion classifies AV blocks by the following degrees (traditional classification).

❏ First-degree AV block
❏ Second-degree AV block Type I
❏ Second-degree AV block Type II
❏ Third-degree AV block

First-Degree AV Block

Description: A *first-degree AV block* is a delay in conduction at the level of AV node rather than an actual block. First-degree AV block is not a rhythm in itself, but a condition superimposed upon another rhythm. The underlying rhythm must also be identified (for example, sinus bradycardia with first-degree AV block).

Etiology: AV block can occur in the healthy heart. However, ischemia at the AV junction is the most common cause.

Rules of Interpretation/Lead II Monitoring (See Figure 21-48.)
   Rate: Depends on underlying rhythm
   Rhythm: Usually regular. However, it can be slightly irregular.
   Pacemaker Site: SA node or atria
   P Waves: Normal
   P-R Interval: Greater than 0.20 sec (diagnostic)
   QRS Complex: Normally, less than 0.12 sec. It may be bizarre in shape if conductive system disease exists in the ventricles.

Clinical Significance: First-degree block is usually no danger in itself. However, a newly developed first-degree block may be a forerunner of a more advanced block.

Treatment: Generally, no treatment is required except observation, unless the heart rate drops significantly. If possible, drugs that slow AV conduction, such as lidocaine and procainamide, should be avoided.

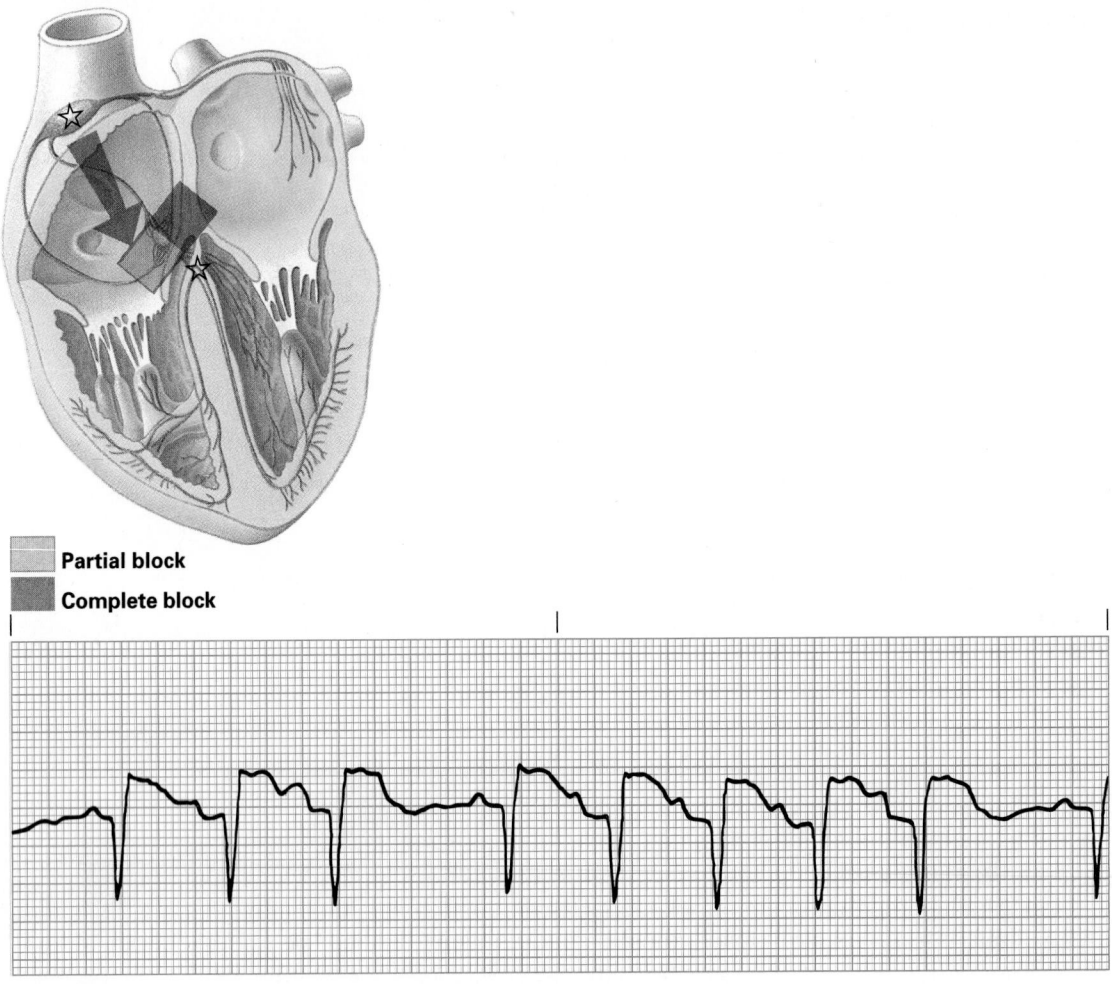

Partial block

Complete block

FIGURE 21-49 Second-degree AV block (Mobitz I) Wenckebach.

Second-Degree AV Block (Mobitz I) Wenckebach

Description: A *second-degree AV block (Mobitz I)* is an intermittent block at the level of the AV node. It produces a characteristic cyclic pattern in which the P-R intervals become progressively longer until an impulse is blocked (not conducted). The cycle is repetitive. The P-P interval remains constant, whereas the P-R interval becomes progressively longer, until a beat is dropped. The ratio of conduction (P waves to QRS complexes) is commonly 5:4, 4:3, 3:2, or 2:1. The pattern may be constant or variable. Second-degree AV block (Mobitz I) is commonly called the *Wenckebach phenomenon*.

Etiology: AV blocks can occur in the healthy heart. However, ischemia at the AV junction is the most common cause. Increased parasympathetic tone and drugs are also common etiologies.

Rules of Interpretation/Lead II Monitoring (See Figure 21-49.)

Rate: Atrial rate is unaffected. The ventricular rate may be normal or slowed.

Rhythm: Atrial rhythm is typically regular. Ventricular rhythm is irregular because of the nonconducted beat.

Pacemaker Site: SA node or atria

P Waves: Normal; some P waves are not followed by QRS complexes.

P-R Interval: It becomes progressively longer until the QRS complex is dropped. The cycle is then repeated.

QRS Complex: Usually less than 0.12 sec. It may be bizarre in shape if conductive system disease exists in the ventricles.

Clinical Significance: If beats are frequently dropped, second-degree block can compromise cardiac output by causing problems such as syncope and angina. This block is often a transient phenomenon that occurs immediately after an inferior wall myocardial infarction.

Treatment: Generally, no treatment, other than observation, is required. If possible, drugs that slow AV conduction, such as lidocaine and procainamide, should be avoided. If the heart rate falls and the patient becomes symptomatic, administer 0.5 mg of atropine IV. This can be repeated every 3–5 minutes until a satisfactory rate has been obtained or 0.04 mg/kg of the drug has been given. If atropine fails, consider transcutaneous cardiac pacing (TCP), if available. Isoproterenol is rarely required.

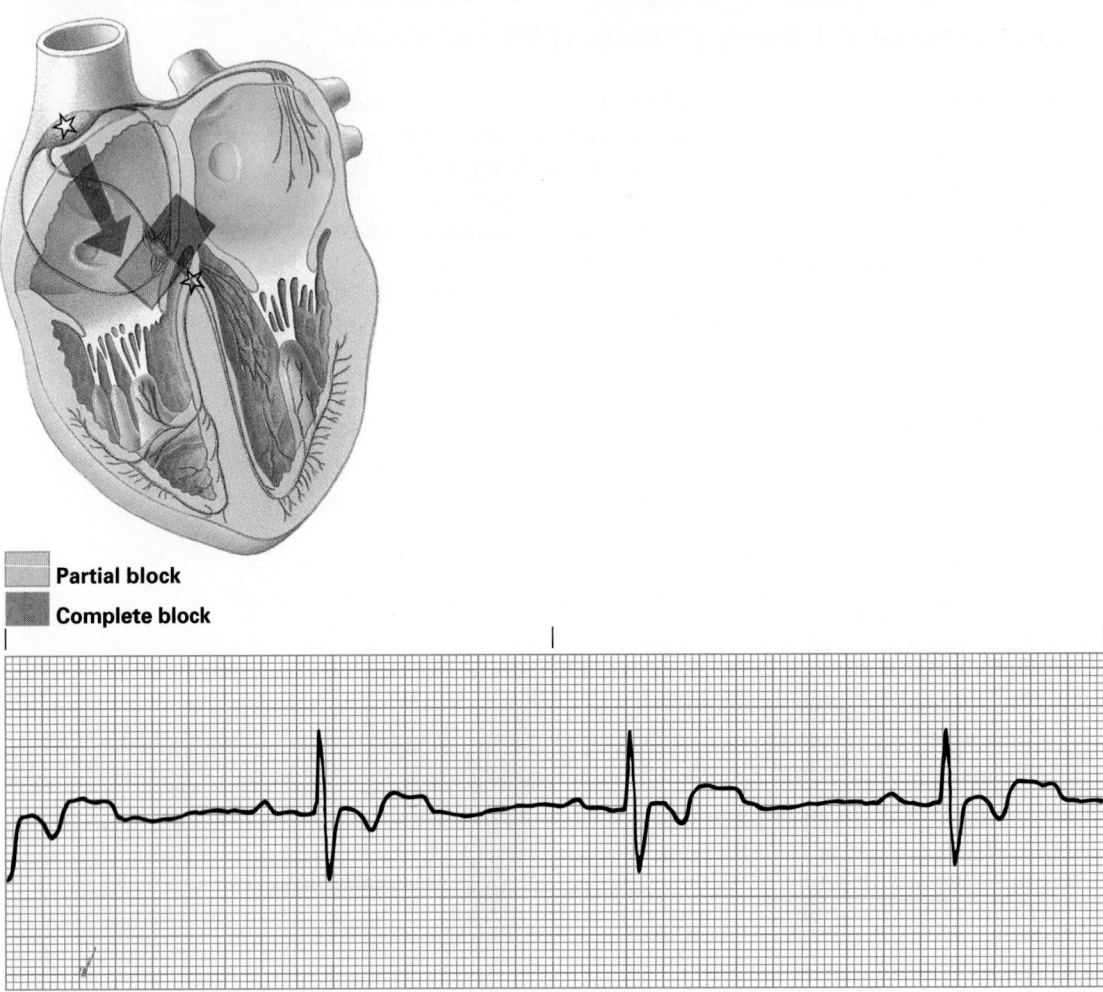

Partial block

Complete block

FIGURE 21-50 Second-degree AV block (Mobitz II).

Second-Degree AV Block (Mobitz II)

Description: A *second-degree AV block (Mobitz II)* is an intermittent block characterized by P waves that are not conducted to the ventricles, but without associated lengthening of the P-R interval before the dropped beats. The ratio of conduction (P waves to QRS complexes) is commonly 4:1, 3:1, or 2:1. The ratio may be constant or may vary. A 2:1 Mobitz II block is often indistinguishable from a 2:1 Mobitz I block.

Etiology: Second-degree AV block (Mobitz II) is usually associated with acute myocardial infarction and septal necrosis.

Rules of Interpretation/Lead II Monitoring (See Figure 21-50.)
   Rate: Atrial rate is unaffected. Ventricular rate is usually bradycardic.
   Rhythm: Regular or irregular, depending upon whether the conduction ratio is constant or varied
   Pacemaker Site: SA node or atria
   P Waves: Normal; some P waves are not followed by QRS complexes.
   P-R Interval: Constant for conducted beats; may be greater than 0.21 sec
   QRS Complex: May be normal. However, it is often greater than 0.12 sec because of abnormal ventricular depolarization sequence.

Clinical Significance: Second-degree block can compromise cardiac output, causing problems such as syncope and angina if beats are frequently dropped. Since this block is often associated with cell necrosis resulting from myocardial infarction, it is considered much more serious than Mobitz I. Many Mobitz II blocks develop into full AV blocks.

Treatment: Pacemaker insertion is the definitive treatment. In the field, if stabilization is required, medications should be administered. If the heart rate falls and the patient becomes symptomatic, you may administer 0.5 mg of atropine IV. This can be repeated every 3–5 minutes until a satisfactory rate has been obtained or 0.04 mg/kg of the drug has been given. *Atropine should be used with caution in patients with high-grade blocks (second-degree Mobitz II and third-degree). The atropine may accelerate the atrial rate, but it may also worsen the AV nodal block.* Consider transcutaneous cardiac pacing (TCP), if available. If the patient remains symptomatic, do not delay application of TCP while awaiting IV access or for atropine to take effect. Isoproterenol is rarely required.

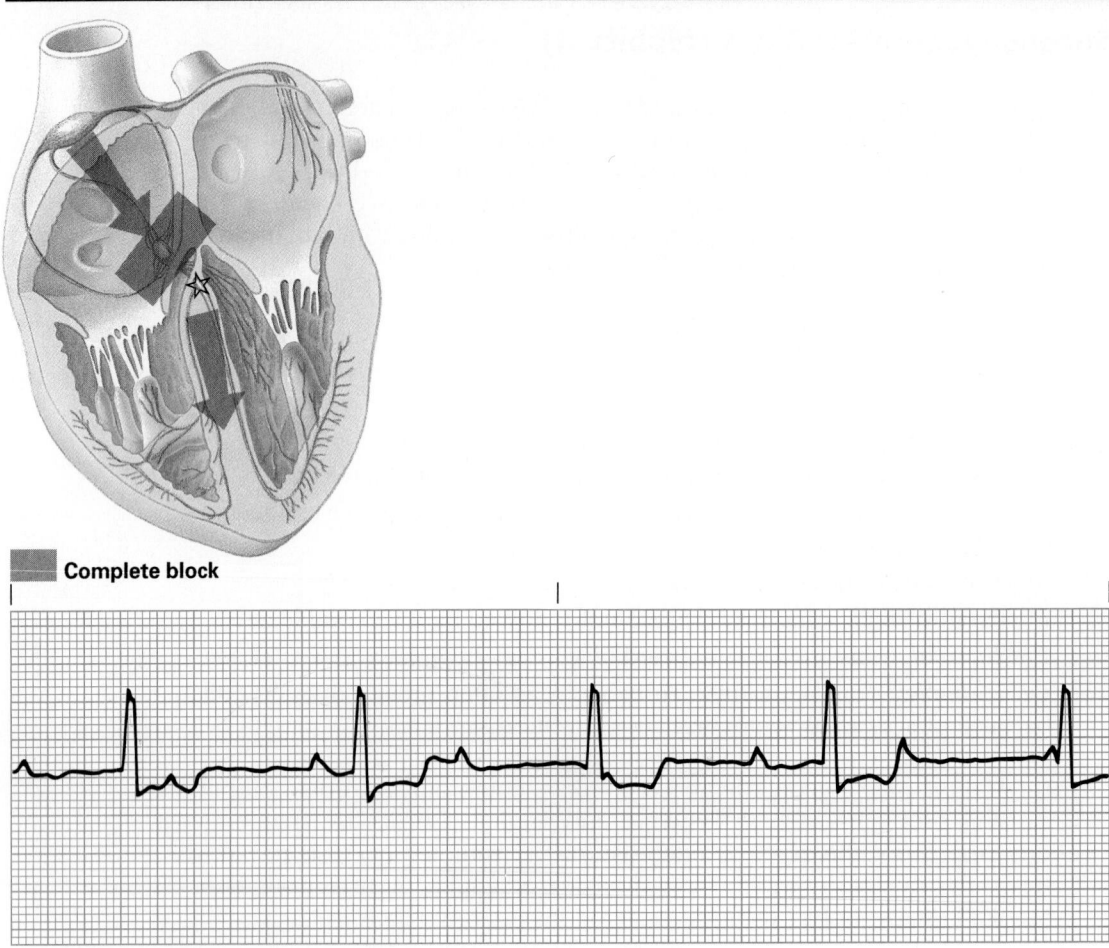

Complete block

FIGURE 21-51 Third-degree AV block.

Third-Degree AV Block

Description: A *third-degree AV block*, or complete block, is the absence of conduction between the atria and the ventricles resulting from complete electrical block at or below the AV node. The atria and ventricles subsequently pace the heart independent of each other. The sinus node often functions normally, depolarizing the atrial syncytium, while the escape pacemaker, located below the atria, paces the ventricular syncytium.

Etiology: Third-degree AV block can result from acute MI, digitalis toxicity, or degeneration of the conductive system, as occurs in the elderly.

Rules of Interpretation/Lead II Monitoring (See Figure 21-51.)

Rate: Atrial rate is unaffected. Ventricular rate is 40–60 if the escape pacemaker is junctional. It is less than 40 if the escape pacemaker is lower in the ventricles.

Rhythm: Both atrial and ventricular rhythms are usually regular.

Pacemaker Site: SA node and AV junction or ventricle

P Waves: Normal. P waves show no relationship to the QRS complex, often falling within the T wave and QRS complex.

P-R Interval: No relationship between P waves and R waves

QRS Complex: Greater than 0.12 sec if pacemaker is ventricular; less than 0.12 second if pacemaker is junctional.

Clinical Significance: Third-degree block can severely compromise cardiac output because of decreased heart rate and loss of coordinated "atrial kick."

Treatment: Pacemaker insertion is the definitive treatment. In the field, if stabilization is required, medications should be administered. If the heart rate falls and the patient becomes symptomatic, you may administer 0.5 mg of atropine IV. This can be repeated every 3–5 minutes until a satisfactory rate has been obtained or 0.04 mg/kg of the drug has been given. *Atropine should be used with caution in patients with high-grade blocks (second-degree Mobitz II and third-degree). The atropine may accelerate the atrial rate, but it may also worsen the AV nodal block.* Consider transcutaneous cardiac pacing (TCP), if available. If the patient remains symptomatic, do not delay application of TCP while awaiting IV access or for atropine to take effect. Isoproterenol is rarely required. NEVER TREAT THIRD-DEGREE HEART BLOCK WITH VENTRICULAR ESCAPE BEATS WITH LIDOCAINE!

Disturbances of Ventricular Conduction

Disturbances in conduction of the depolarization impulse are not limited to the AV node. Problems can arise within the ventricles as well. Certain terms are frequently used in describing disturbances in ventricular conduction. **Aberrant conduction** is a single supraventricular beat that is conducted through the ventricles in a delayed manner. **Bundle branch block** is a disorder in which all supraventricular beats are conducted through the ventricles in a delayed manner. Either the left or right bundle branch can be involved. If both branches are blocked, then a third-degree AV block exists. These terms are used to describe complexes that originate above the ventricles. They should be distinguished from pure ventricular rhythms, which can have a similar QRS morphology.

Two causes have been identified for ventricular conduction disturbances. One is ischemia or necrosis of either the right or left bundle branch, making it unable to conduct the impulse to the ventricle it supplies. The second cause occurs when either a premature impulse (PAC or PJC) reaches the ventricles or one of the bundle branches, usually the right, finding it still refractory and unable to conduct. This is often seen in atrial fibrillation as a result of the varying speed of repolarization related to the highly irregular rhythm.

The ECG features of ventricular conduction disturbances include a QRS complex longer than 0.12 sec. This happens because the blocked side of the heart is depolarized much more slowly than the unaffected side. The impulse passes much more slowly through the myocardium than through the rapid electrical conduction pathway. The QRS morphology is often bizarre. The QRS can be notched or slurred, reflecting rapid depolarization through the normal conductive system and slow depolarization through the myocardium on the blocked side.

The presence of a ventricular conduction disturbance sometimes complicates the interpretation of ECG rhythm strips. In these cases, supraventricular beats can have QRS complexes that are abnormally wide. Because of this, it may be impossible to distinguish between PVCs and aberrantly conducted PACs or PJCs on a Lead II rhythm strip. Also, it is often difficult to distinguish supraventricular tachycardia. A 12-lead tracing is usually necessary to make the diagnosis. The presence of a bundle branch block or aberrancy does not affect management of the patient. When in doubt, treat all premature beats or rhythms with abnormally wide QRS complexes as ventricular in origin.

Pre-excitation Syndromes

The remaining category of cardiac dysrhythmias to be presented is the pre-excitation syndromes, the most common of which is *Wolff-Parkinson-White (WPW) syndrome.* WPW occurs in approximately 3 out of every 1,000 persons. It is characterized by a short P-R interval, generally less than 0.12 sec, and a prolonged QRS duration, generally longer than 0.12 sec. In addition, there is often a slur on the upstroke of the QRS, called the *delta wave.* (See Figure 21-52.) In WPW, there is abnormal conduction of the depolarization impulse from the atria to the ventricles. An extra conduction pathway, the **bundle of Kent**, is present between the atria and ventricles. The AV node is effectively by-passed, resulting in a shortened P-R interval and prolonged QRS complex. Most WPW patients are asymptomatic. However, the disorder is associated with a high incidence of tachydysrhythmias, usually through a reentry mechanism. WPW is also frequently associated with organic heart disease, such as atrial septal defects, mitral valve prolapse, and other problems. Treatment is based on the underlying rhythm.

■ **aberrant conduction** conduction of the electrical impulse through the heart's conductive system in an abnormal fashion.

■ **bundle branch block** a kind of interventricular heart block in which conduction through either the right of left bundle branches is blocked or delayed.

■ **bundle of Kent** an accessory AV conduction pathway that is thought to be responsible for the ECG findings of pre-excitation syndrome.

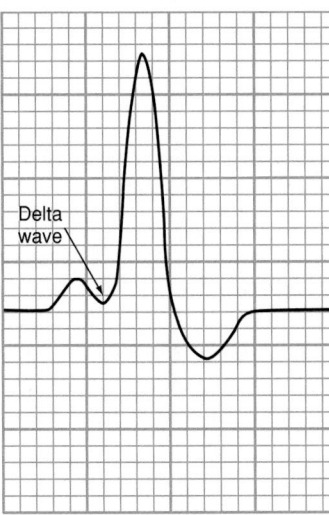

FIGURE 21-52 The delta wave of Wolf-Parkinson-White syndrome.

ASSESSMENT OF THE CARDIAC PATIENT

Assessment of the cardiac patient follows the same principles of patient assessment presented throughout this text. Particular emphasis should be placed upon obtaining the chief complaint and history and conducting a detailed assessment of the cardiovascular system.

Common Chief Complaints and Symptoms

Cardiac disease can manifest itself in several ways. When assessing a patient suspected of suffering cardiac disease, note each presenting complaint. Common presenting symptoms of cardiac disease include:

❑ Chest pain or discomfort
❑ Shoulder pain
❑ Neck pain
❑ Jaw pain
❑ Dyspnea
❑ Syncope
❑ Palpitations

The following sections address the common presenting symptoms of cardiac disease. Tips on pertinent history appear on page 685. (You may conduct part, or all, of the history while ascertaining the chief complaint or symptoms.)

Chest Pain Chest pain or chest discomfort is a common presenting symptom of cardiac disease. Chest pain is the most common presenting symptom of myocardial infarction. When confronted by a patient with chest pain, obtain the following essential elements of the history.

✳ Chest pain is the most common presenting symptom in cases of cardiac disease.

❑ Specific location of the chest pain (midsternal, etc.)
❑ Radiation of the pain, if present (e.g., to the jaw, back, or shoulders)

- ❏ Duration of the pain
- ❏ Factors that precipitated the pain (exercise, stress, etc.)
- ❏ Type or quality of the pain (dull or sharp)
- ❏ Associated symptoms (nausea, dyspnea)
- ❏ Anything that aggravates or alleviates the pain (including medications)
- ❏ Previous episodes of a similar pain (e.g., angina)

It is important to remember that chest pain has many causes other than cardiac disease. The history, therefore, is an important determining factor.

Shoulder, arm, neck, or jaw pain or discomfort may also be an indicator of cardiac disease. Any of these may occur with or without associated chest pain. If the patient has any of these symptoms, and if you suspect heart disease, obtain information similar to that described above for chest pain.

Dyspnea   Because of the close interrelationship between the heart and the respiratory system, many cardiac patients have dyspnea. Dyspnea is often an associated symptom of myocardial infarction. In some patients, it may be the only symptom of myocardial infarction. It may also be a primary symptom of pulmonary fluid congestion due to heart failure. Dyspnea is a subjective symptom and is often difficult to assess. When confronted by a dyspneic patient, try to determine the following essential elements.

- ❏ Duration of dyspnea
- ❏ Onset (sudden or rapid)
- ❏ Anything that aggravates or relieves the dyspnea (including medications)
- ❏ Previous episodes
- ❏ Any associated symptoms
- ❏ Prior cardiac problems

Many illnesses, other than cardiac disease, can cause dyspnea. These include pneumonia, chronic obstructive pulmonary disease, asthma, and pulmonary embolism.

Syncope   Cardiac problems are a major cause of syncope. Syncope, which is caused by an interruption of blood flow to the brain, may be the only presenting symptom of cardiac disease, especially in the elderly. Cardiac causes of syncope usually result from dysrhythmias. These can include transient or prolonged bradycardia, causing decreased cardiac output and, subsequently, decreased cerebral perfusion. Very rapid heart rates, on the other hand, do not allow adequate time for ventricular filling. This also results in decreased cardiac output and can cause syncope. When the primary complaint is syncope, try to establish the following essential elements.

- ❏ Circumstances of occurrence (for example, patient's position)
- ❏ Duration of the episode
- ❏ Any symptoms before the episode of syncope
- ❏ Other associated symptoms
- ❏ Previous episodes of syncope

Syncope will be discussed in detail in Chapter 23, "Nervous System Emergencies."

Palpitations Some patients with cardiac disease complain of an awareness of their own heartbeat. This is termed **palpitation** and is usually related to either an irregular beat ("skipping beats") or a rapid heart rate. When assessing these patients, essential aspects of the history include:

■ **palpitation** a sensation that the heart is pounding, racing, or skipping a beat.

- ❏ Circumstances of occurrence
- ❏ Duration of occurrence
- ❏ Associated symptoms
- ❏ Frequency of occurrence
- ❏ Previous episodes

Significant Past Medical History

You should not spend a great deal of time obtaining the past medical history of a cardiac patient. The patient will be treated based upon current symptoms rather than the history. However, if the patient's condition permits, use the following questions to develop aspects of the medical history.

1. Is the patient taking prescription medications regularly, particularly cardiac medications? Examples include:
   - Nitroglycerin
   - Propranolol (Inderal)
   - Digitalis (Lanoxin)
   - Diuretics (Lasix, Maxzide, Dyazide)
   - Antihypertensives (Vasotec, Prinivil, Capoten)
   - Other antidysrhythmics (Mexitil, Quinaglute, Tambocor)
2. Is the patient currently under treatment for any serious illness?
3. Has the patient ever been known to have any of the below conditions?
   - Heart attack or angina
   - Heart failure
   - Hypertension
   - Diabetes
   - Chronic lung disease
4. Does the patient have any allergies?

Physical Examination

The physical examination of the suspected cardiac patient should begin like the examination of any patient. First, complete the primary survey. (See Figure 21-53.) This should include the mini-neuro examination. Subsequently, after addressing any life-threatening problems detected in the primary survey, begin the secondary assessment. Pay particular attention to the blood pressure, respiratory rate, regularity and rate of the pulse (an irregular pulse may be the first indication of a dysrhythmia), and level of consciousness. Any deviation from the normal level of consciousness may indicate inadequate cerebral perfusion, possibly caused by poor cardiac output.

The secondary survey of the cardiac patient should be systematic and complete. The following tips will help guide the "look," "listen," and "feel" of your secondary assessment.

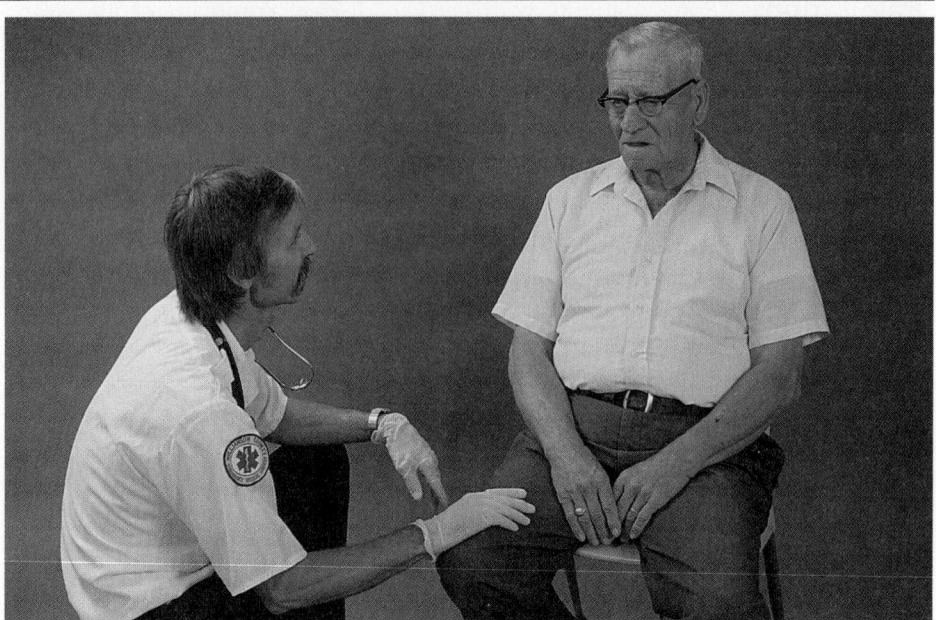

FIGURE 21-53 When treating a potential cardiac patient, always begin with the primary assessment.

Look

❑ *Skin Color and Capillary Refill.* Both skin color and capillary refill are good indicators of red blood cell oxygenation. (See Figure 21-54.) They also indicate pump adequacy, since peripheral perfusion is among the first areas to become compromised in pump failure.

❑ *Jugular Venous Distention.* The internal jugular veins are major vessels of the venous system. Thus, an increase in central venous pressure is often evidenced by jugular venous distention. (See Figure 21-55.) Pump failure can cause backpressure in the systemic circulation and jugular vein engorgement. The patient should be examined while seated at a 45-degree angle, not lying flat. Jugular venous distention is often difficult to assess in the obese patient.

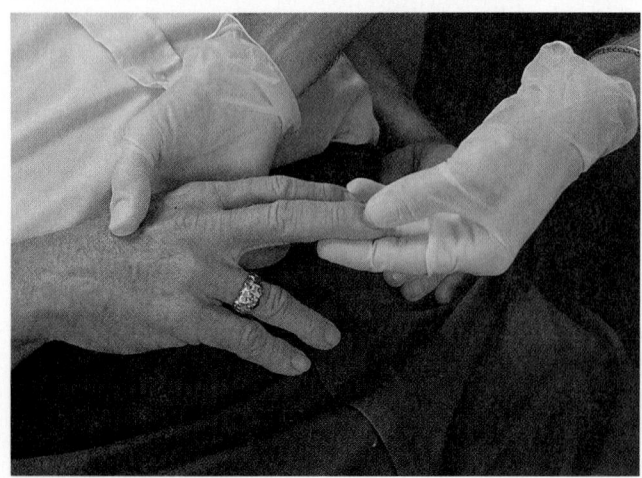

FIGURE 21-54 Assess capillary refill.

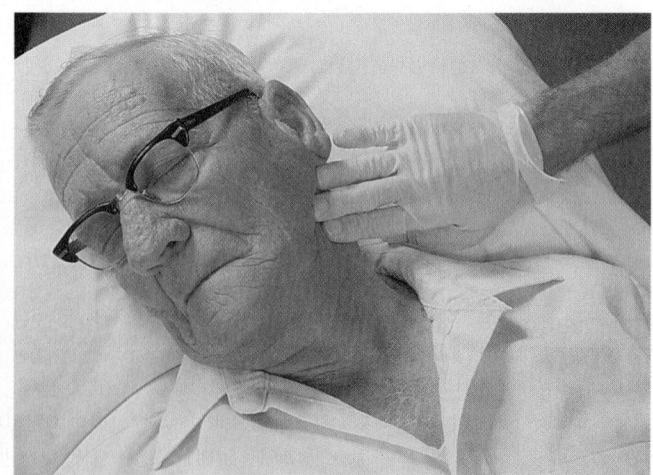

FIGURE 21-55 Look for the presence of jugular venous distension, ideally with the patient elevated at a 45-degree angle.

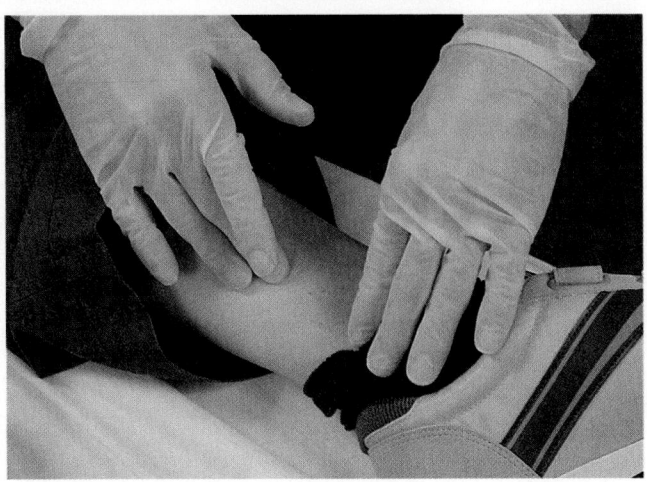

FIGURE 21-56 Check for peripheral edema.

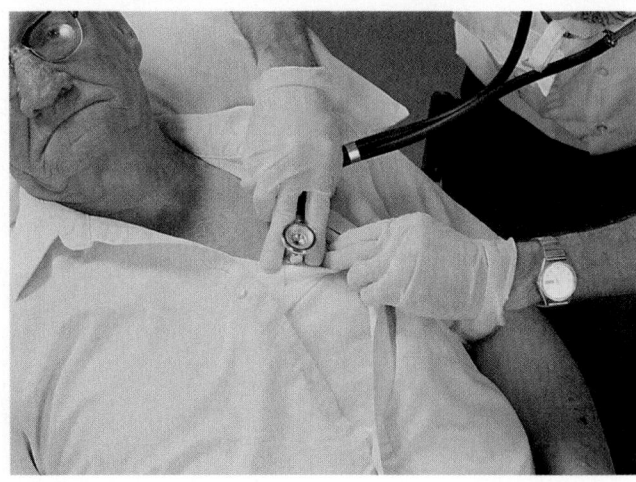

FIGURE 21-57 Auscultate the chest. Listen for heart sounds.

❑ *Peripheral/Presacral Edema.* Peripheral and presacral edema are caused by chronic backpressure in the systemic venous circulation. They are most obvious in dependent parts, such as the ankles. (See Figure 21-56.) In bedridden patients, it is often necessary to inspect and palpate the sacral region for the presence of edema. Edema is generally classified as mild or pitting. The two types can be distinguished by pressing firmly on the edematous part. If, after removal of the pressure, the depression remains, then the edema is said to be pitting.

❑ *Subtle Indicators of Cardiac Disease.* Observe for things that indicate that a patient is being treated for cardiac problems. These include the presence of a midsternal scar from coronary artery bypass surgery, a pacemaker, or a nitroglycerin skin patch.

Listen

❑ *Breath Sounds.* Assessment of breath sounds in the cardiac patient is just as important as it is in the patient with respiratory disease. Assess the lung fields for equality as well as for the presence of adventitious sounds (rales, wheezes, or rhonchi) that may indicate pulmonary congestion or edema.

❑ *Heart Sounds.* Do not spend a great deal of time auscultating heart sounds in the field, as the information obtained will generally not affect patient management. However, you should be familiar with normal heart sounds and be able to distinguish abnormal from normal findings. (See Figure 21-57.) The first heart sound, referred to as S1, is produced by closure of the AV valves (tricuspid and mitral) during ventricular systole. The second heart sound, or S2, is produced by closure of the aortic and pulmonary valves. S1 and S2 are normal findings. Extra heart sounds are abnormal findings. The third heart sound, or S3, is associated with congestive heart failure. Occasionally, the skilled listener can hear the fourth heart sound, or S4, that occurs immediately before S1. It is associated with increased contraction of the atria.

❑ *Carotid Artery Bruit.* A bruit is a sign of turbulent blood flow through a vessel. Auscultation of the carotid arteries may reveal the presence of bruits. (See Figure 21-58.) A bruit indicates partial blockage of the vessel,

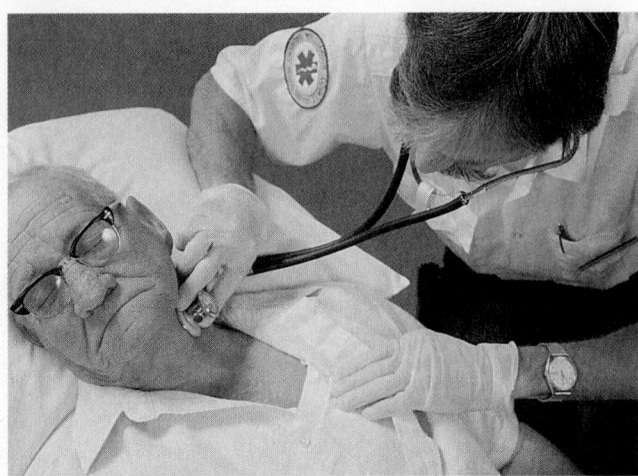

FIGURE 21-58 Listen to the carotid arteries. The presence of noisy blood flow is termed a bruit and may indicate underlying disease in the artery.

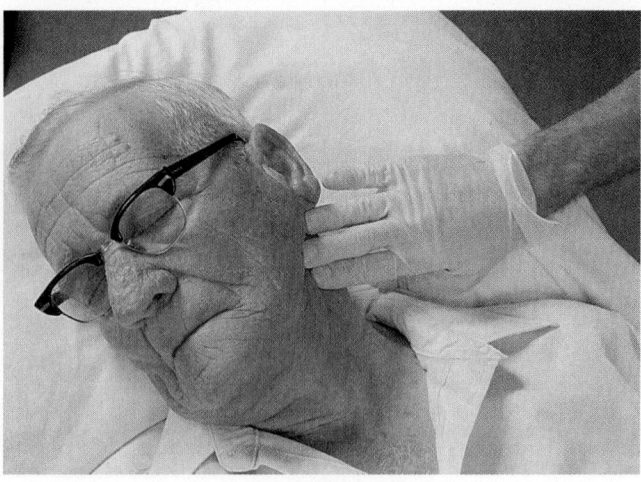

FIGURE 21-59 Check the patient's pulse for both strength and character.

most commonly from atherosclerosis. If a bruit is present, carotid sinus massage should not be attempted. This care step may dislodge plaque, resulting in stroke or other mishap.

Feel

❑ *Pulse.* As mentioned above, the pulse can tell a great deal about the status of the circulatory system. (See Figure 21-59.) Determine the rate and regularity of the pulse. Equality of the pulses should also be noted. Any pulse deficit can indicate underlying peripheral vascular disease and should be reported to the medical control physician.

❑ *Skin.* Several changes in the skin can be associated with cardiovascular disease. A pale and diaphoretic skin is an indicator of peripheral vasoconstriction and sympathetic stimulation. It accompanies heart disease and other problems. A mottled appearance often indicates chronic cardiac failure.

PATHOPHYSIOLOGY OF CARDIOVASCULAR DISEASE

The following sections will detail the pathophysiology of common cardiovascular emergencies, giving special emphasis to life-threatening illnesses.

Atherosclerosis

■ **atherosclerosis** a progressive, degenerative disease of the medium-sized and large arteries.

Cardiovascular disease is the number one cause of death in the United States and most developed countries. The major underlying factor in many cardiovascular emergencies is atherosclerosis. **Atherosclerosis** is a progressive, degenerative disease of the medium-sized and large arteries. It affects the aorta and its branches, the coronary arteries, and the cerebral arteries, among others. It results from the deposition of fats (lipids and cholesterol) under the tunica intima layer of the involved vessels. After fat is deposited, an injury response occurs in the vessel wall, which subsequently damages the tunica media as well. Over time, calcium is deposited, causing the formation of plaques. Small hemorrhages can occur in the plaques, which in turn lead to scarring, fibrosis, and even larger plaques. The involved arteries can become completely blocked, either by additional plaque or by a blood clot. The conditions below increase the risk for developing atheriosclerosis.

Modifiable Risk Factors

- ❏ Hypertension
- ❏ Smoking
- ❏ Elevated blood lipids (cholesterol and triglycerides)
- ❏ Lack of exercise
- ❏ Obesity

Nonmodifiable Risk Factors

- ❏ Male gender
- ❏ Advanced age
- ❏ Family history of heart disease and atherosclerosis
- ❏ Diabetes mellitus (good control reduces risk)

The results of atherosclerosis are evident in many disease processes. First, disruption of the intimal surface of the involved blood vessel causes loss of vessel elasticity. This condition, known as **arteriosclerosis**, can result in hypertension and other related problems. Second, blood flow through the affected vessel can be reduced. Common manifestations of this include angina pectoris and intermittent **claudication**. Frequently, thrombosis and complete obstruction occur, resulting in total obstruction of the vessel or the tissues it supplies. Myocardial infarction is a classic example of this process.

Several conditions are related to atherosclerosis of the coronary arteries. These include angina pectoris and myocardial infarction. As a paramedic, one of your major roles will be the prompt recognition of acute myocardial infarction and initiation of effective prehospital treatment.

Angina Pectoris *Angina pectoris* literally means "pain in the chest." The condition is much more complicated than that, however. Angina occurs when the oxygen demands of the heart are transiently exceeded by the blood supply. In other words, during periods of increased oxygen demand, the coronary arteries cannot deliver an adequate amount of blood to the myocardium. This can result in ischemia of the myocardium and chest pain.

As a rule, the reduction in blood flow through the coronary arteries results from atherosclerosis. However, abnormal spasm of the coronary arteries, commonly called *vasospastic angina* or **Prinzmetal's angina**, can also lead to inadequate blood flow. It is important to remember that blood flow through a vessel is related to its diameter. Reducing the diameter of a vessel by one-half, as can occur in atherosclerosis, causes a major reduction in the amount of blood that can be transported through that vessel.

Angina is generally divided into two types—stable angina and unstable, or preinfarction, angina. *Stable angina* is angina that occurs during activity, when the oxygen demands of the heart are increased. Attacks of stable angina are usually precipitated by physical or emotional stress. They can be of relatively short duration, 3–5 minutes, or prolonged, lasting 15 minutes or more. The pain of stable angina can often be relieved by rest, nitroglycerin, or oxygen. *Unstable angina*, on the other hand, may not respond as readily.

■ **arteriosclerosis** a thickening, loss of elasticity, and hardening of the walls of the arteries from calcium deposits.

■ **claudication** severe pain in the calf muscle due to inadequate blood supply. It typically occurs with exertion and subsides with rest.

■ **Prinzmetal's angina** variant of angina pectoris caused by vasospasm of the coronary arteries; not blockage *per se*.

Unstable angina occurs at rest. Because the condition often indicates severe atherosclerotic disease, it is also called *preinfarction angina.*

Signs and Symptoms. The pain associated with angina is primarily caused by a buildup of lactic acid and CO_2 in the ischemic myocardium. The patient usually complains of substernal chest pain or epigastric discomfort. The patient may describe the discomfort as pain, pressure, squeezing, or tightness. Anginal pain is frequently mistaken for indigestion. One-third of angina patients feel pain only in the chest. Others have pain that radiates to the shoulder, arm, neck, jaw, or through to the back. Some patients have associated symptoms of anxiety, dyspnea, or diaphoresis.

Angina can be accompanied by dysrhythmias that are precipitated by ischemia. For this reason, all patients suspected of suffering angina should be placed on the cardiac monitor.

If a patient has a prior history of angina and is currently taking nitroglycerin, try to determine if the patient has taken nitroglycerin for the present attack. Also find out how much has been taken, and if it has relieved the discomfort. If the patient's nitroglycerin tablets are old, they may be ineffective. It is not uncommon for a patient's symptoms to be relieved because of nitroglycerin therapy by the time EMS arrives.

Management. The patient experiencing angina is often apprehensive. Place the patient at rest, physically and emotionally, to decrease myocardial oxygen demand. Administer oxygen, generally at a high-flow rate, to increase oxygen delivery to the myocardium. Administer nitroglycerin sublingually, either as a tablet or spray. Nitroglycerin decreases myocardial work and, to a lesser degree, dilates coronary arteries. If the patient's symptoms persist after the administration of one or two doses of nitroglycerin, assume that something more serious than angina is occurring, such as myocardial infarction.

Nifedipine (Procardia) is now being used, in addition to nitroglycerin, in the management of angina. It is a vasodilator that works through a different mechanism than nitroglycerin. Patients with first episodes of angina, or episodes that are not relieved by medication, are usually admitted to the hospital for evaluation.

■ **acute myocardial infarction (MI)** death and subsequent necrosis of the heart muscle caused by inadequate blood supply.

Myocardial Infarction   **Acute myocardial infarction (MI)** is the death of a portion of the heart muscle from prolonged deprivation of arterial blood supply. MI can also occur when the oxygen demand of the heart exceeds its supply for an extended period of time. Myocardial infarction is most often associated with *atherosclerotic heart disease (ASHD).* The precipitating event is commonly the formation of a *thrombus,* or blood clot, in a coronary artery already diseased from atherosclerosis. Myocardial infarction can also result from coronary artery spasm, microemboli, acute volume overload, hypotension (from any cause), or from acute respiratory failure (acute hypoxia).

The actual location and size of the infarction depends on the vessel involved and the site of the obstruction. (See Figure 21-60.) Most infarctions involve the left ventricle. Obstruction of the left coronary artery may result in anterior, lateral, or septal infarcts. Right coronary artery occlusions usually result in inferior wall infarctions. The actual infarction is often classified as transmural or subendocardial. In a *transmural infarction,* the entire thickness of the myocardium was destroyed. This lesion is associated with Q wave changes on the ECG and is occasionally called *Q wave infarction.* In a *subendocardial infarction,* only the subendocardial layer is involved. This type of infarction is not usually accompanied by Q wave changes on the ECG. For this reason, it is often called a *non-Q wave infarction.*

The tissues affected by myocardial infarction can exhibit various degrees

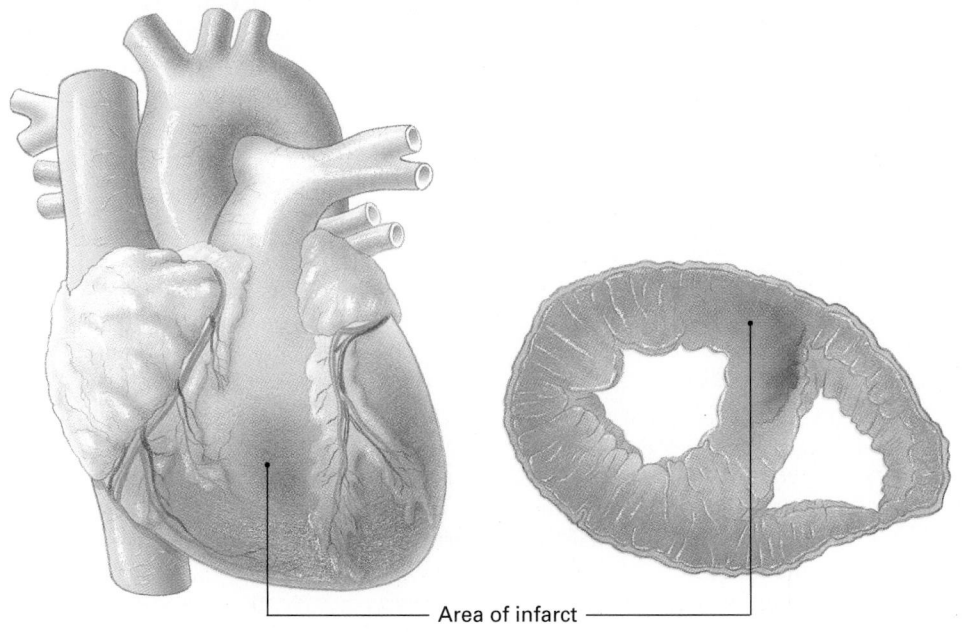

Area of infarct

FIGURE 21-60 Myocardial infarction.

of damage. First, following occlusion of the coronary artery, the affected tissue develops ischemia. If the blockage is not relieved and collateral circulation is inadequate, the tissue will infarct and die. The infarcted tissue becomes necrotic and eventually forms scar tissue. The area of infarcted myocardium is surrounded by a ring of ischemic tissue. This ischemic tissue survives, primarily because of collateral circulation. The ischemic area is often the origin of many dysrhythmias.

Myocardial infarction has several complications, the most common of which is dysrhythmias. Life-threatening dysrhythmias can occur almost immediately and can result in **sudden death**, or death within one hour after the onset of symptoms. This is the most common cause of death resulting from myocardial infarction.

In addition to dysrhythmias, the patient can develop congestive heart failure because of destruction of a portion of the myocardial muscle mass. Such patients may have right heart failure, left heart failure, or both. *Heart failure* is present if the pumping ability of the heart is impaired, but the heart can meet the demands of the body. That is, the heart is inefficient but adequate. If the heart cannot meet the oxygen demands of the body, then *inadequate tissue perfusion* occurs, resulting in **cardiogenic shock**. In cardiogenic shock, the heart is both inefficient and inadequate. Another cause of death from MI is *ventricular aneurysm* of the myocardial wall. The damaged portion of the wall weakens. In some cases, it bursts, resulting in sudden death. *Pump failure*, resulting from extensive myocardial damage, can also result in death.

Signs and Symptoms. The most common presenting sign or symptom of myocardial infarction is substernal chest pain or epigastric pain. The pain generally has the same characteristics and location as anginal pain. It may be severe and is often described as crushing, but it may also be relatively mild. It frequently radiates to other areas, such as the arms, neck, jaw, and back. The pain is present when the patient is at rest and is not necessarily precipitated by exertion. The pain of myocardial infarction is not relieved by sublingual nitroglycerin or other home medications. Frequently, large doses of morphine, or a nitroglycerin drip, are required to alleviate it.

■ **sudden death** death within one hour after the onset of symptoms.

■ **cardiogenic shock** the inability of the heart to meet the metabolic needs of the body, resulting in inadequate tissue perfusion.

✳ The patient with MI may not have chest pain as a symptom.

Patients with MI, especially elderly and diabetic patients, may not have chest pain. Instead, they may complain of pain in the shoulder, arm, neck, jaw, or back. Some patients with MI have no symptoms whatsoever. The MI is diagnosed by ECG changes or elevated cardiac enzyme levels.

Symptoms often associated with MI include:

❑ Diaphoresis
❑ Anxiety or apprehension
❑ Dyspnea
❑ Nausea or vomiting
❑ Pallor
❑ General weakness or malaise

Many patients, especially the elderly, have no pain. Instead, they complain of general malaise or a history of syncope. Many MI patients deny the seriousness of the problem. This often causes them to delay seeking medical care during the first hours following onset of discomfort, the most critical phase of the illness.

The vital signs associated with MI can vary with the extent of pump damage and the degree of autonomic nervous system response. The blood pressure can be normal, elevated due to increased sympathetic tone, or low due to increased parasympathetic tone or pump failure. The pulse rate depends on whether dysrhythmias are present. The rate may be fast or slow, regular or irregular, weak or bounding. Respirations may be either normal or increased.

Dysrhythmias are the most common complication of MI. Some dysrhythmias are warnings of life-threatening dysrhythmias and may require prehospital intervention. Life-threatening dysrhythmias such as ventricular fibrillation can result in sudden death. Non-life-threatening dysrhythmias may not require prehospital intervention.

All patients with chest pain should be transported to the hospital. Any patient with chest pain and a compatible history should be presumed to have a myocardial infarction until proven otherwise. Age and other factors are not good discriminators.

Prehospital Management of MI. Prehospital intervention can mean the difference between life and death to a patient with MI. Goals of prehospital intervention include:

❑ Preventing pain and apprehension
❑ Preventing serious dysrhythmias
❑ Limiting the size of the infarct
❑ Initiating of thrombolytic therapy if transport time is long

✳ With the advent of thrombolytic therapy (drugs that dissolve the blood clot causing a heart attack), prehospital care must be undertaken quickly, with expedient transport to the emergency department.

Time is of the essence. Complete the primary assessment, and begin the secondary survey quickly. Obtain the medical history while conducting the physical examination and initiating treatment. Place the patient physically at rest and reassure him or her. This will help decrease anxiety and apprehension, which in turn will reduce heart rate and myocardial oxygen demand. In addition, place the patient in a position of comfort, ideally reclining with the head elevated 30 degrees. Do not allow the patient to walk. Get the stretcher as near to the patient as possible.

Administer oxygen at high-flow rate, unless there is significant documented chronic obstructive pulmonary disease. This will increase myocardial oxygen delivery and can aid in the reduction of infarct size. Determine baseline vital signs. A slow, fast, or irregular pulse may be the first indication of a dysrhythmia. Repeat the vital signs frequently. As soon as possible, establish an IV at a "to keep open" (TKO) rate to provide venous access. Place the ECG electrodes, and record a baseline ECG. Cardiac monitoring should continue throughout patient assessment and transport. Record any dysrhythmias, and attach the rhythm strip to the patient report. Complete the history and physical examination, including auscultation of the lungs. The presence of basilar rales may indicate early heart failure.

Following patient assessment, administer medications according to written protocols or upon order of the medical control physician. Drugs commonly used for pain relief include:

❑ *Nitroglycerin.* Nitroglycerin dilates peripheral arteries and veins, thus reducing preload and afterload and myocardial oxygen demand. Some coronary artery dilation may occur, increasing blood flow though the collaterals. Nitroglycerin administration often helps distinguish angina from MI. MI symptoms are not relieved by nitroglycerin.

❑ *Morphine Sulfate.* Morphine is an important medication in the management of MI. It reduces myocardial oxygen demand by reducing venous return (preload) and systemic arterial resistance (afterload). It acts directly on the central nervous system to relieve pain. Morphine also reduces sympathetic nervous system discharge, which can further decrease myocardial oxygen demand.

❑ *Nitrous Oxide (Nitronox).* Administration of the fixed combination of nitrous oxide and oxygen is useful in the management of MI. It is purely an analgesic without significant hemodynamic effects. However, delivery of 50 percent oxygen can increase myocardial oxygen supply.

❑ *Diazepam (Valium).* Diazepam may be administered if the patient is extremely apprehensive or agitated. Diazepam is not an analgesic, but it will help relax the patient.

❑ *Nalbuphine (Nubain).* Nalbuphine is used in some EMS systems instead of morphine. It is an effective analgesic but lacks the desirable hemodynamic effects of morphine.

You may also be called upon to administer drugs commonly prescribed for dysrhythmias. Again, check local protocols or confirm with medical control. Drugs used for dysrhythmias include:

❑ *Lidocaine (Xylocaine).* Lidocaine is the first-line antidysrhythmic agent for ventricular dysrhythmias. It can effectively suppress most dysrhythmias associated with acute myocardial infarction.

❑ *Procainamide (Pronestyl).* Procainamide can be used for dysrhythmias refractory to lidocaine or in patients allergic to lidocaine.

❑ *Atropine Sulfate.* Atropine is a parasympatholytic and is effective in bradycardias, especially of atrial origin. It is often useful in the management of asystole.

❑ *Epinephrine.* Epinephrine is used in cardiovascular collapse and life-threatening dysrhythmias such as ventricular fibrillation and asystole.

❑ *Adenosine (Adenocard).* Adenosine is used in the management of symptomatic supraventricular tachydysrhythmias, especially PSVT.

❑ *Verapamil (Isoptin, Calan).* Verapamil is used in the management of supraventricular tachycardias, particularly if the rate is so fast that it compromises cardiac output.

❑ *Bretylium (Bretylol).* Bretylium is used in the management of life-threatening ventricular dysrhythmias. It is not a first-line agent.

Most patients suffering MI can be adequately stabilized in the field. After the patient is stabilized, he or she can be transported calmly, without lights or siren. This will decrease apprehension and improve patient care. However, some patients may require expedient transport.

In-Hospital Management of MI. It is important for you to understand the management of the MI patient after he or she has been delivered to the emergency department. This is especially true if you belong to an EMS system in which paramedics also staff emergency departments as part of their regular assignments.

In the hospital setting, myocardial infarction is usually diagnosed by ECG. The 12-lead ECG can indicate whether an infarction has occurred, its location, and its severity (transmural versus subendocardial).

Elevated cardiac enzyme levels also indicate the presence of mycardial infarction. *Cardiac enzymes* are muscle enzymes released from damaged myocardial cells. Commonly assayed enzymes include lactate dehydrogenase (LDH), creatine phosphokinase (CPK), and serum glutamic oxaloacetic transaminase (SGOT or AST).

Do not administer any medication intramuscularly to a patient suspected of suffering MI. This can cause a release of muscle enzymes from the site of the injection, resulting in elevated enzyme levels. Such an elevation can hinder the emergency physician in determining whether an MI has occurred. Later, the source of the enzyme elevation can be detected in the laboratory, but this is not generally possible in the acute setting.

The current trend in the management of MI is *thrombolytic therapy,* or the administration of agents that can dissolve the blood clot responsible for the infarction. This action prevents death of a significant amount of myocardium. Commonly used thrombolytic agents include streptokinase, urokinase, and tissue plasminogen activator (tPA). These agents are administered intravenously or directly into the obstructed artery. If treatment is successful, blood flow is restored, and, in some cases, significant infarction is averted.

Other treatments used in the hospital include the placement of cardiac pacemakers, dilation of stenotic arteries with balloon angioplasty, emergency bypass surgery, and insertion of the aortic counterpulsation balloon pump.

Left Ventricular Failure With Pulmonary Edema

Left ventricular failure occurs when the left ventricle fails as an effective forward pump, causing back pressure of blood into the pulmonary circulation, often resulting in pulmonary edema. (See Figure 21-61.) This can be caused by various types of heart disease, including MI, valvular disease, chronic hypertension, and dysrhythmias. In left ventricular failure, the left ventricle cannot eject all the blood delivered to it from the right heart. Left atrial pressure rises and is subsequently transmitted to the pulmonary veins and capillaries. When pulmonary capillary pressure becomes too high, the serum (fluid) portion of the blood is forced into the alveoli, resulting in pulmonary edema. Progressive fluid accumulation in the alveoli decreases the oxygenation capacity of the lungs and can result in death from hypoxia. Since MI is a common cause of left ventricular failure, all patients with pulmonary edema should be assumed to have had an MI.

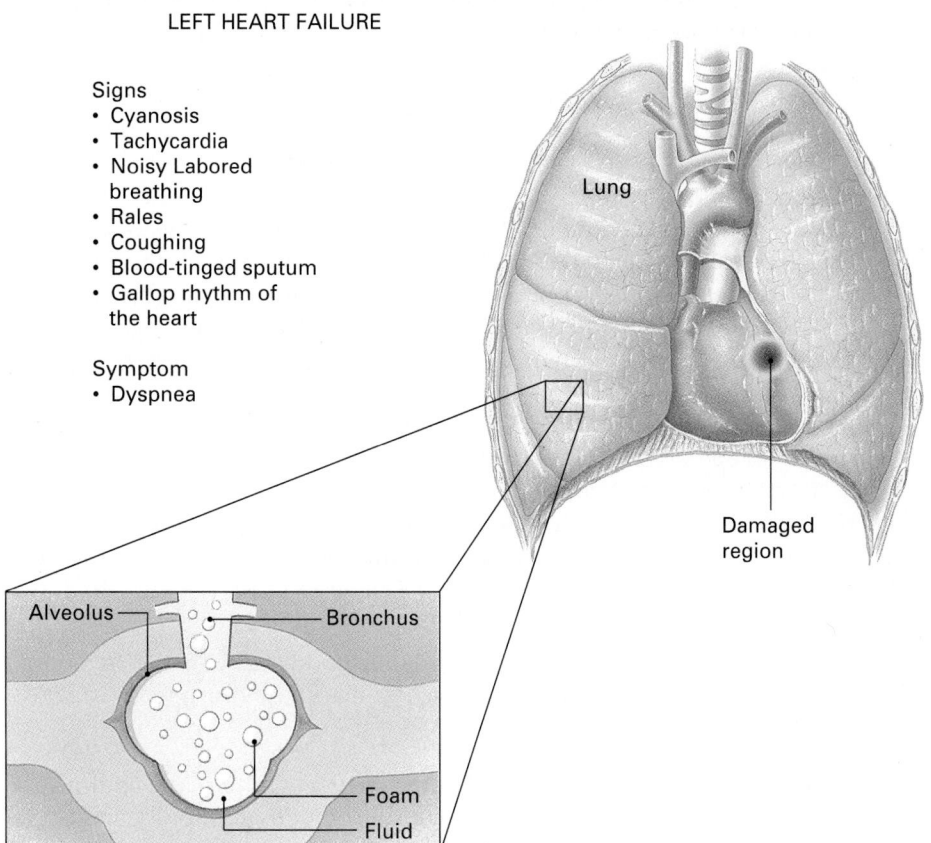

LEFT HEART FAILURE

Signs
• Cyanosis
• Tachycardia
• Noisy Labored breathing
• Rales
• Coughing
• Blood-tinged sputum
• Gallop rhythm of the heart

Symptom
• Dyspnea

Lung

Damaged region

Alveolus — Bronchus

Foam
Fluid

FIGURE 21-61 Left heart failure.

Signs and Symptoms   Signs and symptoms of left ventricular failure and pulmonary edema include the following conditions.

❑ *Severe Respiratory Distress.* Severe respiratory distress is evidenced as orthopnea or dyspnea. Spasmodic coughing, which may be productive of pink, frothy sputum, is a characteristic finding. The patient may report a history of **paroxysmal nocturnal dyspnea (PND)** as well.

❑ *Severe Apprehension, Agitation, and Confusion.* Left ventricular failure and pulmonary edema can result in hypoxia. The patient often has a smothering feeling. He or she becomes apprehensive and frightened. As hypoxia worsens, agitation and confusion can develop.

❑ *Cyanosis.* Cyanosis results from inadequate exchange of oxygen and carbon dioxide in the lungs, resulting from pulmonary edema. Thus the PaO_2 level falls and the $PaCO_2$ level increases.

❑ *Diaphoresis.* Diaphoresis often results from sympathetic stimulation, either from apprehension associated with pulmonary edema or from MI.

❑ *Adventitious Lung Sounds (Pulmonary Congestion).* Adventitious lung sounds are often present in pulmonary edema. These include:

• *Rales.* Rales, especially at the bases of the lungs, result from fluid in the alveoli. Severe rales can be heard all the way up to the scapulae and do not clear with coughing.

• *Rhonchi.* Rhonchi are associated with fluid in the larger airways and often indicate severe pulmonary edema.

✱ The most common presenting symptom of left heart failure is respiratory distress.

■ **paroxysmal nocturnal dyspnea (PND)** a sudden episode of difficult breathing that occurs after lying down; most commonly caused by left heart failure.

- *Wheezes.* Wheezes occur in response to reflex airway spasm. The presence of fluid in the alveoli is misinterpreted by the protective mechanisms of the lungs, resulting in bronchoconstriction in an attempt to keep additional fluid from entering. The wheezing seen in pulmonary edema and congestive heart failure is often called "cardiac asthma," which is a confusing term that should be avoided.
- ❑ *Jugular Venous Distention.* Jugular venous distention does not result directly from left ventricular failure. However, it may be present when backpressure from left ventricular failure extends through the right heart to the venous circulation. Examine the patient for jugular venous distention with the patient seated and the head elevated at a 45-degree angle.
- ❑ *Vital Signs.* There is usually a significant increase in sympathetic discharge to help the body compensate for the left heart failure. The blood pressure is often elevated. The pulse is rapid to compensate for the low stroke volume. The pulse may be irregular if dysrhythmias are present. Respirations are rapid and labored.
- ❑ *Level of Consciousness.* The level of consciousness may vary. The patient may be extremely anxious or apprehensive. As cerebral perfusion decreases and hypoxia increases, the patient may become agitated, confused, and, finally, unresponsive.
- ❑ *Chest Pain.* The presence of chest pain depends on whether myocardial infarction has occurred. The pain may be masked by respiratory distress.

Prehospital Management Left ventricular failure and pulmonary edema is a true emergency. The patient can decompensate rapidly and unpredictably. The goals of management should include:

- ❑ Decreasing venous return to the heart (preload)
- ❑ Decreasing myocardial oxygen demands
- ❑ Improving ventilation and oxygenation

Obtain pertinent medical history, and complete the physical exam while initiating treatment. Seat the patient with the feet dangling. This will promote venous pooling, thus decreasing preload. DO NO LIE THE PATIENT FLAT AT ANY TIME. Administer high-flow oxygen. If necessary, provide positive-pressure assistance with either a demand valve or bag-valve-mask unit if the patient can assist or is unresponsive.

If possible, establish an IV of D5W at a TKO rate. It is imperative that fluids be limited. Therefore, use a minidrip set to avoid the accidental infusion of excessive amounts of fluid.

Place ECG electrodes. If the patient is extremely diaphoretic, apply tincture of benzoin first. Record a baseline ECG. Keep the monitor in place throughout care.

Administer medications according to written protocols or on the order of the medical control physician. Some cases of left ventricular failure result from very rapid dysrhythmias. If you suspect a dysrhythmia as a cause, treat it according to established protocols. Medications frequently used in left ventricular failure and pulmonary edema include:

- ❑ *Morphine Sulfate.* Morphine is administered primarily for its hemodynamic properties, since the patient may not be in pain. Morphine decreases venous return (preload), reduces myocardial work, and helps alleviate anxiety.

- *Nitroglycerin.* Nitroglycerin may be used for peripheral vasodilation. This will decrease preload and afterload and can lessen the symptoms of left ventricular failure.
- *Furosemide (Lasix).* Furosemide is a potent loop diuretic with a relaxant effect on the venous system. Effects are often seen within 5 minutes. Also, through its diuretic effect, it decreases intravascular fluid volume. Increased doses of furosemide may be required if the patient has been taking this medication, or another diuretic, at home.
- *Dobutamine (Dobutrex).* Like dopamine, dobutamine increases cardiac output by increasing stroke volume. It has little effect on heart rate and is occasionally used in isolated left heart failure until other medications, such as digitalis, have taken effect. Dobutamine is administered by intravenous infusion.

Rapid transport to the hospital is essential in all cases involving left ventricular failure and pulmonary edema.

Right Ventricular Failure

Right ventricular failure is failure of the right ventricle as an effective forward pump, resulting in backpressure of blood into the systemic venous circulation and venous congestion. (See Figure 21-62.) The most common cause of right ventricular failure is left ventricular failure. This is because myocardial infarc-

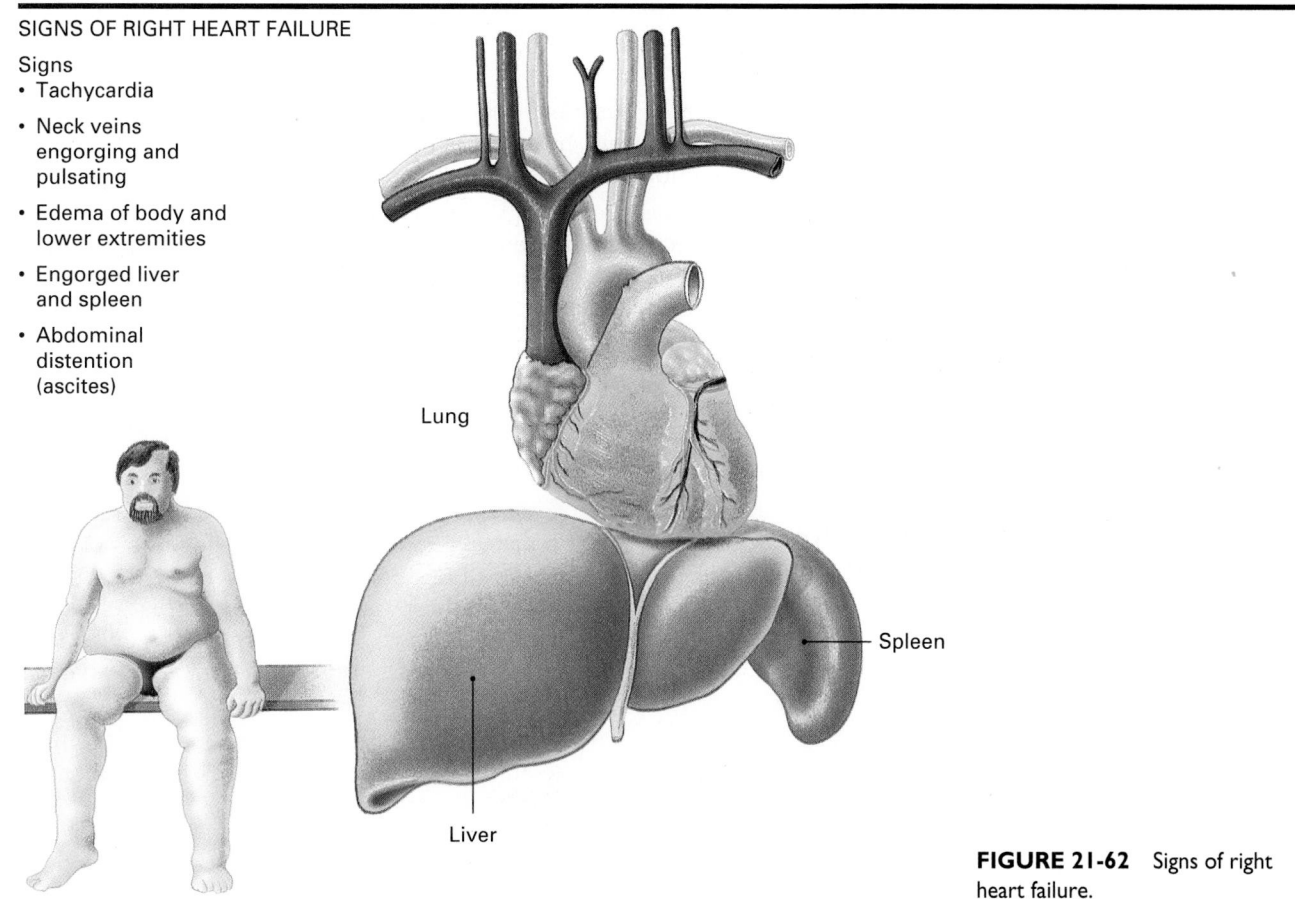

SIGNS OF RIGHT HEART FAILURE

Signs
- Tachycardia
- Neck veins engorging and pulsating
- Edema of body and lower extremities
- Engorged liver and spleen
- Abdominal distention (ascites)

Lung

Spleen

Liver

FIGURE 21-62 Signs of right heart failure.

tion is more common in the left ventricle than in the right and because the left ventricle is more adversely affected by chronic hypertension than is the right.

However, right ventricular failure has other causes as well. Systemic hypertension can affect both sides of the heart and can cause pure right ventricular failure. Pulmonary hypertension and *cor pulmonale* result from the effects of chronic obstructive pulmonary disease (COPD). These problems are related to increased pressure in the pulmonary arteries. Increased pressure results in right ventricular enlargement, right atrial enlargement, and, if untreated, right heart failure.

Pulmonary embolism, the presence of a blood clot in one of the pulmonary arteries, is another cause of right heart failure. If the clot is large enough, a major vessel can be occluded, increasing the pressure against which the right ventricle must pump. This can throw the right ventricle into failure in much the same manner as pulmonary hypertension. In fact, it can be considered an acute form of pulmonary hypertension. Infarct of the right atrium or ventricle, although rare, can also cause right ventricular failure.

From a pathophysiological standpoint, right heart failure develops when the right ventricle cannot keep up with venous return. As the stroke volume decreases, right atrial pressure rises and backpressure is transmitted to the vena cava and the rest of the venous system. When the systemic venous pressure becomes too high, the liquid portion of the blood (serum) is forced into the interstitial space, resulting in edema.

Signs and Symptoms   The signs and symptoms of right heart failure depend upon the degree of failure and the patient's general condition. Common findings include:

❑ *Tachycardia.* Tachycardia results from the body's attempts to maintain cardiac output by increasing heart rate to compensate for the fall in stroke volume.

❑ *Venous Congestion.* Systemic venous congestion is the hallmark of right heart failure. This results from the leakage of fluid into interstitial spaces. Symptoms of venous congestion include:

• *Peripheral Edema.* Peripheral edema is usually noted in the ankles and the pretibial area. In the bedridden patient, it may be present only in the presacral region. Severe pitting edema may occur. Generalized edema affecting virtually the entire body, or *anasarca*, is often an ominous finding.

• *Jugular Venous Distention.* Jugular venous distention results directly from an increase in systemic venous pressure. Examine the patient for jugular venous distention with the patient seated and the head at a 45-degree angle.

• *Fluid Accumulation in Serous Cavities.* The leakage of fluid out of the intravascular space can result in fluid accumulation in serous cavities. Fluid can accumulate in the abdominal cavity (ascites), the pleural space (pleural effusion), and in the pericardium (pericardial effusion). The amount of fluid in a serous cavity can be quite large. Patients often tolerate even large quantities of effusion that develop over an extended period.

❑ *Liver Engorgement.* Increased venous pressure causes edema of the liver. This may be evident only to the skilled examiner. Liver enlargement is a common finding in right heart failure.

❑ *History.* Patients with right heart failure often have histories of prior MIs and may have chronic pump failure. Often, these patients are taking digoxin (Lanoxin) and furosemide (Lasix). Such medications will provide a clue to the patient's underlying problem. Occasionally, patients use lay terms such as "dropsy," "enlarged heart," or "weak heart" to describe their disease.

Prehospital Management   Right heart failure is usually not an emergency, unless it is accompanied by left heart failure and pulmonary edema. Administer high-flow oxygen. If possible, establish an IV of D5W at a TKO rate. It is imperative that fluids be limited. Use a minidrip set to avoid the accidental infusion of excessive amounts of fluid.

Place ECG electrodes. If the patient is extremely diaphoretic, apply tincture of benzoin first. Record a baseline ECG, and leave the monitor in place throughout care. Rapid transport to the hospital is usually not necessary, unless left heart failure develops. Left heart failure should be treated as previously described.

Cardiogenic Shock

Cardiogenic shock, the most severe form of pump failure, occurs when left ventricular function is so compromised that the heart cannot meet the metabolic demands of the body and compensatory mechanisms are exhausted. Cardiogenic shock is shock that remains after correction of existing dysrhythmias, hypovolemia, or altered vascular tone. It usually occurs after extensive myocardial infarction, often involving more than 40 percent of the left ventricle, or from diffuse ischemia.

✳ Cardiogenic shock is the most severe form of pump failure.

Signs and Symptoms   Myocardial infarction often precedes cardiogenic shock, and symptoms are initially the same as would be expected with MI. However, as cardiogenic shock develops and compensatory mechanisms fail, hypotension develops. The systolic blood pressure is often less than 80 mmHg. There may be an altered level of consciousness, ranging from restlessness and confusion to coma. The usual heart rhythm is sinus tachycardia, a reflection of the cardiovascular system's attempts to compensate for the decrease in stroke volume. If serious dysrhythmias are present, it may be difficult to determine whether the dysrhythmias are the cause of the hypotension or the result of the cardiogenic shock. Therefore, any major dysrhythmias must be corrected. The patient's skin is usually cool and clammy, reflecting peripheral vasoconstriction. Tachypnea is often present, since pulmonary edema is a common complication.

Management   Management of cardiogenic shock is difficult, even in the hospital. The mortality rate approaches 80–90 percent, even when the best technology is readily available. Therefore, prolonged stabilization in the field is not indicated. Transport should be expeditious. Carry out the primary assessment. Secure the airway and administer high-flow oxygen. Place the patient in a supine position. Initiate an IV of D5W, using a minidrip set. Place ECG electrodes and obtain a baseline ECG. On physical examination, pay particular attention to blood pressure, jugular venous distention, and breath sounds. Administer medications per written protocol or by order of the medical control physician. Remember, always treat the rate and rhythm first. (See Figure 21-63.) Medications to be used include

✳ The mortality of cardiogenic shock approaches 80–90 percent, even when the best technology is readily available.

❑ *Dopamine (Intropin)*. Dopamine increases cardiac output. It stimulates both the α and ß receptors. It offers an advantage over other drugs in that it often maintains renal perfusion at recommended dosages.

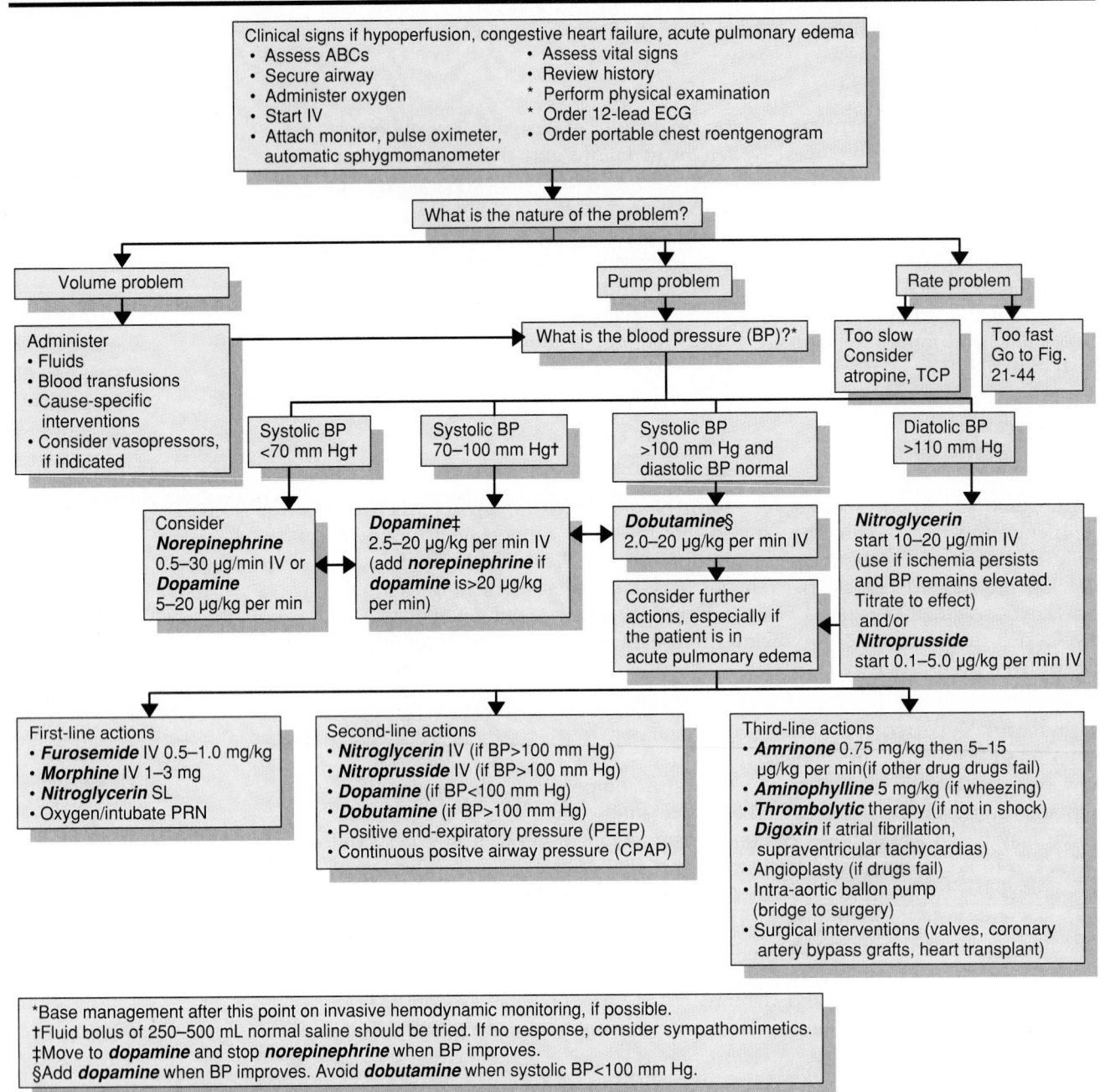

FIGURE 21-63 Management of hypotension, shock, and pulmonary edema.

❑ *Norepinephrine (Levophed)*. For many years, norepinephrine was the standard vasopressor used for cardiogenic shock. With the advent of dopamine, it has fallen into relative disuse, primarily because of its adverse effects on renal perfusion and its lack of significant ß properties.

If left heart failure and pulmonary edema are present (as they often are), they should be treated concurrently. First-line medications include morphine, furosemide, and oxygen with positive pressure ventilation (see above). Some authors have recommended use of the PASG in cardiogenic shock. This device may have a role in treatment of patients without pulmonary edema. Its use is controversial. Therefore, you should check local protocols before using a PASG in the field.

The patient with cardiogenic shock should be transported rapidly. Do not wait to observe the effects of medications administered in the field.

Cardiac Arrest/Sudden Death

Cardiac arrest and sudden death accounts for 60 percent of all deaths from coronary artery disease. *Sudden death* is death that occurs within one hour after the onset of symptoms. At autopsy, actual infarction often is not present. Because severe atherosclerotic disease is common, authorities usually believe that a lethal dysrhythmia is the mechanism of death. The risk factors for sudden death are basically the same as those previously presented for atherosclerotic heart disease (ASHD). In a large number of patients, cardiac arrest is the first manifestation of heart disease. Causes of sudden death other than ASHD include:

❑ Drowning   ❑ Acid-base imbalance
❑ Electrocution   ❑ Drug intoxication
❑ Electrolyte imbalance   ❑ Hypoxia
❑ Hypothermia   ❑ Pulmonary embolism
❑ Trauma   ❑ Cerebrovascular accident

As mentioned above, dysrhythmias are often associated with cardiac arrest. The major offending dysrhythmia is *ventricular fibrillation*, which causes an estimated 60–70 percent of cases. The dysrhythmia may be the cause of the cardiac arrest (primary cause) or may result from another factor (secondary cause). In addition to ventricular fibrillation, cardiac arrest can result from ventricular tachycardia, asystole, severe bradycardias, severe heart blocks, and pulseless electrical activity (PEA)..

The following sections will present basic considerations for managing cases of cardiac arrest. The actual protocol for each type of cardiac arrest is addressed later.

Basic Management Considerations
Basic life support is the mainstay of cardiac arrest therapy. Initiate basic life support promptly, during the primary survey. If basic life support is delegated to assisting personnel, you must continuously monitor its performance and effectiveness.

The airway can be managed by any number of methods. The most sophisticated method is not always the best. Individual circumstances should dictate the form of airway management utilized.

Primary ventricular fibrillation is easier to abolish than secondary ventricular fibrillation. To adequately treat **secondary ventricular fibrillation**, you must often find and correct the underlying cause. Defibrillation should occur as soon as possible, since this gives the best chance of successful resuscitation. External cardiac pacing may be used for bradycardias or asystole, or immediately after defibrillation of ventricular fibrillation.

Some cardiac arrests are managed differently than those occurring due to ASHD because of the underlying mechanism of arrest. Examples include cardiac arrests that result from the following medical emergencies.

❑ Drowning
❑ Hypothermia
❑ Traumatic arrest

The management of these problems is discussed elsewhere in the text.

■ **primary ventricular fibrillation** ventricular fibrillation due to a problem occurring within the heart itself, such as acute myocardial infarction.

■ **secondary ventricular fibrillation** ventricular fibrillation due to a problem elsewhere in the body that secondarily affects the heart (e.g., electrolyte abnormalities, hypoxia, and hypovolemia).

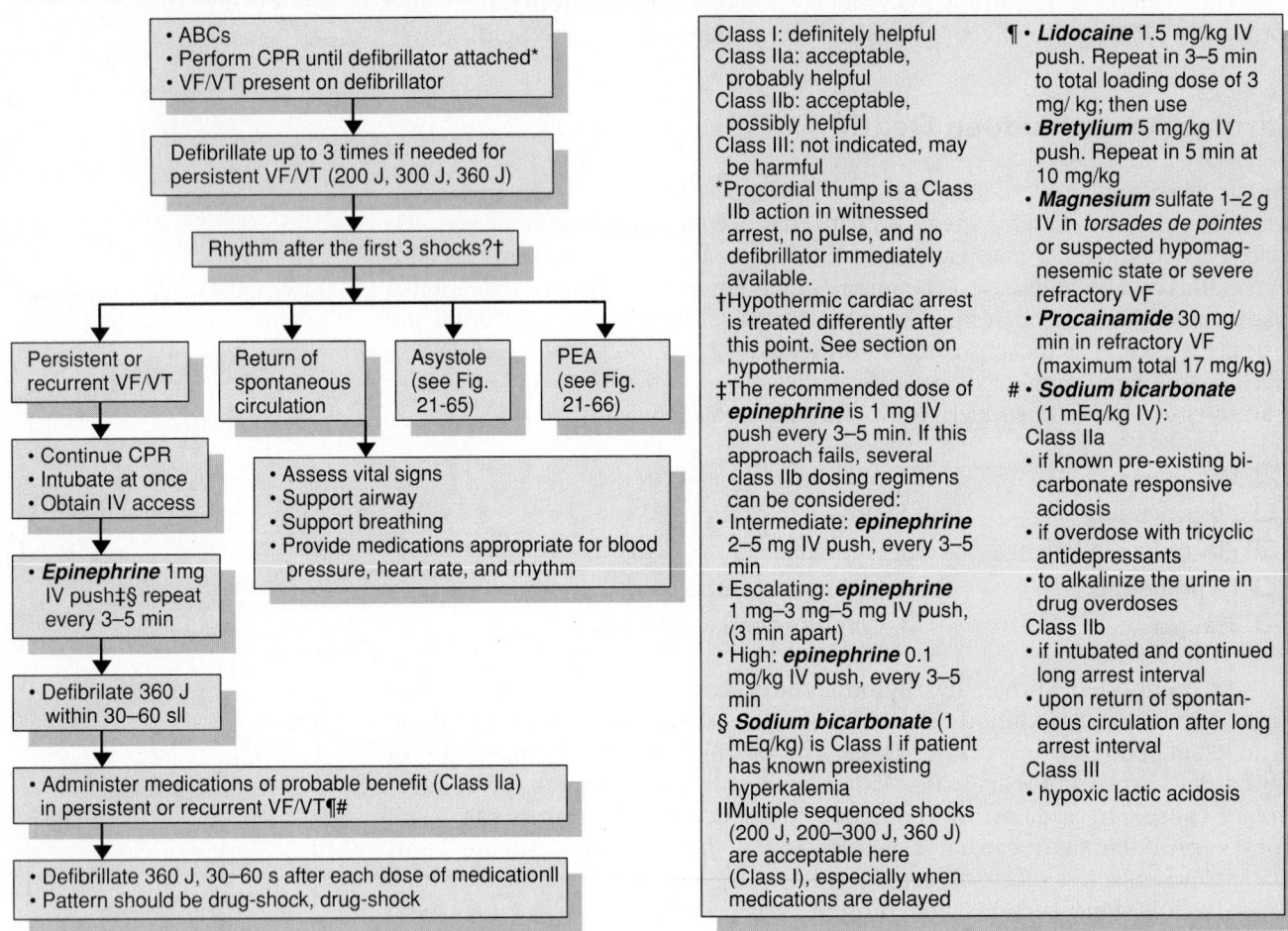

The flowchart contains the following boxes:

- ABCs
- Perform CPR until defibrillator attached*
- VF/VT present on defibrillator

↓

Defibrillate up to 3 times if needed for persistent VF/VT (200 J, 300 J, 360 J)

↓

Rhythm after the first 3 shocks?†

Branches:

Persistent or recurrent VF/VT
- Continue CPR
- Intubate at once
- Obtain IV access

↓

- Epinephrine 1mg IV push‡§ repeat every 3–5 min

↓

- Defibrillate 360 J within 30–60 sll

↓

- Administer medications of probable benefit (Class IIa) in persistent or recurrent VF/VT¶#

↓

- Defibrillate 360 J, 30–60 s after each dose of medicationll
- Pattern should be drug-shock, drug-shock

Return of spontaneous circulation
- Assess vital signs
- Support airway
- Support breathing
- Provide medications appropriate for blood pressure, heart rate, and rhythm

Asystole (see Fig. 21-65)

PEA (see Fig. 21-66)

Right side legend:

Class I: definitely helpful
Class IIa: acceptable, probably helpful
Class IIb: acceptable, possibly helpful
Class III: not indicated, may be harmful
*Procordial thump is a Class IIb action in witnessed arrest, no pulse, and no defibrillator immediately available.
†Hypothermic cardiac arrest is treated differently after this point. See section on hypothermia.
‡The recommended dose of epinephrine is 1 mg IV push every 3–5 min. If this approach fails, several class IIb dosing regimens can be considered:
• Intermediate: epinephrine 2–5 mg IV push, every 3–5 min
• Escalating: epinephrine 1 mg–3 mg–5 mg IV push, (3 min apart)
• High: epinephrine 0.1 mg/kg IV push, every 3–5 min
§ Sodium bicarbonate (1 mEq/kg) is Class I if patient has known preexisting hyperkalemia
llMultiple sequenced shocks (200 J, 200–300 J, 360 J) are acceptable here (Class I), especially when medications are delayed

¶ • Lidocaine 1.5 mg/kg IV push. Repeat in 3–5 min to total loading dose of 3 mg/ kg; then use
• Bretylium 5 mg/kg IV push. Repeat in 5 min at 10 mg/kg
• Magnesium sulfate 1–2 g IV in torsades de pointes or suspected hypomagnesemic state or severe refractory VF
• Procainamide 30 mg/min in refractory VF (maximum total 17 mg/kg)
• Sodium bicarbonate (1 mEq/kg IV):
Class IIa
• if known pre-existing bicarbonate responsive acidosis
• if overdose with tricyclic antidepressants
• to alkalinize the urine in drug overdoses
Class IIb
• if intubated and continued long arrest interval
• upon return of spontaneous circulation after long arrest interval
Class III
• hypoxic lactic acidosis

FIGURE 21-64 Management of ventricular fibrillation and pulseless ventricular tachycardia.

Management of Cardiac Arrest due to Ventricular Fibrillation and Ventricular Tachycardia. The management of cardiac arrest secondary to ventricular tachycardia and ventricular fibrillation follows the guidelines for cardiopulmonary resuscitation and emergency cardiac care as published by the American Heart Association. The algorithm for cardiac arrest secondary to ventricular tachycardia is shown in Figure 21-64.

Management of Cardiac Arrest Secondary to Asystole. Cardiac arrest secondary to asystole carries a poor overall prognosis for resuscitation. Asystole may be the end result of ventricular fibrillation or electromechanical dissociation. Asystole usually indicates extensive myocardial damage, a severe metabolic deficit, or markedly increased parasympathetic tone. Many authorities believe that asystole is a fine ventricular fibrillation. If there is any question whether the rhythm is asystole or fine ventricular fibrillation, then defibrillation should be carried out.

The management of asystole follows the guidelines for cardiopulmonary resuscitation and emergency cardiac care as published by the American Heart Association. The algorithm for asystole is shown in Figure 21-65.

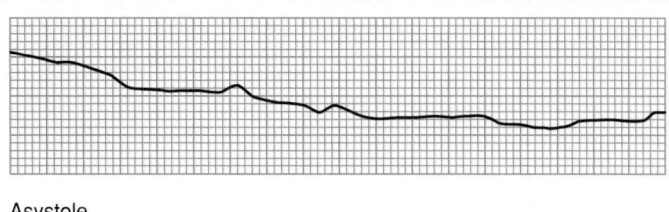

Asystole

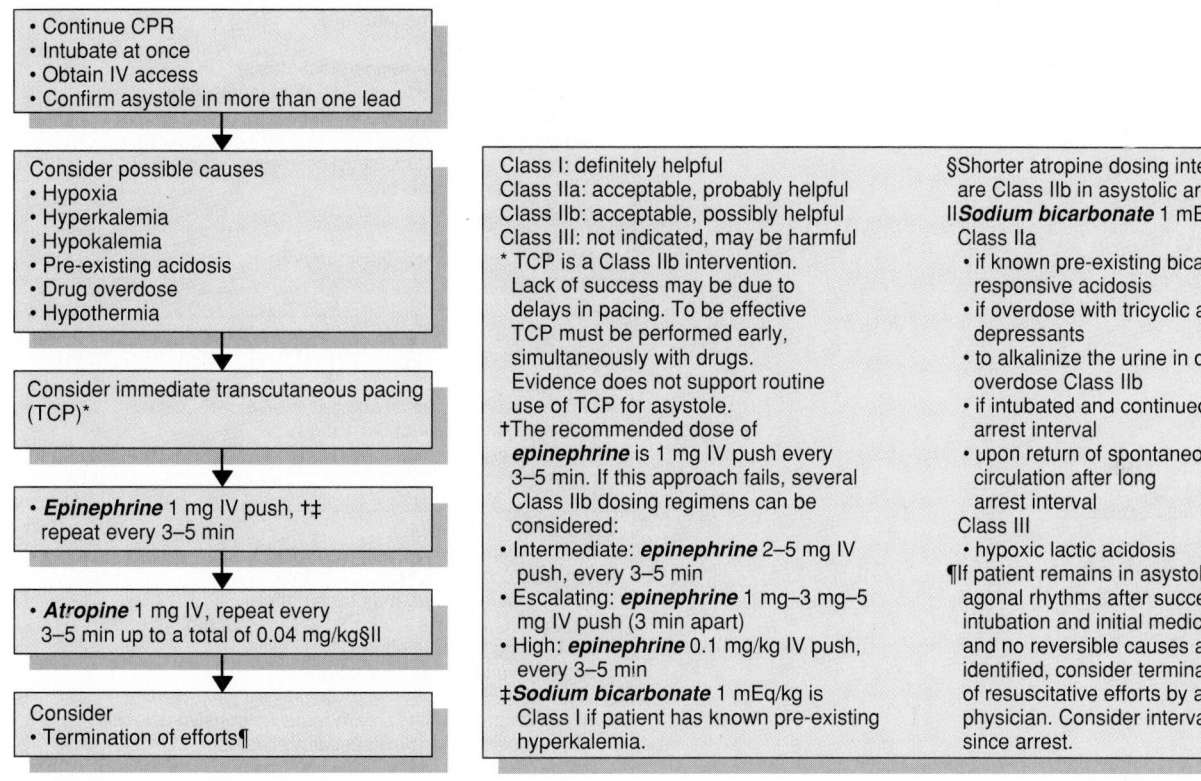

- Continue CPR
- Intubate at once
- Obtain IV access
- Confirm asystole in more than one lead

Consider possible causes
- Hypoxia
- Hyperkalemia
- Hypokalemia
- Pre-existing acidosis
- Drug overdose
- Hypothermia

Consider immediate transcutaneous pacing (TCP)*

- *Epinephrine* 1 mg IV push, †‡ repeat every 3–5 min

- *Atropine* 1 mg IV, repeat every 3–5 min up to a total of 0.04 mg/kg§‖

Consider
- Termination of efforts¶

Class I: definitely helpful
Class IIa: acceptable, probably helpful
Class IIb: acceptable, possibly helpful
Class III: not indicated, may be harmful
* TCP is a Class IIb intervention. Lack of success may be due to delays in pacing. To be effective TCP must be performed early, simultaneously with drugs. Evidence does not support routine use of TCP for asystole.
†The recommended dose of **epinephrine** is 1 mg IV push every 3–5 min. If this approach fails, several Class IIb dosing regimens can be considered:
- Intermediate: **epinephrine** 2–5 mg IV push, every 3–5 min
- Escalating: **epinephrine** 1 mg–3 mg–5 mg IV push (3 min apart)
- High: **epinephrine** 0.1 mg/kg IV push, every 3–5 min
‡**Sodium bicarbonate** 1 mEq/kg is Class I if patient has known pre-existing hyperkalemia.

§Shorter atropine dosing intervals are Class IIb in asystolic arrest.
‖**Sodium bicarbonate** 1 mEg/kg:
Class IIa
- if known pre-existing bicarbonate-responsive acidosis
- if overdose with tricyclic anti-depressants
- to alkalinize the urine in drug overdose Class IIb
- if intubated and continued long arrest interval
- upon return of spontaneous circulation after long arrest interval
Class III
- hypoxic lactic acidosis
¶If patient remains in asystole or agonal rhythms after successful intubation and initial medications and no reversible causes are identified, consider termination of resuscitative efforts by a physician. Consider interval since arrest.

FIGURE 21-65 Management of asystole.

Management of Cardiac Arrest Secondary to Pulseless Electrical Activity (PEA). *Pulseless electrical activity (PEA)*, also called *electro-mechanical dissociation (EMD)*, is any organized ECG rhythm without a pulse. This condition, like asystole, carries a grave prognosis. Causes of pulseless electrical activity include massive myocardial damage, hypovolemia, cardiac rupture, cardiac tamponade, and acute pulmonary embolism. Most of these conditions cannot be diagnosed or managed in the field. Some, however, are treatable in the hospital if detected early. When confronted by a patient in pulseless electrical activity, consider PASG, an IV fluid challenge, and rapid transport if there is a suspicion of any treatable etiology, such as hypovolemia.

The management of cardiac arrest secondary to pulseless electrical activity follows the guidelines for cardiopulmonary resuscitation and emergency cardiac care as published by the American Heart Association. The algorithm for cardiac arrest secondary to pulseless electrical activity (PEA) is shown in Figure 21-66.

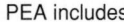

PEA includes
- Electromechanical dissociation (EMD)
- Pseudo-EMD
- Idioventricular rhythms
- Ventricular escape rhythms
- Bradyasystolic rhythms
- Postdefibrillation idioventricular rhythms

- Continue CPR   • Obtain IV access
- Intubate at once • Assess blood flow using Doppler ultasound

Consider possible causes
(Parentheses=possible therapies and treatments)
- Hypovolemia (volume infusion)
- Hypoxia (ventilation)
- Cardiac tamponade (pericardiocentesis)
- Tension pneumothorax (needle decompression)
- Hypothermia
- Massive pulmonary embolism (surgery, thrombolytics)
- Drug overdose such as tricyclics, digitalis, β-blockers, calcium channel blockers
- Hyperkalemia*
- Acidosis†
- Massive acute myocardial infarction

- Epinephrine 1mg IV push, *‡ repeat every 3–5 min

- if absolute bradycardia (<60 beats/min) or relative bradycardia, give atropine 1 mg IV
- Repeat every 3–5 min up to a total of 0.04 mg/kg§

Class I: definitely helpful
Class IIa: acceptable, probably helpful
Class IIb: acceptable, possibly helpful
Class III: not indicated, may be harmful
* Sodium bicarbonate 1 mEq/kg is Class I if patient has known pre-existing hyperkalemia.
† Sodium bicarbonate 1 mEq/kg:
  Class IIa
  - if known pre-existing bicarbonate-responsive acidosis
  - if overdose with tricyclic antidepressants
  - to alkalinize the urine in drug overdoses
    Class IIb
  - if intubated and long arrest interval
  - upon return of spontaneous circulation after long arrest interval
    ClassIII
  - hypoxic lactic acidosis
‡ The recommended dose of epinephrine is 1 mg IV push every 3–5 min. If this approach fails, several Class IIb dosing regimens can be considered.
  - Intermediate: epinephrine 2–5 mg IV push, every 3–5 min
  - Escalating: epinephrine 1 mg–3 mg–5 mg IV push (3 min apart)
  - High: epinephrine 0.1 mg/kg IV push, every 3–5 min
§ Short atropine dosing intervals are possibly helpful in cardiac arrest (Class IIb).

FIGURE 21-66   Management of pulseless electrical activity (PEA).

Peripheral Vascular and Other Cardiovascular Emergencies

In addition to cardiac arrest, other commonly encountered cardiovascular emergencies involve the arterial and venous systems.

Aneurysm

Aneurysm is a nonspecific term meaning dilation of a vessel. The types of aneurysms include:

■ **aneurysm** the ballooning of an arterial wall, resulting from a defect or weakness in the wall.

❑ Atherosclerotic
❑ Dissecting
❑ Infectious
❑ Congenital
❑ Traumatic

Most aneurysms result from atherosclerosis and involve the aorta. The aorta is the vessel commonly involved because the pressure within it is the highest of that of any vessel in the body. This section discusses abdominal, dissecting, and traumatic aneurysms. Infectious aneurysms are most commonly associated with syphilis and are rarely encountered. Congenital aneurysms can occur with several disease states. One is *Marfan's syndrome*, a hereditary disease that affects the connective tissue. People with Marfan's syndrome are often slender and tall with long fingers. Aortic aneurysm occurs in people with Marfan's syndrome because of involvement of the connective tissue within the vessel wall. Those affected may experience sudden death, usually from spontaneous rupture of the aorta, often at a fairly young age.

Abdominal Aortic Aneurysm *Abdominal aortic aneurysm* commonly results from atherosclerosis and occurs most frequently in the aorta, below the renal arteries and above the bifurcation of the common iliac arteries. (See Figure 21-67.) It is 10 times more common in men than in women and most prevalent between ages 60 and 70.

Signs and symptoms of an abdominal aortic aneurysm include:

❑ Abdominal pain
❑ Back and flank pain
❑ Hypotension
❑ Urge to defecate, caused by the retroperitoneal leakage of blood

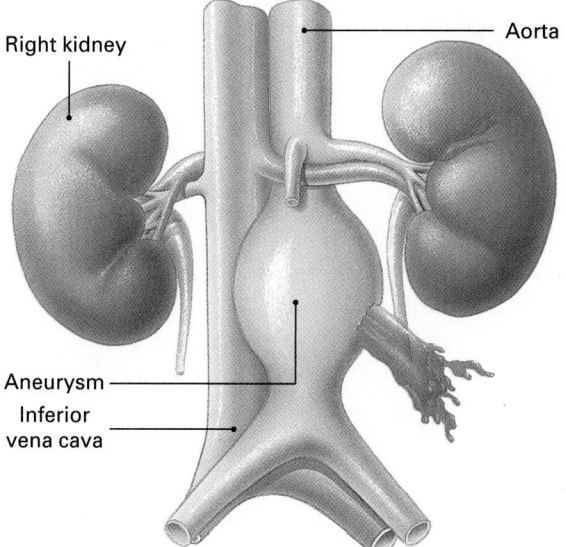

Right kidney

Aorta

Aneurysm

Inferior
vena cava

FIGURE 21-67 Rupture of an abdominal aortic aneurysm.

- Pulsatile mass (the mass can usually be felt when it exceeds 5 cm in diameter)
- Decreased femoral pulse
- GI bleeding if the aneurysm erodes into the bowel

Prehospital management consists of treating the patient for shock. Treatment should consist of oxygen, PASG, and intravenous volume replacement. Suspect abdominal aortic aneurysm when any of the above signs or symptoms are present. If ordered by medical control, palpate the abdomen gently to note the presence of a mass. Do not carry out additional palpation, as rupture can occur. Transport the patient rapidly.

Dissecting Aortic Aneurysm. A *dissecting aortic aneurysm* occurs after a small tear in the inner wall of the aorta allows blood to enter and create a false passage within the wall of the vessel. This can cause hematoma and, subsequently, aneurysm. The original tear often results from **cystic medial necrosis**, a degenerative disease of connective tissue often associated with hypertension, and, to a certain extent, aging. Predisposing factors include hypertension, which is present in 75–85 percent of cases. There is also a family tendency for this disease. It occurs more frequently in patients older than 40–50, although it can occur in younger individuals, especially pregnant women.

■ **cystic medial necrosis** a death or degeneration of a part of the wall of an artery.

Of dissecting aortic aneurysms, 67 percent involve the ascending aorta. Once dissection has started, it can extend to all of the abdominal aorta as well as its branches, including the coronary arteries, aortic value, subclavian arteries, and carotid arteries. The aneurysm can rupture at any time, usually into the pericardial or pleural cavity.

The signs and symptoms of dissecting aortic aneurysm include pain, which is commonly characterized as ripping or tearing. The pain is usually substernal and may radiate to the back between the scapulae. Pulses in the lower extremities may be markedly diminished or absent. The blood pressure is often elevated, yet the patient will usually look "shocky" as a result of impaired perfusion. Dissection into other arteries and structures may cause the following conditions.

- Syncope
- Stroke
- Absent or reduced pulses
- Heart failure
- Pericardial tamponade
- Acute myocardial infarction

Prehospital management consists of rapid transport for definitive care. Rupture can occur, even into another body cavity. Keep the patient quiet and administer high-flow oxygen. Start an IV of a crystalloid solution, such as lactated Ringer's solution, preferably en route to the hospital. If the diagnosis is fairly definite, the medical control physician may order the administration of morphine sulfate. Transport the patient rapidly. The survival rate is fairly good if the aneurysm has not ruptured and the patient is treated promptly.

In-hospital management may be medical or surgical. Occasionally, the tear heals, creating a double lumen in the vessel.

Traumatic Aortic Aneurysm (Rupture). *Traumatic aortic aneurysm* or rupture can result from blunt or penetrating trauma to the vessel. If rupture occurs, the prognosis is grave. If the aneurysm is detected before it ruptures, it can occasionally be treated surgically. Additional discussion of traumatic aortic aneurysm and rupture is presented in the trauma chapters.

Acute Arterial Occlusion   An *acute arterial occlusion* is the sudden occlusion of arterial blood flow to an area as a result of trauma, thrombosis, tumor, embolus, or idiopathic means. Embolus is probably the most common cause. Emboli can arise from within the chamber (*mural emboli*), a thrombus in the left ventricle, an atrial thrombus secondary to atrial fibrillation, or a thrombus from abdominal aortic atherosclerosis. Arterial occlusions most commonly involve vessels in the abdomen or extremities.

The signs and symptoms of an acute arterial occlusion include sudden, excruciating pain. Pain is present in 75–80 percent of cases and peaks within several hours. If pain is absent, there is usually paresthesia in the involved extremity. The area distal to the obstruction is often pale. The occluded extremity may have a mottled, cyanotic appearance. It is often cool to the touch because of loss of blood flow. The pulses distal to the occlusion are absent. An easy way to remember the signs and symptoms of arterial occlusion are the "5 P's" shown below.

- ❑ Pallor
- ❑ Pain
- ❑ Pulselessness
- ❑ Paralysis
- ❑ Paresthesia

If the occlusion involves the *mesentery*, or blood supply to the intestines, shock can develop. The prehospital management of a mesenteric occlusion consists of typical shock treatment: oxygen, IV fluids, and PASG. Morphine sulfate may be ordered by the medical control physician for relief of pain. Extremity occlusion is serious, but not life-threatening. Blood flow must be established within 4–8 hours. This is usually accomplished by surgical removal of the clot. If acute arterial occlusion is present, the affected extremity should be protected from injury. The patient should not be allowed to walk on it.

Acute Pulmonary Embolism   *Acute pulmonary embolism* is a blood clot or other particle that lodges in a pulmonary artery, blocking blood flow through that vessel. Sources of pulmonary emboli include air emboli, fat emboli, amniotic fluid, and blood clots. Factors that predispose a patient to blood clots include prolonged immobilization, thrombophlebitis, use of certain medications, and atrial fibrillation.

When a pulmonary embolism occurs, the blood flow through the affected vessel is blocked, causing the right heart to pump against increased resistance. This results in increased pulmonary capillary pressure. The area of the lung supplied by the occluded vessel ceases to function, resulting in decreased gas exchange.

The signs and symptoms of pulmonary embolism depend upon the size of the obstruction. The patient suffering acute pulmonary embolism may report a sudden onset of severe and unexplained dyspnea, which may or may not be associated with chest pain. There may be a recent history of immobilization, such as hip fracture, surgery, or other debilitating illness.

The physical examination may reveal labored breathing, tachypnea, and tachycardia. Patients with massive pulmonary emboli may have signs of right heart failure, such as jugular venous distention and, in some cases, falling blood pressure.

If you suspect that a patient has a pulmonary embolism, establish and maintain an airway. Assist the patient's ventilations as required. Administer supplemental oxygen at the highest possible concentration. Establish an IV and transport the patient immediately.

Pulmonary embolism is often difficult to diagnose. Therefore, you should suspect this condition in patients with associated signs and symptoms. Patients with acute pulmonary embolism can present in a similar fashion to those with hyperventilation syndrome. Do not assume that all cases of hyperventilation are caused by anxiety. If in doubt, always administer oxygen.

Noncritical Peripheral Vascular Conditions   Several peripheral vascular conditions are not immediately life-threatening, but worthy of discussion. These include deep venous thrombosis, varicose veins, and peripheral arterial atherosclerotic disease.

Deep Venous Thrombosis.   *Deep venous thrombosis* is a blood clot in a vein. It most commonly occurs in the larger veins of the thigh and calf. Predisposing factors include a recent history of trauma, inactivity, pregnancy, or varicose veins.

The patient often complains of gradually increasing pain and calf tenderness. Often the leg and foot are swollen because of occlusion of venous drainage. The signs and symptoms may improve with leg elevation. In some cases, the patient may be asymptomatic. Gentle palpation of the calf and thigh may reveal tenderness and, on some occasions, cordlike clotted veins. Dorsiflexion of the foot may cause discomfort behind the knee. This is referred to as *Homan's sign* and is associated with deep venous thrombosis. The skin may be warm and red.

Prehospital management is primarily supportive. Deep vein thrombosis is not a life-threatening emergency, but patients are prone to develop pulmonary emboli. Palpate the calf and thigh gently. Elevate the leg, and do not allow the patient to walk.

Varicose Veins.   *Varicose veins* are the dilation of the superficial veins, usually in the lower extremity. Predisposing factors include pregnancy, obesity, and a genetic tendency. Signs and symptoms include the visible distention of the leg veins, lower leg swelling and discomfort (especially at the end of the day), and skin color and texture changes in the legs and ankles. If the condition is chronic, venous stasis ulcers can develop. Venous stasis ulcers are a noncritical condition. However, rupture can occur. The bleeding, which occasionally is significant, can usually be controlled by direct pressure.

Peripheral Arterial Atherosclerotic Disease.   Atherosclerosis, as discussed previously, can involve any of the major arteries. *Peripheral atherosclerotic disease* results from atherosclerosis of the aorta and its tributaries. It is a gradual, progressive disease, often associated with diabetes mellitus. Signs and symptoms include trophic changes in the feet, pretibial hair loss, and red skin color in the extremities when dependent. In extreme cases, there may be significant arterial insufficiency leading to ulcers and gangrene. *Intermittent claudication* occurs after exercise and is comparable to angina in the heart. It is characterized by pain and cramping in the affected leg when tissue demands are in excess of the blood supply. Peripheral arterial disease is not a medical emergency unless arterial occlusion occurs.

Hypertensive Emergency

A hypertensive emergency is a life-threatening elevation of blood pressure. It occurs in one percent or less of patients with **hypertension**, usually when the hypertension is poorly controlled or untreated. A **hypertensive emergency** is characterized by a rapid increase in diastolic blood pressure (usually >130 mmHg) accompanied by restlessness, confusion, blurred vision, and nausea and vomiting. It is often accompanied by **hypertensive encephalopathy**, which is characterized by severe headache, vomiting, visual disturbances (including transient blindness), paralysis, seizures, stupor, and coma. On occasion, this condition may cause left ventricular failure, pulmonary edema, or stroke.

Prehospital management varies with the patient. Keep the patient quiet, and administer oxygen. In cases where frank hypertensive encephalopathy has not yet developed, the medical control physician may request the administration of sublingual nifedipine (Procardia). This is a calcium channel blocker that causes vasodilation of peripheral and coronary vessels, thus reducing blood pressure. In severe cases, especially if hypertensive encephalopathy is present, the medical control physician may order one of the three medications listed below:

❑ *Sodium Nitroprusside (Nipride).* Sodium nitroprusside is a popular agent for use in hypertensive crisis. It is a potent arterial and venous vasodilator. It is administered as an IV infusion, thus making administration more controlled and the patient's response more predictable.

❑ *Labetolol (Trandate, Normodyne).* Labetolol is a beta blocker that effectively decreases blood pressure. It is given by IV bolus and infusion.

❑ *Morphine Sulfate.* Morphine sulfate can lower blood pressure through vasodilation and alleviation of anxiety and headache.

If heart failure or pulmonary edema develops, the patient should be treated with appropriate medications.

Hypertension-Related Emergencies   Hypertension is a related factor in other emergencies. These include such things as pulmonary edema from left ventricular failure, dissecting aortic aneurysm, toxemia of pregnancy, and cerebrovascular accident. In these cases, hypertension often results from the primary problem. Treatment should be directed at the primary problem.

MANAGEMENT OF CARDIOVASCULAR EMERGENCIES

After you have an understanding of the pathophysiology of the most commonly encountered cardiac emergencies, you can more effectively decide upon the best management method. Choices include use of cardiovascular drugs and/or one of several management techniques. Remember that prompt and efficient prehospital care often means the difference between life and death in cardiac emergencies. Therefore, you should become thoroughly familiar with the various drugs and management techniques suggested by local protocol.

■ **hypertension** a common disorder characterized by a persistent elevation of the blood pressure above 140/90 mmHg.

■ **hypertensive emergency** an acute elevation of blood pressure that requires the blood pressure to be lowered within one hour; characterized by end-organ changes such as hypertensive encephalopathy, renal failure, or blindness.

■ **hypertensive encephalopathy** a cerebral disorder of hypertension indicated by severe headache, nausea, vomiting, and altered mental status. Neurological symptoms may include blindness, muscle twitches, inability to speak, weakness, and paralysis.

Drugs Used in Cardiovascular Emergencies

Medications used in the prehospital care of cardiovascular emergencies were discussed in detail in Chapter 13. This section reviews these medications in preparation for the following sections on Advanced Cardiac Life Support.

Antidysrhythmics   *Antidysrhythmic medications* are those used to control or suppress cardiac dysrhythmias. They include:

- ❑ *Atropine Sulfate.* Atropine sulfate is a parasympatholytic agent used in the treatment of symptomatic bradycardias, especially those arising from the atria. It also plays a role in the management of asystole. It is given by IV bolus or through an endotracheal tube.
- ❑ *Lidocaine.* Lidocaine is a first-line antidysrhythmic agent used in the treatment and prophylaxis of life-threatening ventricular dysrhythmias. It is administered by IV bolus, IV drip, or through an endotracheal tube.
- ❑ *Procainamide.* Procainamide is a second-line antidysrhythmic drug to lidocaine, used for ventricular dysrhythmias refractory to lidocaine or in patients who are allergic to lidocaine. It is administered by slow IV bolus and IV drip.
- ❑ *Bretylium.* Bretylium is a second-line antidysrhythmic agent used in the treatment of life-threatening ventricular dysrhythmias, especially ventricular fibrillation. It is administered by IV bolus and IV drip.
- ❑ *Adenosine.* Adenosine is used in the management of supraventricular tachydysrhythmias. It is administered by IV rapid bolus.
- ❑ *Verapamil.* Verapamil is a calcium channel blocker that is effective in slowing heart rate in symptomatic atrial tachycardias. It is used to terminate paroxysmal supraventricular tachycardia and to control the rapid ventricular response often seen with atrial fibrillation or flutter. It is administered by slow IV bolus.

Sympathomimetic Agents   *Sympathomimetic agents* are drugs similar to the naturally occurring hormones epinephrine and norepinephrine. They duplicate or mimic stimulation of the sympathetic nervous system. They act either on alpha or beta adrenergic receptors. Stimulation of alpha receptors causes peripheral vasoconstriction. Stimulation of beta receptors causes an increase in heart rate, cardiac contractile force, bronchodilation, and peripheral vasodilation. Dopaminergic receptors are located in renal and mesenteric blood vessels. Stimulation of these receptors causes dilation. Sympathomimetic agents include:

- ❑ *Epinephrine.* Epinephrine is the mainstay of cardiac arrest resuscitation. It acts on both alpha and beta adrenergic receptors. It is used in ventricular fibrillation, asystole, and electromechanical dissociation. It is also sometimes used in bradycardias refractory to atropine. It is given by IV bolus, subcutaneously, and through the endotracheal tube.
- ❑ *Norepinephrine.* Norepinephrine is a sympathomimetic with enhanced alpha agonist properties as compared to epinephrine. It also acts, to a lesser degree, on beta receptors. It is used occasionally in hemodynamically significant hypotension and cardiogenic shock, although dopamine is considered the first-line agent for those conditions. It may be effective if total peripheral resistance is low, such as in neurogenic shock. It is administered by intravenous infusion.
- ❑ *Isoproterenol.* Isoproterenol is a potent beta agonist. It increases heart

rate and cardiac contractile force. It is used in bradycardias refractory to atropine and in the management of asystole. Transcutaneous pacing is preferred to isoproterenol usage. When the drug is used, it is administered by intravenous infusion.

❑ *Dopamine.* Dopamine is a vasopressor with both alpha and beta properties that are dose-related. In the appropriate dosage range, it maintains renal and mesenteric perfusion. It is used in the management of cardiogenic shock and given by intravenous infusion.

❑ *Dobutamine.* Dobutamine has a more pronounced effect on cardiac contractility than on heart rate. It is used in the treatment of significant left heart failure and administered by intravenous infusion.

Drugs for Myocardial Ischemia and Pain   Drugs used in the treatment of myocardial ischemia and the relief of pain include:

❑ *Oxygen.* Oxygen is an important agent in emergency cardiac care. It increases the oxygen content of the blood and aids in the oxygenation of peripheral tissues. It is indicated in any situation in which hypoxia or ischemia is possible.

❑ *Nitrous Oxide (Nitronox).* Nitronox is a fixed combination of 50 percent nitrous oxide and 50 percent oxygen. It is an effective analgesic, at the same time providing 50 percent oxygen. The effects dissipate within 2–5 minutes after the cessation of administration.

❑ *Nitroglycerin.* Nitroglycerin is an arterial and venous vasodilator that decreases myocardial workload. It is used in the management of angina pectoris and MI. In addition, it can be used for pulmonary edema because of its vasodilatory effect. Nitroglycerin is administered sublingually or intravenously.

❑ *Morphine Sulfate.* Morphine is a narcotic and a potent analgesic. In addition to its sedative effects, it causes peripheral vasodilation. It is used in MI, pulmonary edema, and other cardiovascular emergencies. It is administered intravenously.

Other Prehospital Drugs   In some situations, other drugs may be recommended by medical control or local protocol. These include:

❑ *Furosemide.* Furosemide is a potent loop diuretic that inhibits sodium reabsorption in the kidneys. It is also thought to cause venous dilation, thus decreasing venous return (preload). Furosemide is used in the management of congestive heart failure and cardiogenic shock. It is administered by intravenous bolus.

❑ *Aminophylline.* Aminophylline is a bronchodilator that acts through a different mechanism than the sympathomimetic drugs. It is occasionally given to cardiac patients if bronchospasm is suspected. It is administered by intravenous infusion.

❑ *Diazepam (Valium).* Diazepam is an anxiolytic. It is used to calm the extremely anxious patient suffering MI and as a sedative prior to cardioversion in the conscious patient. It is administered by slow intravenous bolus.

Infrequently Used Drugs in the Prehospital Setting   Many medications are not routinely used in the prehospital setting. These are described here because many paramedics also work in the emergency department. In addition, many patients take these medications on a chronic basis.

❏ *Digitalis (Digoxin, Lanoxin)*. Digitalis is a cardiac glycoside. It increases the force of the cardiac contraction and cardiac output. It slows impulse conduction through the AV node and decreases the ventricular response to certain supraventricular dysrhythmias, such as atrial fibrillation, atrial flutter, and paroxysmal supraventricular tachycardia. It is used in the treatment of heart failure and the dysrhythmias mentioned above. Digitalis toxicity can result in almost any dysrhythmia that often is refractory to traditional antidysrhythmic drugs.

❏ *Beta Blockers*. Beta blockers are frequently used to control dysrhythmias, high blood pressure, and angina. Many beta blockers, such as propranolol (Inderal), are nonselective, while others are selective for β_1 or β_2 receptors. Beta blockers may precipitate congestive heart failure, heart block, and asthma in patients who are predisposed to these conditions.

❏ *Calcium Channel Blockers*. The calcium channel blockers are a relatively new class of medication. They include verapamil (Isoptin, Calan), diltiazem (Cardizem), and nifedipine (Procardia). These agents are being used increasingly for angina pectoris, dysrhythmias, hypertension, and other cardiovascular problems.

Management Techniques

The following section will address, and in some cases review, management techniques frequently used in cardiac emergencies. You should become familiar with local protocols and procedures, since these can vary from system to system.

✱ Basic life support is the mainstay of prehospital cardiac care.

Basic Life Support   Basic life support is the primary skill for the management of serious cardiovascular problems. The techniques of basic life support should be frequently reviewed.

ECG Monitoring   ECG monitoring in the field is accomplished mainly with a combination ECG monitor/defibrillator that operates on a direct current (DC) battery source. (See Procedure 21-1.) The ECG monitor/defibrillator consists of the following parts.

❏ Paddle electrodes
❏ Defibrillator controls
❏ Synchronizer switch
❏ Oscilloscope
❏ Paper strip recorder
❏ Patient cable and lead wires
❏ Controls for monitoring
❏ Special features (data recorders, etc.)

Monitoring requires the placement of three leads on the chest, corresponding to the bipolar leads described earlier in this chapter. One lead is positive, another negative, and the last a ground. The placement of the leads varies according to the brand of equipment used. As a rule, Lead II is usually monitored. However, lead MCL_1 is occasionally used and is often better at determining the site of ectopic beats.

The patient can be monitored either through the defibrillator paddles ("quick-look") or through chest electrodes. The quick-look paddles are more frequently used in cases of cardiac arrest, in which there is no time to place

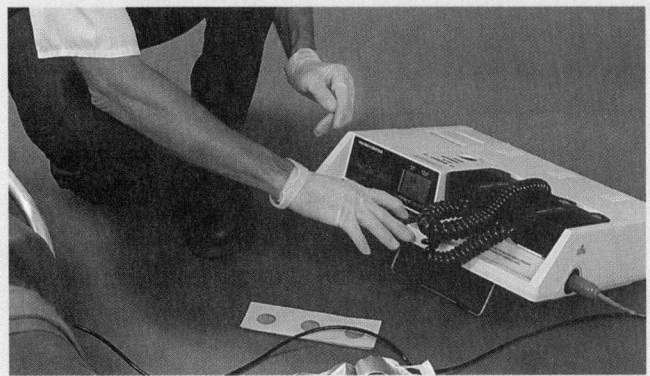

21-1A. Turn the machine on.

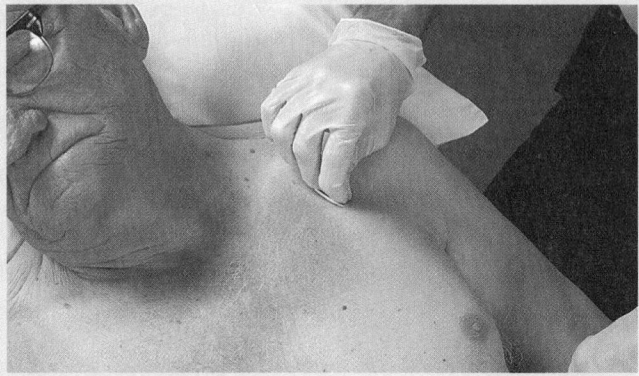

21-1B. Prepare the skin.

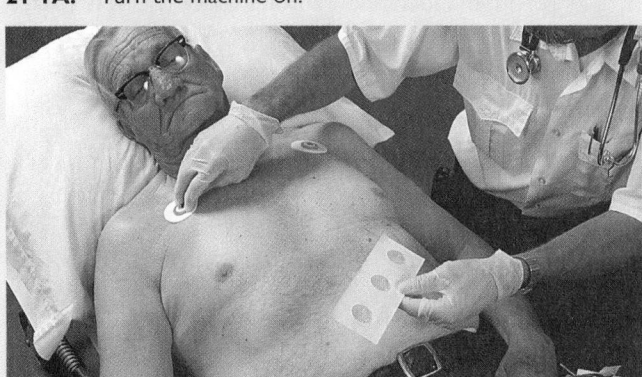

21-1C. Apply the electrodes.

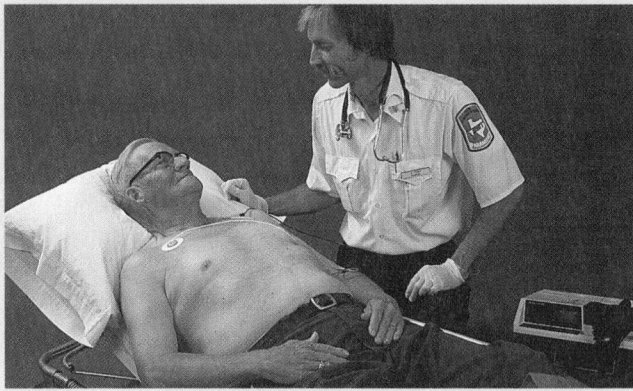

21-1D. Ask the patient to relax and remain still.

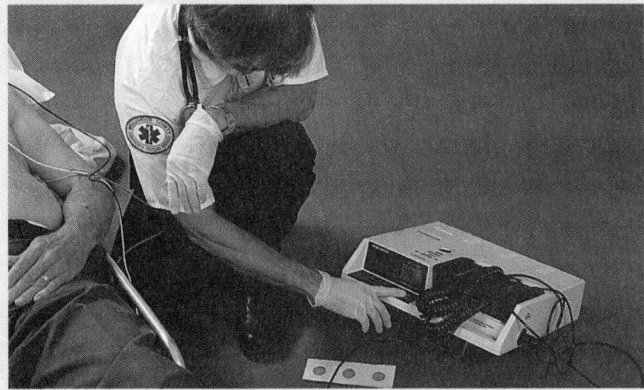

21-1E. Check the ECG.

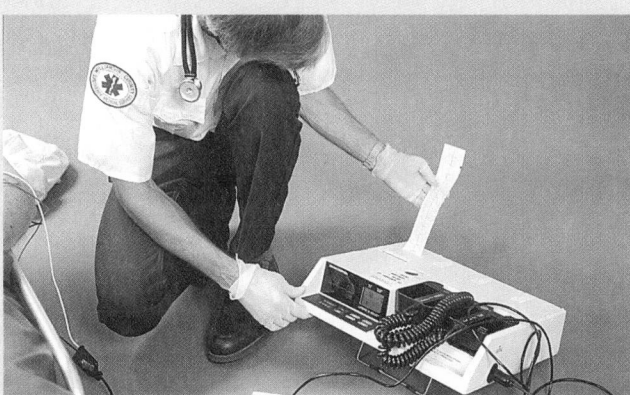

21-1F. Obtain tracing.

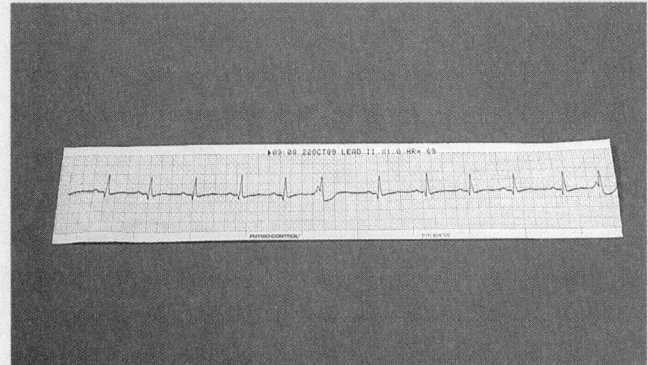

21-1G. ECG strip.

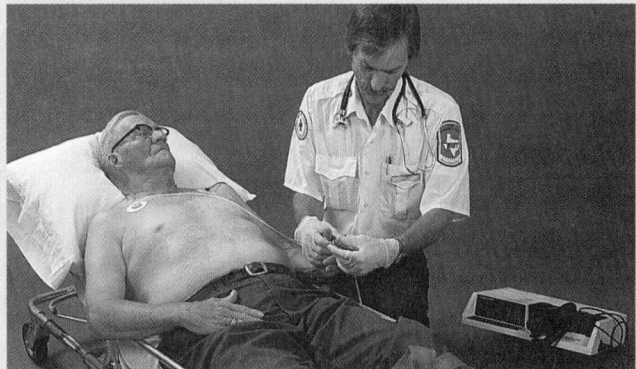

21-1H. Continue ALS care.

chest electrodes. This system can also be used when the patient cable is inoperative. "Quick-look" paddle electrodes have several disadvantages. First, they tend to pick up more artifact than chest electrodes. Second, in order to monitor, they must be held in continuous contact with the chest.

The procedure for using quick-look paddles involves the following steps.

❑ Turn on oscilloscope power.
❑ Apply conducting gel or other medium liberally to the paddle surface.
❑ Hold the paddles firmly on the chest wall with the negative electrode on the right upper chest and the positive electrode on the left lower chest. This closely simulates Lead II.
❑ Observe the monitor and obtain a tracing if desired.

The type of chest leads varies from manufacturer to manufacturer. Usually, to mimic Lead II, the positive electrode is placed on the left lower chest and the negative electrode on the right upper chest. Placement of the ground wire varies. For MCL_1, the positive electrode is placed on the right lower chest wall and the negative electrode on the left upper chest wall. Placement of the ground wire varies.

Electrodes should be placed to avoid large muscle masses, large quantities of chest hair, or anything that keeps the electrodes from being flat on the skin. Also, avoid placing electrodes where defibrillator paddles would be placed if required. The procedure for placing electrodes involves the following steps.

❑ Cleanse the skin with alcohol or abrasive pad. This removes dirt and body oil for better skin contact. If there is a lot of chest hair, shave small amounts before placing the electrodes. If the patient is extremely diaphoretic, tincture of benzoin may be applied.
❑ Apply electrodes to the skin surface.
❑ Attach wires to the electrodes.
❑ Plug the cable into the monitor.
❑ Adjust gain or sensitivity to the proper level.
❑ Adjust the QRS volume. Be aware that the continual beep of the ECG may disturb the patient.
❑ Obtain a baseline tracing.

A poor ECG signal is useless and should be corrected. The most common cause is poor skin contact. Whenever you spot a poor signal, check for one of the following possible causes.

❑ Excessive hair
❑ Loose or dislodged electrode
❑ Dried conductive gel
❑ Poor placement
❑ Diaphoresis

An initially poor tracing may improve as the conductive gel breaks down skin resistance. Other causes of poor tracings include:

❑ Patient movement or muscle tremor
❑ Broken patient cable
❑ Broken lead wire

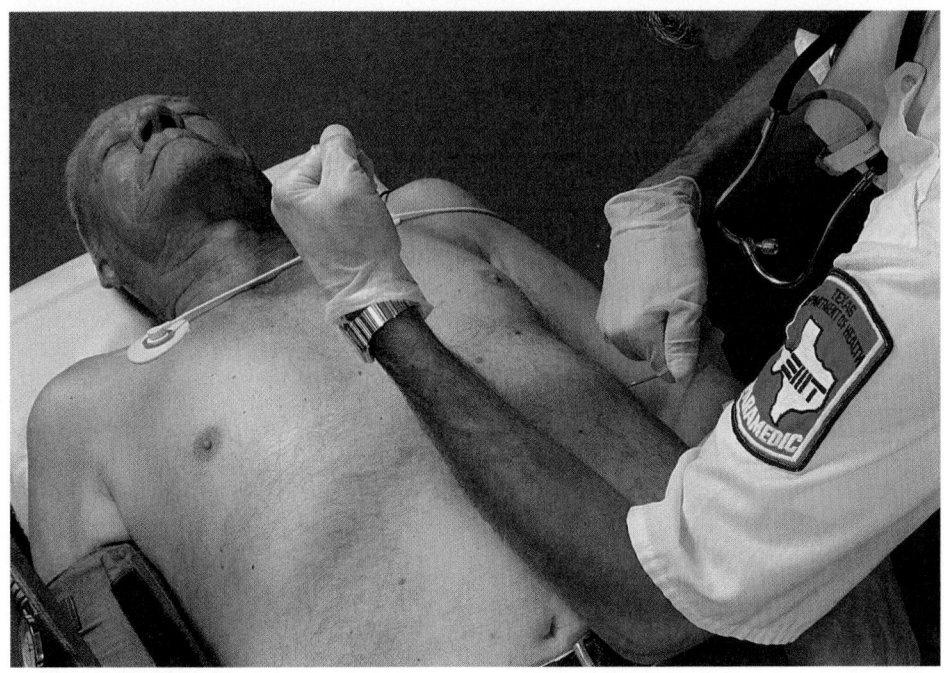

FIGURE 21-68 The precordial thump.

❑ Low battery
❑ Faulty grounding
❑ Faulty monitor

A paper printout should be obtained from each monitored patient. Be sure the stylus heat is adjusted properly. Each strip should be calibrated at the beginning of monitoring. A 1 mV calibration curve should deflect the stylus 10 mm (2 large boxes).

Precordial Thump The precordial thump still has a role in advanced prehospital care. The precordial thump is used to stimulate a depolarization within the heart. It is also sometimes effective in causing ventricular depolarization and resumption of an organized rhythm. Conversions from ventricular tachycardia, complete AV block, and, occasionally, ventricular fibrillation, have been reported. The technique should be used only in cases of monitored ventricular fibrillation or when a defibrillator is not readily available. It is not recommended in pediatric patients.

The thump is delivered to the midsternum with the heel of the fist from a height of 10–12 in. (See Figure 21-68.) The arm and wrist should be parallel to the long axis of the sternum to avoid rib fractures and other problems.

Defibrillation **Defibrillation** is the process of passing a current through a fibrillating heart to depolarize the cells and allow them to repolarize uniformly, thus restoring an organized cardiac rhythm. A critical mass of the myocardium must be depolarized in order to suppress all of the ectopic foci. The critical mass is related to the size of the heart but cannot be calculated for a given individual or situation.

The *defibrillator* is an electrical capacitor that stores energy for delivery to the patient at a desired time. It consists of an adjustable high-voltage power supply, energy storage capacitor, and paddles. The capacitor is connected to the paddles by a current-limiting inductor.

■ **defibrillation** the process of passing an electrical current through a fibrillating heart to depolarize a "critical mass" of myocardial cells. This allows them to depolarize uniformly, resulting in an organized rhythm.

Most defibrillators use direct current (DC). Alternating current (AC) models should not be used. Direct current is more effective, more portable, and causes less muscle damage. The electrical charge consists of several thousand volts delivered over a very short time interval, generally 4–12 milliseconds. The strength of the shock is commonly expressed in energy according to the following formula:

$$\text{Energy (joules)} = \text{power (watts)} \times \text{duration (seconds)}$$

The chest wall offers resistance to the electrical charge, which lowers the actual amount of energy delivered to the heart. Therefore, it is important to lower the resistance pathway between the defibrillator paddles and the chest. Factors that influence chest wall resistance include:

❑ Paddle pressure
❑ Paddle-skin interface
❑ Paddle surface area
❑ Number of previous countershocks
❑ Inspiratory versus expiratory phase at time of countershock

The following factors influence the success of defibrillation.

❑ *Duration of Ventricular Fibrillation.* In conjunction with effective CPR, defibrillation begun within 4 minutes after the onset of fibrillation will yield significantly improved resuscitation rates, as compared with defibrillation begun within 8 minutes.

❑ *Condition of the Myocardium.* It is more difficult to convert ventricular fibrillation in the presence of acidosis, hypoxia, hypothermia, electrolyte imbalance, or drug toxicity. Secondary ventricular fibrillation (ventricular fibrillation that results from another cause) is more difficult to treat than primary ventricular fibrillation.

❑ *Heart Size and Body Weight.* This is controversial. It is known that pediatric and adult energy requirements differ. However, it is not entirely clear whether a relationship exists between size and energy level settings in adults.

❑ *Previous Countershocks.* Repeated countershocks decrease transthoracic resistance, thereby allowing more energy to be delivered to the heart at the same energy level.

❑ *Paddle Size.* Larger defibrillator paddles are thought to be more effective and cause less myocardial damage. The ideal size for adults, however, has not been established. It is recommended that the paddles be 10–13 cm in diameter. In infants, 4.5 cm paddles are adequate.

❑ *Paddle Placement.* The placement of the paddles on the chest (transthoracic) is recommended for the emergency setting in both adults and children. One paddle is positioned to the right of the upper sternum, just below the clavicle. The other is placed to the left of the left nipple in an anterior axillary line, which is immediately over the apex of the heart. Paddles should not be placed over the sternum. The paddles may be marked as apex (positive electrode) and sternum (negative electrode). Reversing polarity does not affect defibrillation. It does, however, invert the ECG tracing.

❑ *Paddle-Skin Interface.* Paddle-skin interface should have as little electrical resistance as possible. Increased resistance decreases energy delivery to the heart and increases heat production on the skin. Many materials are available to decrease resistance. These include gels, creams, pastes, saline-soaked pads, and prepackaged gel pads. Any creams used should be made specifically for defibrillation, not for ECG monitoring. When using cream, make sure that the cream does not run, thus forming a bridge between paddles. NEVER use alcohol-soaked pads. These pads can cause fire.

❏ *Paddle Contact Pressure.* The paddle contact pressure is important. Firm, downward pressure decreases transthoracic resistance. Do not lean on the paddles; they may slip.

❏ *Properly Functioning Defibrillator.* The machine should deliver the amount of energy that it indicates. Therefore, frequent inspection and testing of the machine are necessary. Change and cycle the batteries as directed by the manufacturer.

Procedure 21-2 shows the steps involved in defibrillation. In performing these steps, keep in mind the basic energy recommendations for defibrillation. Defibrillation should initially be attempted at 200 joules in an adult. This should be increased to a maximum of 360 joules in 1–2 repeat countershocks. The pediatric dosage is generally 2 joules/kg initially, repeated at 4 joules/kg if required.

Emergency Synchronized Cardioversion   Emergency synchronized cardioversion is the delivery of an electrical shock to the heart, synchronized so as to coincide with the R wave of the cardiac cycle, thus avoiding the relative refractory period. Synchronization reduces the energy required and the potential for secondary complicating dysrhythmias.

Indications for emergency synchronized cardioversion include:

❏ Perfusing ventricular tachycardia
❏ Paroxysmal supraventricular tachycardia
❏ Rapid atrial fibrillation
❏ 2:1 atrial flutter

■ **cardioversion** the passage of an electric current through the heart during a specific part of the cardiac cycle to terminate certain kinds of dysrhythmias.

The energy requirements are based on the type of dysrhythmia being treated. Some dysrhythmias, especially those of atrial origin, can be treated with as little as 10 joules.

The procedure for synchronized cardioversion is the same as for defibrillation. (See Procedure 21-3.) Conscious patients should be sedated with diazepam. Turn on the synchronizer switch, and verify that the machine is detecting the R waves. If is not, the electrodes may need repositioning. The discharge buttons must be pressed and held until the machine discharges (on the next R wave). If ventricular fibrillation occurs, the synchronizer switch should be turned off. The machine should then be used in the defibrillation mode. In ventricular fibrillation, there is no R wave, so the machine will not discharge.

Carotid Sinus Massage (Optional Skill)   Carotid sinus massage is used to convert paroxysmal supraventricular tachycardia into sinus rhythm by stimulation of the baroreceptors in the carotid bodies. This results in an increase in vagal tone and a decrease in heart rate.

The technique involves the following steps. (See Procedure 21-4.)

1. Initiate IV, oxygen, and ECG monitoring.
2. Position patient on the back, slightly hyperextending the head.
3. Gently palpate each carotid pulse SEPARATELY. Auscultate each side for

(continued on p. 721)

Management of Cardiovascular Emergencies   **717**

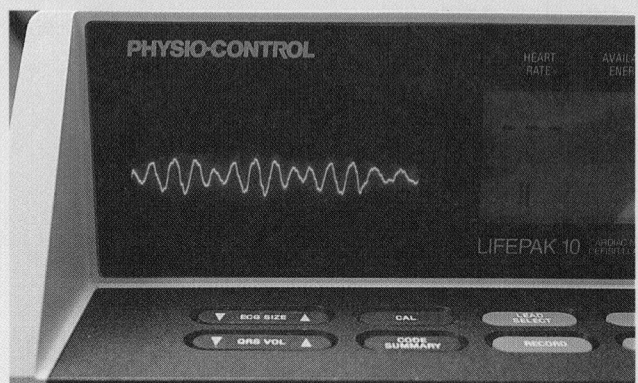

21-2A. Confirm rhythm.

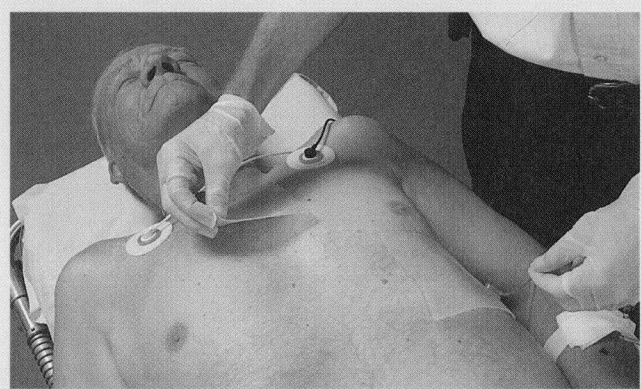

21-2B. Place conductive pads.

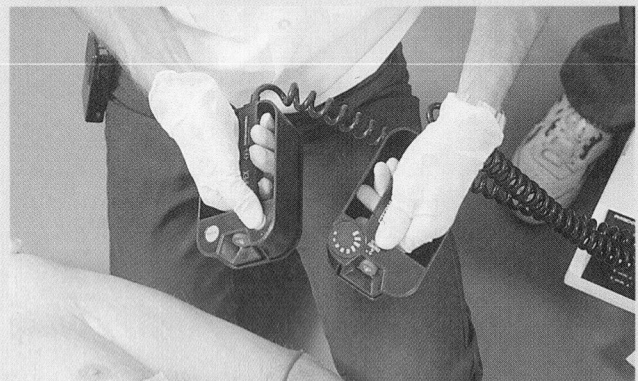

21-2C. Charge the defibrillator.

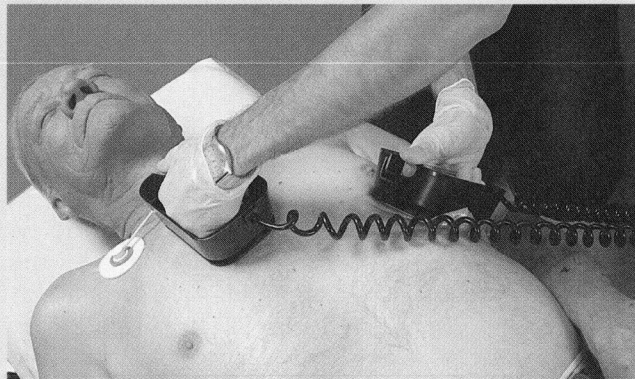

21-2D. Apply the paddles.

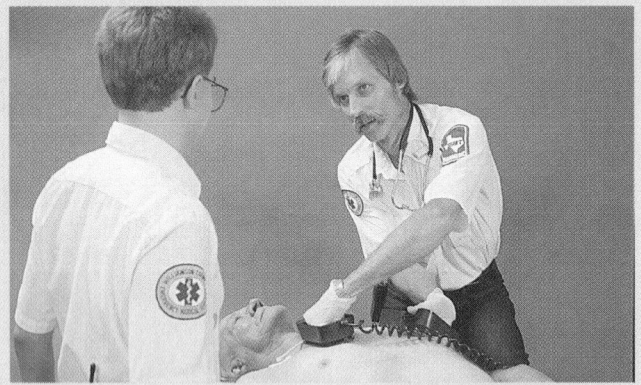

21-2E. Ensure that everyone is clear of the patient.

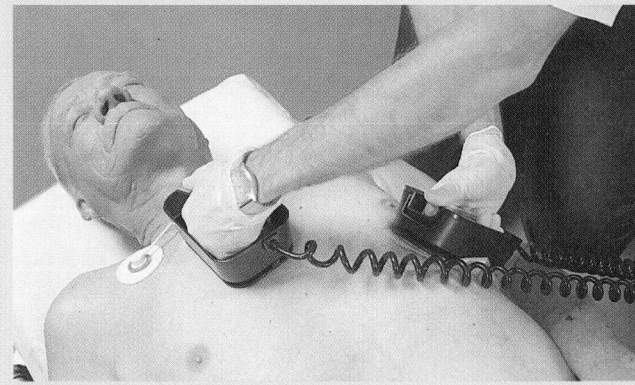

21-2F. Discharge the machine.

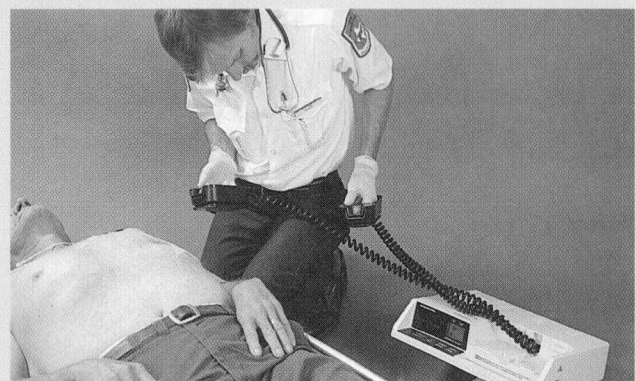

21-2G. Check the ECG.

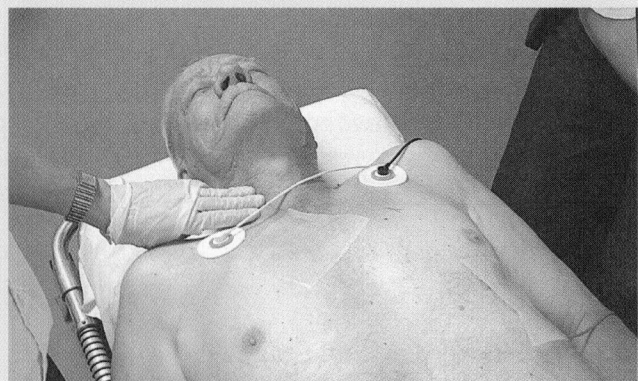

21-2H. Check the pulse.

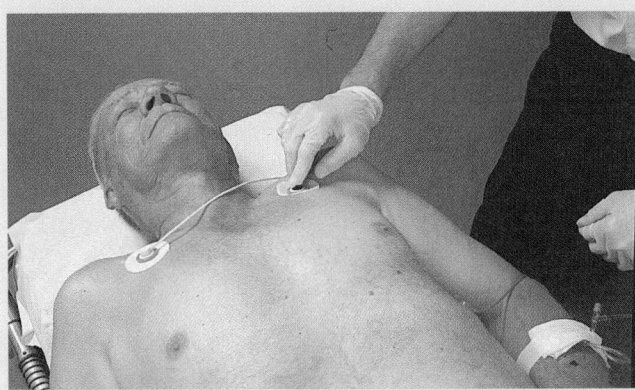

21-3A. Place the patient on the monitor.

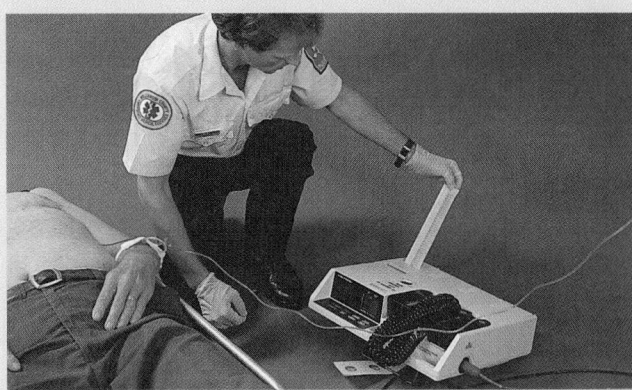

21-3B. Confirm the rhythm.

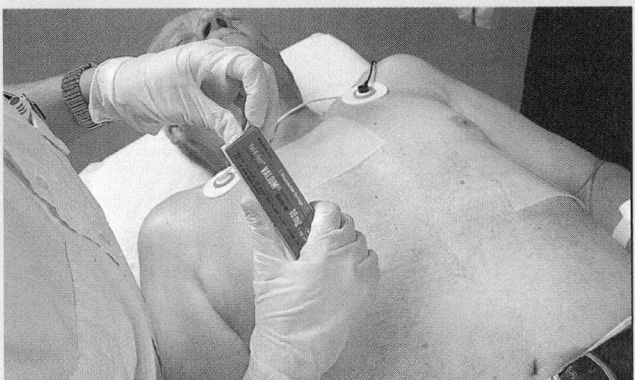

21-3C. Sedate the patient, if necessary.

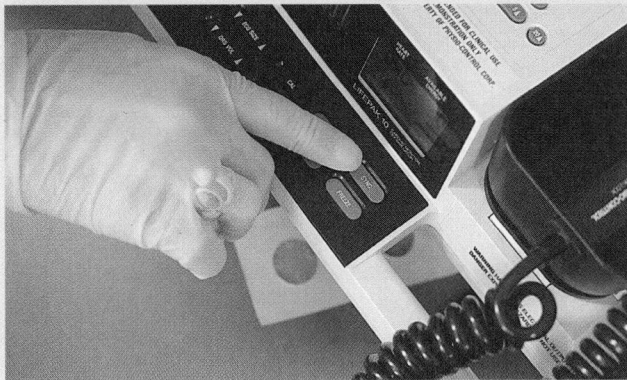

21-3D. Activate the synchronizer.

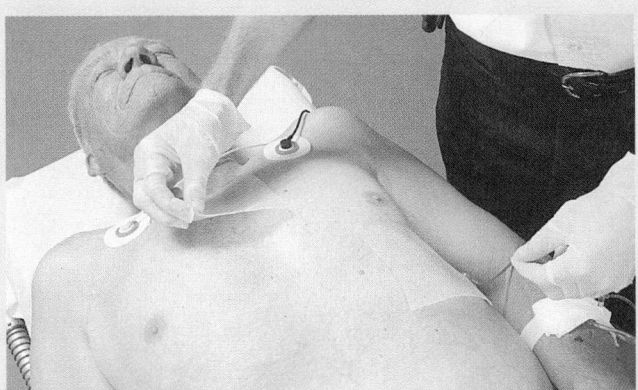

21-3E. Place the conductive pads.

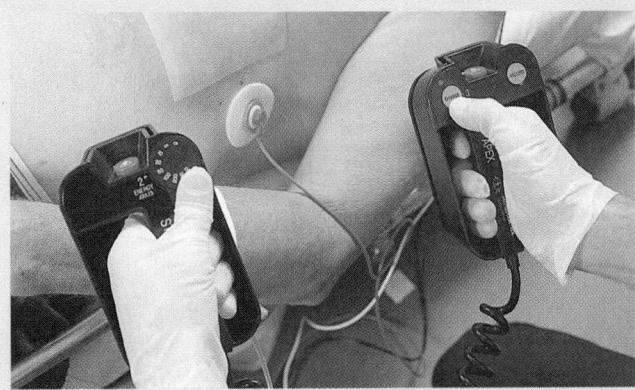

21-3F. Select the appropriate energy level.

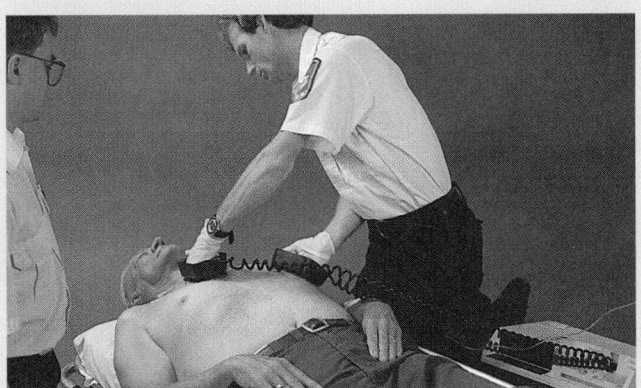

21-3G. Discharge the machine.

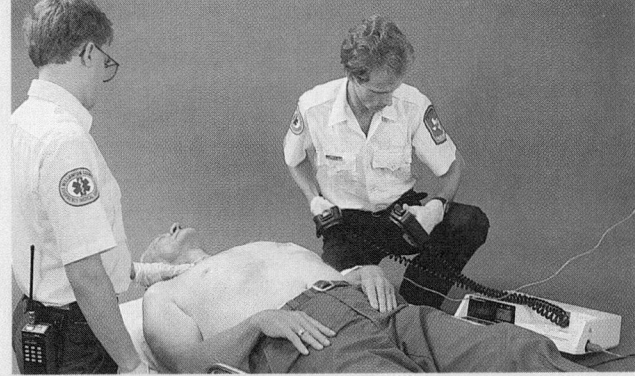

21-3H. Monitor the patient.

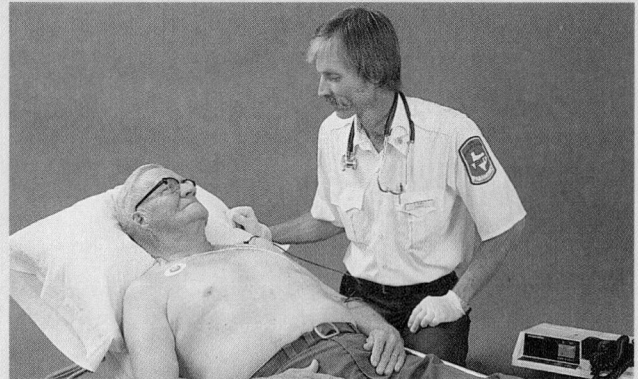

21-4A. Assess the patient.

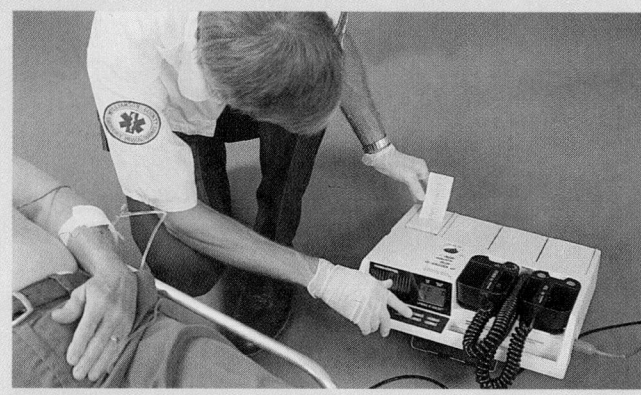

21-4B. Turn on the monitor.

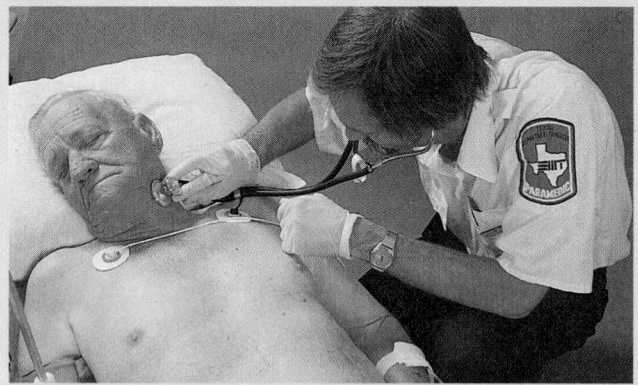

21-4C. Listen to both carotids for the presence of bruits.

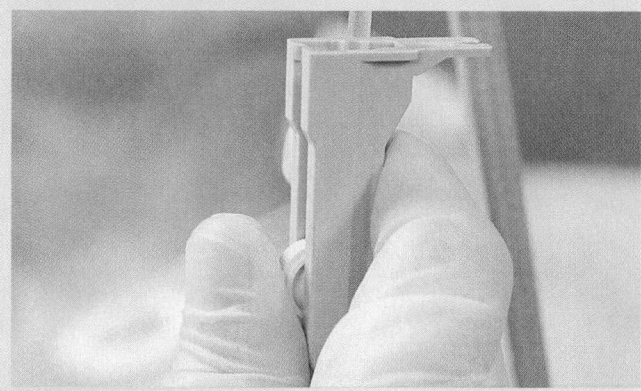

21-4D. Start an IV line.

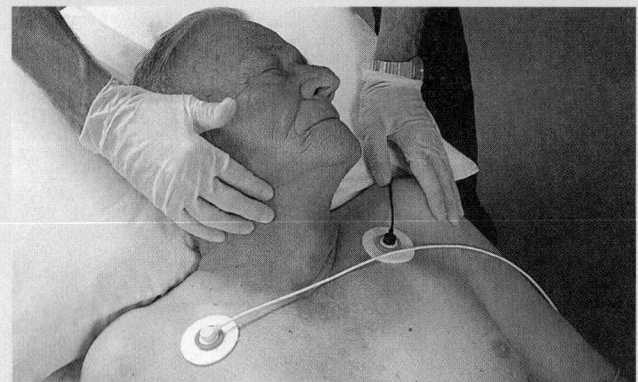

21-4E. Rub the right carotid. Wait.

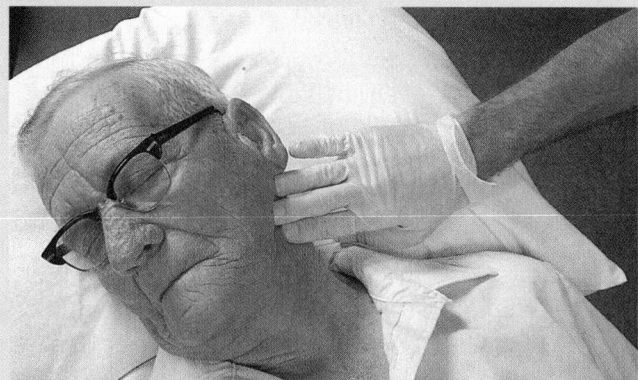

21-4F. If unsuccessful, rub the left carotid.

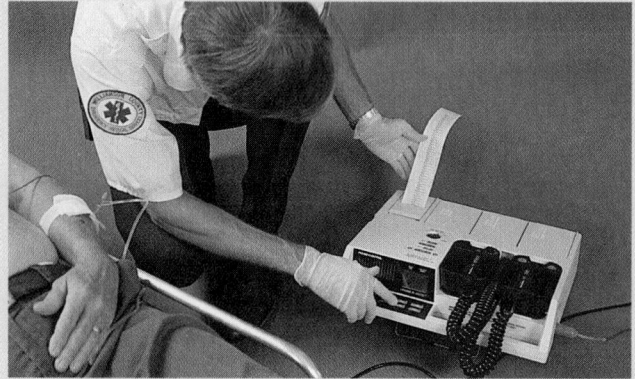

21-4G. Check the rhythm

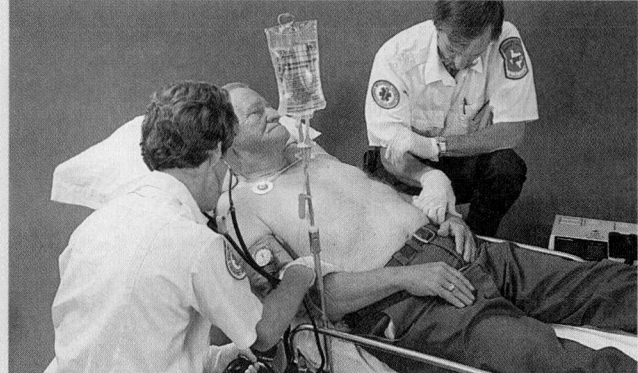

21-4H. Re-evaluate the patient.

the presence of carotid bruits. If the pulse is diminished, or if carotid bruits are present, DO NOT attempt carotid sinus massage.

4. Tilt the patient's head to either side, and place your index and middle fingers over one artery below the angle of the jaw and as high up on the neck as possible.
5. Firmly massage the artery by pressing it against the vertebral body and rubbing.
6. Monitor the ECG, and obtain a continuous readout. Terminate massage at the first sign of slowing or heart block.
7. Maintain pressure no longer than 15–20 seconds.
8. If it is ineffective, the massage may be repeated, preferably on the other side of the patient's head.
9. Have atropine sulfate readily available.

Complications include dysrhythmias such as asystole, PVCs, ventricular tachycardia, or fibrillation. In addition, carotid sinus massage can interfere with cerebral circulation, causing syncope, seizure, or even stroke. Increased parasympathetic tone can cause bradycardias, nausea, or vomiting.

Transcutaneous Cardiac Pacing (TCP) Many paramedic units now have the capability to perform external cardiac pacing. External cardiac pacing is beneficial in cases of symptomatic bradycardia such as that which occur with high-degree AV blocks, atrial fibrillation with slow ventricular response, and other significant bradycardias.

The technique for external cardiac pacing involves the following steps. (See Procedure 21-5.)

1. Initiate IV, oxygen, and ECG monitoring.
2. Place the patient in a supine position.
3. Confirm symptomatic bradycardia, and confirm medical control order for external cardiac pacing.
4. Apply the pacing electrodes per the manufacturer's recommendations. Assure that there is a good electrode/skin interface.
5. Connect the electrodes.
6. Set the desired heart rate on the pacemaker. This will typically be in the range of 60–80 beats per minute.
7. Turn the voltage setting down to 0.
8. Turn the pacer on.
9. Slowly increase the voltage until you note ventricular capture.
10. Check the pulse and blood pressure, and adjust the rate and voltage as ordered by medical control.
11. Monitor the patient's response to treatment.

Occasionally, external cardiac pacing may cause patient discomfort. If this occurs, the medical control physician may request the administration of an analgesic.

SUMMARY

Cardiovascular disease is the number one cause of death in the United States today. Many deaths from heart attack occur within the first 24 hours—many within the first hour. Therefore, prompt and efficient prehospital care can literally mean the difference between life and death.

External cardiac pacing is now possible in the prehospital setting. External pacing is of benefit in bradycardias and heart blocks which are symptomatic. The electrodes are placed on the chest as shown. The desired heart rate is selected. The current is then adjusted until "capture" of the heart's conductive system is obtained.

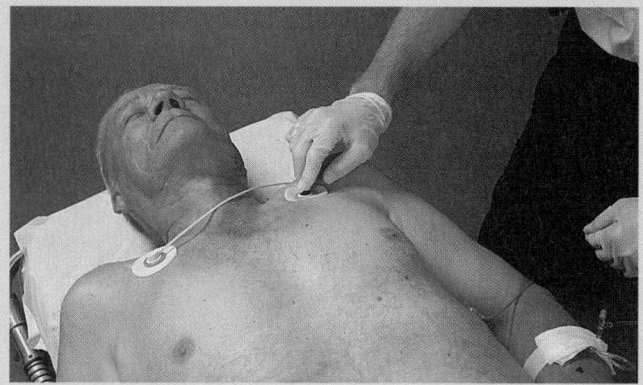

21-5A. Place ECG electrodes.

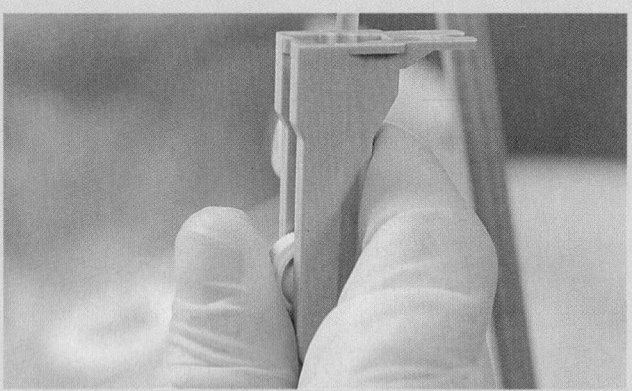

21-5B. Establish an IV line.

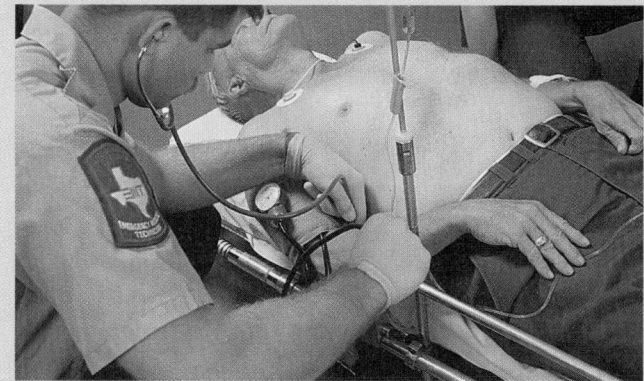

21-5C. Carefully assess vital signs and contact medical control.

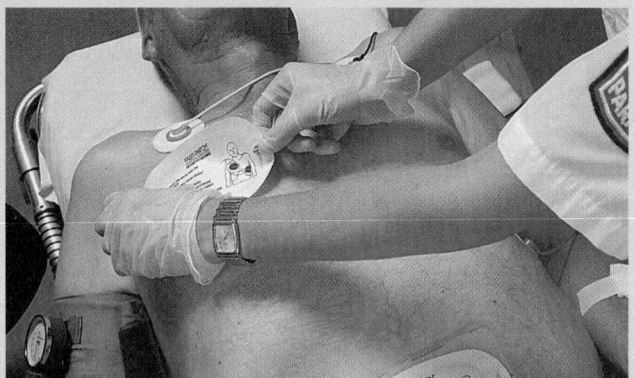

21-5D. If external pacing ordered, apply the pacing electrodes per the manufacturer's recommendations.

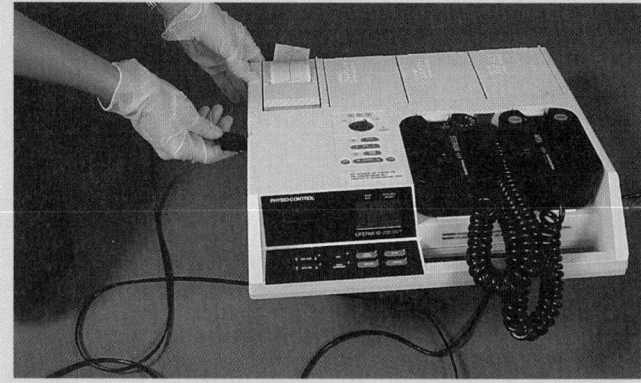

21-5E. Establish an IV line.

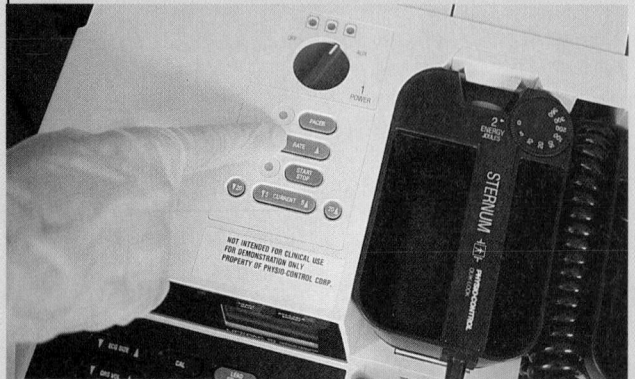

21-5F. Select the desired pacing rate and current.

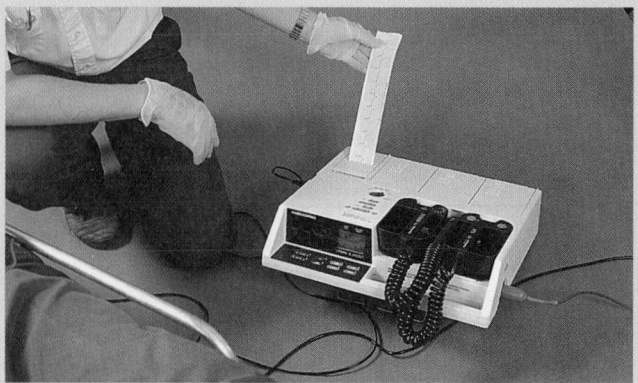

21-5G. Monitor the patient's response to treatment.

FURTHER READING

American Heart Association. *Textbook of Advanced Cardiac Life Support*, 3rd Ed. Dallas: American Heart Association, 1993.

Bledsoe, Bryan E. "Hypertensive Emergencies: Performing Under Stress." *JEMS* April, 1990.

Bledsoe, Bryan E., Gideon Bosker, and Frank J. Papa, *Prehospital Emergency Pharmacology*, 3rd Ed. Englewood Cliffs, NJ: Prentice-Hall, 1992.

Guyton, Arthur C. *Textbook of Medical Physiology*, 8th Ed. Philadelphia: W.B. Saunders, 1991.

Walraven, Gail. *Basic Arrhythmias*, 2nd Ed., Rev. Englewood Cliffs, NJ: Prentice-Hall, 1986.

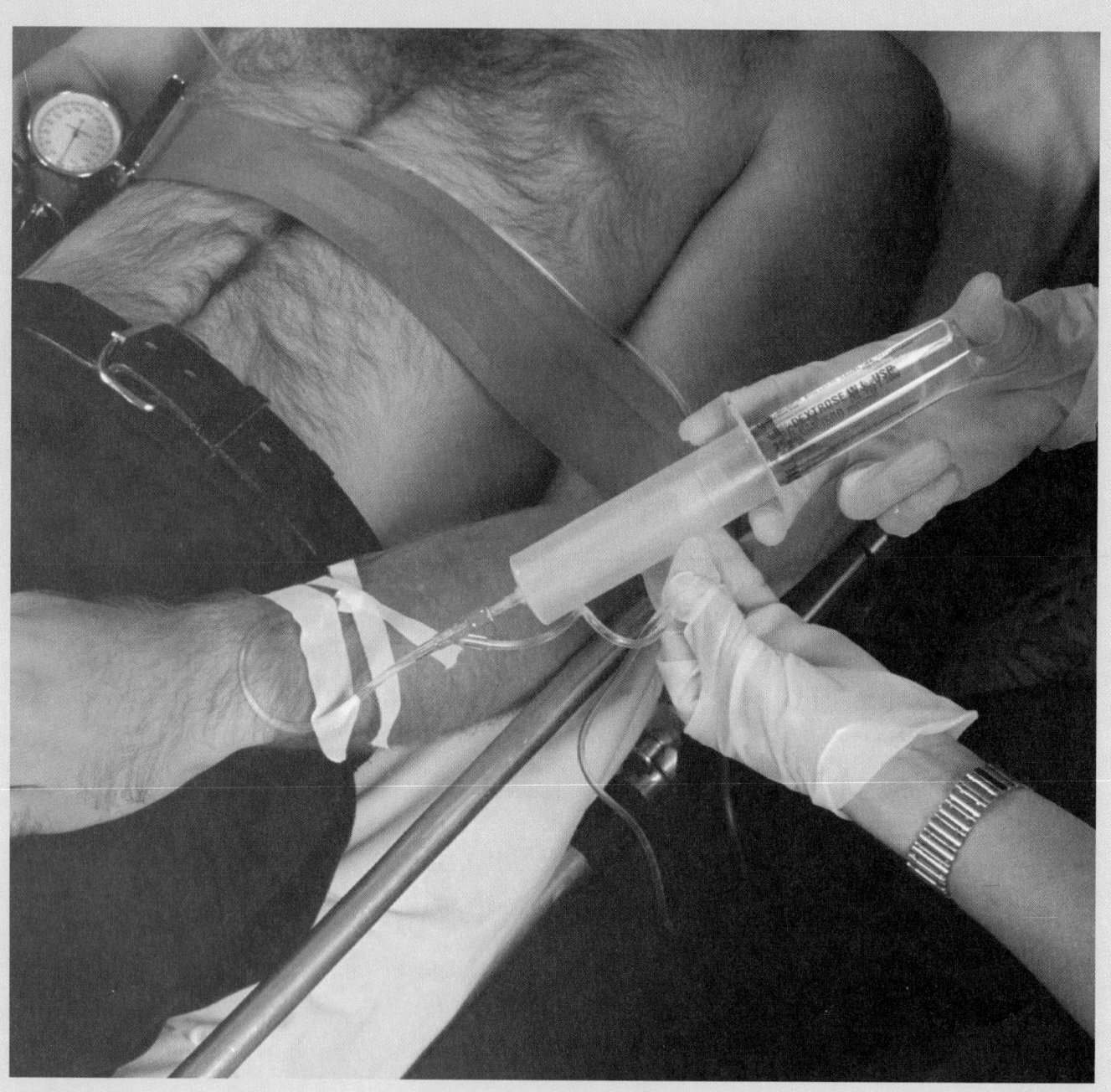

22

ENDOCRINE AND METABOLIC EMERGENCIES

Objectives for Chapter 22

After reading this chapter, you should be able to:

1. Define the term hormone. (See p. 726.)

2. Discuss the location and function of the following endocrine glands. (See below pages.)
- pituitary (pp. 726–728)
- thyroid (p. 728)
- parathyroid (p. 728)
- pancreas (p. 729)
- adrenal (pp. 729–730)
- gonads (p. 730)

3. List two functions of the islets of Langerhans. (See p. 729.)

4. Discuss the function of glucagon. (See p. 729.)

5. Define diabetes mellitus. (See p. 730.)

6. Discuss the function of insulin and its relation to glucose metabolism. (See pp. 730–731.)

7. Compare and contrast Type I (insulin-dependent) and Type II (non-insulin-dependent) diabetes mellitus. (See pp. 731–732.)

8. Discuss the osmotic diuresis occurring in diabetes. (See pp. 731–732.)

9. Discuss the presentation, assessment, and management of diabetic ketoacidosis. (See pp. 732–733.)

10. Discuss the presentation, assessment, and management of hypoglycemia. (See pp. 733–736.)

The dispatcher sends Rescue 21 to a "medical emergency" in the suburb where the unit is stationed. Upon arrival, the crew finds a 31-year-old male lying unconscious on the couch. His wife says that she discovered him upon returning home to pick up her clothes after a domestic quarrel. She adds that she has not seen her husband for four days. The man's wife states that he is diabetic, and she heads to the refrigerator for his insulin.

The paramedics now go to work. While one paramedic obtains the patient's history, the other completes the primary assessment. The patient is breathing deeply at a rate of 30 breaths per minute. His pulse rate is 100, his skin is warm and dry, and he is unresponsive. The paramedic in charge then completes the secondary assessment, locating no other problems. She notices, however, a sweet odor on the patient's breath. ECG reveals sinus tachycardia. Pulse oximetry shows an oxygen saturation of 96 percent on room air. She obtains a blood sample and determines the blood glucose level with a rapid glucose determination device. The device shows a reading of "HIGH."

The crew alerts medical control, and the on-line physician orders an IV of normal saline established. The first two liters of normal saline are to be administered rapidly, then the infusion slowed to 200 mL per hour. One paramedic begins oxygen administration with a nonrebreather oxygen mask, while the other starts the IV. Blood is drawn for the hospital per protocol. The paramedics again contact medical control and update the physician as they prepare to transport.

The patient's status remains the same en route. At the hospital, he is admitted to the ICU. His blood glucose was 840 mg percent in the sample drawn by the paramedics (normal = 70–110). The attending physician begins an insulin drip and continues fluids. Ultimately, the patient recovers. The paramedics learn later that he was intoxicated virtually the entire time after his wife's departure and forgot to take his insulin.

INTRODUCTION

Closely tied to the nervous system, the *endocrine system* controls many body functions. The system exerts its control by releasing special chemical substances called **hormones**. Hormones are chemicals that, when secreted by endocrine glands into the blood stream, affect other **endocrine glands** or body systems. The endocrine system derives its name from the fact that the various glands release hormones directly into the blood, which in turn transports the hormones to their target tissue. Exocrine glands, on the other hand, transport their hormones to target tissues via ducts. Emergencies involving the endocrine system range from the very common, such as diabetes, to the unusual, such as **thyrotoxicosis**.

ANATOMY AND PHYSIOLOGY

The endocrine system consists of several glands located in various parts of the body. (See Figure 22-1.) They include the glands discussed in the following sections.

Pituitary

The *pituitary gland* is a small gland located on a stalk hanging from the base of the brain. Sometimes referred to as the "master gland," its primary function is to control the other endocrine glands. The pituitary produces many hor-

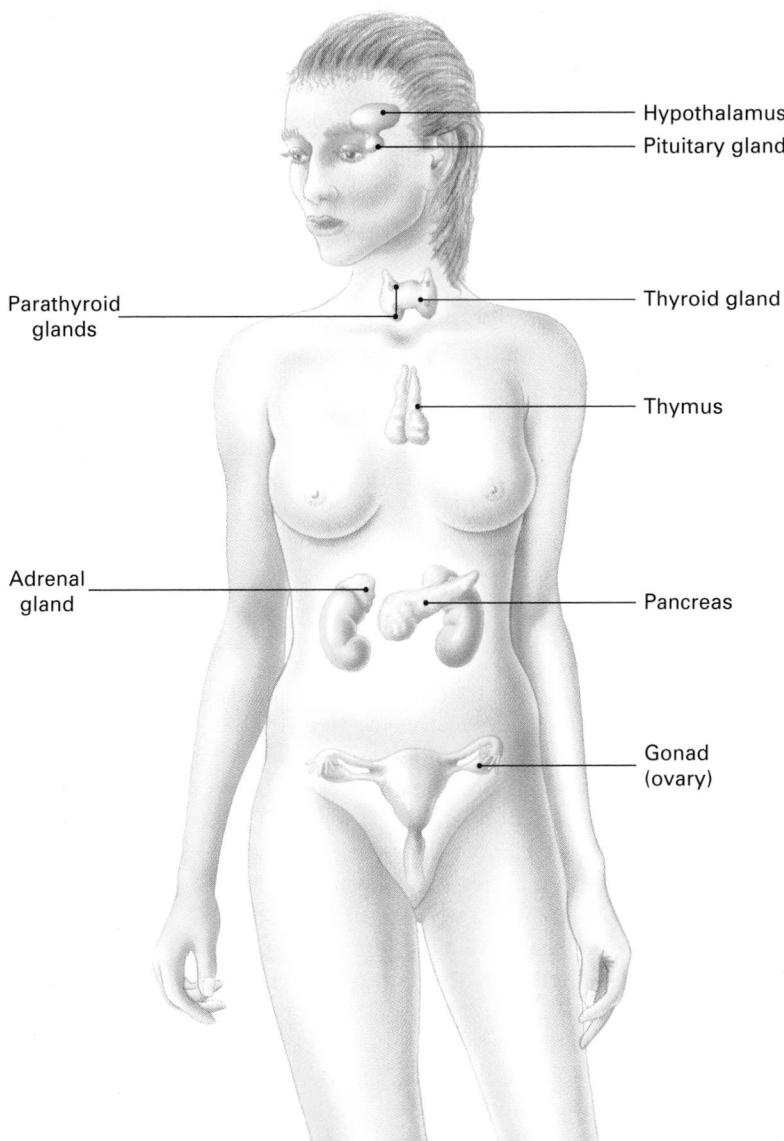

FIGURE 22-1 The endocrine system.

mones. Their secretion is controlled by the hypothalamus in the base of the brain. The pituitary gland is divided into two areas, differing both structurally and functionally. Each area has separate types of hormone production. The *posterior pituitary* produces oxytocin and antidiuretic hormone (ADH). The *anterior pituitary* produces thyroid-stimulating hormone (TSH), growth hormone (GH), adrenocorticotropin (ACTH), follicle-stimulating hormone (FSH), luteinizing hormone (LH), and prolactin. The function of these various hormones is discussed below.

Posterior Pituitary   *Oxytocin*, the natural form of the drug pitocin, stimulates contraction of the gravid uterus and "let down" of milk from the breast. *ADH*, sometimes called vasopressin, causes the kidney to retain water. The interrelationship of these two hormones is significant in emergency medicine. For example, women suffering preterm labor are often administered a bolus of IV fluid to suppress their labor. When the IV fluid is administered, it increases the intravascular fluid volume. Detecting this increase, the kidney sends a message to the pituitary that there is now adequate intravascular fluid volume, and therefore, it is time to release some fluid by filtration through the kidney. The kidney's message causes the pituitary to decrease secretion of ADH, thereby allowing the kidney to produce more urine. Inhibition of ADH by the fluid bolus, however, also causes inhibition of oxytocin, as the two hormones are quite similar and secreted from the same portion of the pituitary. Thus, by using a fluid bolus, it is sometimes possible to suppress preterm labor.

Anterior Pituitary   The anterior pituitary hormones primarily regulate other endocrine glands and are rarely a factor in endocrinological emergencies. *TSH* stimulates the thyroid gland to release its hormones, thus increasing metabolic rate. When released by the pituitary, *growth hormone* has several effects. In adults, the most important is to decrease glucose usage and to increase consumption of fats as an energy source. *ACTH* stimulates the adrenal cortex to release its hormones. *FSH* and *LH* each have specific roles in stimulating maturation and release of eggs from the ovary.

Thyroid Gland

The *thyroid gland* lies in the anterior part of the neck just below the larynx. It has two lobes, located on either side of the trachea, connected by a narrow band of tissue called the *isthmus*. Sacs inside the gland contain a thick material called *colloid*. Within the colloid are the thyroid hormones *thyroxine* (T4) and *triiodothyronine* (T3). When stimulated, either by TSH from the anterior pituitary or by cold, the thyroid gland releases these two hormones into the circulatory system. Their release increases the overall metabolic rate.

The thyroid gland also contains specialized cells called "C-cells" that produce the hormone *calcitonin*. Calcitonin, when released, lowers the amount of calcium in the blood. Calcitonin and parathyroid hormone (discussed below) are important in regulating the levels of calcium in the body.

Inadequate levels of the thyroid hormones produce *hypothyroidism*, or myxedema. Symptoms of this disorder include facial bloating, weakness, cold intolerance, lethargy, and altered mental states. Additionally, the skin and hair are quite oily. Treatment is by replacement of thyroid hormone.

Increased thyroid hormone release causes *hyperthyroidism*, commonly called *Graves' disease*. Signs and symptoms include insomnia, fatigue, tachycardia, hypertension, heat intolerance, and weight loss. If the hyperthyroidism has existed fairly long, there will be exophthalmos, or bulging of the eyeballs. In severe cases, a medical emergency, called *thyrotoxicosis*, can result. Discussion of these conditions is not within the scope of this text.

Parathyroid Glands

The *parathyroid glands* are small, pea-shaped glands, located in the neck near the thyroid. There are usually four of them, although the number can vary. The parathyroid glands regulate the level of calcium in the body. They produce a hormone called *parathyroid hormone* that, when released, causes the level of calcium in the blood to increase.

The parathyroid glands rarely cause problems. Sometimes they are accidentally removed with the thyroid. They may also be destroyed if the thyroid is irradiated. Removal or destruction of the parathyroid glands causes loss of parathyroid hormone, and hypocalcemia may then occur.

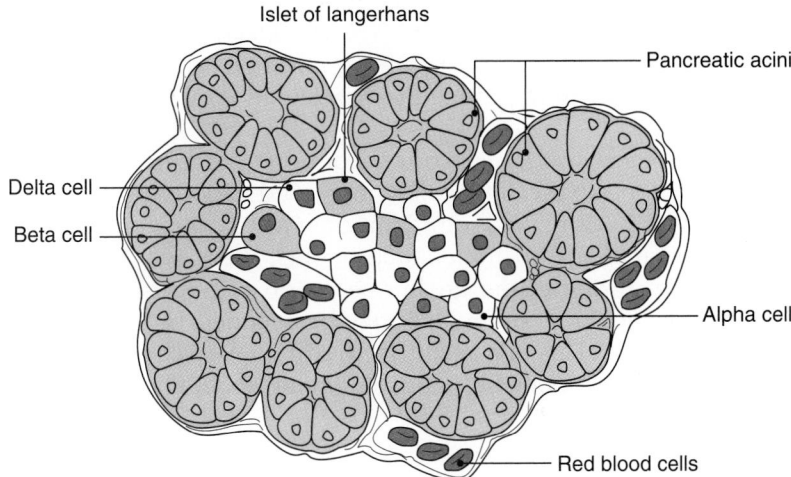

Islet of langerhans

Pancreatic acini

Delta cell

Beta cell

Alpha cell

Red blood cells

FIGURE 22-2 The internal anatomy of the pancreas.

Pancreas

The *pancreas* is a key gland located in the folds of the duodenum within the abdominal cavity. It has both exocrine and endocrine functions. (See Figure 22-2.) Exocrine functions include secretion of several key digestive enzymes.

Within the pancreas are specialized tissues, referred to as the *islets of Langerhans*. Here the pancreas' endocrine functions occur. The islets of Langerhans include three types of cells: alpha (α) cells, beta (ß) cells, and delta (∂) cells. Each secretes an important hormone.

The alpha cells release *glucagon*, essential for controlling blood glucose levels. Whenever glucose levels fall, the alpha cells increase the amount of glucagon in the blood. The surge of glucagon stimulates the liver to release glucose stores from glycogen and additional glucose storage sites. It also stimulates the liver to manufacture glucose from other substances in a process called *gluconeogenesis*. Together, both processes effectively raise the blood glucose level.

The beta cells release *insulin*, which is antagonistic to glucagon. Insulin increases the rate in which various body cells take up glucose. Thus, insulin effectively lowers the blood glucose level. Insulin is rapidly broken down by the liver and must be secreted constantly. The role of insulin in the disease diabetes mellitus will be discussed later in this chapter.

The third type of pancreatic endocrine cell, the delta cell, produces *somatostatin*. This hormone inhibits both glucagon and insulin. Its role in regulating the blood glucose level is incompletely understood.

Adrenal Glands

The *adrenal glands* are two small glands that sit atop both kidneys. These glands have two distinct divisions, each with different functions. The *adrenal medulla*, closely related to the sympathetic component of the autonomic nervous system, secretes the catecholamine hormones *norepinephrine* and *epinephrine*. The *adrenal cortex* secretes three classes of hormones, all of them steroid hormones. They include the *glucocorticoids*, the *mineralocorticoids*, and the *androgenic hormones*.

The glucocorticoids account for 95 percent of adrenal cortex hormone production. Like glucagon, they increase the level of glucose in the blood. But they perform many other functions, such as anti-inflammatory actions and immune suppression. They are released—like the hormones from the adrenal medulla—in response to stress, trauma, or serious infection. The mineralocorticoids play an important role in regulating the concentration of potassium and sodium in the body.

A prolonged increase in adrenal cortex hormone secretion results in *Cushing's disease.* Patients typically exhibit increased blood sugar levels, unusual body fat distribution, and rapid mood swings. Additionally, if there is an associated increase in mineralocorticoids, there will be a serious electrolyte imbalance due to the greater secretion of potassium by the kidney, causing hypokalemia. Sodium also may be retained by the kidney, resulting in hypernatremia. This can result in dysrhythmias, coma, or even death. A tumor is usually responsible, and treatment generally consists of removing it.

Gonads

The gonads are the endocrine glands associated with human reproduction. The female's ovaries produce eggs, and the male's testes produce sperm. However, both ovaries and testes also have endocrine functions.

Ovaries   The *ovaries,* or the female gonads, are located in the abdominal cavity adjacent to the uterus. As described, they produce eggs for reproduction. Under the control of LH and FSH from the anterior pituitary, they also manufacture *estrogen* and *progesterone.* These hormones have several functions, including sexual development and preparation of the uterus for implantation of the egg.

Testes   The testes, or the male gonads, are located in the scrotum and, as indicated, produce sperm for reproduction. They also manufacture testosterone, which promotes male growth and masculinization. Like the female ovary, the testes are controlled by the anterior pituitary hormones FSH and LH.

ENDOCRINE EMERGENCIES

By far the most common endocrine emergencies that you can expect to treat will involve the disease known as diabetes mellitus. Frequent complications include diabetic ketoacidosis and hypoglycemia.

Diabetes Mellitus

■ **diabetes mellitus** endocrine disorder characterized by inadequate insulin production by the beta cells of the islets of Langerhans in the pancreas.

Diabetes mellitus is one of the most common diseases in North America. It is characterized by decreased insulin secretion by the beta cells of the islets of Langerhans in the pancreas. The complications of this disease are numerous. Among others, it contributes to heart disease, stroke, kidney disease, and blindness. To understand the pathophysiology of diabetes, you need to explore the mechanics of glucose metabolism.

Glucose Metabolism   Glucose, also called *dextrose,* is a simple sugar required by the body to produce energy. Sugars, also called *carbohydrates,* are one of the three major food sources used by the body. The other two include proteins and fats. Most sugars in the human diet are classified as *complex* and must be broken down into *simple* sugars—glucose, galactose, and fructose—before they can be used by the body for energy. This breakdown is carried out by enzymes in the gastrointestinal system. Once broken down into simple sugars, they are absorbed from the gastrointestinal system into the body. By the time the various sugars enter the bloodstream, more than 95 percent are in the form of glucose.

For the body to convert glucose to energy, glucose first must be transported through the cell membrane. However, the glucose molecule is large and does not readily diffuse through the cell membrane. Instead, it must pass into the cell by binding to a special carrier protein on the cell's surface. This process is called *facilitated diffusion* and does not utilize energy. Once bound to the special carrier protein, the molecule is transported through the cell membrane into the cell. Here it is released and subsequently converted to energy.

The rate at which glucose can enter the cell is dependent upon insulin levels. Insulin acts as a messenger. When released by the pancreas, it travels through the blood to the target tissues. On reaching its destination, insulin combines with specific insulin receptors on the surface of the cell membrane, allowing glucose to enter the cell. The rate at which glucose can be transported into the cells can be accelerated 10 or more times by insulin. Without insulin, the amount of glucose that can be transported into the cells is far too small to meet the body's energy demands.

Diabetes mellitus results from inadequate amounts of circulating insulin. Generally, the disease can be divided into two different categories. Type I diabetes, or insulin-dependent diabetes, usually begins in the early years. Patients who have Type I diabetes must take insulin. Type II, or non-insulin-dependent diabetes, usually begins later in life and tends to be associated with obesity. Type II diabetes can often be controlled without using insulin. It is important for you to understand the difference between these two forms of diabetes.

Type I Diabetes Mellitus

Type I diabetes mellitus is a serious disease characterized by inadequate production of insulin by the endocrine pancreas. The cause of Type I diabetes is not well understood. One theory is that a viral infection attacks the pancreatic beta cells, thus slowing or stopping insulin production. Another theory proposes that the body's immune system mistakenly targets the pancreatic beta cells as foreign and attacks them. In either case, heredity appears to be a factor in increasing a person's chance in contracting the disease.

With Type I diabetes mellitus, the patient must take daily doses of insulin. In the normal state, the intake of glucose, such as in a meal, results in the release of insulin. Insulin promotes the uptake of glucose by the cells. Type I diabetes generally begins with decreased insulin secretion, subsequently leading to elevated blood glucose levels. However, since insulin is required for glucose to enter into the various body cells, they become glucose-depleted despite increased blood glucose levels.

In diabetes, a drop in insulin levels is accompanied by a steady accumulation of glucose in the blood. As the cells become glucose-depleted, they begin to use other sources of energy. Therefore, various harmful by-products, such as *ketones* and *organic acids*, are produced. When these start to accumulate, several of the classic findings of diabetic **ketoacidosis** appear. If the various acids and ketones continue to collect in the blood, severe metabolic acidosis occurs and coma ensues. Severe acidosis can result in serious brain damage or death.

■ **ketoacidosis** complication of diabetes due to decreased insulin secretion or intake. It is characterized by high levels of glucose in the blood, metabolic acidosis, and, in advanced stages, coma. Ketoacidosis is often called *diabetic coma.*

As the concentration of glucose in the blood continues to rise, the kidneys will begin excreting glucose in the urine. When glucose is spilled into the urine, it takes water with it, resulting in an *osmotic diuresis*, which dehydrates the patient.

Type II Diabetes Mellitus   *Type II diabetes mellitus* occurs more commonly than Type I does. Like Type I, it is characterized by decreased insulin production by the endocrine pancreas. As mentioned previously, Type II diabetes usually begins in later life. It is often associated with obesity, but can occur in non-obese patients. Increased body weight causes a relative decrease in the number of available insulin receptors. In addition, the insulin receptors become defective and less responsive to insulin. The pancreas also becomes less responsive to stimulation from increased blood glucose levels. Thus, insulin is not secreted as needed, increasing blood glucose levels even further.

The first approach in treating Type II diabetes is to reduce the intake of carbohydrates by encouraging the patient to lose weight. Physicians may also prescribe oral hypoglycemic agents. These medications tend to stimulate increased insulin secretion from the pancreas and to promote an increase in the number of insulin receptors on the cells. Both actions tend to lower blood glucose levels. If diet and oral agents fail, insulin may be required.

Type II diabetes does not usually result in diabetic ketoacidosis. It can, however, develop into a life-threatening emergency termed *nonketotic hyperosmolar coma*. In Type II diabetes, when blood glucose levels exceed 600 mg/dL, the high osmolality of the blood causes an osmotic diuresis and dehydration of body cells. In non-ketotic hyperosmolar coma, sufficient insulin is produced. This prevents the manufacture of ketones and the complications of metabolic acidosis. In this respect, the condition differs from diabetic ketoacidosis. However, it is difficult to distinguish diabetic ketoacidosis from non-ketotic hyperosmolar coma in the field. Therefore, the prehospital treatment of both emergencies is identical.

Diabetic Ketoacidosis (Diabetic Coma)

Diabetic ketoacidosis is a serious complication of diabetes mellitus. It occurs when insulin levels become inadequate to meet the metabolic demands of the body.

Pathophysiology   *Diabetic ketoacidosis* develops as blood glucose levels increase and individual cells become glucose-depleted. The body begins spilling sugar into the urine. This causes a significant osmotic diuresis and serious dehydration, evidenced by dry, warm skin and mucous membranes. As cellular glucose-depletion continues, ketone and acid production occur. Subsequently, the blood becomes acidotic. Deep respirations begin as the body tries to compensate for the metabolic acidosis. If the ketoacidosis is uncorrected, coma will follow.

✱ The symptoms of diabetes include:

- Polyuria
- Polyphagia
- Polydipsia

Clinical Presentation   The onset of diabetic ketoacidosis is slow, lasting from 12 to 24 hours. In its early stages, the signs and symptoms include increased thirst, excessive hunger, urination, and malaise. Increased urination results from the osmotic diuresis accompanying glucose spillage into the urine. Intensified thirst is caused by the body's attempt to replace the fluids lost by increased urination. Diabetic ketoacidosis is characterized by nausea, vomiting, marked dehydration, tachycardia, and weakness. The skin is usually warm and dry. Coma is not uncommon. The breath may have a sweet or acetone-like

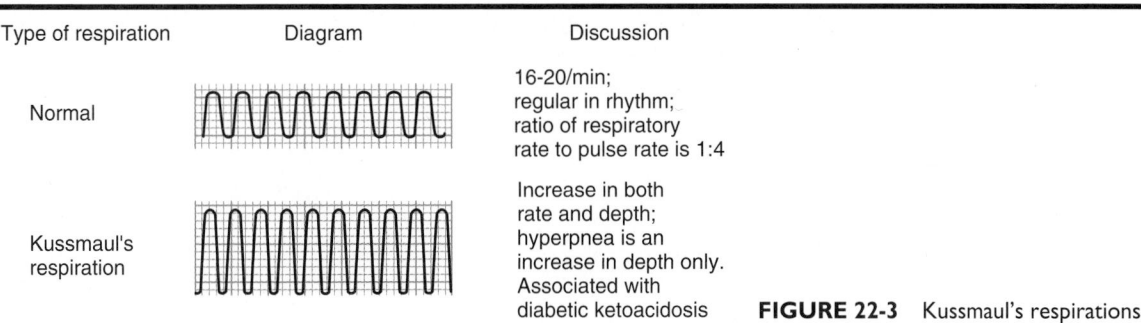

Type of respiration	Diagram	Discussion
Normal		16-20/min; regular in rhythm; ratio of respiratory rate to pulse rate is 1:4
Kussmaul's respiration		Increase in both rate and depth; hyperpnea is an increase in depth only. Associated with diabetic ketoacidosis

FIGURE 22-3 Kussmaul's respirations.

character due to the increased ketones in the blood. Very deep, rapid respirations, called *Kussmaul's respirations*, also occur. (See Figure 22-3.) Kussmaul's respirations represent the body's attempt to compensate for the metabolic acidosis produced by the ketones and organic acids present in the blood.

Diabetic ketoacidosis is often associated with infection or decreased insulin intake. It may be complicated by several electrolyte imbalances. The most significant is decreased potassium. Decreased potassium (hypokalemia) can lead to serious dysrhythmias or even death.

Ketoacidosis can occur in patients who fail to take their insulin or who take an inadequate amount over an extended period. Persons not previously diagnosed as diabetic will occasionally present in ketoacidosis.

Assessment The approach used with the patient suffering from diabetic ketoacidosis is essentially the same as with any unconscious patient. You should first complete the primary assessment of airway, breathing, and circulation. You will then undertake the secondary assessment. Pay particular attention to the presence of Medic-Alert bracelets and/or insulin in the refrigerator. Also, take a history from bystanders. The fruity odor of ketones occasionally can be detected on the breath. If available, complete the rapid test for blood glucose. (See Procedure 22-1.)

Emergency Intervention If you can estimate the blood glucose level in the field, a hi gh blood glucose can alert you to the classical signs and symptoms of diabetic ketoacidosis. In such cases, treatment should consist of drawing a red top tube (or the tube specified by local protocols) of blood. Following this, you should administer one to two liters of 0.9 percent sodium chloride. If transport time is lengthy, the medical control physician may request intravenous or subcutaneous administration of regular insulin.

If the blood glucose level cannot be quickly determined, draw a red top tube of blood for analysis and start an IV of normal saline. Following this, administer 50 mL of 50 percent dextrose solution. If the patient is alcoholic, consider administering 100 mg of thiamine. This additional glucose load will not adversely affect the ketoacidotic patient because it is negligible compared to the total quantity present in the body.

Hypoglycemia (Insulin Shock)

Hypoglycemia occurs when insulin levels are excessive. Hypoglycemia is an urgent medical emergency as a prolonged hypoglycemic episode can result in serious brain injury.

■ **hypoglycemia** complication of diabetes characterized by low levels of blood glucose. This often occurs from too high a dose of insulin or from inadequate food intake following a normal insulin dose. Sometimes called *insulin shock*, hypoglycemia is a true medical emergency.

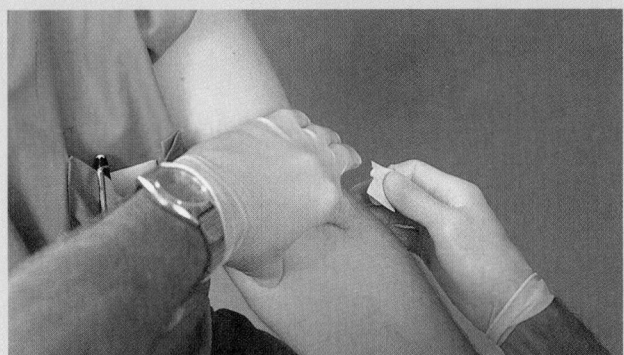

22-1A. Choose a vein, and prep the site.

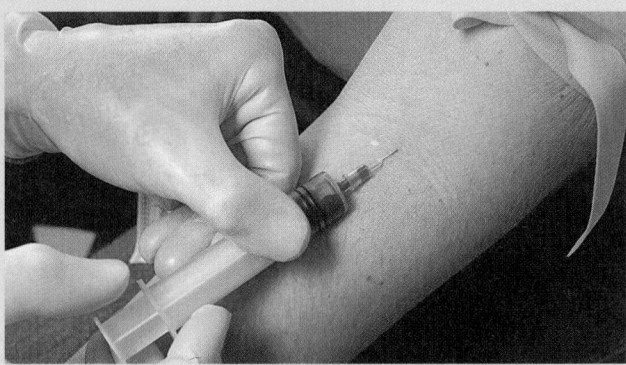

22-1B. Perform the venipuncture.

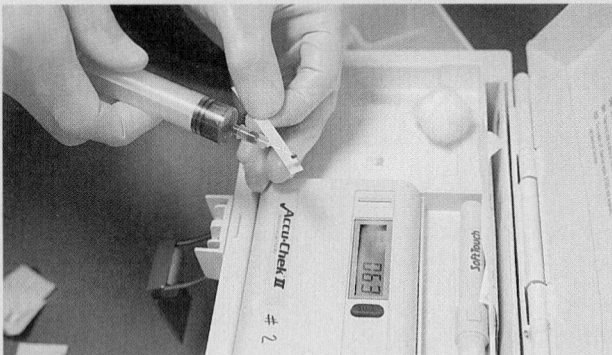

22-1C. Place a drop of blood on the reagent strip. Activate the timer.

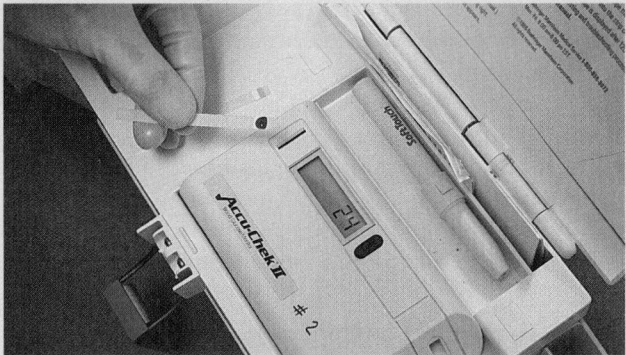

22-1D. Wait until the timer sounds.

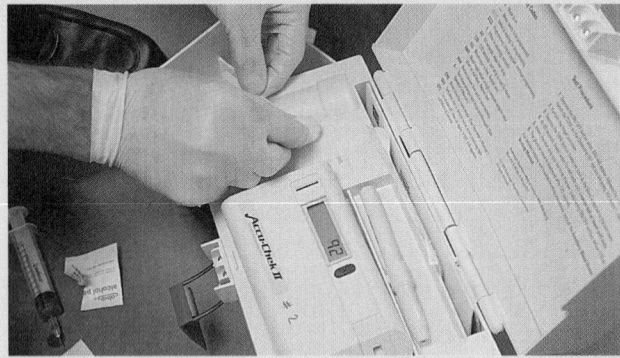

22-1E. Wipe the reagent strip.

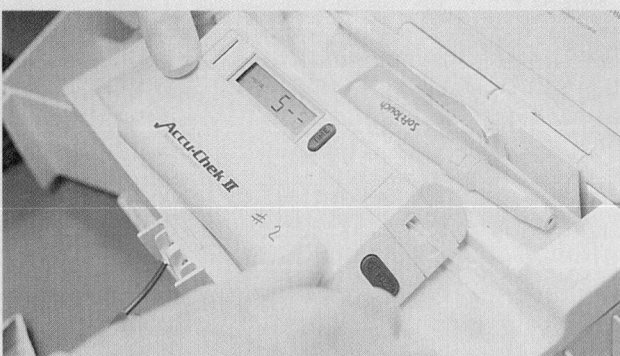

22-1F. Place the reagent strip in the glucometer.

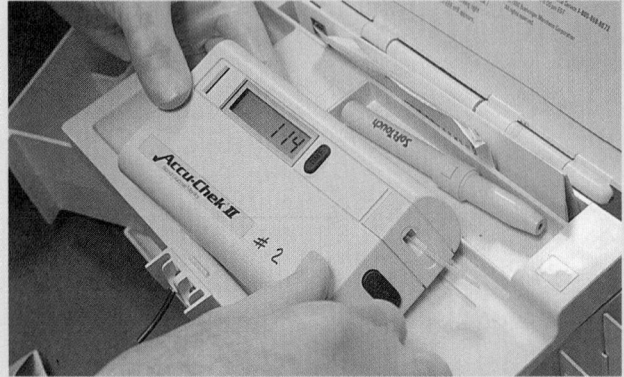

22-1G. Read the blood glucose level.

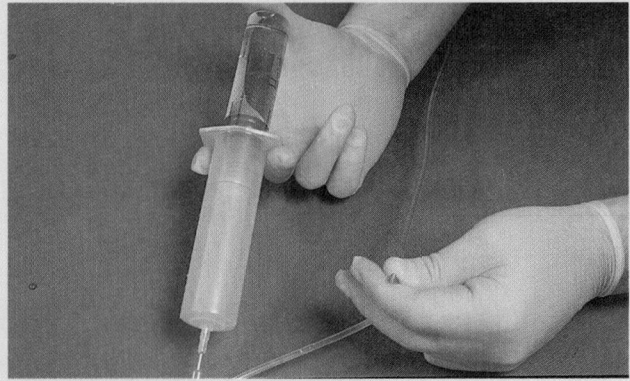

22-1H. Administer 50 percent dextrose intravenously, if the blood glucose level is less than 80 mg.

Pathophysiology   Hypoglycemia, sometimes called insulin shock, lies at the other end of the spectrum from diabetic ketoacidosis. Hypoglycemia can occur if a patient accidentally or intentionally takes too much insulin or eats an inadequate amount of food after taking insulin. If the patient is untreated, the insulin will cause the blood glucose level to drop to a very low level. THIS IS A TRUE MEDICAL EMERGENCY. If the patient is not treated quickly, he or she can sustain serious injury to the brain since it receives most of its energy from glucose metabolism.

Clinical Presentation   The clinical signs and symptoms of hypoglycemia are many and varied. An abnormal mental status is the most important. In the earliest stages of hypoglycemia, the patient may appear restless or impatient or complain of hunger. As the blood sugar falls lower, he or she may display inappropriate anger (even rage) or display a variety of bizarre behaviors. Sometimes the patient may be placed in police custody for such behaviors or be involved in an automobile accident.

Physical signs may include diaphoresis and tachycardia. If the blood sugar falls to a critically low level, the patient may sustain a **hypoglycemic seizure** or become comatose.

■ **hypoglycemic seizure** seizure that can occur when blood glucose levels fall dangerously low, seriously altering the brain's energy supply.

In contrast to diabetic ketoacidosis, hypoglycemia can develop quickly. A change in mental status can occur without warning. When encountering a patient behaving bizarrely, you should always consider hypoglycemia. (See Tables 22-1 and 22-2.)

Assessment   In suspected cases of hypoglycemia, perform the primary assessment quickly. Inspect the patient for Medic-Alert bracelets. If possible,

TABLE 22-1 Diabetic Emergencies	
Diabetic Ketoacidosis	**Hypoglycemia**
Causes	**Causes**
Patient has not taken insulin.	Patient has taken too much insulin.
Patient has overeaten, flooding the body with carbohydrates.	Patient has overexerted, thus reducing glucose levels.
Patient has infection that disrupts glucose/insulin balance.	
Signs and Symptoms	**Signs and Symptoms**
Polyuria, polydypsia, polyphagia	Weak, rapid pulse
Nausea/vomiting	Cold, clammy skin
Tachycardia	Weakness/uncoordination
Deep, rapid respirations	Headache
Warm, dry skin	Irritable, nervous behavior
Fruity odor on breath	May appear intoxicated
Abdominal pain	Coma (severe cases)
Falling blood pressure	
Fever (occasionally)	
Decreased LOC	
Management	**Management**
Fluids, insulin	Dextrose

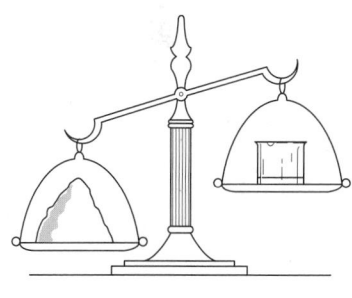

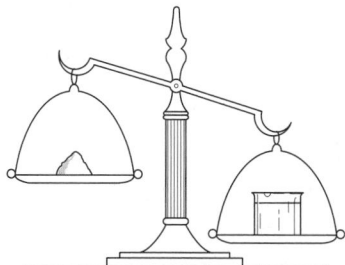

TABLE 22-2 Diagnostic Signs by System

System	Diabetic Ketoacidosis	Hypoglycemia
Cardiovascular		
Pulse	Rapid	Normal (may be rapid)
Blood Pressure	Low	Normal
Respiratory		
Respirations	Exaggerated air hunger	Normal or shallow
Breath odor	Acetone (sweet, fruity)	
Nervous		
Headache	Absent	Present
Mental state	Restlessness → unconsciousness	Apathy, irritability → unconsciousness
Tremors	Absent	Present
Convulsions	None	In late stages
Gastrointestinal		
Mouth	Dry	Drooling
Thirst	Intense	Absent
Vomiting	Common	Uncommon
Abdominal pain	Frequent	Absent
Ocular vision	Dim	Double vision (diplopia)

determine the blood glucose level. Because of the seriousness of the emergency, most paramedic units need to have the capability to perform this task or to rush a blood sample to the hospital along with the patient.

Emergency Intervention If the blood glucose level is noted to be less that 60 mg/dl, draw a red top tube of blood and start an IV of normal saline. Next, administer 50–100 milliliters of 50 percent dextrose intravenously. If the patient is conscious and able to swallow, complete glucose administration with orange juice, sodas, or commercially available glucose pastes.

If the blood glucose cannot be obtained and if the patient is unconscious, you should start an IV of normal saline and administer 50–100 milliliters 50 percent dextrose. Transport to a medical facility is also indicated. (See Table 22-1.) If you suspect alcoholism, administer 100 mg of thiamine.

SUMMARY

Like the nervous system, the endocrine system regulates many body functions. With the exception of complications from diabetes mellitus, endocrine emergencies tend to be quite rare and probably would be undetected in the prehospital setting.

Prehospital personnel should always suspect diabetes. Hypoglycemia, the most urgent diabetic emergency, must be quickly treated to prevent serious nervous system damage. When the exact type of diabetes is undetermined, prehospital personnel should treat the emergency as if it were hypoglycemia. Keep in mind that treatment of diabetic ketoacidosis is primarily a hospital procedure.

FURTHER READING

Bledsoe, B.E. "Dealing With Diabetic Emergencies." *JEMS*. 16(12), December 1991 (pp. 40-50).

Hamburger, S., D.R. Rush, and G. Bosker. *Endocrine and Metabolic Emergencies.* Bowie, MD:Brady Communications, 1984.

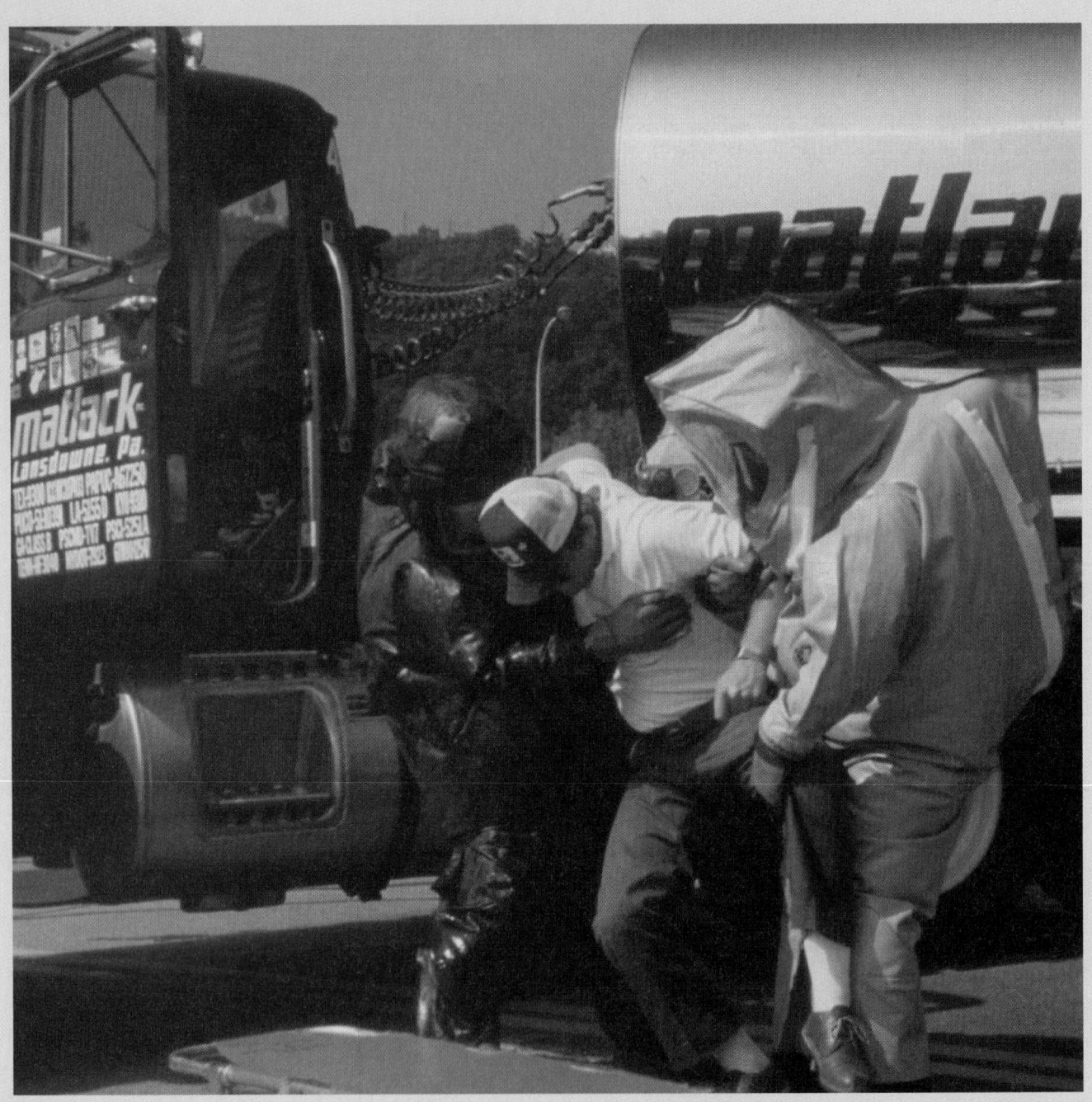

23

NERVOUS SYSTEM EMERGENCIES

Objectives for Chapter 23

After reading this chapter, you should be able to:

1. Identify the parts of the neuron, and give their function. (See pp. 741–742.)

2. Describe the process of nerve impulse transmission. (See pp. 741–742.)

3. Identify the protective structures of the brain and the spinal cord. (See pp. 742–744.)

4. List the major divisions of the brain, and briefly state the function of each. (See pp. 744–746.)

5. Identify the functions of the spinal cord. (See pp. 746–747.)

6. Identify the location of the *brachial plexus*. (See p. 747.)

7. Identify the factors to be elicited when evaluating the nervous system, including trauma and non-trauma related problems. (See pp. 749–754.)

8. Identify the following specific observations and physical findings to be evaluated in a patient with a nervous system disorder. (See below pages.)

   a. primary assessment (p. 749)

   b. secondary assessment (p. 749)

      i. pupils (p. 750)

      ii. respiratory status (pp. 750–751)

      iii. spinal evaluation (pp. 751–752)

      iv. vital signs (p. 752)

   c. neurological evaluation (pp. 752–753)

9. Describe the Glasgow Coma Scale. (See pp. 753–754.)

10. Describe the use of the following drugs in relation to CNS problems. (See below pages.)

- D-50-W (p. 757)
- naloxone (p. 757)
- thiamine (pp. 758–759)
- dexamethasone (p. 759)
- diazepam (pp. 763–764)

11. Describe the pathophysiology, assessment, and management of the following nervous system disorders. (See below pages)

- altered mental status (pp. 754–760.)
- seizure (pp. 760–763.)
- status epilepticus (p. 763.)
- CVA and TIA (pp. 763–767.)

12. List the possible causes of altered mental status. (See p. 755.)

13. Describe and differentiate the major types of seizures. (See pp. 760–761.)

14. Describe the different phases of a grand mal seizure. (See p. 760.)

15. Differentiate between syncope and seizures. (See p. 762.)

A call comes into Paramedic Engine Company 10 and Ambulance 17. The dispatcher reports an apparent "seizure" at a run-down hotel usually frequented by the homeless. The units respond in approximately three minutes. Upon arrival, the hotel clerk leads emergency personnel to a ramshackle room where they see an elderly male lying on a mattress on the floor. The room smells of urine and feces.

Paramedics quickly perform a primary assessment. The patient has a good airway. Respirations are adequate, and the pulse is strong. The secondary survey reveals a thin male with many of the stigmata of alcoholism. As paramedics attempt to arouse the patient and assess the level of consciousness, his body goes into intense spasm. This is followed by alternating contraction and relaxation of the skeletal muscles. The seizure lasts approximately 45 seconds.

Following the seizure, the patient remains postictal. Paramedics quickly administer oxygen to the patient with a non-rebreathing mask. They then establish an IV of normal saline. Per standing orders, the paramedics administer 100 mg of thiamine and 50 mL of 50 percent dextrose. As the paramedic is pushing the dextrose, the patient has another seizure, within 2 minutes of the last. The paramedics now administer 5 mg of diazepam intravenously, and the seizure ends. The patient remains postictal while the ambulance crew prepares for transport to the hospital.

Upon arrival at the emergency department, the patient's condition remains unchanged. A routine laboratory profile is normal. Blood levels of the patient's seizure medications (Dilantin and phenobarbital) are subtherapeutic. Because of the patient's sluggish arousal from the seizure, the emergency department physician orders a CT scan of the brain. The CT scan reveals a rather large subdural hematoma on the left side. The patient is taken to the operating room where a neurosurgeon evacuates the subdural hematoma. The patient's postoperative course is unremarkable, and the hospital transfers him to the Veterans Administration hospital. Here the patient's rehabilitation continues.

INTRODUCTION

Emergencies involving the nervous system are often difficult to recognize and to treat. Nervous system emergencies are generally categorized as traumatic or medical. This chapter will address the relevant anatomy and physiology of the nervous system. It will also present common medical neurological emergencies as well as the recommended prehospital management.

ANATOMY AND PHYSIOLOGY

✱ The nervous system is the body's control system.

The *nervous system* is the body's control system. It regulates nearly all bodily functions via electrical impulses transmitted through nerves. The endocrine system is closely related to the nervous system. It too exerts bodily control via hormones. Yet a third system, the circulatory system, assists in regulatory functions by distributing hormones and other chemical messengers.

■ **autonomic nervous system** part of the nervous system controlling involuntary bodily functions. It is divided into the sympathetic and the parasympathetic systems.

The nervous system is customarily divided into the central nervous system and the peripheral nervous system. The *central nervous system* consists of the brain and the spinal cord. In contrast, the *peripheral nervous system* is composed of the cranial nerves and the peripheral nerves. The **autonomic nervous system**, a part of the peripheral nervous system, is divided functionally into the *sympathetic* and the *parasympathetic* nervous systems. (See Figure 23-1.)

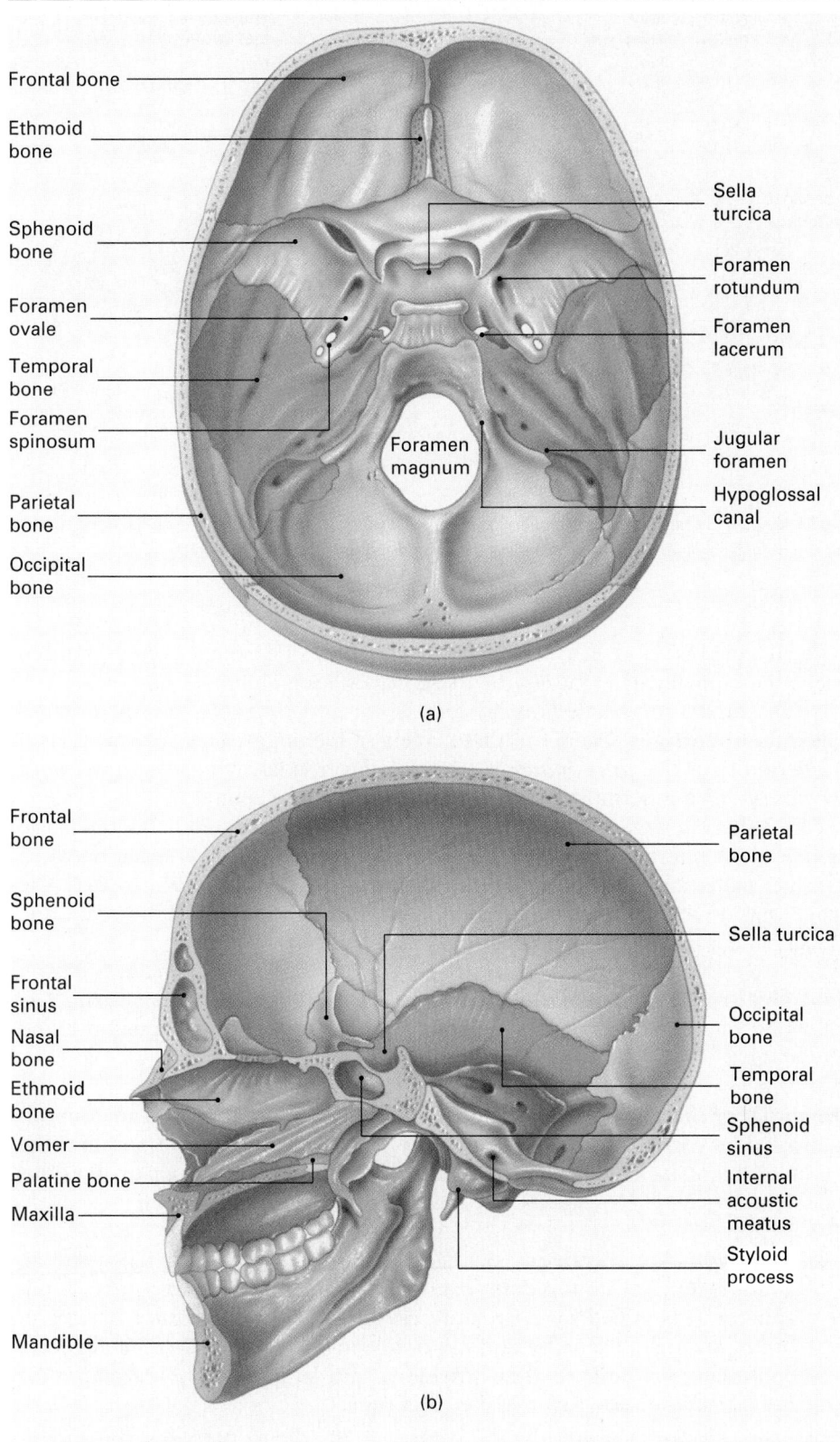

Frontal bone

Ethmoid bone

Sphenoid bone

Foramen ovale

Temporal bone

Foramen spinosum

Parietal bone

Occipital bone

Sella turcica

Foramen rotundum

Foramen lacerum

Foramen magnum

Jugular foramen

Hypoglossal canal

(a)

Frontal bone

Sphenoid bone

Frontal sinus

Nasal bone

Ethmoid bone

Vomer

Palatine bone

Maxilla

Mandible

Parietal bone

Sella turcica

Occipital bone

Temporal bone

Sphenoid sinus

Internal acoustic meatus

Styloid process

(b)

FIGURE 23-4 The bones of the skull.

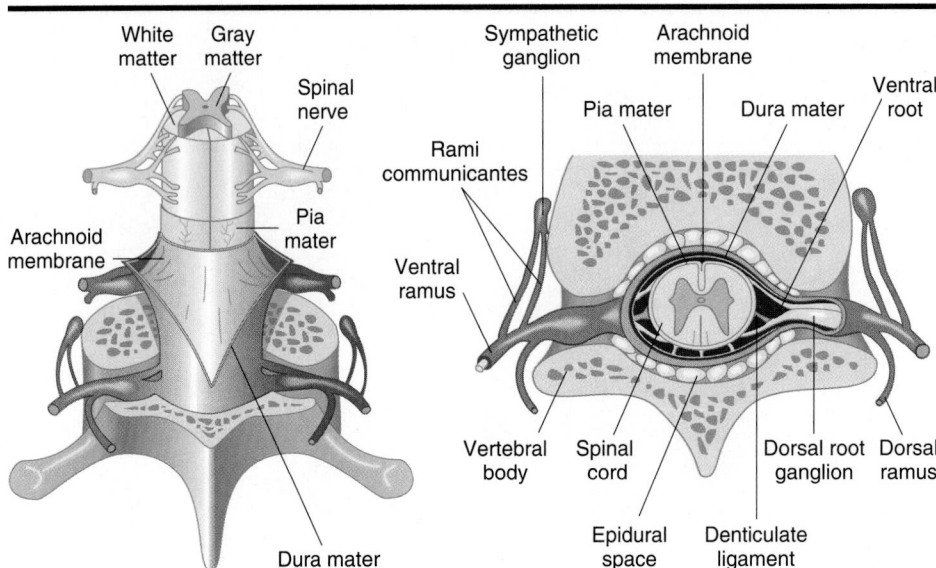

FIGURE 23-5 The spinal cord and spinal meninges: (a) posterior view of the spinal cord showing the meningeal layers; (b) sectional view showing distribution of spinal nerves.

■ **meninges** membranes covering and protecting the brain and spinal cord. They consist of the pia mater, arachnoid membrane, and dura mater.

■ **cerebrospinal fluid** watery, clear fluid that acts as a cushion, protecting the brain and spinal cord from physical impact. The cerebrospinal fluid also serves as an accessory circulatory system for the central nervous system.

■ **brainstem** that part of the brain connecting the cerebral hemispheres with the spinal cord. It is comprised of the medulla oblongata, the pons, and the midbrain.

■ **cerebrum** largest part of the brain. It consists of two hemispheres separated by a deep longitudinal fissure. The cerebrum is the seat of consciousness and the center of the higher mental functions such as memory, learning, reasoning, judgement, intelligence, and the emotions.

5 sacral vertebra, and 3 to 5 coccygeal vertebra. The spinal cord is housed inside the "spinal canal" formed by these bones. (See Figure 23-5.)

The entire central nervous system is covered by protective membranes called the **meninges**. There are three layers of meninges. The outermost layer is referred to as the *dura mater*. The middle layer is known as the *arachnoid membrane*. The innermost layer, directly overlying the central nervous system, is called the *pia mater*. The space between the pia mater and the arachnoid membrane is referred to as the *subarachnoid space*, while the space between the dura mater and the arachnoid membrane is called the *subdural space*. The space outside the dura mater is called the *epidural space*. Both the brain and the spinal cord are bathed in **cerebrospinal fluid**.

The Brain　The brain is the largest part of the central nervous system. The following information provides a general profile of the brain's anatomy and physiology.

Divisions of the Brain.　Filling the cranial vault, the brain can be anatomically divided into six major parts. (See Figure 23-6.) The midbrain, pons, and the medulla oblongata collectively form the **brainstem**. The six main divisions include:

❑ *Cerebrum.* The **cerebrum**, occasionally referred to as the telencephalon, is in the anterior and middle fossa of the cranium. Containing two hemispheres, it is joined by a structure called the *corpus callosum*. The cerebrum governs all sensory and motor actions. It is the seat of intelligence, controlling learning, analysis, memory, and language. The *cerebral cortex* is the outermost layer of the cerebrum.

❑ *Diencephalon.* Covered by the cerebrum, the diencephalon is the superior most portion of the brainstem. Inside it are the *thalamus, hypothalamus*, and the *limbic system*. This area is responsible for many involuntary actions such as temperature regulation, sleep, water balance, stress response, and emotions. It plays a major role in regulating the autonomic nervous system.

es from the body to the brain. Efferent fibers carry impulses from the brain to the body. Each nerve root has a corresponding area of the body, called a **dermatome**, to which it supplies sensation. The amount of paralysis incurred in a spinal cord injury depends on the location of the injury. The nearer the brainstem, the more serious it is.

■ **dermatome** areas of the skin innervated by spinal nerves.

Anatomy and Physiology of the Peripheral Nervous System

Consisting of the cranial and the peripheral nerves, the peripheral nervous system has both voluntary and involuntary components. The twelve pairs of cranial nerves originate in the brain and supply nervous control to the head, neck, and certain thoracic and abdominal organs. (See Figure 23-8.) The peripheral nerves, as described previously, originate in the spinal cord and also supply nervous control to the periphery.

Categories of Peripheral Nerves   The four categories of peripheral nerves include:

- ❏ *Somatic Sensory*. These nerves transmit sensations involved in touch, pressure, pain, temperature, and position (proprioception).
- ❏ *Somatic Motor*. These fibers carry impulses to the skeletal muscles.
- ❏ *Visceral Sensory*. These tracts transmit sensations from the visceral organs. Sensations such as a full bladder or the need to defecate are mediated by visceral sensory fibers.
- ❏ *Visceral Motor*. These fibers leave the central nervous system and supply nerves to the viscera, such as glands and other organs.

Many of the nerves innervating the upper extremity come from the cervical and thoracic portion of the spinal cord. They enter a network of nerves at the posterior part of the neck called the *brachial plexus*. This system can be injured either at birth or with trauma to the upper extremity, causing permanent disability.

Autonomic Nervous System   The involuntary component of the peripheral nervous system, commonly called the *autonomic nervous system*, is responsible for the unconscious control of many body functions. There are two functional divisions of the autonomic nervous system—the sympathetic nervous system and the parasympathetic nervous system.

The Sympathetic Nervous System.   The **sympathetic nervous system**, often referred to as the "fight-or-flight" system, prepares the body for stressful situations. It is located near the thoracic and lumbar part of the spinal cord. Stimulation causes increased heart rate and blood pressure, pupillary dilation, rise in the blood sugar, as well as bronchodilation. The neurotransmitters epinephrine and norepinephrine mediate its actions. The sympathetic nervous system is closely associated with the adrenal gland of the endocrine system.

■ **sympathetic nervous system** division of the autonomic nervous system that prepares the body for stressful situations.

The Parasympathetic Nervous System.   The **parasympathetic nervous system**, sometimes called the "feed-or-breed" system, is responsible for controlling vegetative functions. Associated with the cranial nerves and the sacral plexus, it is mediated by the neurotransmitter acetylcholine. When stimulated, it causes a decrease in heart rate, an increase in digestive activity, pupillary constriction, and a reduction in blood glucose.

■ **parasympathetic system** division of the autonomic nervous system that is responsible for controlling vegetative functions.

The sympathetic and parasympathetic systems are antagonistic. In their normal state, they exist in balance with each other. During stress, the sympathetic system dominates. During rest, the parasympathetic system dominates. (For additional discussion of the autonomic nervous system, see Chapter 13).

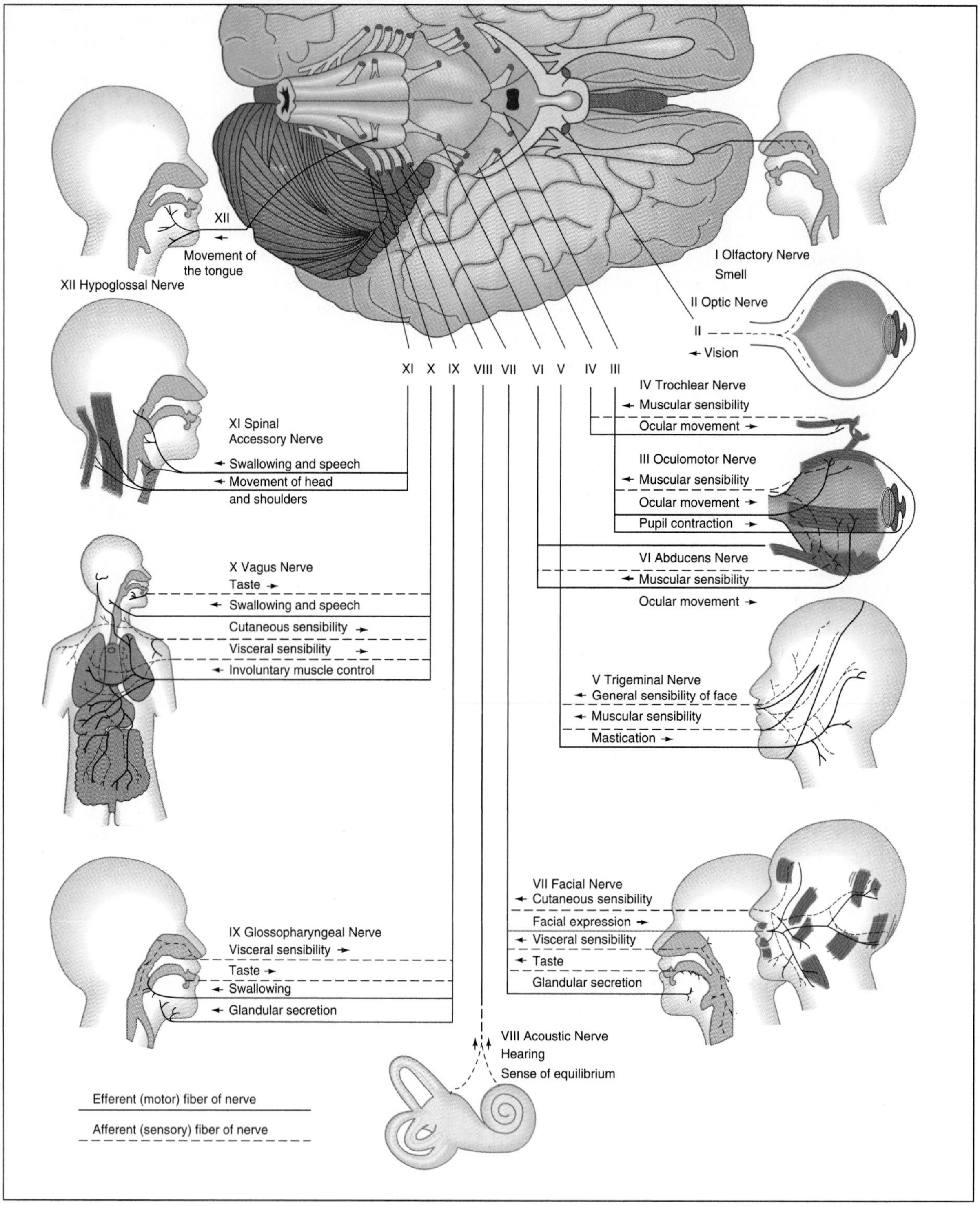
XII
Movement of the tongue
XII Hypoglossal Nerve
I Olfactory Nerve
Smell
II Optic Nerve
II
Vision
XI X IX VIII VII VI V IV III
IV Trochlear Nerve
Muscular sensibility
Ocular movement
XI Spinal Accessory Nerve
Swallowing and speech
Movement of head and shoulders
III Oculomotor Nerve
Muscular sensibility
Ocular movement
Pupil contraction
VI Abducens Nerve
Muscular sensibility
Ocular movement
X Vagus Nerve
Taste
Swallowing and speech
Cutaneous sensibility
Visceral sensibility
Involuntary muscle control
V Trigeminal Nerve
General sensibility of face
Muscular sensibility
Mastication
VII Facial Nerve
Cutaneous sensibility
Facial expression
Visceral sensibility
Taste
Glandular secretion
IX Glossopharyngeal Nerve
Visceral sensibility
Taste
Swallowing
Glandular secretion
VIII Acoustic Nerve
Hearing
Sense of equilibrium
Efferent (motor) fiber of nerve
Afferent (sensory) fiber of nerve

FIGURE 23-8 The cranial nerves.

ASSESSMENT OF THE NEUROLOGICAL SYSTEM

Assessment of the neurological system is often difficult. Many of the signs and symptoms of nervous system dysfunction are subtle. Initial evaluation of the patient with a nervous system emergency should begin with the primary assessment. This should be followed by a thorough secondary assessment, with particular emphasis on the neurological examination.

Primary Assessment

When you perform the patient assessment, first check for responsiveness. Place the greatest emphasis on maintenance of the airway and alignment of the cervical spine. If the patient is unconscious, assume that a cervical spine injury exists, and treat it appropriately. Use the chin-lift and jaw-thrust maneuvers to open the airway. Once opened, insert the appropriate airway adjunct. In unresponsive patients, the tongue may be all that is occluding the airway. In such cases, you may only need to place an oropharyngeal or nasopharyngeal airway to maintain the airway. (For more on these techniques, see Chapter 11.)

In any patient with CNS injury, it is essential to observe for respiratory arrest that can result from increased intracranial pressure. Remain alert for an absent gag reflex and vomiting. In addition, blood from facial injuries and possible aspiration of gastric contents further threaten the patient's airway.

Secondary Assessment

Following completion of the primary assessment and correction of any immediate threats to the patient's life, turn your attention to the secondary assessment. The secondary assessment should include a brief history, head-to-toe examination, vital signs, and a pertinent neurological evaluation.

History   One of the first steps in assessment involves attempts to establish whether the CNS problem is traumatic or medical. Clarification will help determine the plan for subsequent prehospital treatment. The initial history may be hard to obtain because of the patient's impaired mental functioning. In these cases, it is critical for you to obtain information from bystanders, if available.

If the neurological emergency is due to trauma, the following questions will help you gather relevant information.

- ❑ When did the incident occur?
- ❑ How did the incident occur, and what is the mechanism of injury?
- ❑ Was there any loss of consciousness?
- ❑ What is the patient's chief complaint?
- ❑ Has there been any change in symptoms?
- ❑ Are there any complicating factors?

If the neurological emergency is due to non-traumatic problems, you might use the following questions as a guide.

- ❑ What is the chief complaint?
- ❑ What are the details of the present illness?
- ❑ Is there a pertinent underlying medical problem such as:
  - • Cardiac disease
  - • Chronic seizures
  - • Diabetes
  - • Hypertension

❑ Have these symptoms occurred before?
❑ Are there any environmental clues? These may include:
  • Evidence of current medications
  • Medic-Alert identification
  • Alcohol bottles or drug paraphernalia

Head-to-Toe Survey   The head-to-toe survey of a patient with a neurological emergency should include the standard examination and a more detailed neurological assessment. Pay particular attention to the pupils, respiratory status, and spinal evaluation.

Pupils. The pupils are controlled by the third cranial nerve. This nerve follows a long course through the skull and is easily compressed by brain swelling. Thus, it can be an early indicator of increasing intracranial pressure. If both pupils are dilated and do not react to light, the patient probably has a brainstem injury or has suffered serious brain anoxia. If the pupils are dilated but still react to light, the injury may be reversible. However, the patient must be transported quickly to an emergency facility capable of treating CNS injuries. A unilaterally dilated pupil that remains reactive to light may be the earliest sign of increasing intracranial pressure. The patient who presents with or develops a unilaterally dilated pupil is in the "immediate transport" category. Slight pupillary inequality is normal.

A common method of assessing extraocular movement is to have the patient follow finger movements. For example, ask the patient to follow your finger to the extreme left, then up, then down. Repeat the same motions to the extreme right. These positions are referred to as the *Cardinal Positions of Gaze.* Because extraocular movements are controlled by the cranial nerves (III, IV, VI), inability to look in all directions with both eyes can be an early indication of a CNS problem.

When examining a patient's pupils, it is important to check for contact lenses. Contact lenses, if present, should be removed and placed into their container or a saline solution and transported with the patient.

Respiratory Status. Respiratory derangements can occur with CNS illness or injury. Five common respiratory patterns may be observed in patients with CNS injury. (See Figure 23-9.)

❑ *Cheyne-Stokes Respiration.* A breathing pattern characterized by a period of apnea lasting 10–60 seconds, followed by gradually increasing depth and frequency of respirations.
❑ *Central Neurogenic Hyperventilation.* Hyperventilation caused by a lesion in the central nervous system, often characterized by rapid, deep, noisy respirations.
❑ *Ataxic Respirations.* Poor respirations due to CNS damage, causing ineffective thoracic muscular coordination.
❑ *Apneustic Respirations.* Breathing characterized by prolonged inspiration unrelieved by expiration attempts. This is seen in patients with damage to the upper part of the pons.
❑ *Diaphragmatic Breathing.* A breathing pattern caused by intercostal muscle dysfunction.

There may be several other respiratory patterns, depending on the injury. As a terminal event, the patient may present with *central neurogenic hyperventilation.* His or her respirations can be affected by so many factors—fear,

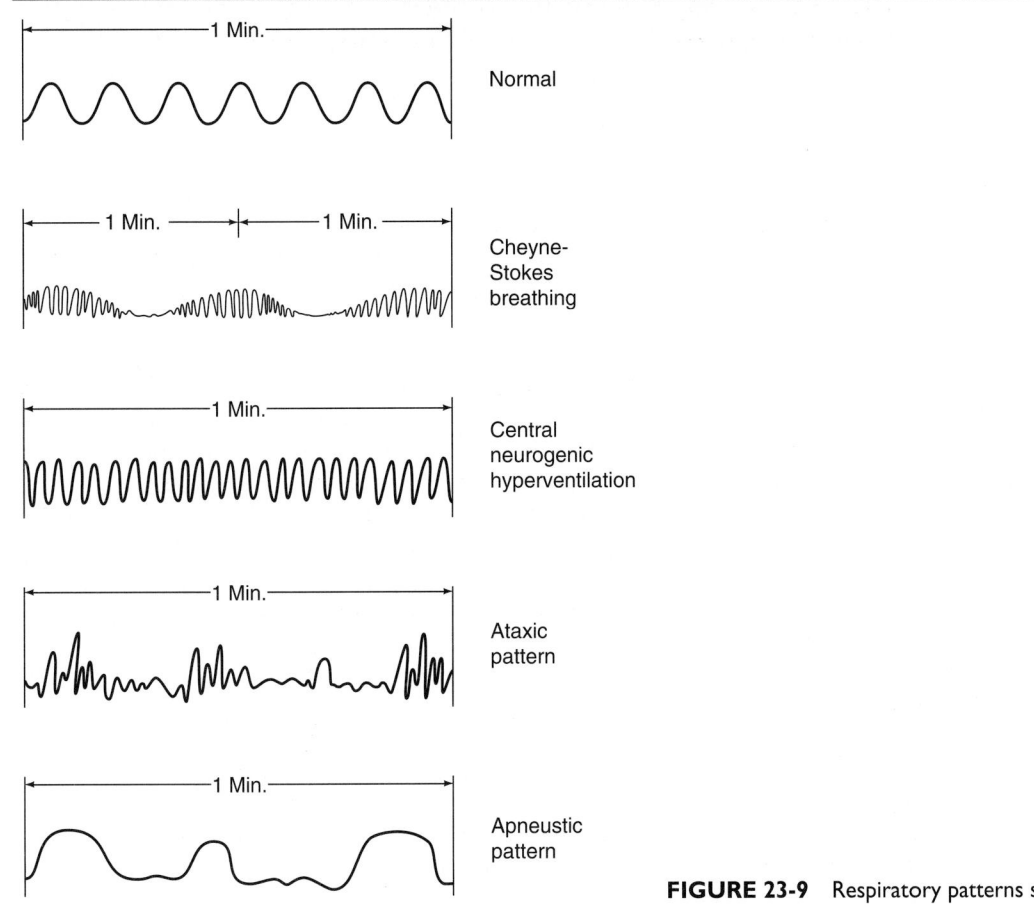

Normal

Cheyne-
Stokes
breathing

Central
neurogenic
hyperventilation

Ataxic
pattern

Apneustic
pattern

FIGURE 23-9 Respiratory patterns seen with CNS dysfunction.

hysteria, chest injuries, spinal cord injuries, or diabetes—that they are not as useful as other signs in monitoring the course of CNS problems.

The blood level of carbon dioxide ($PaCO_2$) has a critical effect on cerebral vessels. The normal blood $PaCO_2$ is 40 mmHg. Increasing the $PaCO_2$ causes cerebral vasodilatation, while decreasing it results in cerebral vasoconstriction. If the patient is poorly ventilated, the $PaCO_2$ will increase, causing even further vasodilatation with a subsequent increase in intracranial pressure. Hyperventilation can decrease the $PaCO_2$ to nearly 25 mm/Hg, effectively causing vasoconstriction of the cerebral vessels. This will help minimize brain swelling. Therefore, any patient suspected of having increased intracranial pressure should be hyperventilated at a rate of 24 breaths per minute or greater.

Spinal Evaluation. The purpose of spinal evaluation is to document loss of sensation and/or motor function. The spinal evaluation does not have to be detailed in the field. To initially assess the patient with a possible spinal injury, perform the following steps.

1. Evaluate for pain and tenderness.
2. Observe for bruises.
3. Observe for deformity.
4. Check for motion, sensation, and position (proprioception) in each extremity. Ask the patient to move his or her toes and push them against resistance. Also, check bilateral grip strength.

TABLE 23-1	Comparison of Vital Signs in Shock and Increased ICP	
Vital Signs	**Shock**	**Increased ICP**
Blood Pressure	Decreased	Increased
Pulse	Increased	Decreased
Respirations	Increased	Decreased
LOC	Decreased	Decreased

5. If the patient is unconscious, you will need to determine the response to pain.

6. Note any urinary or rectal incontinence.

If you suspect spinal injury, place the patient on a long spine board with the PASG in place. A patient with spinal injury may develop spinal shock. He or she is also likely to vomit. Therefore, it must be possible for you to roll the patient on a long spine board to one side or the other to prevent aspiration of vomitus.

Vital Signs. Vital signs are crucial in following the course of CNS problems. Such signs can indicate changes in intracranial pressure. Patients suspected of having a CNS injury should have vital signs taken and recorded every five minutes. Increased intracranial pressure is characterized by the following changes in vital signs (*Cushing's Reflex*).

❑ Increased blood pressure
❑ Decreased pulse
❑ Decreased respirations
❑ Increased temperature

Table 23-1 compares vital signs of a patient in shock versus those of a patient with head injury and increased intracranial pressure. A patient in the early stages of increased intracranial pressure usually shows a decrease in pulse rate and a rise in blood pressure and temperature. Later, if the intracranial pressure continues to rise without correction, the pulse will increase, the blood pressure will fall, and the body temperature will remain elevated. Dysrhythmias are common with increased intracranial pressure. Continuous ECG monitoring and pulse oximetry, if available, should be utilized to spot early signs of CNS lesions.

Neurological Evaluation   Prehospital assessment of the patient with a CNS injury cannot be comprehensive. Nevertheless, an effective neurological examination depends upon a thorough knowledge of the range of normal responses. An orderly neurologic examination will provide the most information in the briefest time. A baseline neurological examination is necessary during the initial patient assessment for comparison with later examinations to determine whether the patient's condition is improving or worsening. To document the progress of the neurologic deficit, you must repeat the examination frequently.

The most significant sign in the evaluation of the patient with a CNS injury is the level of consciousness. You can best assess the level of consciousness through what is known as the "AVPU" method. AVPU is rapid and easy to understand.

ther examination. Alterations may vary from minor thought disturbances to unconsciousness. Unconsciousness, also called **coma**, is a state in which the patient cannot be aroused, even by powerful external stimuli.

There are generally only two mechanisms capable of producing alterations in mental status. They include:

1. Structural lesions that depress consciousness by destroying or encroaching upon the substance of the brain.
2. Toxic-metabolic states, involving either the presence of circulating toxins or metabolites or the lack of metabolic substrates (oxygen, glucose, or thiamine). These states produce diffuse depression of both cerebral hemispheres, with or without depression within the brainstem.

Within the two general mechanisms, there are many difficult-to-classify causes of altered mental status. Some of the more common causes are listed in the following six general categories.

❏ *Structural:* Trauma
Brain tumor
Epilepsy
Intracranial hemorrhage
Other space-occupying lesions

❏ *Metabolic:* Anoxia
Hypoglycemia
Diabetic ketoacidosis
Hepatic failure
Renal failure
Thiamine deficiency

❏ *Drugs:* Barbiturates
Narcotics
Hallucinogens
Depressants (including alcohol)

❏ *Cardiovascular:* Hypertensive encephalopathy
Shock
Anaphylaxis
Dysrhythmias
Cardiac arrest
CVA

❏ *Respiratory:* COPD
Inhalation of toxic gas

❏ *Infectious:* Meningitis
Encephalitis
AIDS Encephalitis

When evaluating a patient, you may find mnemonic devices useful as assessment aids. A mnemonic that may help you remember some of the common causes of altered mental status is "AEIOUTIPS."

A = Acidosis, alcohol
E = Epilepsy
I = Infection
O = Overdose
U = Uremia (kidney failure)
T = Trauma, tumor
I = Insulin (hypoglycemia or diabetes ketoacidosis)
P = Psychosis
S = Stroke

Primary Assessment   During the primary assessment, pay special attention to the cervical spine and airway. Early placement of an endotracheal tube in an unresponsive patient will help protect the airway from aspiration and will facilitate hyperventilation to minimize increased intracranial pressure.

Secondary Assessment   The initial assessment should help you to determine the severity and cause of the CNS disorder. To assess the patient suffering altered mental status, take the following steps.

History. While performing the secondary assessment, try to gather information from the patient's relatives, friends, or bystanders. Data regarding the patient's past history is especially valuable, including whether he or she is a diabetic or substance abuser. Also, find out if a fall or head trauma was involved. Note any medications used by the patient or mention of previous episodes of a similar nature. The following questions can serve as a guide.

❑ What is the length of the alteration in mental status?
❑ Was it of sudden or gradual onset?
❑ Is there a history of recent head trauma within the last four weeks?
❑ Is the patient under medical care?
❑ Is there any alcohol or drug use or abuse?
❑ Were there any preceding symptoms or complaints?
❑ What medications is the patient taking?
❑ Is there Medic-Alert identification?

In addition to such questions, you may obtain clues about the mechanism of the problem by quickly surveying the environment.

Physical Examination. Of primary importance is the patient's breathing and cardiovascular status. Your initial evaluation of the patient should include:

❑ Breathing
❑ Response to stimuli
❑ Eye response
❑ Pupil response

Further examination of the patient may explain why he or she is unresponsive. While performing an assessment on the patient presenting with a CNS problem, focus on the following signs or symptoms.

❑ *Pupillary Reflexes.* Constriction of the pupils is controlled by parasympathetic fibers. These originate in the midbrain and accompany the oculomotor nerve (III). Dilatation of the pupils involves fibers that descend the entire brainstem and ascend in the cervical sympathetic chains. Failure in the midbrain interrupts both pathways, usually resulting in fixed, midsized pupils. Lesions within the pons can interfere with sympathetic tone alone, producing pinpoint pupils barely reactive to light. Third-nerve compression interrupts parasympathetic tone. This presents itself by a unilateral fixed and dilated pupil. Fixed or asymmetric pupils strongly imply structural lesions. In contrast, reactive pupils generally indicate toxic-metabolic states.
❑ *Extraocular Movements.* Dysconjugate gaze at rest usually implies the patient has received a structural brainstem injury.
❑ *Motor Findings.* Motor responses to noxious stimuli mark the level and

asymmetry of brain dysfunction. Asymmetry generally implies structural lesions. Appropriate responses by the patient that localize or withdraw from pain indicate normal or minimally impaired cortical function. Decorticate and decerebrate posturing are ominous signs of deep cerebral hemispheric or upper brainstem injury. Flaccid paralysis usually indicates spinal injury.

❏ *Respiratory Patterns.* As already noted, a number of factors can affect respiratory patterns. Therefore, they may not be as clinically useful as pupillary reactivity, extraocular movements, and motor responses. For example, Kussmaul respirations are virtually indistinguishable from central neurogenic hyperventilation. Kussmaul respirations are commonly seen with deep bilateral dysfunction of the cerebral hemispheres. In contrast, central neurogenic hyperventilation results from dysfunction at a level anywhere from the forebrain to the upper pons. Apnea places the CNS dysfunction in the medulla.

❏ *Vital Signs.* Determine vital signs early in the secondary assessment. Signs and symptoms of CNS dysfunction include:

- Hypertension
- Bradycardia
- Abnormal respiratory patterns

❏ Elevation or depression of body temperature

Management   Your initial priority is to assure that the patient's cervical spine is immobilized (in cases of suspected head/neck injury). Following this, secure his or her airway and administer supplemental oxygen. If the patient is breathing inadequately, then support respirations. An unresponsive patient requires an appropriate airway adjunct.

After the airway is secured, management should include the following steps.

1. Draw blood, and determine the blood glucose using a reagent strip or glucometer. A serum glucose determination will tell you if the altered mental status is due to hypoglycemia.

2. Establish an IV of normal saline or lactated Ringer's at a keep open rate.

3. Monitor the cardiac rhythm.

4. If the blood glucose level is low or if you are unable to determine the level, administer 50 percent dextrose. This will correct hypoglycemia, which may be the cause of the altered mental status. Even if the patient is an uncontrolled diabetic, hyperglycemia produced by administration of glucose will not do any harm. If, however, the patient is hypoglycemic from too much insulin, the administration of glucose can be life-saving, and he or she may immediately respond. For the alcoholic patient who is hypoglycemic, the glucose may be life-saving as well. The field dosage for 50 percent dextrose is set below. (For more information, see Table 23-2.)

    Adult: 50 mL (25 gm) IVP. May be repeated as necessary.

    Pediatric: 0.5 to 1.0 gm/kg IVP. Dilute D-50-W 1:1 with sterile water or normal saline to yield a 25 percent (D-25-W) solution.

5. Administer naloxone (see Table 23-3) in the patient suspected of having a narcotic overdose. Naloxone, a narcotic antagonist, has proven effective in the management and reversal of overdose caused by narcotics or synthetic narcotic agents. Field dosage for naloxone is set below.

    Adult: 1–2 mg IV, ET, IM, or SQ. This may be repeated at 2–3-minute intervals for 2–3 doses, if no response is noted. Darvon overdoses may require larger doses of naloxone.

TABLE 23-2 50% Dextrose

Class:	Carbohydrates
Actions:	Elevates blood glucose level rapidly
Indications:	Hypoglycemia
	Coma of unknown origin
Contraindications:	None in the emergency setting
Precautions:	Dextrostix must be performed and blood sample drawn before administration
Side Effects:	Local venous irritation
Dosage:	25 grams (50 ml)
Route:	IV
Pediatric Dosage:	0.5–1 gm/kg slow IV

TABLE 23-3 Naloxone (Narcan®)

Class:	Narcotic antagonist
Actions:	Reverses effects of narcotics
Indications:	Narcotic overdoses including:
	Morphine Demerol® heroin
	Dilaudid® Paregoric Percodan®
	fentanyl methadone
	Synthetic analgesic overdose including:
	Nubain® Talwin®
	Stadol® Darvon®
	Alcoholic coma
	To rule out narcotics in coma of unknown origin
Contraindications:	Patients with a history of hypersensitivity to the drug
Precautions:	Should be administered with caution to patients dependent on narcotics as it may cause withdrawal effects
Side effects:	None
Dosage:	1–2 mg up to a total dose of 10 mg (larger doses may be required to reverse effects of Darvon®)
Routes:	IV
	IM
Pediatric Dosage:	0.01 mg/kg

Pediatric: 0.01 mg/kg/dose. Maximum dose = 0.8 mg IV or ET. If no response in 10 minutes, 2 mg should be given.

6. If the patient is a suspected alcoholic, administer 100 mg of thiamine (Vitamin B1). (See Table 23-4.) It is required for the conversion of pyruvic acid to acetyl-coenzyme-A. Without this step, a significant amount of energy available in glucose cannot be obtained. The brain is extremely sensitive to thiamine deficiency.

Chronic Alcoholism. Chronic alcoholism interferes with the absorption, intake, and use of thiamine. A significant percentage of alcoholics have thiamine deficiency that can cause Wernicke's syndrome or Korsakoff's psychosis. **Wernicke's syndrome** is an acute and reversible encephalopathy characterized by ataxia,

■ **Wernicke's syndrome** condition characterized by loss of memory and disorientation, associated with chronic alcohol intake and a diet deficient in thiamine.

TABLE 23-4   Thiamine (Vitamin B1)

Class:	Vitamin
Actions:	Allows normal breakdown of glucose
Indications:	Coma of unknown origin (especially if alcohol or malnourishment may be involved)
Contraindications:	None
Precautions:	Occasional anaphylactic reactions have been reported
Side Effects:	Rare, if any
Dosage:	100 mg
Route:	IV
Pediatric Dosage:	Rarely used

eye muscle weakness, and mental derangement. Of even greater concern is **Korsakoff's psychosis**, characterized by memory disorder. Once established, Korsakoff's psychosis may be irreversible. Therefore, unresponsive patients, especially those who are suspected alcoholics, should receive intravenous thiamine as well as 50 percent dextrose and naloxone. The field dosage of thiamine is 100 mg IV push. When an IV cannot be started, thiamine can be given IM.

Increased Intracranial Pressure. If an increase in intracranial pressure is likely, as occurs in a closed head injury, the patient should be hyperventilated. Decreasing the carbon dioxide level will cause cerebral vasoconstriction and will minimize brain swelling. In addition, the medical control physician may request administration of a steroid. The most commonly used steroid is dexamethasone (Decadron), which may help reduce cerebral edema. (See Table 23-5.) Many systems also use the osmotic diuretic mannitol (Osmotrol). Mannitol causes diuresis, eliminating fluid from the intravascular space through the kid-

■ **Korsakoff's syndrome** psychosis characterized by disorientation, muttering delirium, insomnia, delusions, and hallucinations. Symptoms include painful extremities, bilateral wrist drop (rarely), bilateral foot drop (frequently), and pain on pressure over the long nerves.

✱ Always consider the administration of thiamine in the alcoholic patient.

TABLE 23-5   Dexamethasone (Decadron®, Hexadrol®)

Class:	Steroid
Actions:	Decreases cerebral edema
	Anti-inflammatory
	Suppresses immune response (especially in allergic/anaphylactic reactions)
Indications:	Cerebral edema
	Possibly effective as an adjunctive agent in the management of shock
Contraindications:	None in the emergency setting
Precautions:	Should be protected from heat
	Onset of action may be 2–6 hours and thus should not be considered to be of use in the critical first hour following an anaphylactic reaction
Side Effects:	GI bleeding
	Prolonged wound healing
Dosage:	4–24 mg
Route:	IV
Pediatric Dosage:	1 mg/kg

neys. Many authorities feel that its oncotic effect also causes a fluid shift from the substance of the brain to the circulation, thus reducing brain edema. As with all drugs, you should follow local protocols for these medications.

Seizures

A **seizure** is a temporary alteration in behavior due to the massive electrical discharge of one or more groups of neurons in the brain. Seizures can be clinically classified as generalized or partial. *Generalized seizures* include grand mal and petit mal and involve the entire cortex. *Partial seizures* may be either simple or complex (**psychomotor**) and may remain confined to a limited portion of the brain or spread, thereby becoming generalized.

Seizures may occur in any individual when placed under the "right" stress, such as hypoxia, sudden elevation of temperature, or a rapid lowering of blood sugar. Seizures also are caused by structural diseases of the brain such as tumors, head trauma, eclampsia, and vascular disorders. The most common cause is due to *idiopathic epilepsy*. The terms epilepsy or epileptic indicate nothing more than the potential to develop seizures in circumstances that would not induce them in most individuals.

Types of Seizures
Seizures can provoke a great deal of anxiety, both in yourself and in bystanders. To assess seizures quickly under such conditions, you need to be thoroughly familiar with their various forms.

Grand Mal. A **grand mal seizure** is a generalized major motor seizure, producing a loss of consciousness. The grand mal seizure also causes alternating **tonic** (contractions) and **clonic** (successive contractions and relaxations) movements of the extremities beyond the patient's control. During the seizure episode, a patient's intercostal muscles and diaphragm become temporarily paralyzed, interrupting respirations and producing cyanosis. The patient's neck, head, and face muscles may also jerk. Once respirations resume, there will be copious amounts of oral secretions (frothing). Incontinence and mental confusion are also common during the seizure episode. The seizure may be followed by coma or drowsiness.

Grand mal seizures have a specific progression of events. It is descriptively convenient to refer to this progression as ranging from warning phase to period of recovery.

1. *Aura.* An aura is a subjective sensation preceding seizure activity. The aura may precede the attack by several hours or by only a few seconds. An aura may be of a psychic or a sensory nature, with olfactory, visual, auditory, or taste hallucinations. Some common types include hearing noise or music, seeing floating lights, smelling unpleasant odors, feeling an unpleasant sensation in the stomach, or experiencing tingling or twitching in a given body area. Not all seizures are preceded by an aura.

2. *Loss of Consciousness.* The patient will become unconscious after the aura sensations.

3. *Tonic Phase.* This is a phase of continuous muscle tension, characterized by tension and contraction of the patient's muscles.

4. ***Hypertonic Phase***. The patient experiences extreme muscular rigidity, including hyperextension of the back.

5. *Clonic Phase.* The patient experiences muscle spasms marked by muscular rigidity and then relaxation.

6. *Post-Seizure.* The patient progresses into a coma.

7. *Postictal.* The patient will awaken confused and fatigued. He or she may complain of a headache and may experience some neurological deficit.

■ **seizure** a disorder of the nervous system due to a sudden, excessive, disorderly discharge of brain neurons.

■ **psychomotor** mental processes causing or associated with physical activity.

■ **grand mal seizure** form of seizure characterized by tonic-clonic muscle contractions. It may occur with or without coma.

■ **tonic** phase of a seizure characterized by tension or contraction of muscles.

■ **clonic** alternating contraction and relaxation of muscles.

■ **hypertonic phase** phase of a seizure when muscles are in a state of greater than normal tension or of incomplete relaxation.

Focal Motor. Focal motor seizures are characterized by dysfunction of one area of the body. When there is electrical discharge from a small portion of the brain, only those functions served by that area will have dysfunction. Focal seizures begin as localized tonic/clonic movements. They frequently spread and appear as generalized major motor seizures. It is crucial that you document how such seizures begin and the course that they subsequently take.

Psychomotor. **Psychomotor seizures**, occasionally called temporal lobe seizures, are characterized by distinctive auras. They include unusual smells, tastes, sounds, or the tendency of objects to look either very large and near or small and distant. Sometimes a seizure patient may visualize scenes that look very familiar (*deja vu*) or very strange. A metallic taste in the mouth is a common psychomotor seizure aura. These are focal seizures, lasting approximately 1–2 minutes. The patient experiences a loss of contact with his or her surroundings. Additionally, the patient may act confused, stagger, perform purposeless movement, or make unintelligible sounds. He or she may not understand what is said. The patient may even refuse medical aid. Some patients develop automatic behavior or show a sudden change in personality, such as abrupt explosions of rage.

■ **psychomotor seizure** type of seizure usually originating in the temporal lobe characterized by an aura and focal findings such as alterations in mental status or mood.

Petit Mal. **Petit mal seizures** are brief, generalized seizures that usually present with a 10- to 30-second loss of consciousness, eye or muscle fluttering and an occasional loss of muscle tone. Unconsciousness may be so brief that the patient or observers may be unaware of the episode. Petit mal seizures are idiopathic disorders of early childhood and rarely begin after age twenty. They may not respond to normal treatment modalities.

■ **petit mal seizure** form of seizure where consciousness may or may not be lost.

Hysterical. Hysterical seizures stem from psychological disorders. The patient presents with sharp and bizarre movements that can often be interrupted with curt commands. The seizure is usually witnessed, and there will not be a postictal period. Very rarely do patients experiencing an hysterical seizure injure themselves. Aromatic ammonia may help differentiate an hysterical from a true seizure.

Assessment   Your initial contact with the patient and bystanders will offer a unique opportunity to obtain a history that may influence your plan of management. What an untrained observer calls a seizure may be a simple fainting spell. Therefore, you need to ascertain exactly what the patient may recall or what bystanders witnessed.

Obtaining a History. Many other problems can suggest that a seizure has occurred. Examples of conditions that may mimic seizures include: migraine headaches, cardiac dysrhythmias, hypoglycemia after exercise or drug ingestion, and the tendency to faint due to orthostatic hypotension. Stiffness of the extremities can be caused by hyperventilation, meningitis, intracranial hemorrhage, or certain tranquilizers. Decerebrate movements, if present, are often associated with increased intracranial pressure. If you are unsure whether the patient has had a seizure, it may be more harmful than beneficial to administer an anticonvulsant medication. When obtaining a history, remember to include the following points.

- ❏ History of seizures. This data should include: length of the seizure; whether it was generalized or focal; presence of auras, incontinence, or trauma to the tongue.
- ❏ Recent history of head trauma.
- ❏ Any alcohol and/or drug abuse.
- ❏ Recent history of fever, headache, or stiff neck.
- ❏ History of diabetes, heart disease, or CVA.

TABLE 23-6 Differentiation between Syncope and Seizure	
Syncope	**Seizure**
Usually begins in a standing position.	May begin in any position.
Patient will usually remember a warning or fainting.	Begins without warning.
Patient regains consciousness almost immediately on becoming supine.	Results in jerking during unconsciousness.
Patient initially has a slow, weak pulse and is clammy and pale.	Often preceded by an aura.

❑ Current medications. Most chronic seizure patients take anticonvulsant medication on a regular basis. Common anticonvulsant medications include: phenytoin (Dilantin), phenobarbital, carbazepine (Tegretol), and valproic acid (Depakote).

Identifying a True Seizure. It is also important to try to distinguish between syncope and true seizure. (See Table 23-6.) **Syncope** is caused by insufficient blood flow to the brain, resulting from ineffective cardiac activity, relaxation of peripheral blood vessels, or insufficient blood volume. Initially, syncope patients will have a short period of seizure-like activity, but this is not followed by a postictal state. The most common cause of fainting is vasovagal syncope associated with fatigue, emotional stress, or cardiac disease.

■ **syncope** transient loss of consciousness due to inadequate flow of blood to the brain; fainting.

Management
The physical examination of the seizure patient should include the following steps.

❑ Note any signs of head trauma or injury to the tongue.
❑ Note any evidence of alcohol and/or drug abuse.
❑ Document dysrhythmias.

Remember that seizures tend to provoke anxiety in patients, families, and paramedics. However, from a medical standpoint, most of these situations only require nasal oxygen and turning the patient to the side to prevent aspiration. Because the patient may become hypo- or hyperthermic if exposed, protecting body temperature is also crucial. Field management of the seizure patient generally includes the following procedures.

✱ Airway maintenance, administration of supplemental oxygen, and protection of the patient from injury are the principle treatments for an uncomplicated seizure.

❑ Maintain airway. Do not force objects between the patient's teeth—this includes padded tongue blades. Pushing objects into the patient's mouth may cause him or her to vomit or to aspirate. It can also cause laryngospasm.
❑ Administer oxygen.
❑ Establish intravenous access. Normal saline or lactated Ringer's solution should be initiated at a keep open rate. Dextrose solutions should not be used. Emergency department personnel may later administer phenytoin (Dilantin), and phenytoin is incompatible with dextrose solutions.
❑ Determine the blood glucose level. If hypoglycemic, administer 50 percent dextrose. If unable to determine the blood glucose level, consider administering 50 percent dextrose solution empirically.
❑ Never attempt to restrain the patient. This may injure him or her. The patient should, however, be protected from hitting objects in the environment.
❑ Maintain body temperature.

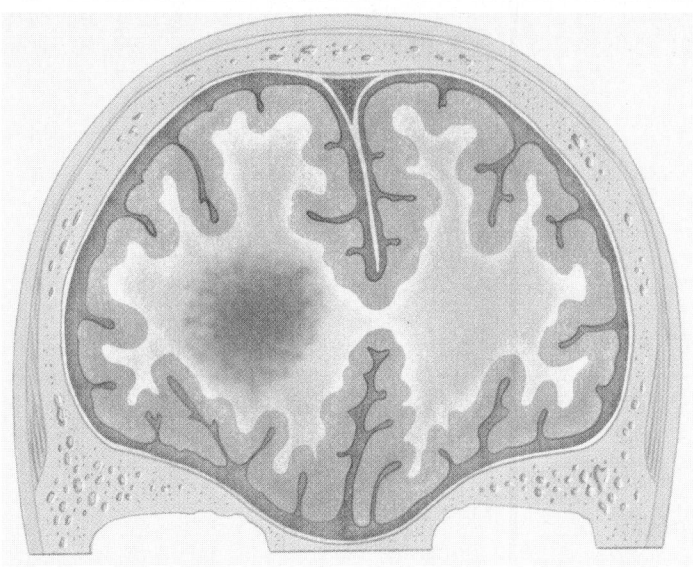

FIGURE 23-14 Intracerebral hemorrhage.

within the brain tissue ruptures. Subarachnoid hemorrhages most often result from congenital blood vessel abnormalities or from head trauma. The congenital abnormalities are known as aneurysms (weakened vessels) and arteriovenous malformations (collections of abnormal blood vessels). Aneurysms tend to be on the surface and may hemorrhage into the brain tissue or the subarachnoid space. Arteriovenous malformations may be within the brain, subarachnoid space, or both.

Hemorrhage inside the brain often tears and separates normal brain tissue. The release of blood into the cavities containing spinal fluid within the brain may paralyze vital centers. If blood in the subarachnoid space impairs drainage of cerebrospinal fluid, it may cause a rise in the intracranial pressure. Herniation (protrusion) of brain tissue through a narrow opening in the skull may then occur.

In infarction, the tissue that has died will swell, causing further damage to nearby tissue, which only has a marginal blood supply. If swelling is severe, herniation may result.

Clinical Presentation of a Stroke Symptoms of the patient who has experienced a stroke will depend upon the area of the brain damaged. Those areas commonly affected are the motor, speech, and sensory centers. The onset of symptoms will be acute, and the patient may experience unconsciousness. There may be stertorous breathing (laborious breathing accompanied by snoring) due to paralysis of a portion of the soft palate. Respiratory expiration may be puffs of air out of the cheeks and mouth. The patient's pupils may be unequal, with the larger pupil on the side of the hemorrhage. Paralysis will usually involve one side of the face, one arm, and one leg. The eyes often will be turned away from the side of the body paralysis. The patient's skin may be cool and clammy. Speech disturbances, or aphasia, also may be noted.

Predisposing factors that possibly contribute to the stroke include: hypertension, diabetes, abnormal blood lipid levels, oral contraceptives, sickle cell disease, and some cardiac dysrhythmias.

Distinguishing Transient Ischemic Attacks (TIAs) Some patients may have small emboli that cause transient stroke-like symptoms known as **TIAs**, or **transient ischemic attacks**. These emboli temporarily interfere with

■ **TIA (transient ischemic attack)** temporary interruption of blood supply to the brain.

the blood supply to the brain, producing symptoms of neurological deficit. These symptoms may last for only a few minutes or for several hours. After the attack, the patient will show no evidence of residual brain or neurological damage. The patient who experiences a TIA may, however, be a candidate for an eventual CVA.

The onset of a transient ischemic attack is usually abrupt, with the patient experiencing giddiness or a light-headed sensation. The specific signs and symptoms depend upon the area of the brain affected. Any one or a combination of the following conditions may be present.

- ❏ Monocular blindness (blindness in one eye)
- ❏ Hemiplegia (paralysis on one side)
- ❏ Inability to recognize by touch
- ❏ Staggering
- ❏ Difficulty in swallowing
- ❏ Hemiparesis (weakness on one side)
- ❏ Aphasia (inability to speak)
- ❏ Dizziness
- ❏ Numbness
- ❏ Paresthesia (numbness or tingling)

Probably the most common cause of a TIA is carotid artery disease. Other causes can be decreasing cardiac output, hypotension, overmedication with antihypertensive agents, or cerebrovascular spasm.

While obtaining the history of the patient suspected of sustaining a TIA, you should try to collect information on or take note of the following factors.

- ❏ Previous neurological symptoms
- ❏ Initial symptoms and their progression
- ❏ Changes in mental status
- ❏ Precipitating factors
- ❏ Dizziness
- ❏ Palpitations
- ❏ History of hypertension, cardiac disease, sickle cell disease, or previous TIA or CVA

During the physical examination, focus attention on the following signs and symptoms.

- ❏ Hemiparesis or hemiplegia noted during neurologic exam
- ❏ Unilateral facial droop
- ❏ Speech disturbances, including dysarthria (impairment of the tongue and muscles essential to speech) and motor and receptive aphasia
- ❏ Confusion and agitation
- ❏ Gait disturbances or uncoordinated fine motor movements
- ❏ Vision problems
- ❏ Inappropriate behavior with excessive laughing or crying
- ❏ Coma

Management of CVA and TIA   Because of impaired blood flow to the patient's brain, he or she should be kept supine with the head elevated approximately 15 degrees. This allows for adequate venous drainage. If the patient has

✱ The prehospital management of stroke and TIA is primarily supportive.

congestive heart failure, he or she should be maintained in a semi-upright position.

As you continue management of the CVA or TIA patient, keep in mind the following points.

- ❏ Assure patient safety.
- ❏ Establish and maintain cervical spine support if trauma is suspected.
- ❏ Establish and maintain an adequate airway. Have suction equipment readily available.
- ❏ Administer oxygen, and assist ventilation when required. If the patient's airway is adequate and air exchange is present, administer oxygen via a face mask or a nasal cannula, as appropriate.
- ❏ Hyperventilate if unresponsive.
- ❏ Draw blood sample for glucose determination.
- ❏ Start an IV of normal saline or lactated Ringer's at a TKO rate.
- ❏ Monitor the cardiac rhythm.
- ❏ If it appears that hypoglycemia may be a factor, the physician may order 25 gm of 50 percent dextrose.
- ❏ Protect paralyzed extremities.
- ❏ Give the patient reassurance—all procedures should be explained to him or her. The patient may be unable to speak, but he or she still may be able to hear.
- ❏ Transport without excessive movement or noise. Otherwise, the patient may feel nauseated and vomit.

SUMMARY

Nervous system emergencies include a complex variety of injuries and illnesses. Your assessment and neurologic checks will help guide your care and will prove invaluable for subsequent hospital management. Initial field management is directed at ensuring an adequate airway and ventilation. The brain requires a constant supply of oxygen, glucose, and vitamins. After 10–20 seconds without blood flow, the patient becomes unconscious. Significant loss of oxygen (anoxia) or low blood sugar (hypoglycemia) can cause coma or seizures. In patients with brain disorders, adequate blood, glucose, and oxygen supplies must be ensured.

CNS injuries need treatment as soon as possible to prevent progressive damage. Signs of central nervous system compromise include: headache, dizziness; fainting; vomiting; partial to full loss of consciousness; personality, pupillary, and respiratory changes; loss of motor function; and altered response to pain. Elevated blood pressure, bradycardia, and convulsions may also occur.

Treatment of CNS injuries includes: airway maintenance, support of the neck and spine, control of hemorrhage, careful neurologic exam, care for any other injuries, and transport to the appropriate emergency facility.

FURTHER READING

Langfitt, D.E. *Critical Care: Certification Preparation and Review.* Bowie, MD: Robert J. Brady Company, 1984.

Lanros, N.E. *Assessment and Intervention in Emergency Nursing*, 3rd ed. Norwalk, CT: Appleton and Lange, 1988.

Tintanelli, J.E., Krome, R.L., and E. Ruiz. *Emergency Medicine: A Comprehensive Study Guide*, 2nd ed. New York, NY: McGraw-Hill Book Company, 1988.

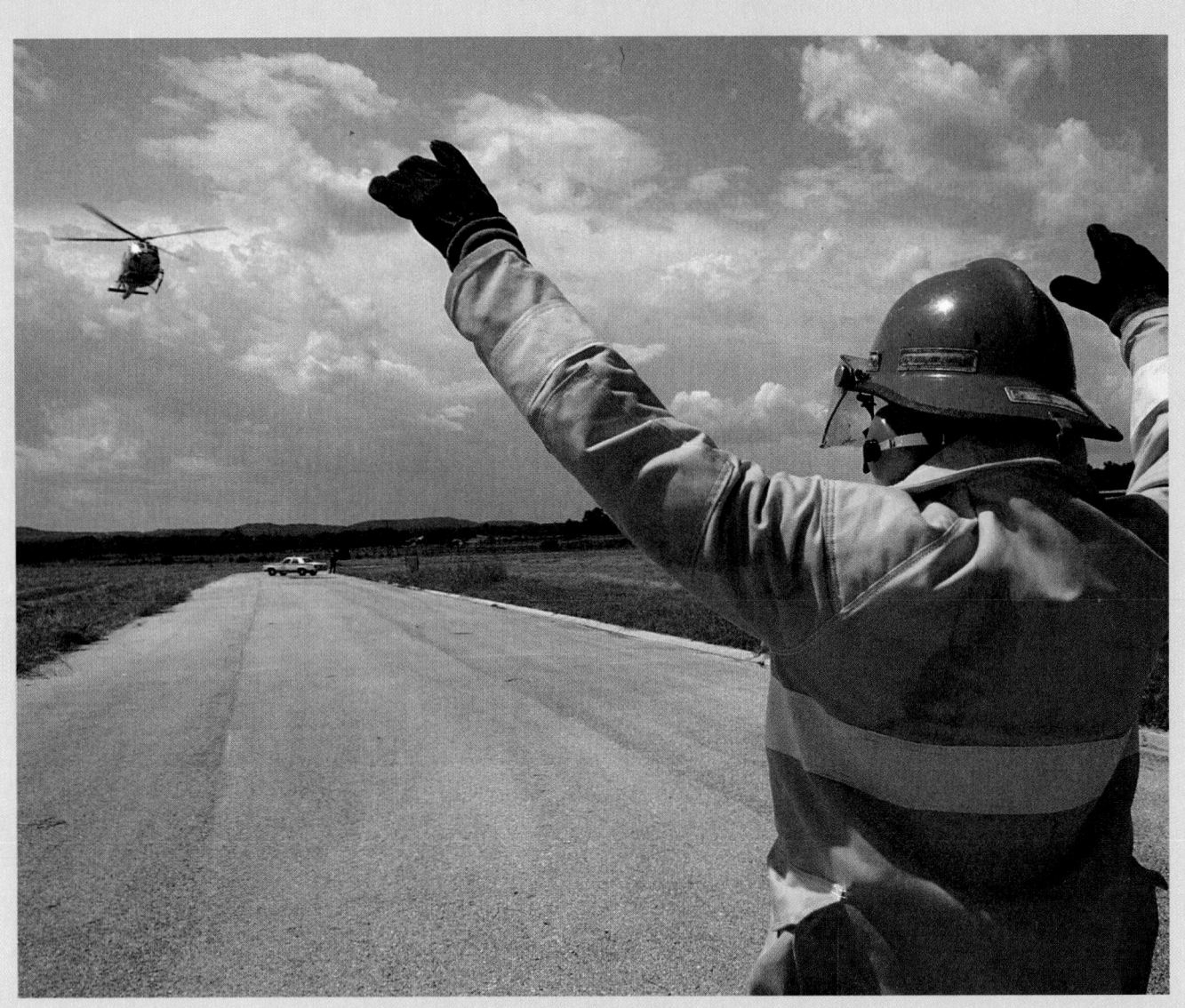

24

GASTROINTESTINAL, GENITOURINARY, AND REPRODUCTIVE SYSTEM EMERGENCIES

Objectives for Chapter 24

After reading this chapter, you should be able to:

1. Describe the structures of the abdominal cavity. (See p. 771.)

2. Discuss the topographical anatomy of the abdomen, and name the organs that lie within each quadrant. (See p. 771.)

3. Describe the organs of the gastrointestinal system. (See pp. 772–773.)

4. Name the two major blood vessels found within the abdominal cavity. (See p. 773.)

5. Describe the organs of the genitourinary system. (See p. 774.)

6. Describe the organs of the male and the female reproductive systems. (See pp. 775–776.)

7. Discuss the causes of acute abdominal pain originating in the gastrointestinal system. (See pp. 776–779.)

8. Describe the signs and symptoms of upper and lower gastrointestinal hemorrhage. (See p. 778.)

9. Discuss the causes of acute abdominal pain originating in the genitourinary system. (See pp. 779–781.)

10. Discuss the causes of acute abdominal pain originating in the reproductive system. (See pp. 781–782.)

11. Describe the method of assessment for patients complaining of abdominal pain. (See pp. 783–786.)

12. Discuss the field management of acute abdominal pain. (See pp. 786–787.)

13. Discuss hemodialysis and peritoneal dialysis. (See pp. 787–788.)

14. Discuss assessment, management, and complications of the dialysis patient. (See pp. 788–790.)

On Sunday afternoon, Steve Fletcher, EMT-P, shifts uneasily in his chair as he tries to watch a baseball game on TV. Steve "just hasn't felt right" ever since he got up. He managed to get through his planned activities for the morning. But, by noon, Steve began to detect a vague abdominal pain around the navel. At first, Steve brushed it off, attributing his discomfort to the beer and nachos that he had consumed the evening before with some other paramedics. Now, as Steve watches the game, the pain worsens. Although he hasn't eaten all day, he finds himself running to the bathroom to vomit.

After throwing up twice, Steve begins to feel feverish. He notices that the pain is moving toward the lower right abdominal quadrant. He sits on the couch, leaning forward, and thinks about what could be wrong. The idea that he might have acute appendicitis suddenly hits him. "No," he reassures himself, "I'm not that sick." But, as he continues to watch the game, he becomes increasingly ill.

Steve finally calls the EMS station to see if anybody else who had been out with him is sick. Steve describes his symptoms to Glen, another paramedic. Glen shoots back, "Hey buddy, you've got appendicitis. Don't go anywhere, we'll be right over." Steve lies down on the couch to wait. Soon he hears a siren. "Surely they didn't respond Code 3," he muses to himself.

With siren on, the ambulance pulls to a halt. The next minute, Glen strides into the room and immediately takes charge of the situation. Steve soon finds himself on the patient side of EMS. Riding in his own ambulance, he is whisked off to the hospital.

That afternoon, Steve undergoes an emergency appendectomy. After three days in the hospital, he returns home. Ten days later, supervisors allow Steve to return to light duty. Best of all—he never gets an ambulance bill.

INTRODUCTION

■ **acute** having a rapid onset and a short course.

■ **acute abdomen** a rapid onset of severe abdominal pain.

■ **guarding** voluntary or involuntary contraction of the abdominal muscles in response to severe abdominal pain.

Abdominal pain is a frequent complaint. Yet it is one of the most difficult problems in medicine to diagnose and treat. As a paramedic, you usually will not be able to determine the cause of most abdominal pain in the field. Nonetheless, an understanding of medical conditions that may produce **acute** pain in the abdomen is essential.

The term **acute abdomen** refers to abdominal pain of relatively sudden onset. It is often accompanied by nausea and vomiting, tenderness, **guarding** (voluntary or involuntary contraction of the abdominal muscles in response to severe abdominal pain), rigidity, and, in some cases, shock. Emergency surgical intervention is frequently required.

Most cases of abdominal pain arise from problems within the abdomen itself. However, approximately 10–15 percent result from pathology elsewhere in the body. Other conditions such as a fracture of the lumber spine, myocardial infarction, pulmonary embolism, and pneumonia may present with abdominal pain as the primary symptom.

Your primary responsibility in dealing with a patient suffering an abdominal emergency consists of detection and stabilization. The patient with an acute abdomen can deteriorate quite rapidly. Therefore, the patient must be constantly reassessed and managed accordingly.

This chapter will describe abdominal anatomy and physiology. It will also cover the pathophysiology, patient assessment, and specific management of acute abdominal emergencies. Within this context, you will learn about gastrointestinal disorders, genitourinary disorders, disorders of the reproductive system, and complications associated with hemodialysis.

ANATOMY AND PHYSIOLOGY OF THE ABDOMEN

The **abdomen** is the largest body cavity. It is separated from the chest by the diaphragm and from the pelvis by an artificial plane extending through the pelvic inlet. It is bordered posteriorly by the spine and back and anteriorly by the abdominal wall. The abdominal cavity contains the organs of the gastrointestinal system and a portion of the organs of the genitourinary system. The pelvic cavity is below the abdominal cavity and contains most of the reproductive organs as well as portions of the genitourinary system.

The anterior surface of the abdomen is divided topographically into four divisions, or quadrants. They are delineated by drawing a vertical line from the symphysis pubis to the xiphoid process and a horizontal line through the umbilicus. Each quadrant contains the following organs. (See Figure 24-1.)

❑ *Left Upper:* spleen, tail of the pancreas, stomach, left kidney, and splenic flexure of the colon.
❑ *Right Upper:* liver, gall bladder, head of the pancreas, part of the duodenum, right kidney, and hepatic flexure of the colon.
❑ *Right Lower:* appendix, ascending colon, small intestine, and the right ovary and fallopian tube.
❑ *Left Lower:* small intestine, descending colon, the left ovary, and fallopian tube.

The lateral portion of the abdomen, often referred to as the *flank,* is associated with the kidneys. Immediately inferior to the xiphoid process is the **epigastrium**. A common location of abdominal pain, the epigastrium is frequently associated with peptic ulcer disease, gastritis, and esophagitis.

The abdomen is lined with a membrane called the **peritoneum**. Most organs are located within the peritoneum. Some, however, are located behind it and are referred to as being *retroperitoneal.* These include the kidneys, por-

■ **abdomen** portion of the body located between the thorax and the pelvis; the superior portion of the abdominopelvic cavity.

■ **epigastrium** portion of the abdomen immediately below the xiphoid process.

■ **peritoneum** serous membrane covering the viscera of the abdomen and lining the interior of the abdominal cavity.

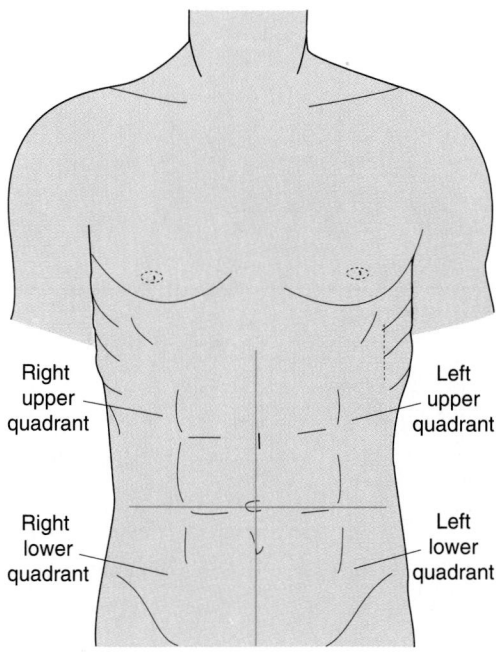

Right upper quadrant

Left upper quadrant

Right lower quadrant

Left lower quadrant

FIGURE 24-1 Topographical anatomy of the abdomen.

tions of the duodenum, and portions of the pancreas. In certain disease states, the peritoneum can become inflamed—a condition known as *peritonitis*. This medical condition is characterized by generalized abdominal pain and **rebound tenderness**.

■ **rebound tenderness** tenderness on release of the examiner's hands, allowing the patient's abdominal wall to return to its normal position. Rebound tenderness is associated with peritoneal irritation.

Anatomically, the organs of the abdominal cavity can be divided into two categories—solid and hollow. These categories appear below.

❑ *Solid Organs:* liver, spleen, pancreas, kidneys, adrenals, and ovaries (in the female).
❑ *Hollow Organs:* stomach, intestines, gall bladder, urinary bladder, and uterus (in the female).

The Gastrointestinal System

Most of the organs in the abdomen belong to the gastrointestinal system. The gastrointestinal system is responsible for converting raw food into an energy form that the body can use. The gastrointestinal system includes the following organs. (See Figure 24-2.)

❑ *Mouth.* The mouth, or oral cavity, consists of the lips, cheeks, gums, teeth, and tongue. It plays an essential role in digestion, breaking down food into smaller particles. Also, through salivary gland secretions, primarily amylase, digestion begins in the mouth.

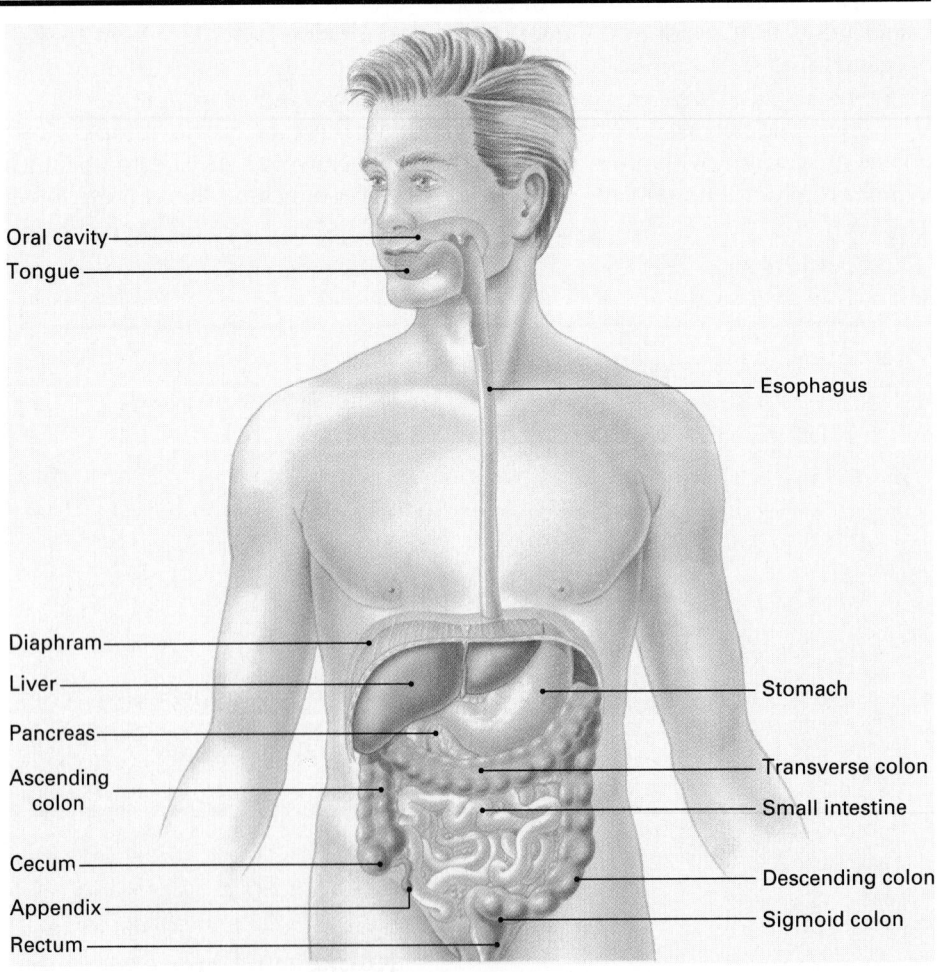

FIGURE 24-2 The gastrointestinal system.

- *Esophagus.* A hollow, muscular tube, the esophagus transports food between the mouth and the stomach.
- *Stomach.* The stomach is a hollow organ in the left upper quadrant of the abdomen. After receiving food from the esophagus, it continues the process of digestion. Covered by a mucous membrane to protect itself from the low pH, the stomach secretes hydrochloric acid.
- *Intestines.* The intestines are the major sites of digestion and absorption. Food moves through the intestines through a process called **peristalsis**. Partially digested food enters from the stomach and is absorbed, primarily in the small intestine. Waste products are also cleared through this system, which has two major intestinal divisions. The longer division, and more proximal, is the *small intestine*, which receives food from the stomach. The small intestine itself has three anatomical divisions: the *duodenum*, *jejunum*, and *ileum*. The food leaves the ileum through the *ileocecal valve* and enters the large intestine, which is also divided into three sections. The proximal division is called the *cecum*. The middle division is the *colon*. And the terminal division is the *rectum*, connecting to the outside via the anus.

Besides these major organs, a number of accessory organs play a part in digestion. These include:

- *Salivary Glands.* Located in the head, the salivary glands produce saliva to lubricate food passage and amylase to initiate digestion.
- *Teeth.* The teeth play a major role in processing food into a form usable by the digestive system.
- *Liver.* Located in the right upper quadrant, the liver is the largest organ in the body. It secretes bile necessary for the digestion of fats. Additionally, the liver produces essential proteins, detoxifies many substances, and stores glucose, in the form of glycogen, for immediate use.
- *Gall Bladder.* The gall bladder is a hollow organ immediately below the liver that stores bile for later use. Following ingestion of a fatty meal, the gall bladder contracts and excretes bile, through the *cystic duct*, into the duodenum.
- *Pancreas.* The pancreas lies in both the right and left upper abdominal quadrants. It secretes several digestive enzymes. The pancreas also has endocrine function, secreting glucagon, insulin, and somatostatin.
- *Appendix.* The appendix is a hollow, finger-like structure attached to the cecal area of the large intestine. Virtually without any function, it is probably a remnant from an earlier stage of evolutionary development.

The Circulatory System

Major blood vessels travel through the abdomen. The descending *aorta* is the largest artery in the abdomen and supplies blood to all of the abdominal viscera. The *superior mesenteric* and *inferior mesenteric arteries* supply blood to most of the intestines. The aorta divides into the *iliac arteries* to supply the lower extremities. The *inferior vena cava*, the largest vein in the abdomen, drains the lower extremities and certain abdominal viscera. The **portal system** is a specialized circulatory system within the abdomen. This system drains blood from parts of the intestines and transports it to the liver, where it is filtered and processed.

The Genitourinary System

Much of the genitourinary system is also located in the abdominal cavity. The system is composed of the following organs. (See Figure 24-3.)

❑ *Kidneys.* The kidneys are paired organs located in the retroperitoneal space. They filter blood and produce urine. Additionally, they perform several endocrine functions, help regulate blood pressure, and maintain fluid and electrolyte balance.

❑ *Ureters.* The ureters are tubes connecting the kidneys with the urinary bladder. They also are retroperitoneal. A kidney stone can sometimes enter a ureter, causing intense pain. These stones often lodge at the pelvic brim where the ureter enters the pelvis.

❑ *Urinary Bladder.* Located in the pelvis, the bladder receives and stores urine from the kidneys.

❑ *Urethra.* The urethra is the tube connecting the bladder to the outside. It is considerably shorter in the female than in the male.

The Reproductive System

The reproductive system allows for continuation of the species. The female and male reproductive organs are detailed in the following sections.

Female   The female reproductive system is located in the pelvic cavity and includes the following organs. (See Figure 24-4.)

❑ *Ovaries.* The ovaries, or female gonads, are small, walnut-sized organs adjacent to the uterus. They are responsible for producing a portion of

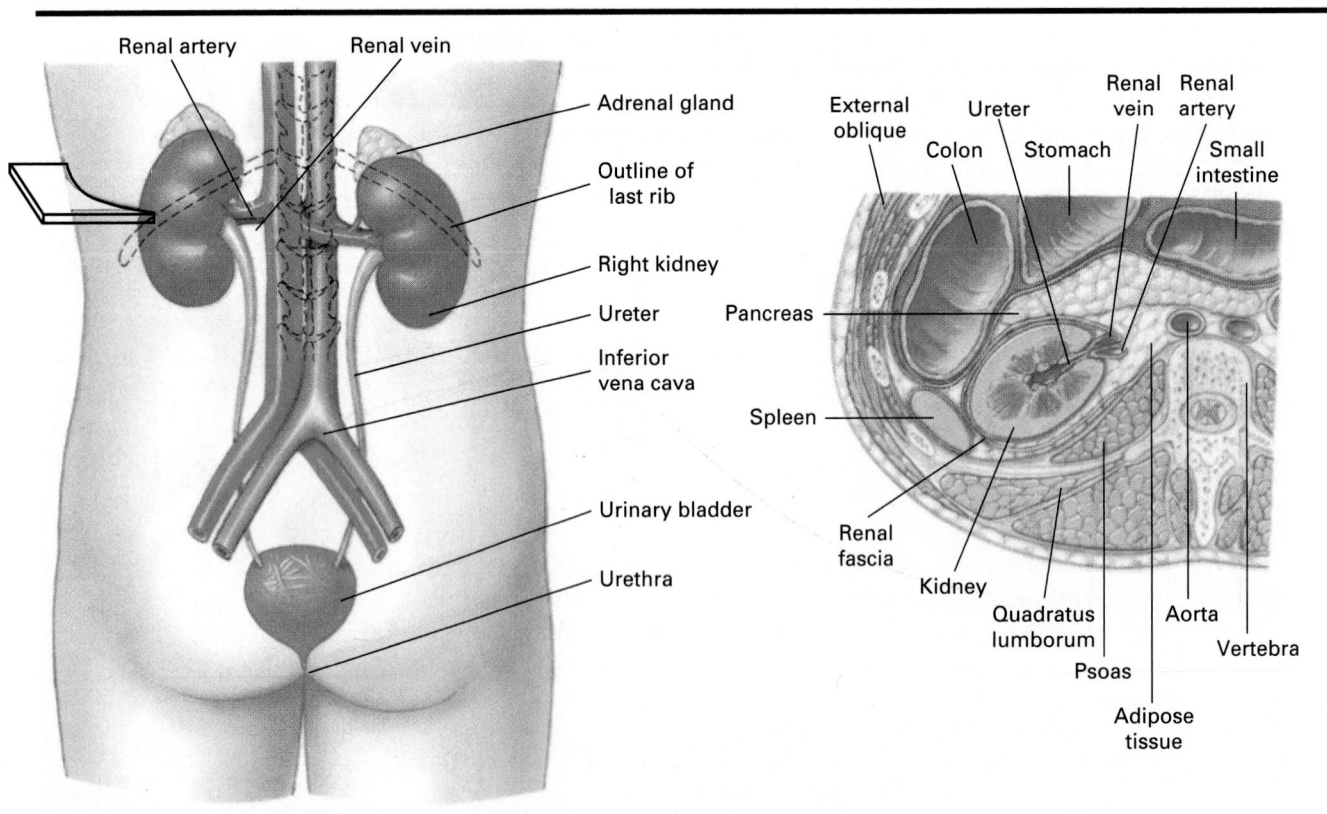

(a)   (b)

FIGURE 24-3   Anatomy of the genitourinary system: (a) posterior view; (b) cross-section.

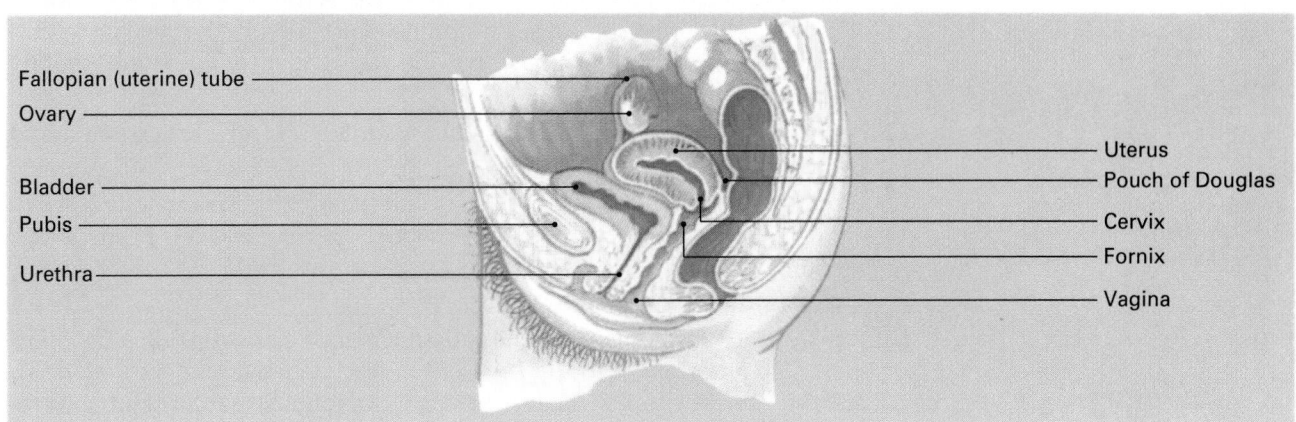

FIGURE 24-4 The female reproductive system.

the female hormones and for production of the female component of reproduction, the ovum.

❑ *Fallopian Tubes.* The fallopian tubes are hollow tubes connecting the ovary to the uterus. They transport the ovum to the uterus. Fertilization usually occurs in the fallopian tube, which is open at the end adjacent to the ovary. This provides direct access to the abdominal cavity and to the uterus. The fallopian tube is a source of infection (salpingitis), especially in pelvic inflammatory disease (PID).

❑ *Uterus.* The uterus is a hollow, muscular organ, situated low in the pelvis. A portion of it, the *cervix*, extends into the vagina. The superior part of the uterus is called the *fundus*. The uterus is the site of implantation and development of the fetus.

❑ *Vagina.* The vagina extends from the uterus to the vulva. It is the female organ of copulation and the birth canal. The external opening of the vagina is called the *introitus*.

❑ *Vulva.* The vulva is the external female genitalia. It consists of the *labia majora, labia minora,* and accessory glands.

Male The male reproductive organs are located in the lower portion of the pelvic cavity, and outside the pelvic cavity in the scrotum. These organs include the following structures. (See Figure 24-5.)

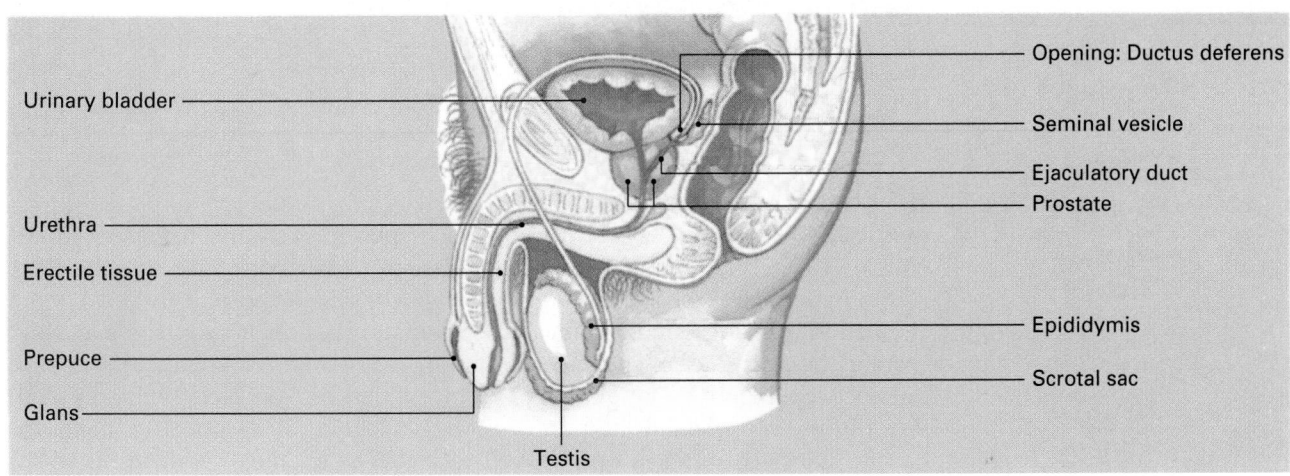

FIGURE 24-5 The male reproductive system.

- *Testes.* The testes, or male gonads, lay in the scrotum. They are responsible for production of the male hormones and sperm. To facilitate sperm production, the scrotum maintains the testes at a temperature slightly lower than that of the body.
- *Epididymis.* The epididymi are small appendages on the testes that act as a reservoir for sperm.
- *Prostate.* A small gland at the base of the bladder, the prostate is responsible for production of fluid to transport sperm. In older men, it can become enlarged (benign prostatic hypertrophy) and, at certain times, obstruct urine flow.
- *Vas Deferens.* The vas deferens are small muscular tubes that transport sperm from the testes to the urethra for discharge during ejaculation. To achieve sterility in the male, they are sometimes cut in a procedure called *vasectomy.*
- *Urethra.* The urethra is a canal that drains urine from the bladder to the outside. In the male, it also discharges sperm during ejaculation.
- *Penis.* The male organ of copulation, the penis is covered by loose skin, thus allowing for erection. The skin overlying the end of the penis (glans) is often surgically removed in a procedure called *circumcision.* Because of its location, the penis is vulnerable to trauma.

ABDOMINAL PATHOPHYSIOLOGY

The "acute abdomen" refers to the relatively sudden onset of abdominal pain. As you have read, it is often associated with other signs and symptoms such as nausea, vomiting, guarding, and rebound tenderness. Many conditions producing the acute abdomen are potentially fatal unless treated promptly by surgery. Therefore, it is essential to assess the severity of the patient's complaints. Every patient with abdominal pain should be transported to the emergency department for evaluation by a physician.

Abdominal emergencies can be divided into gastrointestinal system emergencies, genitourinary system emergencies, or reproductive system emergencies. Because it is difficult to determine the source of an abdominal problem in the field, your approach to the patient with acute abdominal pain should be the same regardless of the system involved.

Gastrointestinal System Emergencies

Problems can arise from virtually any organ of the gastrointestinal system. The following is a discussion of common gastrointestinal system problems, beginning proximally at the esophagus.

Esophageal Varices   Esophageal **varices** are swollen veins in the lower third of the esophagus. They result from increased pressure in the portal circulation (portal hypertension). The portal circulation drains from the intestines to the liver. Diseases of the liver, such as alcoholic cirrhosis, can slow portal circulation, causing engorgement of the veins in the lower esophagus and the rectum (hemorrhoids). The most common presentation is painless gastrointestinal bleeding. Massive quantities of blood can be vomited. Treatment consists of fluid replacement and transfusion. If bleeding does not stop, the veins can be injected—via a scope passed into the esophagus—with an agent to constrict them. A specialized tube (Sengstaken-Blakemore) may occasionally

■ **varices** an enlarged and tortuous vein, artery, or lymphatic vessel.

be placed to tamponade the bleeding vessels. Patients with significant bleeding esophageal varices tend to do poorly.

Gastritis   Gastritis is an inflammation of the lining of the stomach. It results from increased gastric acid secretion and is associated with alcohol ingestion, drugs, stress, and other factors. The patient will often complain of epigastric pain, belching, and indigestion. The pain often improves after eating. If allowed to progress untreated, the protective lining of the stomach will eventually be destroyed and a gastric ulcer (erosion) may develop. Treatment involves administration of antacids and H_2 blocking drugs such as cimetidine (Tagamet).

Peptic Ulcer Disease   Peptic ulcer disease is caused by ulcers (erosions) in the lining of the esophagus, stomach, or duodenum. It often results from excess secretion of hydrochloric acid from glands in the lining of the stomach. The breakdown of the protective mucous lining of these organs by drugs, alcohol, and other agents is another cause. Aspirin and the non-steroidal anti-inflammatory class of drugs (Motrin, Advil, Naprosyn) are common offending agents. Abdominal pain associated with peptic ulcer disease is usually located in the epigastrium or the left upper quadrant. It is often improved following meals or following usage of antacids such as Maalox, Mylanta, or Riopan. Severe ulceration can cause significant gastrointestinal bleeding. The ulcer can sometimes erode through the wall of the organ, resulting in an acute abdomen.

Diverticulitis   **Diverticula** are pouches that develop, usually with age, on the large intestine, particularly on the descending segment (left side). These diverticula can become inflamed in much the same manner as the appendix. In fact, most cases of **diverticulitis** present like a left-sided appendicitis. The patient has abdominal pain, fever, vomiting, **anorexia**, and tenderness. Treatment includes antibiotics, dietary modifications, and, in certain cases, surgery.

■ **diverticula** small finger-like pouches on the colon associated with degeneration of the muscular layer of the organ.

■ **diverticulitis** an inflammation or infection of a diverticulum.

Bleeding Diverticulosis   Bleeding **diverticulosis** is hemorrhage from diverticula on the large intestines. It usually presents as painless rectal bleeding. Left-sided abdominal plain, however, can be present. The primary concern is prevention of shock.

■ **anorexia** lack of or loss of appetite.

■ **diverticulosis** the presence of diverticula on the colon.

Carcinoma of the Colon   **Carcinoma** of the colon is a malignant growth occurring anywhere in the colon. The presentation may be diverse. It can begin as painless rectal bleeding, weight loss, or abdominal pain. Prevention of shock is the primary concern if the bleeding is severe.

■ **carcinoma** malignant (cancerous) growth arising from epithelial cells.

Appendicitis   Appendicitis is the inflammation of the *vermiform appendix.* A piece of hard stool (fecalith) or a similar substance will occasionally obstruct the **lumen** of the appendix. This can result in inflammation of the appendix itself. Often, however, no identifiable cause can be found.

■ **lumen** the cavity or channel within a tube or organ.

The patient suffering appendicitis will usually complain of right lower quadrant abdominal pain. The onset of the pain is usually acute, often beginning in the area around the umbilicus. As the process develops, the pain migrates to the right lower quadrant. Nausea, vomiting, fever, and anorexia are common. The peritoneum will generally become inflamed and rebound tenderness will be present. If the appendix ruptures, the pus will leak into the abdominal cavity. The result is severe peritonitis characterized by guarding, rebound tenderness, and, occasionally, a rigid abdomen. Prehospital treatment should include fluid replacement and prevention of shock. Definitive treatment is surgical removal of the appendix.

Perforated Abdominal Viscus   Perforation of a hollow abdominal organ, most commonly the stomach, duodenum, or colon, can cause loss of the stomach or intestinal contents into the abdominal cavity. This can result in inflammation and infection of the peritoneum and other abdominal organs. Common causes of perforation include perforated ulcers or a perforated diverticulum. The patient will present with sudden onset of abdominal pain and generalized tenderness. Rebound is often present. In many cases, the abdomen is rigid from sympathetic contraction of the muscles of the abdominal wall. Treatment includes IV fluids, antibiotics, and emergency surgery to repair the perforation.

Bowel Obstruction   A bowel obstruction is the blockage of a portion of the intestines. The most common site is the small intestine, resulting in a *small bowel obstruction.* Causes include tumors, ingested foreign bodies, or most commonly, prior abdominal surgery. Large intestine obstructions are less common. Causes of large intestine obstruction include tumors and fecal impactions. The patient will often give a history of progressive anorexia, abdominal bloating, diffuse abdominal pain, nausea, and vomiting. If the obstruction has been present for a prolonged period of time, the patient may have fever, chills, and peritonitis. Prolonged bowel obstruction can cause death of the affected portion of the intestine. Prehospital treatment includes fluid replacement and prevention of shock. Definitive treatment often involves surgery.

Gastrointestinal Hemorrhage   Bleeding from the gastrointestinal system can be massive and exhibit very few outward signs. Gastrointestinal hemorrhage is usually classified as either an upper GI hemorrhage or a lower GI hemorrhage.

Upper GI Hemorrhage.   Bleeding that arises from the esophagus, stomach, or duodenum is referred to as an *upper GI hemorrhage.* Causes of upper GI hemorrhage include peptic ulcer disease (stomach or duodenum), gastritis, esophagitis, tumors, and esophageal varices. Signs and symptoms of an upper GI hemorrhage include **hematemesis** (vomiting of blood), dark stools resembling coffee grounds, or both. The stools appear dark because the blood is partially digested as it passes through the gastrointestinal tract. The presence of dark stools tends to indicate an upper GI hemorrhage as opposed to a lower GI hemorrhage. Blood in the intestinal tract acts as a **cathartic**. Thus, most patients with a GI hemorrhage will complain of increasingly frequent stools or frank **melanotic** diarrhea. Pain, if present, usually manifests as epigastric or left upper quadrant pain.

Lower GI Hemorrhage.   Bleeding that arises from the distal small intestine, colon, or rectum is referred to as a *lower GI hemorrhage.* Causes include tumors, bleeding from diverticula on the colon (diverticulosis), hemorrhoids, or rectal fissures. Signs and symptoms include rectal bleeding (either bright red or wine-colored, depending on the source of the bleeding) and increased stool frequency. Pain may or may not be present. If present, it usually presents as crampy, diffuse abdominal pain.

Assessment of GI Hemorrhage.   Often patients with GI hemorrhage will have few symptoms. Weakness is a common complaint. GI hemorrhage can be severe, causing frank shock. Orthostatic vital signs should be obtained. Vital signs indicative of a significant GI hemorrhage include increased heart rate, decreased blood pressure, orthostatic changes (positive **tilt test**), and normal to increased respirations. Prehospital treatment includes supplemental

■ **hematemesis** the vomiting of blood.

■ **cathartic** an agent or substance that causes evacuation of the bowels.

■ **melena** black, tar-like feces due to gastrointestinal bleeding.

■ **tilt test** drop in the systolic blood pressure of 15 mmHg or an increase in the pulse rate of 15 beats per minute when a patient is moved from a supine to a seated position. Such a condition is considered positive and suggestive of a relative hypovolemia. Also called orthostatic vital signs.

oxygen administration and fluid replacement. Because it is impossible to determine the amount of hemorrhage, two IVs of normal saline or lactated Ringer's should be established. Rapid transport is indicated.

Pancreatitis Pancreatitis, an inflammation of the pancreas, is frequently associated with chronic alcohol abuse. It can also occur in persons with marked elevations of blood lipids (cholesterol and triglycerides). In some cases, the cause is unclear. Patients with pancreatitis will often complain of abdominal pain that begins abruptly. Located in the mid-abdomen, the pain tends to radiate through to the back and shoulders. Nausea and vomiting are common. Treatment of the condition includes IV fluids, pain medications, and placement of a nasogastric tube to rest the patient's digestive system and to control vomiting.

Cholecystitis Inflammation of the gall bladder is called *cholecystitis*. It usually occurs when gall stones lodge in the cystic duct that drains the gall bladder. A stone may also lodge in the common bile duct, causing congestion of the liver, inflammation of the gall bladder, and, in severe cases, pancreatitis. The usually colicky pain of cholecystitis is located in the upper right quadrant. It generally worsens following meals, especially those containing high amounts of fats (fried foods, cheeses, etc.). Antacids usually do not lessen this pain. Treatment often includes surgical removal of the gall bladder.

Hepatitis Hepatitis is an inflammation or infection of the liver. It results from viral infections most commonly, and alcohol or other substance abuse. The patient will often complain of dull right upper quadrant abdominal tenderness, usually unrelated to digestion of food. Many cases involve associated malaise, decreased appetite, clay-colored stools, and jaundice (yellow tint to sclera and skin). In non-viral cases, treatment of hepatitis involves removing the offending agent. But, in viral-induced hepatitis, the patient is simply observed and treated symptomatically.

Aortic Aneurysm Weakness in the wall of the descending aorta can occur with age and result in a ballooning of the wall of the vessel. This ballooning may increase in size and eventually rupture. The patient with an abdominal aortic aneurysm is usually an older person who complains of diffuse abdominal pain and severe back pain. Such patients will occasionally report a tearing sensation if the artery is dissecting (loosening of the layers of the artery wall, allowing blood to flow in between). A pulsatile abdominal mass may be noted. Prehospital treatment consists of supplemental oxygen administration and initiation of two large bore IVs with normal saline or lactated Ringer's. The PASG should be placed and inflated if shock is evident. Definitive treatment consists of surgical repair or replacement of the diseased blood vessel.

Genitourinary System Emergencies

There are four general causes of genitourinary disorders: inflammation, infection, obstruction, and hemorrhage. These conditions usually present in the following forms.

Kidney Stone A kidney stone is the result of crystal aggregation in the collecting system of the kidney. Urinary stone formation is more common in men than in women. The usual age range is 20–50 years, although it can occur at any age. Kidney stones may form anytime during the year, but they seem to form more often in the spring and the fall.

Many factors predispose a patient to kidney stone formation. These include urinary tract infections, immobilization, certain metabolic disorders (increased calcium), gout (increased uric acid), and tumors. Sometimes these stones will break loose and enter the ureter. Since their diameter is usually greater than that of the ureter, the passage is quite painful. Some kidney stones will not pass completely through the ureter and will obstruct urine flow from the kidney on the involved side.

The kidney stone is one of the most painful conditions known to humans. The pain typically starts acutely as the stone enters the ureter. Initially colicky (intermittent), the pain appears either in the back or in the flank. As the stone moves down the ureter, the pain also appears to move down. When the stone approaches the bladder, the pain may actually seem as though it is in the testicle (in male patients). Patients with a kidney stone are often restless and cannot get comfortable. They change positions frequently or pace around the room. Many patients will have difficulty urinating. When urinating, the urine is often bloody (**hematuria**). Nausea and vomiting are also common.

Initial therapies for kidney stones include intravenous fluids, which often facilitate stone movement into the bladder, and analgesics. Kidney stones unable to pass remain lodged in the ureter and require surgical removal. Sometimes they can be broken up by sound waves generated through extracorporeal shock wave lithotripsy. Complications from urinary stone formation include inflammation, infection, and partial or total urinary obstruction.

Urinary Tract Infections

Urinary tract infections (UTI) occur frequently. The most common UTI is bladder infection (cystitis), seldom a medical emergency. UTI occurs more often in females because of the relatively short urethra compared to that in males. Such infections are extremely rare in the male and less common in the female who is sexually inactive. The UTI can sometimes infect the kidney, causing pyelonephritis. This is usually characterized by fever, chills, and flank pain. Symptoms of urinary tract infection include dysuria (painful or burning urination), hesitancy (difficulty starting urine stream), discolored urine, and lower abdominal pain (especially during urination).

Pyelonephritis

Pyelonephritis is infection of the kidney. Because it often results from infection ascending from the bladder, it appears more commonly in women than in men. Women's bladders are more prone to infection because of the shortness of the urethra. The patient will typically be febrile and complain of flank or low back pain. Chills are also common. There may be tenderness at the area below where the 12th rib attaches to the 12th thoracic vertebra (costovertebral angle). Urinary burning and frequency may or may not be present. Treatment usually requires intravenous antibiotics.

Renal Failure

The kidneys normally maintain body fluid volume, blood pH, and the composition of body fluids within a very narrow range. They also continuously eliminate metabolic waste products. However, the kidneys can sometimes quit working or work less efficiently. This condition is often referred to as renal failure or renal insufficiency. Depending on its duration and potential reversibility, renal failure can be classified as acute or **chronic**.

Acute Renal Failure. *Acute renal failure* is characterized by rapid and potentially reversible deterioration of kidney function. Acute renal failure can be caused by several conditions. These include:

❑ *Prerenal*: reduced renal blood flow (shock, dehydration, and use of vasopressor agents).

❑ *Renal*: injury to the substance of the kidney itself (trauma, nephrotoxic drugs, or infection).

❑ *Postrenal*: obstruction of the flow of urine (enlarged prostate or tumor obstructing the ureters or bladder).

As renal failure progresses, metabolic waste products accumulate. These can have a toxic effect on virtually every body organ. Urea is an end-product of protein metabolism and is usually cleared by the kidneys. In renal failure, the level of urea in the blood increases, producing a condition known as **uremia**.

■ **uremia** toxic condition caused by the retention of nitrogen-based substances (urea) in the blood, normally excreted by the kidneys.

Chronic Renal Failure. *Chronic renal failure* refers to long-standing renal failure associated with loss of nephron (kidney cell) mass and is usually irreversible. Many disease processes can destroy the kidneys or the renal arteries, resulting in chronic renal failure.

Presentation. Renal failure can produce fluid overload, dangerously elevated potassium levels, uremic pericarditis, pericardial tamponade, and uremic encephalopathy. In patients with severe renal failure and low urine output, the ability to excrete electrolytes and water is markedly diminished, predisposing them to fluid overload and episodes of noncardiac pulmonary edema. These patients present with severe dyspnea, neck vein distention, **ascites**, and rales at the lung bases.

■ **ascites** accumulation of fluid within the peritoneal cavity.

Patients with chronic renal failure will often appear wasted. Their skin will be pasty yellow and their extremities thin. The latter is due to the protein loss accompanying chronic renal failure and poor nutrition. In the later stages, urea crystals may form on the skin, producing a frostlike appearance (uremic frost). Edema (due to decreased protein, jaundice, and low urine output) is frequently present.

Management. Many medications are eliminated through the kidneys. Because patients with renal failure do not clear medications as rapidly as normal patients do, they are susceptible to toxic drug concentrations despite relatively low medication doses.

Reproductive System Emergencies

Occasionally, the reproductive organs may be the source of acute abdominal pain. The next sections present common reproductive system emergencies that can cause acute abdominal pain.

Female   Reproductive emergencies arising in the female patient include the following conditions.

Pelvic Inflammatory Disease (PID). PID is an infection of the female reproductive organs that is usually sexually transmitted. As an ascending infection, PID spreads from the vagina or cervix to the uterus, the fallopian tubes, and the broad ligament. The patient usually presents with fever, chills, lower abdominal pain, and vaginal bleeding or discharge. In addition, the patient may complain of pain on walking or pain with intercourse. (See Chapter 31 for additional discussion of PID.)

Ovarian Cyst. An ovarian cyst is a fluid-filed sac that forms intermittently on the ovaries. If the cyst ruptures, blood will be spilled into the abdominal cavity causing pain and tenderness. The patient will often present with abdominal pain, occurring with either a rapid or a gradual onset. Often, intercourse will cause the cyst to rupture and the pain will begin acutely. On rare occasions, the patient may experience syncope and develop shock.

Mittelschmerz. Mittelschmerz is abdominal pain that may accompany ovulation. It occurs half-way through the menstrual cycle and is associated with release of the ovum from the ovary. In rare cases, pain can be severe.

Ectopic Pregnancy. An ectopic pregnancy is the implantation of a developing fetus outside of the uterus. It must be considered as a cause in any female of childbearing age with lower abdominal pain. The most common location is in the fallopian tube (hence the name "tubal pregnancy"). The fetus continues to grow until it exerts pressure on the wall of the fallopian tube. If the pregnancy is allowed to progress, the fallopian tube can rupture, causing significant bleeding into the abdomen and pelvis.

Upon questioning, a patient often will report a missed menstrual period or irregular periods. She also may have already had a positive pregnancy test. The patient will usually present with tenderness on the affected side. She will often show pallor, weak pulse, and signs of shock or hemorrhage. Pain may be referred to the shoulder, and the umbilicus may appear bluish in color. Prehospital treatment includes the administration of supplemental oxygen, initiation of 1–2 IVs of normal saline or lactated Ringer's. If shock is present, consider application of the PASG and emergent transport. (See Chapters 31 and 32 for additional information on ectopic pregnancy.)

Male Reproductive system emergencies in the male are relatively uncommon. The most serious male reproductive system emergency is testicular torsion. If undetected, it can result in loss of the testicle. Male reproductive system emergencies include the following conditions.

Testicular Torsion. Torsion of testes occurs when the testicle rotates in the scrotum. This rotation twists the spermatic cord and can stop blood flow to the testicle. Testicular torsion usually occurs in children and teenagers. However, it can occur in older patients as well. Patients who have a history of testicular torsion have a tendency to have the problem recur on the opposite side. The patient will present with severe testicular pain and may feel as though he has received an injury to his testicles. There may be associated lower abdominal pain as well. Often the affected testicle is swollen, tender, and appears higher in the scrotum than the other. Occasionally, a knot can be palpated in the spermatic cord immediately above the affected testicle. Prehospital treatment includes reassurance and possibly administration of analgesics.

Epididymitis. Epididymitis is the inflammation of the epididymis. It may occur secondary to gonorrhea, syphilis, tuberculosis, mumps, prostatitis, urethritis, or following prolonged use of an indwelling catheter. The patient with epididymitis will present with fever and chills, pain in his inguinal region, and a swollen epididymis.

Prostatitis. Infection of the prostate is called *prostatitis*. Male patients tend to develop prostate infections instead of bladder infections. Signs and symptoms of prostatitis include urinary frequency, burning, pain with ejaculation, and occasionally pain with defecation. Sometimes a patient with prostatitis will present with fever, chills, nausea, and vomiting. Prehospital treatment is primarily supportive.

ASSESSMENT OF THE ACUTE ABDOMEN

You should not attempt to discern the cause of abdominal pain in the prehospital setting. This is a difficult enough process for the emergency department with laboratory, X-ray, and other diagnostic facilities available. However, you still need to perform a complete assessment in order to detect obvious threats to life, including impending shock.

✱ The paramedic should not attempt to discern the cause of abdominal pain in the prehospital setting.

Primary Assessment

As with any other emergency, you should begin with the primary assessment. You should deal immediately with any threats to life. Unstable vital signs, or shock, warrant emergent transport with care provided en route.

Secondary Assessment

If the patient is stable, you should proceed with the secondary assessment, including the standard head-to-toe survey. Pay particular attention to the abdomen. First, you need to inspect it, noting any obvious asymmetry or distention. (See Figure 24-6.) Also, observe the position of the patient. Patients

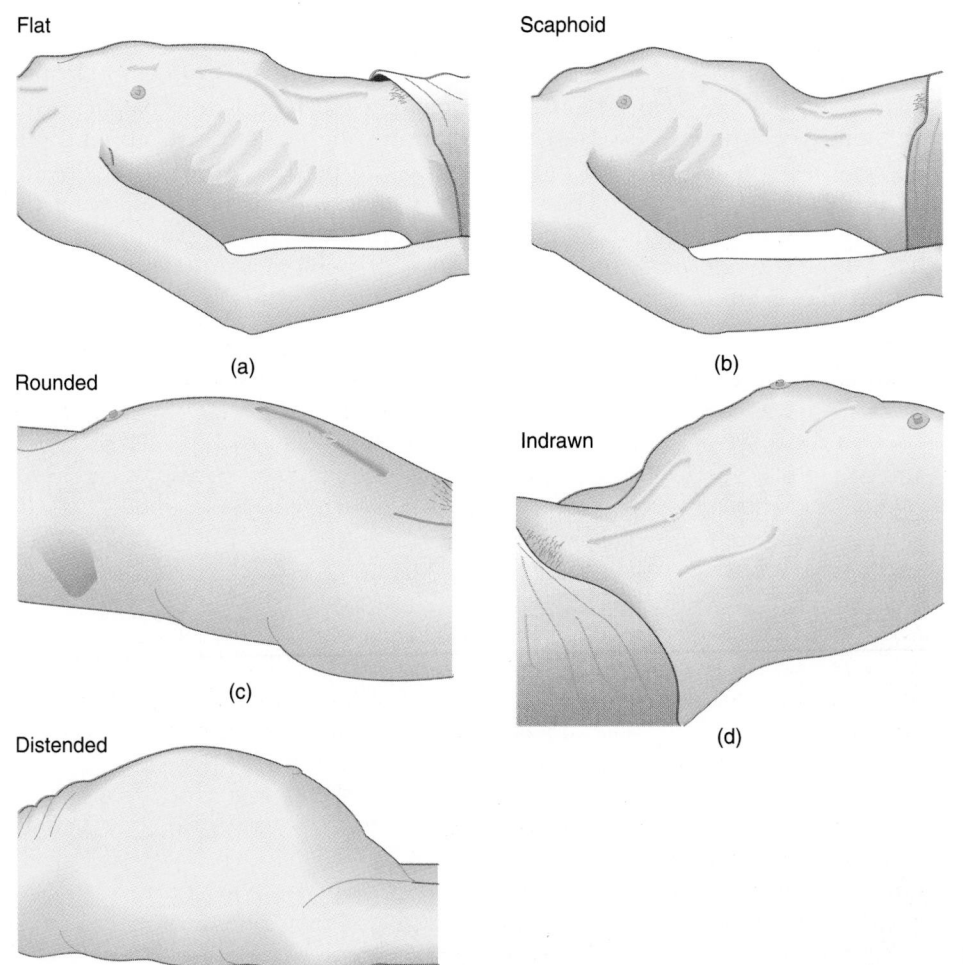

Flat

(a)

Scaphoid

(b)

Rounded

(c)

Indrawn

(d)

Distended

FIGURE 24-6 Various abdominal appearances.

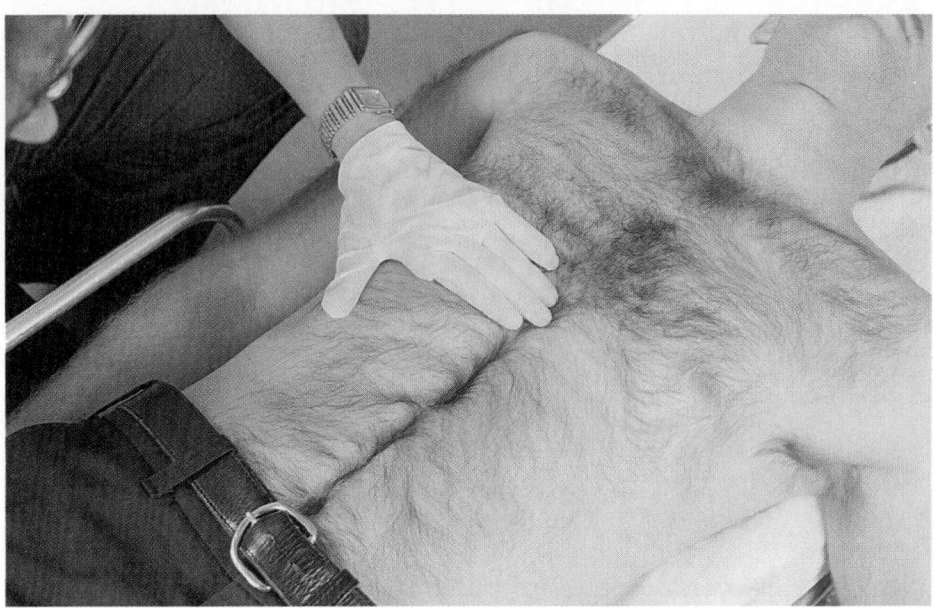

FIGURE 24-7   Inspection of the abdomen.

presenting with acute abdominal pain will frequently have the knees drawn up toward the chest to lessen tension on the peritoneum and to decrease intra-abdominal pressure.

The abdomen should be gently palpated. (See Figure 24-7.) First, ask the patient to point to the location of the pain. (See Figure 24-8.) Begin palpation away from the site of the pain. Each quadrant must be lightly palpated and any tenderness noted. Also, test the patient for the presence of rebound tenderness, if permitted by local protocols. This can be done slowly by palpating each abdominal quadrant. Then, quickly withdraw your hand, allowing the abdominal wall to return to its normal position. If this causes pain, the patient has rebound tenderness, usually suggestive of peritoneal irritation. Do NOT repeat the examination for rebound tenderness as this is painful for the

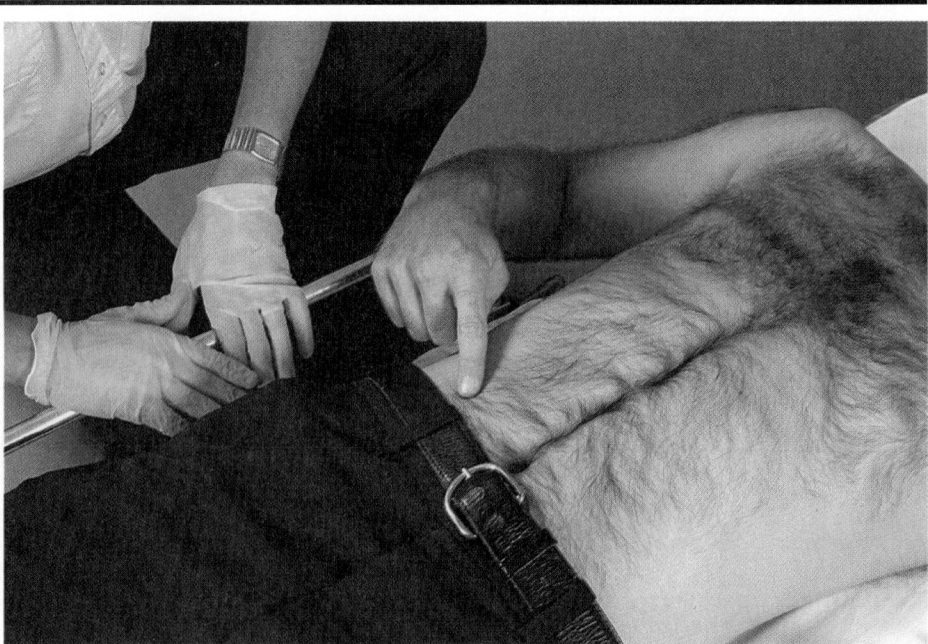

FIGURE 24-8   Have the patient point to the site of the pain. Leave examination of this quadrant until last.

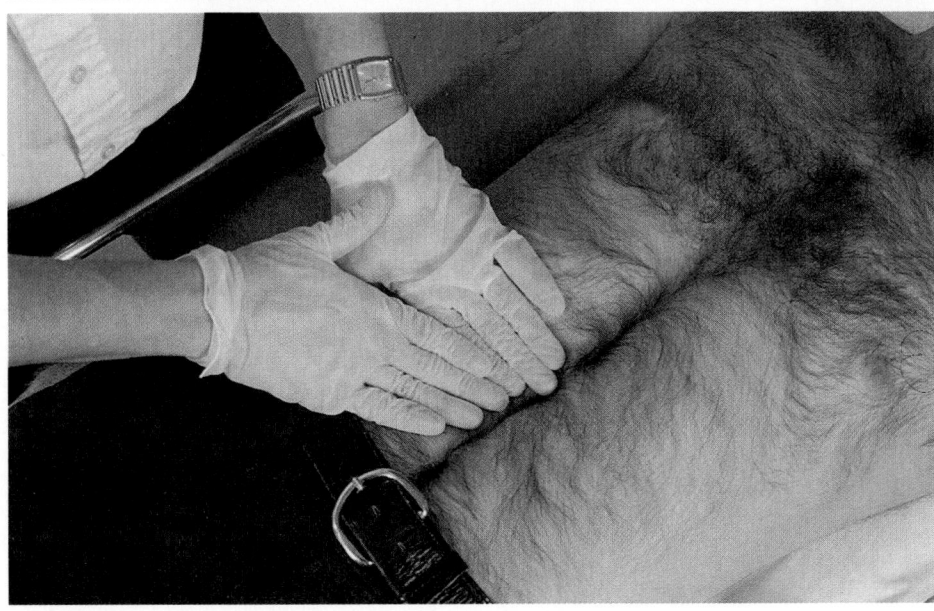

FIGURE 24-9 Soft palpation.

patient and can lead to complications. (See Figure 24–9.) If you locate a pulsatile mass, stop palpation and immediately transport the patient. Prolonged or vigorous palpation of an abdominal aortic aneurysm can result in rupture with disastrous consequences. Remember, do not attempt auscultation and percussion of the abdomen in the prehospital setting.

Determination of vital signs is extremely important in the patient suffering abdominal pain. Take the pulse, blood pressure, respiration, and if possible, the temperature. Additionally, perform a tilt test on all patients with abdominal pain. First, take the patient's blood pressure and pulse in the supine position. Then repeat both with the patient in a seated position. A positive tilt test is an increase in the pulse rate of 15 beats per minute or a drop in the systolic blood pressure of 15 mm/Hg when the patient is moved from the supine to the sitting position. A positive tilt test indicates a relative hypovolemia and necessitates further intervention. (See Figures 24-10 and 24-11.)

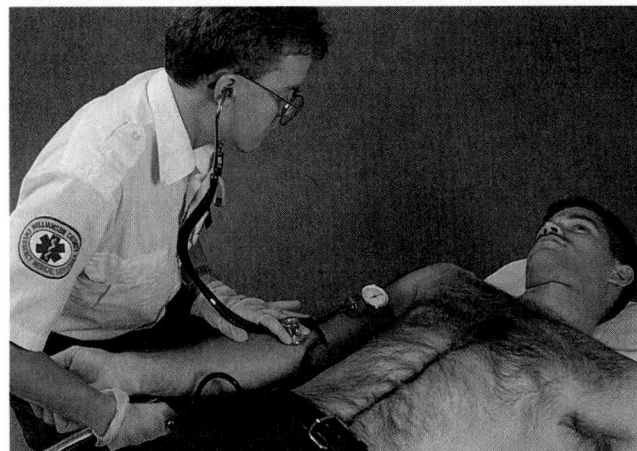

FIGURE 24-10 The tilt test should be performed. First, determine the pulse and blood pressure with the patient supine.

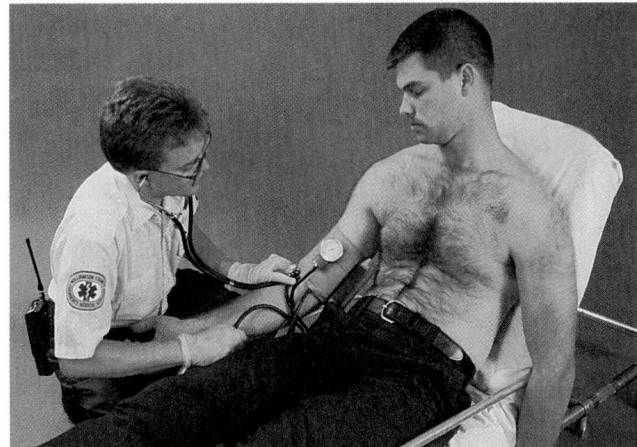

FIGURE 24-11 Then, elevate the patient and repeat the pulse and blood pressure. A fall in the systolic blood pressure of 15 mm/Hg or a rise in the pulse of 15 beats per minute is considered positive.

History

After the primary and secondary assessment, you should obtain a pertinent and brief history. Pain is the most common presentation of the acute abdomen. Elicit information about the quality of the pain. Is it continuous, intermittent, or constant? Does it increase, then decrease, and subsequently increase again?

The patient should be asked where in the abdomen the pain began and whether it radiates or is referred to another area of the body. If the pain moves, determine whether it penetrates through to the back or goes around the abdomen to the back. Also, ask if the pain is associated with or aggravated by food intake, physical activity, or any increase in intra-abdominal pressure (breathing, coughing, or straining). The occurrence of related symptoms such as nausea, vomiting, or diarrhea can be of assistance in localizing the source of the symptoms to a specific site or organ. Many paramedics find the following OPQRST method useful for evaluating pain.

O   **O**nset: *What were you doing when the pain began?*

P   **P**rovocation: *What initiates the pain? What makes it better or worse?*

Q   **Q**uality: *How would you describe the pain?*

R   **R**adiation: *Where is the pain located? Does the pain travel to other body areas?*

S   **S**everity: *How intense is the pain? on a scale from 1 to 10?*

T   **T**ime: *How long ago did the pain begin? When does it occur? Is it intermittent or constant?*

It is crucial to obtain a history of menstrual activity in female patients who present with abdominal pain. Record the date of the last menstrual period (LMP). Also, ask the patient whether her periods have been regular. Question her about the use of oral contraceptives (birth control pills). If she uses them, inquire about any pills that may have been missed. If the LMP was abnormal, note the duration, time of onset, estimated amount of blood loss, or unusual pain associated with menstruation. If the patient's menses are late, question her about possible pregnancy.

Appropriate past medical history is also significant in assessing the patient presenting with abdominal pain. Obtain information concerning any previous illnesses, particularly any abdominal condition or prior surgery, during the patient assessment.

MANAGEMENT OF THE ACUTE ABDOMEN

If the patient shows no evidence of active hemorrhage and if the vital signs are stable without signs of shock, you should consider the following procedures. Your choice of action will, of course, depend upon assessment.

❑ Keep the patient supine.
❑ Supply oxygen via nasal cannula.
❑ Monitor vital signs and cardiac rhythm.
❑ Start an IV of normal saline or lactated Ringer's TKO
❑ Provide immediate transport.

If the patient exhibits active hemorrhage (bloody stools or vomiting

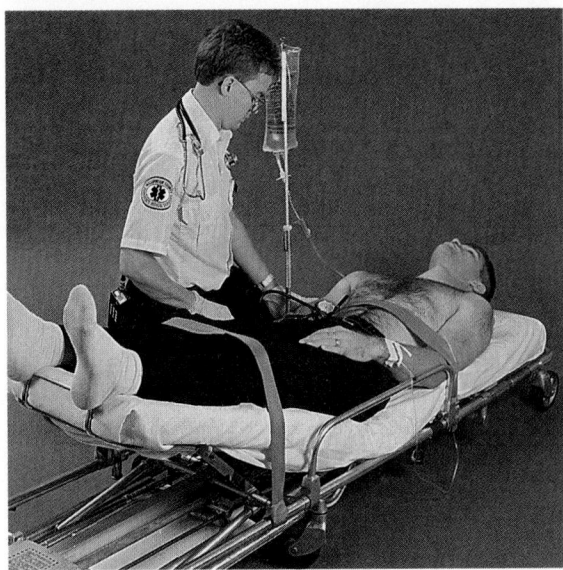

FIGURE 24-12 Management of the patient with an acute abdomen and positive tilt test.

blood) or shows signs of impending shock (positive tilt test), you should initiate the following treatment. (See Figure 24-12.)

- ❏ Keep patient in the shock position (feet elevated).
- ❏ Administer high-flow oxygen (100 percent).
- ❏ Start IV(s), using normal saline or lactated Ringer's wide open.
- ❏ Monitor vital signs and cardiac rhythm.
- ❏ Position PASG (if needed later).
- ❏ Provide rapid transport.

SPECIAL PATIENTS: DIALYSIS

Patients with chronic renal failure require **dialysis** to live. This process helps remove toxic substances from the bloodstream—a function no longer adequately provided by the kidneys.

■ **dialysis** process of exchanging various biochemical substances across a semipermeable membrane to remove toxic substances.

Types of Dialysis

Treatment of renal failure takes one of two forms: hemodialysis or peritoneal dialysis. Choice of procedure depends upon the patient's medical condition.

Hemodialysis   **Hemodialysis** is a medical procedure whereby waste products, normally excreted by the kidneys, are removed by a machine. Patients with renal failure must undergo dialysis two to three times a week. Many patients now have home dialysis units, and you may be called upon to assist them.

■ **hemodialysis** a medical procedure whereby waste products and fluid, normally excreted by the kidneys, are removed by a machine.

The basic principle of dialysis is the diffusion of water and solutes across semipermeable membranes separating two fluid compartments. Solutes tend to migrate from areas of higher concentrations to ones of lower concentrations. Over time, these solutes will equilibrate. This equilibration forms the basis for dialysis treatment. During dialysis, the patient's blood comes in contact with a physiologic solution called **dialysate** across a semipermeable

■ **dialysate** physiologic solution used in renal dialysis.

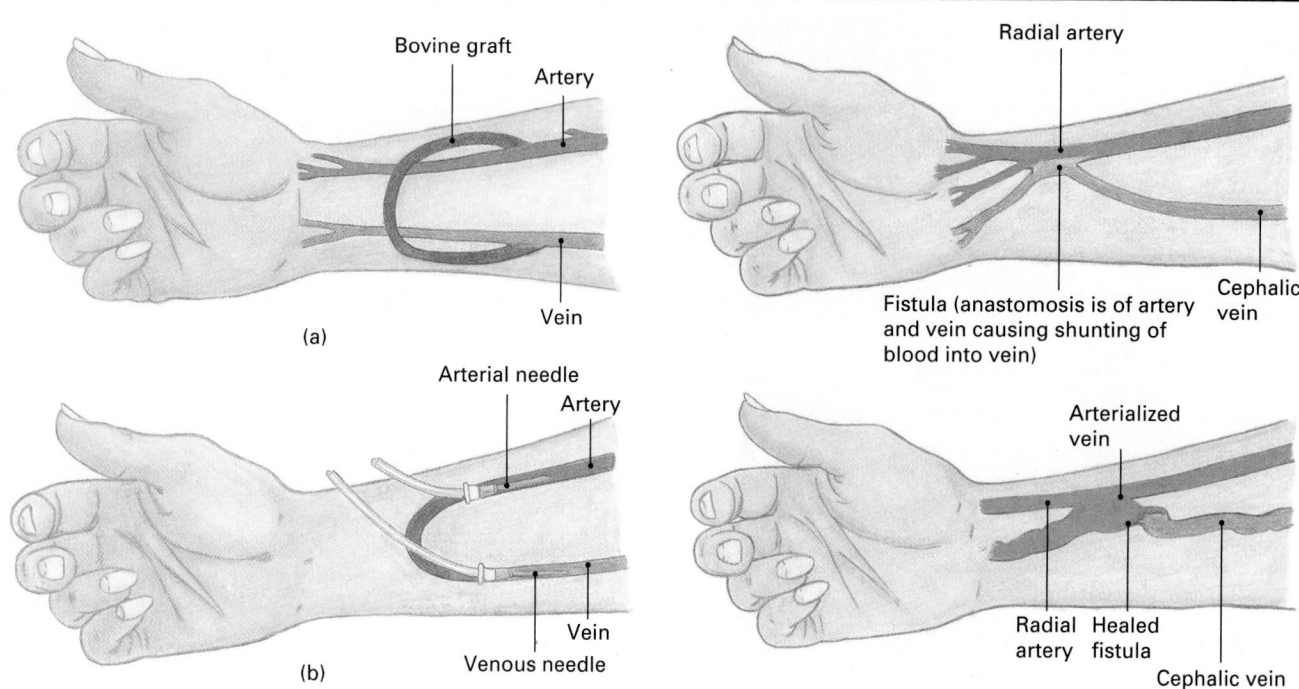

Bovine graft
Artery

Vein

(a)

Radial artery

Fistula (anastomosis is of artery
and vein causing shunting of
blood into vein)

Cephalic
vein

Arterial needle
Artery

Vein
Venous needle

(b)

Arterialized
vein

Radial   Healed
artery   fistula

Cephalic vein

FIGURE 24-13   Dialysis cannula in place.

FIGURE 24-14   Fistula for dialysis access.

membrane. Equilibration of the patient's blood with dialysate normalizes the patient's electrolyte composition and eliminates undesirable waste products that his or her kidneys cannot excrete.

Vascular access must exist to dialyze the patient. The two most common routes of access are external arteriovenous shunts or internal fistulae. An arteriovenous shunt is a surgical connection between the arterial and venous systems. It provides the high flow required for dialysis and to prevent clotting. External arteriovenous shunts are usually placed in the patient's forearm, groin, or ankle. Between treatments, the shunt is wrapped and protected by a dressing to prevent dislodgment or injury. The internal fistula—located in the subcutaneous tissue of the forearm, groin, or upper arm—will have a bruit that can be palpated. It results from turbulent blood flow from the high pressure arterial system to the low pressure venous system. (See Figures 24-13 and 24-14.)

Peritoneal Dialysis   Another method for dialysis is via the peritoneum. Peritoneal dialysis uses the lining of the peritoneal cavity as the dialysis membrane. Dialysate is introduced into the patient's peritoneal cavity, where it is allowed to remain 1–2 hours before removal. If needed, the procedure can be repeated as often as necessary. The major complication of peritoneal dialysis is the development of peritonitis. Therefore, this procedure must be done under aseptic conditions. (See Figure 24-15.)

Complications of Dialysis

There are many complications that can arise from dialysis. Fortunately, they are fairly uncommon and often recognized at the time of dialysis. Complications of dialysis include the following conditions.

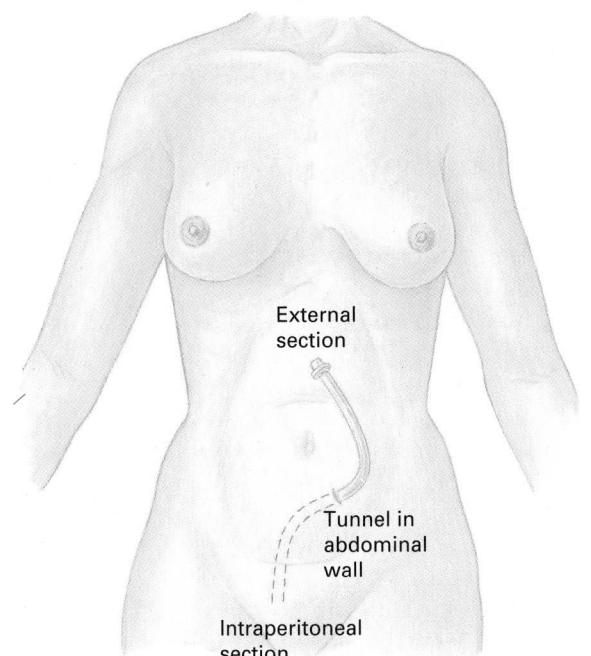

External
section

Tunnel in
abdominal
wall

Intraperitoneal
section

FIGURE 24-15 Peritoneal dialysis.

Hypotension   Hypotension due to dialysis is caused by dehydration, sepsis, or blood loss. The patient who becomes hypotensive will present with lightheadedness, dizziness, weakness, pallor, cold sweats, and syncope. The hypotension is treated by reducing the rate of blood flow through the dialysis machine, lowering the patient's head, elevating the legs, and infusing IV saline.

Chest Pain/Dysrhythmias   Dysrhythmias produced in response to dialysis can be caused by potassium intoxication. Yet, frequently, no specific electrolyte derangement can be identified. Dysrhythmias sometimes may be related to the development of transient myocardial ischemia, which may also cause the patient to experience chest pain. The most commonly seen cardiac abnormalities are PVCs. The dialysis procedure must be discontinued if the dysrhythmia is considered severe or does not respond to treatment.

Disequilibrium Syndrome   Disequilibrium syndrome is characterized by cerebral symptoms in patients with severe renal failure. It can occur at the beginning, during, or immediately following hemodialysis. These patients may present with headache, lethargy, convulsions, and may even lapse into coma. Disequilibrium syndrome may be caused by rapid changes of body fluids, sodium concentrations, and osmolalities. With a rapid decline in the level of blood urea, time is insufficient for an equal lowering of urea across the "blood-brain barrier." This may cause an osmotic diuresis of water from the cerebral blood and from the extracellular fluid in the central nervous system, resulting in cerebral edema and increased intracranial pressure. The major concern is the development of convulsions. Diazepam may be given to the patient with seizures.

Air Embolism   An air embolism can occur when negative pressure develops in the venous side of the dialysis tubing. This negative pressure sucks air in and carries it to the right ventricle of the heart where it mixes with blood, creating a foam. The foam is pumped into the pulmonary artery, blocking the passage of blood to the left side of the heart. This will cause the patient to experience severe dyspnea, cyanosis, hypotension, and respiratory distress. Modern dialysis machines have protective devices that prevent air emboli. If these devices fail, the dialysis machine must be immediately shut off and the patient turned on the left side, with feet elevated, and head down. Oxygen should be administered via nasal cannula.

Complications Related to Vascular Access

Complications may arise related to the venous access devices placed for chronic dialysis. The following are two examples of such conditions.

Clotting   Clotting of the shunt of fistula can occur spontaneously. A clotted shunt is easy to recognize because, in an internal shunt, the bruit will be lost. In an external shunt, clots will be visible in the tubing. Clotting poses no immediate emergency.

Hemorrhage   Massive external hemorrhage can occur with separation of arteriovenous fistulas. Rupture of internal fistulas is possible if an aneurysm has formed and the shunt ruptures through the skin. For the external shunt, clamps are secured to the dressing covering it. The devices allow you to clamp the shunt when necessary. If an internal shunt ruptures, the hemorrhage can be frightening to the patient and difficult for you to stop. The best method to end the hemorrhage is by direct pressure and rapid transport to the emergency department.

Management of the Dialysis Patient

In most EMS systems, the paramedic rarely has an opportunity to deal with a dialysis patient on a regular basis. Listed below are treatment guidelines specific to the dialysis patient.

❑ Review intravenous therapy carefully. IV access may be difficult. The shunt SHOULD NOT be used. The IV, if ordered, should be placed in the arm opposite the shunt. Fluid administration should be at the direction of the medical control physician.
❑ Monitor ECG.
❑ Use the arm opposite the shunt for taking the blood pressure.
❑ Treat medical emergencies the same as for any patient.
❑ Remove the patient from dialysis machine using the below steps.
  • Turn off dialysis machine.
  • Clamp the ends of shunt tubing.
  • Control shunt hemorrhage (internal or external) with either direct pressure or by pinching the shunt ends.

SUMMARY

Determining the origin of an abdominal disorder can be extremely difficult, not only for the paramedic in the field, but for the emergency physician. Most field procedures required for abdominal emergencies can be performed while en route to the emergency department. Excessive time should not be spent in the field since many of these patients may require abdominal surgery.

As a paramedic, you may be called upon to treat the patient on renal hemodialysis. Therefore, you should be familiar with complications and management of dialysis such as hypotension, dysrhythmias, chest pain, disequilibrium syndrome, air embolism, clotting, and hemorrhage.

FURTHER READING

Bledsoe, Bryan E. *Atlas of Paramedic Skills*, 2nd ed. Englewood Cliffs, NJ: Prentice-Hall, Inc., 1993.

Langfitt, D.E. *Critical Care: Certification Preparation and Review.* Bowie, MD: Robert J. Brady Company, 1984.

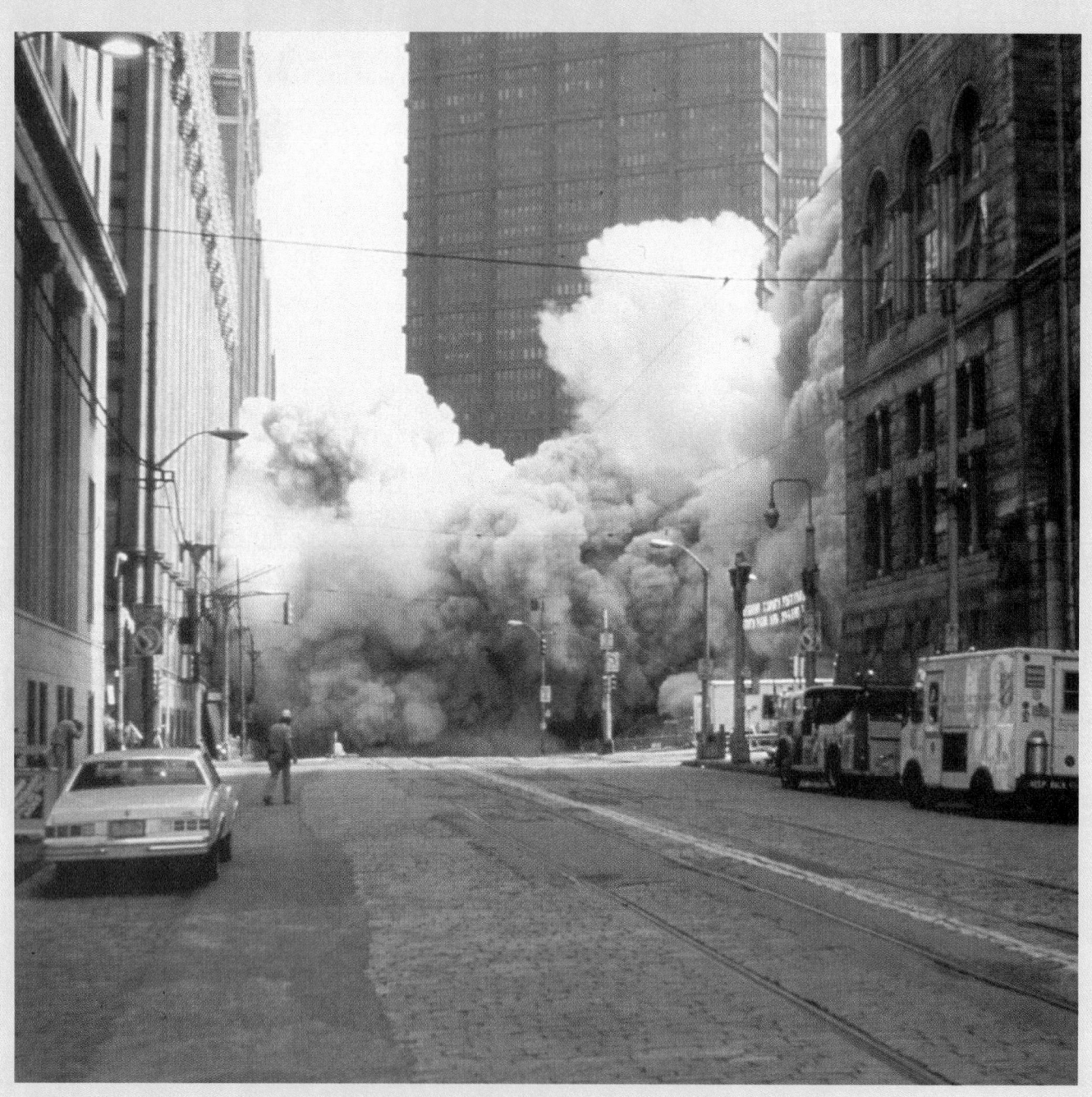

25

ANAPHYLAXIS

Objectives for Chapter 25

After reading this chapter, you should be able to:

1. Define anaphylaxis. (See p. 794.)

2. Define antigen. (See p. 796.)

3. List ways an antigen can be introduced into the body. (See p. 794.)

4. Define antibody. (See p. 796.)

5. Describe the pathophysiology of allergic reactions and anaphylaxis. (See pp. 796–798.)

6. Discuss the effects of allergic reactions and anaphylaxis on the following body systems. (See below pages.)

   - skin (pp. 798–799)
   - respiratory (pp. 798–799)
   - cardiovascular (pp. 798–799)
   - gastrointestinal (pp. 798–799)
   - nervous (p. 798)

7. Describe the clinical presentation of the patient suffering an allergic reaction and anaphylaxis. (See pp. 798–799.)

8. Discuss the assessment of the patient suffering an allergic reaction and anaphylaxis. (See pp. 798–799.)

9. Describe the management of a patient with a severe allergic reaction. (See pp. 799–803.)

10. Describe the actions of the following medications, and relate their usage in the management of allergic reactions and anaphylaxis. (See below pages.)

   - oxygen (p. 799)
   - epinephrine (pp. 800–801)
   - antihistamines (pp. 801–802)
   - corticosteroids (p. 802)
   - beta agonists (pp. 802–803)

Just as the crews sit down to lunch, Medic 1 and Engine 3 are dispatched to a local physician's office for a medical emergency. The emergency medical dispatcher reports that a 45-year-old male patient is having difficulty breathing. Fortunately, the response time for both units is less than three minutes.

Upon arrival at the physician's office, EMS personnel are met by the receptionist who leads them to a treatment room. The patient is a male in his mid-forties who is lying on an examination table. He is very pale and diaphoretic. The office nurse states that the patient had just received his third series of allergy shots immediately before he became ill. She reports that he comes in once a week at lunch time for the shots. Unfortunately, the doctor had already left the office for lunch and was unavailable. The nurse reports that she gave the patient 50 milligrams of diphenhydramine (Benadryl) approximately 5 minutes before the arrival of EMS.

Paramedics from Medic 1 and Engine 3 begin the primary assessment. The patient's airway is open, breathing labored, and pulse weak and rapid. He is responsive, but lethargic and confused.

Supplemental oxygen is administered via a nonrebreather mask. While one member of the team prepares an IV of lactated Ringer's, another obtains the vital signs. The patient's pulse is 130 and weak, respirations are 18 and shallow, and blood pressure 70 mmHg by palpation. A pulse oximeter is attached which reveals an SpO_2 of 93%. ECG leads are placed. The ECG shows a sinus tachycardia without ectopy. The ECG electrodes do not adhere well because of the patient's diaphoresis. Tincture of Benzoin is applied to the skin and the leads adhere much better.

While the IV is started, the secondary assessment is completed. The patient is still pale and very diaphoretic. In addition, there are raised, red blotches on the skin consistent with hives.

INTRODUCTION

anaphylaxis an unusual or exaggerated allergic reaction to a foreign protein or other substance. *Anaphylaxis* means "the opposite of *phylaxis* or protection."

Anaphylaxis is an acute, generalized, and violent antigen-antibody reaction—the most severe form of an allergic reaction—that may be rapidly fatal even with prompt and appropriate emergency medical care. Anaphylaxis develops in seconds to minutes after the ingestion, injection, inhalation, or absorption of an antigenic substance. (See Figure 25-1.) Anaphylaxis is an emergency in which appropriate prehospital intervention by EMS personnel is life-saving. This chapter will address the pathophysiology and management of anaphylaxis, allergies, and related disorders.

THE IMMUNE SYSTEM

immune system the body system responsible for combating infection.

The **immune system** plays a central role in allergies and anaphylaxis. The immune system is a complicated body system responsible for combating infection. Components of the immune system can be found in the blood, the bone marrow, the connective tissues, and in the lymphatic system.

immune response complex of events within the body that works toward the destruction or inactivation of pathogens, abnormal cells, or foreign molecules.

The **immune response** is a complex cascade of events. The goal of the immune response is the destruction or inactivation of pathogens, abnormal cells, or foreign molecules such as toxins. The body can accomplish this through two mechanisms: cellular immunity and humoral immunity. *Cellular immunity* is derived from special leukocytes called *T lymphocytes*. They originate in the *thymus*, a gland located in the upper part of the chest. T lymphocytes are primarily responsible for fighting infections of biological agents living in certain body cells, including tuberculosis, many viral infections, and most fungal infections. Such infections result in movement of white cells to the site of infection, which then attack and eliminate the infection.

Auscultation of the chest reveals fine wheezes throughout. The patient shivers intermittently.

While starting the IV, the paramedics notice that the patient has become more confused and listless. The IV is successfully placed in the right forearm. Following standing orders, 0.4 milligram of epinephrine 1:10,000 is administered intravenously. The IV line is flushed, then 50 milligrams of diphenhydramine are administered intravenously.

Almost immediately, the patient's mental status improves. His heart rate increases to 160 beats per minute. His respirations increase to 28 breaths per minute. The severe diaphoresis improves and the hives begin to clear. The blood pressure is repeated and noted to be 130/90 mmHg.

The patient's physician returns at this time after noticing the emergency equipment in the parking lot in front of the office. He quickly reviews the paramedics' actions and is relieved the patient is doing better. He requests that the para-

medics administer 125 milligrams of methylprednisolone (Solu-Medrol) by intravenous infusion. Because this is not a part of their protocols, the paramedics contact the on-line medical control physician who approves the request. The methylprednisolone infusion is begun.

As the patient is prepared for movement to the ambulance, the vital signs are repeated. His blood pressure is now 130/80 mmHg, pulse is 120, and respirations are 20. The hives are virtually clear and the patient is alert and conversive. The patient is transported to the hospital without incident.

Once at the emergency department the patient is evaluated and monitored by the emergency department staff. Following a two-hour observation period, the patient is discharged with a prescription for an antihistamine (Atarax) and a short course of corticosteroids (Medrol DosePak). He does well following discharge. His family physician decides not to continue the allergy shots.

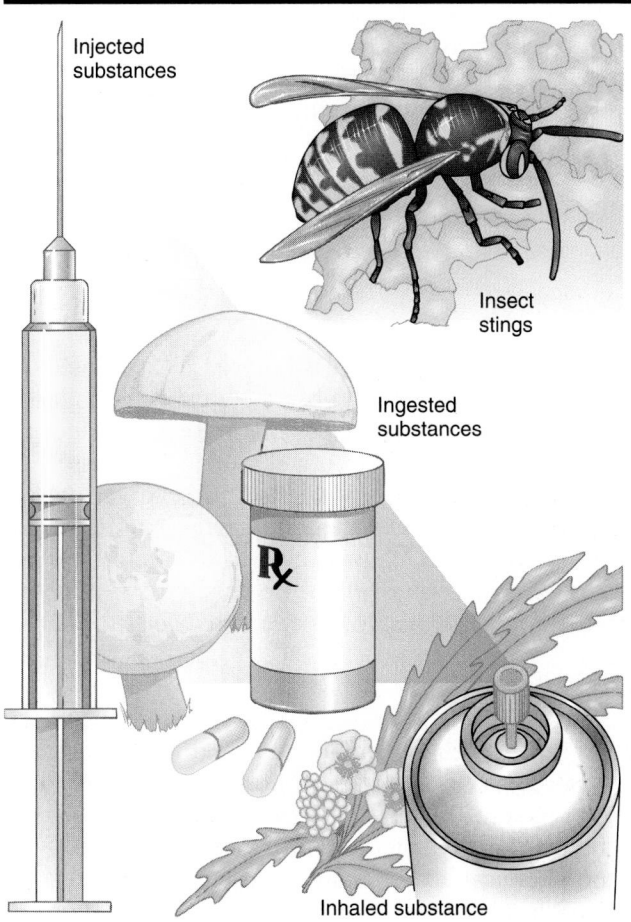

Injected substances

Insect stings

Ingested substances

Inhaled substance

FIGURE 25-1 Anaphylactic reactions can result from a variety of causes.

TABLE 25-1 Agents that May Cause Anaphylaxis
Antibiotics and other drugs
Foreign proteins (e.g., horse serum. Streptokinase)
Foods (nuts, eggs, shrimp)
Allergen extracts (allergy shots)
Hymenoptera stings (bees, wasps)
Hormones (Insulin)
Blood Products
Aspirin
Non-steroidal anti-inflammatory agents (NSAIDS)
Preservatives (sulfiting agents)
X-ray contrast media
Dextran

Humoral immunity is much more complicated. Humoral immunity derives from *B lymphocytes* and results in the formation of special proteins called **antibodies**. There are five classes of human antibodies (also called **immunoglobulins**). They include:

❑ *IgM*—the antibody that responds immediately
❑ *IgG*—the antibody that has "memory" and recognizes a repeatedly invading infection
❑ *IgA*—the antibody present in the mucous membranes
❑ *IgE*—the antibody contributing to allergic and anaphylactic responses
❑ *IgD*—the antibody present in the lowest concentration

The humoral immune response begins with exposure of the body to an **antigen**. Most antigens are proteins; however, an antigen is defined as any substance capable of inducing an immune response. (See Table 25-1.) The antibodies seek out the invading antigen and combine, forming what is commonly called the *antigen-antibody complex*. This large complex is subsequently removed by scavenger cells such as *macrophages*.

If the body has never been exposed to a particular antigen, the response of the immune system is different than if it has been previously exposed to the particular antigen. The initial response to an antigen is called the *primary response*. Following exposure to a new antigen, several days are required before both the cellular and humoral components of the immune system respond. Generalized antibodies (IgG and IgM) are initially released to help fight the antigen.

At the same time, other components of the immune system begin to develop antibodies specific for the antigen. These cells also develop a memory of the particular antigen. If the body is exposed to the same antigen again, the immune system responds much faster. This is called the *secondary response*. As a part of the secondary response, antibodies specific for the offending antigen are released. Antigen-specific antibodies are much more effective in facilitating removal of the offending antigen than the generalized antibodies released during the primary response.

ALLERGIES

The initial exposure of an individual to an antigen is referred to as **sensitization**. Sensitization results in an immune response. Subsequent exposure induces a much stronger secondary response. Generally, a person is not made uncomfortable by, and does not even notice, this kind of normal immune response.

However, some individuals can become *hypersensitive* (overly sensitive) to a particular antigen. **Hypersensitivity** is an unexpected and exaggerated reaction to a particular antigen, which usually results in some kind of discomfort for the individual. *Hypersensitivity* is often used synonymously with the term **allergy**. There are two types of hypersensitivity reactions: delayed and immediate.

Delayed Hypersensitivity

Delayed hypersensitivity is a result of cellular immunity and does not involve antibodies. Delayed hypersensitivity usually occurs in hours and days following exposure and is the sort of allergy that occurs in normal people. Delayed hypersensitivity most commonly results in a skin rash and is often due to exposure to certain drugs and chemicals. The rash associated with poison ivy is an example of delayed hypersensitivity.

Immediate Hypersensitivity

When people use the term "allergy," they are usually referring to immediate hypersensitivity reactions. Examples of immediate hypersensitivity reactions include hay fever, drug allergies, food allergies, eczema, and asthma. Some persons have an allergic tendency, known as **atopy**. This allergic tendency is usually genetic, meaning it is passed from parent to child, and is characterized by the presence of large quantities of **immunoglobulin E (IgE)** antibodies. An antigen that causes release of the IgE antibodies is referred to as an **allergen**.

Following exposure to a particular allergen, large quantities of IgE are released. Among other things, IgE becomes attached to the membranes of basophiles and mast cells. *Basophiles* and *mast cells* are specialized cells of the immune system which contain chemicals that assist in the immune response. When the allergen binds to IgE attached to the mast cells and basophiles, these cells release histamine, heparin, and other substances into the surrounding tissues. Histamine and the other substances are stored in *granules* found within the basophiles and mast cells. In fact, because of this feature, basophiles and mast cells are often called *granulocytes*. The process of releasing these substances from the cells is called *degranulation*. This release results in what people call an *allergic reaction*. An allergic reaction can range from very mild to very severe.

The principal chemical mediator of an allergic reaction is histamine. **Histamine** is a potent substance which causes bronchoconstriction, increased intestinal motility, vasodilation, and increased vascular permeability. Increased vascular permeability causes the leakage of fluid from the circulatory system into the surrounding tissues. Histamine acts on specialized histamine receptors present throughout the body. There are two classes of histamine receptors. H1 receptors, when stimulated, cause bronchoconstriction and contraction of the intestines. H2 receptors cause peripheral vasodilation and secretion of gastric acids.

The goal of histamine release is to minimize the body's exposure to the antigen. Bronchoconstriction decreases the possibility of the antigen entering through the respiratory tract. Increased gastric acid production helps destroy an ingested antigen. Increased intestinal motility serves to move the antigen quickly through the gastrointestinal system with minimal absorption of the antigen into the body. Vasodilation and capillary permeability help remove the allergen from the circulation where it has the potential to do the most harm.

■ **atopy** a clinical hypersensitivity state, or allergy, with a genetic predisposition.

■ **immunoglobulin E (IgE)** the antibody that is released in response to an antigen and that contributes to allergic and anaphylactic reactions.

■ **allergen** a substance capable of inducing allergy of specific hypersensitivity. Allergens may be protein or non-protein, although most are proteins.

■ **histamine** a product of mast cells and basophiles that causes vasodilation, capillary permeability, bronchoconstriction, and contraction of the gut.

ANAPHYLAXIS

As stated at the beginning of this chapter, the most severe type of allergic reaction is termed *anaphylaxis*. Anaphylaxis usually occurs when a specific allergen is injected directly into the circulatory system. This is the reason anaphylaxis is more common following injections of drugs and diagnostic agents and following bee stings.

When the allergen enters the circulation, it is distributed widely throughout the body. The allergen interacts with both basophiles and mast cells, resulting in the massive dumping of histamine and other substances associated with anaphylaxis. The principal body systems affected by anaphylaxis are the skin, the respiratory system, the cardiovascular system, the gastrointestinal system, and the nervous system. Histamine causes widespread peripheral vasodilation, as well as increased permeability of the capillaries. Increased capillary permeability results in "leaking" and a marked loss of plasma from the circulation. People sustaining anaphylaxis can actually die from circulatory shock.

Also released from the basophiles and mast cells is a substance called *slow-reacting substance of anaphylaxis (SRA)*. This causes spasm of the bronchiole smooth-muscle causing an asthma-like attack and occasionally asphyxia. SRA potentiates the effects of histamine, especially on the respiratory system.

Clinical Features of Anaphylaxis

The signs and symptoms of anaphylaxis begin within 30–60 seconds following exposure to the offending allergen. In a small percentage of patients, the onset of signs and symptoms may be delayed over an hour. The severity of the reaction is often related to the speed of onset. Reactions that develop very quickly tend to be much more severe.

The signs and symptoms of anaphylaxis can vary significantly. Patients suffering an anaphylactic reaction often have a sense of impending doom. This is followed by flushing, generalized itching (*pruritus*), and an increase in heart rate. Often there is the immediate development of hives (**urticaria**). Itching and hives are the most common manifestations. As shown in Table 25-2, virtually all body systems may be affected in anaphylaxis or other allergic reactions.

■ **urticaria** the raised areas, or wheals, that occur on the skin, associated with vasodilation due to histamine release; commonly called "hives."

TABLE 25-2 Clinical Presentation of Allergies and Anaphylaxis

Skin
flushing
itching
hives
swelling
cyanosis

Respiratory System
respiratory difficulty
sneezing, coughing
wheezing, stridor
laryngeal edema
laryngeospasm
bronchospasm

Cardiovascular System
vasodilation
increased heart rate
decreased blood pressure

Gastrointestinal System
nausea and vomiting
abdominal cramping
diarrhea

Nervous System
dizziness
headache
convulsions
tearing

ASSESSMENT

As with any emergency, the initial step in the management of suspected anaphylaxis is to complete the primary assessment, particularly evaluation of the patient's airway, breathing, and circulation to detect and correct any immediate threats to the patient's life. The primary assessment should be followed by a more detailed secondary assessment.

Primary Assessment

The first step in the primary assessment is to evaluate the airway. Laryngeal edema is a frequent complication of anaphylaxis and can threaten the airway. Initially, laryngeal edema will cause a hoarse voice. As the edema worsens, the patient may develop stridor. Finally, complete airway obstruction may develop, resulting from either massive laryngeal edema or laryngospasm or both.

Any problems with the airway must be immediately corrected before moving to the next step of the primary assessment. If an airway problem is detected, first apply basic airway maneuvers such as head positioning or the modified jaw-thrust maneuver. Use oropharyngeal and nasopharyngeal airways with caution as they can cause laryngospasm.

If the patient is having severe airway problems, consider early endotracheal intubation to prevent complete occlusion of the airway. It is important to remember that the glottic opening may be smaller than expected due to laryngeal edema. Because of this, a smaller-than-average endotracheal tube may be needed. Also, it is important to remember that the larynx will be very irritable and any manipulation of the airway may lead to laryngospasm. Ideally, the most experienced member of the crew should perform endotracheal intubation, as one attempt may be all that will be possible. Equipment for placement of a surgical airway, such as a needle cricothyrotomy, should be available in case it is needed.

After assessing and managing the airway, evaluate breathing. As detailed earlier in the chapter, anaphylaxis adversely affects the respiratory system. Bronchospasm is a common finding in anaphylaxis. First, evaluate the rate and depth of breathing. Often the patient will be tachypneic, but will have shallow respirations. Quickly auscultate both sides of the chest. Wheezing indicates bronchospasm. Beware of the silent chest as this can indicate severe bronchospasm with minimal air movement. The first step is to administer high-flow oxygen with a nonrebreather mask. If respirations are shallow, consider assisting them with positive-pressure ventilation. Patients with significant dyspnea may require endotracheal intubation and mechanical ventilation.

Next evaluate circulation. Anaphylaxis causes peripheral vasodilation and increased capillary permeability. Both can cause hypotension. The pulse rate may be either fast or slow depending on the stage of the illness. Be prepared to provide CPR if the pulse is absent.

During the primary assessment, be sure to obtain a baseline assessment of the patient's mental status, using the AVPU scale. One of the earliest signs and symptoms of shock is a change in the patient's mental status. The patient's mental status may deteriorate as the condition worsens. Thus it is important to monitor the patient's mental status over time using objective criteria.

Always consider the possibility of trauma in anaphylaxis. If there is any suspicion of coincidental trauma, stabilize the cervical spine. It is not uncommon for people to injure themselves as they try to escape from wasps and bees. They may fall or otherwise cause an injury. The signs and symptoms of trauma may be masked by the signs and symptoms of anaphylaxis. Always err on the side of safety and immobilize if there is any possibility of cervical spine injury.

Secondary Assessment

When performing the secondary assessment on a patient with a severe allergic reaction or anaphylaxis, concentrate on the skin, the respiratory system, the cardiovascular system, and the gastrointestinal system—the body areas most affected by the mediators of anaphylaxis.

Begin at the head and pay particular attention to the airway. A hoarse voice, stridor, or a croupy cough can indicate laryngeal edema or spasm. Quickly evaluate the chest by inspection, palpation, and auscultation. Listen closely for wheezing and reduced airflow. Next turn your attention to the gastrointestinal system. Note particularly any nausea, vomiting, or diarrhea. These are all associated with histamine release. Check peripheral pulses. Also note the presence of edema. Many patients will have hives—raised red blotches across the body. They are primarily due to histamine release which causes plasma leakage resulting in the classic whelps.

The vital signs are an important part of the secondary assessment. Accurately determine the pulse rate, respiratory rate, and blood pressure. The vital signs should be repeated frequently. Use pulse oximetry (if available) and continuous ECG monitoring

MANAGEMENT

Complete the primary and secondary assessment as soon as possible. Apply airway management techniques as needed and administer oxygen via a nonrebreather mask. Place the patient in a supine position with legs slightly elevated and apply a blanket or other covering to maintain body temperature.

Fluid and Pharmacological Therapy

Intravenous fluid replacement is critical in preventing hypovolemia and hypotension. As soon as possible, establish an IV with a crystalloid solution such as lactated Ringer's or normal saline. If the patient is hypotensive, fluids should be administered wide open. If time allows, place a second IV line.

The principal treatment of anaphylaxis is pharmacological. Emergency medications used in the treatment of anaphylaxis include epinephrine, antihistamines, and corticosteroids. Occasionally, inhaled beta agonists, such as albuterol, may be required.

Epinephrine   The primary drug for treatment of severe allergic reactions and anaphylaxis is epinephrine. (See Table 25-3.) Epinephrine is a sympathetic agonist. It causes an increase in heart rate, an increase in the strength of the cardiac contractile force, and peripheral vasoconstriction. Epinephrine also reverses much of the capillary permeability caused by histamine. It acts within minutes of administration and can reverse the effects of anaphylaxis quickly.

In severe anaphylaxis, characterized by hypotension and/or severe airway obstruction, epinephrine 1:10,000 should be administered intravenously.

* Epinephrine is the primary drug for management of anaphylaxis.

TABLE 25-3	Epinephrine
Class:	Sympathomimetic
Actions:	Bronchodilation
	Positive chronotrope
	Positive inotrope
Indications:	Cardiac arrest
	Anaphylaxis
	Allergic Reactions
	Bronchial asthma
	Exacerbation of COPD
Contraindications:	Patients with serious underlying cardiovascular disease
	Hypertension
	Pregnancy
Precautions:	Should be protected from light
	Blood pressure, pulse, and ECG must be constantly monitored
Side Effects:	Palpitations
	Anxiousness
	Headache
Dosage:	*Epinephrine 1:1,000 (1 mg epinephrine in 1 mL solvent)*
	Mild-moderate allergic reaction
	Bronchial asthma
	Exacerbation of COPD
	0.3–0.5 mg (0.3–0.5mL) subcutaneously
	Epinephrine 1:10,000 (1 mg epinephrine in 10 mL solvent)
	Cardiac arrest
	0.5–1.0 mg (5–10 mL) intravenously or endotracheally
	Anaphylaxis
	0.3–0.5 mg (3–5 mL) intravenously or endotracheally
Route:	Subcutaneously (1:1,000)
	Intravenously (1:10,000)
	Endotracheally (1:10,000)
	Intraosseously (1:10,000)
Pediatric Dosage:	0.01 mg/kg up to 0.3 mg

Epinephrine 1:10,000 contains 1 milligram of epinephrine in 10 milliliters of solvent. The standard adult dose of epinephrine is 0.3–0.5 milligrams. The effects of intravenous epinephrine wear off in 3–5 minutes. Repeat boluses may be required. In severe cases of sustained anaphylaxis, medical control may order the preparation and administration of an epinephrine drip.

Lesser allergic reactions and simple urticaria, which are not accompanied by hypotension or airway problems, can be adequately treated with epinephrine 1:1,000 administered subcutaneously. Epinephrine 1:1,000 contains 1 milligram of epinephrine in 1 milliliter of solvent. When administered into the subcutaneous tissue, the drug is absorbed more slowly and the effect is more prolonged when compared to the intravenous route. The subcutaneous dose is the same as the intravenous dose (0.3–0.5 milligram). The subcutaneous route should not be used in severe anaphylaxis. Many physicians prefer to give epinephrine 1:1,000 intramuscularly. This has a faster rate of onset, but a shorter duration of action. Side-effects associated with epinephrine (tremor, palpitations, tachycardia, hypertension) are most pronounced when the drug is given intravenously.

The dosage of epinephrine should be reduced for children. The standard pediatric dose is 0.01 milligram of epinephrine per kilogram of body weight. The 1:10,000 dilution should be used for intravenous administration while the 1:1,000 dilution should be used for subcutaneous administration.

Antihistamines   **Antihistamines** are second-line agents in the treatment of anaphylaxis. They should only be given following the administration of epinephrine. Antihistamines block the harmful effects of histamine by blocking histamine receptors. They do not displace histamine from the receptors, only block additional histamine from binding. They also help reduce histamine release from mast cells and basophiles. Most antihistamines are non-selective and block both H1 and H2 receptors. Others are selective for either H1 or H2 histamine receptors.

Diphenhydramine (Benadryl) is probably the most frequently used antihistamine in the treatment of allergic reactions and anaphylaxis. (See Table 25-4.) It

■ **antihistamine** a substance that counteracts the effects of histamine. Most antihistamines compete with histamine for available histamine receptors.

TABLE 25-4 Diphenhydramine (Benadryl®)	
Class:	Antihistamine
Actions:	Blocks histamine receptors
	Has some sedative effects
Indications:	Anaphylaxis
	Allergic Reactions
Contraindications:	Asthma
	Nursing mothers
Precautions:	Hypotension
Side Effects:	Sedation
	Dries bronchial secretions
	Blurred vision
	Headache
	Palpitations
Dosage:	25–50 mg
Route:	Slow IV push
	Deep IM
Pediatric Dosage:	2–5 mg/kg

TABLE 25-5 Methylprednisolone (Solu-Medrol®)

Class:	Steroid
Actions:	Anti-inflammatory
	Suppresses immune response (especially in allergic/ anaphylactic reactions)
Indications:	Severe anaphylaxis
	Possibly effective as an adjunctive agent in the management of shock
Contraindications:	None in the emergency setting
Precautions:	Must be reconstituted and used promptly
	Onset of action may be 2–6 hours and thus should not be expected to be of use in the critical first hour following an anaphylactic reaction
Side Effects:	GI bleeding
	Prolonged wound healing
	Supression of natural steroids
Dosage:	125–250 mg
Route:	IV
	IM
Pediatric Dosage:	30 mg/kg

is non-selective and acts on both H1 and H2 receptors. The standard dose of diphenhydramine is 25–50 milligrams intravenously or intramuscularly. It should be administered slowly when given intravenously. The pediatric dose of diphenhydramine is 1–2 milligrams per kilogram of body weight. Other non-selective antihistamines frequently used are hydroxyzine (Atarax, Vistaril) and promethazine (Phenergan). Hydroxyzine is a potent antihistamine, but it can only be administered intramuscularly. Promethazine can be administered intravenously or intramuscularly, but it does not appear to be as potent as diphenhydramine.

Selective histamine blockers have been available for the last 15 to 20 years. These are primarily H2 blockers and used to treat ulcer disease. Blockade of the H2 receptors decreases gastric acid secretion. However, H2 receptors are also present in the peripheral blood vessels. Administration of H2 blockers conceivably will help reverse some of the vasodilation associated with anaphylaxis. The two most frequently used H2 blockers are cimetadine (Tagamet) and ranitidine (Zantac). Typically, 300 milligrams of cimetadine or 50 milligrams of ranitidine are administered by slow intravenous push (over 3–5 minutes). Some recent studies have questioned the effectiveness if H2 blockers in allergic reactions and anaphylaxis. These agents are also considerably more expensive than the non-selective antihistamines.

Corticosteroids   The corticosteroids are important in the treatment and prevention of anaphylaxis. However, they are of little benefit in the initial stages of treatment. Commonly used corticosteroids include methylprednisolone (Solu-Medrol) (See Table 25-5), hydrocortisone (Solu-Cortef), and dexamethasone (Decadron). Corticosteroids help suppress the inflammatory response associated with these emergencies.

Beta Agonists   Many patients with severe allergic reactions and anaphylaxis will develop bronchospasm, laryngeal edema, or both. In these cases, an inhaled beta agonist can be useful. The most frequently used beta agonist in prehospital care is albuterol (Ventolin, Proventil). Although usually used in the treatment of asthma, these agents will help reverse some of the bronchospasm and laryngeal edema associated with anaphylaxis. The adult patient should receive 2.5 milligrams of albuterol (0.5 milliliters in 3 milliliters of normal saline) via a hand-held nebulizer. Children should receive 0.15 milligram per kilogram of albuterol based on their weight. Other beta agonists, such as metaproterenol (Alupent) and isoetharine (Bronkosol) may be used instead of albuterol.

Other Agents   Several other drugs are available that are occasionally used in the treatment of anaphylaxis. These include aminophylline and cromolyn sodium. Aminophylline is a bronchodilator unrelated to the beta agonists. It can be administered by slow intravenous infusion to treat the bronchospasm associated with anaphylaxis. Cromolyn sodium (Intal) is not used in the treatment of allergic reactions and anaphylaxis, but is used as a preventative agent. Cromolyn sodium helps to stabilize the membranes of the mast cells, thus reducing the amount of histamine and other mediators released when these cells are stimulated.

SUMMARY

Fortunately, severe allergies and anaphylaxis are uncommon. However, when they do occur, they can progress quickly and result in death within minutes. The central physiological action in anaphylaxis is the massive release of histamine and other chemical mediators. Histamine causes bronchospasm, airway edema, peripheral vasodilation, and increased capillary permeability. The prehospital treatment of anaphylaxis is to reverse the effects of these agents.

Anaphylaxis can rapidly kill. It must be promptly recognized and treated.

The primary, and most important, drug used in the treatment of anaphylaxis is epinephrine. Epinephrine helps reverse the harmful effects of histamine. It also supports the blood pressure and reverses detrimental capillary leakage. Following the administration of epinephrine, potent antihistamines should be used to block the additional effects of the massive histamine release. Inhaled beta agonists are useful in cases of severe bronchospasm and upper airway involvement. Intravenous fluid replacement is crucial in preventing hypovolemia and hypotension.

The key to successful prehospital management of anaphylaxis is prompt recognition followed by the specific treatment described in this chapter.

FURTHER READING

Atkinson, T.P. and M.A. Kaliner. "Anaphylaxis," *The Medical Clinics of North America.*, Volume 6, Number 4, July, 1992.

Barrett, J.T. *Textbook of Immunology: An Introduction to Immunochemistry and Immunobiology*, 4th ed. Saint Louis: C.V. Mosby Company, 1983.

Bayer, Mark J., Barry H. Rumack, and Lee A. Wanke. *Toxicological Emergencies*. Bowie, MD: Brady Communications, 1984.

Bledsoe, Bryan E., Dwayne Clayden , and Frank J. Papa. *Prehospital Emergency Pharmacology, 4th ed.* Upper Saddle River, NJ: Prentice Hall, 1996.

Guyton, A.C. *Textbook of Medical Physiology*, 8th ed. Philadelphia: W.B. Saunders Company, 1991.

Runge, J.W. et. al. "Histamine Antagonists in the Treatment of Acute Allergic Reactions," *Annals of Emergency Medicine*, Volume 21, March, 1992.

Saryan, J.A .and J.M. O'Loughlin: "Anaphylaxis in Children," *Pediatric Annals*, Volume 21, Number 9, September, 1992.

Stoloff, R. et. al. "Emergency Medical Recognition and Management of Idiopathic Anaphylaxis," *The Journal of Emergency Medicine*, Volume 10, 1992.

Yunginger, J.W. "Anaphylaxis," *Current Problems in Pediatrics*, March, 1992.

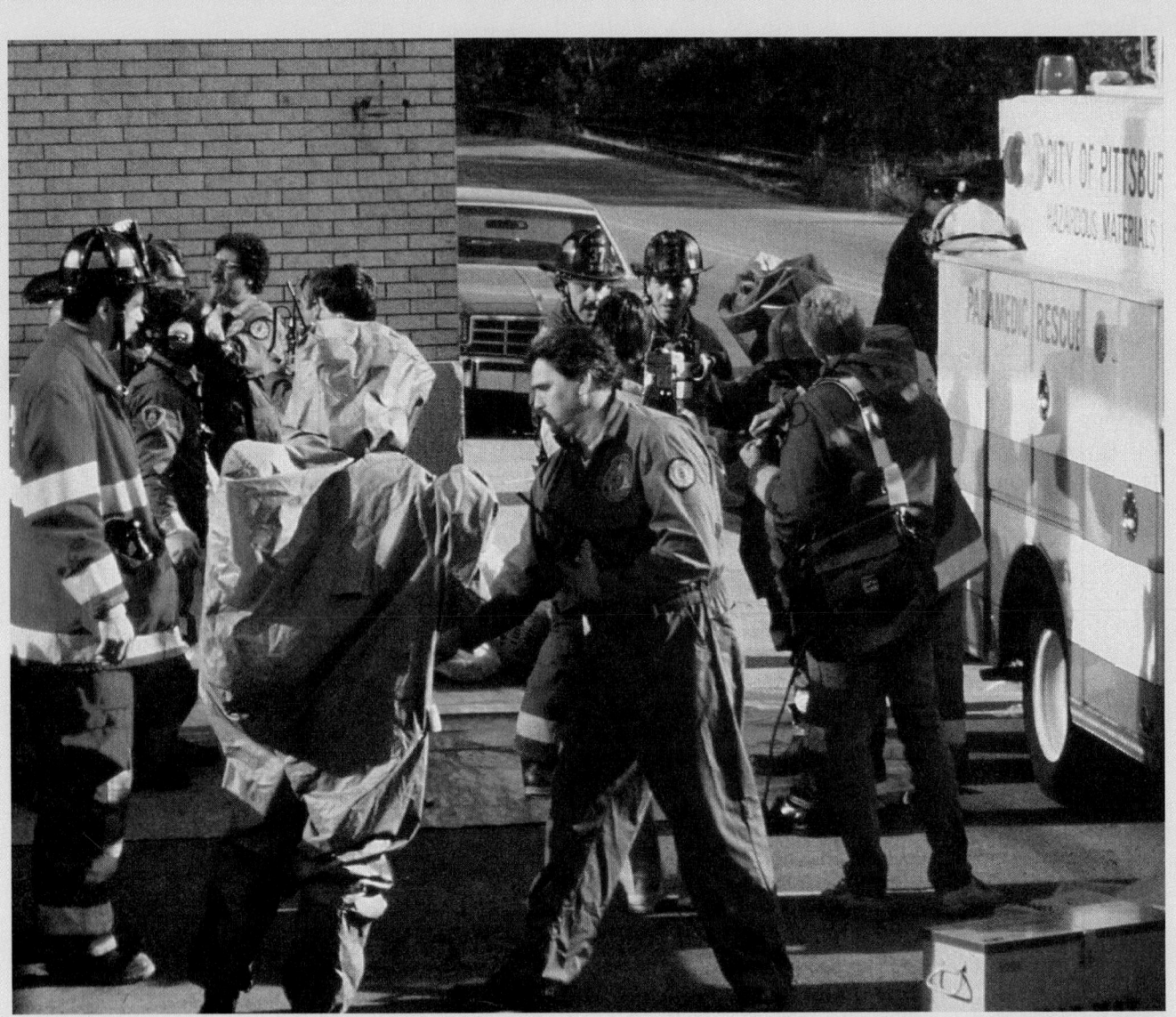

26

TOXICOLOGY AND SUBSTANCE ABUSE

Objectives for Chapter 26

After reading this chapter, you should be able to:

1. Discuss the importance of toxicological emergencies in prehospital care. (See p. 806.)

2. Describe the various entry routes of toxic substances into the body. (See pp. 807–809.)

3. Discuss the role of poison control centers within the EMS system. (See p. 809.)

4. Describe general principles of toxicologic management. (See p. 809.)

5. Relate general principles for assessing and managing patients who have ingested poison. (See pp. 812–817.)

6. Discuss the factors affecting the decision to induce vomiting in a patient who has ingested poison. (See pp. 812–813.)

7. Describe the signs, symptoms, and management of patients who have ingested the following toxins. (See below pages.)

- Antiemetics (pp. 814–815)
- Contaminated food (p. 815)
- Poisonous plants (pp. 815–816)
- Niacin (p. 816)
- Ethylene glycol/methanol (pp. 816–817)

8. Describe the presentation and treatment of the following toxic conditions. (See below pages.)

- Inhaled poisons (pp. 817–821)
- Injected poisons (pp. 821–829)
- Surface absorbed poisons (pp. 829–834)

9. Discuss the presentation and management of the following bites or stings. (See below pages.)

- *Hymenoptera* such as bees, hornets, wasps, or yellow jackets (pp. 821–822)
- Brown recluse spiders (pp. 822–824)
- Black widow spiders (p. 824)
- Scorpions (pp. 824–825)
- Pit vipers such as rattlesnakes, copperheads, or cotton–mouth water moccasins (pp. 826–827)
- Coral snakes (pp. 827–828)
- Marine animals (p. 828)

10. Discuss the general principles regarding the recognition and management of substance abuse. (See pp. 830–836.)

11. Identify some of the physiological signs and effects of chronic alcohol abuse. (See pp. 830–836.)

Paramedics spring to attention as a call comes into Rescue 190. The dispatcher reports an unconscious person at 1311 East Rosedale. The paramedics immediately recognize the address. It lays in a run-down part of town where drug use is rampant.

The paramedics arrive at the scene within a few minutes. Police officers meet paramedics and take them to a young male lying face down on the pavement. Evidently, the police found the patient during a drug raid.

The paramedics quickly complete the primary assessment. The patient is alive but unresponsive. They now start supportive ventilations with a demand valve. The secondary assessment reveals pin-point pupils and needle tracks on both arms.

The paramedics establish an IV and contact medical control. The medical control physician orders 1 mg of naloxone given intravenously at a slow rate. The blood glucose is 83 mg% by glucometer.

Shortly after administration of the naloxone, the patient begins to arouse. At first, he moans and then pushes away the demand valve. When the patient spots the police officers, he tries to get up, as if to run away. Officers quickly subdue him. The patient elects to go to the hospital instead of jail. But he refuses any additional care, including oxygen. The transport to the hospital is uneventful. The patient remains in the emergency department for four hours before being discharged.

INTRODUCTION

■ **toxicology** medical and biological science that studies the detection, chemistry, pharmacological actions, and antidotes of toxic substances.

The study of poisons and their antidotes is referred to as **toxicology**. Physicians or scientists who specialize in the field of toxicology are called *toxi-cologists*. Toxicological emergencies result from the ingestion, inhalation, injection, or surface absorption of toxic substances.

During recent years, toxicological emergencies have become more prevalent in society. The following figures reveal the high potential for involvement of a toxic substance on an EMS call.

❑ Over one million persons are poisoned annually.
❑ Ten percent of all emergency department visits and EMS responses involve toxic exposures.
❑ Seventy percent of accidental poisonings occur in children under the age of six years.
❑ A child who has experienced an accidental ingestion has a 25 percent chance of another, similar ingestion within one year.
❑ Eighty percent of all attempted suicides involve a drug overdose.

■ **poisoning** taking a substance into the body that interferes with normal physiological functions.

■ **overdose** a dose of a drug in excess of that usually prescribed. An overdose can adversely affect the patient's health.

Theoretically, all toxicological emergencies can be classified as **poisoning**. However, in this discussion, the term "poisoning" will be used to describe exposure to non-pharmacological substances. The term **overdose** will be used to describe exposure to pharmacological substances, whether the overdose is accidental or intentional. Substance abuse, although technically a form of poisoning, will be addressed separately.

In this chapter, we will discuss various aspects of toxicological emergencies as they apply to prehospital care. Rather than cover specific poisons in great detail, we will establish general treatment guidelines for each type of toxic exposure. Because of rapid changes in the field of toxicology, it will be virtually impossible for you to stay up-to-date on treatment protocols for each type of toxic exposure. Specific treatment should be directed by medical control in association with a **poison control center**. This system will ensure that the patient is receiving the most current level of care available.

■ **poison control center** information center staffed by trained personnel that provides up-to-date toxicologic information.

POISONING—AN OVERVIEW

The term "poisoning" usually refers to the accidental exposure of the body to toxic substances in an amount sufficient to have a damaging or destructive effect.

Routes of Toxic Exposure

In order to have a destructive effect, poisons must gain entrance into the body. The four portals of entry are ingestion, inhalation, injection, and surface absorption. (See Figure 26-1.) It is important to note that regardless of the portal of entry, toxic substances have both *immediate* and *delayed effects.*

Ingestion   **Ingestion** is the most common route of entry for toxic exposure. Frequently ingested poisons include:

❑ Household products
❑ Petroleum-based agents (gasoline, paint)

■ **ingestion** the entrance of a substance into the body through the gastrointestinal tract.

INHALATION

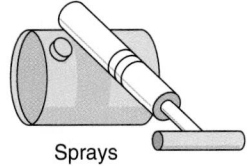

Sprays

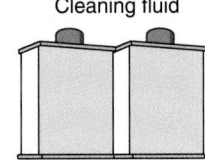

Cleaning fluid

INJECTION

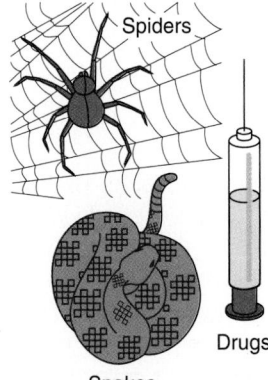

Spiders

Drugs

Snakes

INGESTION

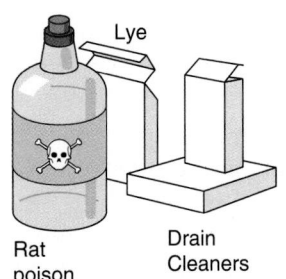

Lye

Rat poison

Drain Cleaners

ABSORPTION

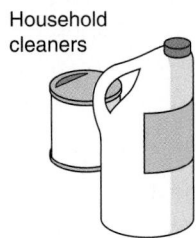

Household cleaners

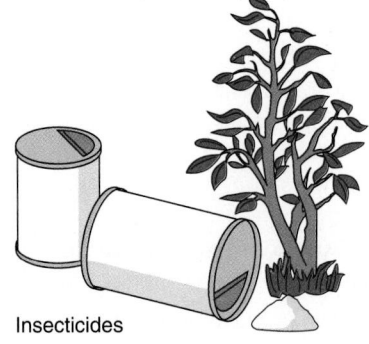

Insecticides

FIGURE 26-1 Routes of toxic exposure.

- Cleaning agents
- Cosmetics
- Medications—prescription, non-prescription, illicit
- Plants
- Foods

Immediate toxic effects of ingestion of corrosive substances such as strong acids or alkalis can involve burns to the lips, tongue, throat, and esophagus. Delayed effects can result from absorption of the poison from the gastrointestinal tract. Most absorption occurs in the small intestine, with only a small amount being absorbed from the stomach. Some poisons may remain in the stomach for up to several hours because the intake of a large bolus of poison can retard absorption. Aspirin ingestion is a classic example of this. When a patient ingests a large number of aspirin tablets, the tablets can bind together to form a large bolus that is difficult to remove.

Inhalation **Inhalation** of a poison results in rapid absorption of the toxic agent through the alveolar-capillary membrane. Inhaled toxins can irritate pulmonary passages causing extensive edema and destroying tissue. When these toxins are absorbed, wider systemic effects can occur. Causative agents can appear as gases, vapors, fumes, or aerosols. Commonly inhaled poisons include:

- Toxic gases
- Carbon monoxide
- Ammonia
- Chlorine
- Freon
- Toxic vapors, fumes, or aerosols
- Carbon tetrachloride
- Methylene chloride
- Tear gas (pepper and non-pepper lacrimators)
- Mustard gas
- Nitrous oxide

Injection **Injection** of a toxic agent under the skin, into muscle, or into the circulatory system also results in both immediate and delayed effects. The immediate local reaction is at the site of the injection. Later, as the toxin is distributed throughout the body by the circulatory system, delayed systemic reactions can occur. In addition, an allergic or anaphylactic reaction may appear.

Other than intentional injection of illicit drugs, most poisonings by injection result from the bites and stings of insects and animals. Most insects that sting and bite belong to the class *hymenoptera*, which includes bees, hornets, yellow jackets, wasps, and ants. Only the females in this group can sting. In addition, spiders, ticks, and other arachnids, such as scorpions, notoriously cause poisonings by injection. Higher life forms that bite and sting include snakes and marine animals. Marine animals with venomous stings include jellyfish (especially the Portuguese man-of-war), stingrays, anemones, coral, hydrae, and certain spiny fish.

Surface Absorption **Surface absorption** is the entry of a toxic substance through the skin. This most frequently occurs from contact with poisonous plants, such as poison ivy, poison sumac, and poison oak. Many toxic chemicals may also be absorbed through the skin. The organophosphates, often used as insecticides, are easily absorbed through dermal contact.

Poison Information Centers

Poison information centers have been set up across the United States and Canada to assist in the treatment of poison victims and to provide information on new products and new treatment recommendations. They are usually based in major medical centers and teaching hospitals that serve a large population. Most poison control centers now have computer systems that access information rapidly.

Poison information centers are usually staffed by physicians, pharmacists, nurses, or poison control specialists trained in toxicology. These experts provide information to callers 24 hours a day. They update information routinely and offer the most current treatment protocols.

Memorize the number of the nearest poison information center and routinely access it. There are several advantages to this practice. First, the poison control center can help you immediately determine potential toxicity based on the type of agent, amount and time of exposure, and physical condition of the patient. Second, in about four out of five cases, the most current, definitive treatment can be started in the field. Finally, the poison information center can notify the receiving hospital of current treatment even before arrival of the patient.

* Paramedics should routinely access their local or state poison information center for additional information regarding a poisoning or overdose.

GENERAL PRINCIPLES OF TOXICOLOGIC MANAGEMENT

Although specific protocols may vary for managing toxicological emergencies, certain basic principles apply to most situations.

Scene Survey

Begin assessment with a thorough evaluation of the scene. Be alert for potential hazards to the rescuer. In toxicological emergencies, put rescuer safety first. Despite a strong desire to assist and treat patients, you will be useless if incapacitated. To ensure rescuer safety, keep the following tips in mind.

❑ Suicidal patients have the potential for violence. Therefore, look for signs of overdose such as empty pill bottles.
❑ In chemical emergencies or spills involving hazardous material, make sure the proper clothing and equipment are available. Assign these materials to rescuers who have been trained in their use.

By taking such precautions, you will avoid turning rescuers into patients.

Primary and Secondary Survey

Once you have evaluated the scene, begin the standard primary survey. Pay particular attention to the airway and respiratory status. Following the primary survey, complete the secondary survey and develop a patient history. (For guidelines on the history, see page 811.) Relay information to the local poison information center. Using the most current treatment, limit absorption and enhance elimination of the poison. If indicated, administer an **antidote**.

* The general principles of poisoning management are to limit absorption and enhance elimination of the poison.

■ **antidote** a substance that neutralizes a poison or the effects of a poison.

TABLE 26-1	Ipecac
Class:	Emetic
Actions:	Irritates the enteric tract
	Stimulates vomiting center
Indications:	Poisoning in conscious patient
Contraindications:	Vomiting should not be induced in any patient with impaired consciousness
	Poisonings involving strong acids, bases, or petroleum distillates
	Vomiting should not be induced in individuals who have ingested an agent that can cause a rapid decrease in consciousness
Precautions:	Monitor and assure a patent airway
Side Effects:	Rare
Dosage:	30 mL (1 ounce) followed by several glasses of warm water
Route:	Oral
Pediatric Dosage:	Less than 1 year of age: 5–10 mL
	Greater than 1 year of age: 15 mL repeated in 20 minutes
	Greater than 12 years of age: 30 mL.

Decontamination

To minimize the extent of toxicity, consider decontamination, especially of the gastrointestinal tract. *Activated charcoal* promotes gastrointestinal decontamination because it has a large surface area that can adsorb molecules from the offending poison. In some cases of ingestion, an emetic agent, such as *syrup of ipecac*, can be used to empty the stomach. (See Tables 26-1 and 26-2.) If the patient is unconscious or uncooperative, syrup of ipecac can be withheld and the stomach can be emptied by inserting a nasogastric tube and aspirating stomach contents. This is often followed by repeated irrigations and aspirations of the stomach with water or a similar solution. Finally, gastrointestinal decontamination can be carried out using a cathartic agent. Cathartics speed passage of the poison through the gastrointestinal system, thereby decreasing absorption.

After decontamination, turn your attention to supportive care. Confirm patient status with the poison control center. Remain alert for respiratory, cardiovascular, or neurological complications—situations that often occur in toxicological patients. (In the following sections, you will find suggestions for managing specific toxicological emergencies.)

INGESTED POISONS

Poisoning by ingestion is the most common route encountered in prehospital care. Prompt and accurate assessment, followed by appropriate prehospital treatment, is essential.

General Principles of Assessment

In cases of ingestion, it takes time for the poison to make its way from the gastrointestinal system into the circulatory system. Therefore, you need to find out not only what was ingested, but when it was ingested. A thorough patient history is essential to patient management.

Taking the History   Begin your history by trying to find out the type of poison ingested, route of intoxication, the quantity of the poison, the time elapsed since ingestion, and whether the patient took any alcohol or other potentiating substance. Ask the victim about drug habituation or abuse. Inquire about underlying medical illnesses and allergies. In cases of poisoning, remember that inaccuracies creep into nearly half the histories because of drug-induced confusion, patient misinformation, or deliberate patient attempts at deception. Therefore, suspect information given by patients in cases of drug overdoses.

✳ The history in a drug overdose patient may be unreliable.

Before leaving a suicidal patient who claims to have been "just kidding," consider the legal ramifications. You may be charged later with patient abandonment. At the same time, be aware of protective custody laws in your state. If in doubt on whether or not to place the patient in protective custody, contact your local law enforcement agency.

The following questions will help you to develop a relevant history.

❑ What did you ingest? (Obtain pill containers and any remaining contents, samples of the ingested substance, or samples of vomitus. Bring with patient to ED.)
❑ When did you ingest the substance? (Time affects your decision to use emesis, gastric lavage, activated charcoal, or an antidote.)
❑ How much did you take (or eat)?
❑ Did you drink any alcohol?
❑ Have you attempted to induce vomiting?
❑ Have you done anything to treat yourself?
❑ Have you been under psychiatric care? If so, why? (Answers may indicate a potential for suicide.)
❑ What do you weigh?

Physical Examination   Since the history can be unreliable, the physical examination assumes an important role. The physical examination of the poisoned patient has two purposes: (1) to provide physical evidence of intoxication, and (2) to find any underlying illnesses that may account for the patient's symptoms or that may affect the outcome of the poisoning. As you complete the primary and secondary assessments, pay attention to the following patient features.

❑ *Skin.* Is there evidence of cyanosis, pallor, wasting, or needle marks? Flushing of the skin may indicate poisoning with an anticholinergic substance. Staining of the skin may occur from chronic exposure to mercuric chloride, bromine, or similar chemicals.
❑ *Eyes.* Pupillary constriction or dilation occurs with various types of poisons (marijuana, methamphetamines, narcotics). Inquire about impaired vision, blurring of vision, or coloration of vision.
❑ *Mouth.* Inspect the mouth for signs of caustic ingestion, presence of gag reflex, amount of salivation, any breath odor, or presence of vomitus.
❑ *Breath.* Breath sounds may reveal evidence of aspiration, atelectasis, or excessive pulmonary secretions.
❑ *Circulation.* Cardiac examination may give clues about the type of poison ingested. For example, the presence of tachydysrhythmias (methamphetamine) or bradydysrhythmias (organophosphates) may suggest specific toxins such as those shown in parentheses.

❏ *Abdomen*. Abdominal pain may result from poisoning by salicylates, methyl alcohol, or caustics.

It is not unusual for a rescuer to be confronted with a patient that has ingested a combination of drugs, either in a suicide attempt or in an effort to get "high." These multiple ingestions present a therapeutic dilemma. Each chemical not only acts by itself, it may also act synergically with the others. A common example of this is the "speedball" (heroin mixed with cocaine). If the narcotic overdose is treated, the rescuer is often presented with a patient that is now in a cocaine-induced catecholamine crisis (tachycardia, hypertension, seizures).

It is important to learn the regional names for street drugs. But this is no guarantee of accuracy. Street terminology changes from area to area. A "hit" of cocaine ("blow," "coke," "snort," or a dozen other names) may mean whatever amount the body can handle—from 2–200 mg.

General Principles of Management

As mentioned previously, priorities in the treatment of the poisoned patient are maintenance of airway, breathing, and circulation. Prevention of aspiration is one of the major objectives of prehospital care. Aspiration pneumonia is a serious concern in the definitive care of the toxic patient.

Assess the adequacy of the patient's airway by observing ventilatory effort, estimating the force and volume of expiration, and detecting any sounds of obstructed breathing. In cases that require more definitive airway management, endotracheal intubation (orally or nasally) may be necessary. Generally, nasal intubation is preferred for patients who have a gag reflex. This may be checked by brushing the eyelashes. If there is a blink reflex, there is probably an intact gag reflex. High-flow oxygen supplementation should be routinely performed.

Inducement of Vomiting

If the patient has ingested the toxic substance within 60–90 minutes of your arrival, contact the local poison control center. Toxicologists at the center or the medical control physician may recommend inducement of vomiting before arrival at the hospital emergency department. When considering decontamination, keep these guidelines in mind.

Vomiting must NOT be induced in the following patients.

❏ Patients with current or potential for decreased level of consciousness
❏ In seizure patients or in patients with the immediate potential for seizures (strychnine)
❏ Patients with possible MI
❏ Patients who have ingested corrosive substances (strong **acids** such as hydrochloric acid or strong **alkalis** such as sodium hydroxide/lye)
❏ Patients who have ingested hydrocarbon substances (petroleum-based products)
❏ Patients who have taken specific drugs such as antiemetics or cyclic/tricyclic antidepressants (due to the rapid onset of unconsciousness and seizures)

However, there are exceptions even in the above circumstances. Vomiting SHOULD be induced if the patient has ingested any of the following substances:

■ **acid** a chemical substance that liberates hydrogen ions (H$^+$) when in solution.

■ **alkali** a strong base; a substance that liberates hydroxyl ions (OH$^-$) when in solution.

TABLE 26-2 Activated Charcoal

Class:	Absorbent
Action:	Absorbs toxins by chemical binding and its large surface area
Indications:	Poisoning following emesis or where emesis is contraindicated
Contraindications:	None in severe poisoning
Precautions:	Should only be administered following emesis in cases where it is so indicated
Side Effects:	Rare
Dosage:	Two tablespoons (50 grams) mixed with a glass of water to form a slurry
Route:	Oral
Pediatric Dosage:	Two tablespoons (50 grams) mixed with a glass of water to form a slurry

❏ Pesticides (NOT organophosphates)
❏ Heavy metals
❏ Halogenated hydrocarbons (carbon tetrachloride, some insecticides)
❏ Aromatic hydrocarbons (benzene, toluene)

Because these substances have such a high toxicity, the risk of aspiration can be justified. If possible, the poison control center should be contacted for assistance. Activated charcoal can often be administered in the field. (See Table 26-2.) If administered, activated charcoal should be given as follows. (The use of premixed preparations such as Actidose is encouraged.)

❏ *Adult:* 50–100 g mixed in tap water to make a slurry
❏ *Pediatric:* 20–50 g (1 g/kg) mixed in tap water to make a slurry

Unless contraindicated, initiate vomiting as soon as possible. If ordered by medical control or the poison center, administer syrup of ipecac in the following doses.

❏ 10 mL in patients < 1 yr of age
❏ 15 mL in patients 1–12 yrs of age
❏ 30 mL in patients over 12 yrs of age

Water should be given in a dose of 15 mL/kg (2–3 glasses in the adult) following the ipecac. If vomiting has not occurred within 20–30 minutes, the ipecac can be readministered. The patient should be appropriately positioned to prevent aspiration. Some toxicologists advocate giving the patient a carbonated beverage after the ipecac because this may stimulate vomiting more rapidly. Also, if water is not available, any acceptable beverage may be given after the ipecac (fruit juice, soda, etc.).

Administration of Fluids and Drugs   As soon as you have assured airway, breathing, and circulation, establish an IV. An IV of LR or NS at a TKO rate is recommended for all potentially dangerous ingestions. Maintenance of blood pressure requires adequate intravascular volume, cardiac function, and systemic vascular resistance. In addition to volume replacement with a crystal-loid solution, cardiac monitoring is necessary. Repeated assessments, including frequent monitoring of vital signs, are mandatory.

Many areas utilize a diagnostic regimen consisting of D50W, naloxone, and thiamine ("coma cocktail"). However, recent research has questioned the role of glucose administration without documented hypoglycemia. As a rule, administer glucose only after determining the presence of hypoglycemia. The unavailability of blood glucose level determining chemstrips or glucometers may alter this procedure. If hypoglycemia is indicated, administer 25–50 g of D50W IV push.

Narcotics affect the respiratory drive. Therefore, respiratory depression is a classic sign of narcotic overdosage. If opiate intoxication is suspected because of respiratory compromise or pinpoint pupils, administer naloxone at 1–2 mg IV push. If chronic alcoholism is suspected, consider administration of 100 mg of thiamine IV.

Physicians sometimes prescribe a group of drugs called the *phenothiazines* for use as antipsychotics, narcotic potentiators, and antiemetics. These drugs may cause *extrapyramidal effects* in patients that are sensitive to them. Adverse reactions have a striking presentation as various muscle groups become dystonic. A patient may report the following signs.

- ❑ Eye deviation
- ❑ Head deviation to one side or the other
- ❑ Difficulty speaking due to a "thick" tongue
- ❑ Involuntary arm or leg twitching/jerking

Fortunately, these reactions may be alleviated with the administration of diphenhydramine. An IV should be established, and 25–50 mg of diphenhydramine (Benadryl) may be given IV push (2 mg/kg in children). Diphenhydramine normally reverses the extrapyramidal effects quickly with great relief to the patient.

Specific Ingested Toxins

A wide range of potentially fatal substances can be swallowed by patients, especially children. It is impossible to cover all the substances that you may encounter in the field (hence the need for regular contact with your local poison control center). The following are some of the most commonly ingested toxins.

Antiemetics A variety of drugs have antiemetic properties and toxicity in larger doses. Management of these ingestions requires an evaluation of location and circumstances of the patient. Contact with the poison control center is highly recommended. If contact cannot be made, you may induce vomiting under the following circumstances.

- ❑ If the patient is conscious.
- ❑ If ingestion has been less than 30 minutes.
- ❑ You have an idea of the amount of antiemetic ingested.

If there will be a short transport time, induction of emesis can be withheld since NG tube placement, lavage, and administration of activated charcoal can be carried out at the hospital. In the event of a prolonged transport time (over 1 hour), NG tube and lavage/activated charcoal may be initiated by the rescuer. This type of ingestion is best discussed ahead of time with the local medical control physician/toxicologist.

Contaminated Food   Food poisoning is caused by a spectrum of different factors. For example, bacteria, viruses, and toxic chemicals notoriously produce varying levels of gastrointestinal distress. The patient may present with nausea, vomiting, and diarrhea. Diffuse abdominal pain is another common complaint.

Bacterial food poisonings range in severity. Bacterial exotoxins or enterotoxins cause the adverse GI complaints noted above. Food contaminated with other bacteria such as *Shigella, Salmonella* or *E. coli* can produce even more severe GI reactions, often leading to electrolyte imbalance and hypovolemia. *Clostridium botulinum*, the world's most toxic poison, presents as severe respiratory distress or arrest. The incubation of this toxin can range from 4 hours to 8 days. Fortunately, *botulism* rarely occurs, except in cases of improper food storage methods such as canning.

A variety of seafood poisonings also occurs. Specific toxins found in dinoflagellate contaminated shellfish such as clams, mussels, oysters, and scallops can produce a syndrome referred to as paralytic shellfish poisoning. This condition can lead to respiratory arrest in addition to standard GI symptoms.

Increased fish consumption by North Americans has also increased the number of cases of fish poisonings from toxins found in many commonly eaten fish. *Ciguatera poisoning* most frequently turns up in fish caught in the Pacific Ocean or along the tropical reefs of Florida and the West Indies. Ciguatera normally takes 2–6 hours to incubate. It may also produce myalgia and paresthesias. *Scombroid (histamine) poisoning* results from bacterial contamination of mackerel, tuna, bonita, and albacore. Both types of poisoning cause the common GI symptoms. Scombroid poisoning will present with an immediate facial flushing as histamines cause vasodilation.

Treatment. Except for botulism, food poisoning is rarely life threatening. Treatment, therefore, is largely supportive. In suspected cases of food poisoning, take the following steps.

- ❏ Perform the necessary primary and secondary assessment.
- ❏ Collect samples of the suspected contaminated food source.
- ❏ Perform the following management actions.
  - Establish and maintain the airway.
  - Administer high-flow oxygen.
  - Intubate and assist ventilations, if appropriate.
  - Use a bag-valve-mask or demand valve.
  - Establish venous access.
  - Contact poison control.
  - Consider the use of syrup of ipecac, if poison control is unavailable.

Poisonous Plants   Plants, trees, and mushrooms contribute heavily to the number of accidental ingestions found in the home. While the vast majority of plants are nontoxic, many of the popular decorative houseplants can present a danger to children who frequently ingest non-food items. Most poison control centers distribute pamphlets that identify toxic household plants. (These pamphlets will help "poison proof" the home.)

It is impossible to cover all the toxic ingestions due to plants and mushrooms. Few rescuers are trained as botanists, and they find it difficult to identify the offending material. Mushrooms are particularly difficult to identify from small pieces. Plus, most people recognize mushrooms by common names rather than scientific species.

A general approach is to obtain a sample of the plant, if possible. Try to find a full leaf, stem, and any flowers. Since many of the ornamental plants contain irritating chemicals or crystals, examine the mouth and throat for erythema, blistering, or edema. Identify other abnormal signs during the secondary evaluation.

Mushroom poisonings generally fall into two categories: people seeking edible mushrooms and accidental ingestions by children. Fortunately, few of the many mushroom species possess extremely dangerous toxins. Toxic mushrooms fall into seven classes. *Amanita* and *Galerina* belong to the deadly *cyclopeptide group.* (*Amanita* accounts for over 90 percent of all deaths.) These mushrooms produce a poison that is extremely toxic to the liver, with a mortality rate about 50 percent. Signs include:

❑ Excessive salivation, lacrimation, diaphoresis
❑ Abdominal cramps, nausea, vomiting, diarrhea
❑ Decreasing levels of consciousness, eventually progressing to coma

For guidance on the treatment of plant poisonings, call the poison control center. If contact cannot be made, refer to the treatment of food poisoning on page 815.

Niacin *Niacin* or *nicotinic acid* is a water soluble B vitamin that is prescribed for hypertriglyceridemia and hypercholesteremia. It is also used as a health food supplement. Unfortunately, some patients will experience a pronounced reaction that consists of the following signs or symptoms.

❑ Profuse flushing
❑ Itching
❑ Burning
❑ Tingling sensations

This is a self-limited reaction. Assure the patient that he or she is not seriously ill. Then suggest that the patient contact his or her physician for a change in dosage or the substitution of niacinamide (which does not produce this reaction).

Ethylene Glycol/Methanol *Ethylene glycol* and *methanol* (methyl alcohol) are used in a variety of automotive products and cooking fuel. Both are toxic when ingested. Consumption of as little as 4 cc of methanol has produced blindness, while 10 cc has caused death. Both are consumed occasionally by chronic alcoholics trying to get intoxicated.

Signs of Methanol Poisoning. The metabolic byproduct of methanol is formic acid and formaldehyde, both of which are extremely toxic to nervous tissue. The signs and symptoms of methanol ingestion include:

❑ Abdominal pain
❑ Nausea, vomiting
❑ Apparent signs of intoxication
❑ Tachypnea/hyperpnea
❑ Blindness

Treatment. In suspected cases of methanol poisoning, take the following steps.

- ❏ Establish and maintain airway.
- ❏ Administer high-flow oxygen.
- ❏ Intubate and assist ventilations, if appropriate.
- ❏ Use bag-valve-mask or demand valve.
- ❏ Establish venous access.
- ❏ Contact poison control.
- ❏ Administer sodium bicarbonate (50 mEq) for lactic acidosis, if poison control is unavailable.
- ❏ Consider 30–60 ml of any 86 proof ethanol (vodka, whiskey, gin, etc.), which delays metabolism.
- ❏ Transport rapidly.

Signs of Ethylene Glycol Poisoning. Ethylene glycol is present in polishes, paints, coolants, and antifreezes. Symptoms progress from an appearance of drunkenness to coma and anuria. Unlike methanol, ethylene glycol leaves little odor on the patient's breath. The signs and symptoms of ethylene glycol ingestion include:

- ❏ Abdominal pain
- ❏ Nausea, vomiting
- ❏ Apparent signs of intoxication
- ❏ Tachypnea/hyperpnea
- ❏ Renal damage

Treatment. In suspected cases of ethylene glycol poisoning, take the following steps.

- ❏ Establish and maintain airway.
- ❏ Administer high-flow oxygen.
- ❏ Intubate and assist ventilations, if appropriate.
- ❏ Use a bag-valve-mask or demand valve.
- ❏ Establish venous access.
- ❏ Contact poison control.
- ❏ Administer sodium bicarbonate (50 mEq) for lactic acidosis, if poison control in unavailable.
- ❏ Consider 30–60 ml of any 86 proof ethanol (vodka, whiskey, gin, etc.), which delays metabolism.
- ❏ Transport rapidly.

INHALED POISONS

Toxic inhalations can result from a poisonous environment or from self-induced inhalations. The following material provides guidelines for assessing and managing common toxic inhalations.

Presentation of Toxic Inhalations

The principal effects of inhaled toxic substances include respiratory disorders such as tachypnea, coughing, hoarseness, stridor, dyspnea, chest pain, chest tightness, chest retraction, and wheezing, rales, or rhonchi. A particularly dangerous form of inhalation results in patients who seek "highs" through the use of the chemical propellants found in many aerosol products. They spray these chemicals into a paper or plastic bag and inhale them. This produces a relative hypoxia, causing the patient to lose consciousness as the chemicals displace oxygen in the lungs. Signs and symptoms of aerosol inhalation include:

❑ *CNS.* Dizziness, headache, confusion, seizures, hallucinations, coma
❑ *Respiratory.* Tachypnea, coughing, hoarseness, stridor, dyspnea, retractions, chest pain, chest tightness, and wheezing, rales, or rhonchi
❑ *Cardiac.* Dysrhythmias

General Management of Toxic Inhalations

✳ Your first concern in any inhalational emergency is personal safety.

The first priority in treating patients who have inhaled toxic gases or powders is safe removal from the source. The following general principles of management apply to most patients exposed to toxic inhalations.

❑ Safely remove the patient from the poisonous environment. In doing so, take the following essential precautions.
 • Wear protective clothing prior to entry.
 • Use appropriate respiratory apparatus.
 • Remove patient's contaminated clothing.
❑ Perform the necessary primary and secondary assessments.
❑ Initiate the following treatment procedures.
 • Establish and maintain airway.
 • Administer high-flow oxygen.
 • Intubate and assist ventilations, if appropriate.
 • Administer CPR, if necessary.
 • Use a bag-valve-mask or demand valve.
 • Establish venous access.
 • Contact poison control.

Specific Inhaled Toxins

Aside from aerosol inhalations, most emergencies that involve inhaled poisons can create a potentially toxic environment for the rescuer. Whenever you come across the following commonly inhaled poisons, survey the scene for hazards to your own safety.

Cyanide Poisoning   Cyanide can enter the body by a variety of routes. It is present in many commercial and household items that can be either ingested or absorbed—rodenticides, silver polish, and fruit seeds (apples, cherries, and so on). It also can be inhaled, especially in fires that release cyanide from products containing nitrogen. A roomful of burning plastics, silks, or synthetic carpeting can also be a roomful of cyanide-filled smoke. Regardless of the entry route, cyanide is an extremely fast-acting toxin. (Suicidal patients have been known to take cyanide salt.) Cyanide inflicts its damage by inhibiting cytochrome oxidase, an enzyme vital to cellular use of oxygen. Once cyanide enters the body, it acts as a *cellular asphyxiant.* To prevent inhalation, you should always wear breathing equipment when entering the scene of a fire.

Signs and symptoms of cyanide poisoning include:

❑ A burning sensation in the mouth and throat
❑ Headache, combative behavior

- Hypertension and tachycardia
- Tachypnea and hyperpnea, rapidly followed by respiratory depression
- Pulmonary edema

Treatment. In suspected cases of cyanide poisoning, take the following steps.

- Protect the airway, and intubate as necessary.
- Administer high-flow oxygen.
- Administer a Cyanide Antidote Kit.
- Transport rapidly to nearest appropriate medical facility.

The Cyanide Antidote Kit contains amyl nitrite ampules, a sodium nitrite, and a sodium thiosulfate solution. Addition of nitrates to blood converts some hemoglobin to methemoglobin, which allows cyanide to bind to it. Thiosulfate also binds with cyanide to form thiocyanate, a nontoxic substance readily excreted renally. Because cyanide is rapidly toxic, you must administer the Cyanide Antidote Kit without delay. If your unit carries this kit, familiarize yourself with its contents and use.

Carbon Monoxide *Carbon monoxide (CO)* is an odorless, tasteless gas that is often the byproduct of incomplete combustion. Because of its chemical structure, it has more than 200 times the affinity of oxygen to bind with the red blood cell's hemoglobin (producing carboxyhemoglobin). Once this molecule has bound with hemoglobin, it is very resistant to removal and causes an effective hypoxia. Because of the variability of the signs and symptoms, people ignore CO poisoning until very toxic levels occur. Common settings for CO poisoning include improperly vented heating systems or the use of a small barbecue to heat a house or camper.

Signs and symptoms of CO poisoning include:

- Headache
- Nausea, vomiting
- Confusion or other altered mental status
- Tachypnea

Treatment. Because of the difficulty in removing CO from hemoglobin, definitive treatment is often performed in a hyperbaric chamber. In this specially designed environment, oxygen under several atmospheres of pressure surrounds the body. In field settings, take the following supportive steps.

- Safely remove the patient from the contaminated area.
- Begin immediate ventilation of the area.
- Initiate the following treatment procedures.
  - Establish and maintain the airway.
  - Administer high-flow oxygen.
  - Intubate and assist ventilations, if appropriate.
  - Administer CPR, if necessary.
  - Use a bag-valve-mask or demand valve.
  - Establish venous access.

Freon *Freon* is used as a common refrigerant and as a chemical solvent in a variety of electrical industry applications. It causes direct cardiac toxicity by the sudden release of endogenous catecholamines. The effect on the heart is a variety of ventricular ectopic activity, including PVCs, ventricular tachycardia, and ventricular fibrillation.

Treatment. In suspected cases of freon inhalation, take the following steps.

- ❏ Safely remove the patient from the contaminated area.
- ❏ Begin immediate ventilation of the area.
- ❏ Initiate the following treatment procedures.
  - Establish and maintain airway.
  - Administer high-flow oxygen.
  - Intubate and assist ventilations, if appropriate.
  - Apply EKG and observe for ventricular ectopic activity.
  - Administer CPR, if necessary.
  - Use a bag-valve-mask or demand valve.
  - Establish venous access.
  - Consider lidocaine (1 mg/kg) for ectopy.

Ammonia   *Ammonia* is a chemical with a distinct odor that is used in a variety of cleaning and agricultural applications. It is a corrosive alkaline chemical that reacts with water to produce a caustic substance. When it is released as a vapor, it is very irritating to eyes and the respiratory tree. Inhalation will produce the following signs or symptoms.

- ❏ Coughing, choking, and respiratory collapse
- ❏ Irritation of the eyes, including excessive tearing
- ❏ Nausea, vomiting, and abdominal pain
- ❏ Seizures

Treatment. In suspected cases of ammonia inhalation, take the following steps.

- ❏ Safely remove the patient from the contaminated area.
- ❏ Begin immediate ventilation of the area.
- ❏ Initiate the following treatment procedures.
  - Establish and maintain airway.
  - Administer high-flow oxygen.
  - Intubate and assist ventilations, if appropriate.
  - Apply EKG monitor.
  - Use a bag-valve-mask or demand valve.
  - Establish venous access.

Methylene Chloride   *Methylene chloride* is a colorless, combustible gas. It has an ether-like odor. Because it can be absorbed dermally, contact with this gas increases its toxicity. Signs and symptoms of methylene chloride poisoning include:

- ❏ Nausea and vomiting
- ❏ Altered level of consciousness, eventually progressing to seizures and coma

Treatment. In suspected cases of methylene chloride inhalation, take the following steps.

- ❏ Safely remove the patient from the contaminated area. Be sure to adhere to the below precautions.
  - • Wear protective clothing prior to entry.
  - • Use appropriate respiratory apparatus.
  - • Remove contaminated clothing.
- ❏ Begin immediate ventilation of the area. AVOID SPARKS!
- ❏ Initiate the following treatment procedures.
  - • Establish and maintain airway.
  - • Administer high-flow oxygen.
  - • Intubate and assist ventilations, if appropriate.
  - • Apply EKG monitor.
  - • Use a bag-valve-mask or demand valve.
  - • Establish venous access.

INJECTED POISONS

Injected poisons can be introduced to the body through accidental or deliberate drug overdose. But most injected poisons result from bites or stings from a variety of land and sea creatures—insects, reptiles, jellyfish, spiny shellfish, and more. The following sections provide some tips on treating the most commonly encountered injected toxins.

General Principles of Management

In treating a patient who has been bitten or stung, you may have to deal with bacterial contamination introduced by the injection or bodily reaction to any injected substances. As a rule, follow the below general principles of field management for bites and stings.

- ❏ Protect rescue personnel—the offending life form may still be around.
- ❏ Remove the patient from repeated injection, especially in the case of yellow jackets, wasps, or hornets.
- ❏ If possible, identify the insect, reptile, or animal that caused the injury. Bring it to the emergency center along with the patient.
- ❏ Perform primary and secondary assessment.
- ❏ Prevent or delay further absorption of poison.
- ❏ Watch for anaphylactic reaction.
- ❏ Transport the patient as rapidly as possible, if indicated.
- ❏ Contact poison control.

Insect and Arthropod Bites and Stings

No matter where anyone lives, they encounter an endless number of insects and arthropods capable of stinging or biting humans. Bites and stings can range from minor irritants to severe toxic reactions. The following sections describe some of the most common offenders.

Insect Stings   Many people die from allergic reactions to the stings from a class of insects known as *hymenoptera*. As mentioned earlier, *hymenoptera* includes wasps, bees, hornets, and ants. Only the common honeybee leaves a stinger. Wasps, yellow jackets, hornets, and fire ants sting repeatedly until removal from contact.

In most cases of insect stings, local treatment is all that is necessary. Unless an allergic reaction occurs, most patients will tolerate the isolated *hymenoptera* sting. Signs and symptoms include:

- ❏ Localized pain
- ❏ Redness
- ❏ Swelling
- ❏ Skin weal

Idiosyncratic reactions may occur to the toxin, resulting in a progressing localized swelling edema. This is not an allergic reaction. However, it responds well to an antihistamine such as diphenhydramine hydrochloride. The major problem resulting from a *hymenoptera* sting is an allergic reaction or anaphylaxis. (See Chapter 25.) Signs and symptoms of allergic reactions or anaphylaxis include:

- ❏ Localized pain, redness, swelling, and a skin weal
- ❏ Allergic reactions such as itching or flushing of the skin, rash, tachycardia, hypotension, bronchospasm, or laryngeal edema
- ❏ Facial edema, uvular swelling

Treatment. In cases of *hymenoptera* stings, take the following supportive steps.

- ❏ Wash the area.
- ❏ Gently remove the stinger by scraping *without* squeezing the venom sac. (This is best accomplished by using a razor blade or knife blade placed flat against the skin and moved in the horizontal plane with the skin.)
- ❏ Apply cool compresses to the injection site.
- ❏ Observe for and treat allergic reactions and/or anaphylaxis.

Brown Recluse Spider Bites
This spider lives in the South and the Midwest. It ranges west to east from Texas to South Carolina and north to south from Indiana to Alabama. It has also been reported in Arizona, Hawaii, California, and Utah. It is found in large numbers in Tennessee, Arkansas, and Oklahoma. If you are uncertain about the presence of this spider, it is advisable to contact a regional college or university biology department.

The brown recluse spider is about 15 mm in length. Its habitat is generally dark, dry locations. It can often be found in and around the house. There is a characteristic violin marking on the back, giving the spider the nickname "fiddleback spider." (See Figure 26-2.) Another identifying feature is the presence of 6 eyes (3 pairs in a semicircle), instead of the usual eight eyes common to most spiders.

The site of the brown recluse spider bite can become ischemic and ulcerate. Most patients are unaware that they have been bitten until after these symptoms develop. (See Figures 26-3 and 26-4.) Severe local symptoms include:

- ❏ Small bleb (erythematous macule) surrounded by a white ring in a few minutes post bite. (This can progress to a blue necrotic lesion after a few days.)
- ❏ Localized pain, redness, swelling 2–8 hours after the bite
- ❏ Localized tissue necrosis (days to weeks later)
- ❏ Chills

- ❏ Fever
- ❏ Nausea and vomiting
- ❏ Joint pain
- ❏ Bleeding disorders (disseminated intravascular coagulation)

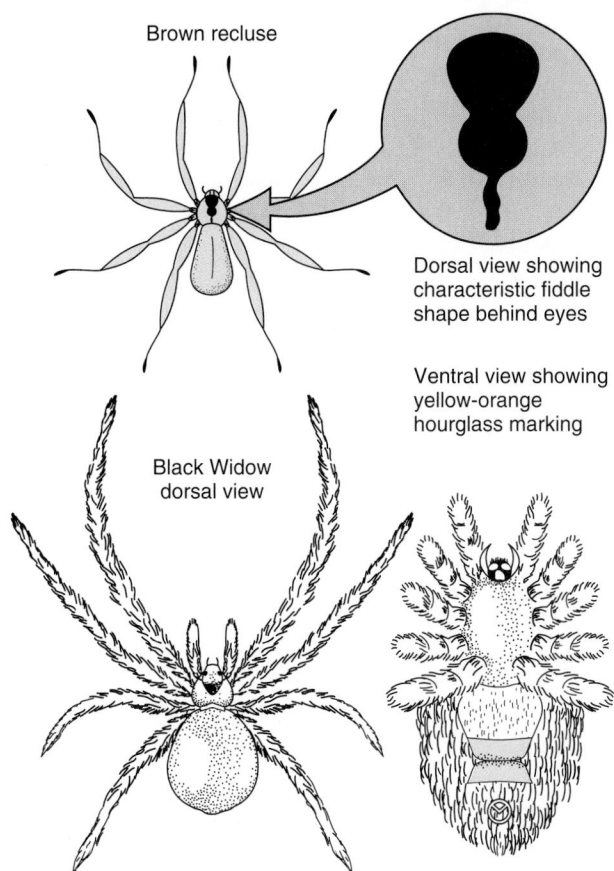

Brown recluse

Dorsal view showing characteristic fiddle shape behind eyes

Ventral view showing yellow-orange hourglass marking

Black Widow dorsal view

FIGURE 26-2 Poisonous spiders.

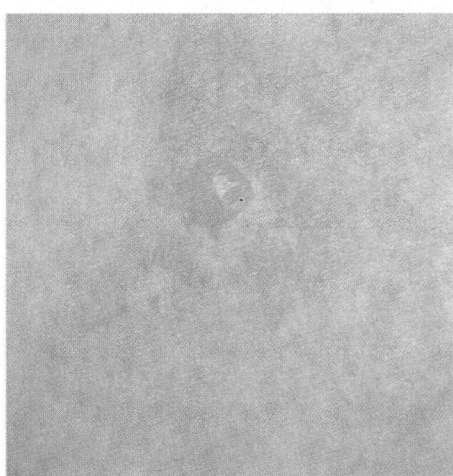

FIGURE 26-3 Brown recluse spider bite 24 hours after bite. Note the bleb and surrounding white halo. (Courtesy of Scott and White Hospital and Clinic.)

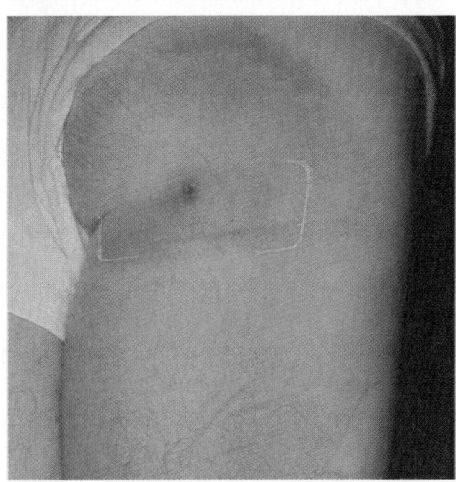

FIGURE 26-4 Brown recluse spider bite 4 days after the bite. Note the spread of erythema and early necrosis. (Courtesy of Scott and White Hospital and Clinic.)

Treatment. Prehospital treatment for the bite of the brown recluse spider is mostly supportive. No antivenom is available. However, if the patient is treated in the emergency department within 24 hours, the prognosis is usually good. Prompt administration of antihistamines may reduce systemic reactions. The patient may require surgical excision of the necrotic tissue. (Similar necrotic lesions, as well as a variety of other medical conditions, are caused by other arthropods, including ticks.)

Black Widow Spider Bites Black widow spiders live in virtually all parts of the continental United States. They are commonly found in brush or wood piles. The female black widow is responsible for bites. It can be recognized by an orange or red hourglass figure against the black abdomen. The venom of the black widow is very potent, probably causing excessive neurotransmitter release at the synaptic junctions. The severity of the symptoms can be influenced by the patient's age, weight, and general health.

Signs and symptoms of the patient bitten by a black widow spider include:

- ❑ Immediate localized pain, redness, and swelling
- ❑ Progressive muscle spasms (usually in the back or abdomen)
- ❑ Progressive spasms of all large muscle groups
- ❑ Severe back, chest, or shoulder pain (bite on upper extremity)
- ❑ Severe abdominal pain (bite on lower extremity)
- ❑ Nausea and vomiting
- ❑ Sweating
- ❑ Seizures
- ❑ Paralysis
- ❑ Hypertension
- ❑ Diminished level of consciousness

Treatment. In suspected cases of black widow spider bites, take the following steps.

- ❑ Reassure the victim.
- ❑ Administer muscle relaxant per physician order to relieve severe muscle spasms. Consider diazepam (2.5–10 mg IV or 10 mL of a 10 percent calcium gluconate IV) solution (calcium chloride is not effective).
- ❑ Monitor blood pressure, and observe for hypertensive crisis.
- ❑ Transport to the emergency department for antivenom.

Scorpion Stings Scorpions are nocturnal arachnids. (See Figure 26-5.) They hide under debris and buildings during the day and move at night. These arthropods live in the arid southwestern United States and Mexico. The scorpion's venom injection structure is located in a bulb-like enlargement at the tip of its long tail. The scorpion stings when provoked and injects only a small quantity of venom. Of the many species of scorpion found in the United States, only the bark scorpion, *Centruroides exilicauda* (formerly *C. sculpturatus*), has caused fatalities.

Fatal scorpion stings are extremely rare. The scorpion's venom acts on the central nervous system by affecting the cardiac and respiratory centers. Scorpion venom is also directly cardiotoxic. It has a direct effect on the neuromuscular junction, causing depolarization of nervous tissue and subsequent

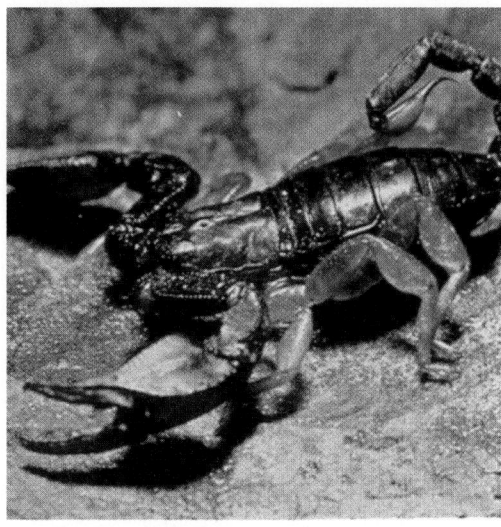

FIGURE 26-5 Scorpion.

muscle twitching and fasiculations. While hyperactivity is found occasionally in adults, it occurs in 80 percent of children under the age of two.

Signs and symptoms of scorpion stings include:

- ❑ Mild to sharp localized pain, which often progresses to numbness
- ❑ Slurred speech
- ❑ Increased restlessness, jerking, writhing, and flailing ("break dancing"); suspect in children when other diagnostic solutions can't be supported (seizures, phenothiazine ingestion, corneal abrasions, etc.)
- ❑ Salivation
- ❑ Muscle twitching
- ❑ Abdominal pain and cramps
- ❑ Nausea and vomiting
- ❑ Seizures

Treatment. In cases of suspected scorpion stings, take the following steps.

- ❑ Reassure the victim (no reported deaths in Arizona since 1970).
- ❑ Apply a constricting band above the wound site no tighter than a watchband to occlude lymphatic flow only.
- ❑ Avoid the use of analgesics, which may increase the toxicity of the venom.
- ❑ If systemic symptoms develop, transport to the emergency department for possible administration of scorpion antiserum.

Snake Bites

There are several thousand snake bites each year in the United States. Even so, these bites rarely result in death. The signs and symptoms of snake bites depend upon the snake, the location of the bite, and the type and amount of venom injected.

There are two families of poisonous snakes native to the United States. One family (*Crotalidae*) includes the pit vipers. Common pit vipers are rattlesnakes (see Figure 26-6), cottonmouths (water moccasins), and copper-

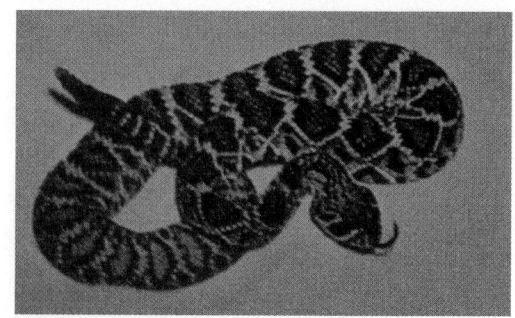

FIGURE 26-6 Rattlesnake.

heads. Pit vipers are so named because of the distinctive pit between the eye and the nostril on each side of the head. These snakes have elliptical pupils, two well-developed fangs, and a triangular-shaped head with a short, thick body. Only the rattlesnake, the most common pit viper, has rattles on the end of its tail. However, one species of rattlesnake doesn't have rattles, and many rattlesnakes lose these sound-producing appendages to predators.

The second family of poisonous snakes is the *Elapidae*, or coral snake, a distant relative of the cobra. Several varieties of coral snakes are found in the United States, primarily the southwest. Because it is a small snake and has small fixed fangs, the coral snake cannot readily attach itself to a large surface, such as an arm or leg. The coral snake has round pupils, a narrow head, and no pit. It has characteristic yellow-banded red and black rings around its body. Several nonpoisonous snakes mimic this coloration pattern. Keep in mind a helpful mnemonic: "red touch yellow, kill a fellow; red touch black, venom lack." This rhyme indicates the distinctive pattern of the coral snake—a pattern that signals danger.

Pit Vipers   Pit viper venom contains destructive proteins, polypeptides, and hydrolytic enzymes that are capable of destroying cell membranes, proteins, and most other tissue components. These toxic venom fractions may produce destruction of red blood cells and other tissue components. They may also affect the body's blood-clotting system within the blood vessels. This will produce infarction and tissue necrosis, especially at the site of the bite.

Signs and Symptoms.   A severe bite of a pit viper can result in death from shock within 30 minutes. However, most deaths from pit-viper bites occur from 6–30 hours after the bite, with 90 percent occurring in the first 48 hours. Signs and symptoms of pit viper bite include:

❑ Fang marks that are often little more than a scratch mark or abrasion (See Figure 26-7.)
❑ Swelling and pain at wound site
❑ Continued oozing at the wound site
❑ Weakness, dizziness, or faintness
❑ Minty, metallic, or rubber taste in mouth and lips
❑ Sweating and/or chills
❑ Thirst
❑ Nausea and vomiting
❑ Diarrhea
❑ Tachycardia and hypotension
❑ Bloody urine and gastrointestinal hemorrhage (late)
❑ Ecchymosis

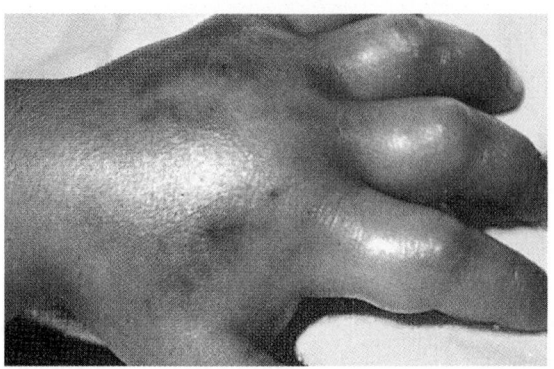

FIGURE 26-7   Rattlesnake bite to the hand.

❏ Necrosis
❏ Shallow respirations, progressing to respiratory failure
❏ Numbness and tingling around face and head (classic)

Treatment. In treating a person who has been bitten by a pit viper, the primary goal is to slow absorption of venom. However, it is important to remember that about 25 percent of all rattlesnake bites are "dry" and no venom is injected. Immediate treatment includes the following steps.

❏ Apply a loose constricting band proximally between bite and heart. This should be no tighter than a watchband.
❏ Keep the patient supine.
❏ Immobilize limb with splint.
❏ Remove tight watches, sleeves, etc.

In planning supportive care, keep the following guidelines in mind.

❏ Apply high-flow oxygen.
❏ Start IV with crystalloid fluid.
❏ Transport to emergency department for management, which may include the administration of antivenom.
❏ DO NOT apply ice, cold pack, or freon spray to the wound.
❏ DO NOT apply an arterial tourniquet.
❏ DO NOT apply electrical stimulation from any device in an attempt to retard or reverse venom spread.

Coral Snake   The venom of the coral snake contains some of the enzymes found in pit viper venom. However, because of the presence of neurotoxin, coral snake venom primarily affects nervous tissue. The classic, severe coral snake bite will result in respiratory and skeletal muscle paralysis.

Signs and Symptoms. After the bite of a coral snake, there may be no local manifestations or even any systemic effects for as long as 12–24 hours. Signs and symptoms of a coral snake bite include:

❏ Localized numbness, weakness, and drowsiness
❏ Ataxia
❏ Slurred speech and excessive salivation
❏ Paralysis of tongue and larynx (produces difficulty breathing and swallowing)
❏ Drooping of eyelids (ptosis), double vision, dilated pupils

✱ Use common sense with snake bites. Apply a constricting band, keep the patient supine, splint the affected limb, administer oxygen, and start an intravenous lifeline.

- ❑ Abdominal pain
- ❑ Nausea and vomiting
- ❑ Loss of consciousness
- ❑ Seizures
- ❑ Respiratory failure
- ❑ Hypotension

Treatment. In cases of suspected coral snake bites, take the following steps.

- ❑ Wash wound with copious amounts of water.
- ❑ Apply constricting band proximally between bite and heart.
- ❑ Immobilize limb with splint.
- ❑ Start IV using crystalloid fluid.
- ❑ Transport to emergency department for administration of antivenom.
- ❑ DO NOT apply ice, cold pack, or freon sprays to the wound.
- ❑ DO NOT incise the wound.
- ❑ DO NOT apply electrical stimulation from any device in an attempt to retard or reverse venom spread.

Marine Animal Injection

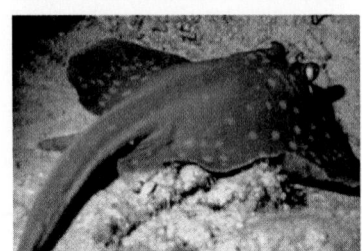

FIGURE 26-8 Sting-ray.

Injection of toxins from marine life can result from stings of jellyfish and corals or from punctures by the bony spines of animals such as sea urchins and sting-rays. (See Figure 26-8.) All venoms of marine animals contain substances that produce pain out of proportion to the size of the injury. These poisonous toxins are unstable and heat labile. Heat will relieve pain and inactivate the venom.

Both fresh water and salt water contain considerable bacterial and viral pollution. Therefore, secondary infection is always a possibility in injuries from marine animals.

Signs and Symptoms   Signs and symptoms of marine animal injection include:

- ❑ Intense local pain and swelling
- ❑ Weakness
- ❑ Nausea and vomiting
- ❑ Dyspnea
- ❑ Tachycardia
- ❑ Hypotension or shock (severe cases)

Treatment   In suspected cases of marine animal injection, take the following steps.

✳ Heat will relieve pain and help inactivate the venom of many marine animals.

- ❑ Establish and maintain airway.
- ❑ Apply constricting band proximally between wound and heart no tighter than a watchband to occlude lymphatic flow only.
- ❑ Apply heat or hot water (110–113°F).
- ❑ Inactivate or remove any stingers. (Jellyfish nematacysts may be inactivated by rubbing alcohol. Scrape off these tentacles with a sharp object such as a knife or razor.)

SURFACE ABSORBED POISONS

Many poisons can be absorbed through the skin. These include the organophosphates, cyanide, and other toxins.

General Principles of Management

Some of the principles for treating absorbed poisons have already been discussed in the management of cyanide (see pages 818–819) and methyl chloride (see pages 820–819). Whenever you suspect absorption of a poison (especially such agents as cyanide or strychnine), take the following steps.

❏ Safely remove the patient from the poisonous environment. Be sure to adhere to the below procedures.
  - Wear protective clothing.
  - Use appropriate respiratory apparatus.
  - Remove patient's contaminated clothing.
❏ Perform primary and secondary assessment.
❏ Initiate the following treatment procedures.
  - Establish and maintain the airway.
  - Administer oxygen.
  - Intubate and assist ventilations, if appropriate.
  - Administer CPR, if necessary.
  - Use a bag-valve-mask or demand value.
  - Establish venous access.
  - Contact poison control.

Organophosphates

Organophosphate compounds are used as insecticides in residential as well as commercial agriculture. Poisoning by the organophosphates is common in agricultural areas where crop dusters are used. Exposure has also been employed as a suicide method. Because of their chemical structure, organophosphates are capable of producing a variety of signs and symptoms affecting both the parasympathetic (muscarinic effects) and the sympathetic (nicotinic effects) nervous systems.

Presentation   Organophosphates inactivate cholinesterase at the synaptic junction, causing elevated levels of the neurotransmitter acetylcholine. This produces excessive salivation, lacrimation, and gastrointestinal problems, including abdominal pain, nausea, vomiting, and incontinence (urine and diarrhea). This cholinergic pattern may be remembered with the mnemonic **SLUDGE** (excessive **S**alivation, **L**acrimation, **U**rination, **D**iarrhea, **G**astrointestinal distress, **E**mesis).

The patient may have constricted pupils (miosis). While bradycardia is often associated with organophosphate poisoning, stimulation of nicotinic receptors will produce a tachycardia instead. The prehospital management of organophosphate poisoning is aimed at reversal of the deleterious excessive cholinergic effects (cholinergic crisis).

Decontamination of a patient with organophosphate poisoning is essential. All clothing should be removed. Repeated washings with copious amounts of water and soap are recommended. All clothing, including all leather items, should be discarded according to Environmental Protection Agency guidelines for hazardous materials.

Treatment   In suspected cases of exposure to organophosphates, take the following steps.

❑ DO NOT INDUCE VOMITING; gastric lavage is the preferred method of decontamination.
❑ Establish and maintain airway. This may require vigorous suctioning due to the excessive secretions caused by the organophosphate.
❑ Administer oxygen at a high concentration.
❑ Intubate and assist ventilations, if appropriate.
❑ Administer CPR, if necessary.
❑ Use a bag-valve-mask or demand value.
❑ Establish venous access.
❑ *ATROPINE.*
   • *Adult*: Administer atropine sulfate 2–5 mg every 10–15 minutes as necessary to dry secretions.
   • *Child*: 0.05 mg/kg.
❑ Seizures may be managed with diazepam (Adult 5–10 mg initially, with repeats per medical protocol; Child 0.25–0.4 mg/kg).
❑ Contact poison control.

DRUG OVERDOSE AND SUBSTANCE ABUSE

In general terms, drug overdose refers to poisoning from a pharmacological substance, either legal or illegal. This can occur by accident, miscalculation, changes in the strength of a drug, suicide, polydrug use, or recreational drug usage. Many overdose emergencies seen in the field occur in the habitual drug abuser. It is difficult to obtain a good history in these cases. However, if you know regional street-drug slang, a more accurate history may be obtained. (See Table 26-3.) It is imperative that you maintain a nonjudgmental attitude in these cases. Addiction is both a physiological and a psychological problem.

The presentation of the drug overdose will vary based on the substance used. Management should be the same as for any ingested, inhaled, or injected poison. *Poison control should be contacted for additional direction.*

As a final word of warning, always survey the ·scene ·in cases of drug overdose. Be alert for possible rescuer danger. Do not go running into a known "crack house" or "shooting gallery" without backup.

ALCOHOL ABUSE

Alcohol (ethyl alcohol, or ethanol) depresses the ˙central nervous system, potentially to the point of stupor, coma, and death. In patients with severe

(continued on page 832)

TABLE 26-3 Common Drugs of Abuse & Overdose

Drug	Symptoms	Routes	Prehospital Management
Alcohol beer whiskey gin vodka wine tequila	•CNS depression •slurred speech •disordered thought •impaired judgment •diuresis •stumbling gait •stupor •coma	•oral	•ABCs •provide respiratory support •oxygenate •establish intravenous access •Administer 100 mg thiamine intravenously •ECG monitor •chemstrip •administer D50W, if hypoglycemic

Cocaine
crack
rock
	•euphoria
	•hyperactivity
	•dilated pupils
	•psychosis
	•twitching
	•anxiety
	•hypertension
	•tachycardia
	•dysrhythmias
	•seizures
	•chest pain
		•snorting
		•injection
		•smoking
		(freebasing)
		•application to skin on
		  mucous membranes
			•ABCs
			•provide respiratory support
			•oxygenate
			•ECG monitor
			•establish intravenous access
			•treat life-threatening
			  dysrhythmias
			•seizure precautions;
			  diazepam 5–10 mg for seizures
			•propanolol 1 mg IV slowly
			  (check local protocol)

Narcotics
heroin
codeine
meperidene
morphine
hydromorphone
pentazocine
Darvon
Darvocet
methadone
	•CNS depression
	•constricted pupils
	•respiratory depression
	•hypotension
	•bradycardia
	•pulmonary edema
	•coma
	•death
		•oral
		•injection
			•ABCs
			•respiratory support
			•oxygenate
			•establish intravenous access
			•administer 1–2 mg naloxone
			  intravenously or endotracheally
			  as ordered by medical control
			  until respirations improve. Larger
			  than average doses (2–5 mg)
			  have been used in the manage-
			  ment of many opiate/opioid
			  overdoses
			•ECG monitor

* With the advent of the opiate antagonist naloxone, narcotic overdosage became easier to manage. It is possible to titrate this effective medication to increase respirations to normal levels without fully awakening the patient. In the case of narcotics addicts, this prevents hostile and confrontive episodes.

Drug	Symptoms	Routes	Prehospital Management
Marijuana grass weed hashish	•euphoria •dry mouth •dilated pupils •altered sensation	•smoked •oral	•ABCs •reassure the patient •speak in a quiet voice •ECG monitor if indicated
Amphetamines Benzedrine Dexedrine Ritalin "speed"	•exhilaration •hyperactivity •dilated pupils •hypertension •psychosis •tremors •seizures	•oral •injection	•ABCs •oxygenate •ECG monitor •establish intravenous access •treat life-threatening dysrhythmias

TABLE 26-3 Common Drugs of Abuse & Overdose *(continued)*

Drug	Symptoms	Routes	Prehospital Management
Hallucinogens LSD STP mescaline psilocybin PCP*	• psychosis • nausea • dilated pupils • rambling speech • headache • dizziness • suggestibility • distortion of sensory perceptions • hallucinations	• oral • smoked	• ABCs • reassure the patient • "talk down" the "high" patient • protect the patient from injury • provide a dark, quiet environment • speak in a soft, quiet voice

While PCP was originally an animal tranquilizer, it manifests hallucinogenic properties when used by humans. In addition to bizarre delusions, it can cause violent and dangerous outbursts of aggressive behavior. The rescuer is advised to remain safe when attempting to treat this type of overdose. PCP patients have been known to have almost superhuman strength and high pain tolerance.

Drug	Symptoms	Routes	Prehospital Management
Sedatives Seconal Valium Librium Xanax Halcion Restoril Dalmane Phenobarbital	• altered mental status • hypotension • slurred speech • respiratory depression • shock • bradycardia • seizures	• oral	• ABCs • respiratory support • oxygenate • establish intravenous access • ECG monitor • medical control may order naloxone

Drug	Symptoms	Routes	Prehospital Management
Benzodiazepines* Valium Librium Xanax Halcion Restoril Dalmane Centrax Ativan Serax	• altered mental status • slurred speech • dysrhythmias • coma	• oral	• ABCs • respiratory support • oxygenate • ipecac and activated charcoal as ordered by medical control • establish intravenous access • ECG monitor • contact poison control

*Deaths due to pure benzodiazepine ingestion are very rare. **Minor** toxicity ranges are 500–1,500 mg. A benzodiazepine antagonist (Mazcicon [flumazenil]) is available. IV Dosage is 1–10 mg, or an infusion of 0.5 mg/hr. It may cause seizures in a benzodiazepine dependent patient.*

■ **benzodiazepines** general term to describe a group of tranquilizing drugs with similar chemical structures.

liver disease, metabolism of alcohol may become impaired, which increases the course and severity of intoxication. At low doses, alcohol has excitatory and stimulating effects, thus depressing inhibitions. At higher doses, alcohol's depressive effect is more obvious. Abuse of, and dependence upon, alcohol is called *alcoholism*. It is a major problem in our society and contributes to many accidents, including automobile collisions, drownings, burns, trauma, and drug overdoses.

TABLE 26-3 Common Drugs of Abuse & Overdose (*continued*)

Drug	Symptoms	Routes	Prehospital Management
Acetaminophen Tylenol Tempra	•asymptomatic •anorexia •nausea •vomiting •malaise •diaphoresis •RUQ pain •ECG monitor	•oral	•ABCs •respiratory support, high-flow oxygen •establish intravenous access •administer ipecac and activated charcoal as ordered by medical control •contact poison control as indicated
Salicylates Bayer Excedrin Bufferin Oil of Wintergreen Aspirin	•nausea •vomiting •confusion •lethargy •seizures •dysrhythmias •coma •death		•ABCs •respiratory support •oxygenate •establish intravenous access •ECG monitor •fluid challenge as ordered •treat life-threatening dysrhythmias •ipecac and activated charcoal as ordered by medical control •administer sodium bicarbonate as ordered by medical control
Tricyclic Antidepressants* Elavil Triavil Norpramin Doxepin Asendin Pamelor Sinequan Tofranil	•CNS depression •tachycardia •dilated pupils •respiratory depression •slurred speech •twitching, jerking •seizures •ST and T wave changes •AV blocks •shock	•oral	•ABCs •respiratory support •oxygenate •establish intravenous access •ECG monitor •activated charcoal as ordered by medical control •administer sodium bicarbonate if ordered by medical control •contact poison contro

*This class of drugs is one of the most dangerous of all the medications that patients overdose on. A one week supply is enough to cause death. Patients that have ingested these antidepressants rapidly loose consciousness and may actively seize. Therefore, following initial evaluation and treatment, rapid transport to a definitive health care facility is necessary.

Alcohol is completely absorbed from the stomach and intestinal tract in approximately 30–120 minutes after ingestion. Once absorbed, alcohol is distributed to all body tissues and fluids. Concentrations of alcohol in the brain rapidly approach the level of alcohol in the blood.

Physiological Effects

Alcohol should always be considered a CNS depressant, despite the initial increased activity as seen with lower doses. In addition, alcohol causes a peripheral vasodilator effect on the cardiovascular system, resulting in flushing

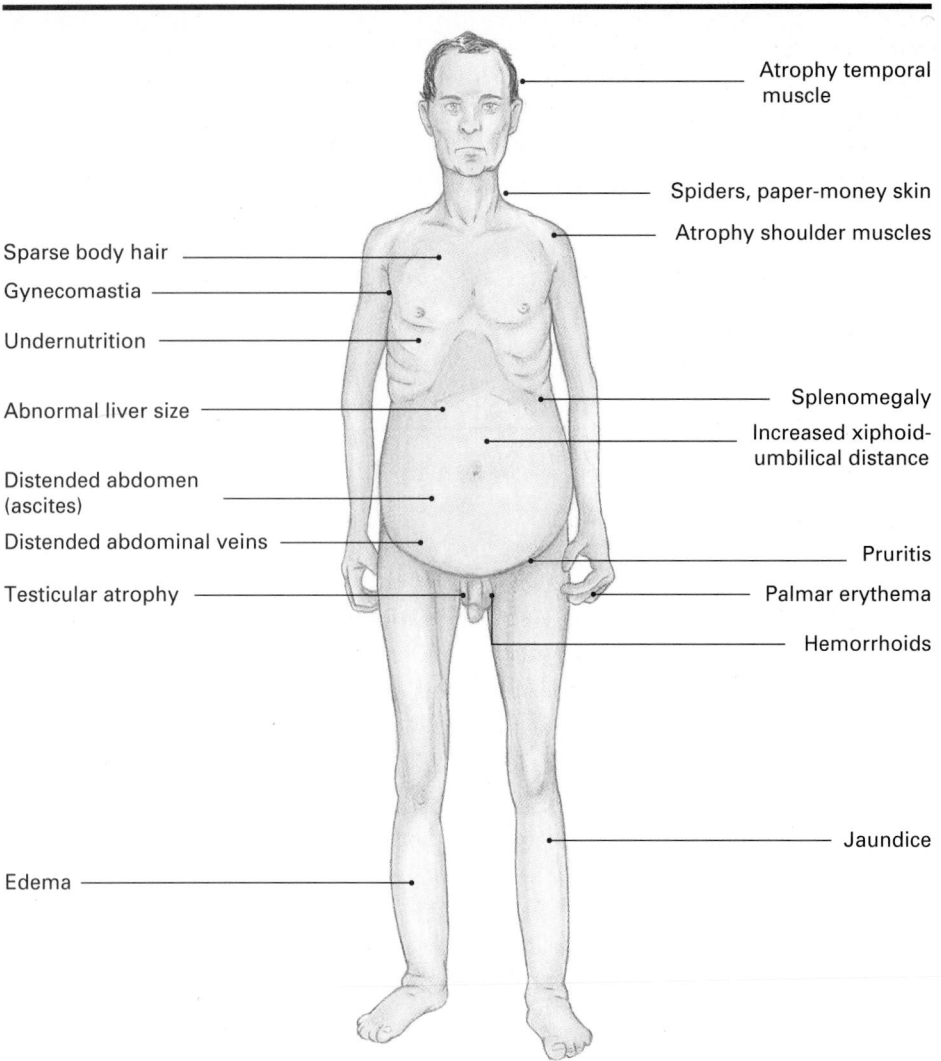

Atrophy temporal muscle

Spiders, paper-money skin

Atrophy shoulder muscles

Sparse body hair

Gynecomastia

Undernutrition

Abnormal liver size

Splenomegaly

Increased xiphoid-umbilical distance

Distended abdomen (ascites)

Distended abdominal veins

Pruritis

Testicular atrophy

Palmar erythema

Hemorrhoids

Jaundice

Edema

FIGURE 26-9   The chronic alcoholic.

and a feeling of warmth. Therefore, in extreme cold conditions, alcohol may cause the blood vessels to dilate, resulting in an increased loss of body heat. The diuretic effect seen when large amounts of alcohol are ingested results from inhibition of vasopressin (antidiuretic hormone). In the absence of vasopressin, urine production increases. The "dry mouth" syndrome experienced after alcohol consumption is thought to be the result of alcohol-induced cellular dehydration. (See Figure 26-9.)

General Alcoholic Profile

Although the symptoms of alcoholism vary from periodic "binge drinker" to daily drinker, the following are warning signs of the disease. (See Figure 26-9.)

❑ Drinks early in the day
❑ Prone to drink alone and secretly

- Periodic binges (may last for several days)
- Partial or total loss of memory ("blackouts") during period of drinking
- Unexplained history of gastrointestinal problems (especially bleeding)
- "Green Tongue Syndrome" (using chlorophyll-containing substances to disguise the odor of alcohol on the breath)
- Cigarette burns on clothing
- Chronically flushed face and palms
- Tremulousness
- Odor of alcohol on breath under inappropriate conditions

Consequences of Chronic Alcoholism

Alcohol abuse adversely affects the body in many ways. Some of the most common effects include:

- Poor nutrition
- Alcohol hepatitis
- Liver cirrhosis with subsequent esophageal varices
- Loss of sensation in hands and feet
- Loss of cerebellar function (balance and coordination)
- Pancreatitis
- Upper gastrointestinal hemorrhage (often fatal)
- Hypoglycemia
- Subdural hematoma (due to falls)
- Rib and extremity fractures (due to falls)

The odor of an alcoholic beverage on the patient's breath should be considered a poor indicator of alcohol intoxication. Insulin shock, subdural hematomas, and other life-threatening disease processes may mimic the signs and symptoms of alcohol intoxication.

Withdrawal Syndrome

The alcoholic may suffer a withdrawal reaction from either abrupt discontinuation of ingestion after prolonged use or from a rapid fall in the blood alcohol level after acute intoxication. Withdrawal symptoms can occur several hours after sudden abstinence and can last up to 5–7 days. Seizures (alcohol withdrawal epilepsy—sometimes called "rum fits") may occur within the first 24–36 hours of abstinence. Signs and symptoms of a withdraw syndrome include:

- Coarse tremor of hands, tongue, and eyelids
- Nausea and vomiting
- General weakness
- Increased sympathetic tone
- Tachycardia
- Sweating

- ❏ Hypertension
- ❏ Orthostatic hypotension
- ❏ Anxiety
- ❏ Irritability or a depressed mood
- ❏ Hallucinations
- ❏ Poor sleep

■ **delirium tremens (DTs)** disorder found in habitual and excessive users of alcoholic beverages after cessation of drinking for 48–72 hours. Patients experience visual, tactile, and auditory hallucinations.

Delirium tremens (DTs) may occur on the second or third day of the withdrawal. Delirium tremens is characterized by a decreased level of consciousness as the patient hallucinates and misinterprets nearby events. Seizures and delirium tremens are ominous signs. There is a significant mortality from delirium tremens. Medical control may order diazepam (Valium) in severe cases.

In-Field Treatment of Alcohol Abuse

Some alcoholics will drink methanol (wood alcohol) or ethylene glycol (a component of antifreeze) if ethanol is unavailable. Ingestion of these chemicals can cause blindness or death. Alcohol intoxication, whether acute or chronic, should not be underestimated as a toxic emergency problem. In cases of suspected alcohol abuse, take the following steps.

- ❏ Maintain airway.
- ❏ Determine if other drugs are involved.
- ❏ Induce emesis using ipecac. Before beginning, consider the age of the victim, amount of alcohol ingested, and vital signs. (Check local protocols or with the poison control center.)
- ❏ Start IV using D5W, LR, or 0.9 percent NS.
- ❏ Administer 100 mg of thiamine.
- ❏ Chemstrip and administer 25 g of D50W if hypoglycemic.
- ❏ Maintain a sympathetic attitude, and reassure the patient of help.

SUMMARY

The effective treatment of poisoning is based upon two factors: (1) prompt recognition of the poisoning and (2) an accurate and thorough initial patient evaluation. The basic concept for prehospital treatment is prompt removal of the poison and the prevention of further absorption. In addition, supportive and specific management should be carried out as indicated based on the route of toxic exposure. Often the initial prehospital treatment will include the administration of activated charcoal and/or syrup of ipecac. If these steps are completed promptly, the need for additional measures will be minimized.

FURTHER READING

Auerbach, Paul S., and Edward C. Geehr, eds. *Management of Wilderness and Environmental Emergencies*, 2nd ed. St. Louis: C.V. Mosby Co., 1989.

Bayer, Mark, J., Barry H. Rumack, and Lee A. Wanke,. *Toxicological Emergencies*. Bowie, MD: Brady Communications, 1984.

Bledsoe, Bryan E., Gideon Bosker, and Frank J. Papa,. *Prehospital Emergency Pharmacology*, 3rd ed. Englewood Cliffs, NJ: Prentice Hall, Inc., 1992.

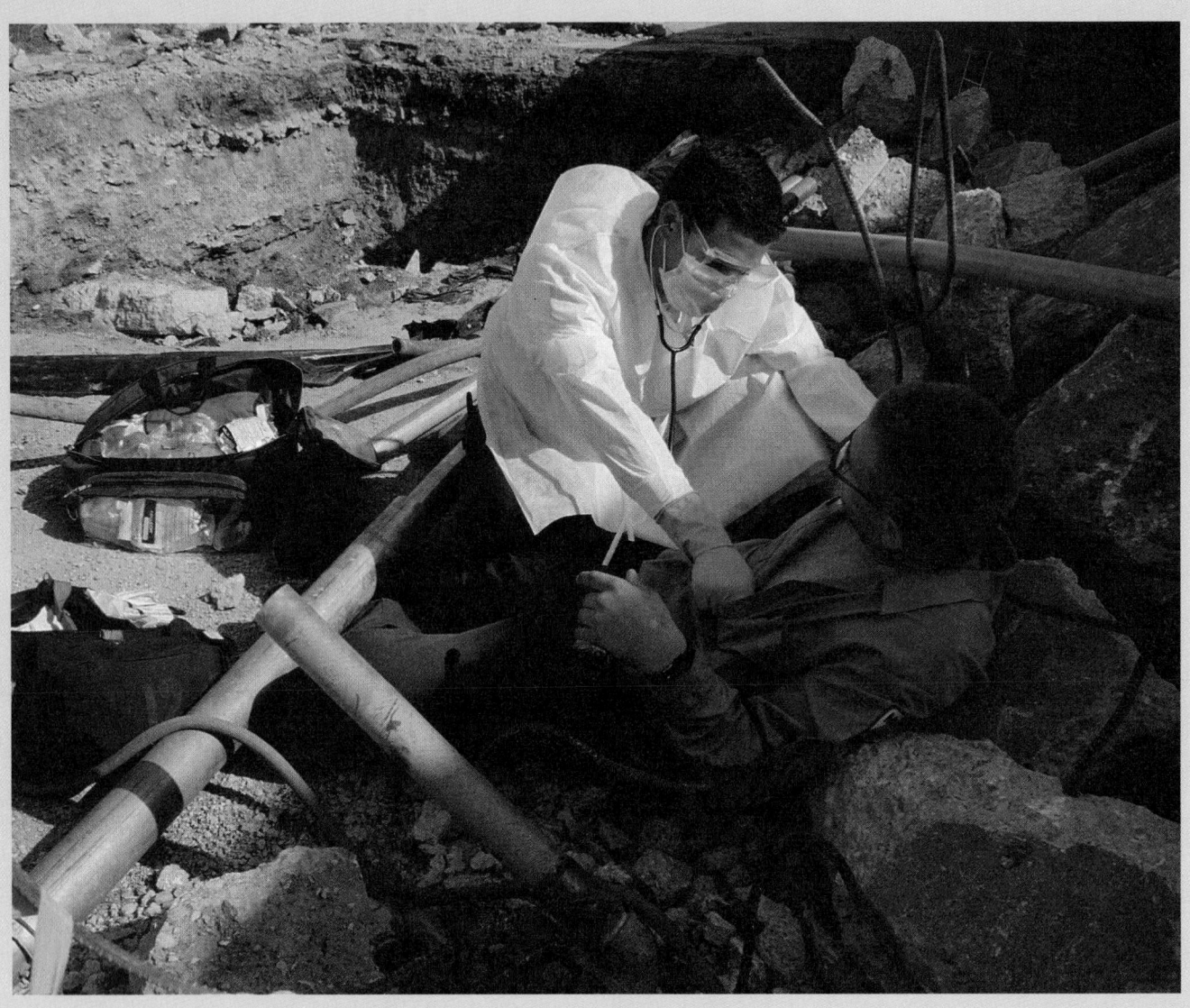

27

INFECTIOUS DISEASES

Objectives for Chapter 27

After reading this chapter, you should be able to:

1. Define the following terms. (See below pages.)
   - bacteria (p. 841)
   - antibiotics (p. 841)
   - virus (p. 841)
   - fungi (p. 842)
   - antigen (p. 842)

2. Define toxin, and give an example of endotoxins and exotoxins. (See p. 841.)

3. Describe the difference between bacterial and viral infections. (See p. 841.)

4. Briefly discuss the body's immune system. (See pp. 842–843.)

5. Define the following terms. (See below pages.)
   - leukocytes (p. 842)
   - cell-mediated immunity (p. 842)
   - humoral immunity (p. 842)
   - macrophages (p. 842)

6. Identify factors that increase the risk of disease. (See pp. 843–844.)

7. Describe meningitis, its presentation, prehospital care, and appropriate safety precautions. (See pp. 850–851.)

8. Describe tuberculosis, its presentation, prehospital care, and appropriate safety precautions. (See pp. 851–853.)

9. Describe scabies and lice. (See pp. 853–854.)

10. Describe common childhood diseases and their implications for prehospital care. (See pp. 854–855.)

11. Describe gastroenteritis, its presentation, prehospital care, and appropriate safety precautions. (See p. 855.)

12. Describe hepatitis, its presentation, prehospital care, and appropriate safety precautions. (See pp. 855–857.)

13. Explain reasons that hepatitis B poses a serious health threat to medical personnel. (See pp. 855–856.)

14. Identify common sexually transmitted diseases, and describe prehospital management. (See pp. 857–861.)

15. Explain acquired immune deficiency syndrome (AIDS). (See pp. 858–859.)

16. Describe methods of HIV transmission. (See pp. 858–859.)

17. List precautions that should be employed to protect prehospital personnel from HBV and HIV. (See pp. 860–861.)

18. Define "Universal Precautions." (See pp. 860–861.)

As usual, Sunday morning begins uneventfully for the paramedics of Station 10. The ambulance and fire engine have been washed and returned to the bay. Also, the patient compartment of the ambulance has been extensively cleaned, as often happens after a busy Saturday night. The paramedics now on duty pay particular attention to cleaning those surfaces frequently contacted by patients.

At approximately 1030 hours, the alarm sounds. The watch officer hands the computer printout to the driver. She states: "Well, your day isn't off to a bang." The printout gives the patient's address and the cross street. Under the comments section, a statement reads: "Patient says his cigarettes don't taste good anymore." The crew of Medic 10 head out, leaving the laughs and comments of the crew from Engine 10 behind.

The trip to the scene takes approximately two minutes. The house is a rundown structure, with all of the windows open and the curtains blowing freely in the summer breeze. Prior to leaving the ambulance, the paramedics don gloves. As they enter the house, they find the patient sitting on the couch, in the dark, with a package of cigarettes beside him. "I just ain't feeling worth a damn," the man says. He explains that he hasn't felt like working and hasn't wanted to drink a beer. Even his cigarettes don't taste good anymore.

The paramedics open the curtains to let in some light. They notice immediately that the patient has a definite yellow hue to his eyes and skin. Adhering to universal precautions, both paramedics complete the patient assessment. The physical examination is essentially unremarkable, except for multiple needle tracks on both forearms and the neck. The patient also exhibits some tenderness in the upper right quadrant of the abdomen. When questioned, the patient states that he has been "shooting up" for several years. He primarily uses heroin and occasionally crack. He states his urine has been dark brown for over a week. His live-in girlfriend, who has left for work at the restaurant where she is a waitress, has had dark urine as well.

The paramedics suspect hepatitis and transport the patient to the hospital. No advanced skills are needed. They leave linen used on the call at the hospital in the infectious linen bag. After delivering the patient, the paramedics immediately wash their hands, and disinfect the ambulance with bleach and water. They then complete a communicable disease exposure report.

Approximately a week later, the paramedics receive a report that the patient not only had hepatitis, but he had hepatitis B. His liver enzymes were markedly elevated, and his blood showed the hepatitis B surface antigen, indicating acute infection. Fortunately, both paramedics had received the hepatitis B vaccine while in school.

INTRODUCTION

Infectious diseases are illnesses caused by infection or infestation of the human body by various biological agents. These diseases account for the majority of known human and animal diseases. Although most infectious diseases seldom prove fatal, you must learn to recognize infectious diseases in the prehospital setting so that you can initiate emergency treatment and take steps to protect emergency personnel. Also, two infectious diseases—acquired immune deficiency syndrome (AIDS) and hepatitis B—present serious hazards to health care workers. The spread of these two diseases has made safety procedures even more important in recent years.

This chapter first addresses the fundamental principles of infectious diseases, including the operation of the immune system. It then examines the various infectious diseases most frequently encountered in the field, with special attention on hepatitis and AIDS.

✳ Infectious diseases, such as hepatitis B and HIV infection, are the number one threat to the health and safety of prehospital personnel today.

PATHOGENESIS OF INFECTIOUS DISEASE

Several biological agents can cause human infection. These include bacteria, viruses, fungi, and parasites. Since treatment and management of the different infections vary significantly, you need to recognize the causative agents of the more commonly encountered infectious diseases.

Bacteria

Bacteria—small, unicellular organisms that live throughout the environment—frequently cause infection. Smaller than human red blood cells, they can only be viewed through the microscope. Bacteria can live without the aid of another organism. They cause many of the common infections in medicine, including middle ear infections in children, many cases of tonsillitis, and meningitis. Most bacterial infections respond to treatment with drugs called **antibiotics**. Once administered, antibiotics kill or inhibit the growth of invading bacteria by one of several mechanisms.

Bacteria can usually be cultured and identified readily in most hospital laboratories. Many bacteria are categorized according to their appearance under the microscope after staining with several dyes referred to as a *Gram stain*. Some bacteria stain blue, while others stain red. Bacteria that stain blue are referred to as *Gram positive bacteria*. They are somewhat similar to each other in their composition. Bacteria that stain red are referred to as *Gram negative bacteria*. They are also somewhat similar to each other in their structure.

Simple infection is not the only consequence of a bacterial infection. Many bacteria release poisonous chemicals, or **toxins**. There are two general categories of toxins: exotoxins and endotoxins. *Exotoxins* are released from living bacteria during infection. They travel throughout the body via the blood or lymph, ultimately causing problems. The life-threatening consequences of tetanus infection are an example of the effects of an exotoxin. Tetanus is caused by the bacterium *Clostridium tetani*. The actual infection by the bacteria is mild and may be limited, for example, to a puncture wound in the foot. Yet, on entering the body, the bacteria release their toxin, called *tetanospasmin*. This toxin then travels through the blood to the skeletal muscles, causing the spastic rigidity classically seen in tetanus. Other bacteria release toxins referred to as endotoxins. *Endotoxins* are usually released upon the death and destruction of the bacterial cell. *Septic shock*, for example, is caused by the release of an endotoxin from several Gram-negative bacteria.

Viruses

Most infections are caused by biological agents called **viruses**. Viruses are much smaller than bacteria and can only be seen with an electron microscope. In addition, they cannot grow without the assistance of another organism. In fact, viruses are referred to as *intracellular parasites*, since they must invade the cells of the organism they infect. Once inside a cell, they take over, using the various cellular enzymes to replicate and produce more viruses. Viruses cannot reproduce outside of the host cell, and, unlike bacteria, they are very difficult to treat. Once a virus infects a cell, it can only be killed by destroying the infected cell. Drugs have not yet been developed that can selectively destroy cells infected by viruses, while simultaneously leaving uninfected cells unharmed. This partially explains the dilemma facing researchers trying to find a cure for AIDS. Fortunately, most viral illnesses are mild and fairly self-limited. Even so, at present, they usually cannot be treated with more than symptomatic care.

bacteria small, unicellular organisms present throughout the environment. They are capable of life independent of other organisms.

antibiotics medications effective in inhibiting the growth of or killing bacteria. They have no impact on viruses.

toxins poisonous chemicals secreted by bacteria or released following destruction of the bacteria.

virus microscopic organism, smaller than bacteria, that requires the assistance of another organism for its survival. Viruses are a common cause of human disease.

Fungi

Another biological agent that can cause human infection are **fungi** (the plural of fungus). More like plants than animals, they include yeasts and molds. Fungi rarely cause human disease other than minor skin infections, such as athlete's foot and some of the more common vaginal infections. Fungi infections are commonly called *mycoses*. Patients with an impaired immune system suffer fungal infection more commonly than healthy people. In such patients, the fungi can invade the lungs, blood, and several organs. Treatment of complicated, deep fungal infections proves difficult even in the hospital setting.

Parasites

Parasites can also cause infection. They range in size from small, unicellular organisms (not much larger than bacteria) to large intestinal worms. Parasites tend to be more common in developing nations than in the United States. Treatment depends upon the organism and the location.

IMMUNITY

The body has a very sophisticated system for fighting disease called the *immune system*. Most viruses and bacteria have proteins on their surface called **antigens**. The human immune system detects these antigens as being foreign and responds to suppress or kill them. Our white blood cells, or *leukocytes*, are primarily responsible for fighting the infection.

Immune Response

There are two general parts to the immune response. One is called *cell-mediated immunity* and the other *humoral immunity*. Cell-mediated immunity is derived from special leukocytes called *T lymphocytes*. They originate in the *thymus*, a gland located in the upper part of the chest. T cells are primarily responsible for fighting infections of biological agents living in certain body cells. Examples of such infections include tuberculosis, many viral infections, and most fungal infections. In these cases, white cells move to the site of infection. Here they attack and attempt to eliminate the invading pathogen.

In contrast, humoral immunity derives from *B lymphocytes* and results in the formation of special proteins called **antibodies**. There are five classes of human antibodies. They include:

❑ *IgM*. The antibody that responds immediately.
❑ *IgG*. The antibody that has "memory" and recognizes a repeatedly invading infection.
❑ *IgA*. The antibody present in the mucous membranes.
❑ *IgE*. The antibody contributing to allergic and anaphylactic responses.
❑ *IgD*. The antibody present in the lowest concentration.

As you have read, antibodies are produced in response to antigens, or proteins that usually appear on the surface of the invading organism. Typically, the antigen is specific for the particular type of invading pathogen. Following exposure to the antigen, the immune system will release *antibodies* that seek out the invading antigen. These antibodies combine with the antigen, forming what is commonly called the *antigen-antibody complex*. This large complex is subsequently removed by scavenger cells such as *macrophages*.

The Lymphatic System

The **lymphatic system** acts as a separate circulatory system. It helps transport materials between the tissues and the blood. As water, solutes, and inactivated or dead infectious agents filter out of the capillaries, they enter the interstitial fluid. (This fluid, as you may recall from Chapter 12, surrounds the body's cells.) The fluid, known as *lymph*, becomes part of the lymphatic system. As the lymph circulates through the system, it enters nodes that filter the fluid and produce additional antibodies. The nodes thus help curb bodily infection.

A key organ in the lymphatic system is the *spleen*. This solid organ lies in the left upper quadrant of the abdomen. It filters red blood cells and participates in the formation of cells that manufacture antibodies. The spleen is quite vulnerable to abdominal trauma. Blood loss from the spleen can be massive and rapidly fatal.

■ **lymphatic system** a complex network of small thin vessels, valves, ducts, lymph nodes, and organs that helps to protect and maintain the fluid environment of the body. The lymphatic system plays a major role in fighting disease. The lymph is restored to the regular circulation by the thoracic duct and the lymphatic duct.

TRANSMISSION OF INFECTIOUS DISEASE

Any of the agents causing infectious disease are transmissible. Infectious diseases can be spread in two ways. *Direct transmission* occurs when the disease is passed from one person to another through contact with infected blood or other body fluids. In addition, it can occur through the transmission of airborne particles. *Indirect transmission* occurs without direct person-to-person contact. Instead, the infectious agent is passed indirectly from one person to another through some contaminated object. For example, blood or another body fluid may be left on an object such as an ambulance stretcher. Later, a second person can contract the disease through contact with the contaminated stretcher.

Routes of Disease Transmission

There are several routes of exposure for infectious diseases. *Bloodborne diseases* are those transmitted by contact with the blood or body fluids of an infected person. Bloodborne diseases include AIDS, hepatitis B, hepatitis C, hepatitis D, and syphilis. Other infectious diseases are transmitted through the air on droplets expelled during a productive cough or sneeze. Examples of *airborne diseases* include tuberculosis, meningitis, mumps, measles, rubella, and chicken pox (varicella). In addition, infections can be transmitted through food, also called the *fecal-oral route*. *Foodborne diseases* include food poisoning, salmonella, staph infections, hepatitis A, and hepatitis E.

Increased Risk of Disease Transmission

It is important to point out that not all disease exposure results in infection. Several factors affect the likelihood that an individual will contract a given disease. Factors that affect the risk potential of contracting a disease include:

❑ *Type of Organism.* Some organisms, particularly bacteria and viruses, are more easily transmitted than others. Parasites and fungi are often more difficult to transmit.

❑ *Virulence.* The virulence is the strength or ability of an organism to infect or overcome the body's defenses. Some organisms, such as the hepatitis B virus (HBV), are very virulent and can remain infectious on a surface for weeks. Other organisms, such as HIV, die when exposed to air and light.

- ❏ *Dosage.* Dosage is the number of live organisms received in an exposure. For most diseases, a certain number of organisms must be received to cause infection. As a rule, the higher the dosage, the greater the likelihood of contracting the disease.
- ❏ *Host Resistance.* Host resistance is the ability of the host to fight off infection. Several factors affect the host's resistance to infection. These include stress, poor hygiene, inadequate nutrition, or living in crowded and unsanitary conditions.

Prehospital personnel should understand the concept of disease transmission. As a paramedic, you will play a major role in curbing infectious diseases by interrupting disease transmission (See Figure 27-1). Such precautions as respiratory isolation, cleaning the ambulance, and protection against bloodborne pathogens help stop the spread of disease.

Post-Exposure Considerations

The presence of specific antibodies in the blood indicates exposure to the disease. Although it is difficult to test for the presence of a specific disease antigen, laboratory tests can often spot the presence of antibodies specific for the disease or antigen. For example, the presence of the human immunodeficiency virus (HIV), which causes AIDS, is detected through the presence of antibodies to HIV.

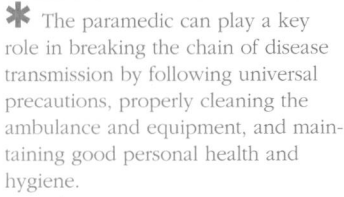 ✱ The paramedic can play a key role in breaking the chain of disease transmission by following universal precautions, properly cleaning the ambulance and equipment, and maintaining good personal health and hygiene.

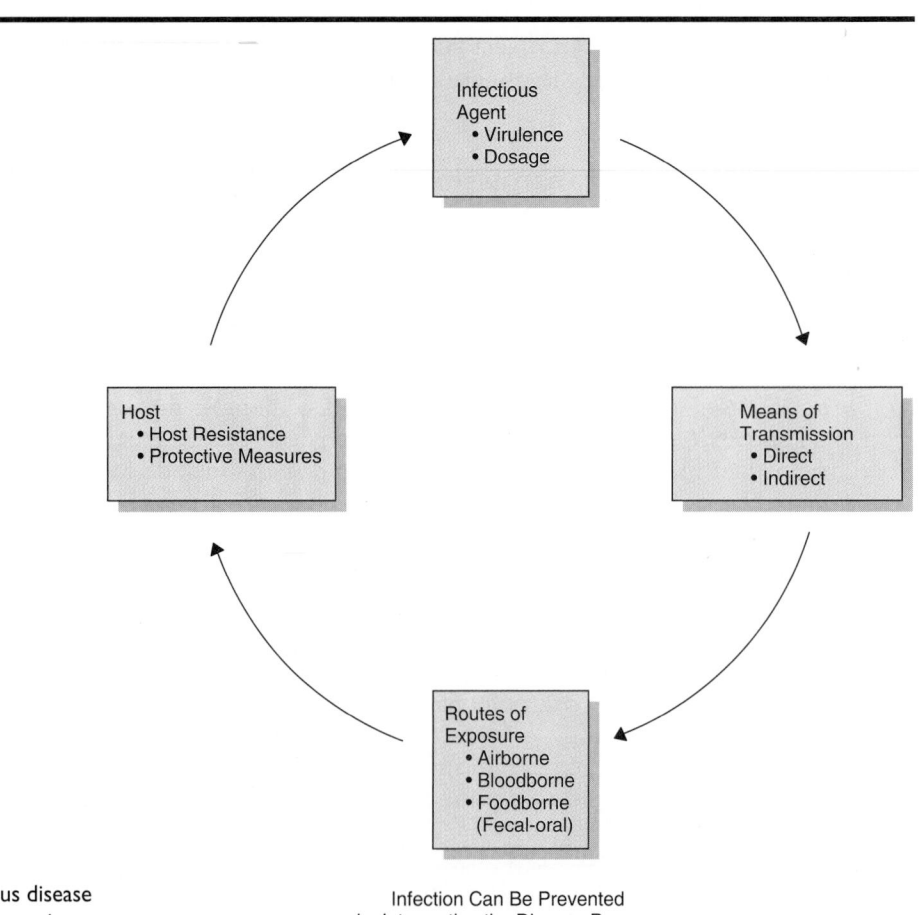

FIGURE 27-1 Interruption of infectious disease transmission is a role of prehospital personnel.

Infection Can Be Prevented by Interrupting the Disease Process

A person who develops antibodies after exposure to a disease is said to *seroconvert*. Seroconversion means that a previously negative test is now positive and disease exposure has occurred. The period of time from exposure to the disease and seroconversion is referred to as the *window phase*. It is important to point out that someone in the window phase may test negative, but may actually be positive and able to spread the disease.

The appearance of symptoms often lags behind exposure to the disease. The time between exposure and presentation is known as the *incubation period*. It may range from a few days, as with the common cold, to months or years, as with AIDS or hepatitis. Because of this delay, prehospital personnel must be notified if any patient subsequently develops a life-threatening infectious disease.

＊ Each EMS system must have a mechanism for tracking exposure to infectious disease and must include post-exposure follow-up.

INFECTION CONTROL IN PREHOSPITAL CARE

There are four phases of infection control in prehospital care. These include:

❑ Preparation for response to emergency incidents
❑ Response to emergency incidents
❑ Actions at emergency incidents
❑ Recovery from emergency incidents

Emergency personnel should have personal protective equipment (PPE) available at all times. (Personal protective equipment is discussed on the pages prior to Chapter 1.) Review this equipment for your own safety.

Preparation for Response to Emergency Incidents

Infection control begins long before an emergency call. To ensure proper protection of patients and personnel from exposure to infectious diseases, each EMS service should complete the following precautions prior to responding to an emergency incident.

❑ Establish and maintain written standard operating procedures (SOPs), and assure that all personnel adhere to these procedures.
❑ Provide adequate infection control training to all personnel.
❑ Ensure that proper personal protective equipment is provided and stored appropriately. Have all equipment checked regularly and maintained properly.
❑ Ensure that all emergency personnel treat and bandage all personal wounds (open sores, cuts, skin breaks, etc.) prior to the emergency response.
❑ Assure that all emergency personnel have a high level of personal hygiene.
❑ Do not allow emergency personnel to deliver patient care if they have a communicable disease such as hepatitis B or influenza.
❑ Assure that all emergency personnel obtain appropriate vaccinations to protect them from contracting communicable diseases.
❑ Do not allow emergency personnel to eat, drink, or have open food in any part of the ambulance.

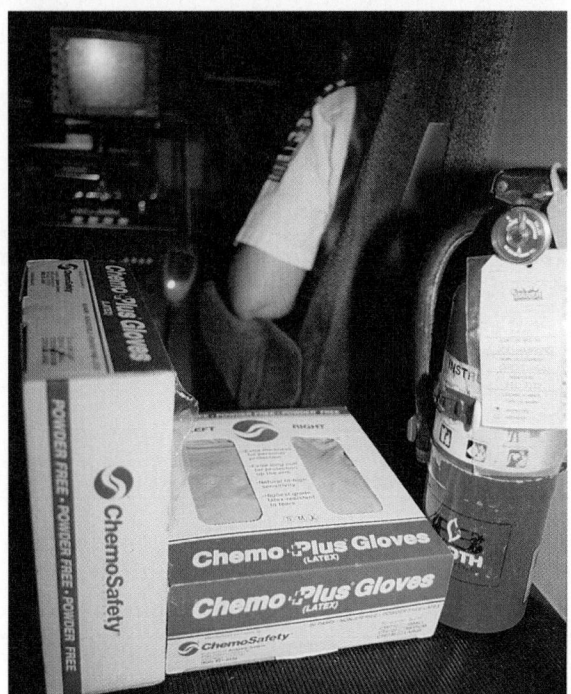

FIGURE 27-2 Preparation for immediate patient care should begin while en route. Protective gloves, eyewear, gowns, and masks should be immediately available.

Response to Emergency Incidents

While en route to an emergency incident, all prehospital personnel should begin preparation for immediate patient care. This can be facilitated by the following actions.

- ❑ Obtain as much information as possible from dispatch regarding the nature of the call.
- ❑ Prepare for patient contact en route. Put on gloves and don eye and face protection as soon as practical. (See Figure 27-2.)
- ❑ Prepare mentally for the call. THINK INFECTION CONTROL!

Actions at Emergency Incidents

Your actions at an emergency scene pose the highest risk for acquiring an infectious disease. You should have all personal protective equipment with you prior to leaving the emergency vehicle. In addition, you should adhere to the following guidelines. (Also, see Table 27-1.)

- ❑ Isolate all body substances. Do not come into contact with any of them.
- ❑ Wear appropriate personal protective equipment. (See Figure 27-3.)
- ❑ Allow only necessary personnel to make patient contact. Limit the risk to as few people as possible, thus minimizing exposure.
- ❑ Use airway adjuncts such as a pocket mask or bag-valve-mask unit to minimize exposures.
- ❑ Properly dispose of biohazardous waste.
- ❑ Use extreme caution with sharp instruments. *DO NOT BEND, RECAP, OR REMOVE NEEDLES.* Dispose of all contaminated sharps in puncture-resistant, properly labeled containers. (See Figure 27-4.)

Task or Activity	Disposable Gloves	Gown	Mask*	Protective Eyewear
Bleeding control with spurting blood	YES	YES	YES	YES
Bleeding control with minimal bleeding	YES	NO	NO	NO
Emergency childbirth	YES	YES	YES	YES
Blood drawing	YES	NO	NO	NO
Starting an IV	YES	NO	NO	NO
Endotracheal intubation	YES	NO	YES	YES
EOA insertion	YES	NO	YES	YES
Oral/nasal suctioning; manually clearing airway	YES	YES	YES	YES
Handling/cleaning instruments with possible contamination	YES	YES	YES	YES
Measuring blood pressure	YES	NO	NO	NO
Giving an injection	YES	NO	NO	NO
Measuring temperature	YES	NO	NO	NO
Rescuing from a building fire	YES	NO	NO	NO
Cleaning back of ambulance after a medical call	YES	NO	NO	NO

*Protective face shields can serve as both mask and eyewear to protect
 against blood splashes.

Reprinted with permission of: United States Fire Administration, National Fire Academy. Emmitsburg, MD (1993)

❏ Allow no smoking, eating, or drinking at the scene.
❏ Do not apply cosmetics or lip balm or handle contact lenses where a reasonable likelihood of exposure exists.

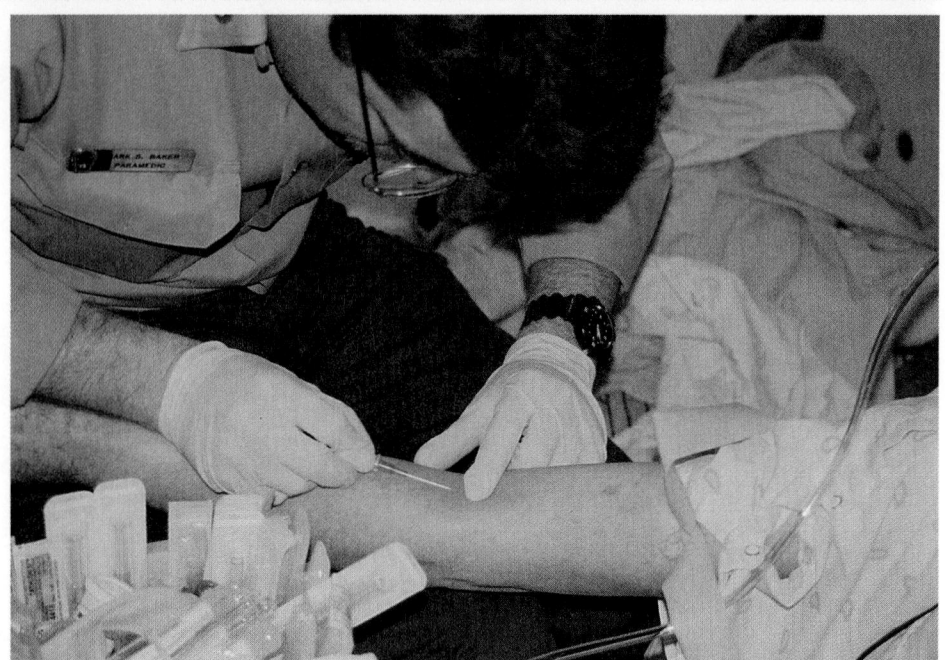

FIGURE 27-3 Always utilize personal protection recommended for the degree of exposure anticipated.

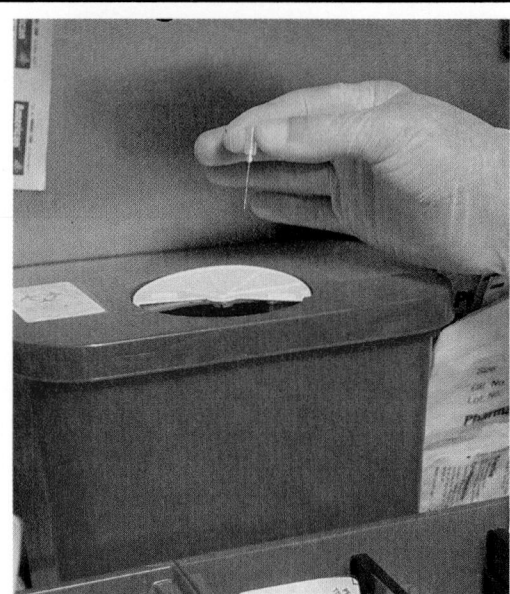

FIGURE 27-4 Dispose of needles and other sharp objects properly.

✳ Proper hand-washing between each call will decrease the likelihood of disease transmission.

❏ Wash hands immediately after patient contact. On-scene, hands can be washed with a waterless, hand-cleansing solution. Upon returning to quarters or at the hospital, thorough hand-washing with soap and water must be carried out. *PROPER AND FREQUENT HAND-WASHING CANNOT BE OVERSTRESSED!*

Recovery From Emergency Incidents

Infection control does not end at the scene. Upon arrival at the hospital, or upon return to quarters, infection control procedures continue. The following actions are necessary.

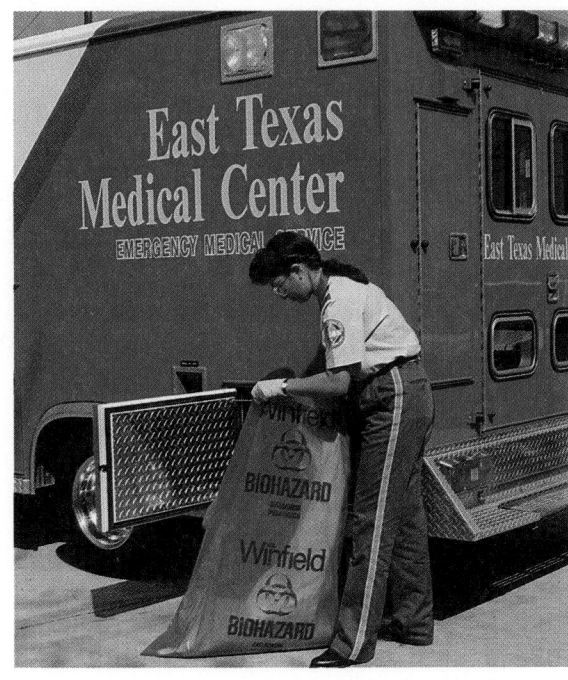

FIGURE 27-5 Bag all linen, and label it infectious.

❏ Dispose of all biohazardous wastes in accordance with local laws and regulations.

❏ Transport infectious wastes in leak-proof containers. Bag any soiled linen, and label for laundry personnel. (See Figure 27-5.)

❏ Decontaminate all contaminated clothing and reusable equipment. (This last point is detailed below.)

Decontamination Methods and Procedures All emergency equipment should be decontaminated following protocols and standard operating procedures established by the EMS service or department. Take equipment to a designated decontamination area, which should be a properly marked, secured, separate room. Ensure that the room has a proper ventilation system and adequate drainage. Be sure to wear gloves, gowns, boots, protective eyewear, and a facemask during decontamination. Begin decontamination cleaning with soap and water to remove surface dirt and debris. Then, carry out disinfection, and if required, sterilization. Various levels of decontamination exist. These include:

❏ *Low-Level Disinfection.* Low-level disinfection destroys most bacteria and some viruses and fungi. It does not destroy *Mycobacterium tuberculosis* or bacterial spores. Low-level disinfection is used for routine housekeeping and cleaning, as well as for removal of visible body fluids. All EPA-registered disinfectants can be utilized for low-level disinfection. (See Figure 27-6.)

❏ *Intermediate-Level Disinfection.* Intermediate level disinfection is used for all equipment that has come into contact with intact skin such as stethoscopes, splints, and blood pressure cuffs. Intermediate-level disinfection destroys *Mycobacterium tuberculosis* and most viruses and fungi. It does not, however, destroy bacterial spores. A 1:10 to 1:100 dilution of water and chlorine bleach can be used. In addition, hard surface germicides and EPA-registered disinfectants/chemical germicides can also be used.

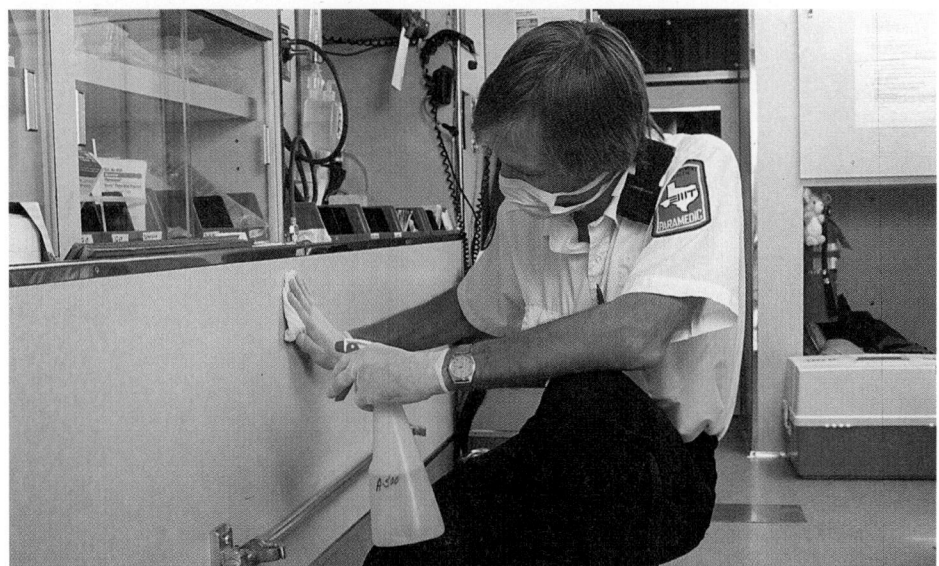

FIGURE 27-6 Routine cleaning and other "housekeeping" chores should be completed after each patient encounter.

❑ *High-Level Disinfection*. High-level disinfection destroys all forms of microorganisms except certain bacterial spores. High-level disinfection is required for all reusable devices that have come into contact with mucous membranes, including laryngoscopes, Magill forceps, and airway adjuncts. High-level disinfection can be accomplished by immersion is an EPA-approved chemical sterilizing agent for a short period of time (10–45 seconds depending upon the manufacturers instructions). Alternatively, immersion in hot water (176° to 212° F) for 30 minutes can be used.

❑ *Sterilization*. Sterilization destroys all microorganisms and is required for all contaminated invasive instruments. This can be accomplished in an autoclave using steam under pressure or with ethylene-oxide gas. These methods, however, are rarely available outside of a hospital setting. Alternatively, immersion in an EPA-approved chemical sterilizing agent for prolonged periods (6–10 hours depending on the manufacturer's instructions) is usually adequate. When possible, any invasive instruments should be disposable.

INFECTIOUS DISEASES AND EMERGENCY CARE

This section will detail the infectious diseases of the various organ systems and their management in the prehospital emergency setting. Particular emphasis will be on protection of the paramedic, since antibiotic therapy and diagnosis of infectious disease lie outside of the scope of standard prehospital care.

Infections of the Nervous System

Infections of the nervous system, although uncommon, can be life threatening. Most cause fever, headache, and alteration in mental status. Examples of central nervous system infections include meningitis, encephalitis, and brain abscess.

■ **meningitis** infection of the lining of the brain and the spinal cord; most commonly caused by bacteria or viruses.

Meningitis **Meningitis** is the most common central nervous system infection encountered in prehospital care. The disease infects the lining of the brain and spinal cord. It occurs more frequently in children, but adults can also be victims. Meningitis can be caused by bacteria, viruses, and occasionally, fungi. Bacterial infections tend to be more severe than viral infections. Common bacterial agents causing meningitis include *Streptococcus pneumoniae*, *Haemophilus influenza*, and *Neisseria meningitis*. Meningitis frequently begins as a cold, sinus infection, or middle ear infection. It subsequently spreads to the brain. Because prompt diagnosis and treatment are essential, suspect meningitis in any patient with these symptoms.

Meningitis is primarily transmitted through airborne droplets expelled by a productive cough or sneeze. The clinical presentation of meningitis depends upon the patient's age. Infants usually show no symptom other than fever, irritability, or poor feeding. Thus, when confronted by an infant under three months of age with a documented fever, physicians tend to assume the child has meningitis until proven otherwise. In older children and adults, meningitis often begins as malaise, low-grade temperature, headache, and a stiff or sore neck. Nausea and vomiting—occasionally projectile vomiting—will also be present. Some patients will exhibit a reddish rash. In more serious or more advanced infections, patients with meningitis will present as acutely confused, in a seizure state, or by unconsciousness. If untreated, meningitis may quickly progress to coma, shock, and, ultimately, death.

Paramedic Safety   When treating or transporting a patient who may have meningitis, take the following recommended precautions.

- ❑ Wear disposable gloves to avoid contact with body fluids.
- ❑ Put on disposable masks to prevent respiratory spread.
- ❑ Bag and label all linen for protection of laundry personnel.
- ❑ Decontaminate the ambulance.
- ❑ Perform medical follow-up, since some cases of meningitis may require antibiotic prophylaxis.
- ❑ Notify emergency department personnel.

Infections of the Respiratory System

Infections of the respiratory system are probably the most common infectious diseases encountered in the prehospital setting. Most of these diseases do not pose a life threat. Even so, a few respiratory infections, particularly tuberculosis, can seriously harm the health of prehospital personnel.

The majority of respiratory infections are viral in origin and involve the upper respiratory tract. On the other hand, lower respiratory tract infections, such as pneumonia, are generally bacterial. While upper respiratory tract infections are fairly easily transmitted, pneumonias are difficult to transmit.

Tuberculosis   Tuberculosis (TB) is a lower respiratory tract infection caused by the bacterium *Mycobacterium tuberculosis*. Generally found in those who are in poor health or who live in crowded areas, tuberculosis is spread through airborne water droplets. The incubation period is fairly long, ranging from 4–12 weeks.

In the last several years, the incidence of tuberculosis has been on the increase. This is particularly true in urban areas, especially in the lower socioeconomic classes. In fact, tuberculosis commonly infects the homeless. Unfortunately, many strains of the tuberculosis bacteria have developed resistance to a number of drugs routinely used in treatment. These new strains of *drug-resistant* tuberculosis pose a significant risk to prehospital personnel and the public at large.

Patients infected with the tuberculosis bacteria initially develop a cough. Chills, fever, fatigue, and weight loss later become common. Most patients will give a history of profuse night sweats, which literally soak their clothing. They also may report coughing up of blood, or hemoptysis. In some instances, the infection can spread outside of the respiratory tract and involve other body systems such as the gastrointestinal and genitourinary systems.

Diagnosis of tuberculosis can usually be done through a chest X-ray. The diagnosis is then confirmed by growing the bacteria on special cultures. It often takes four to six weeks to culture the tuberculosis bacterium. The most common screening test for tuberculosis is the so-called *PPD* skin test. It consists of placing a small amount of protein from the tuberculosis bacteria into the skin. After 72 hours, the site is examined. If there is a firm raised area greater than 10 millimeters in diameter, the patient is said to have "converted," indicating prior exposure to tuberculosis. A positive PPD test does not mean that the patient has tuberculosis, only that additional testing is required. Prehospital personnel should undergo routine testing for TB. It is also important to ask patients suspected of having TB if they have converted.

In addition to infections from the standard tuberculosis bacteria, there has been an increase in infections due to the so-called *atypical bacteria*. These infections most commonly occur in AIDS patients whose altered immune systems make them more susceptible to infection.

Paramedic Safety   When treating or transporting a patient suspected of having tuberculosis, take the following recommended precautions.

❏ Wear disposable gloves to avoid contact with body fluids.
❏ Put on disposable masks to prevent respiratory spread. (See Figure 27-7.)
❏ Place a disposable mask on the patient.
❏ Open the windows of the ambulance to allow a maximum exchange of fresh air.
❏ Avoid prolonged contact with the patient, especially in confined spaces.

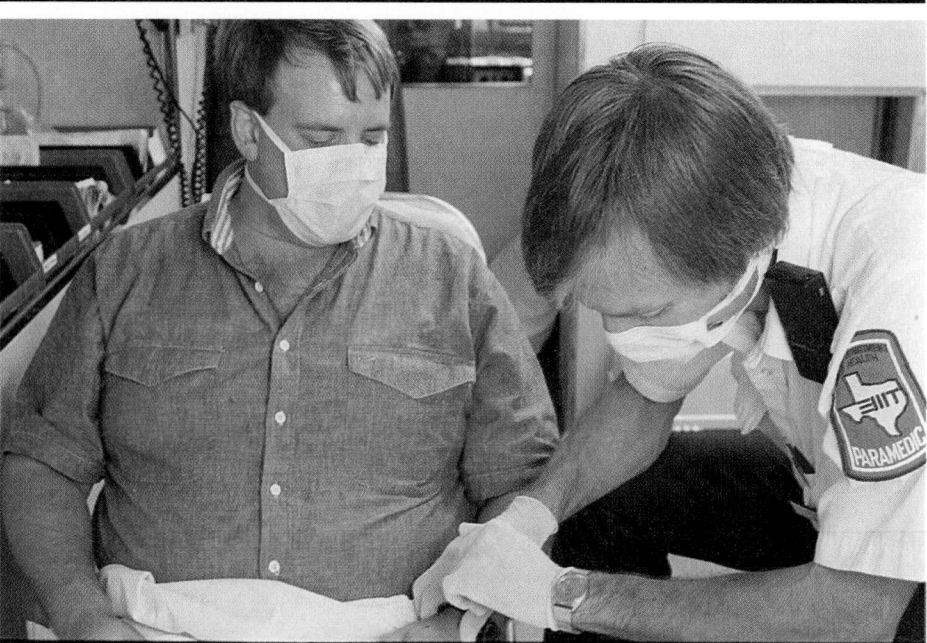

FIGURE 27-7   Use respiratory protection if a respiratory infectious disease, such as tuberculosis, is suspected.

❑ Avoid contact with the sputum.

❑ Bag and label all linen for protection of laundry personnel.

❑ Decontaminate the ambulance.

❑ Perform medical follow-up, since some of the cases encountered may require antibiotic prophylaxis.

❑ Notify emergency department personnel.

Skin Infections

There are many types of skin infections. Although most do not threaten health care workers, you should be familiar with two common skin parasites—scabies and lice.

Scabies   Scabies is a highly communicable skin disease caused by a species of mite. This infection, commonly called "the seven year itch," results from burrowing of the mite into the skin. The webs of the fingers and toes are among the most common sites of infections. Close inspection may reveal the small mite burrows. Besides these burrows, papules may be present. Both are associated with intense itching.

Lice   Lice are parasites slightly larger than mites. Becoming attached to hair follicles, they ultimately lay their eggs, or "nits," there. Patients infested with lice usually experience severe itching and have small white specks in the hair. Close inspection will frequently reveal the parasite itself. As with scabies, lice infestation is highly communicable and precautions should be taken.

Paramedic Safety   When treating or transporting patients suspected of having scabies or lice, take the following recommended precautions.

❑ Wear gloves at all times. (See Figure 27-8.)

❑ Wash hands following contact with the patient.

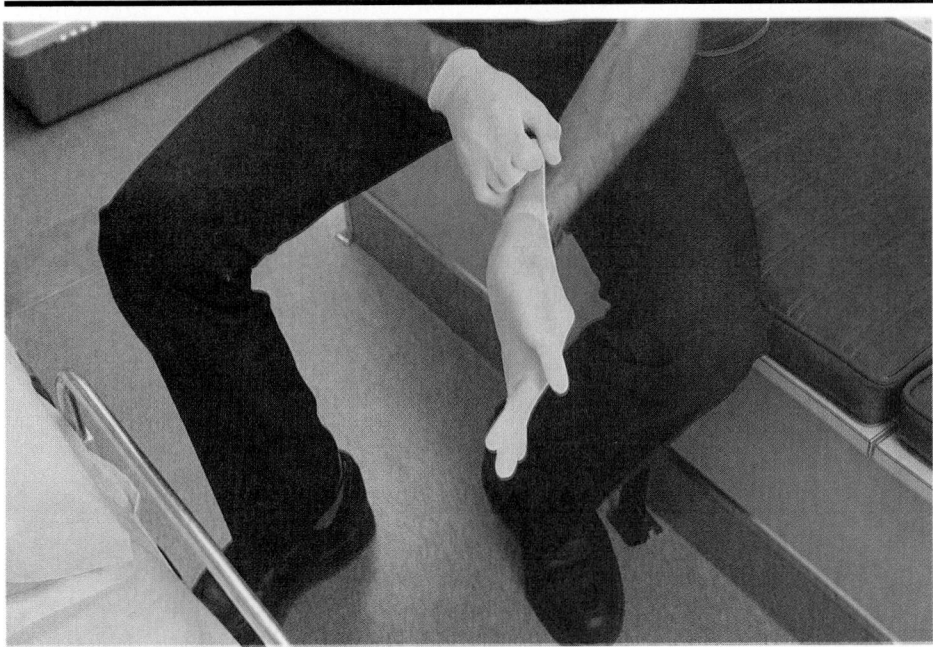

FIGURE 27-8 Anytime you suspect a tear in your gloves, remove them and replace them immediately with a new pair.

❏ Notify emergency department personnel.
❏ Dispose of or sterilize all instruments used.
❏ Bag and label all linen.

Childhood Diseases

Most children are required by law to have vaccinations against the common childhood diseases. Vaccines now exist for mumps, measles, German measles, polio, diphtheria, whooping cough, and tetanus. Some children also receive a vaccine against *Haemophilus influenza* meningitis. Nevertheless, most children are not vaccinated against chicken pox (varicella).

Measles   Widespread vaccination has greatly reduced measles, commonly called red measles. Caused by the measles (rubeola) virus, the infection is primarily transmitted through the respiratory tract. In rare epidemic situations, persons born since 1956 and not vaccinated after 1968 are at risk for developing measles due to changes that have occurred in the vaccine.

    The incubation period for measles is 8–13 days. Usually, the initial fever is accompanied by a reddish rash that typically appears first on the face and then spreads to the rest of the body. Measles is usually self-limited and treatment is symptomatic. The high fever occasionally may cause febrile seizures.

Mumps   Like measles, vaccinations have greatly reduced cases of mumps. The infection results from the mumps virus. Transmission usually occurs through the saliva of an infected person. The incubation period is 12–26 days. The disease begins as a fever, with later swelling of the salivary glands under the jaw and around the cheek area. In males, the testes can sometimes become involved. In females, the ovaries are subject to involvement. The disease is self-limited and treatment is symptomatic.

Varicella   Chicken pox, or varicella, is still quite common. Technically, varicella is a herpes infection. Although a vaccine now exists, it has not been used extensively in this country. The varicella zoster virus, a member of the herpes class, causes the infection. Transmission is primarily through the respiratory tract. The incubation period is approximately 10–21 days. Chicken pox initially begins as a fever. Shortly afterwards, "crops" of reddish skin eruptions appear over the body. The lesions first appear on the trunk and usually move to the extremities. Several crops will typically appear, each associated with itching. While the eruptions are still oozing, transmission is possible.

    Treatment is symptomatic and the infection is self-limited. Once a person has been infected, he or she is usually immune for life. But the virus may remain in the body dormant for many years, generally living in nerves along the back. In later life, or during periods of stress, the virus may become active. Spreading through the distribution of the nerve in which it resides, the virus causes the illness known as *shingles*. Unlike chicken pox, shingles is not contagious.

Paramedic Safety   When you treat or transport a patient suspected of having a childhood infectious disease, take the following recommended safety precautions.

❏ Wear masks at all times for respiratory isolation.
❏ Wear gloves at all times.
❏ Wash hands following contact with any body secretions.

❑ Notify emergency department personnel.

❑ Dispose of or heat sterilize all instruments used.

❑ Bag all linen and trash for protection of others.

❑ Always follow-up with the emergency department to determine what sort of infection the person had.

Infections of the Gastrointestinal System

Infections of the gastrointestinal system—like infections of the respiratory system—are fairly common. Most gastrointestinal infections result from viruses. These infections rarely cause little more than vomiting and diarrhea. Few people summon EMS unless the infection becomes severe and serious dehydration develops.

Gastroenteritis It is not uncommon for paramedics to answer calls for suspected cases of "food poisoning." Food poisoning usually refers to an infection of the stomach and intestines, commonly called *gastroenteritis*. It occurs within minutes or hours after eating food that has been infected by either a bacterium or virus. Food poisoning is especially common in developing countries.

Treatment of gastroenteritis consists of identifying a possible source of infection and treating it according to the causative agent. If dehydration is evident, IV fluid replacement should be carried out.

Hepatitis Hepatitis is one of the most dangerous infections that you may encounter in a prehospital setting. Hepatitis is an infection or inflammation of the liver. Most cases are caused by viruses. Five specific types of hepatitis have been identified.

Hepatitis A. Hepatitis A is the most common form of hepatitis. This infection, formerly called infectious hepatitis, is caused by the hepatitis A virus (HAV). The route of transmission is usually fecal-oral. Patients become infected by eating food contaminated with stool from someone infected with the disease. Isolated outbreaks of hepatitis A occasionally may be traced to a particular restaurant, where a worker is identified as the source.

The mean incubation period for hepatitis A is approximately 30 days. The initial symptom typically is malaise. Later, the patient will experience weakness and loss of appetite. Smokers may remark that cigarettes do not taste good to them anymore. Still later, the patient will develop the characteristic yellow tint to the skin called *jaundice*. He or she may also complain of dark-colored urine and stools.

Hepatitis A is usually self-limited and the patient recovers uneventfully. A carrier state does *not* exist. Once a person has been infected, he or she is then immune for life.

Hepatitis B. Commonly called serum hepatitis, hepatitis B is a much more severe infection than hepatitis A. Hepatitis B poses a serious risk to prehospital personnel. Hepatitis B is caused by the hepatitis B virus (HBV), sometimes called the *Dane particle*. This infection is bloodborne, transmitted only through blood or contact with other body secretions. Persons at risk include homosexuals, prostitutes, intravenous drug abusers, hemophiliacs, patients on chronic hemodialysis, and health care workers.

Following infection, the mean incubation period for hepatitis B is approximately 50 days. Its presentation is virtually identical to that described

✳ All prehospital personnel should consider receiving vaccination against hepatitis B.

for hepatitis A. But hepatitis B tends to last longer, and patients have a more pronounced jaundice. Moreover, it can result in a *carrier state*. The liver infection resolves, but the body does not clear the virus. Therefore, the patient can transmit the disease throughout his or her lifetime. In other cases, the hepatitis B virus is not cleared and the liver involvement persists causing a chronic infection called *chronic hepatitis*. This can sometimes evolve into cirrhosis of the liver, eventually leading to death.

Hepatitis C. Hepatitis C is a bloodborne disease caused by the hepatitis C virus (HCV). It was the major cause of post-transfusion hepatitis. Now, with routine testing of the nation's blood supply for hepatitis C, the incidence of hepatitis C is declining. Hepatitis C is transmitted in much the same manner as hepatitis B. Most patients with confirmed hepatitis C report a prior history of blood transfusion, accidental needlestick injury, or parenteral (needle-injected) drug abuse.

The mean incubation period for hepatitis C is 50 days. Both a carrier state and a chronic hepatitis can develop following infection with the hepatitis C virus. The signs and symptoms of hepatitis C infection are similar to hepatitis A and B. However, the jaundice is typically not as severe as with other types of infectious hepatitis.

Hepatitis D. Hepatitis D, formerly called *delta hepatitis*, is caused by the hepatitis D virus (HDV). The hepatitis D virus is a "defective virus," which means that it requires a helper virus to replicate. Thus, hepatitis D usually occurs as a co-infection with hepatitis B. Hepatitis D is a bloodborne infection. The mean incubation period is not known. However, following infection with hepatitis D, a chronic carrier and chronic hepatitis state can develop.

Co-infection with hepatitis B and hepatitis D may cause more severe and prolonged signs than infection with hepatitis B alone. However, simultaneous infection of HBV and HDV is usually self-limited. Superinfection of hepatitis D in a patient with chronic hepatitis B often leads to chronic hepatitis D. Chronic hepatitis D has a poor prognosis with many patients rapidly developing fatal cirrhosis of the liver.

Hepatitis E. Hepatitis E is transmitted by the fecal-oral route and is responsible for occasional outbreaks of hepatitis. Caused by the hepatitis E virus (HEV), the infection is most common in Central America, Africa, and the Indian subcontinent. The mean incubation period is 40 days. A chronic carrier and chronic hepatitis state does not appear to exist. Signs and symptoms are identical to other forms of hepatitis previously presented.

Paramedic Safety
When treating or transporting a patient suspected of having hepatitis, take the following recommended precautions.

❑ Wear gloves at all times.
❑ Wear a gown, goggles, and mask (or face shield) in the presence of spurting blood, during childbirth, or while performing mechanical airway maneuvers (especially endotracheal intubation).
❑ Wear a gown, goggles, and mask (or face shield) while cleaning instruments or equipment.
❑ Wash hands following contact with any body secretions.
❑ Notify emergency department personnel.
❑ Dispose of or heat sterilize all instruments used.
❑ Bag all linen and trash for protection of others.

❑ Always follow-up with the emergency department to learn what type of hepatitis was diagnosed.

If you do not take these precautions and the patient later tests positive for hepatitis A, consult a physician to determine whether gamma globulin is indicated. If the patient tests positive for hepatitis B, the physician may recommend that you receive Hepatitis B Immune Globulin (HBIG).

Hepatitis B Vaccine, a safe vaccine, provides protection against hepatitis B. When injected three times over a six-month period, the vaccine offers significant protection against hepatitis B. All prehospital personnel should receive this vaccine. Hepatitis B vaccine presents no risk of acquiring AIDS.

Sexually Transmitted Diseases

Sexually transmitted diseases are infectious illnesses caused by the transmission of an infectious agent from one person to another as a result of sexual intercourse or other sexual acts. Most sexually transmitted diseases are caused by either viruses or bacteria. Many sexually transmitted diseases result from heterosexual intercourse and are initially limited to the genitourinary tract. Persons who practice homosexual intercourse, oral sex, or anal sex may also contract infections that involve the gastrointestinal tract or other body systems.

Syphilis　Syphilis is an infectious sexually transmitted disease whose history dates back to pre-biblical times. The bacterium *Treponema palladium* causes it. Syphilis is a bloodborne disease. People contract it through sexual intercourse with somebody already infected. The disease initially involves the genitourinary system, but later spreads to virtually every body system. If untreated, it is ultimately fatal. Syphilis may also be transmitted from an infected mother to her fetus. The baby born of such a mother will have multiple anomalies. Syphilis is usually divided into three distinct stages. They include:

❑ *Primary Stage.* The primary stage usually occurs two to four weeks after exposure and is characterized by the appearance of a *chancre*. The chancre, a painless ulcer located in the genital region, can also appear on any mucous membrane. If untreated, the chancre will ultimately disappear, and the patient may become asymptomatic.

❑ *Secondary Stage.* Approximately six to eight weeks after the appearance of the chancre, the patient will develop headache, malaise, anorexia, fever, and often a sore throat. A reddish rash develops on both the palms of the hands and the soles of the feet. Often referred to as the *latent stage*, this stage will end even if untreated. The patient may again become asymptomatic.

❑ *Tertiary Stage.* Months or years after the secondary stage, the patient will enter the tertiary phase of syphilis. In this stage, the bacteria invade various blood vessels, especially the aorta, and the central nervous system. The spinal cord is particularly vulnerable, and a syndrome called *tabes dorsalis* develops. *Tabes dorsalis* is characterized by a wide gait, slapping of the feet on the ground, and ataxia. Tertiary syphilis is also characterized by psychosis. If untreated, especially in the tertiary stage, the disease will be fatal. A common cause of death is rupture of the aorta due to weakening of the aortic wall from infection by syphilis bacteria.

Gonorrhea and Chlamydia　Gonorrhea is another common sexually transmitted disease that has been a public health problem for many years.

Caused by the bacterium *Neisseria gonorrhea*, it exists throughout the world. In the male, gonorrhea is characterized by burning urination and yellowish penile discharge. In the female, it is not always symptomatic. When symptomatic, the female may complain of lower abdominal pain, yellowish vaginal discharge, and pain with intercourse. Often, walking or movement will cause pain, and the patient will begin to walk with a shuffled gait.

Recently, gonorrhea has been surpassed in frequency of infection by chlamydia. Caused by the bacteria *Chlamydia trachomatous*, chlamydia has symptoms quite similar to those of gonorrhea. Both gonorrhea and chlamydia are common causes of pelvic inflammatory disease in the female.

Herpes Herpes is a sexually transmitted disease caused by the herpes virus. The herpes class of viruses is a common source of human disease. There are two general categories of herpetic infections. They include:

❑ *Herpes Simplex, Type I.* Herpes simplex, Type I causes thin-walled vesicles, usually around the mouth and lips. Commonly called "cold sores," these infections tend to be self-limited.
❑ *Herpes Simplex, Type II.* Herpes simplex, Type II causes genital herpes. This infection is quite painful, resulting in thin-walled vesicles on the genitalia. Other signs and symptoms include burning, itching, tingling, and tenderness. In some cases, these symptoms may be accompanied by fever, swollen lymph glands, and general malaise. The infection is recurrent and no curative treatment is currently available. If the patient is pregnant, she should be asked when the most recent recurrence of the infection occurred. This information should be noted on the patient report form and relayed to emergency department personnel. Women who have active herpes lesions are typically delivered by Caesarean section to prevent infection of the baby as it passes through the birth canal.

✱ Herpes Whitlow, a herpes infection of the finger, can occur following contact with a person who has an active herpes lesion.

Paramedic Safety When treating or transporting a patient suspected of having a sexually transmitted disease, take the following precautions.

❑ Wear gloves at all times.
❑ Wash hands following contact with any body secretion.
❑ Notify emergency department personnel.
❑ Dispose of or sterilize all instruments used.
❑ Bag and label all linen.

HIV Infection

■ **acquired immune deficiency syndrome (AIDS)** fatal illness caused by infection with the Human Immunodeficiency Virus (HIV). Because AIDS destroys the ability of the immune system to fight infection, patients die from overwhelming infection. Also called HIV infection.

Acquired immune deficiency syndrome (AIDS) is a world-wide epidemic and a virtual threat to every individual. AIDS is caused by the *Human Immunodeficiency Virus (HIV)*.

Transmission The HIV virus is transmitted through body secretions. These include:

❑ Blood
❑ Vaginal secretions
❑ Semen
❑ Cerebrospinal fluid

Although not common, the virus may *theoretically* be transmitted by contact with the following fluids.

- ❏ Tears
- ❏ Saliva
- ❏ Breast milk
- ❏ Amniotic fluid
- ❏ Urine

People at high risk include those who have increased exposure to blood or body secretions. Initial high-risk groups included homosexual and bisexual males, IV drug abusers, and hemophiliacs. But now AIDS is occurring with increasing frequency in the heterosexual population. Health care workers are at high risk because of potential contact with contaminated blood or body secretions. Yet infection of those who work with AIDS patients has been exceedingly rare.

The virus can enter the body via breaks in the skin, through mucous membranes or the eyes, or by transmission through the placenta from an infected mother to her fetus. In health care workers, accidental needlestick injuries are the most frequent source of infection. Once in the blood, the virus affects the T lymphocytes of the immune system. This weakens the entire immune system, making the body susceptible to infection.

Presentation   Following exposure to HIV, some patients will develop antibodies and seroconvert. The blood test for antibodies to HIV is now easy to obtain and accurate. It is important to point out that there is a window phase following exposure to the virus. During this time, the patient can transmit the virus, but has yet to seroconvert. The time from exposure to seroconversion varies as does the time from exposure to initial disease symptoms. The incubation period varies from 6 months to 10 years. The average period is about 2 years.

The HIV infected patient may initially develop vague symptoms such as fatigue, fever, chronic diarrhea, and weight loss. These symptoms may seem so trivial to the patient that he or she will not seek health care. As the disease progresses, many patients will develop a severe, often life-threatening pneumonia. The most common cause of pneumonia in AIDS patients is the parasite *Pneumocystis carinii*. Often, pneumonia is the first presenting symptom of AIDS. At this point, many patients will seek health care and learn they are HIV-positive. In addition, there may also be secondary infection with atypical bacteria related to the causative agent of tuberculosis.

The patient with AIDS may show generalized swelling of the lymph nodes, which becomes quite striking in conjunction with the weight loss. Many patients will develop unusual, purplish skin tumors (known as *Kaposi's sarcoma*) anywhere on the body. As the disease progresses, the central nervous system becomes involved and a psychosis, commonly called *AIDS encephalopathy*, will develop. Death usually results from overwhelming infection, loss of respiratory function due to pneumonia, and, often, suicide. (See Figure 27-9.)

Treatment   At present there is no cure or vaccine for AIDS. There are several drugs, such as AZT, which are being used in treatment. These drugs alleviate many of the symptoms, but have little effect on the overall course of the disease.

AIDS patients are obviously difficult to treat. Despite some recent changes in societal attitudes, they are often shunned and condemned. Even if medicine has little to offer them in terms of treatment, it is tremendously important for prehospital personnel to be compassionate, understanding, and nonjudgmental. As a paramedic, you must take precautions to prevent disease transmission. But you should do this in a humane, compassionate manner.

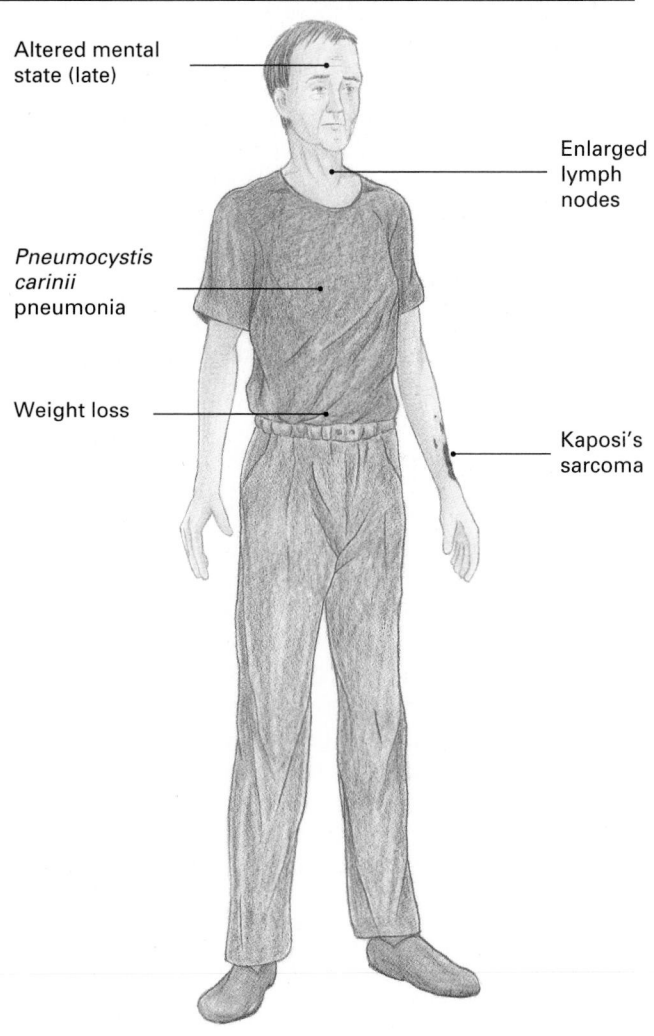

Altered mental state (late)

Enlarged lymph nodes

Pneumocystis carinii pneumonia

Weight loss

Kaposi's sarcoma

Figure 27-9 Clinical features of acquired immune deficiency syndrome (AIDS).

■ **universal precautions** set of procedures and precautions published by the Centers for Disease Control to assist health care personnel in protecting themselves from infectious disease.

✱ Universal precautions should be just that; you should assume every patient is infected and follow the universal precautions detailed here.

Paramedic Safety The Centers for Disease Control has recommended the **universal precautions** for persons, such as EMS personnel, who are at increased risk for exposure to blood-bone infections such as AIDS. Since it is impossible to determine reliably which patients have a blood-borne infection, the following precautions are recommended *FOR ALL PATIENTS*.

❑ All health-care workers should routinely use appropriate barrier precautions to prevent exposure of the skin and mucous membranes to any contact with blood, or other body fluids, from ANY patient. Gloves should be worn whenever touching blood and body fluids, mucous membranes, or nonintact skin; handling items or surfaces soiled with blood or body fluids; and performing venipuncture or other vascular access procedures. After contact with each patient, gloves should be changed and discarded. To prevent exposure of the mucous membranes of the mouth, nose, and eyes, masks and protective eye wear or protective face shields should be worn during procedures likely to generate droplets of blood or other body fluids. If a glove is torn or a needlestick occurs, the glove should be removed and replaced as soon as possible. The needle or instrument should also be discarded and another obtained. Gowns or aprons should be worn during any procedure likely to generate splashes of bloods or other body fluids.

- Hands and other skin surfaces should be washed immediately and thoroughly if contaminated with blood or other body fluids. Hands should also be washed immediately after removal of gloves.
- All health-care workers should take precautions to prevent injuries caused by needles, scalpels, or other sharp instruments or devices whenever performing procedures, cleaning instruments, or disposing of instruments. To prevent needlestick injuries, needles SHOULD NOT be recapped, purposely bent, broken by hand, removed from disposable syringes, or otherwise manipulated by hand. After they are used, disposable syringes and needles, scalpel blades, and other sharp items should be placed in puncture-resistant containers for disposal. These containers should be placed as close as possible to work areas.

  * Needles should never be recapped.

  * Never reuse equipment labeled as disposable.
- Although saliva has not been directly implicated in HIV transmission, paramedics should still have mouth pieces, resuscitation bags, or ventilation devices immediately available for use in areas in which the need for resuscitation is predictable. This will avoid mouth-to-mouth ventilation.
- Health-care workers who have exudative or weeping skin lesions should refrain from direct patient care and from handling patient care equipment until the condition resolves.
- Pregnant health care workers are not known to be at greater risk of contracting HIV infection than health care workers who are not pregnant. If, however, a health care worker develops HIV infection during pregnancy, the infant is at risk from perinatal transmission. Therefore, pregnant health care workers should be especially familiar with, and strictly adhere to, precautions to minimize the risk of HIV transmission.

SUMMARY

Prehospital personnel generally will not be directly involved in the treatment of infectious disease. Nevertheless, you should suspect infectious disease and take proper precautions. Appropriate protective devices should be immediately available for every paramedic in your unit. These devices include disposable gloves, eye protection, face masks, and gowns or aprons. A mouth shield or mouth-to-mask ventilation device should also be readily available. Moreover, because the spectrum of infectious disease is changing rapidly, you must keep up to date with the latest recommendations on prevention of infectious disease. The key to infectious disease management is prevention.

FURTHER READING

Centers For Disease Control. "Guidelines for Prevention of Transmission of Human Immunodeficiency Virus and Hepatitis B Virus to Health-Care and Public Safety Workers," *MMWR*, June 23, 1989, vol. 38, No. 5–6.

Hauptman, William, Robert Hitscherich, and Paul Miskovitz. "Update on Acute and Chronic Hepatitis." *Hospital Medicine*, January, 1993 (pp. 83–106).

U. S. Department of Labor, OSHA. *Worker Exposure to AIDS and Hepatitis B*. Washington, DC, OSHA, 1988.

United States Fire Administration, National Fire Academy. *Infection Control for Emergency Response Personnel: The Supervisor's Role*. National Fire Academy, Emmitsburg, MD, 1992.

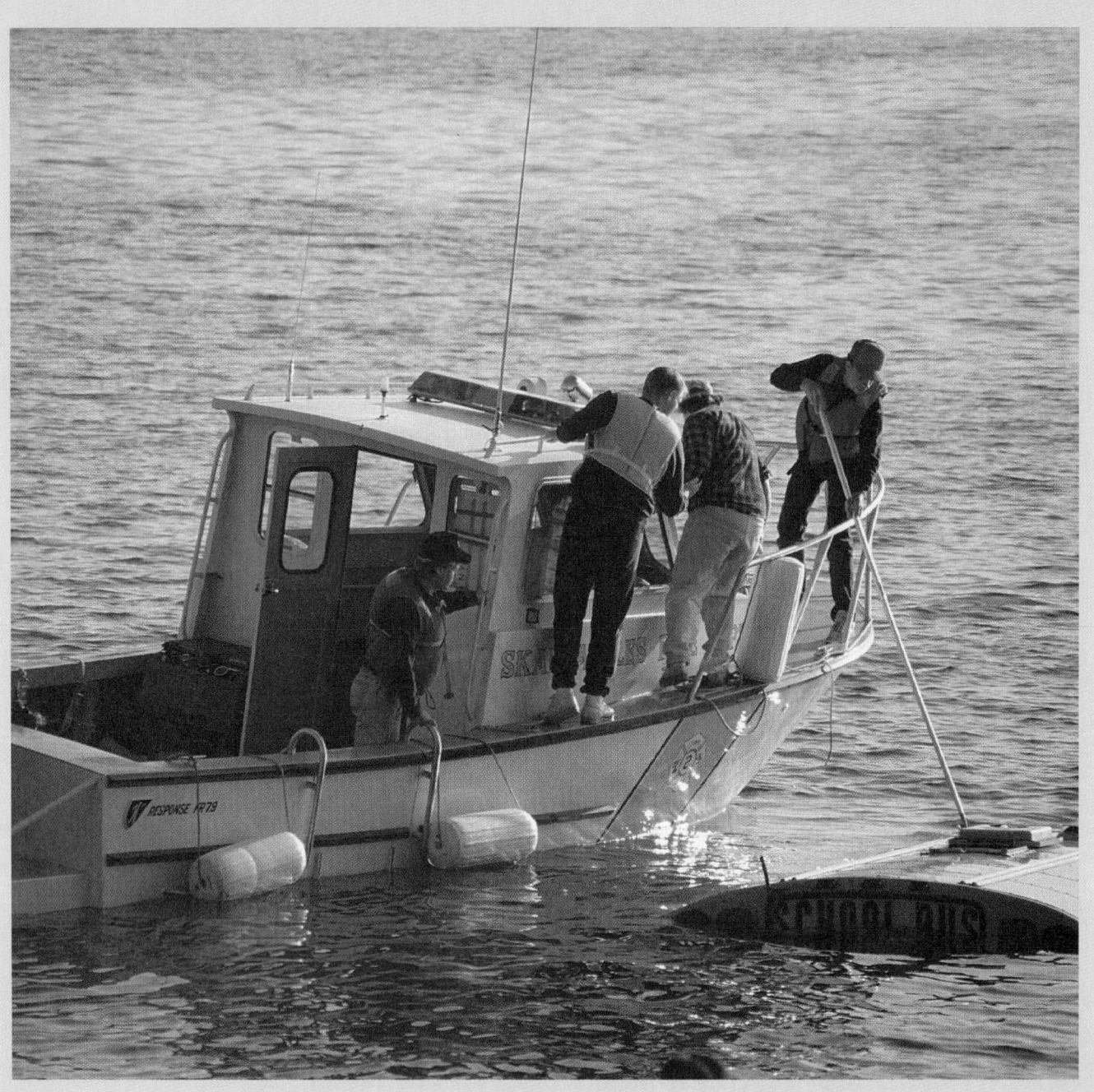

28

ENVIRONMENTAL EMERGENCIES

Objectives for Chapter 28

After reading this chapter, you should be able to:

1. Describe the four ways in which the body loses heat. (See p. 865.)

2. Describe mechanisms used by the body to maintain a core temperature in both warm and cold environments. (See pp. 865–867.)

3. Distinguish between hyperthermia and hypothermia. (See pp. 867–876.)

4. Identify the signs, symptoms, and recommended management techniques for heat cramps, heat exhaustion, water intoxication and heat stroke. (See pp. 869–871.)

5. Discuss the pathology of hypothermia and cold-related injuries. (See pp. 871–877.)

6. Identify the stages of systemic hypothermia, and describe the physical signs and symptoms associated with them. (See pp. 874–876.)

7. Identify non-environmental causes of hypothermia. (See p. 874.)

8. Discuss the concerns and precautions involved in rewarming a hypothermia patient in the field. (See pp. 874–876.)

9. Describe the events that occur during the near-drowning emergency. (See pp. 877–879.)

10. Identify the sources of ionizing radiation, and relate their relative penetrating potential. (See pp. 880–881.)

11. Name some of the factors that can help reduce exposure to a radiation source. (See pp. 881–882.)

12. Identify prehospital management of a patient who has been exposed to ionizing radiation. (See pp. 883–884.)

13. Identify common diving/hyperbaric emergencies. (See pp. 884–886.)

14. Describe the signs and symptoms of diving-related emergencies. (See pp. 886–890.)

15. Describe the management of the patient with a diving-related emergency. (See pp. 889–890.)

Central dispatch sends Engine 21, Rescue 10, and EMS 10 to a "possible drowning" at a local apartment complex. En route to the scene, the dispatcher reports that another dispatcher is giving telephone CPR instructions to bystanders. Upon arrival, paramedics find a 15-year-old male lying beside the pool in cardiac arrest. Although two bystanders are attempting CPR, patient vomiting hinders their efforts.

With the aid of the EMTs, the paramedics perform a primary survey. The "quick-look" paddles reveal fine ventricular fibrillation. Paramedics apply a 200 joule shock. Ventricular fibrillation persists. So paramedics charge the paddles again and deliver another 300 joule shock. When this proves unsuccessful, paramedics try a third time at 360 joules. They then initiate CPR with 100 percent oxygen via demand valve. With the patient still in ventricular fibrillation, paramedics establish an IV and place an endotracheal tube. They administer one milligram of epinephrine intravenously. The next defibrillation converts the patient to an idioventricular rhythm. Paramedics soon detect a carotid pulse.

During transport, paramedics continue respirations. At the hospital, the patient never regains consciousness. He remains alive for three days before dying from multiple organ failure.

INTRODUCTION

The *environment* can be defined as all of the surrounding external factors that affect the development and functioning of a living organism. Human beings obviously require the environment for life. But they also must be protected from its extremes.

As a paramedic, you will frequently be called upon to treat medical emergencies related to environmental conditions. Most of these emergencies occur during the summer or winter. Understanding their causes and underlying pathophysiologies can help you recognize these emergencies promptly and manage them effectively. Although many environmental factors can result in medical emergencies, this chapter will focus primarily on problems related to temperature extremes, drowning or near-drowning, nuclear radiation, and diving accidents.

THERMOREGULATION

The human body functions within a very small temperature range. The body temperature of the deep tissues, commonly called the *core temperature*, usually does not vary more than a degree or so from its normal 37° Celsius (98.6° F). This characteristic of warm-blooded animals is called *steady-state metabolism*. The various biochemical reactions occurring within the cell are most efficient when the body temperature is within this narrow temperature range. A naked person can be exposed to an external environment ranging anywhere from 55–144° F and still maintain a fairly constant internal body temperature. The production, loss, and physiological regulation of heat form the subject of this section.

Generation and Loss of Heat

The amount of heat in the body continually fluctuates between the heat generated and the heat lost. The following information explains some of the ways in which the body produces or loses heat.

Heat Generation   The human body gains heat through either internal or external sources. In addition to the heat generated by energy-producing chemical reactions, the body also absorbs heat from the environment.

Internal Heat. Internal heat comes from routine cellular metabolism and a process called **thermogenesis**. In producing energy, the cell gives off heat. Sympathetic stimulation, including an increase in circulating norepinephrine and epinephrine, can cause an immediate increase in the rate of cellular metabolism, which in turn increases heat production. Besides routine cellular metabolism, the body can stimulate certain cells to generate heat through thermogenesis. This primarily occurs in fatty tissue. Shivering can further generate heat through skeletal muscle contraction. Finally, heat can be generated through strenuous exercise, which greatly increases metabolic rates.

■ **thermogenesis** the production of heat, especially within the body.

Environmental Heat.   Our body receives external heat from the environment via the thermal gradient. The **thermal gradient** is the difference in temperature between the environment and the body. The environment is usually at a different temperature than the body. If the environment is warmer than the body, heat flows from it to the body. If the body is warmer than the environment, heat flows from the body to it. Several factors affect the thermal gradient. They include ambient air temperature, infrared radiation, and relative humidity. Ambient air temperature is simply the temperature of the surrounding air. Infrared radiation is radiation with a wavelength longer than that of visible light. Relative humidity is the percentage of water vapor present in air.

■ **thermal gradient** the difference in temperature between the environment and the body.

Heat Loss   The heat generated by the body is constantly lost to the environment. This occurs because the body is usually warmer than the surrounding environment. These heat transfers occur through the following methods. (See Figure 28-1.)

Radiation.   An unclothed person will lose approximately 60 percent of total body heat by radiation at normal room temperature. This heat loss is in the form of infrared rays. All objects not at absolute zero temperature will radiate heat.

Conduction.   Direct contact of the body's surface to another, cooler object causes the body to lose heat by **conduction**. Heat flows from higher temperature matter to lower temperature matter. The law of thermodynamics states that if **ambient** air temperature is higher than the skin temperature, then heat will flow from the air to the skin.

■ **conduction** moving electrons, ions, heat, or sound waves through a conductor or conducting medium.

■ **ambient** surrounding on all sides.

Convection.   Heat loss to air currents passing over the body is called **convection**. Heat, however, must first be conducted to the air before being carried by convection currents.

■ **convection** transferring of heat via currents in liquids or gases.

Evaporation.   Evaporative heat loss occurs as water evaporates from the skin. Additionally, a great deal of heat loss occurs through **evaporation** of fluids in the lungs. Water evaporates from the skin and lungs at approximately 600 mL/day.

■ **evaporation** change from liquid to a gaseous state.

Heat-Controlling Mechanisms

The body must maintain a balance between the production and loss of heat. Nervous or negative feedback mechanisms regulate the body's temperature almost entirely. Most of these mechanisms operate through temperature-regu-

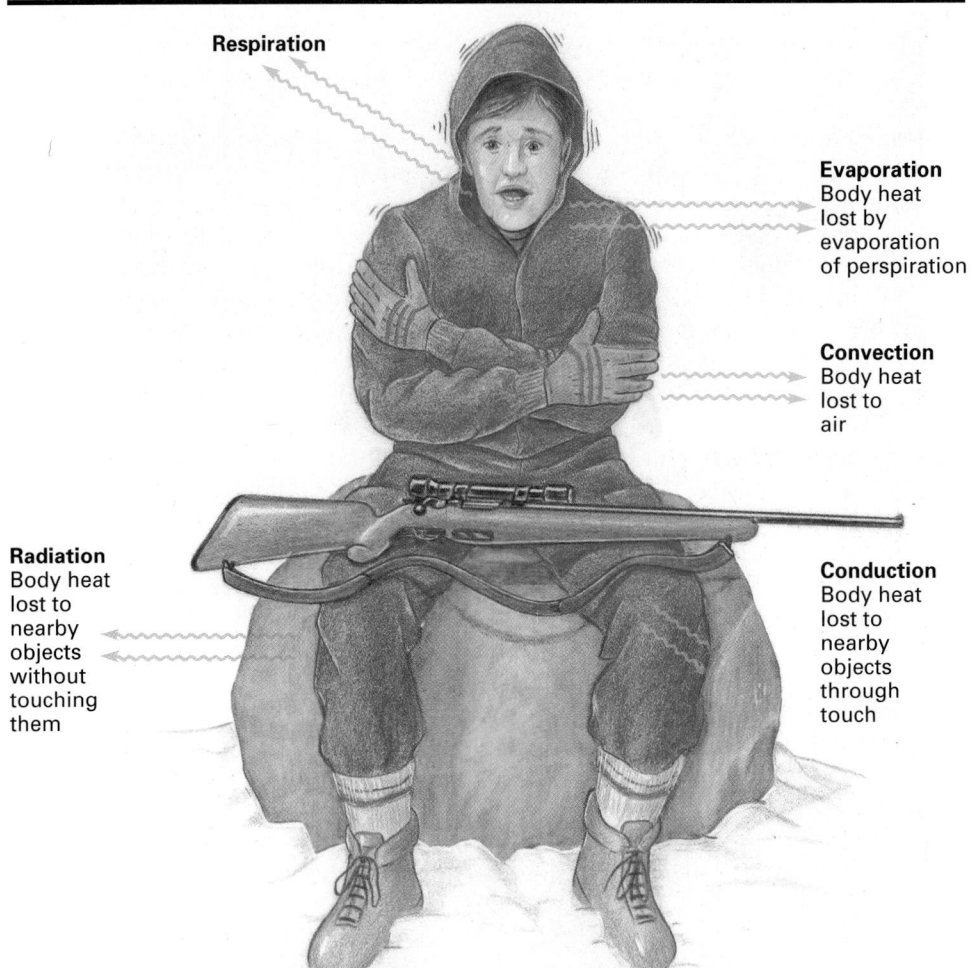

Respiration

Evaporation
Body heat
lost by
evaporation
of perspiration

Convection
Body heat
lost to
air

Radiation
Body heat
lost to
nearby
objects
without
touching
them

Conduction
Body heat
lost to
nearby
objects
through
touch

FIGURE 28-1 Heat loss by the body.

■ **hypothalamus** portion of the diencephalon producing neurosecretions important in the control of certain metabolic activities, including body temperature regulation.

lating centers located in the **hypothalamus** at the base of the brain. This area functions like a thermostat. It produces neurosecretions important in the control of many metabolic activities, including temperature regulation.

Although the hypothalamus plays a key role in body temperature regulation, temperature receptors in other parts of the body also help to moderate temperatures. Temperature receptors in the skin, certain mucous membranes, and selected deep tissues of the body are especially significant. The skin has both cold and warm receptors. Because cold receptors outnumber warm receptors, peripheral detection of temperature consists mainly of detecting cold instead of warmth. Deep body temperature (afferent) receptors lay mostly in the spinal cord, abdominal viscera, and in or around the great veins. These receptors are exposed to the body's core temperature rather than the surface temperature. They respond mainly to cold rather than warmth. Both skin and deep temperature receptors act to prevent hypothermia.

Heat Elimination   When the body becomes too hot, the *hypothalamic thermostat* and associated temperature receptors attempt to eliminate body heat through five mechanisms. These include:

❑ *Vasodilation.* The blood vessels in the skin become dilated due to the inhibition of the sympathetic centers in the hypothalamus. Heat is then lost through the skin by sweating and other mechanisms.

❑ *Perspiration.* Perspiration occurs when the core temperature rises above "normal" (98.6° F or 37° C). This mechanism is ineffective if the relative humidity is 75 percent or greater due to decreased evaporation of perspiration from the skin surface.

❑ *Decrease in Heat Production.* Shivering and chemical thermogenesis are inhibited, causing decreased heat production.

❑ *Increased Cardiac Output.* Increased cardiac output aids in increasing blood flow through the skin, thus aiding in the elimination of heat.

❑ *Increased Respiratory Rate.* An increase in respiratory rate results in elimination of warm air and in water evaporation.

Heat Preservation   When the body becomes too cold, the hypothalamic thermostat reacts in exactly the opposite fashion. To preserve heat, the body engages the following mechanisms.

❑ *Vasoconstriction.* Caused by stimulation of the hypothalamic sympathetic centers, *vasoconstriction* diverts the flow of blood from the skin to the body's core to maintain heat.

❑ *Piloerection* (hairs standing on end). This response developed millions of years ago when humans had a great deal more body hair than now. Piloerection increased the insulating ability of body hair and decreased heat loss.

❑ *Increased Heat Production.* Heat production is increased by the metabolic systems in the following ways.

   • *Thermogenesis (shivering).* The hypothalamus has an area called the *primary motor center* that controls shivering. It is excited by cold signals from the skin and spinal cord.

   • *Sympathetic Stimulation.* Norepinephrine and epinephrine are released following sympathetic stimulation, which causes an immediate increase in the rate of cellular metabolism and generates heat.

Heat Fluctuations   In summary, if the body temperature gets too high, the various cooling mechanisms are engaged. If the body becomes too cool, heat-preserving mechanisms are engaged. An increase in the body temperature is called **hyperthermia**, while a decrease is called **hypothermia**. Hyperthermia and fever are different. Fever occurs when the hypothalamus "resets" the "thermostat" in the brain. This purposeful increase in body temperature helps the body's various defense mechanisms clear itself of the infectious agent (i.e., bacteria or virus).

■ **hyperthermia** unusually high body temperature.

■ **hypothermia** having a body temperature below normal.

THERMAL DISORDERS

Disruption of the body's normal thermoregulation can produce a number of heat-related disorders. Some of these include hyperthermia, fevers, hyperpyrexia, hypothermia, and frostbite.

Hyperthermia

Hyperthermia is an increase in the body temperature caused by heat transfer from the external environment. It can manifest either as heat cramps, heat exhaustion, water intoxication, or heat stroke. (See Figure 28-2 and Table 28-1.)

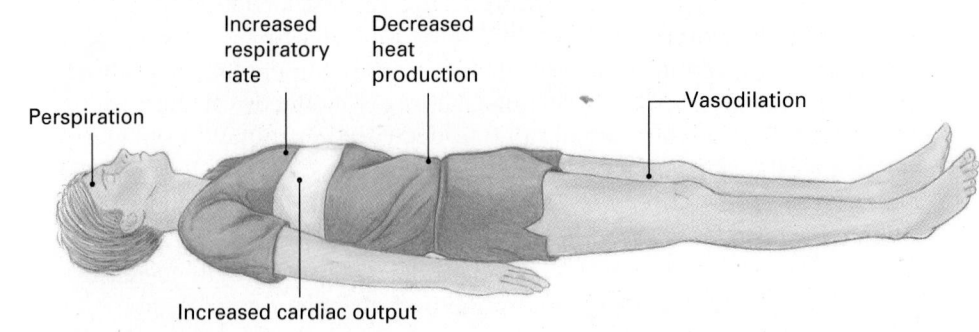

FIGURE 28-2 The victim of a heat emergency.

Perspiration

Increased respiratory rate

Decreased heat production

Vasodilation

Increased cardiac output

TABLE 28-1 Algorithm for Heat-Related Illnesses

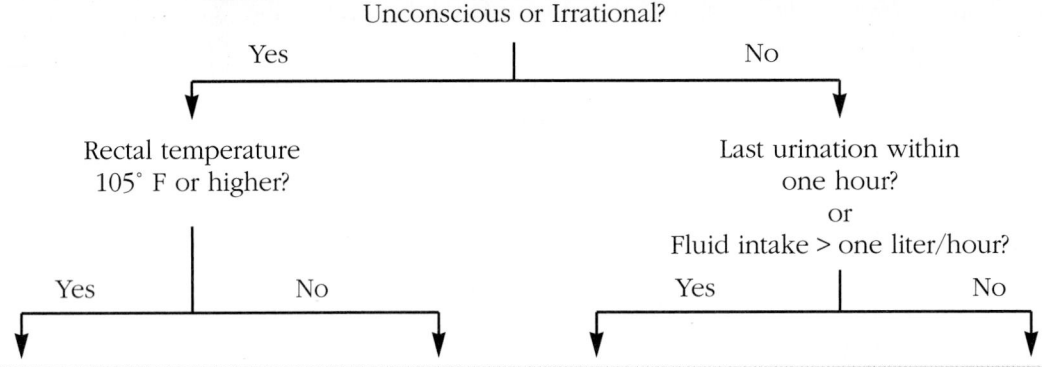

Unconscious or Irrational?

Yes — Rectal temperature 105° F or higher?

No — Last urination within one hour? or Fluid intake > one liter/hour?

Rectal temperature 105° F or higher? → Yes: Heat Stroke / No: Water Intoxication*

Last urination within one hour? or Fluid intake > one liter/hour? → Yes: Water Intoxication* / No: Heat Exhaustion

Heat Stroke	**Water Intoxication***	**Heat Exhaustion**

1. Initiate cooling measures.
2. Administer high-flow oxygen.
3. Incidental findings include:
  • Tachycardia
  • Bradycardia
  • Hypotension with low or absent diastolic reading
  • Rapid, shallow respirations
4. Be prepared for airway problems, seizures, and cardiac arrest.
  • Establish 1–2 IVs and run wide open.
  • Administer diazepam to control seizures.
5. Transport rapidly.
	1. Findings include:
	  • Nausea/vomiting
	  • Urinary frequency or incontinence
	  • Normal vital signs with negative orthostatic vital signs
	  • Chills
	  • Loss of coordination
	  • Headache
	  • Dizziness
	2. Significant neurological changes?
	
	Yes → Monitor and transport.
	No → Withhold fluids and encourage foods high in sodium.
		1. Findings include:
		  • Nausea/vomiting
		  • Diarrhea
		  • Muscle cramps
		  • Headache
		  • Tachycardia
		  • Positive orthostatic vital signs
		  • Dizziness
		  • Syncope
		  • Headache
		2. Evaluate the victim's ability to take oral fluids.
		3. Administer high-flow oxygen.
		4. Initiate 1–2 IVs.
		5. Transport.

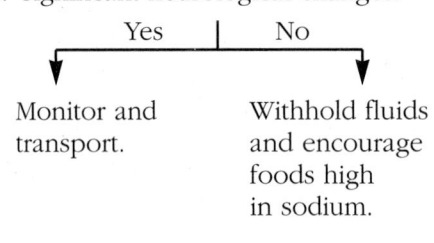

*In the unresponsive patient, water intoxication needs to be differentiated from other causes of unresponsiveness, including diabetic emergencies, stroke, and alcohol or drug intoxication.

Heat (Muscle) Cramps

Heat cramps are extremely common in hot climates. They result in intermittent, painful contractions of various skeletal muscles. Heat cramps are caused primarily by a rapid change in extracellular fluid osmolarity resulting from sodium and water losses. Sweating occurs as sodium is transported to the skin. Because "water follows sodium," it is deposited on the skin surface. Here evaporation occurs, thus aiding in the cooling process. Sweating not only involves the loss of water, but the loss of electrolytes (such as sodium) as well.

The patient with heat cramps will present with cramps in the fingers, arms, legs, or abdominal muscles. He or she will be generally mentally alert, with hot sweaty skin, tachycardia, normal blood pressure, and a normal core temperature.

Prehospital Management. The treatment of heat cramps is usually easily accomplished by removing the patient from the hot environment. Fluid and sodium intake should be increased. Severe cases of heat cramps may require IV fluid replacement with a balanced salt solution such as 0.9 percent sodium chloride or lactated Ringer's.

Heat Exhaustion

Heat exhaustion is the most common heat-related illness seen clinically by prehospital personnel. Dehydration and salt loss due to sweating account for the presenting symptoms. However, these signs and symptoms are not exclusive to heat exhaustion. Instead, they mimic those of an individual suffering from fluid and sodium loss. A history of exposure to hot weather is needed to obtain an accurate assessment. Signs and symptoms that you may encounter include:

- ❑ A history of low-fluid intake
- ❑ Decreased urine output
- ❑ Positive orthostatic vital signs
- ❑ Tachycardia
- ❑ Nausea and vomiting
- ❑ Dizziness and transient syncope
- ❑ Headache
- ❑ Muscle cramps
- ❑ Diarrhea

An individual performing work in a hot environment will lose 1–2 liters of water an hour. Each liter lost contains 20–50 milliequivalents of sodium. The loss of water and sodium, combined with general vasodilation, leads to a decreased circulating blood volume, venous pooling, and reduced cardiac output.

Prehospital Management. Prehospital treatment of heat exhaustion consists of removing the patient from the hot environment and providing intravenous replacement with a solution such as 0.9 percent sodium chloride or lactated Ringer's. If untreated, heat exhaustion can progress to heat stroke. (See pages 870–871)

Water Intoxication

Water intoxication occurs when an individual in a hot environment drinks water at a rate that exceeds fluid loss from sweating and fails to replace associated sodium losses. In water intoxication, sodium levels drop causing signs and symptoms similar to those seen with heat exhaustion. Common signs and symptoms of water intoxication include nausea, vomiting, headache, and alterations in mental status. Generally, the

■ **heat cramps** acute painful spasms of the voluntary muscles following strenuous activity in hot environment without adequate fluid or salt intake.

■ **heat exhaustion** acute reaction to heat exposure. Blood pools in the vessels as the body attempts to give off excessive heat. It can lead to collapse due to inadequate blood return to the heart.

patient will report water intake of greater than one liter per hour and may exhibit urinary frequency and dilute urine. Untreated water intoxication may lead to alterations in mental status and coma.

Prehospital Management. Patients suffering water intoxication should be encouraged to eat foods high in sodium and to restrict further water intake. Unresponsive patients should receive standard care and an IV of 0.9 percent sodium chloride at a "to keep open" rate.

Heat Stroke

Heat stroke occurs when the body's hypothalamic temperature regulation is lost, causing uncompensated hyperthermia. This in turn causes cell death and physiologic collapse. Heat stroke is generally characterized by a body temperature of at least 105° F (40.6° C), CNS disturbances, and usually the cessation of sweating. Sweating is thought to stop due to destruction of the sweat glands or when sensory overload causes them to temporarily dysfunction. However, the patient's skin may be either dry or covered with sweat. If the patient has not been exercising, the skin will be dry. But if the heat stroke occurred during strenuous exercise, sweating may be profuse. The patient may also present with the following signs and symptoms.

- ❏ Increased core temperature
- ❏ Tachycardia followed by bradycardia
- ❏ Hypotension with low or absent diastolic reading
- ❏ Rapid, shallow respirations, which may later slow
- ❏ Confusion or disorientation
- ❏ Seizures
- ❏ Coma

If the patient develops heat stroke due to exertion, he or she may go into severe metabolic acidosis caused by lactic acid accumulation. Hyperkalemia may also develop because of the release of potassium from injured muscle cells, renal failure, or metabolic acidosis.

Prehospital Management. Prehospital management of the shock patient is aimed at immediate cooling and replacement of fluids. Steps include:

1. *Rapid Patient Cooling.* This can be accomplished en route to the hospital by removing the patient's clothing and covering the patient with sheets soaked in ice-water. Body temperature must be lowered to 102° F. (39° C). A target of 102° is used to avoid an overshoot. Ice packs and fans may also be used.
2. *Administer Oxygen.* High-flow oxygen should be administered with a nonrebreather mask. If respirations are shallow, they should be assisted with a bag-valve-mask unit supplied with 100 percent oxygen. Pulse oximetry, if available, should be utilized.
3. *Establish IV(s).* Begin 1–2 IVs, using lactated Ringer's or normal saline. Initially infuse them wide open.
4. *Monitor ECG.* Cardiac dysrhythmias may occur at any time. S-T segment depression, non-specific T wave changes with occasional PVCs, and supraventricular tachycardias are common.
5. *Avoid Vasopressors and Anticholinergic Drugs.* These agents may potentiate heat stroke by inhibiting sweating. They can also produce a hypermetabolic state in the presence of high environmental temperatures and relatively high humidity.

■ **heat stroke** acute, dangerous reaction to heat exposure, characterized by a body temperature usually above 106° F (41.1° C). The body ceases to perspire.

✳ The patient with heat stroke should be cooled as soon as possible.

6. *Monitor Core Temperature.* EMS systems operating in extremely warm climates should carry some device to record the body temperature, whether a simple rectal thermometer or a sophisticated electronic device. Simple glass thermometers generally do not measure above 106° F or below 95° F. This may become significant during long transport when it is essential to detect changes in the patient's condition. (See Procedure 28-1.)

Fever (Pyrexia)

A fever (**pyrexia**) is the elevation of the body temperature above the normal temperature (0.5–1.0° higher for rectal temperatures) for that person. In other words, fever is essentially a resetting of the hypothalamic thermostat. The body develops a fever when pathogens enter and cause infection, which in turn stimulates the production of pyrogens. **Pyrogens** are any substances that cause fever. They reset the hypothalamic thermostat to a higher level. Metabolism is therefore increased, producing a fever. The increased body temperature wards off infection by making the body a less hospitable environment for the invading organism. The hypothalamic thermostat will reset to normal when pyrogen production stops or when pathogens end their attack on the body.

■ **pyrexia** fever, or above normal body temperature.

■ **pyrogen** any substance causing a fever.

Prehospital Management   The underlying cause of the fever must be treated before the fever can be arrested. Do not attempt to treat fever unless it is very high (>105° F) or unless changes in mental status exist or febrile seizures appear imminent. If requested by medical control, prehospital treatment of fever includes the oral or rectal administration of acetaminophen (Tylenol). Additional cooling may be obtained by removing all extra clothing and allowing the patient to lose heat to the environment by convection. Sponge baths are generally not recommended as these can drop the body's core temperature too much. The cooling will induce shivering and additional heat production.

✱ Sponge baths are not recommended in the management of fever.

Hyperpyrexia

Hyperpyrexia is the elevation of body temperature above 106° F (41.1° C). It can be produced by physical agents such as hot baths or hot air or by reaction to infection caused by microorganisms. Some people develop hyperpyrexia in the hospital within 24 hours after surgery. A rare cause of hyperpyrexia is *malignant hyperthermia*, which can occur following a general anesthetic in patients genetically predisposed. This, however, is rarely seen outside of the hospital setting.

■ **hyperpyrexia** elevation of body temperature, due to fever, above 106° F (41.1° C).

Hypothermia

Hypothermia is a state of low body temperature, specifically low body core temperature. When the core temperature of the body drops below 95° F (35° C), an individual is considered to be in a hypothermic state. Hypothermia can be attributed to either a decrease in heat production, an increase in heat loss, or a combination of both.

Exposure to cold normally causes shivering and increased muscle tone, resulting in increased metabolism to maintain the body temperature. Initial signs of hypothermia are peripheral vasoconstriction with an increase in cardiac output and respiratory rate. When this additional heat production can no longer keep up with heat lost from the body surface, the body temperature

Condition	Muscle Cramps	Breathing	Pulse	Weakness	Skin	Perspiration	Loss of Consciousness
Heat cramps	Yes	Varies	Varies	Yes	Moist-warm No change	Heavy	Seldom
Heat Exhaustion	No	Rapid Shallow	Weak	Yes	Cold Clammy	Heavy	Sometimes
Heat-Stroke	No	Deep, then shallow	Full Rapid	Yes	Dry-hot	Little or none	Often

1 HEAT CRAMPS

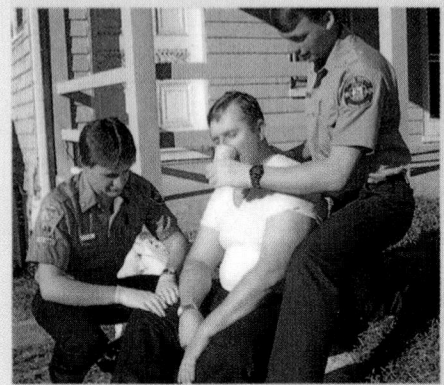

SYMPTOMS AND SIGNS:
Severe muscle cramps (usually in the legs and abdomen), exhaustion, sometimes dizziness or periods of faintness.

EMERGENCY CARE PROCEDURES:
- Move patient to a nearby cool place.
- Give patient salted water to drink or half-strength commercial electrolyte fluids.
- Massage the "cramped" muscle to help ease the patient's discomfort, massaging with pressure will be more effective than light rubbing actions. (Optional in some EMS systems).
- Apply moist towels to the patient's forehead and over cramped muscles for added relief.
- If cramps persist, or if more serious signs and symptoms develop, ready the patient for transport.

2 HEAT EXHAUSTION

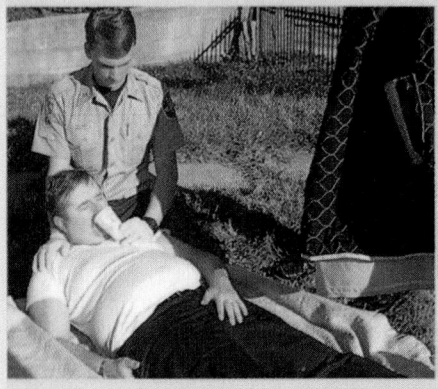

SYMPTOMS AND SIGNS:
Rapid and shallow breathing, weak pulse, cold and clammy skin, heavy perspiration, total body weakness, and dizziness that sometimes leads to unconsciousness.

EMERGENCY CARE PROCEDURES:
- Move patient to a nearby cool place.
- Keep the patient at rest.
- Remove enough clothing to cool the patient without chilling him (watch for shivering).
- Fan the patient's skin.
- Give the patient salted water or half-strength commercial electrolyte fluids. Do not try to administer fluids to an unconscious patient.
- Treat for shock, but do not cover to the point of overheating the patient.
- Provide oxygen if needed.
- If unconscious, fails to recover rapidly, has other injuries, or has a history of medical problems, transport as soon as possible.

3 HEATSTROKE

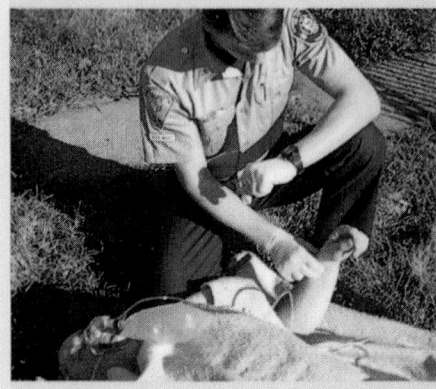

SYMPTOMS AND SIGNS:
Deep breaths, then shallow breathing; rapid strong pulse, then rapid, weak pulse; dry, hot skin; dilated pupils; loss of consciousness (possible coma); seizures or muscular twitching may be seen.

EMERGENCY CARE PROCEDURES:
- Cool the patient—in any manner—rapidly, move the patient out of the sun or away from the heat source. Remove patient's clothing and wrap him in wet towels and sheets. Pour cool water over these wrappings. Body heat must be lowered rapidly or brain cells will die!
- Treat for shock and administer a high concentration of oxygen.
- If cold packs or ice bags are available, wrap them and place one bag or pack under each of the patient's armpits, one behind each knee, one in the groin, one on each wrist and ankle, and one on each side of the patient's neck.
- Transport as soon as possible.
- Should transport be delayed, find a tub or container—immerse patient up to face in cooled water. Constantly monitor to prevent drowning.
- Monitor vital signs throughout process.

falls. As the body temperature falls, so does the metabolic rate and cardiac output. Hypovolemia results from the shift of fluid from the vascular to the extravascular compartment, allowing the body to preserve energy and prevent cell death. However, if the hypothermic state is not corrected, cell ischemia and necrosis eventually result in death.

As discussed, the major sources of heat production are exercise and cold-weather shivering. The major sources of body heat loss are conduction, radiation, evaporation, and convection. Heat loss can be increased by the removal of clothing, the wetting of clothing by rain or snow, increased air movement around the body (increased convection), or increased conduction such as cold-water immersion.

Presentation   Hypothermia patients can be divided into three categories: mild, moderate, and severe. A core temperature between 94° and 97° F (34–36° C) is considered mild hypothermia. A core temperature between 86° and 94° (30–34° C) is considered moderate hypothermia. A core temperature less than 86° F (30° C) is classified as severe hypothermia. Patients who experience body temperatures above 86° F will usually have a favorable prognosis. Those with temperatures below 86° F show a significant increase in mortality rate. Remember that most thermometers used in medicine do not register below 96° F. EMS systems in colder areas should carry special thermometers for recording subnormal temperature readings.

Patients experiencing mild to moderate hypothermia (core temperature >86° F) will generally exhibit shivering. (See Figure 28-3.) The patient may be lethargic and somewhat dulled mentally. (But, in some cases, they may be fully oriented.) Muscles may be stiff and uncoordinated, causing the patient to walk with a stumbling, staggering gait.

Patients experiencing severe hypothermia (core temperature <86° F) may be disoriented and confused. As their temperatures continue to fall, they will proceed into stupor and complete coma. Shivering will usually stop, and physical activity becomes uncoordinated. Muscles may be stiff and rigid. Continuous cardiac monitoring is indicated for anyone experiencing hypothermia. The ECG will frequently show pathognomonic (indicative of a disease) **J waves**, also called Osborn waves, associated with the QRS complexes. Atrial fibrillation is the most common presenting dysrhythmia seen in hypothermia. As the body cools, however, the myocardium becomes progressively more irritable and may develop a variety of dysrhythmias. In severe hypothermia, bradycardia is inevitable. Ventricular fibrillation becomes more probable as the body's core

■ **J wave** ECG deflection found at the junction of the QRS complex and the ST segment. It is associated with hypothermia and seen at core temperatures below 32° C, most commonly in leads II and V_6. Also called the Osborn wave.

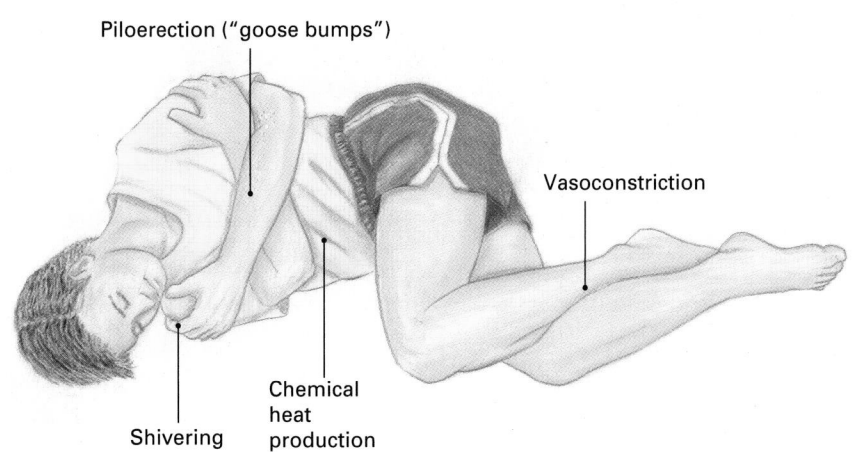

Piloerection ("goose bumps")

Vasoconstriction

Shivering

Chemical heat production

FIGURE 28-3 The victim of hypothermia.

temperature falls below 86° F (30° C). The severely hypothermic patient requires assessment of pulse and respirations for at least 30 seconds every 1–2 minutes.

Metabolic Factors in Hypothermia

Not all hypothermia cases are caused by environmental conditions. For example, hypothyroidism depresses the body's heat-producing mechanisms. Brain tumors or head trauma can depress the hypothalamic temperature control center, causing hypothermia. Other conditions—myocardial infarction, diabetes, hypoglycemia, drugs, poor nutrition, sepsis, or old age—can also contribute to metabolic and circulatory disorders that predispose to hypothermia.

Any patient thought to have hypothermia, but with no history of exposure to the environment, should be assessed for any predisposing factors that may have led to it. Evaluate the patient for level of consciousness, cool skin, and shivering. Also, evaluate the rectal temperature. A rectal temperature of less than 97° F indicates hypothermia.

Prehospital Management

✳ Rewarming of the hypothermic patient should be deferred until the patient is in the emergency department unless transport time is long and rewarming is ordered by medical control.

Rewarming of the hypothermic patient is best carried out by a team using a prearranged protocol in the hospital. Most patients who die during rewarming die from ventricular fibrillation. Rewarming should not be attempted in the field unless travel to the emergency department will take more than 15 minutes.

External application of heat by warmed blankets is a safe and effective means of rewarming the hypothermic patient. Application of external heat, however, results in peripheral vasodilatation. This, in turn, may cause the blood pressure to fall, especially when there is also volume depletion. An IV volume expander should be used to manage volume depletion. Another excellent means of rewarming the hypothermic patient is by administering heated and humidified oxygen. The hypothermic patient should be moved gently. Unnecessary rough handling may stimulate the return of cool blood and acids from the extremities to the core. This causes an "afterdrop" core temperature decrease and may induce cardiac dysrhythmias.

Specific care steps should take place after an adequate primary survey of the hypothermic patient. Mild or moderate hypothermia is treated slightly different than severe hypothermia. (See Figure 28-4.)

Mild/Moderate Hypothermia. In caring for the patient with mild/moderate hypothermia, take the following recommended steps.

❑ Remove all wet clothes.
❑ Protect against heat loss and wind chill.
❑ Maintain horizontal position.
❑ Avoid rough movement and excess activity.
❑ Monitor the core temperature.
❑ Monitor the cardiac rhythm.
❑ Add heat to the patient's head, neck, chest, and groin. Respiratory warmers may also be used.
❑ Do not give alcohol, coffee, or nicotine.
❑ Provide warm oral fluids and sugar sources AFTER uncontrolled shivering stops and the patient exhibits evidence of rewarming.

Severe Hypothermia (Vital Signs Present). In caring for the patient with severe hypothermia, take the following recommended steps.

❑ Remove all wet clothes.

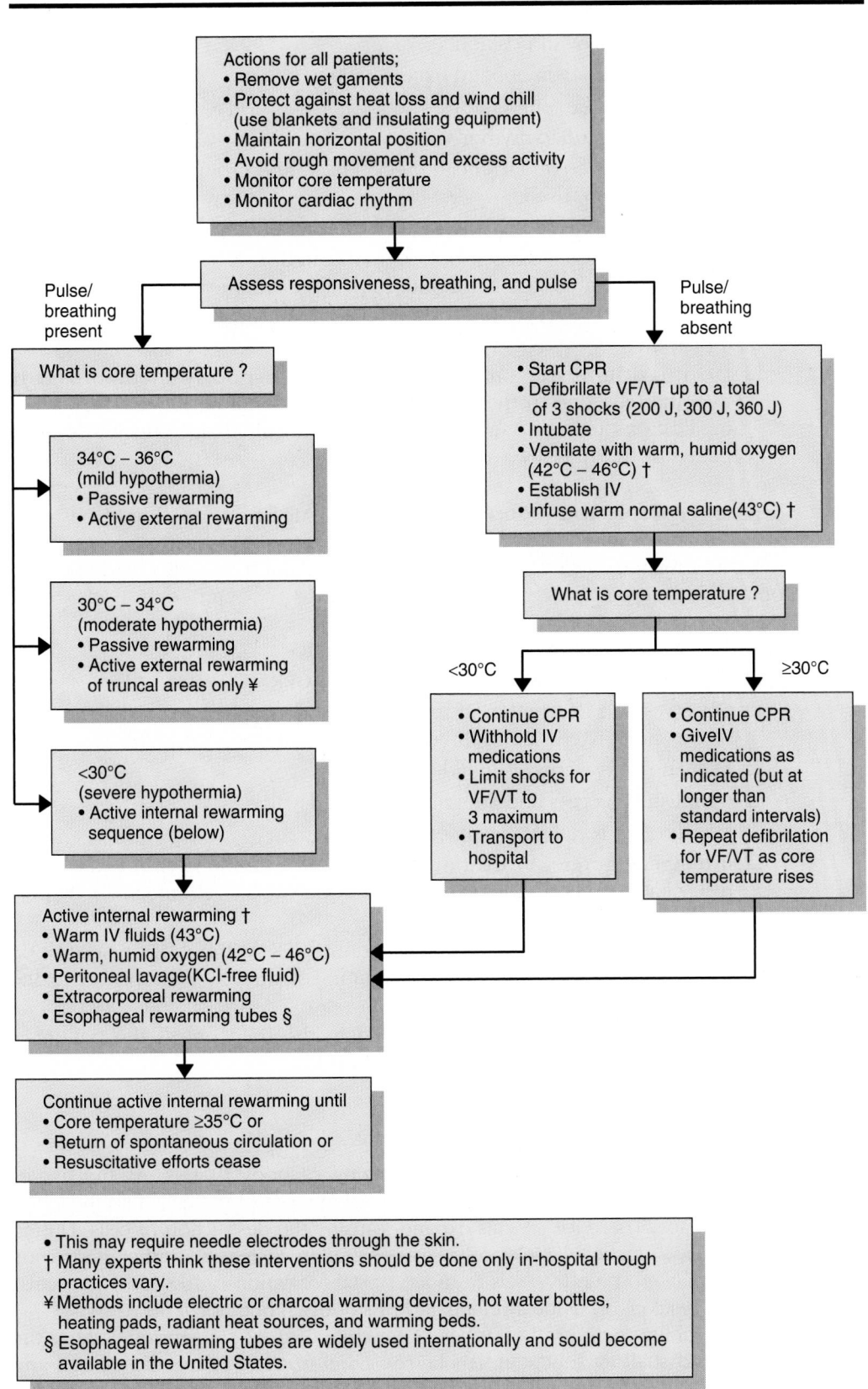

Actions for all patients;
• Remove wet gaments
• Protect against heat loss and wind chill
  (use blankets and insulating equipment)
• Maintain horizontal position
• Avoid rough movement and excess activity
• Monitor core temperature
• Monitor cardiac rhythm

Assess responsiveness, breathing, and pulse

Pulse/breathing present

Pulse/breathing absent

What is core temperature ?

34°C – 36°C
(mild hypothermia)
• Passive rewarming
• Active external rewarming

30°C – 34°C
(moderate hypothermia)
• Passive rewarming
• Active external rewarming
  of truncal areas only ¥

<30°C
(severe hypothermia)
• Active internal rewarming
  sequence (below)

• Start CPR
• Defibrillate VF/VT up to a total
  of 3 shocks (200 J, 300 J, 360 J)
• Intubate
• Ventilate with warm, humid oxygen
  (42°C – 46°C) †
• Establish IV
• Infuse warm normal saline(43°C) †

What is core temperature ?

<30°C

≥30°C

• Continue CPR
• Withhold IV
  medications
• Limit shocks for
  VF/VT to
  3 maximum
• Transport to
  hospital

• Continue CPR
• GiveIV
  medications as
  indicated (but at
  longer than
  standard intervals)
• Repeat defibrilation
  for VF/VT as core
  temperature rises

Active internal rewarming †
• Warm IV fluids (43°C)
• Warm, humid oxygen (42°C – 46°C)
• Peritoneal lavage(KCI-free fluid)
• Extracorporeal rewarming
• Esophageal rewarming tubes §

Continue active internal rewarming until
• Core temperature ≥35°C or
• Return of spontaneous circulation or
• Resuscitative efforts cease

• This may require needle electrodes through the skin.
† Many experts think these interventions should be done only in-hospital though
  practices vary.
¥ Methods include electric or charcoal warming devices, hot water bottles,
  heating pads, radiant heat sources, and warming beds.
§ Esophageal rewarming tubes are widely used internationally and sould become
  available in the United States.

FIGURE 28-4 Algorithm for treatment of hypothermia.

- ❑ Protect against heat loss and wind chill.
- ❑ Maintain horizontal position.
- ❑ Avoid rough movement and excess activity.
- ❑ Monitor the core temperature.
- ❑ Monitor the cardiac rhythm.
- ❑ Add heat to the patient's head, neck, chest, and groin. Respiratory warmers may also be used.
- ❑ Give nothing by mouth.
- ❑ Do not administer oxygen unless it is heated to > 99° F. If warmed oxygen is unavailable, use the mouth-to-mask technique for ventilations.
- ❑ Establish an IV of D5W or D5NS at 75 mL/hr (with fluids warmed to 43° C, if possible).
- ❑ Do not administer medications. They are poorly metabolized in hypothermia, due to the hypometabolic state. Administration may cause medications to persist in the body, resulting in toxic drug levels upon patient rewarming.

Severe Hypothermia (Vital Signs Absent). Modifications should be made in advanced cardiac life support of cardiac arrest victims with core temperatures less than 86° (30° C). In such cases, you should take the following recommended steps.

- ❑ Assess pulse and respirations for 1–2 minutes.
- ❑ If pulse and respirations are absent, begin CPR.
- ❑ Observe the ECG rhythm. If the patient is in ventricular fibrillation, defibrillate immediately (up to three shocks) at 200, 300, 360 joules.
- ❑ Ventilate with warmed humidified oxygen.
- ❑ Establish IV access and administer warmed saline.
- ❑ Measure the rectal core temperature.
- ❑ If temperature greater than or equal to 86° F, continue CPR and give IV resuscitation medications as indicated (but at longer intervals). Repeat defibrillation as temperature rises.
- ❑ If temperature is less than 86° F, continue CPR, withhold IV resuscitation medications, limit shocks to a maximum of three, and transport to the hospital.
- ❑ Rewarming should not be attempted in the field unless the patient is more than 15 minutes from a medical facility.

Frostbite

Frostbite is environmentally induced freezing of body tissues. As the tissues freeze, ice crystals form within and water is drawn out of the cells into the extracellular space. These ice crystals expand, causing the destruction of cells. During this process, intracellular electrolyte concentration increases, further destroying cells. Damage to blood vessels from ice crystal formation causes loss of vascular integrity, resulting in tissue swelling and loss of distal nutritional flow.

Generally there are two types of frostbite. *Superficial frostbite* affects the dermis and shallow subcutaneous layers. *Deep frostbite* affects the dermal and subdermal layers of tissue.

Assessment   Frostbite mainly occurs in the extremities and in areas of the head and face exposed to the environment. Subfreezing temperatures are required for frostbite to occur, although they are not necessary to produce hypothermia. Many patients who have frostbite will also have hypothermia.

Most patients will describe the clinical sequence of events for frostbite in the following order: extremities become cold → then become painful → pain gradually changes to numbness. The skin may initially have the appearance of reddening. This will change to a white or gray with full freezing. There can be tremendous variation of how an individual can present with frostbite. For example, some patients do not feel a great deal of pain at onset. Others will report severe pain. A certain degree of compliance may be felt beneath the frozen layer in superficial frostbite. But in deep frostbite, the frozen part will be hard and non-compliant.

Prehospital Management   In treating frostbite, take the following recommended steps.

- ❏ Do not thaw affected area if there is any possibility of refreezing.
- ❏ Do not massage the frozen area or rub with snow. Rubbing the affected area may cause ice crystals within the tissues to damage the already injured tissues more seriously.
- ❏ Administer analgesia prior to thawing.
- ❏ Thaw frozen part by immersion rewarming in a 100–106° F water bath. Water temperature will fall rapidly, requiring additional warm water throughout the process.
- ❏ Cover the thawed part with loosely applied, dry, sterile dressings.
- ❏ Elevate the thawed part.
- ❏ Do not puncture or drain the blisters.
- ❏ Do not allow the patient to ambulate on frozen feet.

✳ Frostbite should be rewarmed in water between 100° F and 106°F.

✳ Do not allow the patient to ambulate on frozen feet.

NEAR-DROWNING AND DROWNING

It is estimated that in the United States, approximately 8,000 persons die annually due to drowning. Approximately 40 percent of these (3,200) are under 5 years of age. Drowning is the second leading cause of accidental death in people ages 1–44. Approximately 85 percent of near-drowning victims are male, and two-thirds of these do not know how to swim. There has been an attempt made to differentiate between the terms drowning and near-drowning. The term *drowning* means that death occurred within 24 hours of submersion, while the term *near-drowning* indicates that death either did not occur or occurred more than 24 hours after submersion.

Pathophysiology

As a paramedic, you will need to understand the sequence of events in drowning or near-drowning. Following submersion, if the victim is conscious, he or she will undergo a period of complete apnea for up to three minutes. This apnea is an involuntary reflex as the victim strives to keep the head above water. During this time, blood is shunted to the heart and brain, in a fashion similar to the primitive "diving reflex" present in certain lower animals.

When the victim is apneic, the $PaCO_2$ in the blood rises to greater than 50 mmHg. Meanwhile, the PaO_2 of the blood falls below 50 mmHg. The stimulus from the hypoxia ultimately overrides the sedative effects of the hypercarbia, resulting in central nervous system stimulation.

Until unconscious, the victim experiences a great deal of panic. During this stage the victim makes violent inspiratory and swallowing efforts. At this point, copious amounts of water enter the mouth, posterior pharynx, and stomach, stimulating severe laryngospasm and bronchospasm. In approximately 10 percent of drowning victims, and in a much greater percentage of near-drowning victims, this laryngospasm prevents the influx of water into the lungs. If a significant amount of water does not enter the lungs, it is referred to as a *dry drowning*. Conversely, if a laryngospasm does not occur, and a significant quantity of water does enter the lungs, it is referred to as a *wet drowning*. The laryngospasm, or airway obstruction due to aspirated water, further aggravates the hypoxia, with coma ultimately ensuing. Persistent anoxia results in a deeper coma.

Following unconsciousness, reflex swallowing continues, resulting in gastric distention and increased risk of vomiting and aspiration. If untreated, hypotension, bradycardia, and death result in a short period.

Drowning and near-drowning are primarily due to asphyxia from airway obstruction in the lung secondary to the aspirated water or laryngospasm. If, in a near-drowning episode this process does not end in death, the fluid may cause lower airway disease. Expect different physiological reactions in cases of fresh-water and sea-water drownings or near-drownings.

Fresh-Water Drowning   In fresh-water drowning or near-drowning, the large surface area of the alveoli and small airways allow a massive amount of hypotonic water to diffuse across and into the vascular space. This results in *hemodilution*. Hemodilution produces a thickening of the alveolar walls with inflammatory cells, hemorrhagic pneumonitis, and destruction of surfactant. **Surfactant** is a substance in the alveoli responsible for keeping the alveoli open. When the capillaries of the alveoli are damaged, plasma proteins leak back into the alveoli, resulting in the accumulation of fluid in the small airways. This in turn leads to multiple areas of atelectasis with shunting and hypoxemia. (See Figure 28-5.)

■ **surfactant** a compound secreted by cells in the lungs that contributes to the elastic properties of the pulmonary tissue.

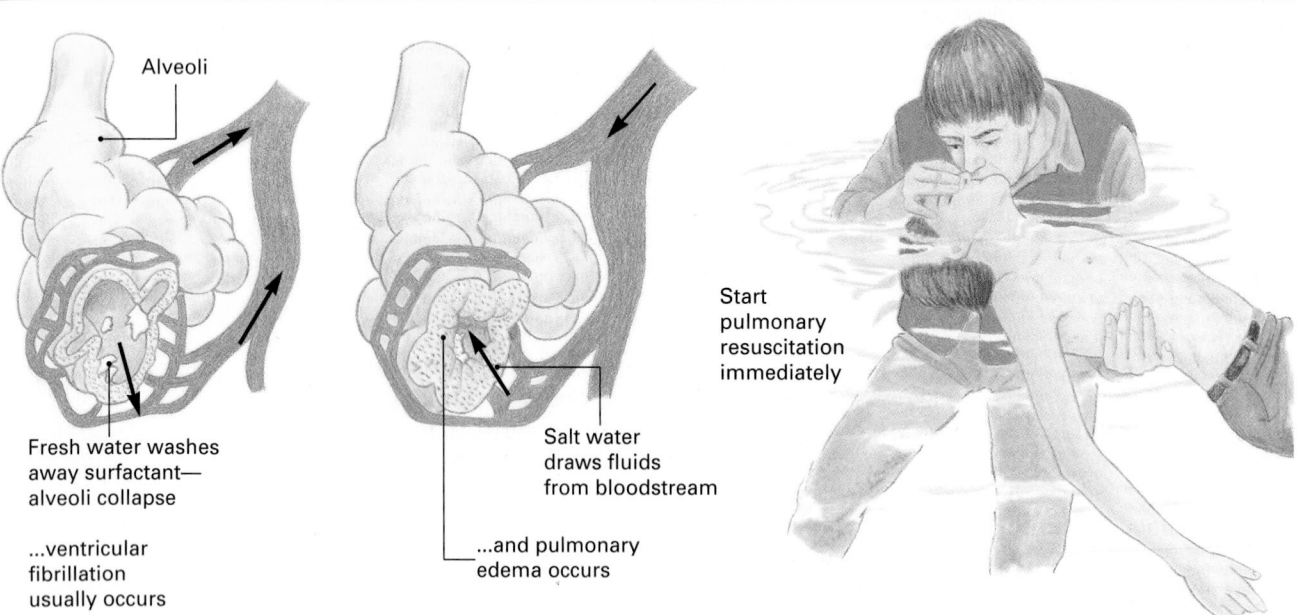

Alveoli

Fresh water washes away surfactant— alveoli collapse

...ventricular fibrillation usually occurs

Salt water draws fluids from bloodstream

...and pulmonary edema occurs

Start pulmonary resuscitation immediately

FIGURE 28-5 Pathophysiological effects of drowning.

Sea-Water Drowning In sea-water drowning, the hypertonic nature of the fluid draws water from the bloodstream into the alveoli. In near-drowning, the hypertonic nature of sea water, which is 3–4 times more hypertonic than plasma, draws water from the bloodstream into the alveoli. This produces pulmonary edema, leading to profound shunting. The result is failure of oxygenation, producing hypoxemia, since the blood is traveling through the lung tissues without being oxygenated. Additionally, respiratory and metabolic acidosis develop due to the retention of CO_2 and developing anaerobic metabolism. Since all of the above factors disrupt normal pulmonary function, initial field treatment must be directed toward correcting the profound hypoxia.

Factors Affecting Survival

There are other factors that may have an impact on drowning and near-drowning survival rates. These include such things as the cleanliness of the water, the length of time submerged, and the age and general health of the victim. Children have a longer survival time and a greater probability of a successful resuscitation. Even more significant is the water temperature. The concept of developing brain death after four to six minutes without oxygen is not applicable in cases of near-drowning in cold water. Some patients in cold water (below 68° F) can be resuscitated after 30 minutes or more in cardiac arrest. However, persons under water 60 minutes or longer usually cannot be resuscitated.

A possible contribution to survival may be the **mammalian diving reflex**. When a person dives into cold water, he or she reacts to the submersion of the face. Breathing is inhibited, the heart rate becomes bradycardic, and vasoconstriction develops in tissues relatively resistant to asphyxia. Meanwhile cerebral and cardiac blood flow is maintained. In this way, oxygen is sent and used only where it is immediately needed to sustain life. The colder the water, the more oxygen is diverted to the heart and brain. A common saying in emergency medicine states: "The cold water drowning victim is not dead until he or she is warm and dead."

■ **mammalian diving reflex** a complex cardiovascular reflex, resulting from submersion of the face and nose in water, that constricts blood flow everywhere except to the brain. It decreases cardiac output and rate and produces stable or slightly increased arterial blood pressure.

Prehospital Management

The patient should be removed from the water as soon as possible by a trained rescue swimmer. Ventilation should be initiated while the patient is still in water. Rescue personnel should wear protective clothing if water temperature is less than 70° F. In addition, a safety line should be attached to the rescue swimmer. In fast water, it is essential to use personnel specifically trained for this type of rescue. (See Chapter 5.)

Suspect head and neck injury if the patient experienced a fall or was diving. Rapidly place the victim on a long backboard and remove him or her from the water.

Examine the near-drowning victim for airway patency, breathing, and pulse. If indicated, begin CPR. Airway management should include proper suctioning and use of airway adjuncts. C-spine injury should be considered and treated accordingly. Administer oxygen at a 100 percent concentration. If available, and if transport time is longer than 15 minutes, respiratory rewarming should take place. The Heimlich maneuver is *contraindicated*.

Next, establish an IV of lactated Ringer's or normal saline for venous access and run at 75 mL/hour. If indicated, carry out defibrillation. ACLS protocols should be followed if the patient is normothermic. If the patient is hypothermic, treat him or her according to the hypothermia protocol presented earlier in the chapter. Unless hypothermia is present, resuscitation is not indicated if there is evidence of putrefaction (decomposition) or if immersion has been extremely prolonged.

More than 90 percent of near-drowning patients survive without sequelae. All near-drowning patients should be admitted to the hospital for observation. Some of these patients have problems with pulmonary parenchymal injury, destruction of surfactant, aspiration pneumonitis, or pneumothorax. A number require an extended hospital stay due to hypoxia, hypercarbia, and mixed metabolic and respiratory acidosis. Treatment of the effects of cerebral hypoxia occasionally continues throughout and even after hospitalization.

NUCLEAR RADIATION

Injury due to exposure to ionizing radiation occurs infrequently. However, the incidence of radiation emergencies has increased in recent years due to the expansion of nuclear medicine procedures and commercial nuclear facilities.

Radiation is a general term applied to the transmission of energy. This energy can include nuclear energy, ultraviolet light, visible light, heat, sound, and X-rays. A radioactive substance emits ionizing radiation. Such a substance is referred to as a *radionuclide* or *radioisotope*.

Basic Nuclear Physics

To understand nuclear radiation, you might begin by taking a look at the structure of an atom and by becoming familiar with some of the basic terms associated with nuclear physics. The atom consists of various subatomic particles. These include:

❑ *Protons.* Positively charged particles that form the nucleus of hydrogen and that are present in the nuclei of all elements. The atomic number of the element indicates the number of protons present.

❑ *Neutrons.* Subatomic particles that are equal in mass to a proton, but lack an electrical charge. As a free particle, a neutron has an average life of less than 17 minutes.

❑ *Electrons.* Minute particles with negative electrical charges, revolving around the nucleus of an atom. When emitted from radioactive substances, electrons are called *beta particles*.

You should also be familiar with two basic terms associated with nuclear medicine. These include:

❑ *Isotopes (radioisotope).* Atoms in which the nuclear composition is unstable. That is, they give off **ionizing radiation**.

❑ ***Half-life.*** The time required for half the nuclei of a radioactive substance to lose their activity due to radioactive decay.

A radioactive substance is one that emits ionizing radiation. There are four types of radiation. These include:

❑ *Alpha Particles.* Alpha particles are slow-moving, low-energy particles that usually can be stopped by such things as clothing and paper. When they contact the skin, they only penetrate a few cells deep. Because they can be absorbed (stopped) by a layer of clothing, a few inches of air, or the outer layer of skin, alpha particles constitute a minor hazard. However, they can produce serious effects if taken internally by ingestion or inhalation.

✱ Radiation emergencies should only be handled by those with proper protective equipment and adequate training.

■ **ionizing radiation** electromagnetic radiation (e.g., X-ray) or particulate radiation (e.g., alpha particles, beta particles, and neutrons) capable of producing ions by direct or secondary processes.

■ **half-life** time required for half of the nuclei of a radioactive substance to lose activity by undergoing radioactive decay.

- *Beta Particles.* Smaller than alpha particles, beta particles are higher in energy. Although beta particles can penetrate air, they can be stopped by aluminum and similar materials. Beta particles generally cause less local damage than alpha particles, but they can be harmful if inhaled or ingested.
- *Gamma Rays.* Gamma rays are more highly energized and penetrating than alpha and beta particles. The origin of gamma rays is related to that of X-rays. Gamma radiation is extremely dangerous, carrying high levels of energy capable of penetrating thick shielding. Gamma rays easily pass through clothing and the entire body, inflicting extensive cell damage. They also create indirect damage by causing internal tissue to emit alpha and beta particles. Protection from gamma radiation can be provided by lead shielding.
- *Neutrons.* Neutrons are more penetrating than the other types of radiation. The penetrating power of neutrons is estimated to be 3–10 times greater than gamma rays, but less than the internal hazard associated with ingestion of alpha and beta particles. Exposure to neutrons causes direct tissue damage. However, in nuclear accidents, neutron exposure is not normally a problem for paramedics because neutrons tend to be present only near a reactor core.

Effects of Radiation on the Body

Ionizing radiation cannot be seen, felt, or heard. Therefore, a detection instrument is required to measure the radiation given off by the radiation source. The most commonly used device is the *Geiger counter.* The rate of radiation is measured in roentgens per hour (R/hr) or milliroentgens per hour (mR/hr) (1,000 mR = 1R).

The unit of local tissue energy deposition is called *radiation absorbed dose (RAD). Roentgen equivalent in man (REM)* provides a gauge of the likely injury to the irradiated part of an organism. For all practical purposes, RAD and REM are equal in clinical value. When neutrons or other high-energy radiation sources are used, a *quality factor (QF)* is applied to determine the equivalent dose.

Simply stated, ionizing radiation causes alterations in the body's cell, primarily the genetic material (DNA). Depending upon the dosage received, the changes can be in cell division, cell structure, and cellular biochemical activities. Cell damage due to ionizing radiation is cumulative over a lifetime. If a person is exposed to ionizing radiation long enough, there will be a decreased number of white blood cells. Additionally, there may be defects in offspring, an increased incidence of cancer, and various degrees of bone marrow damage.

Detection of the first biological effects of exposure to ionizing radiation occurs at varying times. (See Table 28-2.) Biological effects include:

- *Acute.* Effects appearing in a matter of minutes or weeks.
- *Long-Term.* Effects appearing years or decades later.

Principles of Safety

There are three basic principles that allow rescue personnel and patients to limit exposure to ionizing radiation. These include: time, distance, and shielding. Determining exposure, absorption, and damage done by radiation requires specialized training. The amount of radiation received by a person depends upon the source of radiation, the length of time exposed, the distance from the

✱ Limiting radiation exposure is based on three principles: time, distance, and shielding.

TABLE 28-2 Dose-Effect Relationships to Ionizing Radiation

Whole Body Exposure

Dose (RAD)	Effect
5–25	Asymptomatic. Blood studies are normal.
50–75	Asymptomatic. Minor depressions of white blood cells and platelets in a few patients.
75–125	May produce anorexia, nausea, and vomiting, and fatigue in approximately 10–20% of patients within two days.
125–200	Possible nausea and vomiting. Diarrhea, anxiety, tachycardia. Fatal to less than 5% of patients.
200–600	Nausea and vomiting, diarrhea in the first several hours, weakness, fatigue. Fatal to approximately 50% of patients within six weeks without prompt medical attention.
600–1,000	Severe nausea and vomiting, diarrhea in the first several hours. Fatal to 100% of patients within two weeks without prompt medical attention.
1,000 or more	"Burning sensation" within minutes, nausea and vomiting within 10 minutes, confusion ataxia, and prostration within one hour, watery diarrhea within 1–2 hrs. Fatal to 100% within short time without prompt medical attention.

Localized Exposure

Dose (RAD)	Effect
50	Asymptomatic.
500	Asymptomatic (usually). May have risk of altered function of exposed area.
2,500	Atrophy, vascular lesion, and altered pigmentation.
5,000	Chronic ulcer, risk of carcinogenesis.
50,000	Permanent destruction of exposed tissue.

source, and the shielding between the exposed person and the source. For example, the amount of radiation at the patient's initial location may be 300 R/hr. If exposure is for 20 minutes, this is the same radiation equivalent as working one hour at a 100 R/hr scene. The amount of radiation may drop off rapidly as the patient is decontaminated and moved away from the exposure. The distance from an ionizing radiation source is crucial since exposure is determined by the inverse square relationship. Doubling the distance away from a radiation source reduces the exposure by a factor of four. Conversely, halving the distance to a radiation source, increases exposure by a factor of four.

There are basically two types of ionizing radiation accidents—clean and dirty accidents. In a *clean accident*, the patient is exposed to radiation but is not contaminated by the radioactive substance, particles of radioactive dust, or radioactive liquids, gases, or smoke. If he or she is properly decontaminated before arrival of rescue personnel, there will be little danger, provided the source of the radiation is no longer exposed at the scene. After exposure to ionizing radiation, the patient is not radioactive. Therefore, he or she poses no hazard to rescue personnel. In contrast, the *dirty accident*—often associated

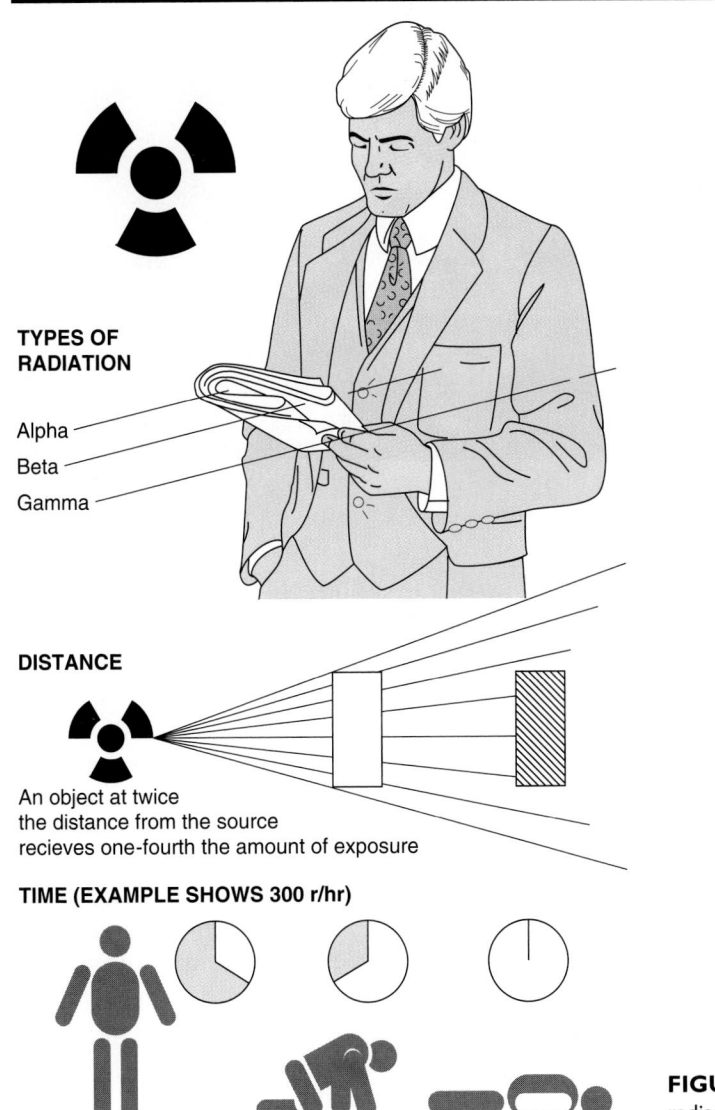

TYPES OF RADIATION

Alpha
Beta
Gamma

DISTANCE

An object at twice
the distance from the source
recieves one-fourth the amount of exposure

TIME (EXAMPLE SHOWS 300 r/hr)

FIGURE 28-6 Nuclear radiation.

with fire at the scene of a radiation accident—exposes the patient to radiation and contaminates him or her with radioactive particles or liquids. The scene may be highly contaminated, although the primary source of radiation is shielded when rescue personnel arrive. Unless you are properly trained in dealing with this type of emergency, you may have to delay rescue procedures until properly trained technical assistance arrives. (See Figures 28-6.)

Prehospital Management

If you find yourself involved in a radioactive emergency, take the following precautionary steps.

❑ Park the rescue vehicle upwind to minimize contamination.
❑ Look for signs of radiation exposure. Radioactive packages are marked by clearly identifiable color-coded labels. (See Figure 28-7.)
❑ Use portable instruments to measure the level of radioactivity. If dose estimates are significant, rotate rescue personnel.

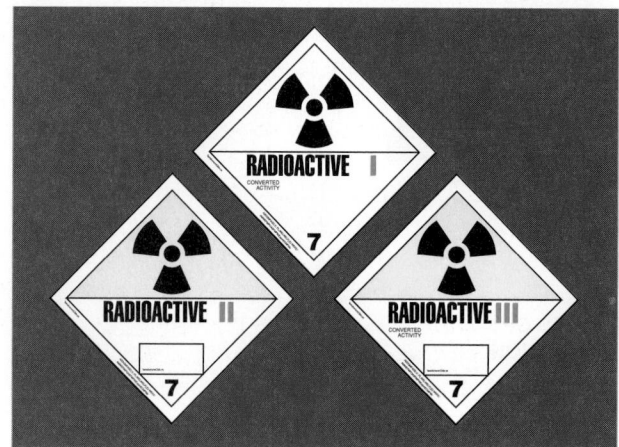

FIGURE 28-7 Radioactive warning labels.

❑ Normal principles of emergency care should be applied—i.e., ABCs, shock management, and trauma care.

❑ Externally radiated patients pose little danger to rescue personnel. Initiate normal care procedures for injuries other than radiation.

❑ Internally contaminated patients (ingested or inhaled) pose little danger to rescue personnel. Normal care procedures should be undertaken. Collect body wastes. If artificial respiration is required, use a bag-valve-mask unit or demand valve. If radioactive particles are inhaled, swab the nasal passages and save the swabs.

❑ Externally contaminated patients (liquids, dirt, smoke) require decontamination. Following decontamination, initiate normal emergency care procedures. Decontamination of paramedic personnel and equipment is required after the call is complete.

❑ Patients with open, contaminated wounds require normal emergency care procedures. Avoid cross-contamination of wounds.

DIVING EMERGENCIES

■ **SCUBA** abbreviation for Self-Contained Underwater Breathing Apparatus.

SCUBA diving has become an extremely popular recreational sport. Although SCUBA diving accidents are fairly uncommon, inexperienced divers have a higher incident rate of injury. SCUBA diving emergencies can occur on the surface, in three feet of water, or at any depth. The more serious emergencies usually follow a dive. To better assess and care for diving injuries, you need to understand a few principles of pressure.

Physical Principles of Pressure

Water is an incompressible, colorless liquid. Fresh water has a density, or weight per unit of volume, of 62.4 pounds per cubic foot. Salt water has a density of 64.0 pounds per cubic foot. This density can be equated to pressure, which is defined as the weight or force acting upon a unit area. Thus, the weight of a cubic foot of fresh water exerts a pressure (weight) of 62.4 pounds over an area of one square foot. This measurement is typically stated in pounds per square inch (psi).

Humans at sea level live in an atmosphere of air, or a mixture of gases. These gases weigh and exert a pressure of 14.7 pounds per square inch. This pressure, however, may vary within the environment. For example, ascending to an altitude of one mile will decrease the weight of air (the atmospheric pressure) by 17 percent to approximately 12.2 pounds. To understand how air pressure affects diving accidents, you need to look at two physical laws—Boyle's Law and Henry's Law.

Boyle's Law   *Boyle's Law* states that the volume of a gas is inversely proportional to its pressure if the temperature is kept constant. For example, doubling the pressure of a gas mixture will decrease its volume by one-half. The pressure of air at sea level is 14.7 lb./sq.in. or 760 mmHg. This pressure is called one atmosphere absolute or one "ata." Two ata occur at a depth of 33 feet of water, three ata occur at a depth of 66 feet of water, and so on. Therefore, one liter of air at the surface is compressed to a 500 mL at 33 feet. At 66 feet one liter of air would be compressed to 250 mL.

Henry's Law   *Henry's Law* states that the amount of gas dissolved in a given volume of fluid is proportional to the pressure of the gas with which it is in equilibrium. The body is made up primarily of liquid. Therefore, gases that are inhaled will be dissolved in the body in proportion to the partial pressure of each breath. The body uses oxygen, but it does not use nitrogen. Therefore, the primary gas dissolved in the body is nitrogen because it is inert and not used by the body. At 33 feet below the surface, the quantity of oxygen and nitrogen dissolved in the tissues will be twice that at sea level.

Gas molecules will be absorbed into a given quantity of liquid until a condition of equilibrium is reached. That is, the gas in the liquid will reach a value equal to the partial pressure of the gas (saturation). A diver's body can also become saturated if he or she breathes gases long enough under pressure. As long as the pressure is maintained, gases dissolved in liquids will remain in solution. However, if the pressure is gradually reduced, the gases in the solution can escape with no noticeable effect. For example, carbon dioxide is held in solution in a carbonated soda by pressure of that gas in the space above the liquid. When the soda can or bottle is opened, the carbon dioxide is released from the solution into the atmosphere.

Gases are dissolved in the diver's blood under pressure. During controlled ascent, dissolved gases escape through respiration or else bubbles can form within the body. The ascending diver who comes to the surface too rapidly, not adhering to safety measures, is at risk of becoming a veritable "living" can or bottle of soda.

Common Diving Injuries

SCUBA diving injuries are due to either barotrauma (mechanical effect of the pressure differential), cerebral air embolism, compression illness, cold, panic, or a combination of the above. Accidents generally occur at one of the following four stages of a dive.

Injuries on the Surface   Surface injuries can involve entanglement of lines or entanglement in kelp fields while swimming to the area of the dive. Divers in these situations may panic, become fatigued, or drown. Additionally, the water may be cold producing shivering and blackout. Boats in the area are another potential source of injury to the diver. To prevent such accidents, divers will usually mark the area of their dive with a flag. Maritime rules require boat operators to stay clear of a flagged area.

Injuries During Descent   Barotrauma, commonly called the "squeeze," becomes a concern during the descent. If the diver cannot equilibrate the pressure between the nasopharynx and the middle ear through the eustachian tube, he or she can experience middle ear pain. Besides pain, signs and symptoms include ringing in the ears, dizziness, and hearing loss. In severe cases, rupture of the ear drum can occur. A diver who has an upper respiratory infection, and who therefore cannot clear the middle ear through the eustachian tube, should not dive. A similar lack of equilibration can occur in the sinuses, producing severe frontal headaches or pain beneath the eye in the maxillary sinuses.

Injuries on the Bottom Major diving emergencies while at the bottom of the dive involve nitrogen narcosis, commonly called "raptures of the deep." This is due to nitrogen's effect on cerebral function. The diver may appear to be intoxicated and may take unnecessary risks. If the diver runs low or out of air, he or she may suddenly panic, causing increased oxygen consumption and further carbon dioxide production.

Injuries During Ascent Serious and life-threatening emergencies can occur during the ascent. The causes may be related to barotrauma and the diver's inability to equilibrate his or her inner ear pressure with nasopharyngeal pressure. Dives below 40 feet require staged ascent to prevent the "bends." (See pages 887–889.)

The most serious barotrauma that occurs during the ascent is injury to the lung. This can occur at as little as three feet below the surface, or it can occur during a deep dive. The injury results from the diver holding his or her breath during the ascent. As the diver ascends, the air in the lung, which has been compressed, expands. If it is not exhaled, the alveoli may rapture. If this occurs, the result will be structural damage to the lung and **air embolism**. There may also be mediastinal and subcutaneous emphysema due to diffusion of the gas through the lung into the mediastinum and the neck. Pneumothorax is possible if the alveoli rupture into the pleural cavity. Air embolism can occur if the air ruptures into the pulmonary veins or arteries and returns to the left atrium and finally into the left ventricle and out the systemic circulation.

■ **air embolism** presence of an air bubble in the circulatory system.

General Assessment of Diving Emergencies

In the early assessment of diving accidents, all symptoms of air embolism and decompression sickness are considered together. Early assessment and treatment of a diving injury is of more importance than trying to distinguish the exact problem. One of your most important tasks in a diving-related injury is elicitation of a *diving history* or *profile*. There are several essential factors to consider. These include:

❑ Time at which the signs and symptoms occurred
❑ Type of breathing apparatus utilized
❑ Type of hypothermia protective garment worn
❑ Parameters of the dive
  • Depth of dive
  • Number of dives
  • Duration of dive
❑ Aircraft travel following a dive
❑ Rate of ascent
❑ Associated panic forcing rapid ascent
❑ Experience of the diver—i.e., student, inexperienced, or "pro"

- ❏ Properly functioning depth gauge
- ❏ Previous medical diseases
- ❏ Old injuries
- ❏ Previous episodes of decompression illness
- ❏ Use of medications
- ❏ Use of alcohol

From a quick assessment of the patient's diving profile, you can rapidly determine if the diver is a likely candidate for a pressure disorder.

Pressure Disorders

Pressure disorders are known as barotrauma, meaning injuries caused by pressure. In the case of diving accidents, most barotrauma results from a pressure imbalance between the external environment and gasses within the body's cavities. the following sections describe some of the most common forms of barotrauma involved in diving accidents.

Decompression Sickness (Caisson Disease or "Bends")

Decompression sickness is a condition that develops in divers subjected to rapid reduction of air pressure after ascending to the surface following exposure to compressed air. A number of general and individual factors can contribute to the development of the bends. (See Table 28-3.)

Pathophysiology. Decompression sickness results as nitrogen bubbles enter the tissue spaces and small blood vessels. Symptoms present when a diver rapidly ascends after being exposed to a depth of 33 feet or more for a time sufficient enough to allow the body's tissues to be saturated with nitrogen. The effects of nitrogen bubbles on the body can be direct or indirect.

Direct Effects

- ❏ *Intravascular.* Blood flow will be decreased, leading to ischemia or infarct.

■ **decompression sickness** condition, commonly known as "the bends," in which nitrogen bubbles develop within the tissues due to a rapid reduction of air pressure after a diver returns to the surface following exposure to compressed air.

TABLE 28-3 General and Individual Factors Relating to the Development of Decompression Sickness	
General Factors	**Individual Factors**
Cold water dives	Age—older individuals
Diving in rough water	Obesity
Strenuous diving conditions	Fatigue—lack of sleep prior to dive
History of previous decompression dive incident	Alcohol—consumption before or after dive
Overstaying time at given dive depth	History of medical problems
Dive at 80 feet or greater	
Rapid ascent—panic, inexperience, unfamiliarity with equipment	
Heavy exercise before or after dive to the point of muscle soreness	
Flying after diving (24 hour wait is recommended)	
Driving to high altitude after dive	

❑ *Extravascular.* Tissues will be displaced, which further results in pressure on neutral tissue.

❑ *Audiovestibular.* Air can diffuse into the **audiovestibular system**, causing vertigo.

Indirect Effects

❑ Surface of air emboli may initiate platelet aggregation and intravascular
coagulation.

❑ Extravascular plasma loss may lead to edema.

❑ Electrolyte imbalances may occur.

❑ Lipid emboli are released.

The bubbles produced by rapid decompression are thought to produce
obstruction of blood flow and lead to local ischemia, subjecting tissues to
anoxic stress. In some cases, this stress may lead to tissue damage.

Presentation. Decompression sickness can be divided into two types based
upon the presenting signs and symptoms.

❑ *Type I.* The historical term for Type I decompression sickness is the
"bends." Patients with it experience extremity pain, usually localized to
larger joints, such as the shoulders or elbows. The bends is caused by
expansion of gases present in the joint space. Skin manifestations of
Type I decompression sickness usually consists only of pruritus (the
itch). However, a rash, spotted pallor or cyanosis, or pitting edema may
also occur. The treatment for Type I decompression sickness mainly consists of oxygen inhalation, occasional **recompression**, and observation
for signs of more serious decompression sickness. Prognosis for Type I
decompression sickness is good.

❑ *Type II.* Patients who develop Type II decompression sickness may present with a broad spectrum of complaints. The patient may exhibit any
of the signs and symptoms of Type I decompression sickness plus any
one or more of the following.

• Paresthesias   • Paralysis
(numbness/tingling)   • Headache

• Dizziness or vertigo   • Dyspnea

• Nausea   • Chest pain

• Auditory disturbances   • Loss of consciousness

• Vestibular disturbances   • Hemoptysis

Decompression sickness has been called the "Great Imitator" due to its
variety of presentations. The pulmonary complications of decompression sickness, referred to as "the chokes," are extremely serious. In summary, the general symptoms of decompression sickness include:

❑ Extreme fatigue (early sign)

❑ Joint pain

❑ Headache

❑ Lower abdominal pain

❑ Chest pain

❑ Urinary dysfunction

❑ Vertigo and ataxia

- ❏ Pruritus (severe itching)
- ❏ Nausea/vomiting
- ❏ Back pain
- ❏ Priapism
- ❏ Paresthesias
- ❏ Paralysis
- ❏ Dysarthria (difficult speech)
- ❏ Frothy, reddish sputum
- ❏ Dyspnea

Prehospital Management. Patients with decompression sickness usually seek medical treatment within 12 hours of ascent from a dive. Some patients may not seek treatment for as long as 24 hours after the last dive. It is generally safe to assume that signs or symptoms developing more than 36 hours after a dive cannot reasonably be attributed to decompression sickness.

Decompression sickness may require urgent recompression for complete treatment. However, prompt stabilization at the nearest emergency department should be accomplished before transportation to a recompression chamber.

Early oxygen therapy may reduce symptoms of decompression sickness substantially. Divers who are administered high concentrations of oxygen have a considerably better treatment outcome. The following list outlines some of the steps in the prehospital management of decompression sickness.

1. Assess ABCs.
2. Administer CPR, if required.
3. Administer oxygen at 100 percent concentration with a nonrebreathing mask. An unconscious diver should be intubated.
4. Keep the patient in left lateral Trendelenburg position (10–15 degrees), if possible (considered optional).
5. Protect the patient from excessive heat, cold, wetness, or noxious fumes.
6. Give the conscious, alert patient nonalcoholic liquids such as fruit juices or oral balanced salt solutions.
7. Evaluate and stabilize the patient at the nearest emergency department prior to transport to a recompression chamber. Begin IV fluid replacement with electrolyte solutions for unconscious or seriously injured patients. You may use Ringer's lactate, normal saline, or 5 percent dextrose in normal saline. Do not use 5 percent dextrose in water.
8. If there is evidence of CNS involvement, administer dexamethasone, heparin, Dextran, or Valium as ordered by medical control.
9. If air evacuation is used, do not expose the patient to decreased barometric pressure. Cabin pressure must be maintained at sea level, or fly at the lowest possible safe altitude.
10. Send diving equipment with the patient for examination. If impossible, arrange for local examination and gas analysis.

Pulmonary Overpressure Accidents

Lung overinflation due to rapid ascent is the common cause of a number of emergencies. A pressure buildup in the lung can damage the lung and allow air to escape into the circulation, leading to air embolism. Air expansion on ascent can rupture the alveolar membranes. This can result in hemorrhage, reduced oxygen and carbon dioxide transport, and capillary and alveolar inflammation. Air can also escape from the lung into other nearby tissues and cause pneumothorax and tension pneumothorax, subcutaneous emphysema, or **pneumomediastinum**.

Air Embolism. If any person using SCUBA equipment presents with neurologic deficits during or immediately after ascent, an air embolism should be suspected. As death or serious disability can result, prompt medical treatment is crucial.

Air embolism is a form of barotrauma of ascent. It is a very serious condition in which air bubbles enter the circulatory system through rupture of small pulmonary vessels. Air can also be trapped in blebs, or air pockets, within the pulmonary tissue. These bubbles can then be transported to the heart and the brain, where they may lodge and obstruct blood flow, causing ischemia and possibly infarct.

Signs and symptoms of air embolism include: a rapid and dramatic onset; sharp, tearing pain; paralysis (frequently hemiplegia); cardiac and pulmonary collapse; unequal pupils; and wide pulse pressure. Prehospital management of air embolism should include the following steps.

1. Assess ABCs.
2. Administer oxygen by nonrebreathing mask at 100 percent.
3. Place patient in left lateral Trendelenburg position.
4. Monitor vital signs frequently.
5. Administer IV fluids at a TKO rate.
6. Administer a corpicosteroid agent, if ordered by medical control.
7. Transport to recompression chamber ASAP.

If air transport is utilized, it is very important to use pressurized aircraft or to fly at a low altitude.

Pneumomediastinum. A *pneumomediastinum* is the release of gas (air) through the visceral pleura into the mediastinum and pericardial sac. Signs and symptoms of a pneumomediastinum include substernal chest pain, irregular pulse, abnormal heart sounds, reduced blood pressure and narrow pulse pressure, and a change in voice. There may or may not be evidence of cyanosis. The field management of pneumomediastinum includes:

❑ Administration of high-concentration oxygen via nonrebreathing face mask.
❑ Start of IV lactated Ringer's or normal saline per physician order.
❑ Transport to the emergency department.

Treatment generally ranges from observation to recompression to relief of acute symptoms. The patient should be observed for 24 hours for any other signs of lung overpressure. He or she should not be recompressed unless air embolism or decompression sickness are also present.

SUMMARY

Basic knowledge of common environmental, recreational, and exposure injuries is necessary in order for you to administer prompt and proper treatment in the prehospital setting. Familiarity with such subjects as hyperthermia, hypothermia, near-drowning, diving, and radiation emergencies is not easy to retain since they are not usually encountered on a daily basis. There are too many cases where paramedics have lost their lives when attempting a rescue for which they were not properly trained. Rapid action is always necessary when performing an environmental rescue. However, common sense must prevail.

FURTHER READING

Bledsoe, Bryan E., Gideon Bosker, and Frank J. Papa. *Prehospital Emergency Pharmacology*. 3rd ed. Englewood Cliffs, NJ: Prentice Hall, Inc., 1990.

Danzl, D.F., R.S. Pozos, and M.P. Hamlet. "Accidental Hypothermia," from Auerbach and Geehr. *Management of*

Wilderness and Environmental Emergencies, 2d ed, St. Louis, MO: C. V. Mosby Co., 1989.

Guyton, A.C. *Textbook of Medical Physiology*. 8th ed. Philadelphia, PA: W.B. Saunders Company, 1990.

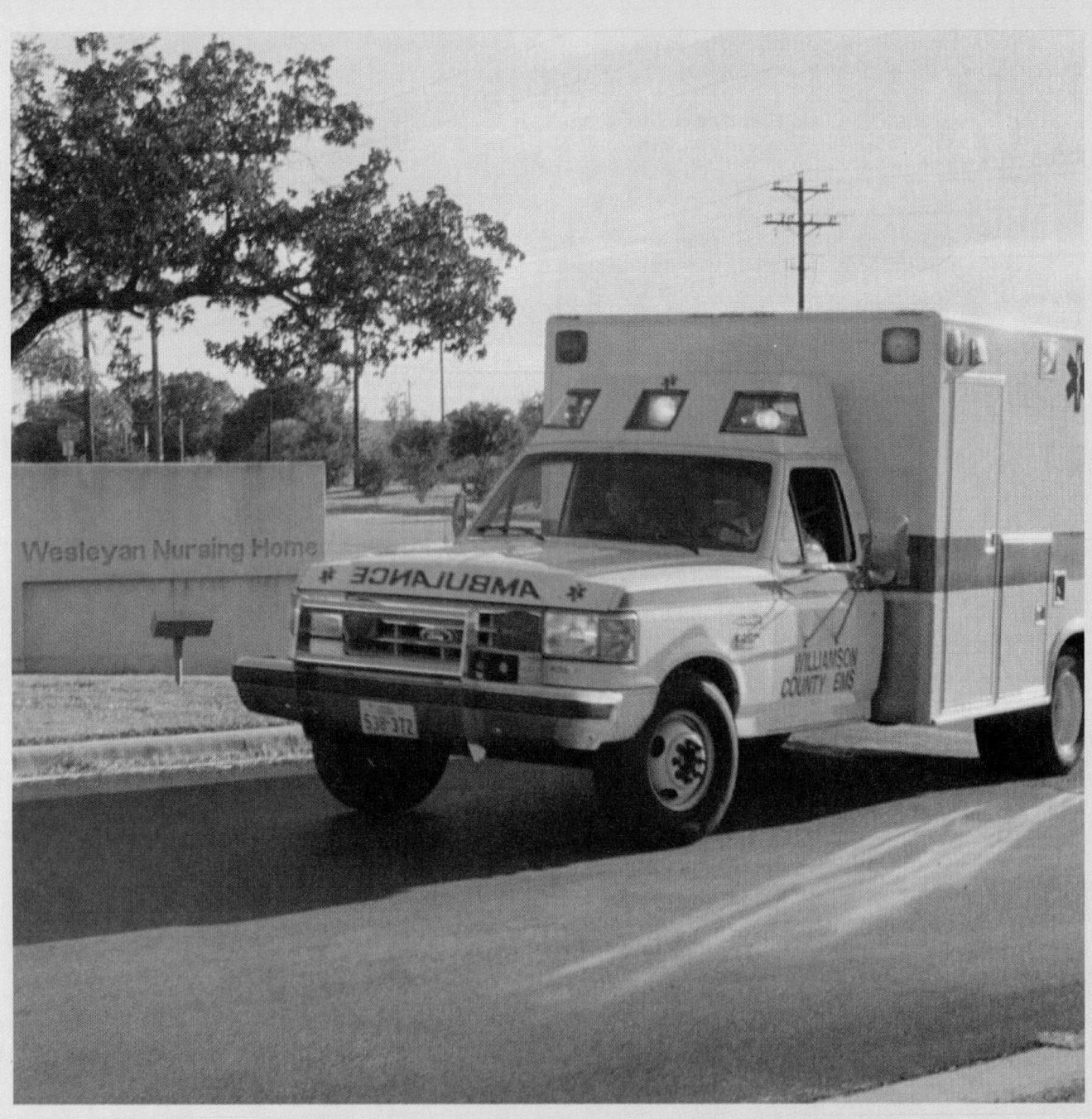

29

EMERGENCIES IN THE ELDERLY PATIENT

Objectives for Chapter 29

After reading this chapter, you should be able to:

1. Discuss statistics on aging and the elderly population in the United States. (See p. 894.)

2. Discuss age-related systemic decline as it relates to the following body systems. (See below pages.)

- respiratory system (p. 896)
- cardiovascular system (p. 896)
- renal system (p. 896)
- nervous system (p. 896)
- musculoskeletal system (p. 896)
- gastrointestinal system (p. 896)

3. Explain the need to distinguish the chief complaint from the primary problem among the elderly. (See p. 897.)

4. List four factors that complicate the clinical evaluation of an aged patient. (See p. 897.)

5. List some factors that complicate gathering a history from an aged patient. (See pp. 898-899.)

6. Describe reasons the elderly are more susceptible to trauma. (See p. 899.)

7. Discuss common respiratory problems among the aged. (See pp. 899–900.)

8. List two causes of cardiac dysrhythmias in the elderly. (See p. 902.)

9. Define syncope. (See p. 902.)

10. Discuss the following kinds of syncope. (See below pages.)

- vasodepressor syncope (pp. 902–903)
- orthostatic syncope (p. 903)
- cardiac syncope (p. 903)

11. Define vertigo, and discuss the progression of events associated with it. (See p. 904.)

12. Define dementia as it applies to the elderly. (See p. 905.)

13. Define Alzheimer's Disease. (See p. 905.)

14. Identify causes of gastrointestinal bleeding in the elderly. (See p. 906.)

15. Discuss the general management of gastrointestinal bleeding in elderly patients. (See pp. 906–907.)

16. Discuss the impact of environmental changes on the elderly. (See pp. 907–908.)

17. Discuss abuse and neglect of the elderly, and determine resources available in your community to address this problem. (See p. 909.)

18. Recognize the need to be familiar with state and local laws regarding abuse or neglect of the elderly. (See p. 909.)

Althea Robertson, a 76-year-old female, lives alone. Her husband died several years ago. But her children visit occasionally. Today, her daughter notices that her mother is quite pale. "I haven't been feeling well," explains Mrs. Robinson. She starts to get up for some coffee, but faints on the floor. Although she soon arouses, her frightened daughter summons EMS.

Within five minutes, a paramedic ambulance arrives. The paramedics complete the primary and secondary assessment. The patient is indeed pale. Her blood pressure is 100/60 and pulse is 110 when supine. The ECG shows atrial fibrillation. The paramedics repeat the vitals signs with the patient seated. The blood pressure drops to 80/60, and the pulse increases to 130. A brief review of

the history reveals that the patient has been having diarrhea, with black stools. She also has had some occasional epigastric pain. Because her arthritis has been acting up, she has been taking a lot more aspirin than usual.

The paramedics administer oxygen and begin an IV of lactated Ringer's. The paramedics place the patient on the PASG, but they do not inflate it. Transport to the hospital goes without problem. In the emergency department, a nasogastric tube is inserted and bloody material aspirated. The patient's hemoglobin is found to be 6.6 grams (normal is 12–14). Emergency endoscopy shows a bleeding duodenal ulcer. The patient is transfused with blood and given anti-ulcer medications. She is discharged seven days later and does well.

INTRODUCTION

■ **elderly** a person age 65 years or older.

Today, people over age 65 represent approximately 12 percent of the population. Persons 65 years of age and older are typically referred to as **elderly**. Although arbitrary, this age represents the time in life when people generally become eligible for Medicare and retirement. Patients 75 years of age and older are often referred to as the "**old-old**."

■ **"old-old"** an elderly person age 75 years or older.

In the 1990s and early 2000s, the elderly promise to be the fastest-growing segment of our population, a trend popularly called "the greying of America." There are several reasons for this trend.

❏ The mean survival of older persons is increasing.
❏ The birth rate is declining.
❏ There has been an absence of major wars and other catastrophes.
❏ Health care has improved significantly since World War II.

■ **geriatrics** the study and treatment of diseases of the aged.

In recent years, physicians and other health care workers have increasingly specialized in care of the elderly. This aspect of medicine, known as **geriatrics**, is essential in caring for our aging population.

Nearly 36 percent of all EMS calls involve the elderly. Therefore, you will need to be familiar with the health-care considerations of this age group. This chapter will present the fundamental principles of geriatrics, especially those related to advanced prehospital care.

ANATOMY AND PHYSIOLOGY OF AGING

Aging is a lifelong process. Many anatomical and physiological changes become evident as we grow older. (See Figure 29-1.)

General Age-Related Changes

As people age, there is a general decline in the function of virtually every organ system. The decline and change begins at the cellular level. The total amount of body water significantly decreases. Also, total body fat decreases by as much as 15–30 percent. Although the metabolic rate remains fairly constant, there is a sharp reduction in the total number of body cells, often up to 30 percent, by age 65.

One of the important changes involves the progressive reduction in the efficiency of the body's homeostatic control systems. The homeostatic systems are those body control systems that keep the internal environment of the body constant. These systems play a major role in aiding the body in recovery from illness or injury, as well as in the prevention of illness and injury. Inhibition of these control systems produces delayed healing and delayed recuperation.

Systemic Age-Related Changes

As mentioned previously, every body system is affected by the aging process. Many of these processes begin early in life, but become detectable in the sixth, seventh, and eighth decades of life.

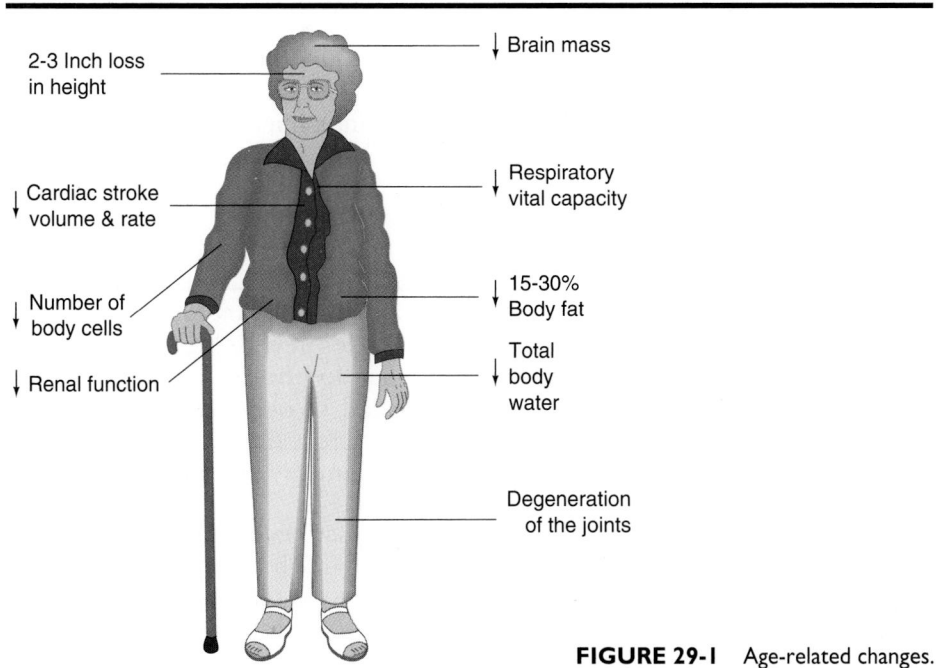

FIGURE 29-1 Age-related changes.

Respiratory System   The effects of aging on the respiratory system begin as early as age 30. Age-related changes in the respiratory system include increased chest wall stiffness, loss of lung elasticity, increased air trapping due to collapse of the smaller airways, and reduced strength and endurance of the respiratory muscles.

Functionally, by the time we reach age 65, vital capacity may decrease by as much as 50 percent. In addition, the maximum breathing capacity may decrease as much as 60 percent, while the maximum oxygen uptake may decrease up to 70 percent. These changes ultimately result in decreased ventilation and progressive hypoxemia. The presence of underlying pulmonary diseases, such as emphysema and chronic bronchitis, further reduces respiratory function.

Cardiovascular System   The cardiovascular system is also affected by aging. The wall of the left ventricle may thicken (**hypertrophy**), often by as much as 25 percent. This is even more pronounced if there is associated hypertension. In addition, **fibrosis** develops in the heart and peripheral vascular system, resulting in hypertension, arteriosclerosis, and decreased cardiac function. The conductive system of the heart degenerates, often causing dysrhythmias and various degrees of heart block. Ultimately, the stroke volume declines and the heart rate slows, leading to decreased cardiac output. Because of this, the heart's ability to respond to stress diminishes.

Renal System   The effects of aging are also evident in the renal system, where the number of functioning **nephrons** may be decreased 30–40 percent. Renal blood flow may decrease by as much as 45 percent, thus increasing the amount of waste products in the blood. In the male, the prostate often becomes enlarged (benign prostatic hypertrophy), causing difficulty in urination or urinary retention.

Nervous System   The brain can lose as much as 45 percent of its cells in certain areas of the cortex. Overall, there is an average 6–7 percent reduction in the weight of the brain. Blood flow to the cerebral areas is also decreased, due to increased resistance and the presence of arteriosclerosis. The amount of oxygen the brain uses, especially in the cortical areas, may decrease. Peripherally, there may be up to a 15 percent reduction in **nerve conduction velocity**, thus slowing reflexes, as well as sensory and motor function.

A steady deterioration of hearing and vision is also associated with aging. Although the degree varies among individuals, impairment may create a sense of confusion in the hearing or visually impaired.

Musculoskeletal System   An aging person may lose as much as 2–3 inches of height from narrowing of the intervertebral discs and **osteoporosis**. Osteoporosis is the loss of mineral from the bone, resulting in softening of the bones. This is especially evident in the vertebral bodies, thus causing a change in posture. The posture of the aged individual often reveals an increase in the curvature of the thoracic spine, commonly called **kyphosis**, and slight flexion of the knee and hip joints. The demineralization of bone makes the patient much more susceptible to hip and other fractures. In addition to skeletal changes, a decrease in skeletal muscle weight commonly occurs with age.

Gastrointestinal System   Age affects the gastrointestinal system in various ways. The volume of saliva may decrease as much as 33 percent. Gastric secretions may decrease to as little as 20 percent of the quantity present in youth. Esophageal motility decreases, thus making swallowing less effective and more difficult.

■ **hypertrophy** an increase in the size or bulk of an organ.

■ **fibrosis** the formation of fiber-like connective tissue, also called scar tissue, in an organ.

■ **nephrons** the functional units of the kidney.

■ **nerve conduction velocity** the rate at which a nervous impulse is transmitted along a nerve.

■ **osteoporosis** softening of bone tissue due to the loss of essential minerals, principally calcium.

■ **kyphosis** exaggeration of the normal posterior curvature of the spine.

ASSESSMENT OF THE GERIATRIC PATIENT

The assessment of the geriatric patient is essentially the same as that for any adult. However, several factors complicate the clinical evaluation. It is often difficult to separate the effects of aging from the consequences of disease. For example, it is hard to discern whether a patient's subjective dyspnea is due to normal age-related changes in the respiratory system or to underlying diseases such as emphysema.

Complicating Factors

Often, the chief complaint of the elderly patient may seem trivial or vague at first. Also, the patient may fail to report important symptoms. Therefore, you should try to distinguish the patient's chief complaint from the patient's primary problem. The chief complaint is the symptom the patient is most concerned about, whereas the primary problem may be entirely different. A patient may complain about nausea, which is the chief complaint. The primary problem, however, may be the rectal bleeding the patient neglected to mention.

Another complicating factor is that elderly patients often suffer from more than one disease at a time. The presence of chronic problems may make it more difficult to assess an acute problem. Often, it is easy to confuse symptoms of a chronic illness with those of an acute problem. When confronted with an elderly patient who has chest pain, for example, it is difficult to determine whether the presence of frequent premature ventricular contractions is acute or chronic. Lacking access to the patient's medical record, you should treat the patient on a "threat-to-life" basis.

Another important complication in managing the elderly patient is that aging changes an individual's response to illness and injury. Pain may be diminished or absent, thus causing both you and the patient to underestimate the severity of the illness. In addition, the temperature-regulating mechanism may be altered or depressed. This can result in the absence of fever, or a minimal fever, even in the face of severe infection. The alteration in the temperature-regulating mechanism makes the elderly more prone to environmental thermal problems. Social and emotional factors may have a greater impact on health in the elderly than in any other age group. A common example is the rapidity of death or serious illness in a previously healthy individual soon after the death of his or her spouse.

Because of such factors, the chief complaint of an elderly patient should not be trivialized. It may mask or be symptomatic of a more serious underlying disease. Common complaints in the elderly include:

* One factor complicating assessment of geriatric patients is that they are more apt to suffer from more than one disease at a time.

- ❏ Fatigue and weakness
- ❏ Dizziness, vertigo, or syncope (to be discussed later)
- ❏ Falls
- ❏ Headache
- ❏ Insomnia (trouble sleeping)
- ❏ Dysphagia (difficulty in swallowing)
- ❏ Loss of appetite
- ❏ Inability to void
- ❏ Constipation or diarrhea

When presented with any of these complaints, you must probe for significant symptoms and, ultimately, the primary problem. Patience, respect, and kindness will elicit the answers needed for a pertinent medical history.

History

In gathering a medical history, keep in mind the complications that arise from multiple diseases and multiple medications. Medications can be an especially important indicator of the patient's diseases. Therefore, you should find all of the patient's medications and take them to the hospital with the patient. You should try to determine which of the medications, including over-the-counter ones, are current. In cases of multiple medications, there is increased incidence of medication errors, drug interactions, and noncompliance.

Communications may be more difficult when dealing with the aged. **Cataracts** and **glaucoma** can diminish sight. Blindness, often resulting from diabetes and stroke, is more common in the elderly. The level of anxiety increases when a patient is unable to see his or her surroundings clearly. As a result, you should talk calmly to the visually impaired patient. Yelling does not help. Instead, position yourself near the patient where he or she can see or touch you.

Age also affects hearing. Diminished hearing or deafness can make it virtually impossible to obtain a history. In such cases, try to determine the history from a friend or family member. Do not shout at the patient. This will not help if the patient is deaf, and it may distort sounds and make it difficult for the patient who has some hearing to understand you. Write notes if necessary. If the patient can lip-read, speak slowly and directly toward the patient. Whenever possible, verify the history with a reliable friend or relative. Also, because loss of hearing may result from other causes, confirm that deafness is a pre-existing condition.

Finally, remember that age sometimes diminishes mental status. The patient can be confused and unable to remember details. In addition, the noise of radios, ECG equipment, and strange voices may add to the confusion. Both senility and organic brain syndrome may manifest themselves similarly. Common symptoms include:

- ❑ Delirium
- ❑ Confusion
- ❑ Distractibility
- ❑ Restlessness
- ❑ Excitability
- ❑ Hostility

When confronted with a confused patient, try to determine whether the patient's mental status represents a significant change from normal. DO NOT assume that a confused, disoriented patient is "just senile," thus failing to assess for a serious underlying problem. Alcoholism, for example, is more common in the elderly than was once recognized. It can further complicate taking the history.

Another complication results from depression, which can be mistaken for many other diseases. It can often mimic senility and organic brain syndrome. Depression may also inhibit patient cooperation. The depressed patient may be malnourished, dehydrated, overdosed, contemplating suicide, or simply imagining physical ailments for attention. If you suspect depression, question the patient regarding drug ingestion or suicidal ideation. It is important to remember that suicide is now the fourth-leading cause of death among the elderly in the United States.

After obtaining the history, and if time allows, try to verify the patient's history with a reliable family member or neighbor. This will often be less offensive to the patient if done out of his or her presence. While at the scene, it is important to observe the surroundings for indications of the patient's ability to care for himself or herself. Look for evidence of drug or alcohol inges-

■ **cataracts** medical condition in which the lens of the eye loses its clearness.

■ **glaucoma** medical condition where the pressure within the eye increases.

✱ Never assume that a confused elderly patient is "just senile." Always assess for an underlying problem.

✱ Depression is more common in the elderly than once thought.

tion and for Medic-Alert and Vial-of-Life items. It is also important to look for signs of abuse or neglect.

Physical Examination

Certain considerations must be kept in mind when examining the elderly patient. Remember that some patients are often easily fatigued and cannot tolerate a long examination. Also, because of the problems with temperature regulation, the patient may be wearing several layers of clothing, which can make examination difficult. Be sure to explain all actions clearly before initiating the examination, especially in patients with impaired vision. Be aware that the patient may minimize or deny symptoms because he or she fears being bedridden or institutionalized or forced to give up self-sufficiency.

Peripheral pulses may be difficult to evaluate, because of peripheral vascular disease and arthritis. Try to distinguish signs of chronic disease from an acute problem. For example, the elderly may have non-pathological rales. There is often an increase in mouth breathing and a loss of skin elasticity, which may be easily confused with dehydration. Dependent edema may be caused by inactivity, not congestive heart failure. Only experience and practice will allow you to distinguish acute from chronic physical findings.

PATHOPHYSIOLOGY AND MANAGEMENT

Because of age-related changes, the elderly are more vulnerable to trauma and disease. You should be familiar with medical and traumatic problems that frequently occur in the elderly. In addition, you should always maintain a high index of suspicion for serious injury when treating an injured elderly person.

Trauma in the Elderly Patient

The elderly are more at risk from trauma than younger people, especially from falls.

> ✱ The elderly are at increased risk for more serious injuries due to trauma than their younger counterparts.

Contributing Factors Contributing factors to increased trauma in the elderly include:

- ❏ Slower reflexes
- ❏ Diminished eyesight and hearing
- ❏ Arthritis
- ❏ Loss of elasticity in the peripheral blood vessels, making them more subject to tearing
- ❏ More fragile tissues and bones

The elderly, because of their physical state and vulnerability, are at high risk from trauma caused by criminal assault. Purse-snatching, armed robbery, and assault occur all too frequently in the elderly.

As a group, the elderly experience more head injuries, even from relatively minor trauma, than their younger counterparts. A major factor is the difference in proportion between the brain and the skull. As mentioned earlier, the brain decreases in size and weight with age. The skull, however, remains constant in size, allowing the brain more room to move, thus increasing the likelihood of brain injury. Because of this, signs of brain injury may develop more slowly in the elderly, sometimes over days and weeks. In fact, the patient may often have forgotten the offending injury.

The cervical spine is also more susceptible to injury due to osteoporosis and spondylolysis. **Spondylolysis** is a degeneration of the vertebral body. The elderly often have a significant degree of this disease. In addition, arthritic changes can gradually compress the nerve rootlets or spinal cord. Thus, injury to the spine in the elderly makes the patient much more susceptible to spinal-cord injury. In fact, sudden neck movement, even without fracture, may cause spinal-cord injury. This can occur with less than normal pain, due to the absence of fracture.

Falls often result in a fracture of the hip or pelvis. Osteoporosis and general frailty contribute to this. The older patient who has fallen should be assumed to have a hip fracture until proven otherwise. Signs and symptoms of a hip fracture include tenderness over the affected joint and shortening and external rotation of the leg. The patient is unable to bear weight on the affected leg. If the patient lives alone, he or she may not be able to get to a phone to summon help. Because of this, they may remain on the floor for a prolonged period of time. This can lead to hypothermia, hyperthermia, and/or dehydration.

Trauma Management in the Elderly Patient   The priorities of care for the elderly trauma patient are similar to those for any trauma patient. However, you must keep in mind the age-related decline of body systems and presence of chronic diseases. This is especially true of the cardiovascular, respiratory, and renal systems. Recent or past myocardial infarctions may contribute to the risk of dysrhythmia or congestive heart failure in the trauma patient. In addition, there may be a decreased response of the heart, in adjusting heart rate and stroke volume, to hypovolemia. An elderly trauma patient may require higher than usual arterial pressures for perfusion of vital organs, due to increased peripheral vascular resistance and hypertension. Care must be taken in intravenous fluid administration because of decreased myocardial reserves. As a result, hypotension and hypovolemia are poorly tolerated. In addition, the geriatric patient's physical response to drugs may be altered.

Physical changes in the elderly can decrease chest wall movement and vital capacity. To complicate matters, age reduces the tolerance of all organs for anoxia. Chronic obstructive pulmonary disease is common. Therefore, you must properly attune airway management and ventilation to provide adequate oxygenation and appropriate CO_2 removal. It is important to remember that use of 50 percent nitrous oxide (Nitronox) for persons of this age group may result in more respiratory depression than would occur in a younger person. Positive pressure ventilation should be used cautiously in the geriatric patient—there is an increased danger of resultant alkalosis and rupture of emphysematous bullae, resulting in pneumothorax. The decreased ability of the kidney to maintain normal acid/base balance, and to compensate for fluid changes, can further complicate the management of the elderly trauma patient. Any pre-existing renal disease can also decrease the kidney's ability to compensate. The decrease in renal function, along with a decreased cardiac reserve, places the injured elderly patient at risk for fluid overload and pulmonary edema.

Positioning, immobilization, and packaging of the elderly patient before transportation may have to be modified. Be attentive to physical deformities such as arthritis, spinal abnormalities, or frozen limbs that may cause pain or require special care.

Respiratory Emergencies in the Elderly Patient

Respiratory emergencies are one of the most common reasons elderly persons summon EMS or seek emergency care. Most elderly patients with a respiratory emergency will present with a chief complaint of dyspnea. However, coughing, congestion, and wheezing are also common chief complaints.

Common Causes of Respiratory Distress   Many factors can cause respiratory distress in the elderly patient. Common causes include pneumonia, pulmonary embolism, pulmonary edema, and exacerbation of chronic obstructive pulmonary disease.

Pneumonia.   Pneumonia is an infection of the lung usually caused by a bacteria or virus. The elderly develop pneumonia much more frequently than younger patients for several reasons. These include an abnormal or ineffective cough reflex, decreased effectiveness of the mucociliary cells of the upper respiratory system, and altered immunity. Residents of nursing homes are at increased risk of developing pneumonia due to immobility and exposure to other patients in relatively closed quarters. Pneumonia in the elderly has a much higher mortality compared to younger patients. It is characterized by increasing dyspnea, congestion, fever, chills, and sputum production.

Pulmonary Embolism.   Pulmonary embolism should always be considered as a possible etiology of respiratory distress in the elderly. Pulmonary emboli usually originate in the deep veins of the thigh and calf and are most apt to occur following a period of immobilization. In addition, atrial fibrillation predisposes patients to develop a pulmonary embolism. Atrial fibrillation causes a dilation of the atria that can lead to clot formation, resulting in a pulmonary embolism. Pulmonary embolism should be suspected in any patient with the acute onset of dyspnea. Often, it is accompanied by pleuritic chest pain and right heart failure. If the pulmonary embolus is massive, you can expect severe dyspnea, cardiac dysrhythmias, and ultimately cardiovascular collapse.

Pulmonary Edema.   Acute pulmonary edema can develop rapidly in the elderly. Although most commonly associated with acute myocardial infarction, it can also occur due to other factors. Pulmonary edema causes severe dyspnea associated with congestion. The patient is usually orthopneic and anxious. Physical examination usually reveals the presence of moist rales and accessory muscle use.

Chronic Obstructive Pulmonary Disease.   Chronic obstructive pulmonary diseases—emphysema, chronic bronchitis, and, to a lesser degree, asthma—are frequent causes of respiratory distress in the elderly. Pneumonia, as well as other respiratory infections, can complicate chronic obstructive pulmonary disease. Associated infection should always be suspect, especially in the face of fever or chills.

Cancer.   Cancer occurs more frequently among the elderly. Often, progressive dyspnea will be the first presentation of a cancerous lesion. Hemoptysis, chronic cough, and weight loss are common symptoms. Cancerous tissue does not have to be present in the lung to cause dyspnea.

Management of Respiratory Distress   The management of respiratory distress in the elderly patient is essentially the same as for all age groups. However, you should be familiar with the altered respiratory function of older patients and plan management strategies accordingly. Many geriatric patients with respiratory disease also have underlying cardiac disease. With this in mind, drugs such as theophylline and the beta agonists should be used with extreme caution.

Cardiovascular Disease in the Elderly Patient

The leading cause of death in the elderly is cardiovascular disease. Cardiovascular disease in the elderly patient is often complicated by disease processes in other organ systems that makes assessment and treatment more difficult.

Cardiac Emergencies   Common cardiac problems that you can expect to encounter in the aged include: myocardial infarction, cardiac dysrhythmias, congestive heart failure, syncope, and aortic disease.

Myocardial Infarction.   The elderly patient with myocardial infarction is less likely to present with classic symptoms than a younger counterpart. Atypical presentations that may be seen in the elderly include: confusion, syncope, dyspnea, neck pain, dental pain, epigastric pain, and fatigue. Many elderly patients will suffer a **silent myocardial infarction**. In addition, the elderly tend to have larger myocardial infarctions than younger patients. The majority of deaths that occur in the first hours following myocardial infarction are due to dysrhythmias. Because of the high mortality associated with myocardial infarction in the older patient, early detection and emergency management are critical.

■ **silent myocardial infarction** a myocardial infarction that occurs without exhibiting obvious signs or symptoms.

Dysrhythmias.   Many cardiac dysrhythmias develop with age. These occur primarily as a result of degeneration of the heart's conductive system. To complicate matters, the elderly patient does not tolerate extremes in heart rate as well as a younger person would. For example, a heart rate of 140 in an older patient may cause syncope, while a younger patient can often tolerate a heart rate greater than 180. A dysrhythmia may be the only clinical finding in an elderly patient suffering acute myocardial infarction.

Congestive Heart Failure.   Congestive heart failure, both acute and chronic, is also common in the elderly patient. It results from myocardial changes that normally occur with age, as well as disease factors such as hypertension, arteriosclerotic disease, and diabetes. It commonly presents with confusion or an alteration in mental status. Congestive heart failure may be hard to diagnose in the elderly, as chronic pedal edema and basilar rales may be normal findings.

■ **aortic dissection** a degeneration of the wall of the aorta.

Aortic Dissection.   **Aortic dissection** is a degeneration of the wall of the aorta, either in the thoracic or abdominal cavity. It can result in an aneurysm or in rupture of the vessel. In younger persons, it is associated with syphilis, connective-tissue diseases, and congenital defects. In older patients, it is almost always due to arteriosclerosis. These patients will often present with tearing chest or abdominal pain or, if rupture occurs, cardiac arrest.

■ **syncope** a transient loss of consciousness caused by inadequate blood flow to the brain.

Syncope.   Cardiovascular conditions are more common in older persons, primarily due to progressive atherosclerotic disease. **Syncope** is a common presenting complaint, yet a difficult one to assess. However, syncope has a much higher morbidity in elderly patients than in younger individuals. Syncope results when blood flow to the brain is temporarily interrupted or decreased. It is most often caused by problems with either the nervous system or the cardiovascular system. The following are some of the common presentations that you may encounter.

❑ *Vasodepressor Syncope.* Vasodepressor syncope is the common faint. It may occur following emotional distress; pain; prolonged bed rest; mild blood loss; prolonged standing in warm, crowded rooms; anemia; or fever.

❏ *Orthostatic Syncope.* Orthostatic syncope occurs when a person rises from a seated or supine position. There are several possible causes. First, there may be a disproportion between blood volume and vascular capacitance. That is, there is a pooling of blood in the legs, reducing blood flow to the brain. Causes of this include: hypovolemia, venous **varicosities**, prolonged bed rest, and **autonomic dysfunction**. Many drugs, especially blood pressure medicines, can cause drug-induced orthostatic syncope due to the effects of the medications on the capacitance vessels.

❏ *Vasovagal Syncope.* Vasovagal syncope occurs as a result of a **valsalva maneuver**, which happens during defecation, coughing, or similar maneuvers. This effectively slows the heart rate and cardiac output, thus decreasing blood flow to the brain.

❏ *Cardiac Syncope.* Cardiac syncope results from transient reduction in cerebral blood flow due to a sudden decrease in cardiac output. It can result from several mechanisms. Syncope can be the primary symptom of silent myocardial infarction. In addition, many dysrhythmias can cause syncope. Dysrhythmias that have been shown to cause syncope include bradycardias, **Stokes-Adams syndrome**, heart block, tachyarrhythmias, and **sick sinus syndrome**.

❏ *Seizures.* Unlike most cases of syncope, seizures tend to occur without warning and are unpredictable. The differentiation of seizures from syncope is often hard to determine in the prehospital setting.

❏ *Transient Ischemic Attacks.* **Transient ischemic attacks** occur more frequently in the elderly. They are a frequent cause of syncope.

Management of Cardiovascular Disease The elderly patient with cardiovascular disease is managed in much the same manner as a younger patient. However, due to the increased prevalence of congestive heart failure, liver disease, and metabolic problems, the medical control physician may often modify medication dosages, as well as fluid administration orders.

Neurological Emergencies in the Elderly Patient

Elderly patients are at risk for several neurological emergencies. Often, the exact cause is not initially known and may require probing in the hospital.

Neurological Disorders Many neurological disorders that you encounter in the field will exhibit an alteration in mental status. You may discover a range of underlying causes from stroke to degenerative brain disease.

Altered Mental Status. Altered mental status in the elderly patient can have many causes. These include:

❏ Cerebrovascular disease (stroke or transient ischemic attack)
❏ Myocardial infarction
❏ Seizures
❏ Medication-related (drug interactions, drug underdose, and drug overdose)
❏ Infection
❏ Fluid and electrolyte abnormalities (dehydration)
❏ Lack of nutrients (hypoglycemia)
❏ Temperature changes (hypothermia or hyperthermia)
❏ Structural changes (dementia, subdural hematoma)

■ **varicosities** an abnormal dilation of a vein or group of veins.

■ **autonomic dysfunction** an abnormality of the involuntary aspect of the nervous system.

■ **valsalva's maneuver** forced exhalation against a closed glottis. This maneuver increases intra-abdominal and intra-thoracic pressure, which in turn slows the pulse.

■ **Stokes-Adams syndrome** a series of symptoms resulting from heart block, most commonly syncope. The symptoms result from decreased blood flow to the brain caused by the sudden decrease in cardiac output.

■ **sick sinus syndrome** a group of disorders characterized by dysfunction of the sinoatrial node in the heart.

■ **transient ischemic attack** reversible interruption of blood flow to the brain. Often seen as a precursor to major stroke.

It is often impossible in the field to distinguish the cause of altered mental status. Even so, you should carry out a thorough primary and secondary assessment. Administer supplemental oxygen as necessary. As soon as practical, obtain a blood glucose level to exclude hypoglycemia as a possible cause. Overall, the approach to the elderly patient with altered mental status is the same as with any patient presenting with similar symptoms.

Cerebrovascular Disease. **Stroke**, or cerebrovascular accident, is a common problem in the elderly. Occlusive stroke is statistically more common in the elderly and relatively uncommon in younger individuals. Older patients are at higher risk of stroke because of atherosclerosis, hypertension, immobility, limb paralysis, congestive heart failure, and atrial fibrillation. Transient ischemic attacks, commonly called TIAs, are also more common in older patients. More than one-third of patients suffering TIAs will go on to develop a major, permanent stroke. TIAs are a frequent cause of syncope in the elderly.

The signs and symptoms can present in many ways—altered mental status, coma, paralysis, slurred speech, a change in mood, and seizures. The disease should be highly suspect in any patient with a sudden change in mental status. If stroke is suspect, it is essential that you complete the Glasgow Coma Scale for later comparison in the emergency department.

Seizures. Seizures may be easily mistaken for stroke in the elderly. Also, a first-time seizure may occur due to damage from a previous stroke. Not all seizures experienced by the elderly are of the major motor type. Some are more subtle. Many etiologies of seizure activity in the elderly have been identified. Common causes include:

❏ Seizure disorder
❏ Recent or past head trauma
❏ Mass lesion (tumor or bleed)
❏ Alcoholic withdrawal
❏ Diabetic hypoglycemia
❏ Stroke

Often, the cause of the seizure cannot be determined in the field.

Dizziness. Dizziness is a frightening experience and a frequent complaint of older persons. The complaint of dizziness may actually mean the patient has suffered syncope, pre-syncope, light-headedness, or true **vertigo**. Vertigo is a specific sensation of motion perceived by the patient as spinning or whirling. Many patients will report that they feel as though they are spinning, while others may report that they feel the room around them is spinning. Vertigo is often accompanied with sweating, pallor, nausea, and vomiting. **Meniere's disease**, a disease of the inner ear, can cause severe, **intractable** vertigo. It is often, however, associated with a constant "roaring" sound in the ears, as well as ear "pressure."

Vertigo results from so many factors that it is often hard, even for the physician, to determine the actual cause. Any factor that impairs visual input, inner-ear function, peripheral sensory input, or the central nervous system can cause dizziness. In addition, alcohol and many prescription drugs can cause dizziness. It is virtually impossible to distinguish dizziness, syncope, and pre-syncope in the prehospital setting.

■ **stroke** an interruption of blood flow—from emboli, thrombus, or hemorrhage—to an area of the brain.

■ **vertigo** the sensation of faintness or dizziness; may cause a loss of balance.

■ **Meniere's disease** a disease of the inner ear characterized by vertigo, nerve deafness, and a roaring or buzzing in the ear.

■ **intractable** resistant to cure, relief, or control.

Dementia. Unfortunately, many older patients experience a decrease in mental functioning along with physical deterioration. **Delirium** is a global mental impairment of sudden onset and self-limited duration. **Dementia**, on the other hand, is a chronic global mental impairment, often progressive or irreversible. It is usually due to an underlying neurological disease. This mental deterioration is often called "organic brain syndrome," "**senile dementia**," or "senility." It is important to find out whether an alteration in mental status is acute or chronic. Causes of dementia include:

- ❑ Small strokes
- ❑ Atherosclerosis of the cerebral blood vessels
- ❑ Aging
- ❑ Neurological diseases
- ❑ Certain hereditary diseases (e.g., Huntington's chorea)

Etiologies of delirium include:

- ❑ Subdural hematoma
- ❑ Tumors and other mass lesions
- ❑ Drug-induced changes or alcohol intoxication
- ❑ CNS infections
- ❑ Electrolyte abnormalities
- ❑ Cardiac failure

Alzheimer's Disease. **Alzheimer's Disease** is a particular type of dementia. It is a progressive, degenerative disease that attacks the brain and results in impaired memory, thinking, and behavior. It affects an estimated 2.5 million American adults.

Management of Neurological Disorders
Management techniques for elderly patients are similar to those for all other age groups. When confronted with a confused, dangerous, or violent patient, it is important to determine whether the behavior is acute or chronic. In the patient who has suffered a syncopal episode, try to obtain essential historical information so that you may better determine the type of syncope. Factors to consider include:

- ❑ Position of the patient at time of attack
- ❑ Any associated symptoms
- ❑ The duration of the attack
- ❑ Vital signs, including evaluation of orthostatic changes

Treatment for elderly patients suffering a neurological emergency is basically the same as for younger patients.

Psychiatric Disorders in the Elderly Patient

Psychiatric problems are common in the geriatric population. There is more dementia and depression, and less schizophrenia and alcoholism, than in younger patients. It is important to remember that emotional disorders are common due to isolation, loneliness, loss of self-dependence, loss of strength, and fear of the future. Any of these may present as physical disorders. Conversely, many physical disorders can present as psychiatric disorders.

■ **delirium** an acute alteration in mental functioning that is often reversible.

■ **dementia** a deterioration of mental status that is usually associated with structural neurological disease. It is often progressive and irreversible.

■ **senile dementia** general term used to describe an abnormal decline in mental functioning seen in the elderly.

■ **Alzheimer's Disease** a progressive, degenerative disease that attacks the brain and results in impaired memory, thinking, and behavior. It affects an estimated 2.5 million American adults.

✳ As the population ages, Alzheimer's Disease will become an even greater problem.

Classifying Psychiatric Disease   There are several methods of classifying psychiatric disease. Some of the common classifications of psychiatric disorders related to old age include:

❑ Organic brain syndrome
❑ Affective disorders (depression)
❑ Neurotic disorders (anxiety, hypochondriasis, phobias)
❑ Personality disorders (dependent personality)
❑ Paranoid disorders (schizophrenia)
❑ Alcoholism

It is important to keep in mind that individuals over 65 years of age account for 25 percent of all suicides reported.

Management of Psychiatric Disturbances   Management of psychiatric disturbances in the elderly is essentially the same as for other age groups. However, remember that the older patient may have increased susceptibility to the depressant effects, as well as the side-effects, of neuroleptic medications such as Haldol and Thorazine.

Gastrointestinal Emergencies Among Elderly Patients

Gastrointestinal emergencies are common among the elderly. The most frequent emergency is gastrointestinal bleeding. However, other gastrointestinal problems can occur.

Common Gastrointestinal Problems   Older people will describe a variety of gastrointestinal complaints—nausea, poor appetite, diarrhea, and constipation, to name a few. Remember, that like other presenting complaints, these conditions may be symptomatic of other more serious diseases. Bowel problems, for example, may point to cancer of the colon or other abdominal organs. Some of the most critical problems that you may encounter in the field will involve internal hemorrhage and bowel obstruction.

GI Hemorrhage.   Gastrointestinal bleeding falls into two general categories: upper GI bleed and lower GI bleed.

Upper GI Bleed
❑ *Peptic Ulcer Disease.* Injury to the mucous lining of the upper part of the gastrointestinal tract due to stomach acids, digestive enzymes, and other agents such as anti-inflammatory drugs.
❑ *Gastritis.* An inflammation of the lining of the stomach.
❑ *Esophageal Varices.* An abnormal dilation of veins in the lower esophagus; a common complication of cirrhosis of the liver.
❑ *Mallory-Weiss Tear.* A tear in the lower esophagus that is often caused by severe and prolonged retching.

Lower GI Bleed
❑ *Diverticulosis.* The presence of bleeding from small pouches on the colon that tend to develop with age; causes 70 percent of life-threatening lower GI bleeds.
❑ *Tumors.* Tumors of the colon can cause bleeding when the tumor erodes into blood vessels within the intestine or surrounding organs.

❏ *Ischemic Colitis.* An inflammation of the colon due to impaired or decreased blood supply.

❏ *Arterio-Venous Malformations.* An abnormal link between an artery and a vein.

Signs of significant gastrointestinal blood loss include the presence of "coffee ground" emesis; black, tarry stools (**melena**); frank blood in the emesis or stool; orthostatic hypotension; pulse greater than 100 (unless on beta blockers); and confusion. Gastrointestinal bleeding in the elderly may result in such complications as a recent increase in angina symptoms, congestive heart failure, weakness, or dyspnea.

■ **melena** a bloody stool.

Bowel Obstruction. Bowel obstruction in the elderly typically involves the small bowel. Causes include tumors, prior abdominal surgery, use of certain medications, and occasionally the presence of vertebral compression fractures. The patient will typically complain of diffuse abdominal pain, bloating, nausea, and vomiting. The abdomen may feel distended when palpated. Bowel sounds may be hypoactive or absent. If the obstruction has been present for a prolonged period of time, the patient may have fever, weakness, shock, and various electrolyte disturbances.

Management of Gastrointestinal Emergencies
Prompt recognition and management of a GI emergency is essential, regardless of the age group. The elderly patient with a GI bleed is at significant risk for life-threatening hemorrhage and shock. There is a tendency to take such patients less seriously than those suffering moderate or severe external hemorrhage. This is a serious mistake. These patients should be aggressively treated. Management should include:

❏ Airway management
❏ Support of breathing and circulation, if compromised
❏ High-flow oxygen therapy
❏ IV fluid replacement with a crystalloid
❏ PASG placement
❏ Rapid transport

Remember that the elderly tolerate hypotension and anoxia less than younger patients.

Environmental Emergencies Among Elderly Patients

The elderly and infants are highly susceptible to extreme variations in environmental temperature. This occurs in the elderly because of altered or impaired thermoregulatory mechanisms. Predisposing factors for hypothermia in the elderly include:

❏ Accident exposure
❏ Drugs that interfere with heat production
❏ CNS disorders
❏ Endocrine disorders
❏ Poor nutrition
❏ Chronic illness and debilitation
❏ Low or fixed income

Similar factors tend to predispose these same patients toward the other extreme, hyperthermia. These factors include:

❏ Decreased functioning of the thermoregulatory center
❏ Commonly prescribed medications that inhibit sweating
❏ Low or fixed income
❏ Altered sensory input, which would normally warn a person of overheating
❏ Inadequate liquid intake

The management technique for the elderly is the same as for other patients. However, you need to take special precautions against accidental fluid overload—a condition that may cause pulmonary edema or congestive heart failure in the aged.

PHARMACOLOGY IN GERIATRICS

Most older patients are on some form of medication. Elderly persons use 25 percent of all prescribed and over-the-counter drugs sold in the United States. Many patients are on multiple medications, thus causing drug interactions to be fairly common. Adverse drug reactions may be more easily missed in the elderly, because of the overall increase in medical problems and symptoms attributed to normal aging.

Complicating Factors

✻ The dosage of emergency medications administered to elderly patients may need to be reduced. For example, elderly patients should receive 50 percent of the regular dose of lidocaine due to slower rate of elimination.

The pharmacokinetics of drugs are altered in the older patient. Because of decreased excretion and poor nutritional state, many drugs tend to accumulate in the blood with prolonged usage. In addition, the various compensatory mechanisms that help buffer against medication side-effects are less effective in the elderly than in younger patients.

Approximately 30 percent of all hospital admissions are related to drug-induced illness. More than 30 percent of these persons are over the age of 60 years. Accidental overdose may occur more frequently in the aged due to confusion, vision impairment, self-selection of medication, and forgetfulness. Intentional drug overdose also occurs in attempts at self-destruction.

Underdose of medication is also more common in the elderly. In fact, underdosing of medication accounts for about half of all medication errors. This can be attributed to forgetfulness (the patient forgot to take the medication) or to limited income (the patient cannot afford the prescribed medication). Drugs that have been identified as commonly causing toxicity in the elderly include:

❏ Digitalis, leading cause (Lanoxin, etc.)
❏ Anti-Parkinson medications (Symmetrel, carbidopa, etc.)
❏ Diuretics (furosemide, hydrochlorothiazide, etc.)
❏ Anticoagulants (Coumadin)
❏ Lidocaine (very important to prehospital care)
❏ Quinidine (Quinaglute, etc.)
❏ Propranolol (Inderal)
❏ Theophylline (Theo-Dur, Slow-Bid, etc.)
❏ Narcotic analgesics and acetaminophen (meperidine, etc.)
❏ Phenothiazines (Haldol, Thorazine, Mellaril, etc.)
❏ Tricyclic antidepressants (Elavil, Limbitrol, etc.)

GERIATRIC ABUSE/NEGLECT

Geriatric abuse and neglect is as big a problem in our society as child abuse and neglect. **Geriatric abuse** is defined as a syndrome in which an elderly person has received serious physical or psychological injury from his or her children or other care providers. Abuse of the elderly knows no socioeconomic bounds. It often occurs when an older person is no longer able to be totally independent, and the family has difficulty upholding their commitment to care for the patient. It can also occur in nursing homes and other health care facilities. The profile of the potential geriatric abuser may often show a great deal of life stress. There is often sleep deprivation, marital discord, financial problems, and work-related problems. As the abuser's life gets in further disarray, and as the patient further deteriorates, abuse may be the outcome.

Signs and symptoms of geriatric abuse or neglect are often obvious. Unexplained trauma is often the primary presentation. The average abused patient is older than 80 and has multiple medical problems, such as cancer, congestive heart failure, heart disease, and incontinence. Senile dementia is often present. In these cases, it is hard to determine whether the dementia is chronic or acute, especially if there is an increased likelihood of head trauma from abuse.

Whenever you suspect geriatric abuse, obtain a complete patient and family history. Pay particular attention to inconsistencies. *Do not confront the family*. Instead, report your suspicions to the emergency department and the appropriate governmental authority. Many states have very strong laws protecting the geriatric patient from abuse or neglect. In fact, many states consider it a criminal offense *not* to report suspected geriatric abuse. These states also offer legal immunity to those who report geriatric abuse, as long as the report is made in good faith.

■ **geriatric abuse** a syndrome in which an elderly person is physically or psychologically injured by another person.

✳ Many states have laws that require prehospital personnel to report suspected cases of geriatric abuse.

SUMMARY

The paramedic of today will be treating an increasing number of aged patients. It is important to remember that many changes occur—anatomical, physiological, emotional—as we enter **senescence**. Keep these changes in mind when treating elderly patients. Also, certain illnesses and injuries tend to occur more frequently in the older patient. Elderly patients are much more susceptible to medication side-effects and toxicity. They are also more susceptible to trauma and environmental stressors. Abuse of the elderly occurs and should always be kept in mind, especially when injuries do not match the history. Any suspected abuse or neglect of an elderly patient should be reported to the emergency department and the appropriate governmental authorities.

■ **senescence** the process of growing old.

FURTHER READING

Benson, Katy. "The Geriatric Factor," *Emergency* 24(9), September, 1992 (pp. 23–25).

Goddar, Thomas. "Geriatric Respiratory Emergencies," *Emergency* 24(9), September, 1992 (pp. 30–56).

Gorgen, Alice. "Altered Level of Consciousness in the Geriatric Patient," *Emergency* 24(9), September, 1992 (pp. 34–57).

Janing, Judy. "Tarnishing the Golden Years," *Emergency* 24(9), September, 1992 (pp. 40–58).

Judd, Richard. "Acute Disease Assessment in the Elderly," *Emergency* 24(9), September, 1992 (pp. 26–29).

Judd, Richard. "EMS Strategies in the Elderly," *Emergency* 23(2), February, 1991 (pp. 28–54).

Schwartz, George R., Gideon Bosker, and John W. Grigsby. *Geriatric Emergencies*. Bowie, MD: Brady Communications, 1984.

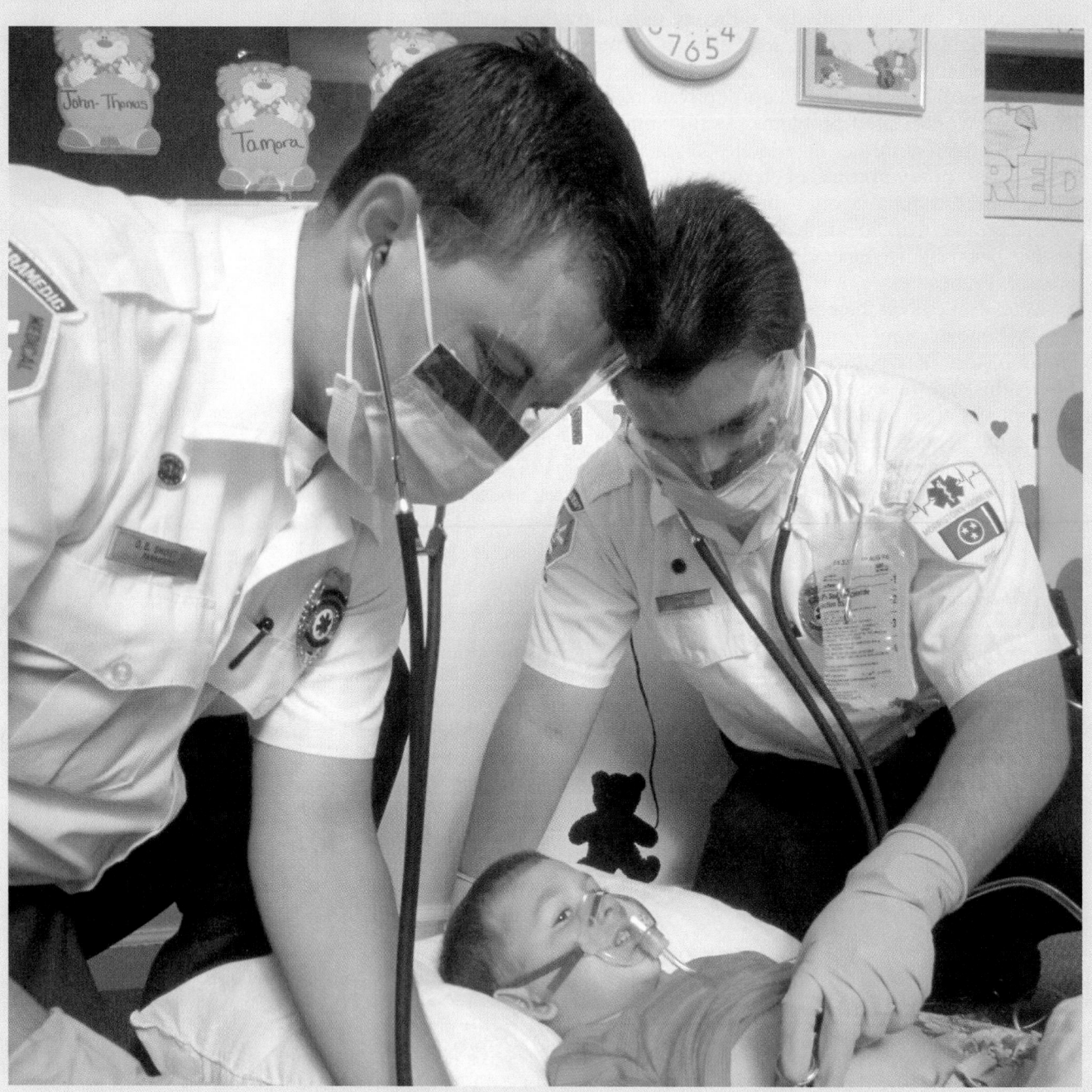

Objectives for Chapter 30

After reading this chapter, you should be able to:

1. Describe a typical child's emotional response to an emergency. (See pp. 912–913.)

2. List appropriate developmental milestones for each age group of children, and relate the appropriate approach to patient assessment. (See pp. 913–917.)

3. Discuss the typical parent's response to a pediatric emergency. (See p. 917.)

4. Describe pediatric patient assessment. (See pp. 917–920.)

5. Describe the normal and abnormal appearance of the anterior fontanelle in the infant. (See pp. 918–919.)

6. Identify normal age-related vital signs in the pediatric patient. (See pp. 919–920.)

7. Describe the role of non-invasive monitoring in prehospital pediatric emergency care. (See p. 920.)

8. Discuss pediatric trauma emergencies, and compare them to trauma emergencies seen in adult patients. (See pp. 921–923.)

9. Describe the characteristics of the abused child and of the child abuser. (See pp. 923–924.)

10. Describe signs and symptoms suggestive of child abuse or neglect. (See pp. 924–926.)

11. List management techniques to use when treating an abused child. (See pp. 926–927.)

12. Discuss the pathophysiology, assessment, and management of the following pediatric neurological emergencies. (See below pages.)

- seizures (pp. 927–928)
- febrile seizures (pp. 927–928)
- meningitis (pp. 928–929)
- Reye's Syndrome (p. 929)

13. Discuss the pathophysiology, assessment, and management of the following pediatric respiratory emergencies. (See below pages.)

- aspirated foreign body (pp. 930–931)
- croup (pp. 931–932)
- epiglottitis (pp. 932–933)
- bronchiolitis (pp. 933–934)
- asthma (pp. 934–935)
- status asthmaticus (p. 935)

14. Discuss the pathophysiology, assessment, and management of the following pediatric gastrointestinal emergencies. (See below pages.)

- nausea and vomiting (p. 935)
- diarrhea (p. 935)

15. Discuss the pathophysiology, assessment, and management of the following pediatric cardiovascular emergencies. (See below pages.)

- dehydration (p. 936)
- sepsis (pp. 936–937)
- dysrhythmias (p. 937)
- congenital heart disease (pp. 938–939)

16. Define Sudden Infant Death Syndrome (SIDS), including the theories of etiology and management in the prehospital setting. (See p. 940.)

17. Describe the concept of Pediatric Advanced Life Support (PALS). (See pp. 941–945.)

18. Describe the modifications required for pediatric advanced life support, including drug dosage, endotracheal intubation, defibrillation, and IV therapy. (See pp. 945–951.)

A call comes into Medic 1 at 5:45 AM. The crew shakes off their sleep to assist "a child with difficulty breathing." The cold, clear morning air snaps them to alertness. The ambulance response time is three minutes.

Arriving at the suburban residence, the paramedics enter the living room. There they see a 2-year-old girl sitting on her mother's lap. The child looks ill and has a barking cough. When she coughs, she becomes somewhat cyanotic. The mother reports they have tried the usual remedies—steamy shower, humidifier, and so on. But the child is getting worse.

Paramedics complete a primary and secondary survey. The child's axillary temperature is 101.2 degrees. However, they do not examine the throat because of the possibility of epiglottitis. The lungs are clear. The brassy stridor is obvious.

The paramedics bundle the child in a blanket and take her to the ambulance. The mother holds the child in the ambulance while paramedics administer humidified oxygen en route to the pediatric emergency room. Arriving at the hospital, the paramedics note the presence of three other children with a similar cough in the emergency room. The emergency physician obtains a soft-tissue X-ray of the neck, which helps exclude epiglottitis. The child is treated and admitted. While in the hospital, she receives intravenous corticosteroids and inhaled bronchodilators. She returns home in improved condition 48 hours later.

INTRODUCTION

The ill or injured child presents special problems for prehospital personnel. First, children often are not be able to describe what is bothering them or what has happened. Second, in addition to the sick or injured child, you must deal with the parents. Finally, the child's size often makes routine procedures more difficult. These and other factors in pediatric emergencies may cause a great deal of stress and anxiety for both you and the parents. Children are not simply "small adults." They have special considerations and needs. This chapter will present the topic of pediatric emergencies as it applies to advanced prehospital care.

✳ Children are not small adults.

GENERAL APPROACH TO PEDIATRIC EMERGENCIES

The approach to the pediatric patient will vary with the age of the patient and the nature of the problem. When obtaining the medical history of the pediatric patient, gather information as quickly and as accurately as possible. The parents are usually the primary source of information. However, as the child becomes older, he or she can also be a good source. You should try to establish a good relationship with the child. Children can often give accurate descriptions of symptoms or details. It is important to let the child express his or her opinion.

The Child's Response to Emergencies

A child's response to an emergency will vary depending on the age of the child. The child's primary emotional response is *fear*. Some common fears of children include:

❑ Fear of being separated from the parents.

- ❑ Fear of being removed from a familiar place, such as home, and never returning.
- ❑ Fear of being hurt.
- ❑ Fear of mutilation or disfigurement.
- ❑ Fear of the unknown.

These fears may be heightened if the child also detects fear or panic from the parents. In addition, the general confusion and panic that surrounds most emergency situations will further distress the child.

Children have a right to know what is being done to them. Be honest with them. If a procedure will hurt, such as IV needle stick, tell them so. Before performing a painful procedure, tell them immediately before doing it. Do not tell them that a procedure will be painful and then take 5 minutes to prepare the equipment. While waiting, the child's anticipation of the pain will steadily build.

✳ Always be honest with a child.

Always use language that is appropriate for the age of the child. Medical and anatomical terms that we routinely use may be completely foreign to younger children. Telling a child that you are going to "apply a cervical collar" means nothing to them. Instead, tell them: "I'm going to put this hard collar around your neck to keep it from moving." "Try and hold your head still." "Tell me if it is too tight."

Development Stages—A Key to Assessment

Your approach to the pediatric patient should be specific for the child's stage of development. The child progresses through several developmental stages on the way to adulthood. These stages are often significantly different, and the approach to the pediatric patient should relate to the appropriate developmental stage.

Neonates (Ages Birth to 1 Month) The **neonate** is generally defined as an infant up to 1 month of age. (See Figure 30-1.) This is a major stage of development. Often, congenital problems and other illnesses will be noted

■ **neonate** an infant up to one month of age.

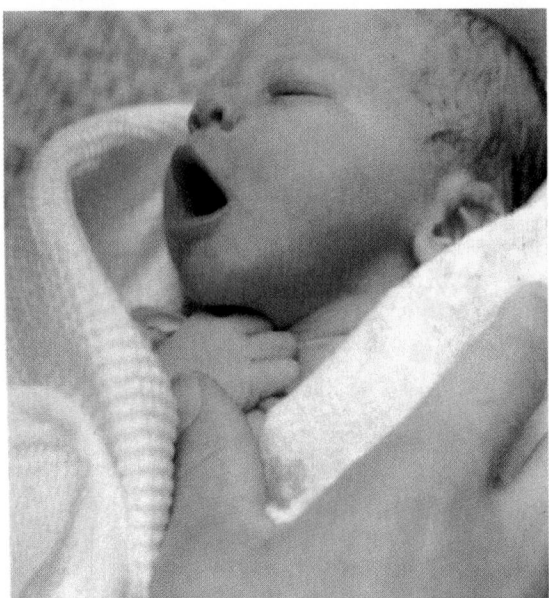

FIGURE 30-1 The neonate.

during this stage. Initially, following birth, there is a weight loss as the neonate adjusts to extrauterine life. It is not uncommon for the infant to lose up to 10 percent of his or her birth weight. This weight loss, however, is routinely recovered in 10 days. Gestational age affects early development. Children born at term (40 weeks) should follow accepted developmental guidelines. Infants born prematurely will not be as developed, both neurologically and physically, as their term counterparts.

This stage of development is one of reflexes. Personality development begins. The infant is close to the mother. He or she may stare at faces and smile. The mother, and occasionally the father, can comfort and quiet the child. Obviously, the history must be obtained from the parents. However, it is also important to observe the child. Common illnesses in this age group include jaundice, vomiting, and respiratory distress. Children of this age generally do not develop fever with minor illnesses. Therefore, the documented presence of fever should raise concern. In fact, many authorities feel that fever in a child under 3 months of age is meningitis, until proven otherwise.

The approach to this age group should include several factors. First, the child should always be kept warm. It is important to observe skin color, tone, and respiratory activity. The absence of tears when crying may indicate dehydration. The lungs should be auscultated early during the exam, while the infant is quiet. It is often helpful to have the child suck on a pacifier during the examination. Allowing the infant to remain in the parent's lap will help keep him or her quiet.

Ages 1 to 5 Months   Children in this age group should have doubled their birth weight by 5 to 6 months of age. They should be able to follow the movements of others with their eyes. Muscle control develops in a cephalocaudal fashion. That is, development of muscular control begins at the head and moves toward the tail. Muscular control also spreads from the trunk toward the extremities during this period. The personality of the child at this stage is still closely centered on the parents. The history must be obtained from the parents, with close observation of illnesses and accidents, including SIDS, vomiting, diarrhea, dehydration, meningitis, child abuse, and household accidents.

The approach to these patients should include keeping the child warm and comfortable. The child should be allowed to remain in the parent's lap. (See Figure 30-2.) A pacifier or bottle can be used to keep the child quiet during the examination.

Ages 6 to 12 Months   Children of this age group may stand or even walk with assistance. They are active and explore their world with their mouths. The personality continues to develop. They have considerable anxiety toward strangers. They don't like lying on their backs. Children in this age group tend to cling to the mother, although the father will "do" most of the time. Common illnesses and accidents include febrile seizures, vomiting, diarrhea, dehydration, bronchiolitis, car accidents, croup, child abuse, poisonings, falls, foreign bodies, and meningitis. These children should be examined in the mother's lap. The exam should progress in a toe-to-head order, since the child may become disturbed if you begin the exam at the face. If time and conditions permit, allow the child to become accustomed to you before beginning the examination.

Ages 1 to 3 Years   Great strides occur in gross motor development during this stage. Children run under or stand on almost everything. They always seem to be on the move. As they grow older, children become braver and more curious or stubborn. They begin to stray away from the parents more.

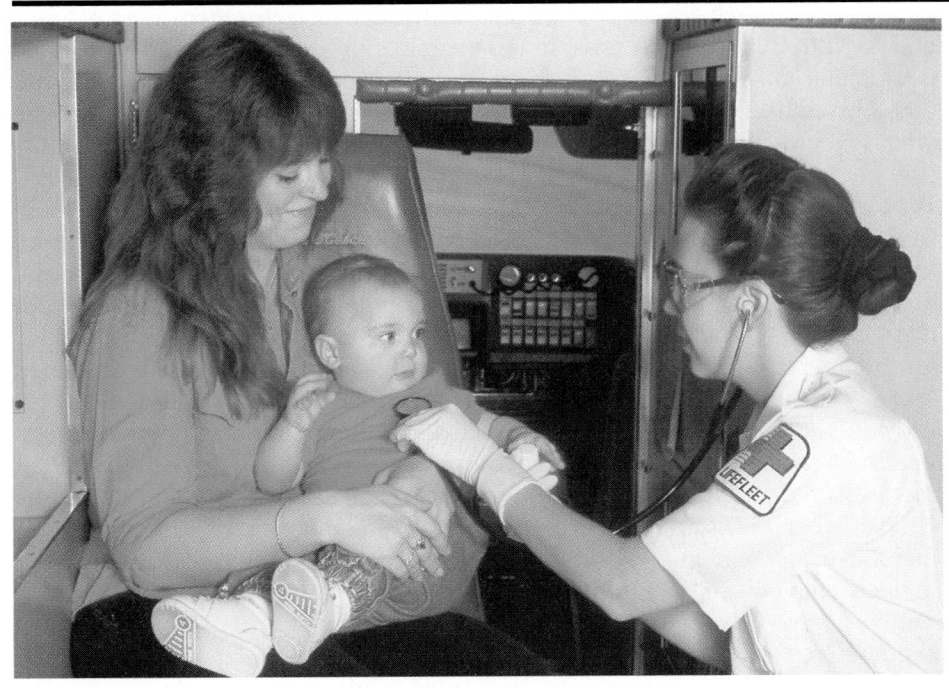

FIGURE 30-2 Young children should be allowed to remain in their mother's arms.

Yet parents remain the only ones who can comfort them quickly, and most children in this age range will cling to parents if frightened.

At ages 1 to 3 years, language development begins. Often children understand better than they can speak. Therefore, the majority of the medical history will come from the parents. But remember that you can ask children some questions.

Accidents of all types are the leading cause of death between the ages of 1 and 15 years. Common illnesses and accidents in this age group include auto accidents, vomiting, diarrhea, febrile seizures, poisonings, falls, child abuse, croup meningitis, and ingestion of foreign bodies. The approach to children in this age group should be more cautious. Approach the child slowly and try to gain his or her confidence. Conduct the exam in a toe-to-head order. The child may be difficult to examine and may resist being touched. Avoid asking questions that allow the child to say "no." Be sure to tell the child if something will hurt.

Ages 3 to 5 Years   Children in this age group show a tremendous increase in fine and gross motor development. Language development continues. Children in this age group know how to talk. However, if frightened, they often won't, especially to strangers. They often have vivid imaginations and may see monsters as a part of their world. Plus they often have tempers and will express them. During this stage of development, children have a fear of mutilation and may view treatment procedures as hostile.

Children in this age group are close to either one parent or the other, depending upon the occasion. They will stick up for their parents and are openly loving. They still look to parents for comfort and support.

When evaluating children in this age group, you should first question the child, keeping in mind that imagination may interfere with facts. The child's time frame is often distorted, and you must rely on the parents to fill in the gaps. Common illnesses and accidents in this age group include croup, asthma, poisonings, auto accidents, burns, child abuse, ingestion of foreign bodies, drowning, epiglottitis, febrile seizures, and meningitis.

The approach to children of this age requires tact. Often, the use of a doll or stuffed animal will assist in the examination. Allow the children to hold equipment and to use it. Let them sit on your lap. Start the examination with the chest and do the head last. Don't trick or lie to the child; always explain what you are going to do.

Ages 6 to 12 Years The children of this age group are active and carefree. Growth spurts sometimes lead to clumsiness. The personality continues to develop. Children of this age are protective and proud of their parents, and they like their parents' attention. Peers are important, but the child also needs home support. When examining children of this age group, it is important to give them the responsibility of providing the history. If an injury was sustained while the child was doing something forbidden, he or she may be reluctant to provide information. The parents can fill in the pertinent details. When assessing children in this age group, it is important to be honest, to protect their modesty, and to tell the child what is wrong. A small toy may help to calm the child. (See Figure 30-3.) Common illnesses and injuries of this age group include drowning, auto accidents, bicycle accidents, fractures, falls, sports injuries, child abuse, and burns.

Ages 12 to 15 Years Youngsters in the 12–15 age group vary significantly in their development. Some are fully mature, while others are not. Teenagers are very concerned with their body image. They are not necessarily adults, but most believe that they are. They have a tremendous desire to be liked and included. The relationships between children and their parents are also changing. This is a time for more independence. Peers are important, as are adolescents of the opposite sex. Generally, these patients are good historians. Their perception of events often differs from that of their parents.

Common illnesses and injuries in this age group include mononucleosis, asthma, auto accidents, sports injuries, drug and alcohol problems, suicide gestures, sexual abuse, and pregnancy. When assessing teenagers, it is important to be honest. Be factual and address the patient's questions. Often, it may

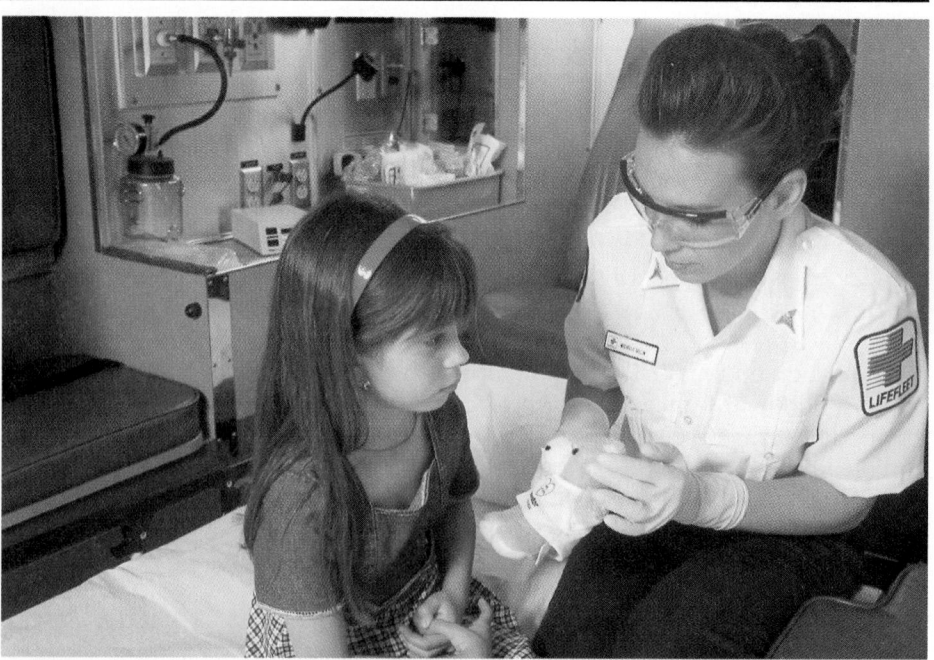

FIGURE 30-3 A small toy may calm a child in the 6–12 years age group.

be wise to interview the child outside of the parents' presence. Pay attention to what the teenager is saying, as well as to what he or she is not saying. Some are very comfortable with their bodies, while others are not. As a paramedic, you should provide support and reassurance.

The Parents' Response to Emergencies

Parents will usually respond to their child's emergency with a grief reaction. Their initial reaction may be shock, denial, anger, guilt, fear, or complete loss of control. The parents' behavior may change during the course of the emergency. As with the child, most parents react to their child's emergency with fear. Parents often express their fears in questions such as the following.

- ❏ "Is my child going to die?"
- ❏ "Did my child suffer brain damage?"
- ❏ "Will my child walk again?"

It is very difficult to answer these questions in the prehospital setting. However, the following actions can help allay parents' fears.

- ❏ Tell them your name and qualifications.
- ❏ Acknowledge their fears and concerns.
- ❏ Reassure them that it is all right to feel the way they do.
- ❏ Redirect their energies to help you care for the child.
- ❏ Remain calm and appear in control of the emergency.
- ❏ Keep the parents informed as to what you are doing.
- ❏ Don't "talk down" to parents.
- ❏ Assure the parents that everything possible is being done for their child.

✱ Redirect the parents' energies to help you care for their child.

If conditions permit, you should allow one of the parents to remain with the child at all times. If the parent is "out of control," have another person take the parent away from the immediate area until he or she settles down. A hysterical parent can cause considerably more anxiety in the ill or injured child.

GENERAL APPROACH TO PEDIATRIC ASSESSMENT

Priorities in management of the pediatric patient, as with all patients, are established on a threat-to-life basis. However, if life-threatening problems are not present, the following general approach is recommended.

History

Questions for the child should be specific and direct. Keep in mind the developmental stages described previously. You should focus on the observed behavior, as well as on what the child or parent says. Visual assessment is very important. Approach the child slowly and gently to encourage cooperation and to gain confidence. (See Figure 30-4, next page.) The approach should be kind, yet firm. The child should not be separated from the parent unnecessarily. Get down to the same visual level as the child. Remember, if the child violated a parental rule, he or she may distort the facts. In addition, children may imagine fantasy as reality and reality as fantasy.

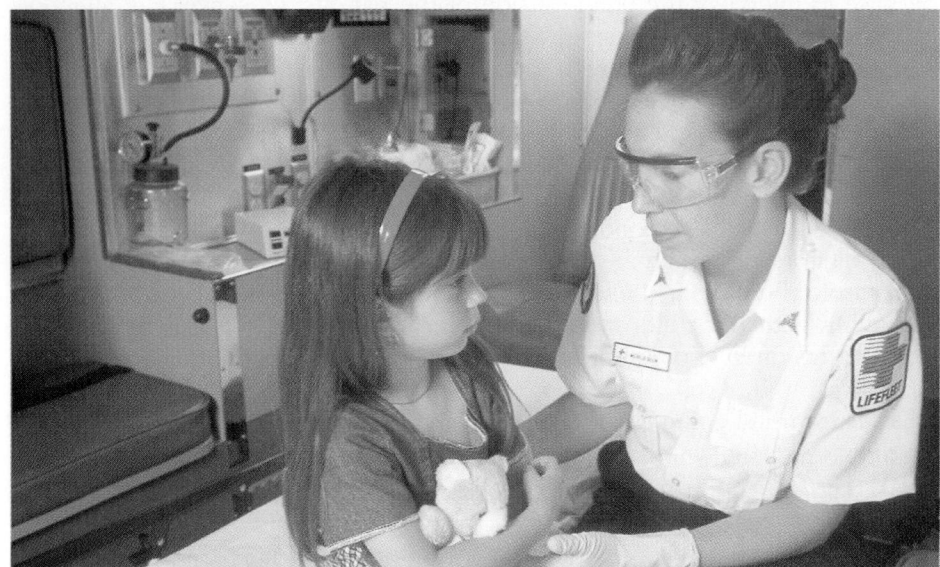

FIGURE 30-4 The approach to the pediatric patient should be gentle and slow.

Always be honest with the patient. Never tell the child that it "won't hurt" if you know it will. Instead, say "This might hurt a little bit, and you can cry if you want to." Children respond to calm reassurance. Converse with the patient in a soft voice, using simple words.

Physical Examination

After the pertinent patient history has been obtained, attention should be turned toward the physical examination. Avoid touching any injured or painful areas until the child's confidence has been gained. (See Figure 30-5.) Begin your examination without instruments. If possible, allow the child to determine the order of the examination.

The physical examination of the child should be systematic and should follow the same format used for adults. In the infant, special attention should

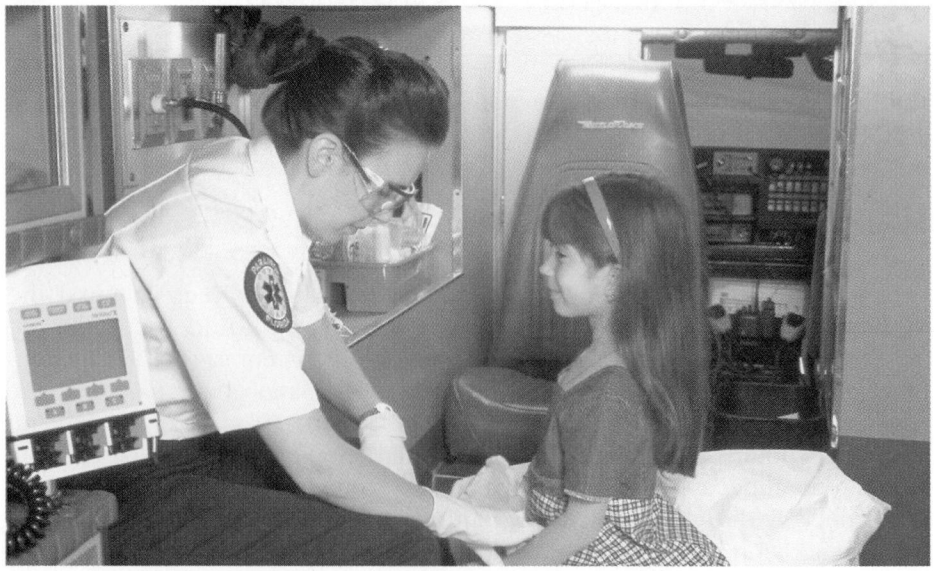

FIGURE 30-5 As confidence is gained, proceed with the secondary survey.

be paid to the anterior fontanelle. The **fontanelles** are areas of the skull that have not yet fused. They allow for compression of the head during childbirth and for rapid growth of the brain during early life. The posterior fontanelle is generally closed by 4 months of age. The anterior fontanelle diminishes after 6 months of age and is generally closed by 9–18 months of age.

The anterior fontanelle should be inspected in all infants. Normally, it should be level with the surface of the skull, or slightly sunken, and it may pulsate. With increased intracranial pressure, such as occurs with meningitis or head trauma, the fontanelle may become tight and bulging. Pulsations may diminish or disappear. With dehydration, the anterior fontanelle may often fall below the level of the skull and appear sunken.

Gastrointestinal disturbances are common in children and can occur with virtually any disorder. When confronted with a child who has been vomiting, it is important to determine how many times the child has vomited, the color of the vomitus, and other associated symptoms. The same procedure holds true for diarrhea.

■ **fontanelles** areas in the infant skull where bones have not yet fused. Posterior and anterior fontanelles are present at birth.

Pediatric Vital Signs

Poorly-taken vital signs in the pediatric patient are of less value than no vital signs at all. The following general guidelines will help you obtain accurate pediatric vital signs.

✱ Poorly-taken, or inaccurate, vital signs are of less value than no vital signs at all.

❑ Take vital signs with the patient in as close to a resting state as possible. If necessary, allow the child to calm down before attempting vital signs. Vital signs in the field should include pulse, respiration, blood pressure, and, if equipment is available, temperature.

❑ Obtain blood pressure with an appropriate-sized cuff. The cuff should be two-thirds the width of the upper arm. Table 30-1 illustrates normal blood pressure readings for children.

❑ Determine the pulse at the brachial artery, carotid artery, or wrist, depending upon the size of the child. There is often a significant variation in pulse rate in children due to respirations. Therefore, it is important to monitor the pulse for at least 30 seconds, a full minute if possible. The range of normal pulse rates is shown in Table 30-1.

❑ It is generally not possible to weigh the child. However, if medications are required, make a good estimate of the child's weight. Often the parents can provide a fairly reliable weight from a recent visit to the doctor. Table 30-2 lists the average weights by age for pediatric patients.

TABLE 30-1	Normal Pediatric Vital Signs by Age		
Age	**Respirations**	**Pulse**	**Blood Pressure (Systolic)**
Newborn	30–60	100–160	50–70
1–6 Wks.	30–60	100–160	70–95
6 Months	25–40	90–120	80–100
1 Year	20–30	90–120	80–100
3 Years	20–30	80–120	80–110
6 Years	18–25	70–110	80–110
10 Years	15–20	60–90	90–120

TABLE 30-2	Pediatric Weights and Pound-Kilogram Conversion	
Age	**Weight (lb)**	**Weight (kg)**
Birth	7	3.5
3 mo	10	5
6 mo	15	7
9 mo	18	8
1 yr	22	10
2 yr	26	12
3 yr	33	15
4 yr	37	17
5 yr	40	18
6 yr	44	20
7 yr	50	23
8 yr	56	25
9 yr	60	28
10 yr	70	33
11 yr	75	35
12 yr	85	40
13 yr	98	44

❑ Observe respiratory rate before beginning the examination. After the examination is started, the child will often begin to cry. It will then be impossible to determine respiratory rate. For an estimate of upper limit of respiratory rate, subtract the child's age from 40. It is also important to identify respiratory pattern, as well as retractions, nasal flaring, or paradoxical chest motion.

❑ Observe the child for level of consciousness. There may be a wide variability in levels of consciousness and activity.

Non-Invasive Monitoring

Electronic monitoring devices are becoming commonplace in modern prehospital care. Pulse oximeters, ECG monitors, and automated blood pressure devices all have application in pediatric emergency care.

Pulse oximetry is particularly useful in pediatric care as many pediatric emergencies are due to respiratory problems. The pulse oximeter gives you immediate information regarding peripheral oxygen saturation. In addition, it allows you to follow trends in the patient's pulse rate and oxygenation status. (See Figure 30-6.)

Any critically ill or injured child should receive continuous ECG monitoring. This will provide essential information regarding the patient's heart rate. It will also help you to monitor the effects of any medications administered.

Monitoring devices may frighten the child. Before applying any monitoring device, explain to the child what you are going to do. Show him or her the display or lights. If the monitoring device makes noise, allow the child to hear the noise before you apply it. Reassure the child that the device will not hurt him or her.

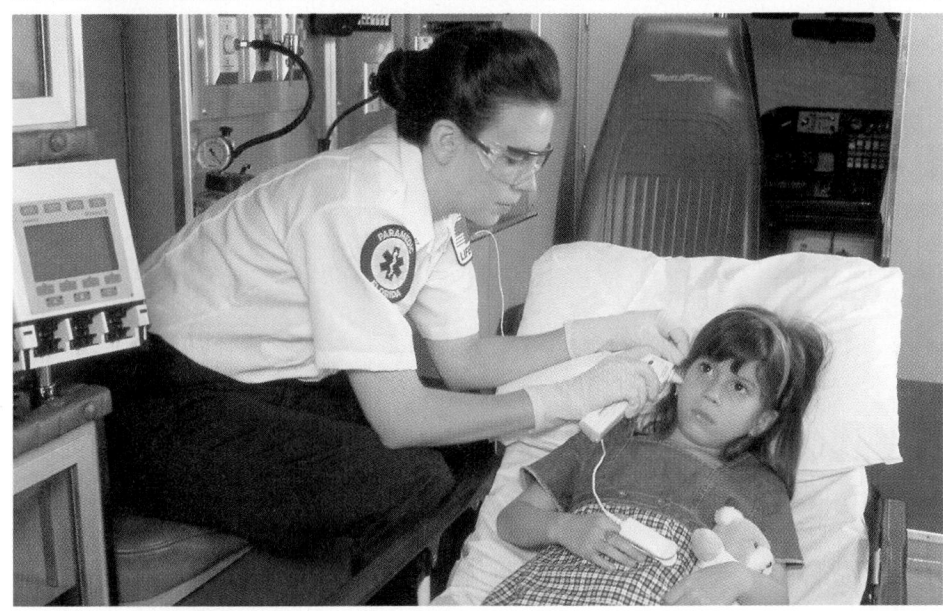

FIGURE 30-6   If available, non-invasive monitoring, including pulse oximetry and temperature measurement, should be utilized in prehospital pediatric care.

PEDIATRIC TRAUMA EMERGENCIES

Trauma is the leading cause of death in children. (See Figure 30-7.) The most common mechanism of injury is motor vehicle accidents, followed by burns, drowning, falls, and firearms. Most pediatric injuries result from blunt trauma. However, if you serve in an urban area, you can expect to see an increasing incidence of penetrating trauma in children. The most common body areas injured in pediatric multiple trauma victims are the head, trunk, and extremities. Your approach to pediatric trauma is much the same as for adult trauma

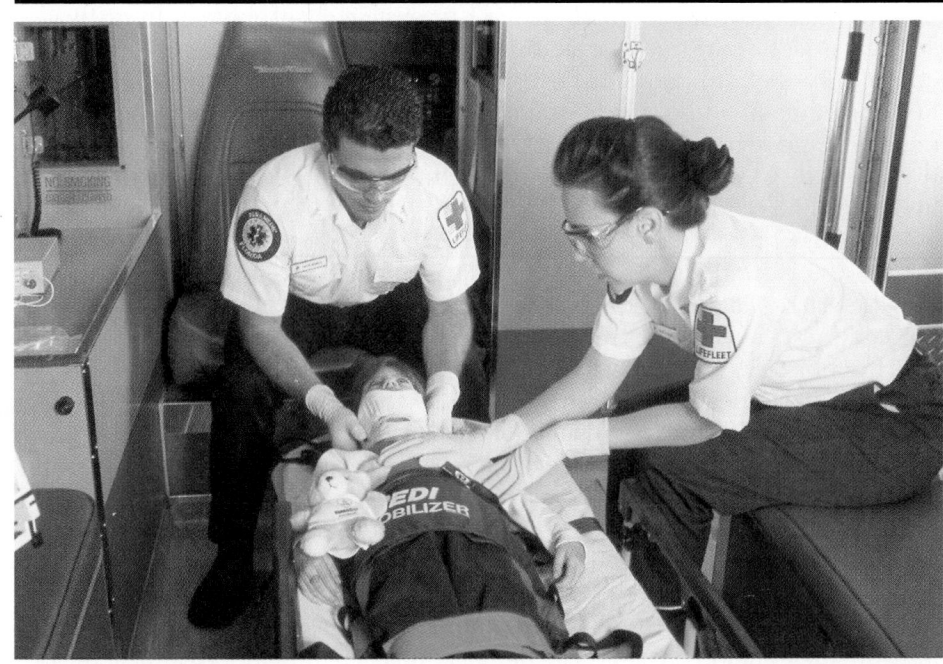

FIGURE 30-7   Injuries account for the majority of pediatric EMS calls.

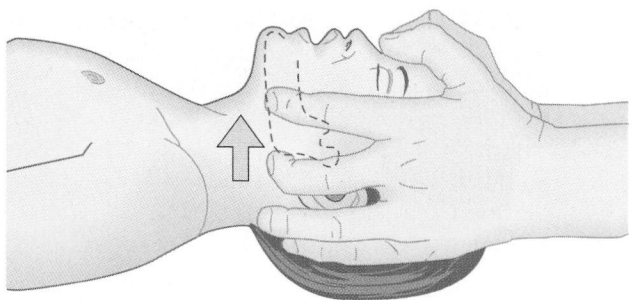

FIGURE 30-8 In the trauma victim, use the combination jaw-thrust/spine stabilization maneuver to open the airway.

victims. You should first complete the A-B-C-D-E steps of primary assessment. These include:

❑ **A**irway with cervical spine stabilization (See Figure 30-8.)
❑ **B**reathing
❑ **C**irculation
❑ **D**isability (neurological examination)
❑ **E**xposure

Any immediate threats to life detected during the primary assessment should be corrected when found. Following this, you should proceed to the secondary assessment, unless the child's condition requires immediate transport. Particular emphasis in the secondary assessment should be on detection of the injuries described in the following discussion.

Head, Face, and Neck Injuries

The majority of children who sustain multiple trauma will suffer an associated head injury. Children are particularly prone to head injuries because their heads are proportionally larger and heavier in comparison to the rest of their body. The mechanism of injury resulting in head trauma varies based upon the age of the child. Infants and small children usually sustain head injuries during a fall. School-age children tend to sustain head injuries from bicycle accidents, falls from trees, or auto-pedestrian accidents. Older children most commonly sustain head injuries in association with sporting events. Remember, child abuse is a frequent cause of head injury. Always be alert for the signs and symptoms of child abuse. Common head injuries seen in children include skin lacerations, skull fractures, contusions, concussions, and intracranial hemorrhage.

Children also frequently injure their faces. The most common facial injuries are lacerations secondary to falls. Young children are very clumsy as they first start walking. A fall onto a sharp object, such as the corner of a coffee table, can result in a laceration. Older children sustain dental injuries in falls from bicycles, skateboard accidents, fights, and sports activities.

Spinal injuries in children are not as common as in adults. However, because of a child's proportionally larger and heavier head, the cervical spine is vulnerable to injury. Any time a child sustains a head injury, always assume that a neck injury may also be present.

Chest and Abdomen Injuries

Chest injuries are the second most common cause of pediatric trauma deaths. Most thoracic injuries result from blunt trauma. Pneumothorax and hemothorax can occur in the pediatric patient, especially if the mechanism of injury was a motor vehicle accident. Tension pneumothorax can also occur in childhood. Pediatric tension pneumothorax results in diminished breath sounds over the affected lung, shift of the trachea to the opposite side, and a progressive decrease in ventilatory compliance. In these cases, a needle thoracostomy may be lifesaving.

Significant blunt trauma to the abdomen can result in injury to the spleen or liver. In fact, the spleen is the most commonly injured organ in children. Signs and symptoms of a splenic injury include tenderness in the left upper quadrant of the abdomen, abrasions on the abdomen, and, occasionally, ecchymosis over the affected area. The liver is also frequently injured in blunt abdominal trauma. Symptoms of liver injury include right upper quadrant abdominal pain and/or right lower chest pain. Both splenic and hepatic injuries can cause life-threatening internal hemorrhage.

Because of the high mortality associated with blunt trauma, children with significant blunt abdominal or chest trauma should be transported immediately to a pediatric trauma center with appropriate care provided en route. Treat for shock with positioning, fluids, maintenance of body temperature, and PASG if indicated.

Extremity Injuries

Extremity injuries in children are typically limited to fractures and lacerations. Children rarely sustain amputations and other serious extremity injuries. An exception includes farm children who may become entangled in agricultural equipment thus causing severe injuries to the extremities.

The most common injuries are fractures, usually resulting from falls. Because children have more flexible bones than adults, they tend to have incomplete fractures such as **bend fractures**, **buckle fractures**, and **greenstick fractures**. In younger children, the bone growth plates have not yet closed. Some types of growth plate fractures can lead to permanent disability if not managed correctly.

Burns

Burns are the second leading cause of death in children. Scald burns are the most common type of burn injury encountered. Children can burn themselves by pulling hot liquids off tables or stoves. Immersion in hot water can also cause a significant scald injury. Chemical burns, flame burns, and electrical burns also occur in children.

Estimation of the burn surface area is slightly different for children. The child's head accounts for a higher percentage of body surface compared to adults. The legs, on the other hand, make up smaller percentage of the child's body surface area. When using the "rule of nines" to calculate the percentage burned in infants and small children, take 4.5 percent from each leg and add it to the head. Thus, each leg is worth 13.5 percent, while the head is worth 18 percent. You might also use the child's palm as a guide. The child's palm is worth 1 percent of the body surface area. This will allow rapid estimation of the percentage of body surface area burned.

Child Abuse and Neglect

Child abuse should always be suspected, especially if injuries are not consistent with the history. There are several characteristics common to abused children. Often, the child is seen as "special" and different from others. Premature

■ **bend fractures** fractures seen in children characterized by angulation and deformity in the bone without obvious break.

■ **buckle fractures** fractures seen in children characterized by a raised or bulging projection at the fracture site.

■ **greenstick fractures** fractures seen in children characterized by an incomplete break in the bone.

infants or a twin stand a higher risk of abuse than other children. Many abused children are less than 5 years of age. Handicapped children, as well as those with special needs, are also at greater risk. So are uncommunicative (i.e., autistic) children. Boys are more often abused than girls. A child who is not what the parents wanted (e.g., the wrong sex) is at increased risk for abuse, too.

The Child Abuser   The child abuser can come from any geographic, religious, ethnic, occupational, educational, or socio-economic group. However, people who abuse children tend to share certain characteristics. The abuser is usually a parent or someone in the role of a parent. When the mother spends most time with the child, she is the parent most frequently identified as the abuser. Most child abusers were abused themselves as children.

Three conditions can alert you to the potential for abuse. They include:

❑ A parent or adult capable of abuse.
❑ A child in one of the high-risk categories.
❑ The presence of a crisis.

Common crises that may precipitate abuse include financial stress, marital or relationship stress, and physical illness in a parent or child.

Sexual Abuse   Sexual abuse can occur at any age. The sexual abuser is almost always someone in the family, someone known to the family, or someone the child trusts. Stepchildren or adopted children face a greater risk for sexual abuse by a parent than biological children. If you suspect the child has been sexually abused, examine the genitalia externally for serious injury. Avoid touching the child or disturbing the clothing. Police may need to examine the child and the clothes for evidence. Your best approach to sexually abused children is one of caring support.

Assessment of the Potentially Abused Child   Signs of child abuse can be startling. As a guide, the following findings should trigger a high index of suspicion. (See Figures 30-9 to 30-12.)

❑ Any obvious or suspected fractures in a child under 2 years of age.
❑ Injuries in various stages of healing, especially burns and bruises.
❑ More injuries than usually seen in children of the same age.
❑ Injuries scattered on many areas of the body.
❑ Bruises or burns in patterns that suggest intentional infliction.
❑ Increased intracranial pressure in an infant.
❑ Suspected intra-abdominal trauma in a young child.
❑ Any injury that does not fit with the description of the cause given.

Information in the medical history may also raise the index of suspicion. Examples include:

❑ A history that does not match the nature or severity of the injury.
❑ Vague parental accounts or accounts that change during the interview.
❑ Accusations that the child injured himself or herself intentionally.
❑ Delay in seeking help.
❑ Child dressed inappropriately for the situation.

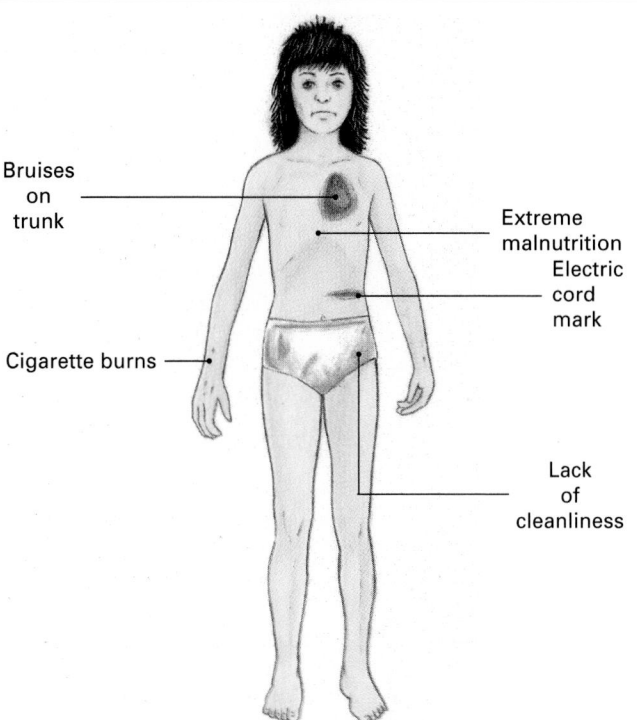

Bruises
on
trunk

Cigarette burns

Extreme
malnutrition
Electric
cord
mark

Lack
of
cleanliness

FIGURE 30-9   The stigmata
of child abuse.

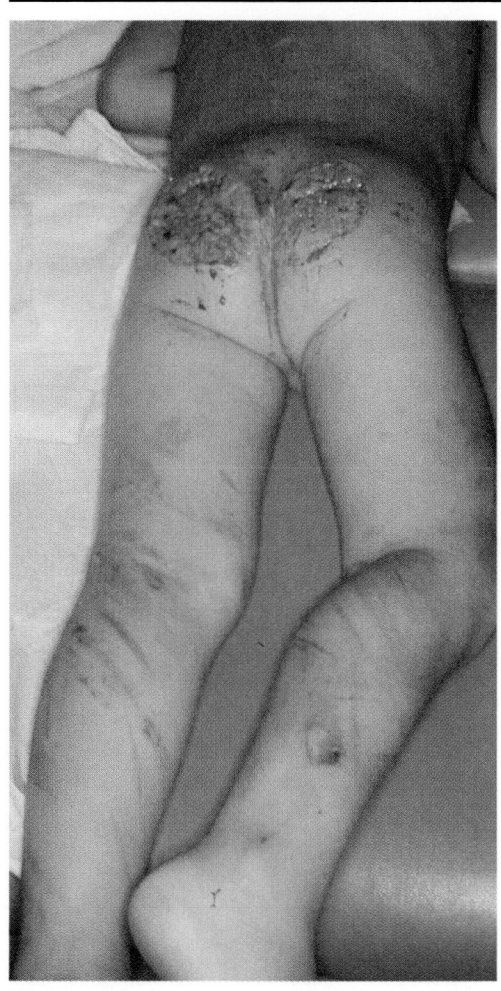

FIGURE 30-10   An abused child. Note
the marks on the legs associated with
beatings with an electrical wire. The burns
on the buttocks are from submersion in hot
water. (Courtesy of Scott and White
Hospital and Clinic)

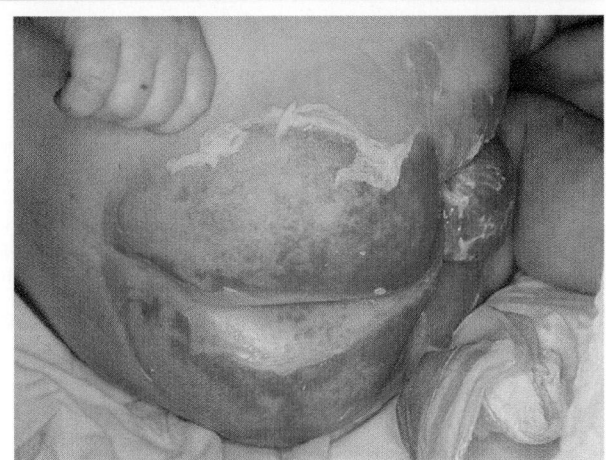

FIGURE 30-11 Burn injury from placing child's buttocks in hot water as a punishment. (Courtesy of Scott and White Hospital and Clinic)

Suspect child neglect if you spot any of the following conditions.

- ❑ Extreme malnutrition.
- ❑ Multiple insect bites.
- ❑ Longstanding skin infections.
- ❑ Extreme lack of cleanliness.

Management of the Potentially Abused Child In cases of child abuse or neglect, the goals of management include: appropriate treatment of injuries, protection of the child from further abuse, and notification of proper authorities. You should obtain as much information as possible, in a non-judgmental manner. Document all findings or statements in the patient report. Don't "cross-examine" the parents; this job belongs to the police. Try to be supportive and non-judgmental toward the parents. However, you should make sure the child is transported to the hospital by the ambulance or by another dependable person. Do not leave the task to the alleged abuser.

✱ Do not confront the parents (or other caregiver) about your suspicion of child abuse. Instead, report it to emergency department personnel or law enforcement officers.

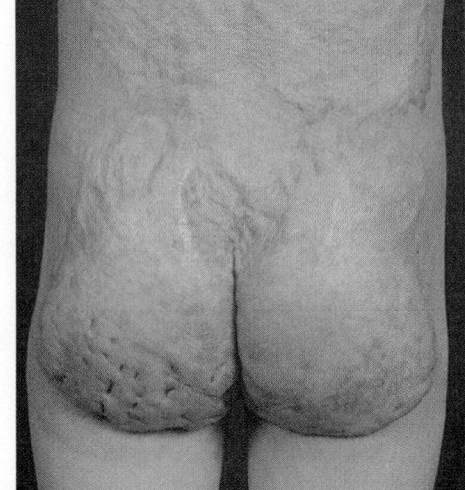

FIGURE 30-12 The effects of child abuse, both physical and mental, can last a lifetime. (Courtesy of Scott and White Hospital and Clinic)

Upon arrival at the emergency department, report your suspicions to the emergency department personnel and the proper authorities. Complete the patient report and all available documentation at this time, since delay may inhibit the accurate recall of data. Child abuse and neglect are particularly stressful aspects of emergency medical services. You must recognize and deal with your feelings, perhaps taking them up at a Critical Incident Stress Debriefing. (See Chapter 7.)

* In many states, prehospital personnel are required by law to report suspected child abuse or neglect to the appropriate authorities.

PEDIATRIC MEDICAL EMERGENCIES

Most childhood medical emergencies involve the respiratory system. However, any body system can be involved. Infections are common during this period in life. Infectious diseases are those illnesses caused by the infection or infestation of the body by an infectious agent such as a virus, bacteria, fungus, or parasite. Childhood is a time of frequent infectious illness due to the relative immaturity of the immune system. Most children will have 5–6 upper respiratory infections per year. Most infections are minor and self-limited. There are, however, several infections that can be life-threatening. These include meningitis, pneumonia, and bacterial septicemia.

Neurological Emergencies

Neurological emergencies in childhood are fairly uncommon. These include seizures, febrile seizures, Reye's syndrome, and meningitis, among others.

Seizures   The topic of seizures has been presented in earlier chapters. However, seizures can and do occur in children. They are a frequent reason for summoning EMS. Several factors have been identified as causing seizures. These include:

❑ Fever
❑ Hypoxia
❑ Infections
❑ Idiopathic epilepsy
❑ Electrolyte disturbances
❑ Head trauma
❑ Hypoglycemia
❑ Toxic ingestions or exposure
❑ Tumor
❑ CNS malformations

Often, however, the etiology is not known. Status epilepticus can also occur in children. *Status epilepticus* is a prolonged seizure or multiple seizures with no regaining of consciousness between them. This is a serious medical emergency. Most pediatric seizures that involve EMS personnel are febrile seizures.

Febrile seizures are those seizures that occur as a result of a sudden increase in body temperature. They occur most commonly between the ages of 6 months and 6 years. Febrile seizures seem related to the rate at which the body temperature increases, not to the degree of fever. Often, the parents will report the recent onset of fever or cold symptoms. The diagnosis of febrile seizure should not be made in the field. All pediatric patients suffering a

* The diagnosis of febrile seizure should not be made in the field.

seizure must be transported to the hospital so that other etiologies can be excluded.

Assessment. The history is a major factor in determining seizure type. Febrile seizure should be suspected if the temperature is above 103° F (39.2° C). The history of a previous seizure may suggest idiopathic epilepsy or other CNS problem. However, there is a tendency for recurrence of febrile seizures in children who are predisposed.

When confronted with a seizing child, determine whether there is a history of seizures or seizures with fever. Has the child had a recent illness? Also, determine how many seizures occurred during the incident. If the child is not seizing upon arrival, elicit a description of the seizure activity. Note the condition and position of the child when found. Question parents or bystanders about the possibility of head injury. A history of irritability or lethargy prior to the seizure may indicate CNS infection. If possible, find out whether the child suffers from diabetes or has recently complained of a headache or a stiff neck. Note any current medications, as well as possible ingestions.

The physical examination should be systematic. Pay particular attention to the adequacy of respirations, the level of consciousness, neurological evaluation, and signs of injury. Also inspect the child for signs of dehydration. Dehydration may be evidenced by the absence of tears or, in an infant, by the presence of a sunken fontanelle.

Management. Management of the pediatric seizure is essentially the same as for the seizing adult. Place the patient on the floor or on the bed. Be sure to lay the child on his or her side, away from the furniture. Do not restrain the child, but take steps to protect him or her from injury. Maintain the airway, but do not force anything, such as a bite stick, between the teeth. Administer supplemental oxygen. Then take and record all vital signs. If the child is febrile, remove excess layers of clothing. If status epilepticus is present, institute the following steps.

❑ Start an IV of NS or RL and perform a Dextrostix.
❑ Administer diazepam as follows:
   Children 1 month to 5 years: 0.2–0.5 mg slowly IV push every 2–5 minutes to a maximum of 2.5 milligrams.
   Children 5 years or older: 1 mg slowly IV push every 2–5 minutes to a maximum of 5 milligrams.
❑ Contact medical control for additional dosing. Diazepam can be administered rectally if an IV cannot be established.
❑ If the seizure appears to be due to fever and a long transport time is anticipated, medical control may request the administration of acetaminophen to lower the fever. Acetaminophen is supplied in an elixir or as suppositories. The initial dose should be 15 mg/kg body weight.

As mentioned previously, all pediatric seizure patients should be transported. Reassure and support the parents; this is a very stressful and frightening situation for them.

✳ Diazepam can be administered rectally to a seizing child when an IV cannot be started.

■ **meningitis** infection and inflammation of the meninges, the covering of the brain and spinal cord.

Meningitis   **Meningitis** is an infection of the meninges, the lining of the brain and spinal cord. Meningitis can result from both bacteria and viruses. Viral meningitis is frequently called *aseptic meningitis*, since an organism cannot be routinely cultured from CSF fluid. Aseptic meningitis is generally less severe than bacterial meningitis and self-limited. Bacterial meningitis most commonly results from *Streptococcus pneumoniae*, *Haemophilus influenza*, and *Neisseria meningitides*. These infections can be rapidly fatal if not promptly recognized and treated appropriately.

Assessment. Meningitis is more common in children than in adults. Findings in the history that may suggest meningitis include: a child who has been ill for one day to several days, recent ear or respiratory tract infection, high fever, lethargy or irritability, a severe headache, or a stiff neck. The child with meningitis may present in various ways. Infants generally do not develop a stiff neck. They will generally become lethargic and will not feed well. Some babies may simply develop a fever. Documented fever in a child less than 3 months of age is considered meningitis until proven otherwise.

On physical examination, the child with meningitis will appear very ill. With an infant, the fontanelle may be bulging or full unless accompanied by dehydration. Extreme discomfort with movement, due to irritability of the meninges, may be present.

✱ Documented fever in a child less than three months of age is meningitis until proven otherwise.

Management. Prehospital care of the infant or child with meningitis is supportive. Rapidly complete the primary survey and secondary assessment. Then transport the infant to the emergency department. If shock is present, treat the child with intravenous fluids (20 mL/kg) and oxygen.

Reye's Syndrome

Reye's syndrome is a disease that was undescribed until 1963. The etiology of Reye's syndrome has not been clearly established. Reye's syndrome affects all ages, with peak incidence between ages 5–15 years. It tends to occur more frequently in younger children. The frequency is higher in fall and winter. After 1 year of age, there is a higher incidence in the suburban and rural populations.

■ **Reye's syndrome** illness of uncertain etiology that results in alteration of mental function in children. Often associated with viral infections and the use of aspirin.

Although no single etiological factor has been identified, several possible toxic and metabolic causes have been postulated. Outbreaks tend to cluster during epidemics of Influenza B. Occasionally, it has been associated with the chicken pox (varicella) virus. Infants often will have a recent history of gastroenteritis. There has also been a correlation between the use of aspirin and the disease, particularly after the flu.

Reye's syndrome typically presents itself in a healthy child who develops severe nausea and vomiting during an unremarkable viral illness. Within hours, the patient may begin to display hyperactive or combative behavior. In addition, there may be personality change, irrational behavior, progressive stupor, restlessness, convulsions, and coma. The sudden onset of vomiting often marks the early stages of the disease. In approximately 10–20 percent of cases, there is a recent history of chicken pox. Other children may have had a recent upper-respiratory infection. Infants may have recently had gastroenteritis.

Assessment. On physical examination, there may be rapid, deep respirations, which may be irregular. The pupils can be dilated and react sluggishly. There also may be signs of increased intracranial pressure, such as deviations in gaze. Unfortunately, Reye's syndrome cannot be diagnosed in the field. The diagnosis is difficult enough to make in the hospital.

Complications that can occur with Reye's syndrome include respiratory failure, cardiac arrhythmias, and acute pancreatitis. Death usually results from CNS complications such as herniation of the brainstem.

Management. Management is general and supportive. Complete the primary survey with particular attention on the respiratory status. Support ventilations, if necessary, and administer supplemental oxygen. Transport should be rapid.

Respiratory Emergencies

Respiratory problems are common in childhood. Children are susceptible to many of the respiratory problems that occur in adults. In addition, there are several problems that are unique to children. Respiratory problems should be identified in the primary assessment and treated appropriately. First, assess the airway. If it is obstructed, clear the airway using BLS techniques, if possible. Second, assess breathing. If the child is not breathing, you should initiate artificial ventilations.

Pediatric respiratory emergencies that deserve special attention include bronchiolitis, croup, epiglottitis, asthma, and aspiration of foreign bodies. Children with any of these disorders can suffer respiratory arrest. This is most often due to airway obstruction or exhaustion.

Aspirated Foreign Body Children, especially 1- to 3-year-olds, are always putting objects into their mouths. These children are at increased risk of aspirating the object, especially when they are running or falling. In addition, many children choke on, or aspirate, food given to them by their parents or other well-meaning adults. Young children have not yet developed coordinated chewing motions in the mouth and pharynx and cannot adequately chew food. Common foods associated with aspiration and airway obstruction in children include chewing gum, hot dogs, grapes, peanuts, and sausages.

✱ Wheezing heard only on one side of a child's chest is suggestive of an aspirated foreign body.

Assessment. The child with a suspected aspirated foreign body may present in one of two ways. If the obstruction is complete, the child will not be breathing. If it is partial, the child may exhibit labored breathing, retractions, chest expansion, and cyanosis. A foreign body aspirated into the respiratory tree will often drop until it lodges. Large objects will lodge in the trachea or the mainstem bronchi. Smaller objects may drop to the bronchioles. Often, the food particle will act as a one-way valve, allowing the entry of air, while restricting its exit. This results in hyperexpansion of the affected lung. If severe, tracheal deviation, away from the involved lung, may be noted.

Management. When confronted with a child suspected of aspirating a foreign body, immediately complete the primary survey. If complete obstruction is noted, clear the airway with accepted basic life support techniques. (See Figure 30-13.) If unsuccessful, visualize the airway with a laryngoscope. If the foreign body is

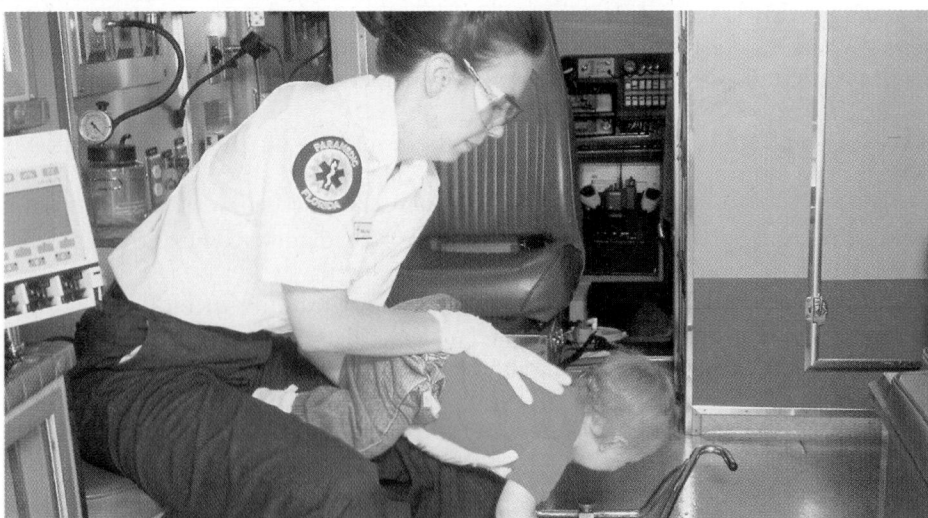

FIGURE 30-13 Attempting to relieve airway obstruction in a baby.

seen, and readily accessible, try to remove it with Magill forceps. If the airway cannot be cleared by routine measures, consider needle cricothyroidotomy.

If the obstruction is partial, make the child comfortable and administer humidified oxygen. Intubation equipment should be readily available since complete airway obstruction can occur. The child should be transported to a hospital, where the foreign body can be removed by fiberoptic bronchoscopy.

Croup

Croup Croup, medically referred to as *laryngotracheobronchitis*, is a viral infection of the upper airway. It most often occurs in children 6 months to 4 years of age and is most prevalent in the fall and winter. The infection causes edema to develop beneath the larynx and glottis, narrowing the lumen of the airway. Severe cases of croup may result in complete airway obstruction.

■ **croup** laryngotracheobronchitis, a common viral infection of young children, resulting in edema of the sub-glottic tissues. Characterized by barking cough and inspiratory stridor.

Assessment. The history for croup is fairly classic. Often, the child will have a mild cold or other infection and be doing fairly well until dark. After dark, however, a harsh, barking cough develops. The attack may subside in a few hours, but can persist for several nights.

The physical exam will often reveal inspiratory stridor. There may be associated nasal flaring, tracheal tugging, or retraction. You SHOULD NEVER examine the oropharynx. Often, in the prehospital setting, it is difficult to distinguish croup from epiglottitis. (See Table 30-3 and Figure 30-14.) If epiglottitis is present, examination of the oropharynx may result in laryngospasm and

TABLE 30-3 Symptoms of Croup and Epiglottitis	
Croup	**Epiglottitis**
Slow onset	Rapid onset
Generally wants to sit up	Prefers to sit up
Barking cough	No barking cough
No drooling	Drooling; painful to swallow
Fever approx. 100–101° F	Fever approx. 102–104° F
	Occasional stridor

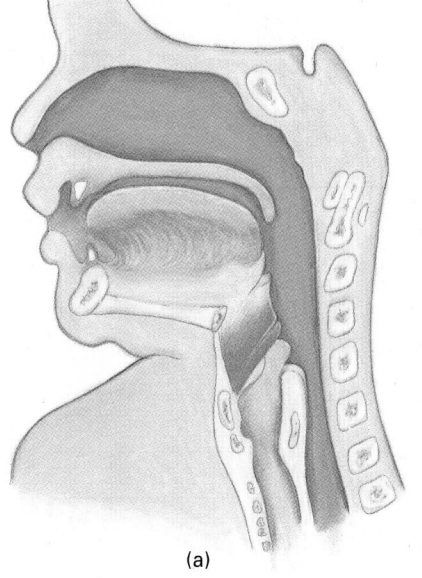

(a)

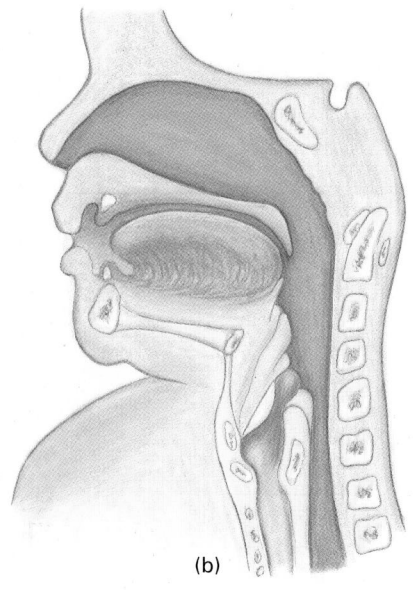

(b)

FIGURE 30-14 Croup (a) and epiglottitis (b).

complete airway obstruction. If the attack of croup is severe and progressive, the child may develop restlessness, tachycardia, and cyanosis. Croup can result in complete airway obstruction and respiratory arrest.

Management. Management of croup should consist of appropriate airway maintenance. Place the child in a position of comfort and administer humidified oxygen by face mask. Then prepare the child for transport to the hospital. The process of transporting the child from the house to the ambulance will often allow him or her to breathe the cool air. Because this cool air causes a decrease in subglottic edema, the child may be clinically improved by the time he or she reaches the ambulance. If the attack of croup is severe, the medical control physician may order the administration of racemic epinephrine or albuterol. Some physicians advocate the use of steroids in croup, because they feel these drugs shorten the course of the illness.

Epiglottitis
Epiglottitis is an acute infection and inflammation of the epiglottis and is potentially life-threatening. The epiglottis is a flap of cartilage that protects the airway during swallowing. Epiglottitis, unlike croup, is caused by a bacterial infection, usually *Haemophilus influenza.* It tends to occur in children 4 years and older. It is characterized by a swollen, cherry red epiglottis.

Assessment. The child with epiglottitis is acutely ill. The presentation is similar to croup. Often, the child will go to bed feeling relatively well, usually with what the parents consider to be a mild infection of the upper respiratory tract. Later, the child awakens with a high fever and a brassy cough. The progression of symptoms can be dramatic. There is often pain upon swallowing, sore throat, high fever, shallow breathing, dyspnea, inspiratory stridor, and drooling.

On physical examination, the child appears toxic. You SHOULD NEVER attempt to visualize the airway. Often, however, when the child is crying, the tip of the epiglottis can be seen posterior to the base of the tongue. In epiglottitis, it is red and swollen. As airway obstruction develops, the child will exhibit retractions, nasal flaring, and pulmonary hyperexpansion. (See Figure 30-15.)

■ **epiglottitis** bacterial infection of the epiglottis, usually occurring in children older than age four. A serious medical emergency.

✱ Epiglottitis is a serious medical emergency.

✱ Never attempt to visualize the pharynx in a child who might have epiglottitis.

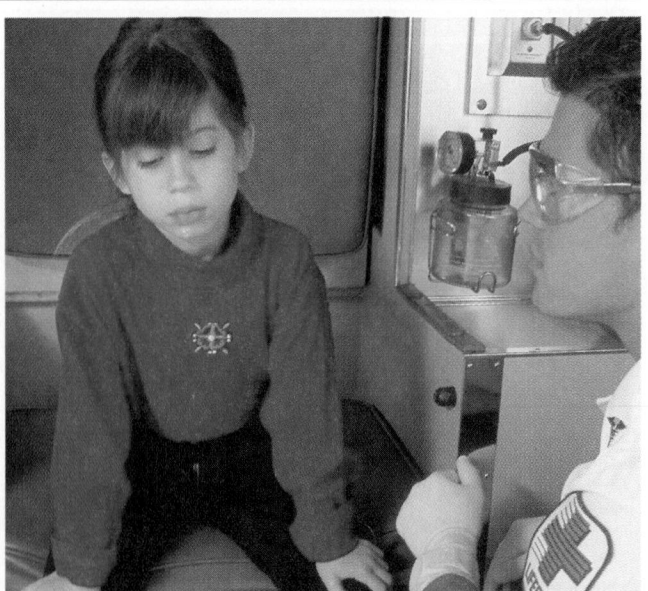

FIGURE 30-15 Posturing of the child with epiglottitis. Often, there will be excessive drooling.

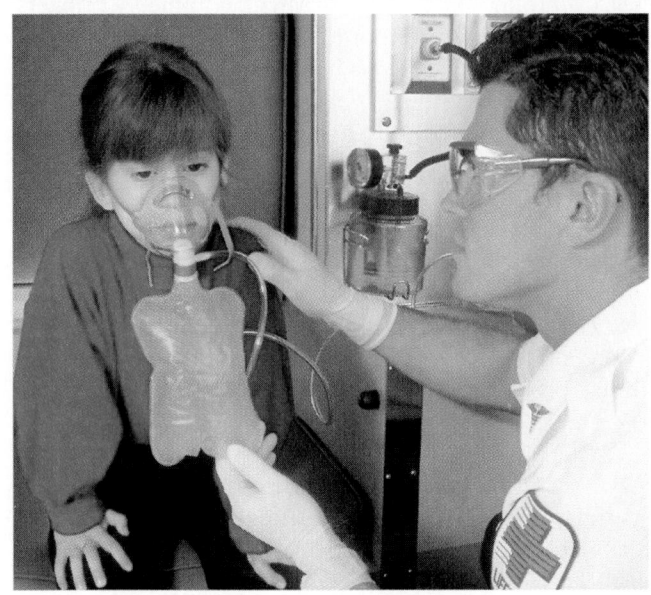

FIGURE 30-16 The child with epiglottitis should be administered humidified oxygen and transported in a comfortable position.

Management. Management of epiglottitis should consist of appropriate airway maintenance. Place the child in a position of comfort and administer humidified oxygen by face mask. (See Figure 30-16.) Racemic epinephrine is contraindicated. Make sure that all intubation equipment is available, including an appropriate-sized endotracheal tube. Remember, however, that intubation is contraindicated, unless complete airway obstruction occurs. In this case, transtracheal ventilation may be required. In cases of epiglottitis, transport the child to the hospital as quickly as possible. If total obstruction develops, attempts should be made to ventilate the patient with high pressures. Often this may require depressing the pop-off valve on the bag-valve-mask device.

Bronchiolitis   Wheezing in a child under one year of age is frequently due to **bronchiolitis**. Bronchiolitis is a respiratory infection of the medium-sized airways—the bronchioles—that occurs in early childhood. It should not be confused with bronchitis, which is an infection of the larger bronchi. Bronchiolitis is caused by a viral infection, most commonly *respiratory syncytial virus (RSV)*, which affects the lining of the bronchioles. Characterized by prominent expiratory wheezing, it clinically resembles asthma.

> ■ **bronchiolitis** viral infection of the medium-sized airways, occurring most frequently during the first year of life.

Assessment. A history is necessary to distinguish bronchiolitis from asthma. Often, with bronchiolitis, there is a family history of asthma or allergies, although neither is yet present in the child. In addition, there often is a low-grade fever. A major distinguishing factor is age. Asthma rarely occurs before the age of one year, whereas bronchiolitis is more frequent in this age group.

The physical examination should be systematic. Pay particular attention to the presence of rales or wheezes. Also, note any evidence of infection or respiratory distress.

> ✳ Wheezing in a child under one year of age, especially in the fall and winter months, is often bronchiolitis.

Management. Prehospital management of suspected bronchiolitis is much the same as with asthma. Place the child in a semi-sitting position, if old enough, and administer humidified oxygen by mask. Ventilations should be supported as necessary. Equipment for intubation should be readily available. If wheezing is present, medical control may request administration of a bronchodilator such as albuterol (Ventolin, Proventil) by small volume nebulizer. The cardiac rhythm should be constantly monitored. Pulse oximetry, if available, should be used continuously.

Asthma   Asthma is a common respiratory disease that affects more than 6 million Americans. It occurs usually before age 10 in approximately 50 percent of the cases, and before age 30 in an additional 33 percent of cases. The disease tends to run in families. It is also commonly associated with atopic conditions, such as eczema and allergies. Although deaths from other respiratory conditions have been steadily declining, asthmatic deaths have increased significantly in the last decade. Hospitalization of children for treatment of asthma has increased by 200 percent or more during the same interval. Because children can die from asthma, prompt prehospital recognition and treatment are essential.

Pathophysiology.   Asthma is a chronic inflammatory disorder of the airways. In susceptible children, this inflammation causes widespread, but variable, airflow obstruction. In addition to airflow obstruction, the airways become hyperresponsive.

Asthma may be induced by one of many different factors, commonly called "triggers." The triggers vary from one child to the next. Common triggers include environmental allergens, cold air, exercise, foods, irritants, and certain medications.

Within minutes of exposure to the trigger, a two-phase reaction occurs. The first phase of the reaction is characterized by the release of chemical mediators such as histamine. These cause bronchoconstriction and bronchial edema that effectively decrease expiratory airflow, causing the classic "asthma attack." If treated early, asthma may respond to inhaled bronchodilators. If the attack is not aborted, or does not resolve spontaneously, a second phase may occur. The second phase is characterized by inflammation of the bronchioles as cells of the immune system invade the respiratory tract. This causes additional edema and further decreases expiratory airflow. The second phase will typically not respond to inhaled bronchodilators. Instead, anti-inflammatory agents, such as corticosteroids are often required.

As the attack continues, and swelling of the mucous membranes lining the bronchioles worsens, there may be plugging of the bronchi by thick mucus. This further obstructs airflow. As a result, there is an increase in sputum production. In addition, the lungs become progressively hyperinflated since airflow is more restricted on exhalation. This effectively reduces vital capacity and results in decreased gas exchange at the alveoli, resulting in hypoxemia. If allowed to progress untreated, hypoxemia will worsen, and unconsciousness and death may ensue.

Assessment.   Asthma can often be differentiated from other pediatric respiratory illnesses by the history. In many cases, there is a prior history of asthma or reactive airway disease. The child's medications may also be an indicator. Children with asthma often have an inhaler or take a theophylline or oral beta agonist preparation.

On physical examination, the child is usually sitting up, leaning forward, and tachypneic. Often, there is an associated unproductive cough. Accessory respiratory muscle usage is usually evident. Wheezing may be heard. However, in a severe attack, the patient may not wheeze at all—this is an ominous finding. Generally, there is an associated tachycardia, and this should be monitored, since virtually all medications used to treat asthma increase the heart rate.

✳ Asthma is a chronic inflammatory disease with a two-phase response. The first phase is characterized by bronchospasm and may be reversed with bronchodilators. The second phase consists of inflammation, requiring anti-inflammatory medications for treatment.

Management. The primary therapeutic goal in the asthmatic is to correct hypoxia, reverse bronchospasm, and decrease inflammation. First, it is imperative that you establish an airway. Next, administer supplemental, humidified oxygen as necessary. The medical control physician may order the administration of an inhaled beta agonist. Many paramedic units have the capability of administering nebulized bronchodilator medications, such as albuterol, terbutaline, or isoetharine. Therefore, administration of these agents may be requested. If there is a prolonged transport time, the medical control physician may also request administration of a steroid preparation.

Status Asthmaticus   Status asthmaticus is defined as a severe, prolonged asthma attack that cannot be broken by repeated doses of epinephrine. This is a serious medical emergency and prompt recognition, treatment, and transport are required. Often, the child suffering status asthmaticus will have a greatly distended chest from continued air trapping. Breath sounds, and often wheezing, may be absent. The patient is usually exhausted, severely acidotic, and often dehydrated. The management of status asthmaticus is basically the same as asthma. However, you should recognize that respiratory arrest is imminent, and remain prepared for endotracheal intubation. Transport should be immediate, with aggressive treatment continued en route.

✱ Status asthmaticus requires immediate transport with treatment administered en route.

Gastrointestinal Emergencies

Childhood gastrointestinal problems almost always present with nausea and vomiting as a chief complaint. As a child gets older, gastrointestinal system emergencies, such as appendicitis, become more common.

Nausea and Vomiting   Nausea and vomiting are symptoms of other disease processes. Virtually any medical problem can cause nausea and vomiting in a child. Fever, ear infections, and respiratory infections are common causes of nausea and vomiting. In addition, many viruses, and certain bacteria, can infect the gastrointestinal system. These infections, collectively called *gastroenteritis*, readily cause vomiting, diarrhea, or both.

The biggest risks associated with nausea and vomiting in children are dehydration and electrolyte abnormalities. Infants and toddlers can quickly become dehydrated from bouts of vomiting. If diarrhea or fever is also present, fluid loss is further accelerated, worsening the situation. Dehydration in infants and toddlers is more difficult to detect compared to older children.

Treatment of pediatric nausea and vomiting is primarily supportive. If the child is dehydrated, and unable to keep oral fluids down, intravenous fluid therapy may be indicated. Severe dehydration, as evidenced by prolonged capillary refill time, should be treated by 20 mL/kg fluid boluses of lactated Ringer's solution or 0.9 percent sodium chloride solution (normal saline).

✱ The dose of fluids for the dehydrated or volume-depleted child is 20 mL/kg of lactated Ringer's or normal saline.

Diarrhea   Diarrhea is a common occurrence in childhood. Often, what parents call diarrhea is actually loose bowel movements. Generally, 10 or more loose stools per day is considered diarrhea. As with nausea and vomiting, the main concern associated with diarrhea is dehydration. Most diarrhea is due to viral infections of the gastrointestinal system or secondary to infections elsewhere in the body. However, certain bacterial infections can cause significant, even life-threatening, diarrhea.

Treatment of the child suffering diarrhea is primarily supportive. If dehydration is evident, administer fluids. Severe dehydration should be treated with 20 mL/kg boluses of intravenous fluids (lactated Ringer's or normal saline).

TABLE 30-4	Signs and Symptoms of Dehydration		
Signs/Symptoms	**Mild**	**Moderate**	**Severe**
Vital Signs			
Pulse	normal	increased	markedly increased
Respirations	normal	increased	tachypneic
Blood Pressure	normal	normal	hypotensive
Capillary Refill	normal	2–3 seconds	> 2 seconds
Mental Status	alert	irritable	lethargic
Skin	normal	dry and ashen	dry, cool, mottled
Mucous Membranes	dry	very dry	very dry/no tears

Cardiovascular Emergencies

Cardiovascular emergencies in children most commonly result from volume depletion due to severe dehydration, hemorrhage, or severe infection. With the exception of congenital heart disease, cardiac emergencies in children are extremely rare. Cardiac arrest in children usually follows respiratory arrest. Lethal dysrhythmias, such as ventricular fibrillation, ventricular tachycardia, or high-grade heart blocks rarely occur in children.

Dehydration   The child is very vulnerable to dehydration. Among the causes are diarrhea, vomiting, poor fluid intake, fever, and burns. Children have a high body-surface-area-to-weight ratio. Therefore, they are very vulnerable to heat loss, and along with it, dehydration. They also have a higher percentage of water to body tissues than adults.

Assessment.   When confronted with a dehydrated child, question the parents about recent infection, diarrhea, vomiting, or fever. Also, ask them about decreased urination. Many parents will notice that their children are wetting fewer diapers than usual.

    Physical examination may show decreased skin turgor, weight loss, and absent tears. Urine may be quite concentrated. The eyes may be dull and sunken-looking. Infants may exhibit a depressed anterior fontanelle. The child may have altered mental status or poor pain response. Table 30-4 will help you determine the severity of dehydration.

Management.   The management of dehydration should first include the primary survey: airway, breathing, and circulation. The vital signs should be determined and monitored. If the child is in shock, start an IV of LR or normal saline. An initial fluid bolus of 20 mL/kg should be administered and repeated as indicated. Do not delay transport, however, if there is difficulty in starting the IV.

■ **sepsis** the presence of an infectious agent, usually bacteria, in the blood stream.

Sepsis   Sepsis is a bacterial infection of the bloodstream. It usually occurs as a complication of an infection at another site such as pneumonia, an ear infection, or a urinary tract infection. Meningitis is frequently associated with sepsis. The etiology can be varied, as can the presenting signs and symptoms. Occasionally, the focus of infection cannot be initially determined. Newborns and small infants are at increased risk for developing sepsis as their immune systems are still relatively immature.

The septic child is critically ill. **Septic shock** may develop due to the release of deadly toxins by the bacteria causing the infection. These toxins cause peripheral vasodilation, leading to a drop in blood pressure and decreased tissue perfusion. Sepsis can be rapidly fatal if not promptly identified and treated.

Assessment. Suspect sepsis in any child who becomes ill or who has been ill for several days, especially if accompanied by fever, lethargy, irritability, or shock. Initial management of the septic child includes the standard primary survey and secondary assessment. Signs and symptoms of sepsis include:

❑ Ill appearance
❑ Irritability or altered mental status
❑ Fever
❑ Vomiting and diarrhea
❑ Cyanosis, pallor, or mottled skin
❑ Nonspecific respiratory distress
❑ Poor feeding

Signs and symptoms of septic shock include:

❑ Very ill appearance
❑ Altered mental status
❑ Tachycardia
❑ Capillary refill time greater than 2 seconds
❑ Hyperventilation, leading to respiratory failure
❑ Cool and clammy skin
❑ Inability of child to recognize parents

Management. The primary survey should be completed. Secure and maintain the airway and assist ventilation as required. Administer supplemental oxygen at a high concentration. Obtain IV access and begin an infusion of lactated Ringer's or normal saline. If the capillary refill time is greater than 2 seconds, administer a 20 mL/kg fluid bolus. Repeat as necessary. Shock can develop and should be anticipated and treated appropriately. Sepsis is a very serious condition that can deteriorate quickly. It must be promptly recognized and treated appropriately. The goal is to prevent the development of septic shock.

Dysrhythmias Dysrhythmias in children are uncommon and usually due to non-cardiac problems. The most common pediatric dysrhythmia is bradycardia. It usually results from hypoxia, hypotension, or acidosis. Supraventricular tachycardia can also occur in children. Although a rare disorder, supraventricular tachycardia can cause sustained heart rates of 200 beats per minute or greater. Heart rates in excess of 200 beats per minute do not allow for adequate ventricular filling. Because of this, cardiac output may fall, resulting in decreased tissue perfusion. Asystole is usually a terminal event, following prolonged, untreated bradycardia. Ventricular fibrillation in children is rare and usually results from serious electrolyte imbalances.

Treatment of pediatric dysrhythmias is much the same as for adults. However, algorithms have been developed for the treatment of pediatric bradycardia and pediatric asystole. (See Figures 30-17 and 30-18, pp. 938 and 939.)

■ **septic shock** type of shock that accompanies a bacterial infection, often due to release of endotoxins by the bacteria.

✳ Sepsis in a child is a medical emergency.

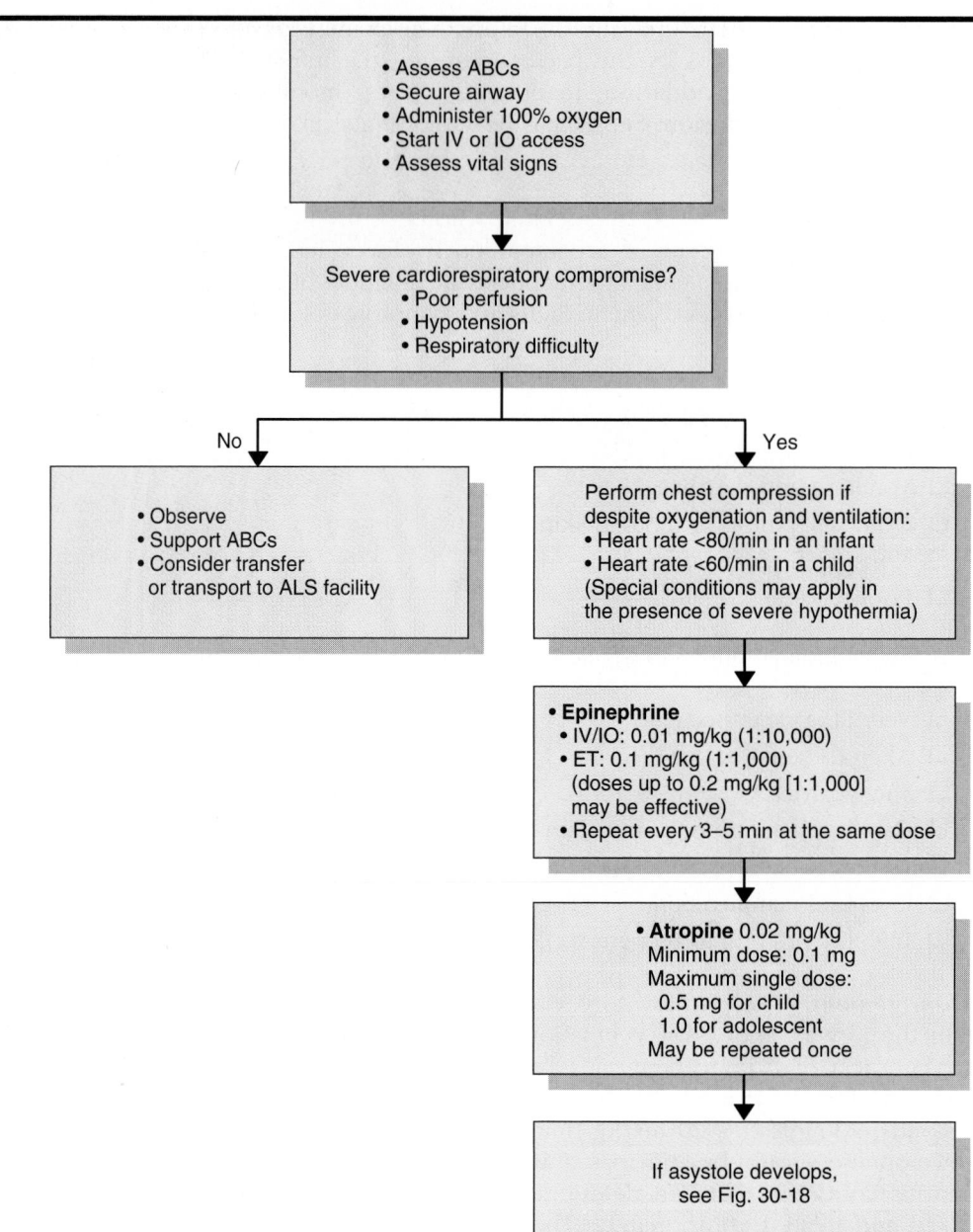

Assess ABCs
• Secure airway
• Administer 100% oxygen
• Start IV or IO access
• Assess vital signs

Severe cardiorespiratory compromise?
• Poor perfusion
• Hypotension
• Respiratory difficulty

No

• Observe
• Support ABCs
• Consider transfer
  or transport to ALS facility

Yes

Perform chest compression if
despite oxygenation and ventilation:
• Heart rate <80/min in an infant
• Heart rate <60/min in a child
(Special conditions may apply in
the presence of severe hypothermia)

• **Epinephrine**
  • IV/IO: 0.01 mg/kg (1:10,000)
  • ET: 0.1 mg/kg (1:1,000)
    (doses up to 0.2 mg/kg [1:1,000]
    may be effective)
  • Repeat every 3–5 min at the same dose

• **Atropine** 0.02 mg/kg
  Minimum dose: 0.1 mg
  Maximum single dose:
    0.5 mg for child
    1.0 for adolescent
  May be repeated once

If asystole develops,
see Fig. 30-18

FIGURE 30-17 Pediatric bradycardia decision tree.

■ **congenital** present at birth.

Congenital Heart Disease   **Congenital** heart disease is an abnormality or defect in the heart present at birth. It is the primary cause of heart disease in children. Most congenital heart problems are detected at birth. Some, however, are not discovered until later in childhood. The most common emergency due to congenital heart disease is cyanosis. This occurs when blood going to the lungs for oxygenation mixes with blood bound for other parts of the body. This may result from holes in the internal walls of the heart or abnormalities of the great vessels.

The child with congenital heart disease may develop respiratory distress, congestive heart failure, or a "cyanotic spell." *Cyanotic spells* occur when oxygen demand exceeds that provided by the blood. It begins as irritability, unconsolable crying, or altered mental status. Severe dyspnea may develop,

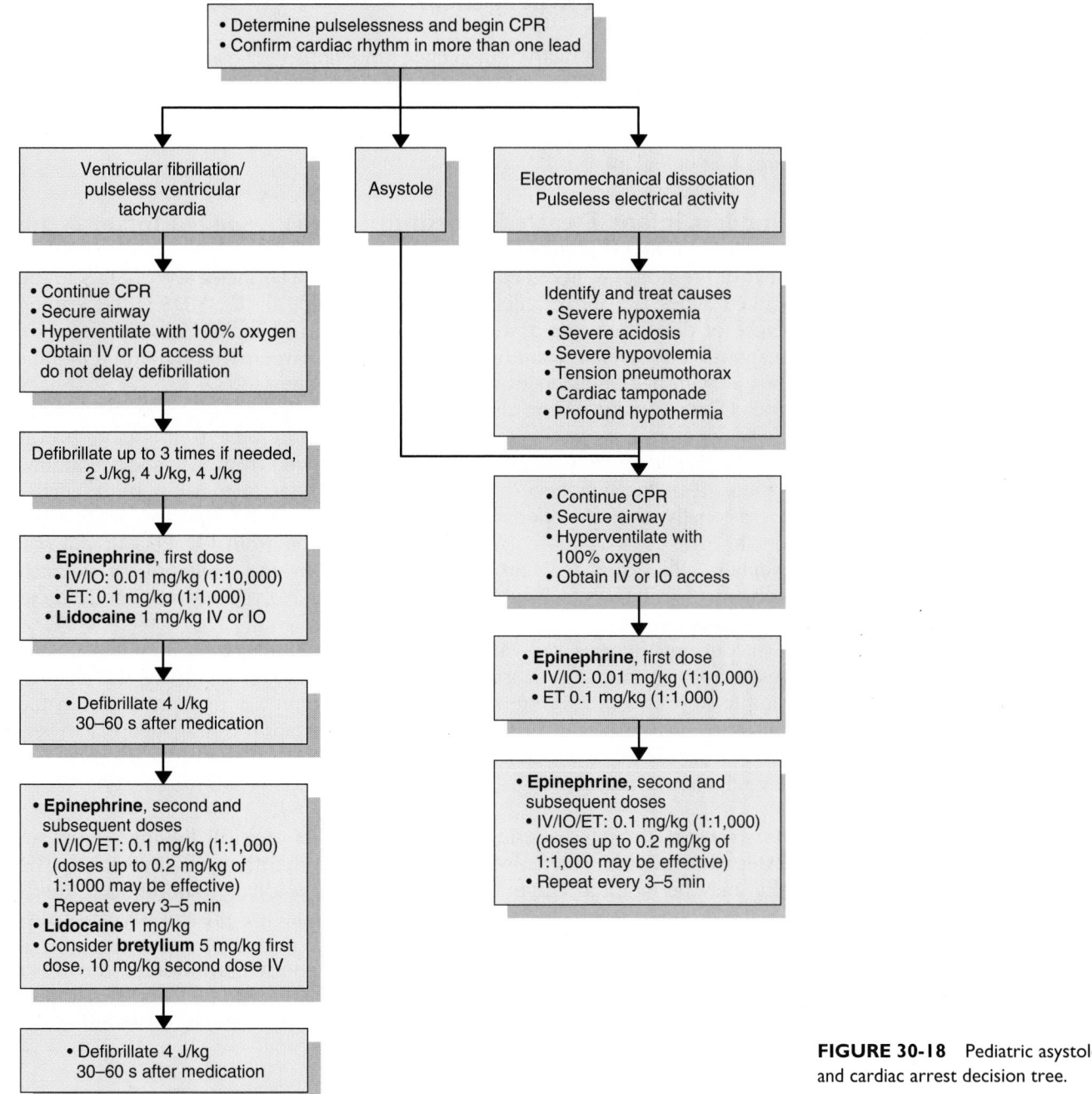

- Determine pulselessness and begin CPR
- Confirm cardiac rhythm in more than one lead

Ventricular fibrillation/ pulseless ventricular tachycardia

- Continue CPR
- Secure airway
- Hyperventilate with 100% oxygen
- Obtain IV or IO access but do not delay defibrillation

- Defibrillate up to 3 times if needed, 2 J/kg, 4 J/kg, 4 J/kg

- **Epinephrine**, first dose
  - IV/IO: 0.01 mg/kg (1:10,000)
  - ET: 0.1 mg/kg (1:1,000)
- **Lidocaine** 1 mg/kg IV or IO

- Defibrillate 4 J/kg 30–60 s after medication

- **Epinephrine**, second and subsequent doses
  - IV/IO/ET: 0.1 mg/kg (1:1,000) (doses up to 0.2 mg/kg of 1:1000 may be effective)
  - Repeat every 3–5 min
- **Lidocaine** 1 mg/kg
- Consider **bretylium** 5 mg/kg first dose, 10 mg/kg second dose IV

- Defibrillate 4 J/kg 30–60 s after medication

Asystole

Electromechanical dissociation Pulseless electrical activity

Identify and treat causes
- Severe hypoxemia
- Severe acidosis
- Severe hypovolemia
- Tension pneumothorax
- Cardiac tamponade
- Profound hypothermia

- Continue CPR
- Secure airway
- Hyperventilate with 100% oxygen
- Obtain IV or IO access

- **Epinephrine**, first dose
  - IV/IO: 0.01 mg/kg (1:10,000)
  - ET 0.1 mg/kg (1:1,000)

- **Epinephrine**, second and subsequent doses
  - IV/IO/ET: 0.1 mg/kg (1:1,000) (doses up to 0.2 mg/kg of 1:1,000 may be effective)
  - Repeat every 3–5 min

FIGURE 30-18 Pediatric asystole and cardiac arrest decision tree.

including progressive cyanosis. In severe and prolonged cases, seizures, coma, or cardiac arrest may result. Non-cyanotic problems associated with congenital heart disease include respiratory distress, tachycardia, decreased end-organ perfusion, drowsiness, fatigue, and pallor.

Treatment includes the standard primary assessment. Administer oxygen at a high concentration. If necessary, provide ventilatory support. If the child is having a cyanotic spell, place him or her in the knee-chest position facing downward. This will help decrease the cardiac workload. Apply the ECG monitor, and start an intravenous line at a TKO rate. Transport immediately.

Other Pediatric Emergencies

In addition to the pediatric emergencies previously discussed, you should be familiar with Sudden Infant Death Syndrome (SIDS). SIDS is a sad and difficult situation for both parents and prehospital personnel. An understanding of SIDS is essential in order to enable you to deal effectively with this heartbreaking emergency.

■ **sudden infant death syndrome (SIDS)** illness of unknown etiology that occurs during the first year of life.

Sudden Infant Death Syndrome (SIDS)   **Sudden Infant Death Syndrome (SIDS)** is defined as the sudden death of an infant during the first year of life from an illness of unknown etiology. The incidence of SIDS in the United States is approximately 2 deaths per 1,000 births. SIDS is the leading cause of death between 1 week and 1 year of age in the United States. It is responsible for a significant number of deaths between 1 month and 6 months of age, with peak incidences occurring at 2–4 months.

Death usually occurs during sleep. The incidence seems to be greater during winter and is more common in males than in females. It is more prevalent in families with younger mothers and in those from low socioeconomic groups. A higher incidence is also reported in infants with a low birth weight. Occasionally, a mild upper respiratory infection will be reported prior to the death. SIDS is not caused by external suffocation from blankets or pillows. Neither is it related to child abuse, regurgitation and aspiration of stomach contents, or allergies to cow's milk. It is not hereditary, but does tend to recur in families.

Current theories vary about the etiology. Some authorities feel it may result from an immature respiratory center in the brain that leads the child to simply stop breathing. Others feel there may be an airway obstruction in the posterior pharynx, as a result of pharyngeal relaxation during sleep, a hypermobile mandible, or an enlarged tongue. There are many other theories and investigation continues.

Assessment. Infants suffering SIDS have similar physical findings. From an external standpoint, there is a normal state of nutrition and hydration. The skin may be mottled. There are often frothy, occasionally blood-tinged, fluids in and around the mouth and nostrils. Vomitus may be present. Occasionally, the infant may be in an unusual position, due to muscle spasm at the time of death. Common findings noted at autopsy include intrathoracic petechia (small hemorrhages) in 90 percent of cases. There is often associated pulmonary congestion and edema. Sometimes, stomach contents are found in the trachea. Microscopic examination of the trachea often reveals the presence of inflammatory changes.

✳ A SIDS death is a very sad event. Provide emotional support for the parents. Active and aggressive care of the infant should continue until delivery to the emergency department.

Management. The immediate needs of the family with a SIDS baby are many. Undertake active and aggressive care of the infant to assure the parents that everything possible is being done. A first responder, or other personnel, should be assigned to assist the parents and to explain the procedures. After arrival at the hospital, direct management and care at the parents, since often nothing can be done for the child. If the infant is dead, allow the family to see the child. Expect a normal grief reaction from the parents. Initially, there may be shock, disbelief, and denial. Other times, the parents may express anger, rage, hostility, blame, or guilt. Often, there is a feeling of inadequacy as a parent, as well as helplessness, confusion, and fear. The grief process may last as long as 1–2 years. SIDS has major long-term effects on family relationships.

PEDIATRIC ADVANCED LIFE SUPPORT (PALS)

Cardiopulmonary arrest in infants and children is usually not a sudden event. Instead, it is the end result of progressive deterioration in respiratory and cardiac function. Because of this, the goal of pediatric advanced life support is to recognize and prevent cardiopulmonary arrest.

Anticipating Cardiopulmonary Arrest

All sick children should undergo a Rapid Cardiopulmonary Assessment. The goal is to answer the question: *"Does this child have pulmonary or circulatory failure that may lead to cardiopulmonary arrest?"* Recognition of the physiologically unstable infant is made by physical examination alone.

Children who should receive the Rapid Cardiopulmonary Assessment include those with the following conditions.

❏ Respiratory rate greater than 60
❏ Heart rate greater than 180 or less than 80 (under 5 years)
❏ Heart rate greater than 180 or less than 60 (over 5 years)
❏ Respiratory distress
❏ Trauma
❏ Burns
❏ Cyanosis
❏ Altered level of consciousness
❏ Seizures
❏ Fever with petechiae (small skin hemorrhages)

✱ The goal of the Rapid Cardiopulmonary Assessment is to answer the question, "Does this child have a pulmonary or circulatory problem that may lead to cardiac arrest?"

Rapid Cardiopulmonary Assessment

The Rapid Cardiopulmonary Assessment is designed to assist you in recognizing respiratory failure and shock, thus anticipating cardiopulmonary arrest. The Rapid Cardiopulmonary Assessment follows the basic ABCs of CPR.

Airway Patency   Inspect the airway using the techniques depicted in Figures 30-19 to 30-22. Ask yourself the following questions.

❏ Is the airway patent?
❏ Is it maintainable with head positioning, suctioning, or airway adjuncts?
❏ Is the airway unmaintainable? If so, what action is required (endotracheal intubation, removal of a foreign body, and so on)?

Breathing   Evaluation of breathing includes assessment of the following conditions.

❏ *Respiratory Rate.* Tachypnea is often the first manifestation of respiratory distress in infants. An infant breathing at a rapid rate will eventually tire. Thus, a decreasing respiratory rate is not necessarily a sign of improvement. A slow respiratory rate in an acutely ill infant or child is an ominous sign.
❏ *Air Entry.* The quality of air entry can be assessed by observing for chest rise, breath sounds, stridor, or wheezing.

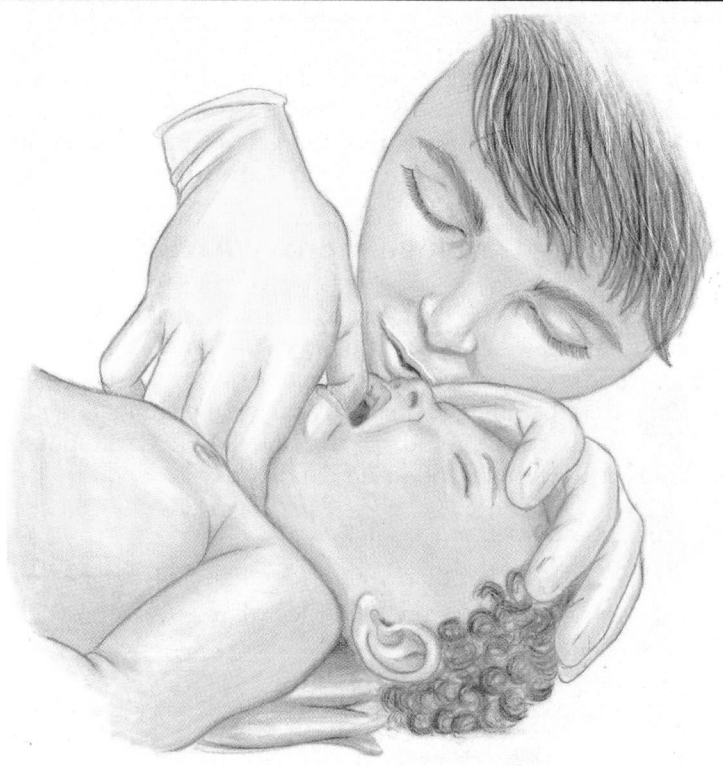

FIGURE 30-19 Opening the airway in a child.

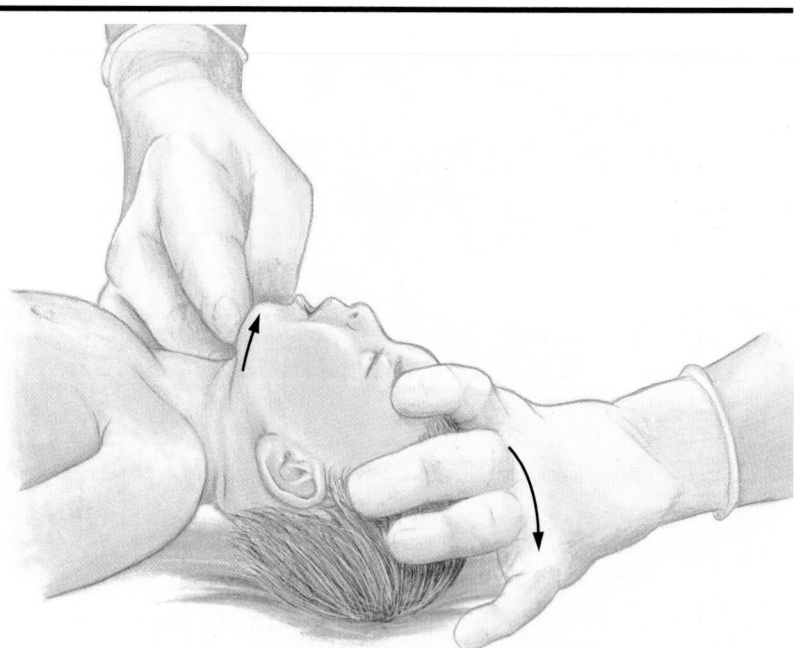

FIGURE 30-20 Chin-lift/Head tilt method.

❑ *Respiratory Mechanics.* Increased work of breathing in the infant and child is evidenced by nasal flaring and use of the accessory respiratory muscles.

❑ *Color.* Cyanosis is a fairly late sign of respiratory failure and is most frequently seen in the mucous membranes of the mouth and the nail beds. Cyanosis of the extremities alone is more likely due to circulatory failure (shock) than respiratory failure.

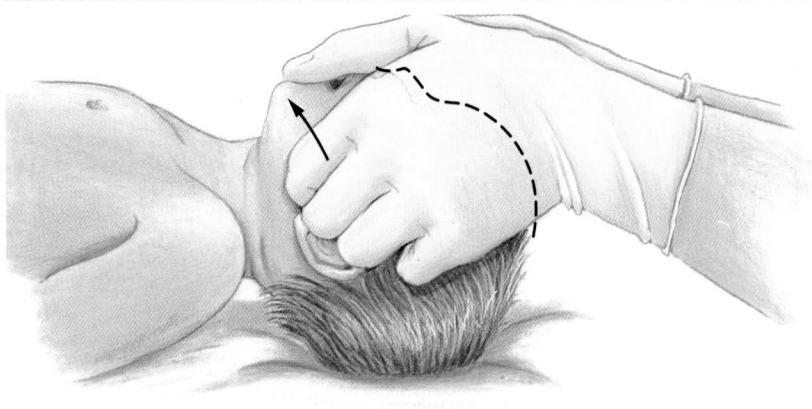

FIGURE 30-21 Jaw-thrust method.

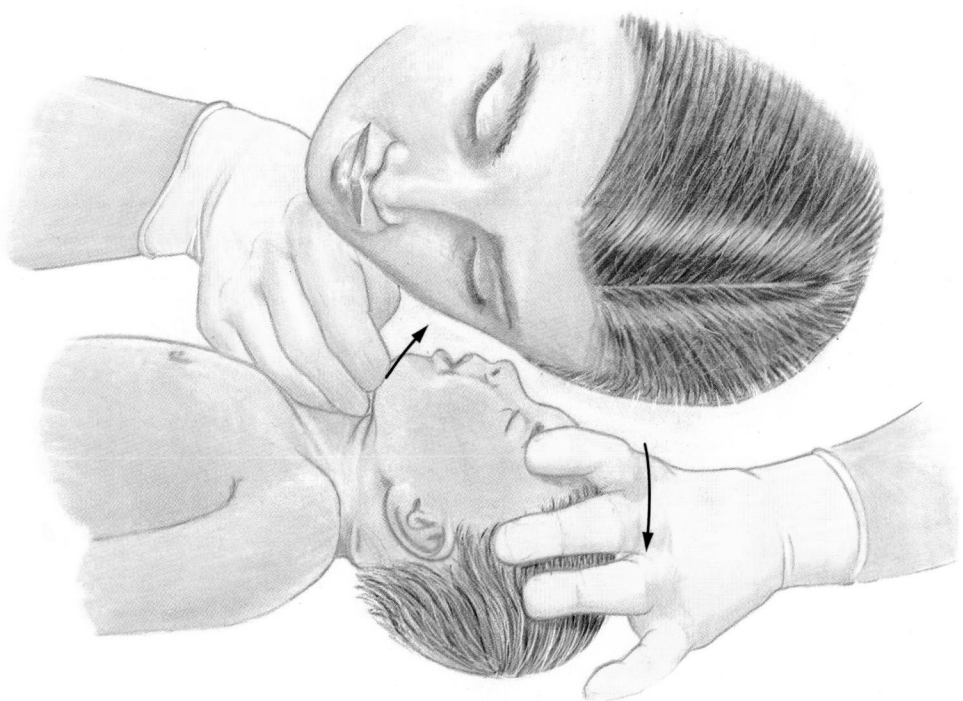

FIGURE 30-22 Assessing the airway.

Circulation   The cardiovascular assessment consists of the following basic procedures.

❑ *Heart Rate.* Normal heart rates for age were presented earlier in the chapter. Infants develop sinus tachycardia in response to stress. Thus, any tachycardia in an infant or child requires further evaluation to determine the cause. Bradycardia in a distressed infant or child may indicate hypoxia and is an ominous sign of impending cardiac arrest.

❑ *Blood Pressure.* Hypotension is a late and often sudden sign of cardiovascular decompensation. Even mild hypotension should be taken seriously and treated quickly and vigorously, since cardiopulmonary arrest is imminent.

❑ *Peripheral Circulation.* The presence of pulses is a good indicator of the adequacy of end-organ perfusion. The pulse pressure (the difference between the systolic and diastolic blood pressure) narrows as shock develops. Loss of central pulses is an ominous sign.

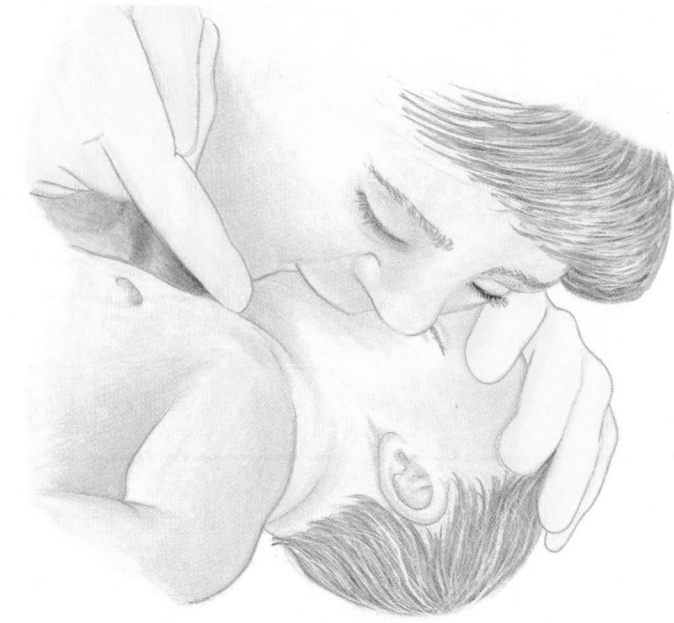

FIGURE 30-23 Artificial ventilation in an infant.

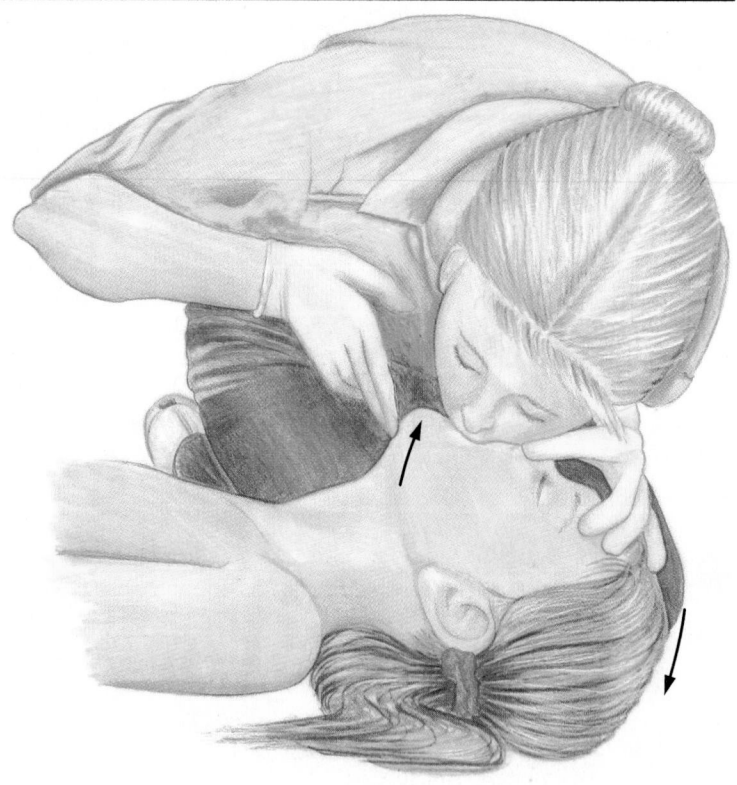

FIGURE 30-24 Artificial ventilation in a child.

❑ *End-Organ Perfusion.* The end-organ perfusion is most evident in the skin, kidneys, and brain. Decreased perfusion of the skin is an early sign of shock. A capillary refill time of greater than 2 seconds is indicative of low cardiac output. Impairment of brain perfusion is usually evidenced by a change in mental status. The child may become confused or lethargic. Seizures may occur. Failure of the child to recognize the parents' faces is often an ominous sign. Urine output is directly related to kidney

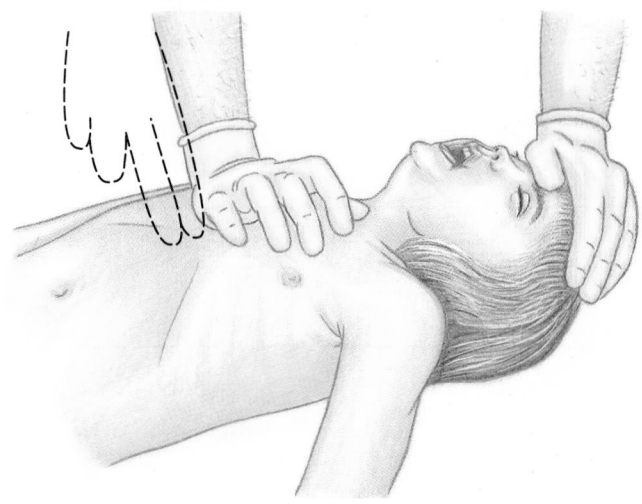

FIGURE 30-25 Hand placement for CPR.

perfusion. Normal urine output is 1–2 mL/kg/hr. Urine flow of less than 1 mL/kg/hr is an indicator of poor renal perfusion.

The Rapid Cardiopulmonary Assessment should be repeated throughout initial assessment and patient transport. This will help you determine whether the patient's condition is deteriorating or improving. Any decompensation or change in the patient's status should be immediately treated.

Management of the Critically Ill Infant or Child

Basic life support (BLS) should be applied according to current standards. It should include maintenance of the airway, artificial ventilation, and, if required, chest compressions. (See Figures 30-23 to 30-25 and Table 30-5.) The following modifications will help you to apply BLS to the pediatric patient.

Pediatric Airway Management   The pediatric airway is somewhat different than that of the adult. Important differences include the following anatomical considerations.

- ❑ A child's larynx is slightly higher in the neck.
- ❑ The epiglottis is U-shaped and extends into the pharynx.
- ❑ The vocal cords are short and concave.
- ❑ The narrowest portion of the airway is at the level of the cricoid cartilage (in children less than 8 years old).

These anatomical differences have several clinical implications in airway management. First, it is slightly more difficult to visualize the airway for endotracheal intubation. Second, the size of the endotracheal tube should be based on size of the cricoid ring, rather than the glottic opening.

Although many of the same airway management techniques for adults are applicable in children, you need to keep in mind some important differences. First, you should not use certain airways in pediatrics because of variations in airway size in children. Avoid esophageal obturator airways (EOA), pharyngeotracheal lumen airways (PtL), and esophageal-tracheal combitubes (ETC). Second, use of nasopharyngeal airways in children is discouraged. Young children have rather large adenoidal tissue and insertion of a nasopharyngeal airway can lacerate these tissues, causing bleeding into the airway.

TABLE 30-5	Summary of BLS Maneuvers in Infants and Children	
Maneuver	**Infant (<1 y)**	**Child (1 to 8 y)**
Airway	Head tilt/chin lift	Head tilt/chin lift
	(unless trauma present)	(unless trauma present)
Jaw thrust	Jaw thrust	
Breathing		
Initial	2 breaths at 1 to	2 breaths at 1 to
	1½ seconds/breath	1½ seconds/breath
Subsequent	20 breaths/minute	20 breaths/minute
Circulation		
Pulse check	Brachial/femoral	Carotid
Compression area	Lower third of sternum	Lower third of sternum
Compression with	2 or 3 fingers	Heel of 1 hand
Depth	Approximately ½ to 1 inch	Approximately 1 to 1½ inch
Rate	At least 100/minute	100/minute
Compression-	5:1 (pause for ventilation)	5:1 (pause for ventilation)
ventilation ratio		
Foreign-body airway obstruction	Back blows/chest thrusts	Heimlich maneuver

Finally, there are several special considerations in endotracheal intubation that must be considered. (See Figures 30-26 and 30-27.) As mentioned, the airway of a child differs from that of an adult. It is, of course, smaller. In addition, it is more flexible. The tongue is also relatively larger, and the glottic opening is higher in the neck. As a rule, in children under 8 years of age, uncuffed endotracheal tubes should be used. Cuffed tubes may be used in older children. Table 30-6 illustrates suggested endotracheal tube and suction catheter sizes for age. Intubation should be preceded by adequate ventilation with 100 percent oxygen. Although either a straight or curved blade may be used, a straight blade is recommended in infants. During intubation, the heart rate should be monitored for the presence of dysrhythmias. Indications for intubation include the inability to ventilate the unconscious patient, cardiac or respiratory arrest, the inability of the patient to protect his or her airway, and the need for prolonged artificial ventilation.

✱ As a rule, uncuffed endotracheal tubes should be used in children under 8 years of age.

Ventilation of the Pediatric Patient
The bag-valve-mask (BVM) device is the ideal device for ventilation of the pediatric patient. Pediatric BVMs should not contain pressure pop-off valves. If they do, the valve should be able to be readily occluded, if necessary, since ventilation pressures required during pediatric CPR may exceed the limit of the pop-off valve. Also, oxygen-powered breathing devices (demand valves) should not be used in pediatric resuscitation.

Vascular Access and Fluid Therapy
The intravenous techniques for children are basically the same as for adults. However, there are additional veins in the infant that may be accessed. These include veins of the neck and scalp, as well as of the arms, hands, and feet. The external jugular vein, however, should only be used for life-threatening situations. Commonly used solutions include normal saline and lactated Ringer's. Intravenous infusions in children should be closely monitored, as it is very easy to fluid-overload the pediatric patient. Minidrip administration sets should be routinely used in pediatric cases.

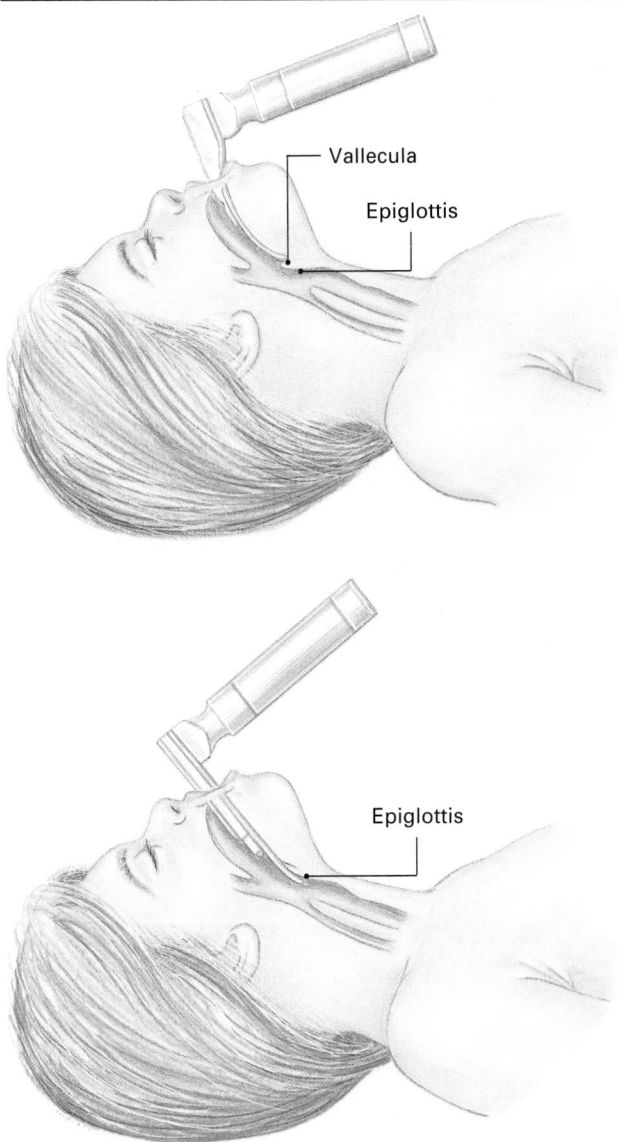

Vallecula

Epiglottis

Epiglottis

FIGURE 30-26 Placement of the laryngoscope in the child.

The use of intraosseous infusion has become popular in the pediatric patient. (See Figures 30-28 and 30-29.) This is especially true when large volumes of fluid must be administered, as occurs in hypovolemic shock, and other means of venous access are unavailable. Certain PALS drugs can be administered intraosseously. These include epinephrine, atropine, dopamine, lidocaine, sodium bicarbonate, and dobutamine. Indications for intraosseous infusion include a child less than 5 years of age, the existence of shock or cardiac arrest, an unresponsive patient, and unsuccessful attempts at peripheral IV insertion.

A standard 16- or 18-gauge needle (either hypodermic or spinal) can be used for intraosseous infusion. However, an intraosseous needle is preferred. The anterior surface of the leg below the knee should be prepped with an antiseptic solution. The needle is then inserted, in a twisting fashion, 1–3 centimeters below the tibial tuberosity. Insertion should be slightly inferior in direction and perpendicular to the skin. Placement of the needle into the marrow cavity can be determined by noting a lack of resistance as the needle passes through the bony cortex. Other indications include the needle standing upright without support, the ability to aspirate bone marrow into a syringe, or free flow of the infusion without infiltration into the subcutaneous tissues.

✱ Always remember the intraosseous route for administering drugs and fluids to the pediatric patient less than five years of age when an IV cannot be placed.

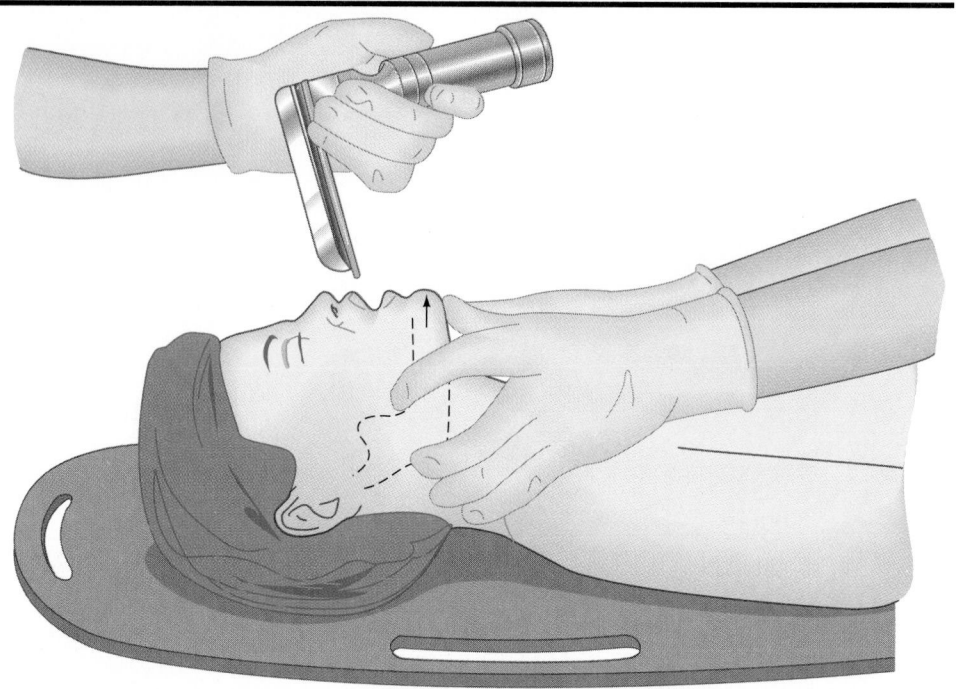

FIGURE 30-27 Simultaneous cervical spine immobilization and intubation in a pediatric trauma victim.

TABLE 30-6 Equipment Guidelines According to Age and Weight

Equipment	Age (50th Percentile Weight)					
	Premie **(1–2.5 kg)**	**Neonate** **(2.5–4.0 kg)**	**6 months** **(7.0 kg)**	**1–2 Years** **(10–12 kg)**	**5 Years** **(16–18 kg)**	**8–10 Years** **(24–30 kg)**
Airway	infant	infant small	small	small	medium	medium large
oral	(00)	(0)	(1)	(2)	(3)	(4.5)
Breathing						
Self-inflating bag	infant	infant	child	child	child	child adult
O₂ ventiliation mask	premature	newborn	infant/child	child	child	small adult
Endotracheal tube	2.5–3.0 (uncuffed)	3.0–3.5 (uncuffed)	3.5–4.0 (uncuffed)	4.0–4.5 (uncuffed)	5.0–5.5 (uncuffed)	5.5–6.5 (cuffed)
Laryngoscope blade	0 (straight)	1 (straight)	1 (straight)	1–2 (straight)	2 (straight or curved)	2–3 (straight or curved)
Suction/stylet (F)	6–8/6	8/6	8–10/6	10/6	14/14	14/14
Circulation						
BP cuff	newborn	newborn	infant	child	child	child adult
Venous access						
Angiocath	22–24	22–24	22–24	20–22	18–20	16–20
Butterfly needle	25	23–25	23–25	23	20–23	18–21
Intracath	—	—	19	19	16	14
Arm board	6″	6″	6″–8″	8″	8″–15″	15″
Orogastric tube (F)	5	5–8	8	10	10–12	14–18
Chest tube (F)	10–14	12–18	14–20	14–24	20–32	28–38

(Reproduced with permission of the American Heart Association)

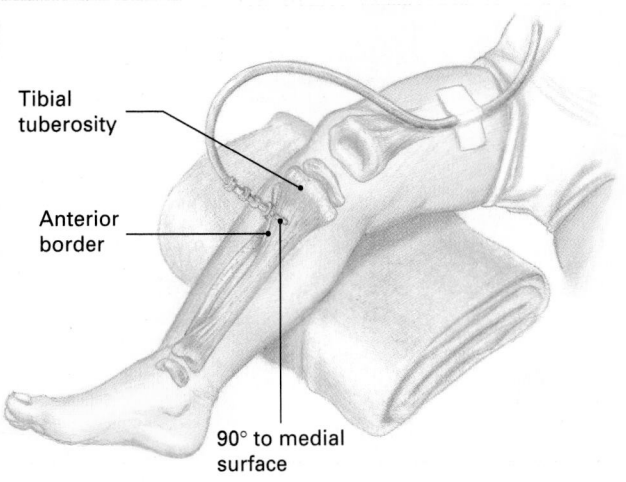

Tibial tuberosity

Anterior border

90° to medial surface

FIGURE 30-28
Intraosseous administration.

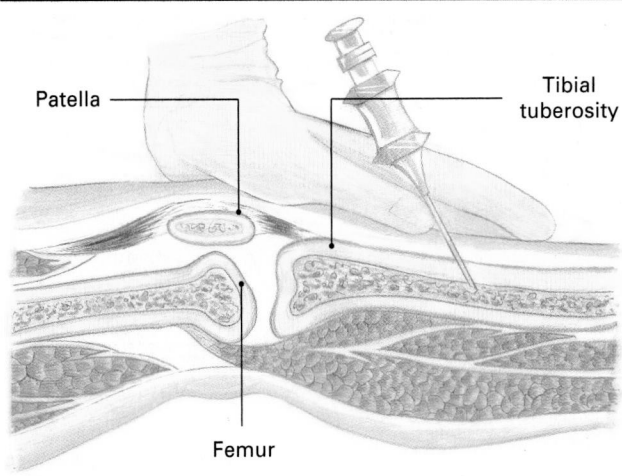

Patella

Tibial tuberosity

Femur

FIGURE 30-29
Correct needle placement for intraosseous administration.

The accurate dosing of fluids in children is crucial. Too much fluid can result in heart failure and pulmonary edema. Too little fluid can be ineffective. The initial dosage of fluid in hypovolemic shock should be 20 mL/kg, given over 10 to 20 minutes as soon as IV access is obtained. After the infusion, the child should be reassessed. If perfusion is still diminished, then a second bolus of 20 mL/kg should be administered. A child with hypovolemic shock may require 40–60 mL/kg, while a child with septic shock may require at least 60–80 mL/kg. Regardless, the most important factor of pediatric fluid therapy is frequent patient reassessment.

Medications   Cardiopulmonary arrest in children is almost always due to a primary respiratory problem, such as drowning, choking, or smoke inhalation. The major aim in pediatric resuscitation is airway management and ventilation, as well as replacement of intravascular volume, if indicated. In certain cases, medications may be required. The objectives of medication therapy in pediatric cardiac arrest include:

❑ Correction of hypoxemia
❑ Increased perfusion pressure during chest compressions

- ❏ Stimulation of spontaneous or more forceful cardiac contractions
- ❏ Acceleration of the heart rate
- ❏ Correction of metabolic acidosis
- ❏ Suppression of ventricular ectopy

TABLE 30-7 Drugs Used in Pediatric Advanced Life Support*

Drug	Dose	Remarks
Adenosine	0.1 to 0.2 mg/kg Maximum single dose: 12 mg	Rapid IV bolus
Atropine sulfate	0.02 mg/kg per dose	Minimum dose: 0.1 mg Maximum single dose: 0.5 mg in child; 1.0 mg in adolescent
Bretylium	5 mg/kg; may be increased to 10 mg/kg	Rapid IV
Calcium chloride 10 percent	20 mg/kg per dose	Give slowly
Dopamine hydrochloride	2–20 µg/kg per minute	Adrenergic action dominates at ≥15–20 µg/kg per minute
Dobutamine hydrochloride	2–20 µg/kg per minute	Titrate to desired effect
Epinephrine *for bradycardia*	IV/IO: 0.01 mg/kg (1:10,000) ET: 0.1 mg/kg (1:1,000)	Be aware of effective dose of preservatives administered (if preservatives are present in epinephrine preparation) when high doses are used
for asystolic or pulseless arrest	First dose: IV/IO:0.01 mg/kg (1:10,000) ET:0.1 mg/kg (1:1,000) Doses as high as 0.2 mg/kg may be effective Subsequent doses: IV/IO/ET: 0.1 mg/kg (1:1,000) Doses as high as 0.2 mg/kg may be effective	Be aware of effective dose of preservatives administered (if preservatives are present in epinephrine preparation) when high doses are used
Epinephrine infusion	Initial at 0.1 µg/kg per minute Higher infusion dose used if asystole present	Titrate to desired effect (0.1–1.0 µg/kg per minute)
Lidocaine	1 mg/kg per dose	
Lidocaine infusion	20–50 µg/kg per minute	
Sodium bicarbonate	1 mEq/kg per dose or 0.3 × kg × base deficit	Infuse slowly and only if ventilation is adequate

*IV indicates intravenous route; IO, intraosseous route; and ET, endotracheal route.

TABLE 30-8 Preparation of Infusions

Drug	Preparation*	Dose
Epinephrine	0.6 × body weight (kg) equals milligrams added to diluent† to make 100 mL	Then 1 mL/h delivers 0.1 µg/kg per minute; titrate to effect
Dopamine dobutamine	0.6 × body weight (kg) equals milligrams added to diluent† to make 100 mL	Then 1 mL/h delivers 0.1 µg/kg per minute; titrate to effect
Lidocaine	120 mg of 40 mg/mL solution added to 97 mL of 5 percent dextrose in water, yielding 1200 µg/mL solution	Then 1 mL/kg per hour delivers 20 µg/kg per minute

*Standard concentration may be used to provide more dilute or more concentrated drug solution, but then individual dose must be calculated for each patient and each infusion rate:

$$\text{Infusion Rate (mL/h)} = \frac{\text{Weight (kg)} \times \text{Dose (µg/kg/min)} \times 60 \text{ min/h}}{\text{Concentration (µg/mL)}}$$

†Diluent may be 5 percent dextrose in water, 5 percent dextrose in half-normal saline, normal saline, or Ringer's lacate.

The dosages of medications must be modified for the pediatric patient. Tables 30-7 and 30-8 illustrate recommended pediatric drug dosage in advanced cardiac life support.

Electrical Therapy   The initial dosage for electrical defibrillation is 2 joules per kilogram of body weight. If this is unsuccessful, it should be increased to 4 joules per kilogram. If this is unsuccessful, attention should be aimed at correcting hypoxia and acidosis.

SUMMARY

Pediatric emergencies can be stressful for both you and the family. Most pediatric emergencies result from trauma, ingestion of poisons, respiratory emergencies, or febrile seizure activity. In addition, you must always be on the lookout for signs and symptoms of child abuse or neglect. The approach and management of pediatric emergencies must be modified for the age and size of the child. Certain skills generally considered routine, such as IV administration and PALS, become more difficult in the pediatric patient due to size and other factors. It is important to remember that children are not "small adults." They have special considerations and needs that must be managed accordingly.

FURTHER READING

American Heart Association and American Academy of Pediatrics. *Textbook of Pediatric Advanced Life Support.* Dallas: American Heart Association, 1993.

Eichelberger, Martin R. *et al. Pediatric Emergencies.* Prentice Hall, Englewood Cliffs, NJ, 1992.

Simon, Joseph E., and Aron T. Goldberg. *Prehospital Pediatric Life Support.* St. Louis, MI, C.V. Mosby Company, 1989.

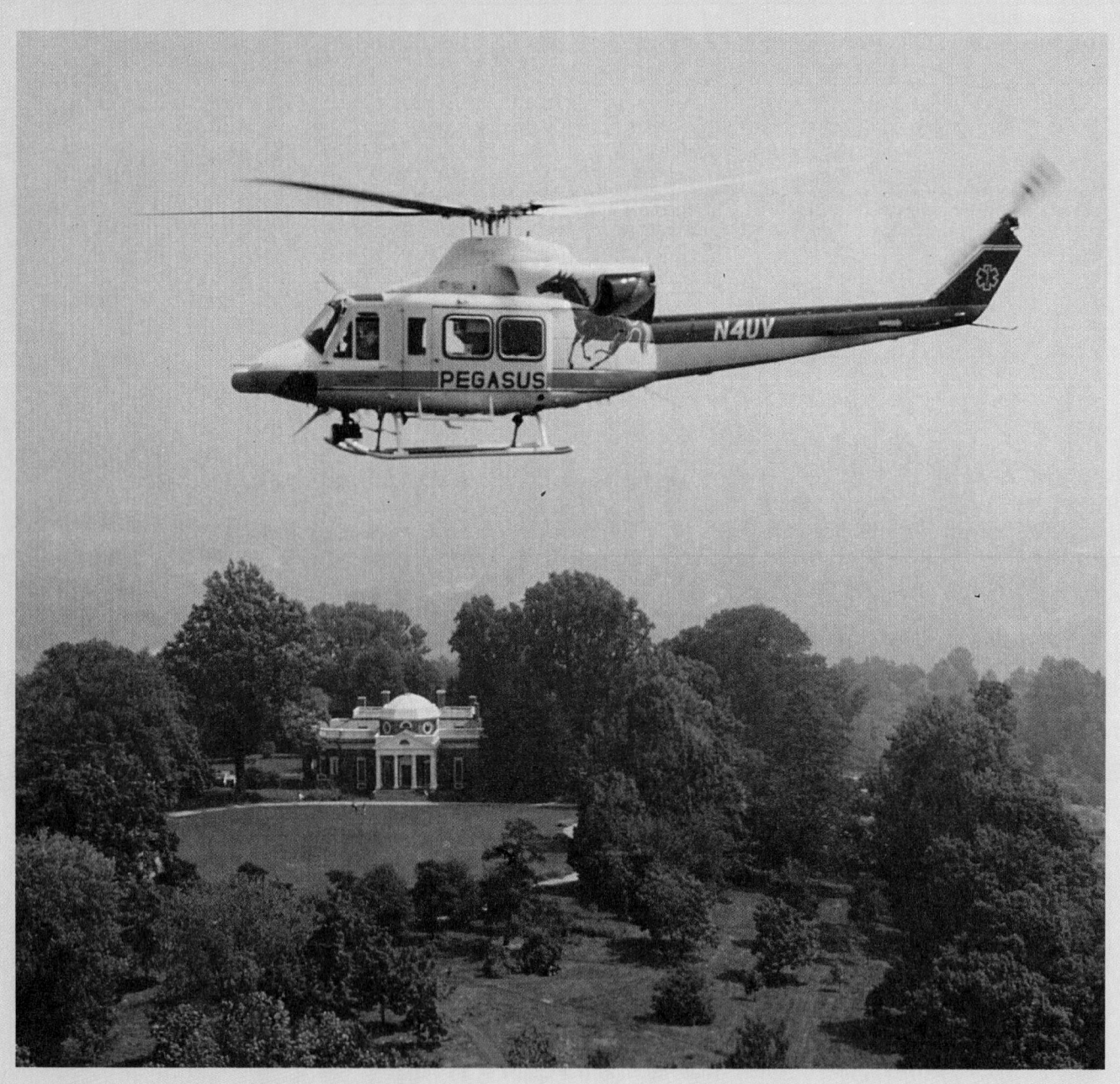

31

GYNECOLOGICAL EMERGENCIES

Objectives for Chapter 31

After reading this chapter, you should be able to:

1. Identify the location and function of the following organs. (See below pages.)

- ovaries (p. 954)
- fallopian tubes (p. 954)
- uterus (pp. 954–956)
- endometrium (p. 956)
- cervix (p. 956)
- vagina (p. 956)
- perineum (p. 956)
- labia (p. 956)

2. Describe the stages of the menstrual cycle. (See p. 957.)

3. Discuss assessment of the gynecological patient. (See pp. 957–958.)

4. Discuss the recognition and management of pelvic inflammatory disease (PID). (See p. 959.)

5. Discuss nontraumatic causes of gynecological abdominal pain in the female. (See pp. 959–960.)

6. Discuss the physical and psychological implications of rape and sexual assault, and describe prehospital management. (See pp. 960–962.)

The dispatcher sends Unit 38 of the Wilmington EMS to a local shopping mall. When the paramedics arrive, a mall security guard escorts them to the administrative office. There, the paramedics find a morbidly obese female patient lying on the couch. The tearful patient complains of excruciating lower abdominal pain.

The paramedics complete a primary and secondary assessment. The patient's vital signs are stable. Her pulse rate is 100. The tilt test is negative. The pain appears to be in the lower left quadrant, but it is difficult to determine because of the patient's obesity. The paramedics administer oxygen and insert an IV of lactated Ringer's solution. With the help of mall security, they take the patient to the ambulance. She remains stable throughout transport.

In the emergency department, a urine sample tests positive for pregnancy. A pelvic ultrasound examination reveals an ectopic pregnancy in the left fallopian tube. Doctors take the patient into surgery where they remove both her left fallopian tube and the ectopic pregnancy. After the operation, the patient has some respiratory problems as a result of her obesity. She spends 24 hours on the ventilator and is then weaned. She is discharged 5 days later.

INTRODUCTION

■ **gynecology** the branch of medicine that treats disorders of the female reproductive system.

Gynecology is the branch of medicine that deals with the female reproductive tract. Therefore, gynecological emergencies involve some part of the female reproductive system. Most gynecological emergency patients that you encounter will experience either abdominal pain or vaginal bleeding. This chapter discusses the nonpregnant patient. The obstetrical patient forms the subject of Chapter 32.

ANATOMY AND PHYSIOLOGY

It is essential that you have a thorough understanding of the anatomy and physiology of the female reproductive system. This knowledge will allow you to better understand, recognize, and treat gynecological emergencies when they arise.

Female Reproductive Organs

The female reproductive organs are located entirely within the pelvic cavity, close to the urinary bladder. (See Figure 31-1.) The female reproductive tract consists of the following organs.

❑ *Ovaries.* The ovaries, located at the lateral aspect of the fallopian tubes, are the female gonads. (See Figure 31-2.) Their function is twofold. First, they produce estrogen and progesterone in response to follicle stimulating hormone (FSH) and luteinizing hormone (LH) secreted from the anterior pituitary gland. Second, they produce eggs for reproduction.

❑ *Fallopian Tubes.* The fallopian tubes, also called the uterine tubes, are hollow tubes that transport the egg from the ovary to the uterus. Fertilization usually occurs in the fallopian tube.

❑ *Uterus.* The uterus is a small, pear-shaped organ that connects with the vagina. The uterus is the organ in which the developing fetus grows. It stretches from a length of about 5 cm, in the nonpregnant state, to a size capable of containing an 8-pound fetus (approximately 40 cm in length).

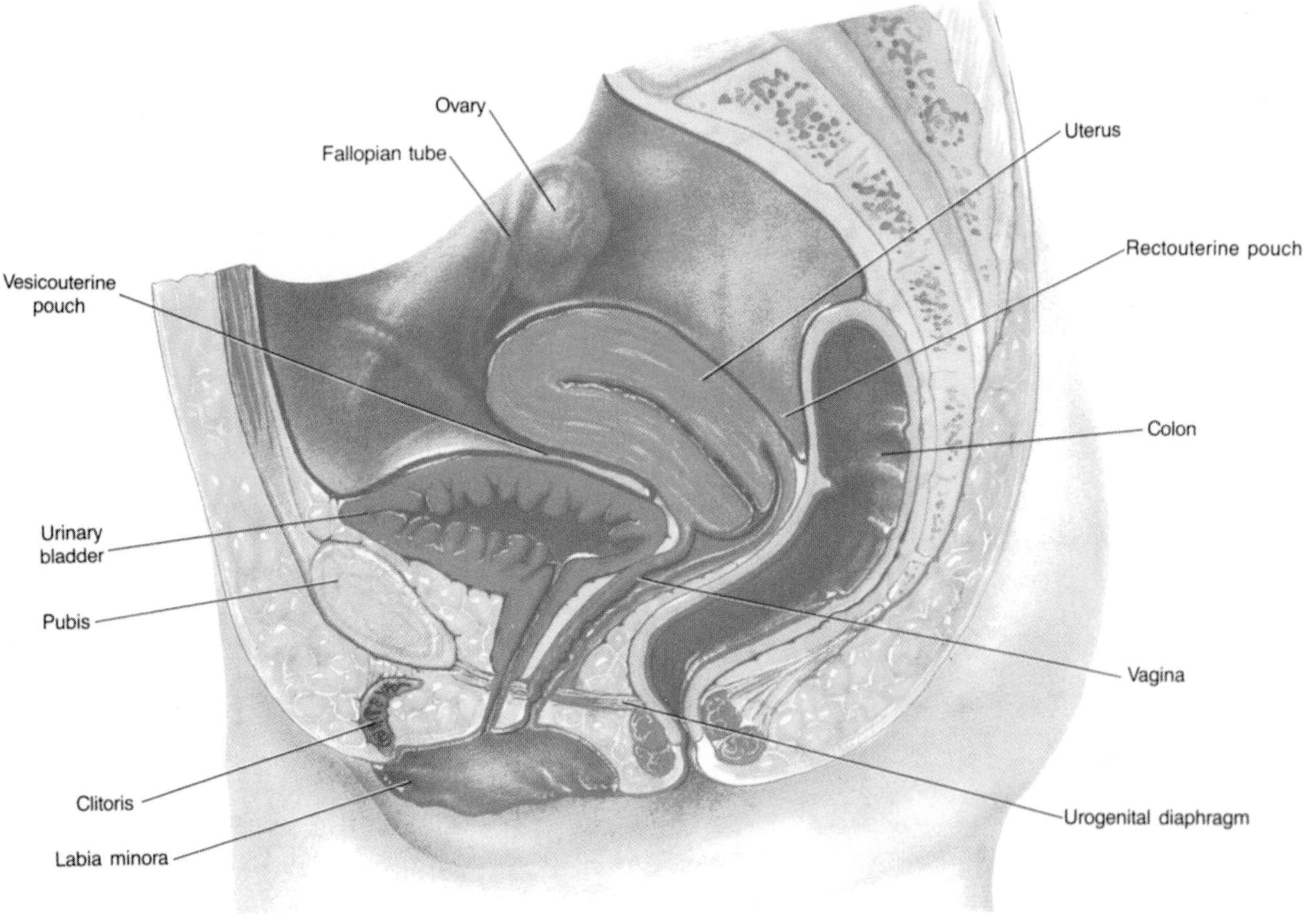

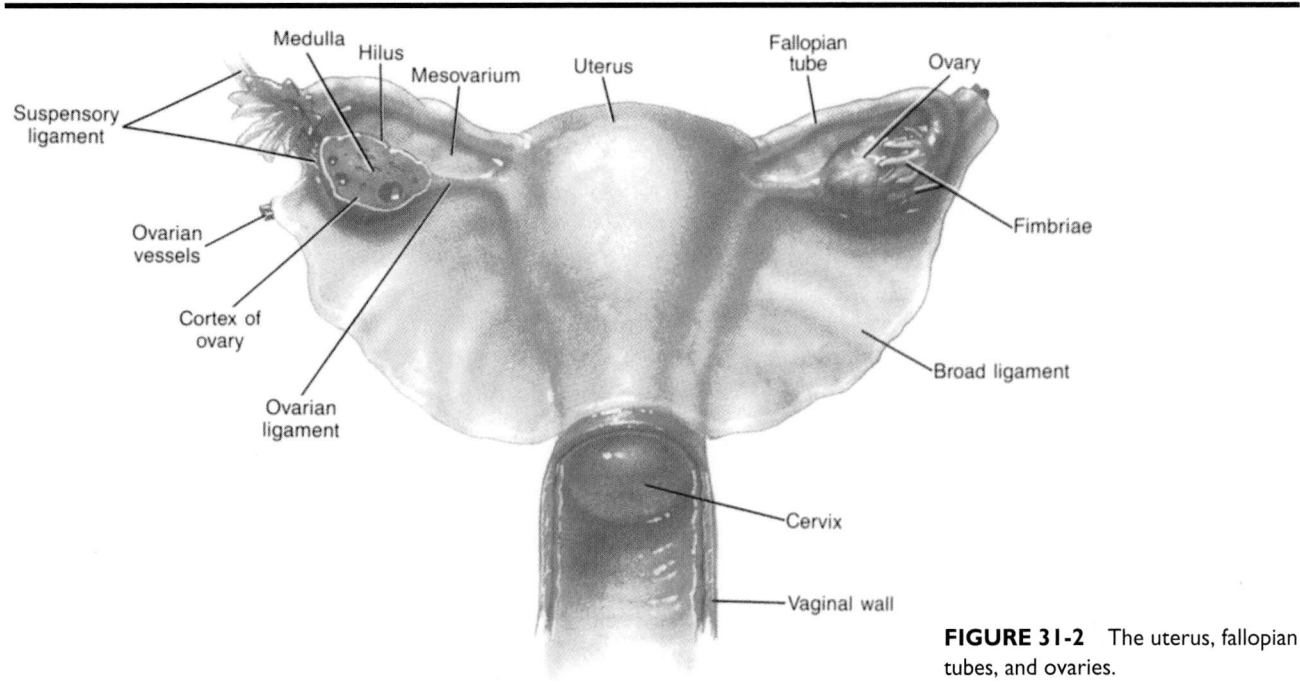

FIGURE 31-1 Cross-sectional anatomy of the female reproductive system.

FIGURE 31-2 The uterus, fallopian tubes, and ovaries.

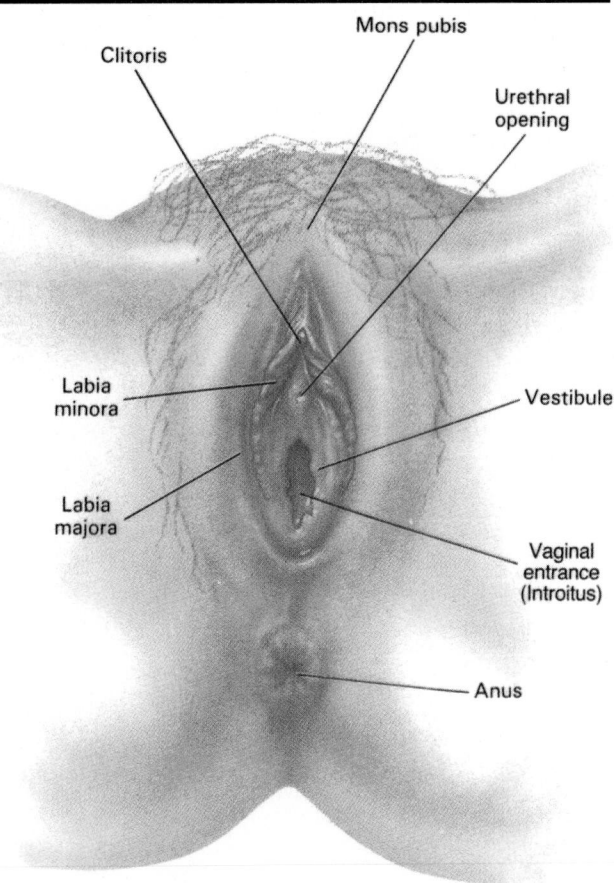

FIGURE 31-3 The vulva.

The upper portion of the uterus is referred to as the *fundus*. The lower portion of the uterus, which extends into the vagina, is referred to as the *cervix*.

■ **endometrium** the inner lining of the uterus where the fertilized egg implants.

❑ *Endometrium.* The **endometrium** is the lining of the uterus. Each month, under the influence of estrogen and progesterone, the endometrium builds up in preparation for the implantation of a fertilized ovum. If fertilization does not occur, the lining simply sloughs off. This sloughing off of the uterine lining is referred to as the *menstrual period.*

❑ *Cervix.* The cervix, or "neck" of the uterus, is visible thorough the vagina. During labor, the cervix dilates from its closed state to a diameter of approximately 10 cm, thus allowing for passage of the baby.

❑ *Vagina.* The vagina is the connection between the uterus and the outside of the body. It is the female sex organ and receives the penis during intercourse.

❑ *Perineum.* The term perineum refers to the area surrounding the vagina and anus. This area is sometimes torn during childbirth.

❑ *Labia.* The labia are the structures that protect the vagina and the urethra. There are two distinct sets of labia. (See Figure 31-3.) The *labia majora* are located laterally. The *labia minora* are more medial. Both sets of labia are subject to injury during trauma to the perineal area, such as occurs with rape.

❑ *Urethra.* The urinary bladder drains through the urethra, which is located superior and anterior to the vagina. In the human female, the urethra is only 2–3 cm in length. Because the female urethra is so short, bacteria travel more easily to the bladder than in the male. Therefore, the female is more susceptible to bladder infections than the male. As a rule, females tend to have more frequent bladder infections once they become sexually active.

Menstrual Cycles

The female undergoes a monthly hormonal cycle that prepares the uterus to receive a fertilized egg. A girl's menses, or menstrual periods, usually begin when she is between 12 and 14 years old. The beginning of the menses is termed **menarche**. At first, the periods are irregular. Later they become more regular and predictable.

■ **menarche** the onset of menses, usually occurring between ages 12 and 14.

The menstrual cycle is influenced by estrogen and progesterone, which are produced by the ovaries. In turn, secretion of estrogen and progesterone is controlled by secretion of FSH and LH from the anterior pituitary.

A "normal" menstrual cycle depends upon the regular pattern in the individual woman. Day 1 of the menstrual cycle is the day on which bleeding begins. The menstrual flow usually lasts from 3 to 5 days. But this number varies from woman to woman. The average menstrual cycle lasts approximately 28 days. But this number also varies from one woman to another.

The first two weeks of the menstrual cycle are dominated by estrogen. Estrogen causes the lining of the uterus to thicken and to become engorged with blood vessels. This is referred to as the *proliferative phase*. At approximately day 14, a sudden surge in LH secretion causes the ovary to release an egg, which matured over the first two weeks of the menstrual cycle. Release of an egg from the ovary is called *ovulation*. The egg is grasped by fine, hairlike structures in the end of the fallopian tube. These structures sweep the egg toward the uterus. If the woman has had sexual intercourse within approximately 24 hours of ovulation, fertilization may take place. If the egg is fertilized, it normally implants in the thickened lining of the uterus, where the fetus subsequently develops. The stage of the menstrual cycle immediately surrounding ovulation is referred to as the *secretory phase*.

If the egg is not fertilized, as normally happens, the woman's estrogen level falls. The uterine lining then sloughs away, starting a new menstrual cycle. The interval immediately preceding and including the menstrual period is referred to as the *menstrual phase*. The absence of a menstrual period, especially in a woman whose periods are usually regular and who is sexually active, should raise the suspicion of pregnancy.

Menstrual periods continue to occur until a woman is in her forties or fifties. At that time, they begin to decline in frequency and length, until they ultimately stop. This stoppage of the menstrual cycle is referred to as **menopause**. Occasionally, physicians use the term *surgical menopause*, which means that a woman's periods have stopped because of surgical removal of her uterus, ovaries, or both.

■ **menopause** the cessation of menses and the end of a woman's reproductive life.

ASSESSMENT OF THE GYNECOLOGICAL PATIENT

Assessment of the gynecological patient should include the standard primary and secondary assessment described earlier in Chapter 10. In addition, you should ask specific questions about the patient's history. Most gynecological patients have lower abdominal pain or discomfort and/or vaginal bleeding. If pain is present, it is important to determine its character. Is it sharp or dull? How did the pain start—suddenly or gradually? How long has the pain lasted? Is it persistent or intermittent? Where is the pain located? Does it radiate anywhere? Is there anything that makes the pain better or worse?

History

Determine if the patient has other medical problems, such as a bladder infection or kidney stones. Quickly gather the obstetric history. The patient should be able to relate the number of times she has been pregnant, or her *gravidity*, and the number of pregnancies that have produced a viable infant, or her *parity*. Also, question the patient about previous cesarean sections, pelvic surgeries, and dilation and curettage (D&C) procedures.

* In the female patient of childbearing age, always document the LMP.

It is important to document the date of the patient's last menstrual period, commonly abbreviated LMP. Ask whether the period was of a normal length and whether the flow was heavier or lighter than usual. An easy way for women to estimate menstrual flow is by the number of pads or tampons used. She can easily compare this number to her routine usage. It is also important to inquire how regular the patient's periods tend to be. Ask the patient what form of birth control, if any, she uses. Also, find out if she uses it regularly.

With the exception of oral contraceptives ("the pill") and intrauterine devices (IUD), side-effects caused by contraceptives are relatively rare. Oral contraceptives have been associated with hypertension, rare incidents of stroke and heart attack, and possibly pulmonary embolism. IUDs can cause perforation of the uterus, uterine infection, or irregular uterine bleeding. This is especially true for IUDs that have remained in place longer than the time recommended by the manufacturer, which rarely exceeds 2 years.

Until proven otherwise, you should assume than any missed or late period is due to pregnancy. If you suspect pregnancy, inquire about other signs, including breast tenderness, bloating, urinary frequency, or nausea and vomiting. Question the patient about the presence or absence of vaginal discharge. It is helpful to ascertain the color of the discharge and the presence of any associated odor or blood. Also, ask the patient about any prior history of trauma to the reproductive tract. Occasionally, it is helpful to ascertain whether the patient, if sexually active, has had pain or bleeding during or after sexual intercourse.

In addition to gynecological symptoms, ask the patient about other associated symptoms such as fever, chills, syncope, diaphoresis, diarrhea, or constipation. It is important to remember that patients with gynecological complaints may be embarrassed or frightened about discussing these problems. Assess the patient's emotional state. If a patient does not care to discuss her complaint in detail, respect her wishes and transport her to the emergency department, where a more detailed assessment can be completed.

Physical Examination

Physical examination of the gynecological patient is limited in the field. Primary and secondary assessment should be completed. Pay particular attention to the abdominal examination. Document and report any masses, distention, guarding, or tenderness. If significant bleeding is reported or evident, it may be necessary to inspect the patient's perineum. Document the character of the discharge, including color, amount, and the presence or absence of clots. DO NOT PERFORM AN INTERNAL VAGINAL EXAM IN THE FIELD.

* Do not perform an internal vaginal exam in the field.

GYNECOLOGICAL EMERGENCIES

Gynecological emergencies can be generally divided into two categories—medical and traumatic.

Medical Gynecological Emergencies

Gynecological emergencies of a medical nature are often hard to diagnose in the field. Probably the most common cause of nontraumatic abdominal pain is pelvic inflammatory disease (PID).

Pelvic Inflammatory Disease. *Pelvic inflammatory disease* is an infection of the female reproductive tract. The organs most commonly involved are the uterus, fallopian tubes, and ovaries. Occasionally, the adjoining structures, such as the peritoneum and intestines, also become involved. The most common causes of PID are gonorrhea and chlamydial infections. In addition, other bacteria, such as staph or strep, can be causative agents. Commonly, gonorrhea or chlamydia progresses undetected in a female until frank PID develops.

PID may be either acute or chronic. If it is allowed to progress untreated, sepsis may develop. In addition, PID may cause the pelvic organs to "stick together," causing adhesions. Adhesions are a common cause of chronic pelvic pain. They also increase the frequency of ectopic pregnancies.

Assessment of the Patient With PID. The most common complaint of patients with PID is abdominal pain. It is often diffuse and located along the lower abdomen. It may be moderate to severe, which occasionally makes it difficult to distinguish from appendicitis. Pain may intensify either before or after the menstrual period. It may also worsen during sexual intercourse, as movement of the cervix tends to cause discomfort. Patients with PID tend to walk with a shuffling gait, since walking often intensifies their pain.

In severe cases, PID may be accompanied by fever, chills, nausea, and vomiting. Occasionally, patients have an associated vaginal discharge, often yellow in color, as well as irregular menses.

Generally, on physical examination, the patient with PID appears acutely ill or toxic. The blood pressure is normal, although the pulse rate may be slightly increased. Fever may or may not be present. Palpation of the lower abdomen generally elicits moderate to severe pain. Occasionally, in severe cases, the abdomen will be tense with obvious rebound tenderness. Such cases may be impossible to distinguish from appendicitis.

Emergency Management of the Patient with PID. The primary treatment for PID is antibiotics, often administered intravenously over an extended period. In the field, the primary goal is to make the patient as comfortable as possible. Generally, the abdominal pain of PID increases when the patient is walking. The patient should be placed on the ambulance stretcher in the position in which she is most comfortable. She may wish to draw her knees up toward her chest, as this decreases tension on the peritoneum. DO NOT PERFORM A VAGINAL EXAMINATION.

Other Nontraumatic Causes of Gynecological Abdominal Pain

In addition to pelvic inflammatory disease, there are other nontraumatic causes of gynecological abdominal pain with which you should be familiar.

Ectopic Pregnancy. Many different problems with the female reproductive system can cause abdominal pain. One problem that emergency department personnel should quickly rule out is ectopic pregnancy. **Ectopic pregnancy** is the implantation of a growing fetus in a place where it does not belong. The most common site is within the fallopian tubes. This is a surgical emergency, because the tube can rupture, triggering massive hemorrhage. Patients with ectopic pregnancy often have one-sided abdominal pain, a late or missed menstrual period, and, occasionally, vaginal bleeding. Additional discussion of ectopic pregnancy is presented in Chapter 32.

Ovarian Cysts. Cysts are fluid-filled pockets. When they develop in the ovary, they can rupture and be a source of abdominal pain. When an egg is released from the ovary, a cyst is often left in its place. Occasionally, cysts develop independent of ovulation. When the cysts rupture, a small amount of blood is spilled into the abdomen. Because blood irritates the peritoneum, it can cause abdominal pain and rebound tenderness.

Appendicitis. As mentioned previously, appendicitis is very difficult to distinguish from PID or even ectopic pregnancy in the field. Patients with appendicitis usually have abdominal pain that begins around the navel and slowly migrates to the right lower quadrant. The pain may be associated with anorexia, fever, nausea, vomiting, or even shock.

Cystitis. Bladder infection, or *cystitis*, is a common cause of abdominal pain. The bladder lies anterior to the reproductive organs and, when inflamed, causes pain, generally immediately above the symphysis pubis.

Other Pelvic Infections. Women who have had recent gynecological surgeries, induced abortions, miscarriages, or delivery of babies can subsequently develop pelvic infections. These infections often present themselves in a manner similar to PID. Therefore, it is important to determine if a woman has recently had any gynecological surgical procedures. An occasional complication of childbirth or gynecological procedures is an infection of the uterine lining. This disorder, *endometritis*, can be quite serious if not quickly treated.

Mittleschmertz. Occasionally, a woman has a day or two of abdominal pain halfway through her menstrual cycle. The pain, referred to as *mittleschmertz*, is associated with release of the egg from the ovary. The pain is usually self-limited and treatment is symptomatic.

Management of Gynecological Abdominal Pain Any woman with significant abdominal pain should be treated and transported to the hospital. Administer oxygen, if indicated. Establish an IV with lactated Ringer's or a similar solution, since rupture of an ectopic pregnancy can cause significant, rapid blood loss into the abdomen.

Traumatic Gynecological Emergencies

Most cases of vaginal bleeding result from obstetrical problems or are related to the menstrual period. However, trauma to the vagina and perineum can also cause bleeding.

Causes of Gynecological Trauma

Causes of gynecological trauma include straddle injuries (such as may occur with a bicycle), blows to the perineal area, foreign bodies inserted into the vagina, attempts at abortion, lacerations following childbirth, and sexual assault. Injuries to the external genitalia should be managed by simple pressure over the laceration. In most cases of vaginal bleeding, the source is not readily apparent. If bleeding is severe, start an IV of lactated Ringer's solution in order to maintain intravascular volume. Monitor the patient's vital signs closely. If required, apply anti-shock trousers. NEVER pack the vagina with any material or dressing, regardless of the severity of the bleeding. Transport the patient to the emergency department rapidly.

Sexual Assault

Sexual assault is one of the fastest-growing crimes in the United States. Unfortunately, it is estimated that more than 60 percent of all sexual assaults are never reported to authorities. Sexual abuse of children is reported even less frequently. There is no "typical victim" of sexual assault. Nobody, from small children to aged adults, is immune.

Sexual assault is sexual contact without the consent of the person assaulted. Definitions vary from state to state; but, as a rule, *rape* is defined as penetration of the vagina or rectum of an unwilling female or the rectum in an unwilling male. In most states, penetration must occur for an act to be classified as rape. Regardless of the legal definition, sexual assault is a crime of violence with serious physical and psychological implications.

Most victims of sexual assault know their assailants. The motivation of the rapist is often unclear. However, humiliation, control of the victim, the desire to inflict pain, or frank aggression, have been implicated as motives.

Assessment of the Victim of Sexual Assault.

Most victims of sexual abuse are female. However, males are not immune, especially male children. As a rule, victims of sexual abuse SHOULD NOT be questioned about the incident in the field. It is not important, from the standpoint of prehospital care, to determine whether penetration took place. Do not inquire about the patient's sexual practices. Even well-intentioned questions may lead to guilt feelings in the patient.

The victim of sexual assault may be withdrawn or hysterical. Some victims use denial, anger, or fear as defense mechanisms. The victim should be approached calmly and professionally. If he or she is incompletely dressed, a cover should be offered. Respect the victim's modesty. Explain all procedures before beginning them. Avoid touching the patient other than to take vital signs or examine other physical injuries. DO NOT examine the genitalia unless there is life-threatening hemorrhage.

Management of the Sexual Assault Patient.

Psychological and emotional support is the most important help you can offer. Maintain a nonjudgmental attitude and assure the victim of confidentiality. If the victim is female, allow her to be cared for by a female EMT or paramedic (if available). If the victim desires, have a female accompany her to the hospital. (See Figure 31-4.) Provide a safe environment, such as the back of a well-lit ambulance. Respond to the victim's feelings and respect his or her wishes. Unless the victim has life-threatening injuries, verbally obtain permission to treat before you begin your assessment.

Preservation of physical evidence is important. When the patient arrives at the hospital, a physician will complete a sexual assault examination. At that

✱ Psychological and emotional support should be afforded the sexual assault victim.

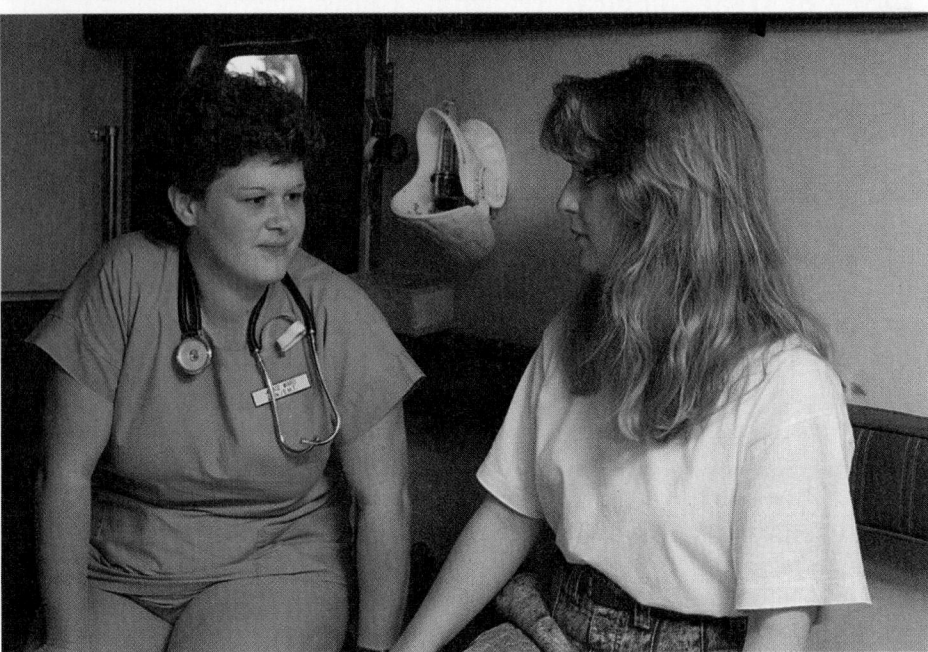

FIGURE 31-4 If possible, have a female EMT or paramedic accompany the victim of alleged sexual assault to the hospital.

time, various legal physical evidence will be gathered. To protect this evidence, it is important that you adhere to the following guidelines.

- ❏ Handle clothing as little as possible, if at all.
- ❏ Do not examine the perineal area.
- ❏ Do not use plastic bags for blood-stained articles.
- ❏ Bag each item separately, if they must be bagged.
- ❏ Do not allow patients to comb their hair or clean their fingernails.
- ❏ Do not allow patients to change their clothes, bathe, or douche (if female) before the medical examination.
- ❏ Do not clean wounds, if at all possible.

SUMMARY

Most gynecological emergency patients have either abdominal pain or vaginal bleeding. The patient with abdominal pain should be made comfortable and transported to the emergency department. The management of vaginal bleeding depends on the severity. Minor bleeding should be simply monitored. Severe bleeding should be treated with IV fluids and/or antishock trousers, if indicated.

In the case of sexual assault, you should first determine if any life-threatening physical injuries exist. Second, respect the victim's wishes and offer emotional support. Third, in treating victims of sexual assault, make every effort to preserve physical evidence. As with any type of emergency care, the primary concern is the patient.

Hafen, Brent, and Keith Karren. *Prehospital Emergency Care and Crisis Intervention*, 4th ed. Englewood Cliffs, NJ: Prentice-Hall, 1992, (Pages 607–609).

Landros, Nedell E. *Assessment and Intervention in Emergency Nursing*, 3rd ed. Norwalk, CT: Appleton and Lange, 1988.

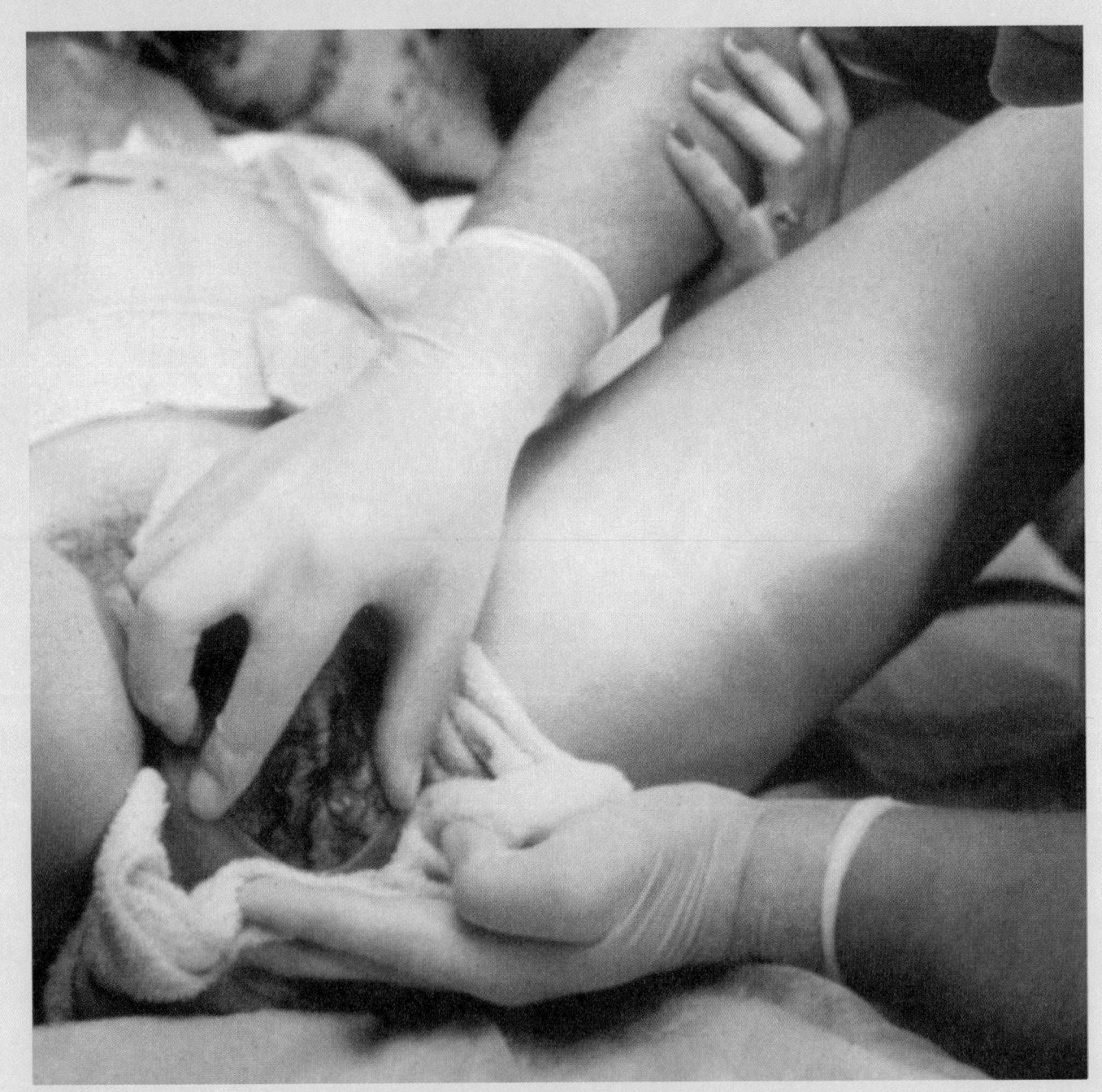

OBSTETRICAL
EMERGENCIES

Objectives for Chapter 32

After reading this chapter, you should be able to:

1. Identify the normal sites of fertilization and implantation of the fertilized egg. (See p. 966.)

2. Describe fetal-maternal blood flow and the role of the placenta. (See pp. 966–967.)

3. Define the following terms. (See below pages.)
- antepartum (p. 970)
- postpartum (p. 970)
- prenatal (p. 970)
- natal (p. 970)
- primigravida (p. 970)
- multigravida (p. 970)
- primipara (p. 970)
- multipara (p. 970)

4. Identify the details of the history that should be obtained from an obstetrical patient. (See pp. 970–971.)

5. Discuss the effects of pregnancy on pre-existing conditions such as diabetes, hypertension, and cardiac problems. (See p. 972.)

6. Define the following terms. (See below pages.)
- spontaneous abortion (p. 974)
- criminal abortion (p. 974)
- therapeutic abortion (p. 974)

7. Describe the management of the patient who has suffered abortion. (See pp. 974–975.)

8. Describe the pathophysiology and management of the following conditions. (See below pages.)
- ectopic pregnancy (p. 975)
- abruptio placentae (pp. 975–977)
- placenta previa (p. 977)

9. Distinguish between pregnancy-induced hypertension, preeclampsia, and eclampsia. (See pp. 977–979.)

10. Describe the pathophysiology and prehospital management of the hypertensive disorders of pregnancy. (See pp. 977–979.)

11. Describe the stages of labor and the approximate length of each stage. (See pp. 981–982.)

12. List and describe the steps of a normal delivery. (See pp. 982–987.)

13. Describe the management, during delivery, of a cord that becomes wrapped around the baby's neck. (See p. 987.)

14. Describe the management of a breech presentation. (See pp. 988–989.)

15. Describe the pathophysiology and management of a prolapsed cord. (See p. 989.)

16. Describe the management of a multiple-birth delivery. (See pp. 989–991.)

17. Describe the pathophysiology and management of the following conditions. (See below pages.)
- postpartum hemorrhage (pp. 991–992)
- uterine inversion (p. 992)
- uterine rupture (p. 992)

As the crew members of Fire Station 29 relax in the television room, they suddenly hear an automobile screech to a halt at the door of the station. The captain rushes to the door and sees an old station wagon parked out front. Beside it, stands a man yelling, "Help! My wife needs help!"

The whole crew spills out the door. In the back seat of the station wagon, they see a 29-year-old pregnant female. She keeps saying, "The baby is coming, the baby is coming!" The ambulance normally based at Station 29 has gone out for gas. The captain notifies fire dispatch, which orders the ambulance to return. Meanwhile, the EMTs assigned to the engine determine that this is the patient's sixth pregnancy and that she feels as though she must move her bowels.

The patient's screams soon change. "I've got to push, I've got to push," she yells. The EMTs don gloves and goggles and check for crowning. They easily spot the top of the baby's head during a contraction. One member of the team retrieves an OB kit and oxygen bottle from the medic box on the fire engine. Shortly thereafter, the patient delivers a viable female infant in the back of the station wagon.

At the time of delivery, the paramedics arrive. They assist the EMT in cutting the cord and wrap the baby in a warming blanket. APGAR scores are 8 at 1 minute and 9 at 5 minutes. The mother receives fundal massage, oxygen, and an IV of lactated Ringer's solution. The paramedics then transport both mother and daughter to the hospital without incident. The next morning, as the Station 29 crew members are walking to their cars, they see a stork artfully painted on the window of the car belonging to the EMT who delivered the baby.

INTRODUCTION

This chapter will address pregnancy and childbirth and the complications associated with them. It is important to remember that childbirth is a natural process and occurs daily. Complications are uncommon, but when they do occur, they must be recognized rapidly and managed accordingly.

THE PRENATAL PERIOD

The prenatal period is the time from conception until delivery of the fetus. During this period, fetal development takes place. In addition, significant physiological changes occur in the mother.

Anatomy and Physiology of the Obstetric Patient

■ **ovulation** the growth and discharge of an egg from the ovary.

Pregnancy begins with ovulation in the female. **Ovulation** is the growth and discharge of an egg, or *ovum*, from the ovary. The ovum develops under the influence of the hormones *estrogen* and *progesterone*. Fourteen days before the beginning of the next menstrual period, the ovum is released from the ovary into the abdominal cavity. It then enters the wide opening of the fallopian tube, where it is transported to the uterus.

If the woman has had intercourse within 24 to 48 hours before ovulation, fertilization may occur in the fallopian tube. *Fertilization* is the combination of the female ovum and the male spermatozoa. (See Figure 32-1.) After fertilization, the ovum begins to divide immediately. The fertilized ovum continues down the fallopian tube to the uterus, where it ultimately attaches itself to the inner lining of the uterus. This process is called *implantation*.

■ **placenta** the organ that supports the fetus during intrauterine development. The placenta is attached to the wall of the uterus and the umbilical cord.

Early in pregnancy, the **placenta** develops. (See Figure 32-2.) The placenta has several important functions for the developing fetus. It provides for

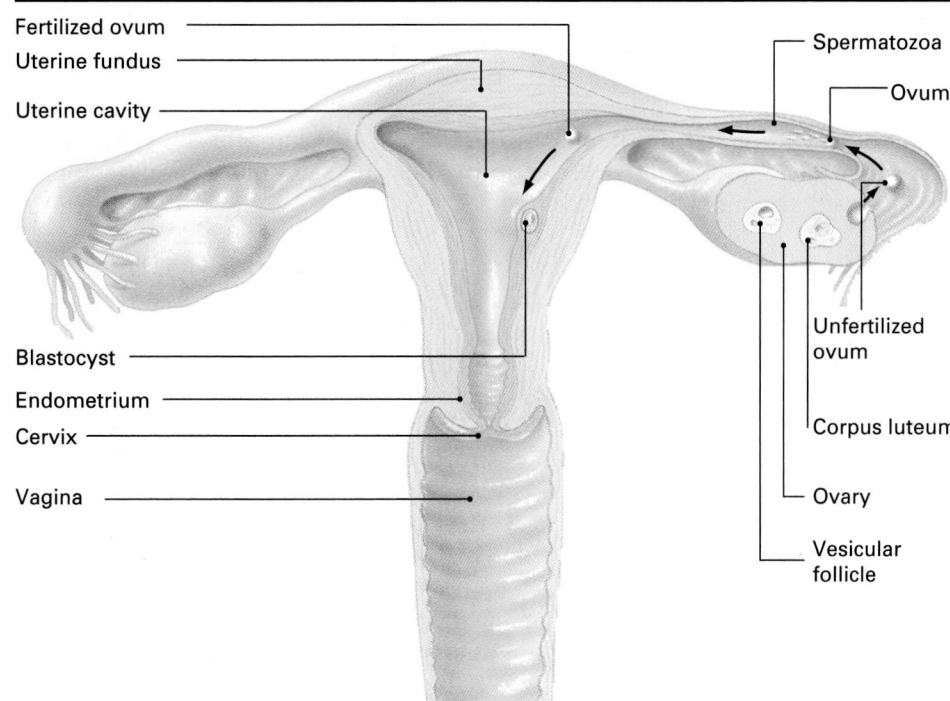

Fertilized ovum
Uterine fundus
Uterine cavity

Spermatozoa
Ovum

Unfertilized ovum

Corpus luteum

Blastocyst
Endometrium
Cervix

Vagina

Ovary

Vesicular follicle

FIGURE 32-1 Fertilization and implantation of the ovum.

the exchange of respiratory gases, transport of nutrients from the mother to the fetus, excretion of wastes, and transfer of heat. In addition, the placenta becomes an active endocrine gland, producing several important hormones.

The placenta is attached to the developing fetus by the **umbilical cord**. This cord normally contains two arteries and one vein. The umbilical vein transports oxygenated blood toward the fetus, while the umbilical arteries return relatively deoxygenated blood to the placenta.

■ **umbilical cord** structure containing 2 arteries and 1 vein that connects the placenta and the fetus.

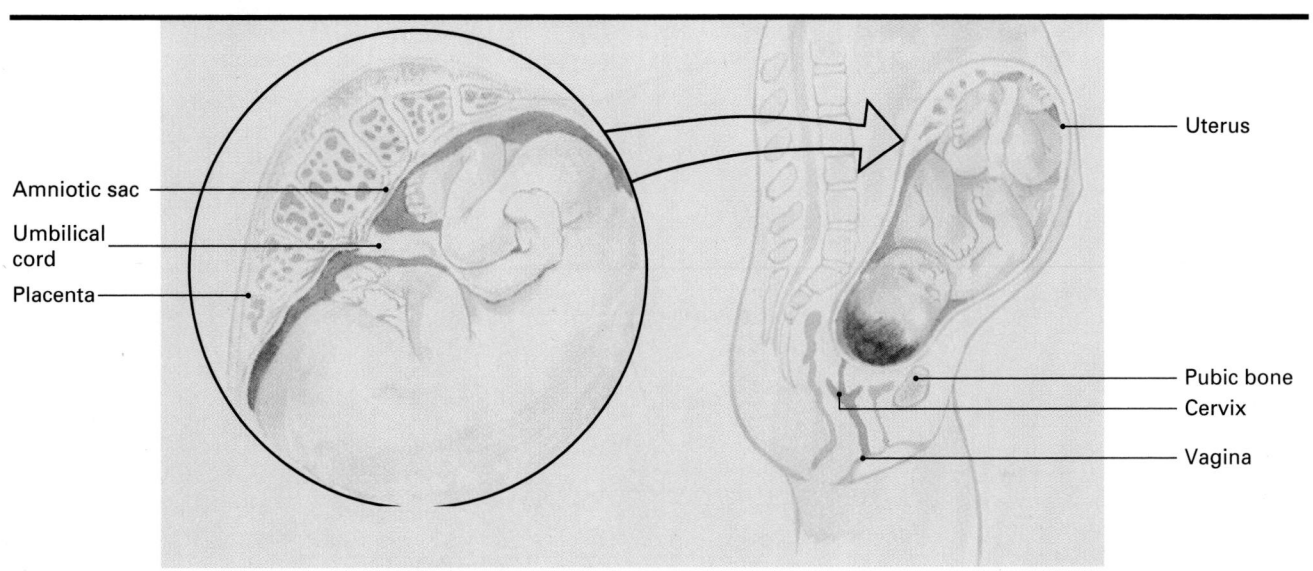

Amniotic sac
Umbilical cord
Placenta

Uterus

Pubic bone
Cervix

Vagina

FIGURE 32-2 Anatomy of the placenta.

The **amniotic sac** also develops early in pregnancy. The amniotic sac consists of membranes that surround and protect the developing fetus throughout intrauterine development. Eventually, the amniotic sac will fill with **amniotic fluid**, which cushions the fetus against trauma and provides a stable environment in which the fetus can develop. The volume of amniotic fluid, approximately 1,000 mL, is maintained by the fetus's continual swallowing of fluid as well as continual urination.

Fetal Development   Fetal development begins immediately after implantation and is quite complex. There are a few developmental milestones with which paramedics should be familiar. First, the normal duration of pregnancy is 40 weeks from the first day of the mother's last menstrual period. This is equal to 10 lunar months or, roughly, 9 calendar months. The time at which fertilization occurs is called *conception*. Conception occurs approximately 14 days after the first day of the last menstrual period. With this knowledge, it is possible to calculate, with fair accuracy, the approximate date the baby should be born. This date is commonly called the *due date*. Medically, it is known as the **estimated date of confinement (EDC)**. The mother is usually told this date on her first prenatal visit.

During normal fetal development, the sex of the infant can usually be determined by the end of the third month. By the end of the fifth month, *fetal heart tones (FHTs)* can be detected by stethoscope. The mother also has generally felt fetal movement. By the end of the sixth month, the baby may be able to survive if born prematurely. Fetuses born after the end of the seventh month have an excellent chance of survival. By the middle of the ninth month the baby is considered *term*, or fully developed. (See Figure 32-3.)

Generally, pregnancy is divided into *trimesters*. Each trimester is approximately 13 weeks, or 3 calendar months. Most of the fetus's organ systems develop during the first trimester. Therefore, this is when the fetus is most vulnerable to the development of birth defects.

Fetal Circulation   The fetus receives its oxygen and nutrients from its mother through the placenta. Thus, while in the uterus, the fetus does not

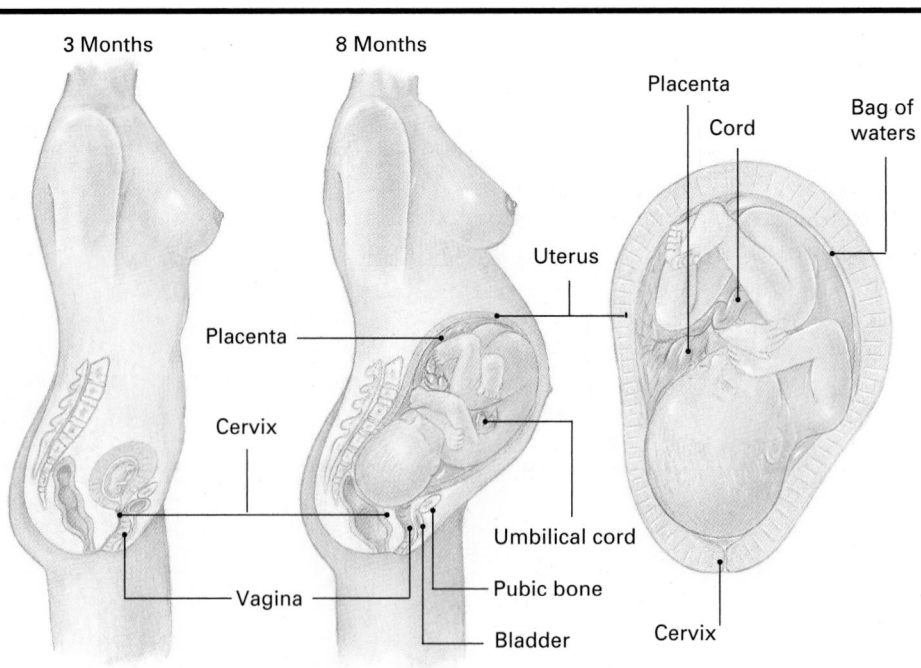

3 Months

8 Months

Placenta
Cord
Bag of waters

Uterus

Placenta

Cervix

Umbilical cord

Pubic bone

Vagina

Bladder

Cervix

FIGURE 32-3   Uterine changes associated with pregnancy.

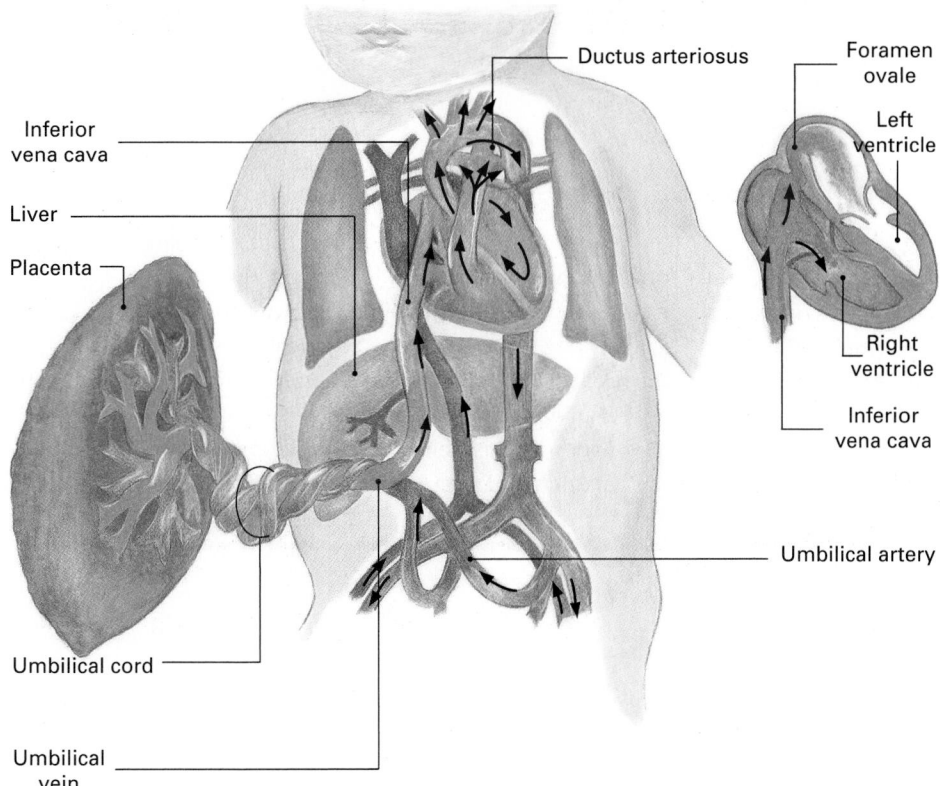

Inferior vena cava

Liver

Placenta

Umbilical cord

Umbilical vein

Ductus arteriosus

Foramen ovale

Left ventricle

Right ventricle

Inferior vena cava

Umbilical artery

FIGURE 32-4 The maternal-fetal circulation.

need to use its respiratory system or its gastrointestinal tract. Because of this, the fetal circulation shunts blood around the lungs and gastrointestinal tract.

The infant receives its blood, from the placenta, by means of the umbilical vein. (See Figure 32-4.) The umbilical vein connects directly to the inferior vena cava by a specialized structure called the *ductus venosus*. Blood then travels through the inferior vena cava to the heart. The blood enters the right atrium and passes through the tricuspid valve into the right ventricle. It then exits the right ventricle, through the pulmonic valve, into the pulmonary artery. The fetus's heart has a hole between the right and left atria, termed the *foramen ovale*, which allows mixing of the oxygenated blood in the right atrium with that leaving the left ventricle bound for the aorta.

At this time, the blood is still oxygenated. Once in the pulmonary artery, the blood enters the *ductus arteriosus*, which connects the pulmonary artery with the aorta. The ductus arteriosus causes blood to bypass the lungs. Once in the aorta, blood flow is basically the same as in extrauterine life. Deoxygenated blood containing waste products exits the fetus, after passage through the liver, via the umbilical arteries.

The fetal circulation changes immediately at birth. As soon as the baby takes his or her first breath, the ambient pressure in the lungs decreases dramatically. Because of this pressure change, the ductus arteriosus closes, diverting blood to the lungs. In addition, the ductus venosus closes, stopping blood flow from the placenta. The foramen ovale also closes as a result of pressure changes in the heart, which stop blood flow from the right to left atrium.

Obstetric Terminology

The field of obstetrics has its own unique terminology. You should be familiar with this terminology, since patient documentation and communications with other health care workers and physicians often require it. (See Table 32-1.)

TABLE 32-1	Common Obstetrical Terminology
Term	**Meaning**
antepartum	the time interval prior to delivery of the fetus
postpartum	the time interval after delivery of the fetus
prenatal	the time interval prior to birth, synonymous with antepartum
natal	literally means birth
gravidity	the number of times a woman has been pregnant
primigravida	a woman who is pregnant for the first time
multigravida	a woman who has been pregnant more than once
nulligravida	a woman who has not been pregnant
parity	the number of times a woman has delivered a viable fetus
primipara	a woman who has delivered her first child
multipara	a woman who has delivered more than one baby
nullipara	a woman who has yet to deliver her first child
grand multiparity	a woman who has delivered at least seven babies

The gravidity and parity of a woman is expressed in the following convention: $G_4 P_2$. "G" refers to the gravidity, and "P" refers to the parity.

Assessment of the Obstetrical Patient

The initial approach to the obstetrical patient should be the same as for the nonobstetrical patient, with special attention paid to the developing fetus. Complete the primary and secondary survey quickly. Next, obtain essential obstetric information.

History   When treating an obstetric patient, obtain information related to the pregnancy, such as the mother's gravidity and parity, the length of gestation, and the estimated date of confinement (EDC), if known. In addition, you should determine whether the patient has had any cesarean sections or any gynecological or obstetrical complications in the past. It is also important to ascertain whether the patient has had any prenatal care.

If the patient is in pain, try to determine when the pain started and whether its onset was sudden or slow. Also, attempt to define the character of the pain—its duration, location, and radiation, if any. It is especially important to determine whether the pain is regular.

The presence of vaginal bleeding or spotting is a major concern in an obstetrical patient. In addition, question the patient about the presence of other vaginal discharges.

A general overview of the patient's current state of health is important. Pay particular attention to current medications and drug and/or medication allergies.

Pregnancy should be highly suspect in a patient who has missed a menstrual period or whose period is late. If the patient is unsure about pregnancy, question her about breast tenderness, urinary frequency, and nausea and vomiting. If pregnancy has been confirmed, then specific questions about **prenatal** care are important. Ask the patient whether a sonogram examination was carried out and what it revealed. A sonogram shows the age of the fetus, the presence of more than one fetus, abnormal presentations, and certain birth defects.

When confronted with a patient in active labor, you should assess whether she feels the need to push or has the urge to move her bowels.

■ **prenatal** means essentially the same thing as "antepartum" and refers to the time period before birth. Health care visits during pregnancy are referred to as "prenatal visits" or "prenatal care."

Determine whether the patient thinks her membranes have ruptured. Patients often sense this as a dribbling of water or, in some cases, a true gush of water.

Physical Examination   Physical examination of the obstetric patient is essentially the same as for any emergency patient. However, you should first estimate the date of the pregnancy by measuring the fundal height. The *fundal height* is the distance from the symphysis pubis to the top of the uterine fundus. Each centimeter of fundal height roughly corresponds to a week of gestation. For example, a woman with a fundal height of 24 cm has a gestational age of approximately 24 weeks. If the fundus is just palpable above the symphysis pubis, the pregnancy is about 12–16 weeks gestation. When the uterine fundus reaches the umbilicus, the pregnancy is about 20 weeks. As pregnancy reaches term, the fundus is palpable near the xiphoid process.

If fetal movement is felt when the abdomen is palpated, the pregnancy is at least 20 weeks. Fetal heart tones can be heard by stethoscope at approximately 18–20 weeks. The normal fetal heart rate ranges from 140–160 beats per minute.

Generally, vital signs in the pregnant patient should be taken with the patient lying on her left side. As pregnancy progresses, the uterus increases in size. Ultimately, when the patient is supine, the weight of the uterus compresses the inferior vena cava, severely compromising venous blood return from the lower extremities. Turning the patient to her left side alleviates this problem. The blood pressure tends to be lower during pregnancy (usually 10–15 Torr), and the pulse rate is faster (10–15 beats per minute). This is because of normal changes occurring in the cardiovascular system.

Occasionally, it may be helpful to perform orthostatic vital signs. First, the blood pressure and pulse rate are obtained after the patient has rested for five minutes in the left lateral recumbent position. Then the vital signs are repeated with the patient sitting up or standing. A drop in the blood pressure level of 15 mm/Hg or more, or an increase in the pulse rate of 20 beats per minute or more, is considered significant and should be reported and documented. When performing this maneuver, it is always important to be alert for syncope. However, remember that this procedure should not be performed if the patient is in obvious shock.

Finally, the patient should be examined for the presence of a *prolapsed cord*, an umbilical cord that comes out of the uterus ahead of the fetus. This can be accomplished simply by looking at the perineum. If, during the physical examination, the patient reports that she feels the need to push, or if she feels as though she must move her bowels, she should be examined for crowning. **Crowning** is the bulging of the fetal head past the opening of the vagina during a contraction. Crowning is an indication of impending delivery. The patient should be examined for crowning only during a contraction. DO NOT CARRY OUT AN INTERNAL VAGINAL EXAMINATION IN THE FIELD.

Complications of Pregnancy

Pregnancy is a normal process. However, women who are pregnant are not immune from other health problems. Several factors, including trauma and pre-existing health problems, complicate pregnancy.

Trauma   Paramedics frequently receive calls to help a pregnant woman who has been in a motor vehicle accident or who has sustained a fall. In pregnancy, syncope occurs frequently. The syncope of pregnancy often results from compression of the inferior vena cava, as described above, or from normal changes in the cardiovascular system associated with pregnancy.

✱ Remember that the blood pressure is normally lower and the pulse rate normally higher throughout pregnancy.

■ **crowning** the bulging of the fetal head past the opening of the vagina during a contraction. Crowning is an indication of impending delivery.

Also, the weight of the gravid uterus alters the patient's balance, making her more susceptible to falls.

Pregnant victims of major trauma are more susceptible to life-threatening injury than are nonpregnant victims, because of the increased vascularity of the gravid uterus. Generally, the amniotic fluid cushions the fetus from blunt trauma fairly well. However, in direct abdominal trauma, the pregnant patient may suffer premature separation of the placenta from the uterine wall, premature labor, abortion, uterine rupture, and possibly, fetal death. The presence of vaginal bleeding or a tender abdomen in a pregnant patient should increase your suspicion of serious injury. Fetal death may result from death of the mother, separation of the placenta from the uterine wall, maternal shock, uterine rupture, or fetal head injury. Any pregnant patient who has suffered trauma should be immediately transported to the emergency department and evaluated by a physician.

Pre-existing or Aggravated Medical Conditions
The pregnant patient is subject to all the medical problems that occur in the nonpregnant state. Abdominal pain is a common complaint. It is often caused by the stretching of the ligaments that support the uterus. However, appendicitis and cholecystitis can also occur. In pregnancy, the abdominal organs are displaced because of the increased mass of the gravid uterus in the abdomen. The pregnant patient with appendicitis may complain of right upper quadrant pain or even back pain. The symptoms of acute cholecystitis may also differ from those in nonpregnant patients. Any pregnant patient with abdominal pain should be evaluated by a physician.

Diabetes. Pregnancy aggravates many medical conditions. One of the most common is diabetes mellitus. Previously diagnosed diabetes can become unstable during pregnancy. Also, many patients develop diabetes during pregnancy (*gestational diabetes*). Pregnant diabetics cannot be managed with oral drugs, since these tend to cross the placenta and affect the fetus. Therefore, all pregnant diabetics are placed on insulin, if their blood sugar levels cannot be controlled by diet alone.

Diabetes also affects the infant. Infants of diabetic mothers, especially those with poorly controlled blood sugar levels, tend to be large. This complicates delivery. Such infants also may have trouble maintaining body temperature after birth and may be subject to hypoglycemia.

Hypertension. Hypertension is also aggravated by pregnancy. Generally, blood pressure is lower in pregnancy than in the nonpregnant state. However, women who were borderline hypertensive before becoming pregnant may become dangerously hypertensive when pregnant. Also, many common blood pressure medications cannot be used during pregnancy. In addition, preeclampsia (discussed later in this chapter) may contribute to maternal hypertension. Persistent hypertension may adversely affect the placenta, thus compromising the fetus as well as placing the mother at increased risk for stroke or renal failure.

Heart Disease. During pregnancy, cardiac output increases up to 30 percent. (See Figure 32-5.) Patients who have serious pre-existing heart disease may develop congestive heart failure in pregnancy. When confronted by a pregnant patient in obvious heart failure, you should inquire about pre-existing heart disease or murmurs. It is important to be aware, however, that most patients develop a quiet systolic flow murmur during pregnancy. This is caused by increased cardiac output and should be documented on the chart. It is rarely a source of concern.

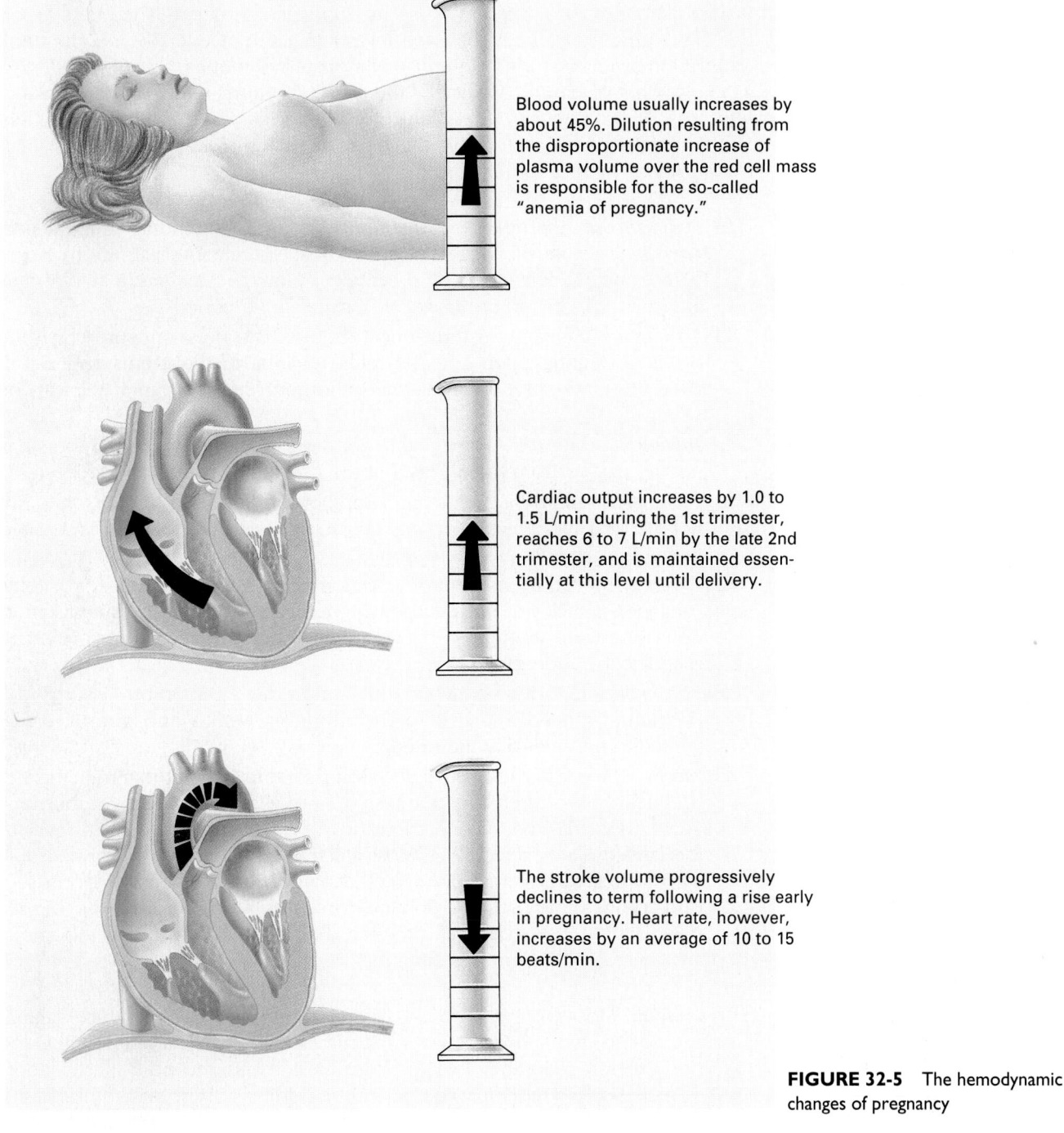

Blood volume usually increases by about 45%. Dilution resulting from the disproportionate increase of plasma volume over the red cell mass is responsible for the so-called "anemia of pregnancy."

Cardiac output increases by 1.0 to 1.5 L/min during the 1st trimester, reaches 6 to 7 L/min by the late 2nd trimester, and is maintained essentially at this level until delivery.

The stroke volume progressively declines to term following a rise early in pregnancy. Heart rate, however, increases by an average of 10 to 15 beats/min.

FIGURE 32-5 The hemodynamic changes of pregnancy

Vaginal Bleeding Vaginal bleeding during pregnancy is always a cause for concern. Bleeding in early pregnancy is often caused by spontaneous abortion, ectopic pregnancy, or vaginal trauma. Third-trimester bleeding can be caused by injury to the vagina or cervix. But it most often results from one of two conditions—*abruptio placentae* or *placenta previa*. Vaginal bleeding can range from simple spotting to life-threatening hemorrhage. Generally, the exact etiology of vaginal bleeding during pregnancy cannot be determined in the field.

Abortion

Abortion is the termination of a pregnancy before the fetus is viable, generally considered to be about 20 weeks gestation. The terms "abortion" and "miscarriage" can be used interchangeably. Generally, people think of abortion as termination of pregnancy at maternal request and of miscarriage as an accident of nature. Medically, the term "abortion" refers to both types of fetal loss. Approximately 15 percent of pregnancies result in abortion. Often, abortion results from defects in the fetus or maternal infection. The several classifications of abortion include:

❏ *Spontaneous Abortion.* A spontaneous abortion, commonly called a *miscarriage*, occurs of its own accord. Most spontaneous abortions occur before the twelfth week of pregnancy. Many occur within two weeks after conception and are mistaken for menstrual periods.

❏ *Threatened Abortion.* A threatened abortion is a pregnancy in which the cervix is slightly open and the fetus remains in the uterus and is still alive. In some cases of threatened abortion, the pregnancy still can be salvaged.

❏ *Inevitable Abortion.* An inevitable abortion is one in which the fetus has not yet passed from the uterus, but the pregnancy cannot be salvaged.

❏ *Incomplete Abortion.* An incomplete abortion is one in which some, but not all, fetal tissue has been passed. Incomplete abortions are associated with a high incidence of infection.

❏ *Criminal Abortion.* A criminal abortion is an attempt to destroy a fetus by a person who is not licensed or permitted to do so. Criminal abortions often are attempted by amateurs. They are rarely performed in aseptic surroundings.

❏ *Therapeutic Abortion.* A therapeutic abortion is an abortion in which the pregnancy posed a threat to the mother's health and abortion was judged to be medically indicated.

❏ *Elective Abortion.* An elective abortion is one in which the termination of pregnancy is desired and requested by the mother. Elective abortions during the first and second trimesters of pregnancy have been legal in the United States since 1973. Most elective abortions are performed during the first trimester of pregnancy. However, some clinics perform second-trimester abortions. Second-trimester abortions have a higher complication rate than first-trimester abortions. Third-trimester abortions are generally illegal in this country.

Assessment. Most women who are having abortions will experience vaginal bleeding. Often, women who have first-trimester miscarriages report passing tissue or excessive clotting. In late first-trimester and second-trimester abortions, a recognizable fetus may be passed. In addition, there will often be significant abdominal cramping and pain. If the abortion was not recent, then frank signs and symptoms of infection may be present.

The physical examination should include orthostatic vital signs, if possible. Examine the external genitalia to determine how much bleeding or tissue is present. Any tissue or large clots should be retained and given to emergency department personnel.

Management. The abortion patient should be treated in the same manner as any patient at risk for hypovolemic shock. Administer oxygen, and establish an IV of normal saline or lactated Ringer's solution to restore lost fluid volume. If the patient is bleeding severely and shock is impending, establish a second IV and apply antishock trousers.

As mentioned above, any tissue or large clots should be retained and given to emergency department personnel. If the abortion occurs during the late first trimester or later, a fetus may be passed. Often, the placenta does not detach, and the fetus is suspended by the umbilical cord. In such a case, place the umbilical clamps from the OB kit on the cord and cut it. Carefully wrap the fetus in linen or other suitable material, and transport it to the hospital with the mother.

An abortion is generally a very sad time. Provide emotional support to the parents. Parents who wish to view the fetus should be allowed to do so. Occasionally, Roman Catholic parents request baptism of the fetus. This can be performed by making the sign of a cross and stating, "I baptize you in the name of the father, the son, and the holy spirit. Amen."

Ectopic Pregnancy   An *ectopic pregnancy*, the implantation of a fertilized ovum outside of the uterus, occurs once in approximately 200 pregnancies. The most common implantation site is in a fallopian tube. However, the ovum can attach to an ovary or anywhere in the abdominal cavity.

✳ Treat any female of childbearing age with lower abdominal pain as pregnant and with an ectopic pregnancy until proven otherwise.

An ectopic pregnancy is a medical emergency. The developing fetus can grow so large that it may rupture the fallopian tube, causing extensive bleeding into the pelvis and abdominal cavity. Women can die from the complications of ruptured ectopic pregnancies.

Several predisposing factors can lead to ectopic pregnancy. They include previous pelvic infections, such as PID, pelvic adhesions from prior abdominal surgery, tubal ligations, or the presence of an IUD. All of these tend to scar the fallopian tube, thus preventing transport of the fetus to its normal implantation site in the uterus.

Most patients with ectopic pregnancy have abdominal pain, which may be severe. Often, there is associated vaginal bleeding. In 15–20 percent of cases, women report shoulder pain, which is probably referred pain. Many patients report a missed period or intermittent spotting over 6–8 weeks. Patients often report pregnancy-associated symptoms, such as breast tenderness, nausea, vomiting, or fatigue. Many patients report a prior history of PID, tubal ligation, previous ectopic pregnancy, or pelvic surgeries.

Assessment. The patient with ectopic pregnancy is at risk for the rapid development of shock. Take vital signs frequently and regularly. Orthostatic vital signs may be helpful, unless the patient is in frank shock. The abdominal examination may reveal significant lower quadrant tenderness, often more pronounced on one side than the other. Rebound tenderness or rigidity may be present. Avoid repeated abdominal examination, as this may cause the ectopic pregnancy to rupture. Vaginal bleeding may range from spotting to profuse hemorrhage. Do not perform a vaginal examination in the field.

Management. Ectopic pregnancy is difficult to diagnose in the field. However, a patient suspected of suffering ectopic pregnancy should be handled like any patient in shock or at risk of hypovolemic shock. The patient should receive high-flow oxygen and ventilatory support as indicated. Start an IV of lactated Ringer's solution or normal saline. Repeat vital signs regularly. If the patient is in shock, apply antishock trousers. Transport should be rapid, as prompt surgical intervention is required.

Third-Trimester Bleeding—Abruptio Placentae   *Abruptio placentae* is the premature separation of the placenta from the wall of the uterus. (See Figure 32-6.) Separation can be either partial or complete. Complete separation almost always results in death of the fetus. Several factors may predis-

Abruptio placentae (premature separation)

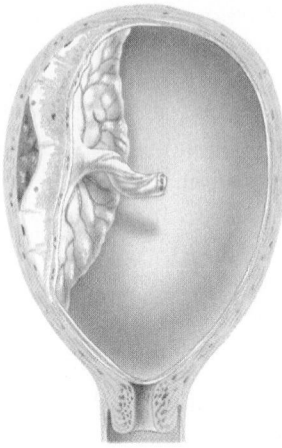 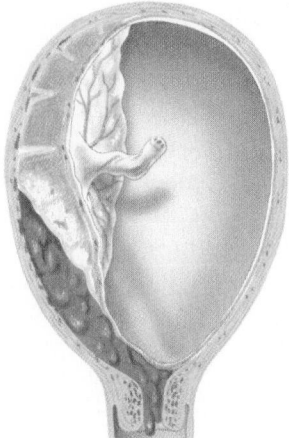 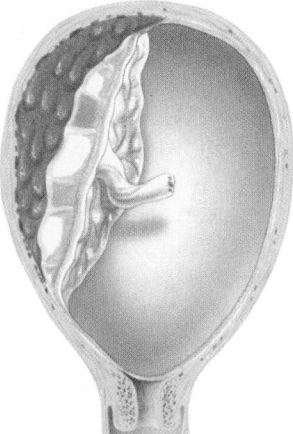

Partial separation
(concealed hemorrhage)
    Partial separation
(apparent hemorrhage)
    Complete separation
(concealed hemorrhage)

Placenta previa (abnormal implantation)

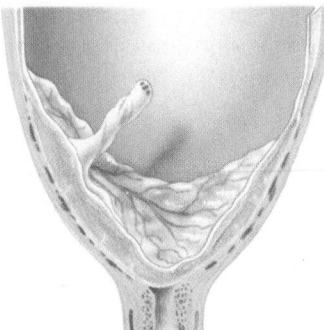 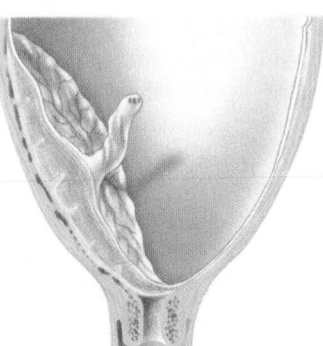

Total placenta
previa
    Partial placenta
previa

FIGURE 32-6 Third-trimester bleeding emergencies.

■ **multiparity** a woman who has delivered more than one baby.

✱ Internal vaginal exams should not be carried out in the prehospital set-

pose a patient to abruptio placentae. These include preeclampsia, maternal hypertension, **multiparity**, abdominal trauma, or an extremely short umbilical cord.

When abruptio placentae occurs, blood tends to collect behind the separating placenta. As a result, vaginal blood loss is minimal. If the placenta is not completely separated, it may apply pressure on the bleeding uterine wall. If the placenta separates completely, this pressure is lost and severe hemorrhage can occur quite suddenly.

Assessment. Most frequently, patients suffering abruptio placenta have constant, severe abdominal pain. Often the patient says that the pain "feels like something is tearing." The abdomen is very tender. Vaginal bleeding may range from absent to very heavy. If present, bleeding will be very dark in color. Occasionally, the patient has a history of abruptio placenta in previous pregnancies.

Physical examination will reveal a very tender uterus that may feel tightly contracted. Fetal heart tones may be slow or absent. Do not perform a vaginal examination in the field.

Management. In abruptio placentae there are two lives at stake. First, administer oxygen at high concentration. The fetus also receives oxygen when it is administered to the mother, unless complete abruption has occurred. Second, establish one or two large-bore IVs with either lactated Ringer's solution or normal saline. Monitor vital signs and fetal heart tones continuously. If shock is impending, apply antishock trousers without inflating the abdominal compartment. Transport the patient rapidly. If the fetus is still viable, the definitive treatment is cesarean section.

Third-Trimester Bleeding—Placenta Previa

Placenta previa is the attachment of the placenta very low in the uterus so that it partially or completely covers the internal cervical *os*, or opening. (See Figure 32-6.) There are three categories of placenta previa: complete, partial, and marginal. *Complete placenta previa* completely covers the internal cervical os and is, fortunately, quite rare. *Partial placenta previa* is partial coverage of the internal cervical os by the placenta. *Marginal placenta previa* occurs when the placenta is adjacent to the cervical os but does not extend over it. Marginal or partial placenta previa occurs in approximately 1 out of every 200 pregnancies. Predisposing factors include multiparity, maternal age greater than 35, and pregnancies in rapid succession.

Implantation of the placenta occurs early in pregnancy. Unless a sonogram is done, placenta previa is usually not detected until the third trimester. At that time, when fetal pressure on the placenta increases, or uterine contractions begin, the cervix **effaces**, or thins out, resulting in placental bleeding. In addition, sexual intercourse or digital vaginal examination can precipitate bleeding from placenta previa.

■ **effacement** the thinning of the cervix during labor.

Assessment. The patient with placenta previa is usually a multigravida in her third trimester of pregnancy. She may have a history of prior placenta previa or of bleeding early in the current pregnancy. She may report a recent episode of sexual intercourse or vaginal examination just before vaginal bleeding began, or she may not bleed until the onset of labor.

✳ Third-trimester bleeding should be attributed to either placenta previa or abruptio placentae until proven otherwise.

The most common sign of placenta previa is painless, bright red vaginal bleeding. In fact, any painless bleeding in pregnancy is considered placenta previa until proven otherwise. The bleeding may or may not be associated with uterine contractions. The uterus is usually soft, and the fetus may be in an unusual presentation. VAGINAL EXAMINATION SHOULD NEVER BE ATTEMPTED, AS AN EXAMINING FINGER CAN PUNCTURE THE PLACENTA, CAUSING FATAL HEMORRHAGE.

✳ A vaginal examination in a patient with placenta previa can cause a fatal hemorrhage.

Management. As with abruptio placentae, there are two lives at stake. Treatment should consist of the following steps. First, administer oxygen at high concentration. Second, establish one or two large-bore IVs with either lactated Ringer's solution or normal saline. Third, monitor vital signs and fetal heart tones continuously. If shock is impending, apply antishock trousers without inflating the abdominal compartment. Transport the patient rapidly. If the fetus is still viable, the definitive treatment is cesarean section.

Hypertensive Disorders of Pregnancy

In addition to vaginal bleeding, you should be aware of several pregnancy-associated problems known collectively as *hypertensive disorders of pregnancy* (formerly called "toxemia of pregnancy"). These disorders are characterized by hypertension, weight gain, edema, protein in the urine, and, in late stages, seizures. Hypertensive disorders of pregnancy occur in approximately 5 percent of pregnancies. They are thought to be caused by abnormal vasospasm in the mother, which results in increased blood pressure and other associated symptoms. The hypertensive disorders of pregnancy generally include:

❑ *Pregnancy-Induced Hypertension (PIH).* PIH is characterized by a blood pressure of 140/90 mmHg or greater in pregnancy in a patient who was previously normotensive. PIH is the early stage of the disease process. It is important to remember that blood pressure usually drops in pregnancy, and a blood pressure reading of 130/80 mmHg may be elevated.

❑ *Preeclampsia.* Preeclamptic patients are those that have hypertension, abnormal weight gain, edema, headache, protein in the urine, epigastric pain, and, occasionally, visual disturbances. If untreated, preeclampsia may progress to the next stage, eclampsia.

✱ Eclampsia is a threat to both the mother's and the baby's life.

❑ *Eclampsia.* Eclampsia is the most serious manifestation of the hypertensive disorders of pregnancy. It is characterized by grand mal seizure activity. Eclampsia is often preceded by visual disturbances, such as flashing lights or spots before the eyes. Also, the development of epigastric pain or pain in the right upper abdominal quadrant often indicates impending seizure. Eclampsia can be distinguished from epilepsy by the history and physical appearance of the patient. Patients who become eclamptic are usually edematous and have markedly elevated blood pressure, while epileptics usually have a prior history of seizures and are taking anticonvulsant medications.

The hypertensive disorders of pregnancy tend to occur most often with a woman's first pregnancy. They also appear to occur more frequently in patients with pre-existing hypertension. Diabetes mellitus is also associated with an increased incidence of this disease process.

Patients who develop PIH and preeclampsia are at increased risk for cerebral hemorrhage, the development of renal failure, and pulmonary edema. Patients who are preeclamptic have intravascular volume depletion, since a great deal of their body fluid is in the third space. If eclampsia develops, death of the mother and fetus frequently results.

Assessment. Developing an accurate history is extremely important whenever you suspect one of the hypertensive disorders of pregnancy. Question the patient about excessive weight gain, headaches, visual problems, epigastric or right upper quadrant abdominal pain, apprehension, or seizures.

On physical exam, patients with PIH or preeclampsia are usually markedly edematous. They are often pale and apprehensive. The reflexes are hyperactive. The blood pressure, which is usually elevated, should be taken after the patient has rested for 5 minutes in the left lateral recumbent position.

Management. Definitive treatment of the hypertensive disorders of pregnancy is delivery of the fetus. However, in the field, use the following management tactics to prevent dangerously high blood pressures or seizure activity.

❑ *PIH.* The patient who is pregnant and has elevated blood pressure, without edema or other signs of preeclampsia, should be closely monitored and transported to the hospital. Record the fetal heart tones and the mother's blood pressure level. If the blood pressure is dangerously high, the medical control physician may request the administration of Apresoline or similar antihypertensives that are safe for use in pregnancy.

❑ *Preeclampsia.* The patient who is hypertensive and shows other signs and symptoms of preeclampsia, such as edema, headaches, and visual disturbances, should be treated quickly. Keep the patient calm, and dim the lights. Place the patient in the left lateral recumbent position, and quickly carry out primary and secondary survey. Begin an IV of lactated Ringer's or normal saline. Transport the patient rapidly, without lights or sirens. If the transport time is long, the medical control physician may request the administration of magnesium sulfate.

❑ *Eclampsia.* If the patient has already suffered a seizure or a seizure appears to be imminent, then, in addition to the above measures, administer oxygen and manage the airway appropriately. Administer 5–10 mg Valium intravenously, as ordered by the medical control physician. In addition, the physician may request the administration of magnesium sulfate, especially if transport time is long. It is important to keep calcium chloride available for use as an antidote to magnesium sulfate.

The Supine-Hypotensive Syndrome   The *supine-hypotensive syndrome* usually occurs in the third trimester of pregnancy. The increased mass and weight of the gravid uterus compresses the inferior vena cava when the patient is supine, markedly decreasing blood return to the heart and reducing cardiac output. (See Figure 32-7.) Some patients are predisposed to this problem because of an overall decrease in circulating blood volume or because of anemia.

Assessment.   As mentioned previously, the supine-hypotensive syndrome usually occurs in a patient late in her pregnancy who has been supine for a period of time. Question the patient about prior episodes of a similar nature and about any recent hemorrhage or fluid loss. The physical examination should be directed at determining whether the patient is volume depleted.

Management.   If there are no indications of volume depletion, such as decreased skin turgor or thirst, place the patient in the left lateral recumbent position. Monitor the fetal heart tones and maternal vital signs frequently. If there is clinical evidence of volume depletion, administer oxygen and start an IV of normal saline or lactated Ringer's solution. Monitor vital signs, fetal heart tones, and ECG. If there is evidence of shock, apply antishock trousers, inflating only the leg compartments. Transport the patient promptly.

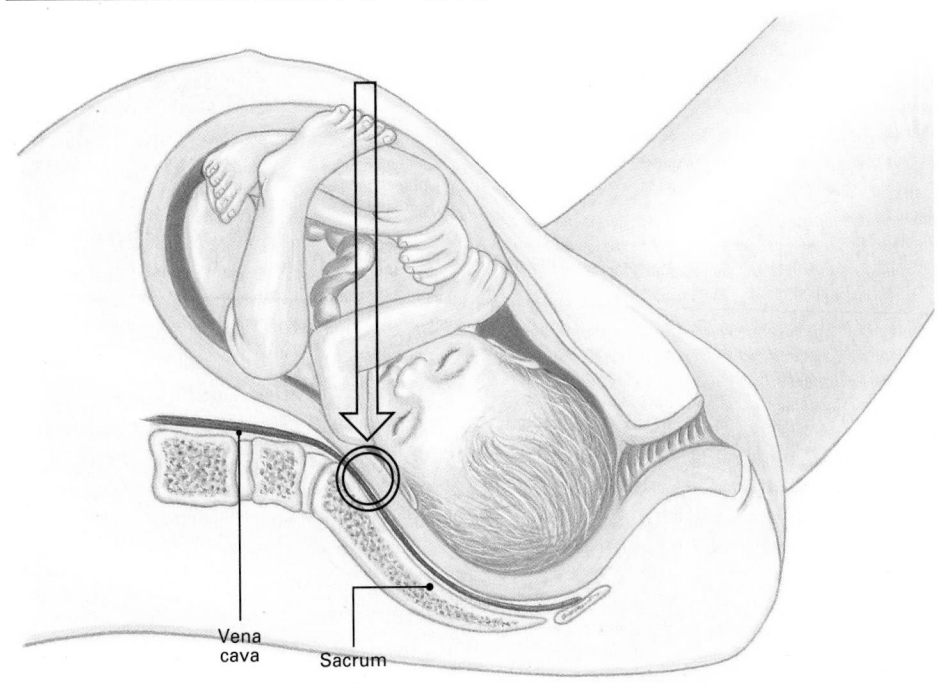

Vena
cava

Sacrum

FIGURE 32-7   The supine-hypotensive syndrome results from compression of the inferior vena cava by the gravid uterus.

Braxton-Hicks Contractions and Preterm Labor   It is occasionally difficult to determine the onset of labor. For many weeks before labor begins, the uterus contracts irregularly, thus conditioning itself for the birth process. As the EDC approaches, these contractions become more frequent. Ultimately, the contractions become stronger and more regular, signaling the onset of labor. *Labor* consists of uterine contractions that change the dilation or effacement of the cervix. The contractions of labor are firm, fairly regular, and quite painful. *Braxton-Hicks contractions*, occasionally called false labor, are generally less intense than labor contractions and do not change the cervix.

It is virtually impossible to distinguish false labor from true labor in the field. Distinguishing the two requires repeated vaginal examinations, over time, to determine whether the cervix is effacing or dilating. This, of course, should not be done in the field. Therefore, all patients with uterine contractions should be transported to the hospital for additional evaluation.

Braxton-Hicks contractions do not require treatment by the paramedic aside from reassurance of the patient and, if necessary, transport for evaluation by a physician. True labor that begins before the 38th week of gestation, referred to as *preterm labor*, may require intervention. Many conditions may lead to preterm labor, including premature rupture of the membranes and abnormalities in the cervix or uterus. In many cases, physicians attempt to stop preterm labor to give the fetus additional time to develop in the uterus.

Assessment.   When confronted by a patient with uterine contractions, first determine the approximate gestational age of the fetus. If it is less than 38 weeks, then preterm labor is suspected. If gestational age is greater than 38 weeks, the patient should be treated as a term patient, as described later in the this chapter.

After determining gestational age, obtain a brief obstetrical history. Then question the mother about the urge to push or the need to move her bowels or urinate. She should also be questioned about the status of her membranes. Any sensation of fluid leakage or "gushing" from the vagina should be interpreted as ruptured membranes until proven otherwise. Next, palpate the contractions by placing your hand on the patient's abdomen. Note the intensity and length of the contractions, as well as the interval between contractions.

✱ The patient with suspected preterm labor should be transported immediately.

Management.   Preterm labor, especially if quite early, should be stopped if possible. The process of stopping labor, or *tocolysis*, is frequently practiced in obstetrics. It is, however, infrequently done in the field.

There are three general approaches to tocolysis. The first is to sedate the patient, often with narcotics or barbiturates, thus allowing her to rest. Often, after a period of rest, the contractions stop on their own. The second approach is to administer a fluid bolus intravenously. The administration of approximately 1 liter of fluid intravenously increases the intravascular fluid volume, thus inhibiting ADH secretion from the posterior pituitary. Since oxytocin and ADH are secreted from the same area of the pituitary, the inhibition of ADH secretion also inhibits oxytocin release, often causing cessation of uterine contractions. Ultimately, if the above methods fail, a beta agonist, such as terbutaline or ritodrine, may be administered to stop labor by inhibiting uterine smooth muscle contraction.

As a rule, tocolysis in the field is limited to sedation and hydration, especially if transport time is long. Paramedics may, however, transport a patient from one medical facility to another with beta agonist administration underway. You should therefore be familiar with its use.

THE PUERPERIUM

The *puerperium* is the time period surrounding birth of the fetus. Childbirth generally occurs in a hospital or similar facility with appropriate equipment. Occasionally, prehospital personnel may be called upon to attend a delivery in the field. Therefore, you should be familiar with the birth process and some of the complications associated with it.

Deliveries

The delivery of the fetus is the culmination of pregnancy. The process by which delivery occurs is called **labor**. Labor is generally divided into three stages (see Figure 32-8):

■ **labor** the time and processes that occur during childbirth.

❑ *First Stage.* The first stage of labor begins with the onset of uterine contractions and ends with complete dilation of the cervix. It lasts approxi-

---

First stage: beginning of contractions to full cervical dilation

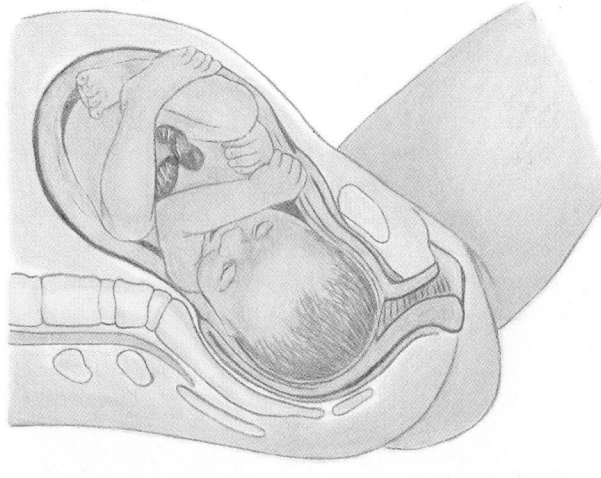

Second stage: baby enters birth canal and is born

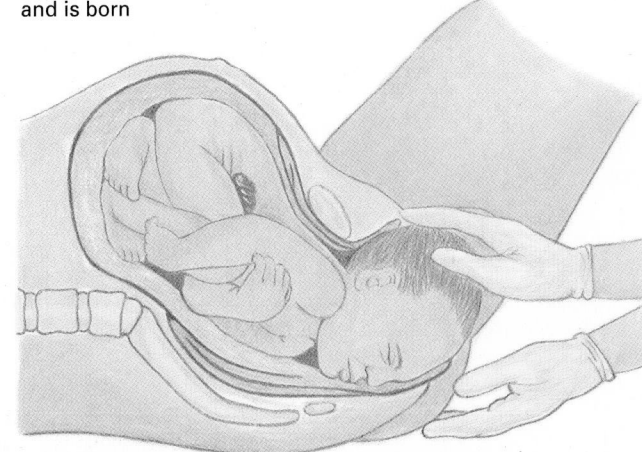

Third stage: delivery of the placenta

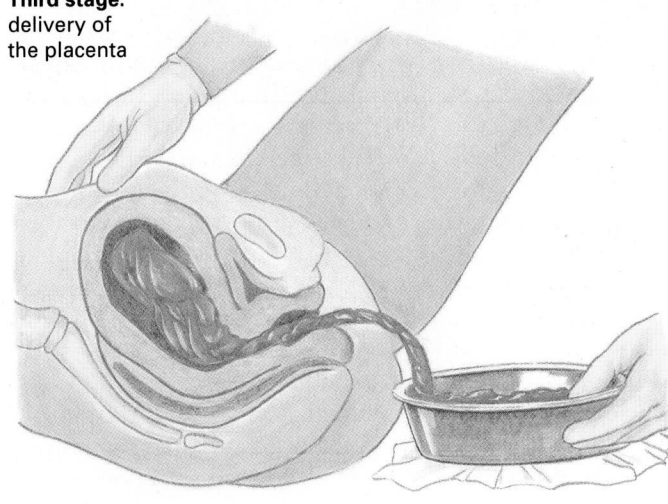

FIGURE 32-8 Stages of labor.

■ **nullipara** a woman who has never delivered a baby.

mately 8 hours in **nulliparous** women and 5 hours in multiparous women. Contractions may be irregular at first. Later in the first stage, the contractions increase in intensity, while the intervals between contractions shorten.

❑ *Second Stage.* The second stage of labor begins with complete dilation of the cervix and ends with delivery of the fetus. In the nulliparous patient, the second stage lasts approximately 50 minutes; in the multiparous patient, it lasts approximately 20 minutes. Contractions are strong, and each one may last 2 or 3 minutes. Often, the patient feels pain in her lower back, as the fetus descends into the pelvis. The urge to push or "bear down" usually begins in the second stage. The membranes usually rupture at this time, if they have not ruptured previously.

❑ *Third Stage.* The third stage of labor begins with delivery of the fetus and ends with delivery of the placenta. Delivery of the placenta usually occurs within 30 minutes after birth.

As discussed earlier, labor is painful. The pain begins in the abdomen. Later, as the fetus moves farther down into the pelvis, the pain may extend to the back. The contractions are regular and generally increase in frequency and intensity. The total length of labor averages 6 to 12 hours, with a great deal of individual variation. Labor usually lasts longer in the nulliparous patient than in the multiparous patient.

The uterus and cervix must undergo several changes to facilitate delivery of the fetus. First, the cervix must efface. *Effacement* is the thinning and shortening of the cervix. Early in pregnancy the cervix is quite thick and long, but after complete effacement it is paper thin. Effacement usually begins several days before active labor ensues. Second, the cervix must dilate. *Dilation* is the progressive stretching of the cervical opening. The cervix dilates from its closed position to 10 cm, which is considered complete dilation.

When dilation and effacement are complete, the baby's head moves down into the vagina. Late in the second stage of labor, the head can be seen at the opening of the vagina during a contraction. This is termed crowning.

The part of the baby that is born first is termed the *presenting part*. In the majority of cases, this is the head. Occasionally, the buttocks or other parts present first. In the field, the presenting part of the baby cannot usually be determined until crowning has occurred, since vaginal examinations should not be performed.

Management of a Patient in Labor

Probably one of the most important decisions you must make with a patient in labor is whether to attempt to deliver the infant at the scene or transport the patient to the hospital. (See Figure 32-9.) There are several factors to take into consideration when making this decision. They include the patient's number of previous pregnancies, the length of labor during the previous pregnancies, the frequency of contractions, the maternal urge to push, and the presence of crowning. Some women have rapid labors and may be completely dilated in a short period of time. Also, as mentioned above, multiparas generally have shorter labors than nulliparas. The maternal urge to push or the presence of crowning indicates that delivery is imminent. In such cases, the infant should be delivered at the scene or in the ambulance.

However, certain factors should prompt immediate transport, despite the threat of delivery. These include prolonged rupture of membranes, since prolonged time between rupture and delivery often leads to fetal infection; abnormal presentation, such as breech or transverse; or fetal distress, as evidenced

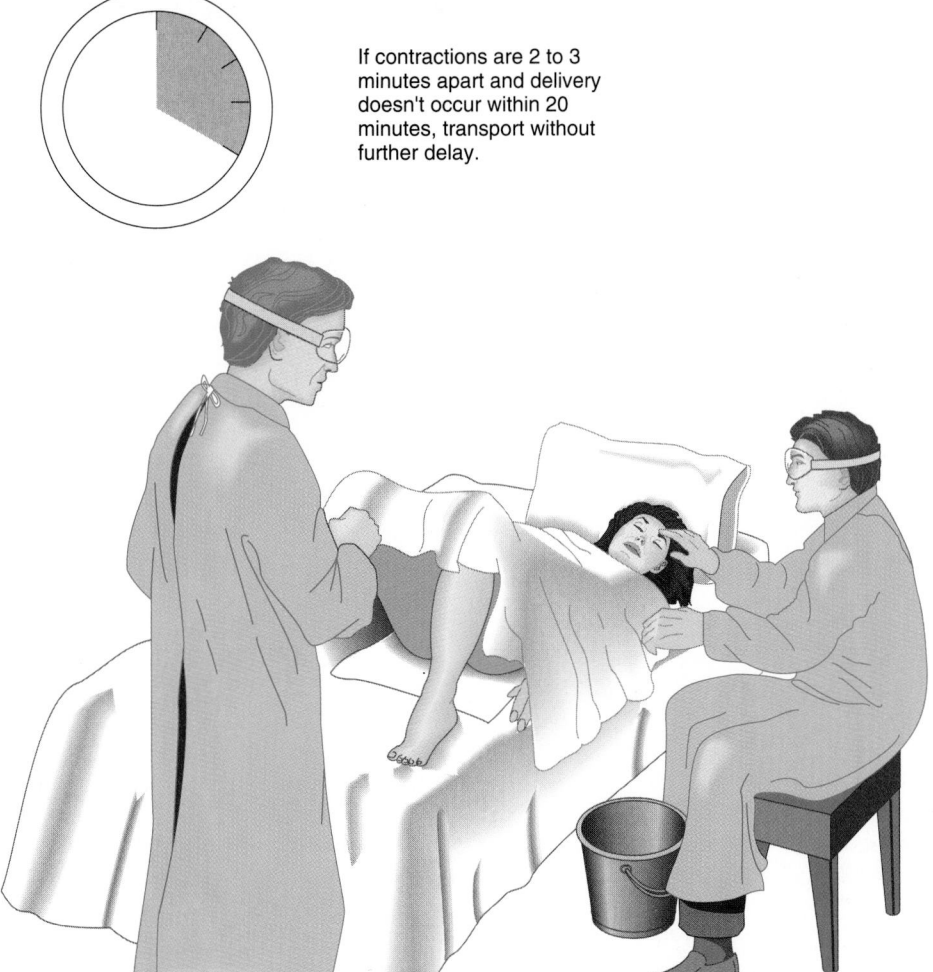

If contractions are 2 to 3 minutes apart and delivery doesn't occur within 20 minutes, transport without further delay.

FIGURE 32-9 The decision to deliver at the scene or to attempt transport is often a difficult one.

by fetal bradycardia or meconium staining (the presence of *meconium*, the first fetal stools, in the amniotic fluid).

Unscheduled Field Delivery

If delivery is imminent, equipment and facilities must be quickly prepared. (See Procedure 32-1.) Set up a delivery area. This should be out of public view, such as in a bedroom or the back of the ambulance. Administer oxygen to the mother. If time permits, establish an IV of lactated Ringer's solution or normal saline. The patient should be placed on her back and, if time permits, draped. Until delivery, the fetal heart rate should be monitored frequently. A drop in the fetal heart rate to less than 90 beats per minute indicates fetal distress and should prompt immediate transport. Coach the mother to breathe deeply between contractions and to push with contractions. Prepare the OB equipment and don sterile gloves and goggles. As the head crowns, control it with gentle pressure. (See Figures 32-10 through 32-20.) An explosive delivery results in increased tearing of maternal tissue. If the membranes are still intact, rupture them with your fingertips to allow leakage of the amniotic fluid.

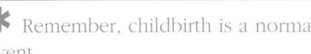 Remember, childbirth is a normal event.

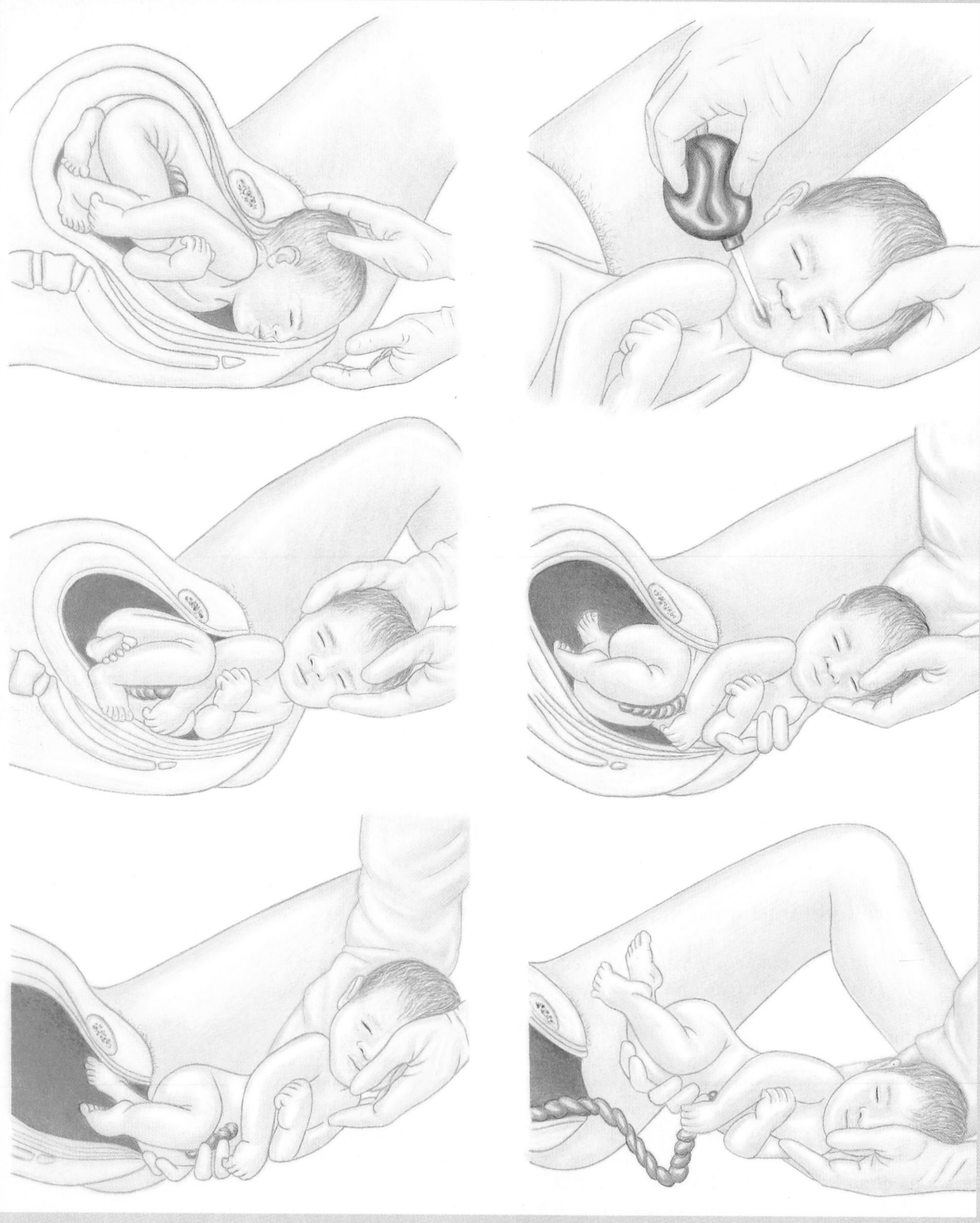

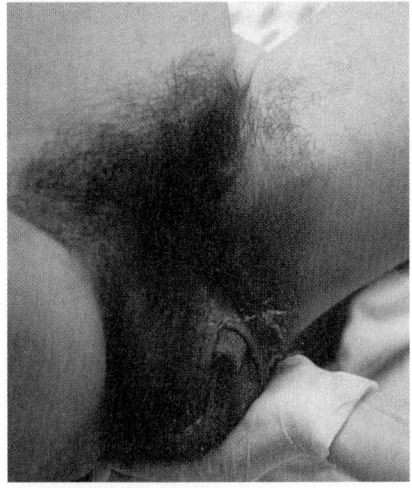

FIGURE 32-10 Crowning.

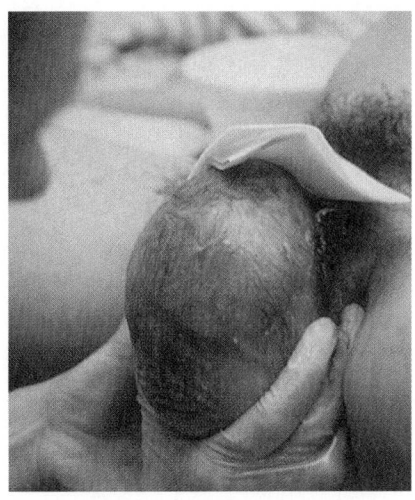

FIGURE 32-11 Delivery of the head.

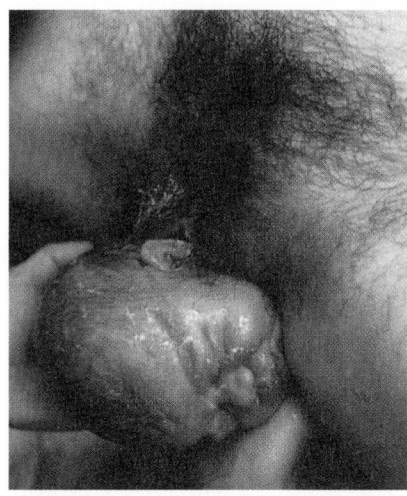

FIGURE 32-12 External rotation of the head.

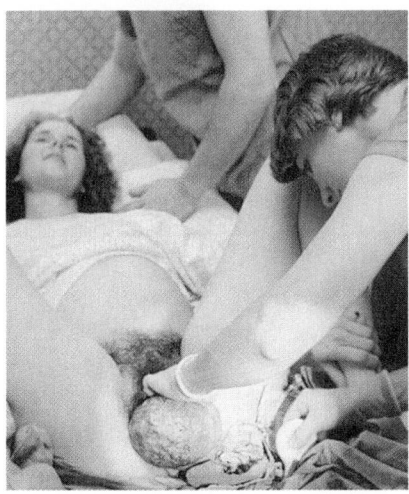

FIGURE 32-13 As soon as possible, suction the mouth, then the nose.

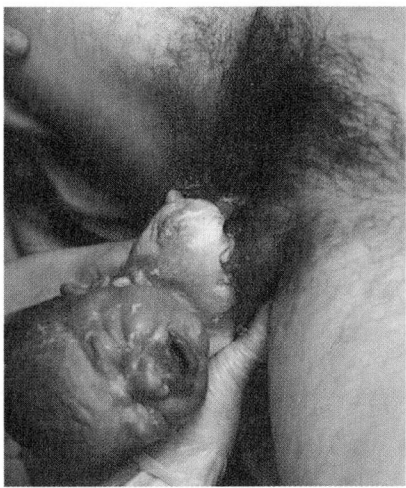

FIGURE 32-14 Delivery of the anterior shoulder.

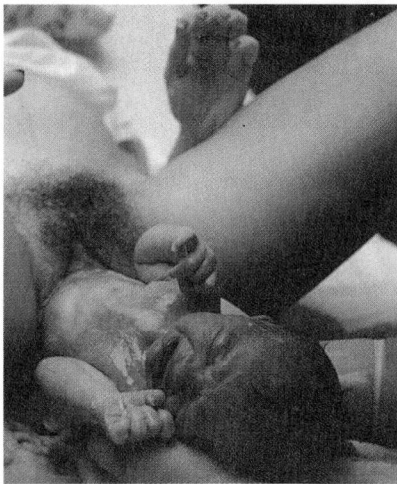

FIGURE 32-15 Complete delivery of the infant.

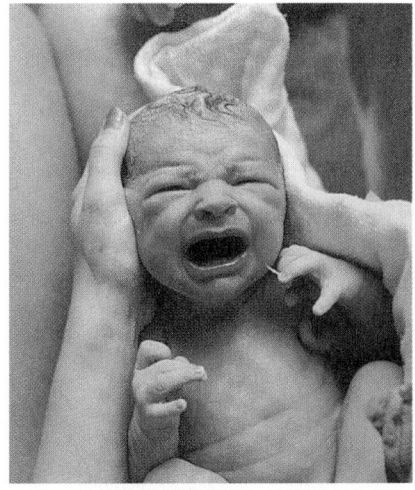

FIGURE 32-16 Dry the infant.

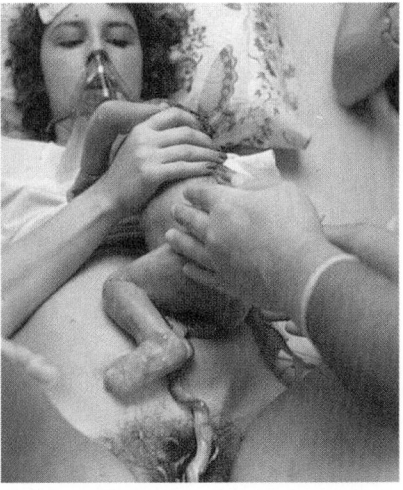

FIGURE 32-17 Place the infant on the mother's stomach.

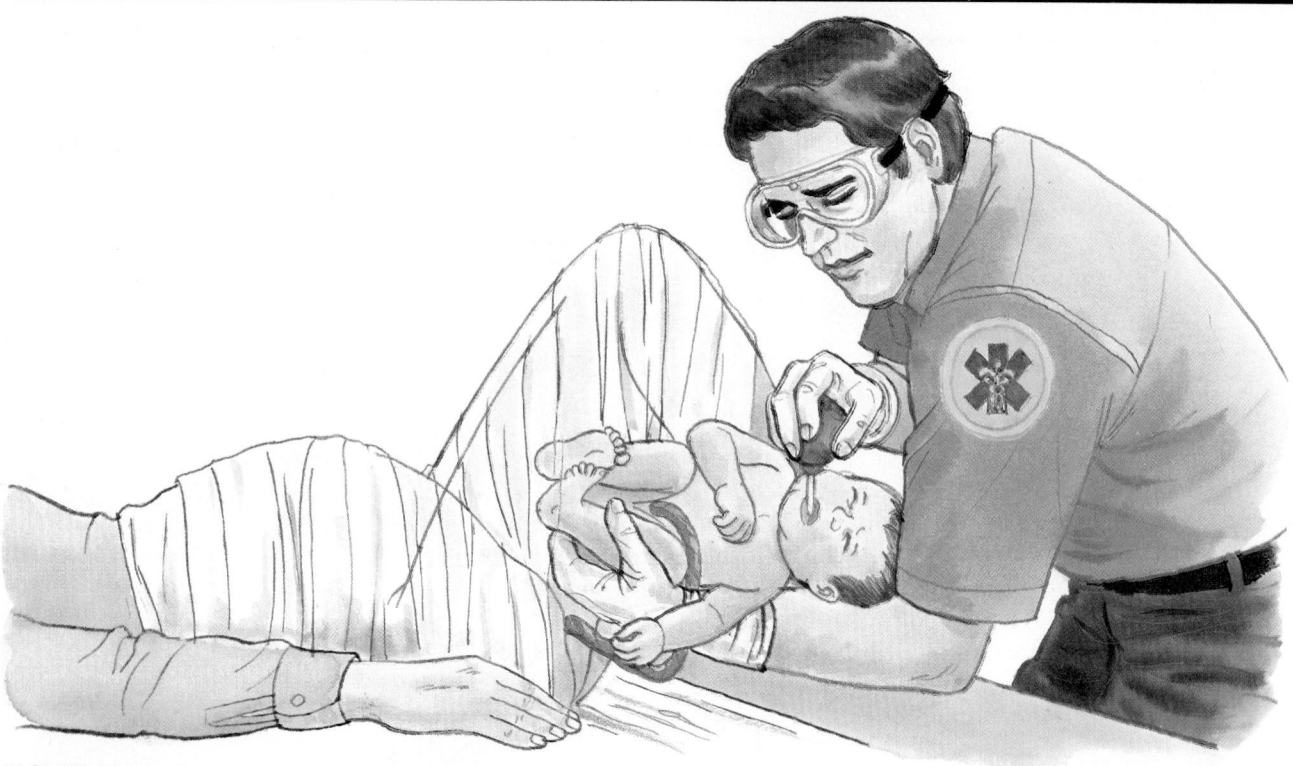

FIGURE 32-18 Re-suction the airway as needed.

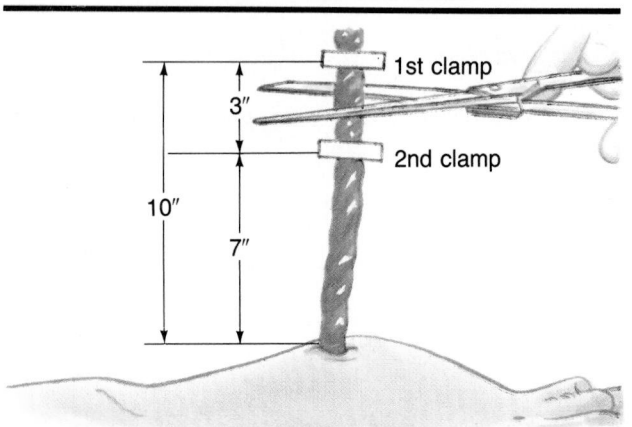

1st clamp

3″

2nd clamp

10″

7″

FIGURE 32-19 Clamp and cut the cord.

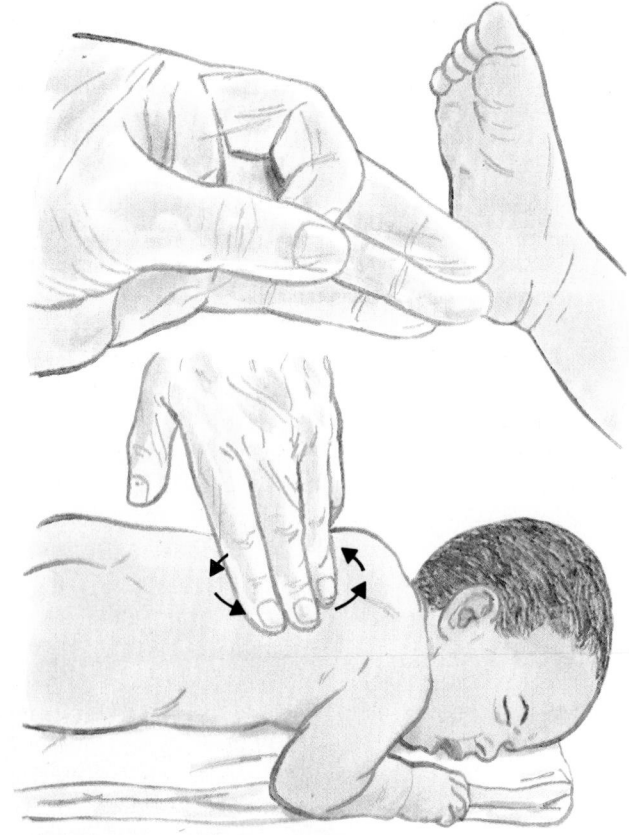

FIGURE 32-20 Stimulate the infant as required.

If the umbilical cord is around the infant's neck during delivery, gently slip it over the infant's head, if possible. If the cord is too tight to slip over the head, apply two umbilical clamps and cut the cord. As soon as the infant's head is clear of the vagina, instruct the mother to stop pushing. Next, suction the infant's mouth and nose with the bulb syringe. Then tell the mother to resume pushing, while you support the infant's head as it rotates. Deliver the anterior shoulder first and then the posterior shoulder. The remainder of the body will follow.

Remember to keep the baby at the level of the vagina to prevent over- or undertransfusion of blood from the cord. Never "milk" the cord. Clamp the cord as follows. Supporting the baby, place the first umbilical clamp approximately 10 cm from the baby. Place the second clamp approximately 5 cm above the first. Then carefully cut the umbilical cord between the clamps.

At this point, suction the infant again, using the bulb suction. Then, wipe the infant dry, and inspect the cord for bleeding. Wrap the baby in a warm blanket, and place it on its side with the head approximately 15 degrees below the torso to facilitate drainage of any aspirated secretions. Note the time of birth.

After birth, the mother's vagina should continue to ooze blood. Do not pull on the umbilical cord. Eventually, the cord will appear to lengthen, which indicates separation of the placenta. The placenta should be delivered and transported with the mother to the hospital. There is no need to delay transport for delivery of the placenta.

At this time, massage the uterine fundus by placing one hand immediately above the symphysis pubis and the other on the uterine fundus. Cup the uterus between the two hands and support it as it is massaged. Continue massage until the uterus assumes a woody hardness. Avoid overmassage.

Following delivery, inspect the mother's perineum for tears. If any tears are present, apply direct pressure. Continuously monitor vital signs. Note the presence of continued hemorrhage, and report it to the medical control physician. Following stabilization, transport the mother and infant to the hospital.

Complications of Delivery

Although most deliveries proceed without incident, complications can arise. Therefore, you should be prepared to deal with them.

Cephalopelvic Disproportion   *Cephalopelvic disproportion* occurs when the baby's head is too big to pass through the maternal pelvis easily. This may be caused by an oversized baby. Large babies are associated with diabetes, multiparity, or postmaturity. Fetal abnormalities such as hydrocephalus, conjoined twins, or fetal tumors may make vaginal delivery impossible. Women of short stature or women with contracted pelvises are at increased risk for this problem. If cephalopelvic disproportion is not recognized and managed appropriately, fetal demise or uterine rupture may occur.

Cephalopelvic disproportion tends to develop most frequently in the primigravida. There may be strong contractions for an extended period of time. On physical examination, the fetus may feel large. Also, labor generally does not progress. The fetus may be in distress, as evidenced by fetal bradycardia or meconium staining.

The usual management of cephalopelvic disproportion is cesarean section. In the field, the mother should be administered oxygen and an IV of lactated Ringer's or normal saline started. Transport should be immediate and rapid.

Abnormal Presentations Most babies present head first, or *vertex*. However, approximately 3 percent of deliveries are *breech presentations*, in which the presenting part is the feet or the buttocks. Breech presentations are more common in premature infants and in mothers with uterine abnormalities. Such deliveries usually carry an increased risk for fetal trauma, anoxia, and cord prolapse.

Because cesarean section is often required, delivery of the breech presentation is best accomplished at the hospital. However, if field delivery is unavoidable, then the following maneuvers are recommended. First, position the mother with her buttocks at the edge of a firm bed. Ask her to hold her legs in a flexed position. Often she will require assistance in doing this. As the infant delivers, do not pull on the legs, simply support them. Allow the entire body to be delivered with contractions only while you support the infant. (See Figure 32-21.)

As the head passes the pubis, apply gentle upward traction until the mouth appears over the perineum. If the head does not deliver, and the baby begins to breathe spontaneously with its face pressed against the vaginal wall, place a gloved hand in the vagina with the palm toward the infant's face. Form a "V" with the index and middle finger on either side of the infant's nose, and push the vaginal wall away from the infant's face to allow unrestricted respiration. (See Figure 32-22.) If necessary, continue during transport.

Other abnormal presentations can complicate delivery. One of the most common is the *occiput posterior position*. Normally, as the infant descends into the pelvis, its face is turned posteriorly. This is important, as extension of the head assists delivery. However, if the baby descends facing forward, or occiput posterior, its passage through the pelvis is delayed. This presentation occurs most frequently in primigravidas. In multigravidas it usually resolves spontaneously.

The presenting part may also be the face or brow, rather than the crown of the head. Occasionally, during these presentations, the face or brow can be seen high in the pelvis during a contraction. Usually, vaginal delivery is impossible in these cases.

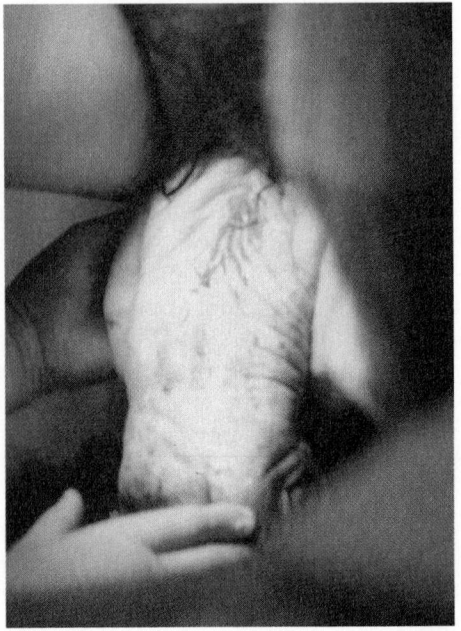

FIGURE 32-21 Breech delivery.

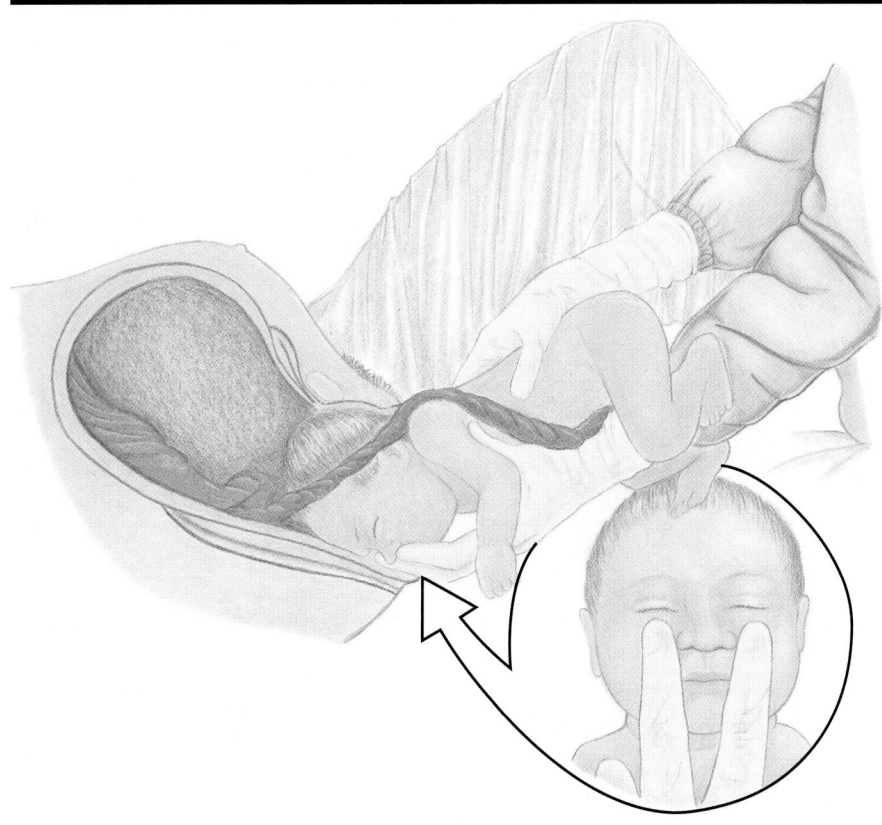

FIGURE 32-22 Placement of the fingers to maintain the airway in a breech birth.

In addition to head-first and breech presentations, the fetus can lie transversely in the uterus. In such a case, the fetus cannot enter the pelvis for delivery. If the membranes rupture, the umbilical cord can prolapse, or an arm or leg can enter the vagina. Vaginal delivery is impossible.

Early recognition of an abnormal presentation is important. If one is suspected, the mother should be reassured, placed on oxygen, and transported immediately, since forceps or cesarean delivery is often required.

Prolapsed Cord A *prolapsed cord* occurs when the umbilical cord falls down into the pelvis and is compressed between the fetus and the bony pelvis, shutting off fetal circulation. (See Figure 32-23.) This tends to occur most frequently in abnormal presentations, with multiple or premature births, or in conjunction with premature rupture of the membranes. It is a serious emergency, and fetal death will occur quickly without prompt intervention.

If the umbilical cord is seen in the vagina, insert two fingers of a gloved hand to raise the presenting part of the fetus off the cord. At the same time, check the cord for pulsations. Place the mother in Trendelenburg or knee-chest position. (See Figure 32-24.) Administer high-flow oxygen to the mother, and transport her immediately, with the fingers continuing to hold the presenting part off the umbilical cord. If assistance is available, apply a dressing moistened with sterile saline to the exposed cord. DO NOT ATTEMPT TO PUSH THE CORD BACK. Definitive treatment is cesarean section.

Multiple Births Multiple births are fairly rare. Usually, the mother knows or at least suspects the presence of more than one fetus. Multiple births should also be suspected if the mother's abdomen remains large after delivery of one baby.

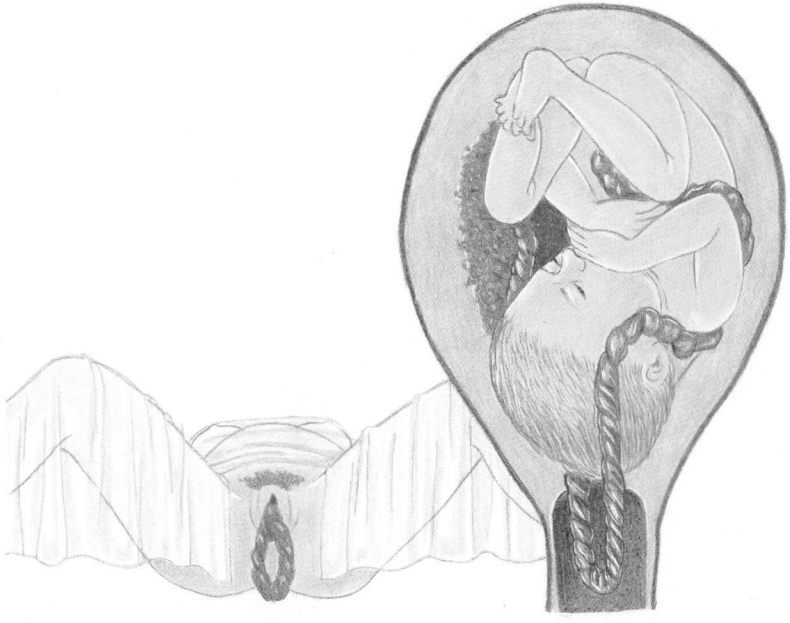

- Elevate hips, administer oxygen and keep warm

- Keep baby's head away from cord

- Do not attempt to push cord back

- Wrap cord in sterile moist towel

- Transport mother to hospital, continuing pressure on baby's head

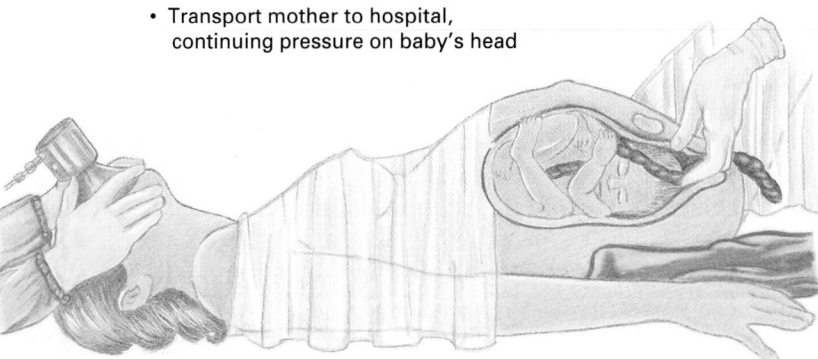

FIGURE 32-23   Prolapsed cord.

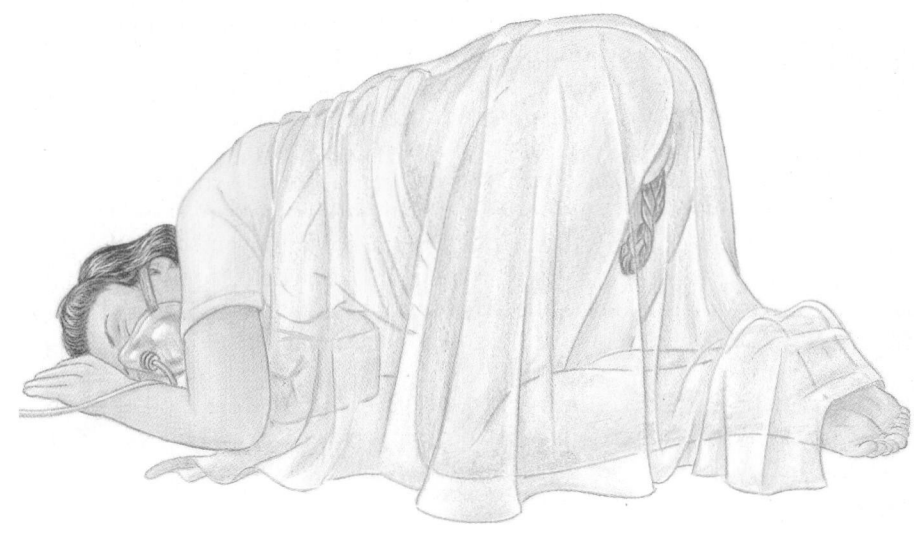

FIGURE 32-24   Patient positioning for prolapsed cord.

In twin births, labor often begins earlier than expected, and the infants are generally smaller than babies born singly. Usually, one twin presents vertex and the other breech. There may be one or two placentas.

After delivery of the first baby, clamp and cut the cord. Then deliver the second baby.

Precipitous Delivery

A *precipitous delivery* is a delivery that occurs after less than 3 hours of labor. This type of delivery occurs most frequently in the **grand multipara** and is associated with a higher-than-normal incidence of fetal trauma, tearing of the umbilical cord, or maternal lacerations.

■ **grand multipara** a woman who has delivered at least seven babies.

The best way to handle precipitous delivery is to be prepared. Do not turn your attention from the mother. Be ready for a rapid delivery, and attempt to control the infant's head. Once delivered, the baby may have some difficulty with temperature regulation and should be kept warm.

Shoulder Dystocia

A *shoulder dystocia* occurs when the infant's shoulders are larger than its head. This occurs most frequently with diabetic and obese mothers and in postmature pregnancies. In shoulder dystocia, labor progresses normally and the head is delivered routinely. However, immediately after the head is delivered, it retracts back into the perineum because the shoulders are trapped between the symphysis pubis and the sacrum ("turtle sign").

If a shoulder dystocia occurs, do not pull on the head. Administer oxygen to the mother and have her drop her buttocks off the end of the bed. Then flex her thighs upward to facilitate delivery, and apply firm pressure with an open hand immediately above the symphysis pubis. If delivery does not occur, transport the patient immediately.

Maternal Complications of Labor and Delivery

Several maternal problems can arise during and after delivery. These include postpartum hemorrhage, uterine rupture, uterine inversion, and pulmonary embolism.

Postpartum Hemorrhage

Postpartum hemorrhage is the loss of 500 mL or more blood in the first 24 hours following delivery. It occurs in approximately 5 percent of deliveries. The most common cause of postpartum hemorrhage is *uterine atony*, or lack of uterine muscle tone. This tends to occur most frequently in the multigravida and is most common following multiple births or births of large infants. Uterine atony also occurs after precipitous deliveries and prolonged labors. In addition to uterine atony, postpartum hemorrhage can be caused by placenta previa, abruptio placentae, retained placental parts, clotting disorders in the mother, or vaginal and cervical tears. Occasionally, the uterus fails to return to its normal size during the postpartum period, and postpartum hemorrhage occurs long after the birth.

■ **postpartum** the time period after delivery of the fetus.

Assessment. Assessment of the patient with postpartum hemorrhage should focus on the history and the predisposing factors described above. You must rely heavily on the clinical appearance of the patient and her vital signs. Often, the uterus will feel boggy and soft on physical examination. Vaginal bleeding is usually obvious.

Management. When confronted by a patient with postpartum hemorrhage, complete the primary and secondary survey immediately. Administer oxygen and begin fundal massage. Administer one or two large-bore IVs of either normal saline or lactated Ringer's solution. If shock is evident, apply antishock trousers. Never attempt to force delivery of the placenta or pack the vagina with dressings. In severe cases, the medical control physician may request the administration of pitocin.

Uterine Rupture   *Uterine rupture* is the actual tearing, or rupture, of the uterus. It usually occurs during labor or at its onset. However, it can also occur before labor with abdominal trauma. During labor, it often results from tetanic uterine contractions or a surgically scarred uterus, such as occurs from previous cesarean section. It can also occur following a prolonged or obstructed labor, as in the case of cephalopelvic disproportion or in conjunction with abnormal presentations.

Assessment. The patient with uterine rupture will often be in shock. There may be a history of continuous abdominal pain that has increased in intensity. Labor may have started, then appeared to have stopped when the uterus ruptured. On physical examination, there is often profound shock without evidence of external hemorrhage. Fetal heart tones are absent. The abdomen is often tender and rigid and may exhibit rebound tenderness.

Management. Management is the same as for any patient in shock. Administer oxygen at high concentration. Next, establish one or two large-bore IVs with either lactated Ringer's solution or normal saline. Monitor vital signs and fetal heart tones continuously. If shock is impending, apply antishock trousers without inflating the abdominal compartment. Transport the patient rapidly. If the fetus is still viable, the definitive treatment is cesarean section with subsequent repair or removal of the uterus.

Uterine Inversion   *Uterine inversion*, a rare emergency, occurs when the uterus turns inside out after delivery. When uterine inversion occurs, the supporting ligaments and blood vessels supplying blood to the uterus are torn, usually causing profound shock. Uterine inversion usually results from pulling on the umbilical cord while awaiting delivery of the placenta or from attempts to express the placenta when the uterus is relaxed.

If uterine inversion occurs, you must act quickly. First, place the patient in a supine position and begin oxygen administration. DO NOT attempt to detach the placenta or pull on the cord. Initiate one or two large bore IVs of normal saline or lactated Ringer's solution. Make one attempt to replace the uterus, using the following technique. With the palm of the hand, push the fundus of the inverted uterus toward the vagina. If one attempt is unsuccessful, cover the uterus with towels moistened with saline and transport the patient immediately.

Pulmonary Embolism   *Pulmonary embolism* is the presence of a blood clot in the pulmonary vascular system. It can occur after pregnancy, usually as a result of venous thromboembolism. It is one of the most common causes of maternal death and appears to occur more frequently following cesarean section than vaginal delivery. Pulmonary embolism can also occur at any time during pregnancy. There is usually a sudden onset of dyspnea and often sharp chest pain. On physical examination, the patient may show tachycardia, tachypnea, and, in severe cases, hypotension.

Management of pulmonary embolism consists of administration of high-flow oxygen and IV of normal saline or lactated Ringer's TKO. Monitor the patient's ECG and vital signs closely and transport her rapidly.

SUMMARY

Obstetrical emergencies are fairly uncommon. However, all pregnant patients are at risk for developing complications, and it is impossible to predict which ones actually will occur. It is therefore important to recognize these complications and act accordingly.

FURTHER READING

Bledsoe, Bryan E. "Trauma During Pregnancy." *Canadian Emergency News*, 15 (3), May, 1992. pp. 14–18.

Cunningham, F., Paul C. MacDonald, and Norman F. Gant. *Williams Obstetrics*, 18th ed. Norwalk, CT: Appleton & Lange, 1989.

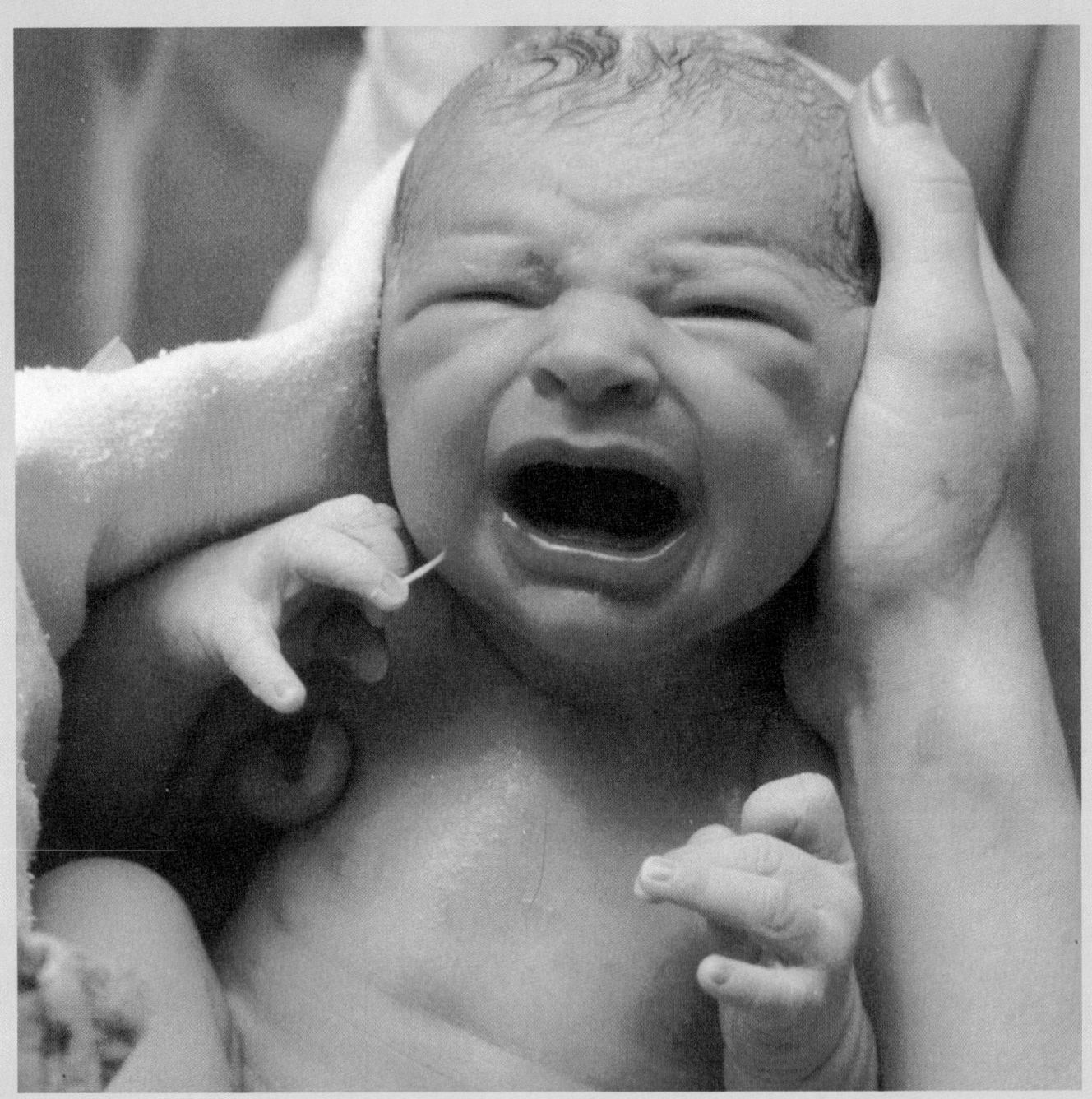

33

EMERGENCY MANAGEMENT OF THE NEONATE

Objectives for Chapter 33

After reading this chapter, you should be able to:

1. Describe the routine care of the newborn. (See pp. 998–999.)

2. List four means by which heat loss occurs in neonates. (See p. 998.)

3. Define the parameters of APGAR scoring and the numerical values used. (See pp. 999–1000.)

4. Identify special considerations in the care of the premature neonate. (See pp. 1000–1001.)

5. Explain the significance of meconium staining. (See p. 1001.)

6. Describe the inverted pyramid approach to neonatal resuscitation. (See pp. 1003–1009.)

7. Describe two methods of stimulating a distressed neonate. (See p. 1005.)

8. Describe the appropriate administration of oxygen to a neonate. (See p. 1007.)

9. Describe the indications for endotracheal intubation of a distressed neonate. (See p. 1008.)

10. Describe methods and problems in ventilating the distressed infant. (See p. 1008.)

11. Describe the technique and rates used in chest compressions in the neonate. (See p. 1009.)

12. List drugs and fluids used in neonatal resuscitation, and give the correct dosages. (See p. 1009.)

A call comes into the paramedics at Bell County Hospital. The dispatcher reports a woman in labor at a location about five minutes from the hospital. Upon arrival, the paramedics find a 24-year-old female who is about to deliver her second baby. They quickly determine that there is not enough time to transport the patient to the hospital. So they prepare equipment for a field delivery.

The delivery proceeds uneventfully. Following birth, however, the baby remains blue and limp, even after the paramedics suction the airway. The paramedics quickly move the infant to the side of the bed where the light is better. There they dry the baby, stimulate, and once again suction the baby. But the baby remains blue and limp despite their efforts. The paramedics now deliver supplemental "blow by" oxygen. Despite this, the neonate's heart rate remains less than 100. The paramedics grab the bag-valve-mask unit and apply artificial ventilation. Almost immediately, the infant "pinks up" and begins to cry. Using the pulse oximeter, the paramedics determine that the oxygen saturation is 95 percent and increasing.

The paramedics ready the baby for transport. They wrap the infant in a blanket with its head covered and give it to the mother to hold. After they load the mother and baby into the ambulance, paramedics continue to administer "blow by" oxygen. The five-minute APGAR score is 9. The trip to the hospital is uneventful. The baby goes home from the hospital one day later than the mother.

INTRODUCTION

■ **neonate** an infant from the time of birth to one month of age.

A **neonate** is an infant less than one month of age. (See Figure 33-1.) After an unscheduled delivery in the field, you have two patients to manage, the mother and the baby. This chapter describes initial care of the neonate. It then discusses the special needs of the distressed neonate and the premature neonate.

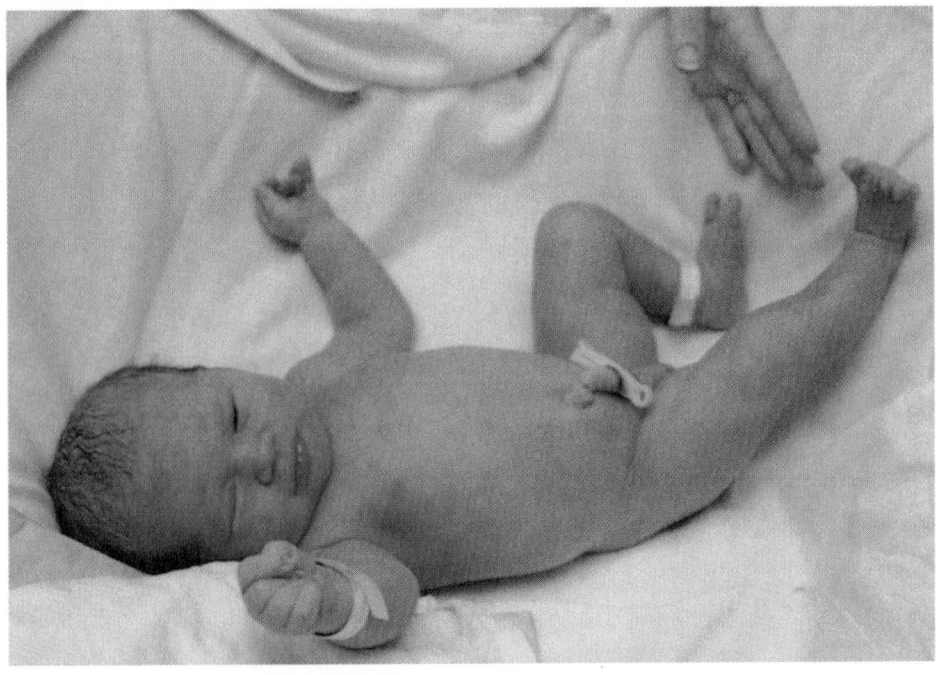

FIGURE 33-1 Term neonate.

ANATOMIC AND PHYSIOLOGIC CHANGES AT BIRTH

At birth, dramatic changes occur within the neonate that prepare it for extrauterine life. The respiratory system, which is essentially non-functional when the fetus is in the uterus, must suddenly initiate and maintain respirations. While in the uterus, fetal lung fluid fills the fetal lungs. The capillaries and arterioles of the lungs are closed. Most blood pumped by the heart bypasses the non-functional respiratory system through the *ductus arteriosus*.

Approximately one-third of fetal lung fluid is removed through chest compression during vaginal delivery. The neonate should take its first breath within a few seconds after delivery. The timing of the first breath is unrelated to the cutting of the umbilical cord. The factors that stimulate the baby's first breath include mild acidosis, initiation of the stretch reflexes in the lung, hypoxia, and hypothermia. (See Figure 33-2.) With the first few breaths, the lungs rapidly fill with air, which in turn displaces the remaining fetal lung

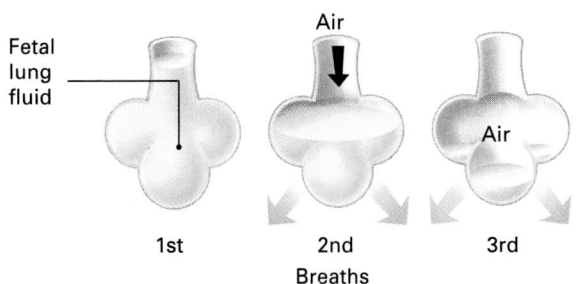

Following birth, the lungs expand as they are filled with air. The fetal lung fluid gradually leaves the alveoli.

Arterioles dilate and blood flow increases

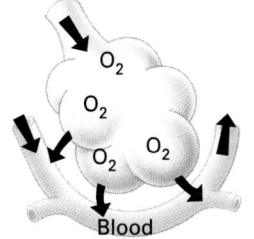

At the same time as the lungs are expanding and the fetal lung fluid is clearing, the arterioles in the lung begin to open, allowing a considerable increase in the amount of blood flowing through the lungs.

Pulmonary blood flow increases

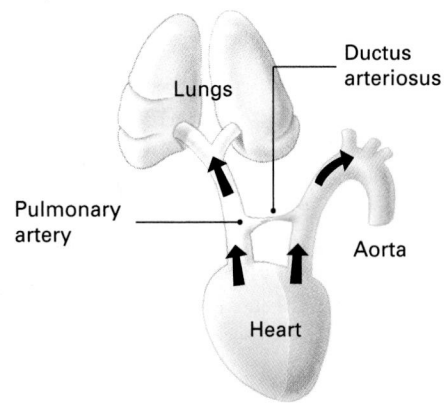

Blood previously diverted through the ductus arteriosus flows through the lungs where it picks up oxygen to transport to tissues throughout the body. Soon there is no need for the ducts, and it eventually closes.

FIGURE 33-2 Hemodynamic changes in the neonate at birth.

fluid. Subsequently, the pulmonary arterioles and capillaries open, decreasing pulmonary vascular resistance. At this point, the resistance to blood flow in the lungs is less than the resistance of the *ductus arteriosus*. Because of this pressure difference, blood flow is diverted from the *ductus arteriosus* to the lungs. Here it picks up oxygen for transport to the peripheral tissues. Soon, there is no need for the *ductus arteriosus*, and it eventually closes.

ROUTINE CARE OF THE NEWBORN

The initial care of the newborn follows the same priorities as all patients. You should complete the primary assessment first. Correct any problem detected during the primary assessment before proceeding to the next step. The vast majority of newborns (approximately 80 percent) require no resuscitation beyond suctioning of the airway, mild stimulation, and maintenance of body temperature.

Establishment of the Airway

The first step in caring for the neonate is airway management. During delivery, fluid is forced out of the baby's lungs, into the oropharynx, and out through the nose and mouth. This fluid drainage is independent of gravity. As soon as the neonate's head is delivered, suction the mouth, and then the nose, with a bulb suction. Always suction the mouth first so that there is nothing for the infant to aspirate if he or she gasps when the nose is suctioned. Repeat suctioning upon delivery of the body.

Immediately following delivery, maintain the neonate at the same level as the mother's vagina, with its head approximately 15 degrees below its torso. This facilitates the drainage of secretions and helps prevent aspiration. If there appears to be a large amount of secretions, a **DeLee suction trap**, attached to a suction source, should be used. First suction the mouth, then the nose. Repeat these steps as necessary until the airway is clear.

Drying and suctioning typically produce enough stimulation to initiate respirations in most newborns. If the neonate does not cry immediately, stimulate it by gently rubbing its back. Vigorous spanking or rubbing is not necessary.

Prevention of Heat Loss in the Neonate

Heat loss is one of the most important risks to the neonate. Heat loss can occur through evaporation, convection, conduction, or radiation. Most heat loss in the neonate occurs through *evaporation*. The neonate is born wet, and the amniotic fluid quickly evaporates, thus cooling the neonate. Immediately after birth, the neonate's core temperature can drop $1°$ C or more from its birth temperature of $38°$ C.

Loss of heat can also occur through *convection*, depending upon the temperature of the room and the movement of air around the neonate. *Conduction* can occur through surfaces in contact with the neonate. In addition, the neonate can lose heat through *radiation* to colder objects nearby.

Heat loss should be minimized. Dry the neonate immediately to prevent evaporative cooling. The *ambient temperature*, the temperature in the delivery room or ambulance, should be at least $23-24°$ C ($74-76°$ F). To prevent drafts, make sure all doors and windows are closed. Discard the towel used to dry

■ **DeLee suction trap** a suction device that contains a suction trap connected to a suction catheter. The negative pressure that powers it can come either from the mouth of the operator or, preferably, from an external vacuum source.

✱ Heat loss is a major risk to the neonate.

the neonate and swaddle the neonate in a warm, dry receiving blanket or other suitable material. In colder areas, place well-insulated hot-water bottles or rubber gloves filled with warm water around the neonate to help maintain a warm body temperature.

Cutting the Umbilical Cord

After you have stabilized the neonate's airway and minimized heat loss, clamp and cut the umbilical cord. You can prevent transfusion of blood by maintaining the baby at the same level as the vagina, as described above. Do not "milk" or strip the umbilical cord, since this increases blood viscosity, or *polycythemia*. Polycythemia can cause cardiopulmonary problems. It can also contribute to excessive red blood cell destruction, which may in turn lead to hyperbilirubinemia (an increased level of bilirubin in the blood that causes jaundice).

* Never "milk" the umbilical cord during a delivery.

Apply the umbilical clamps within 30-45 seconds after birth. Place the first clamp approximately 10 cm from the neonate. Place the second clamp approximately 5 cm farther away from the neonate than the first clamp. Then cut the cord between the two clamps. After the cord is cut, inspect it periodically to be sure that there is no additional bleeding.

Assessment of the Neonate

Assess the neonate immediately after birth. Ideally, if two paramedics are available, one will attend the mother, while the other attends the neonate.

Obtain vital signs quickly. The neonate's respiratory rate should average 40–60 breaths per minute. If asphyxia is present, begin resuscitation at once. Next, check the heart rate. The heart rate is normally 150–180 beats per minute at birth, slowing to 130–140 beats per minute shortly thereafter. A pulse rate of less than 100 beats per minute indicates distress and requires emergency intervention. The skin color should be evaluated as well. Some cyanosis of the extremities is common immediately after birth. However, cyanosis of the central part of the body is abnormal, as is persistent peripheral cyanosis.

The APGAR Score

As soon as possible, the neonate should be assigned an **APGAR score**. Ideally, this is done at 1 and 5 minutes after birth. However, if the neonate is not breathing, DO NOT withhold resuscitation until determining the APGAR score.

■ **APGAR scoring** a numerical system of rating the condition of a newborn. It evaluates the neonate's heart rate, respiratory rate, muscle tone, reflex irritability, and color.

* Never delay resuscitation to determine the APGAR score.

The APGAR scoring system helps to differentiate those neonates who need only routine care from those who need greater assistance. The system also predicts long-term survival. It was developed in 1952 by Dr. Virginia Apgar, an anesthesiologist. The parameters for APGAR scoring include appearance, pulse rate, grimace, activity, and respiratory effort. A score of 0, 1, or 2 is given for each parameter. The minimum total score is 0 and the maximum is 10. (See Table 33-1.) A score of 7–10 indicates an active and vigorous neonate that requires only routine care. A score of 4–6 indicates a moderately depressed neonate that requires oxygenation and stimulation. Severely depressed neonates, those with APGAR scores of less than 4, require immediate resuscitation. By repeating the APGAR score at 1 and 5 minutes, it is possible to determine whether intervention has caused a change in the neonate's status.

TABLE 33-1 The APGAR Score

Sign	0	1	2	Score	
				1 min	5 min
Appearance (Skin color)	Blue, pale	Body pink, extremities blue	Completely pink		
Pulse Rate (Heart Rate)	Absent	Below 100	Above 100		
Grimace (Irritability)	No response	Grimaces	Cries		
Activity (Muscle Tone)	Limp	Some flexion of extremities	Active motion		
Respiratory (Effort)	Absent	Slow and irregular	Strong cry		
			TOTAL SCORE =		

THE PREMATURE NEONATE

The *premature neonate* is one that weighs less than 2500 grams (5.5 pounds) or that is born before the 38th week of gestation. (See Figure 33-3.) Premature neonates are at risk for hypothermia, hypoglycemia, volume depletion, several respiratory problems, and, in some cases, cardiovascular problems related to hypoxia.

Premature neonates are more susceptible to heat loss than full-term neonates for the following reasons.

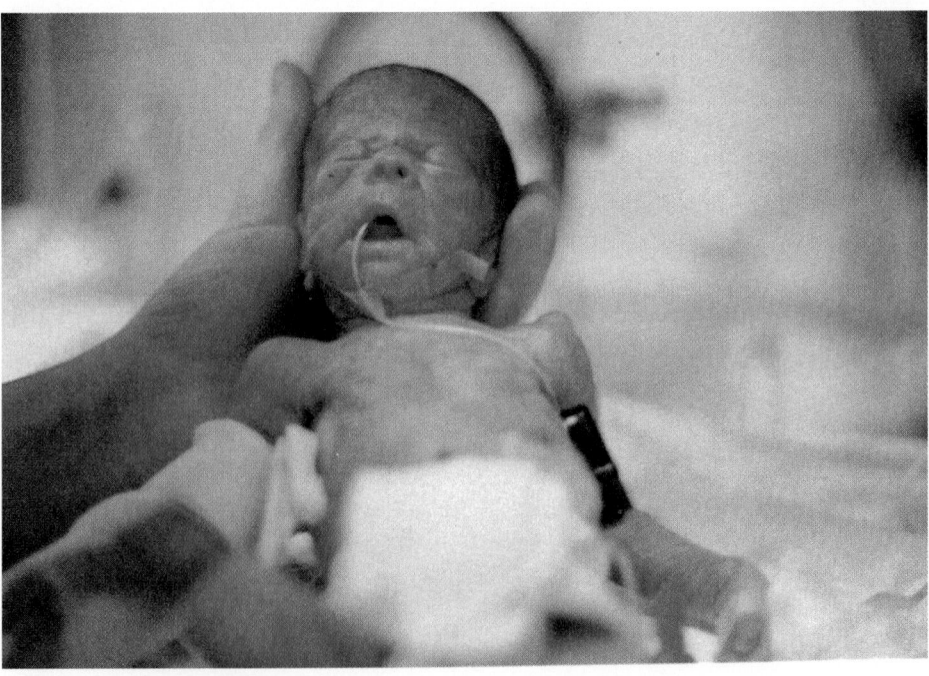

FIGURE 33-3 The premature neonate.

1. The premature neonate tends to lose heat more readily than the term neonate. This is because of its relatively large body surface area and comparatively small weight.
2. The premature neonate has not sufficiently developed the control mechanisms needed to regulate body temperature.
3. The premature neonate has smaller subcutaneous stores of insulating fat.
4. Neonates cannot shiver and must maintain body temperature through other mechanisms.

As with full-term neonates, keep the airway clear. If the premature neonate shows signs or symptoms of respiratory distress, administer supplemental oxygen and, if necessary, carry out ventilation. (Discussion of these techniques follow.) Monitor the umbilical cord for bleeding. If possible, transport the neonate to a facility with a neonatal intensive care unit (NICU).

THE DISTRESSED NEONATE

The neonate in distress may be either full-term or premature. The presence of fetal **meconium** at birth indicates the possibility of fetal respiratory distress. If the neonate is simply meconium stained, then distress may have been remote. But if there is particulate meconium, distress may have occurred recently, and the neonate should be managed accordingly. Aspiration of meconium can cause severe lung inflammation and pneumonia in the neonate. If you spot meconium during delivery, do not induce respiratory effort until you have removed the meconium from the trachea by suctioning under direct visualization with the laryngoscope. (See Figure 33-4.) Report the presence of meconium to the medical control physician.

■ **meconium** dark-green material found in the intestine of the full-term neonate. It can be expelled from the intestine into the amniotic fluid during periods of fetal distress.

✱ The presence of meconium indicates the possibility of fetal distress either recently or some time in the past.

Airway and Ventilation

The most common problems in the period immediately after birth involve the airway and ventilation. Resuscitation of the neonate primarily consists of ventilation and oxygenation. The use of IV fluids, drugs, or cardiac equipment is usually not indicated. Suctioning, drying, and stimulating the distressed neonate are particularly important.

The single most important indicator of neonatal distress is fetal heart rate. The neonate has a relatively fixed stroke volume; thus cardiac output is directly related to heart rate. Bradycardia, as caused by hypoxia, results in decreased cardiac output and, ultimately, poor perfusion. A pulse rate of less than 60 beats per minute in a distressed neonate indicates that CPR should be initiated. In distressed neonates, monitor the heart rate manually.

Resuscitation of the Distressed Neonate

The vast majority of neonates do not require resuscitation beyond stimulation, maintenance of the airway, and maintenance of body temperature. Unfortunately, it is difficult to predict which neonates ultimately will require resuscitation. Each EMS unit should contain a neonatal resuscitation kit that includes the following supplies.

❑ Bag-valve-mask unit
❑ Bulb syringe
❑ DeLee suction trap

When head is delivered

As soon as the baby's head is delivered (prior to delivery of the shoulders) *the mouth, oropharynx, and hypopharynx should be thoroughly suctioned,* using a 10 Fr. DeLee suction catheter or other flexible suction catheter. Any catheter used should be no smaller than a 10 Fr.

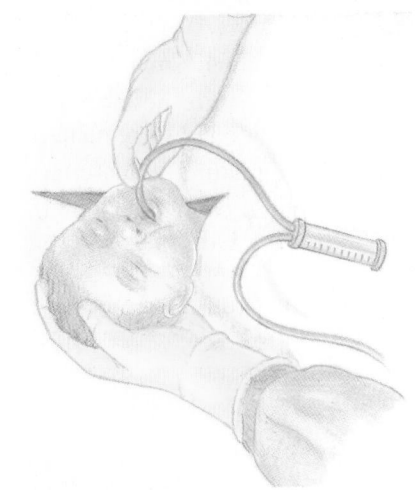

Following delivery

After delivery of the infant, the trachea should be intubated and any residual meconium removed from the lower airway.

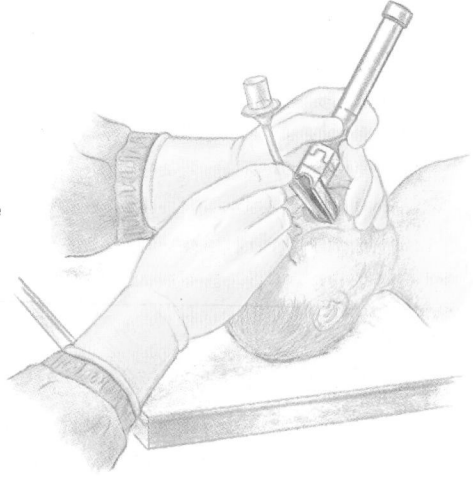

FIGURE 33-4 Management of the infant with meconium staining.

- ❑ Laryngoscope with size 0 and size 1 blades
- ❑ Uncuffed endotracheal tubes (2.5, 3.0, 3.5) with appropriate suction catheters
- ❑ Endotracheal tube stylet
- ❑ Umbilical catheter and 10 mL syringe
- ❑ Three-way stopcock
- ❑ 20 mL syringe and 8 french feeding tube for gastric suction
- ❑ Dextrostix
- ❑ Assorted syringes and needles
- ❑ Towels (sterile)
- ❑ Medications:
  - Epinephrine 1:10,000 and 1:1,000
  - Neonatal Narcan
  - Volume expander (lactated Ringer's solution or saline)
  - Sodium bicarbonate (10 mEq in 10 mL)

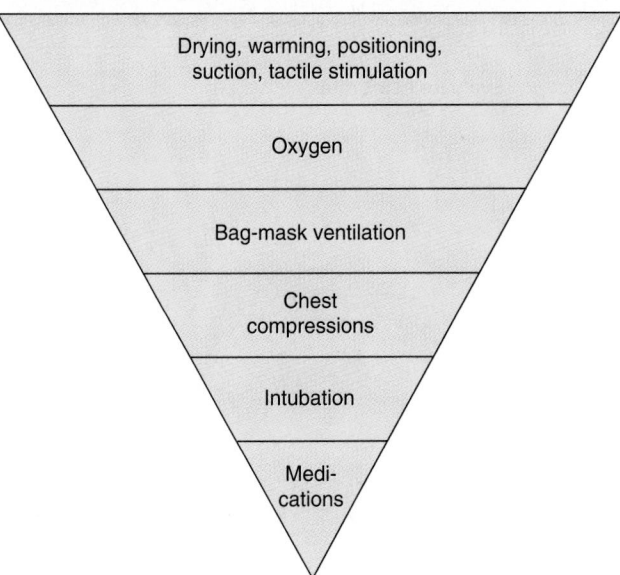

FIGURE 33-5 The Inverted Pyramid for resuscitation of the distressed neonate.

Drying, warming, positioning, suction, tactile stimulation

Oxygen

Bag-mask ventilation

Chest compressions

Intubation

Medications

Inverted Pyramid for Resuscitation The inverted pyramid illustrates the relative frequency with which various steps in neonatal resuscitation are required. (See Figure 33-5.) Procedure 33-1 illustrates the steps involved in resuscitating a neonate.

Step 1: Drying, Warming, Positioning, Suction, and Tactile Stimulation.
The first step in resuscitation involves drying, warming, positioning, suctioning, and stimulating the neonate. (See Figure 33-6.) Immediately upon delivery, minimize heat loss by drying the neonate. Next, place the neonate in a warm, dry blanket. Make sure the environment is warm and free of drafts.

After you have dried the neonate, place the infant on its back with its head slightly below its body and its neck slightly extended. (See Figure 33-7.) This facilitates drainage of secretions and fluid from the lungs. Place a small blanket, folded to a 2 cm thickness, under the neonate's shoulders to help maintain this position.

Next, suction the neonate again, using a bulb syringe or DeLee suction trap. Deep suctioning can cause a vagal response and result in bradycardia.

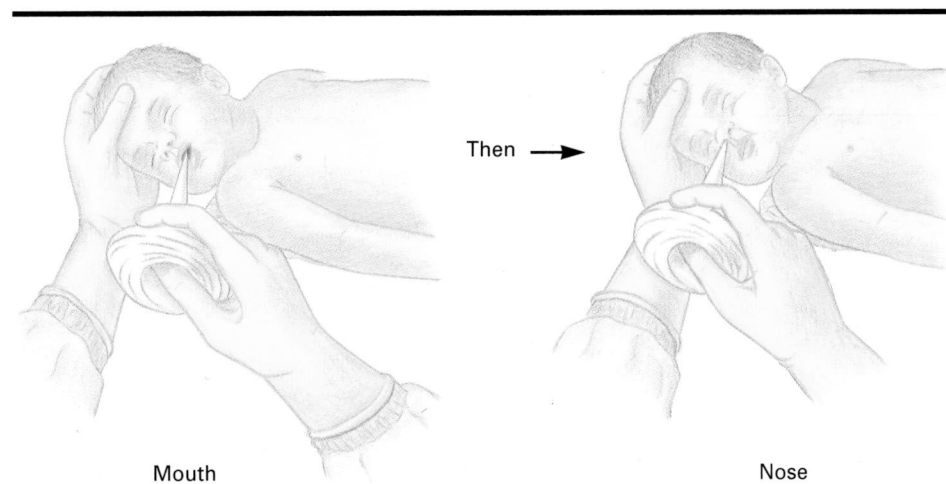

Mouth   Then →   Nose

FIGURE 33-6 Suctioning the mouth, then nose.

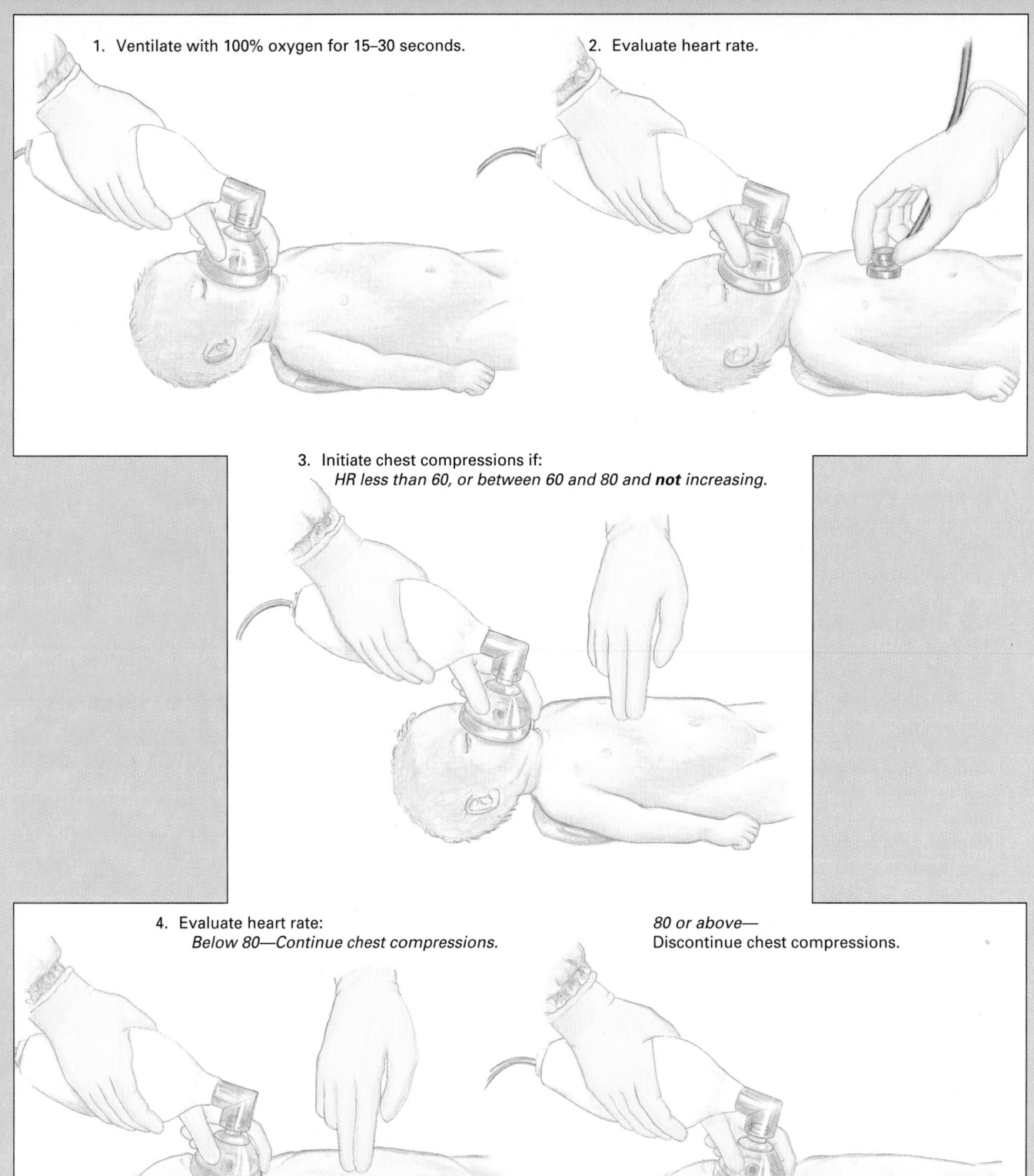

1. Ventilate with 100% oxygen for 15–30 seconds.

2. Evaluate heart rate.

3. Initiate chest compressions if:
   *HR less than 60, or between 60 and 80 and **not** increasing.*

4. Evaluate heart rate:
   Below 80—Continue chest compressions.

   80 or above—
   Discontinue chest compressions.

CORRECT

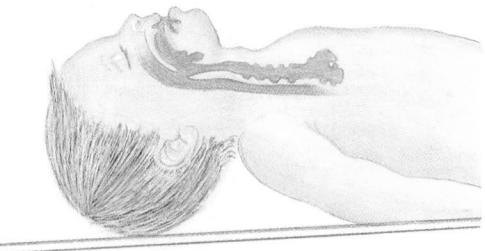

Neck slightly extended

Care should be taken to prevent hyperextension or underextension of the neck since either may decrease air entry.

INCORRECT

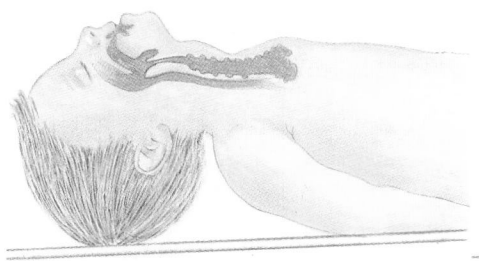 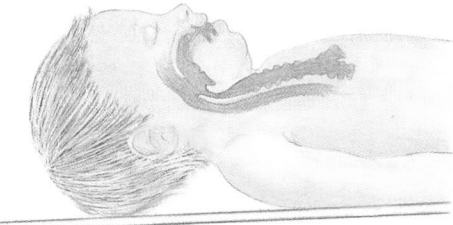

Neck hyperextended   Neck underextended

FIGURE 33-7   Positioning the neonate to open the airway.

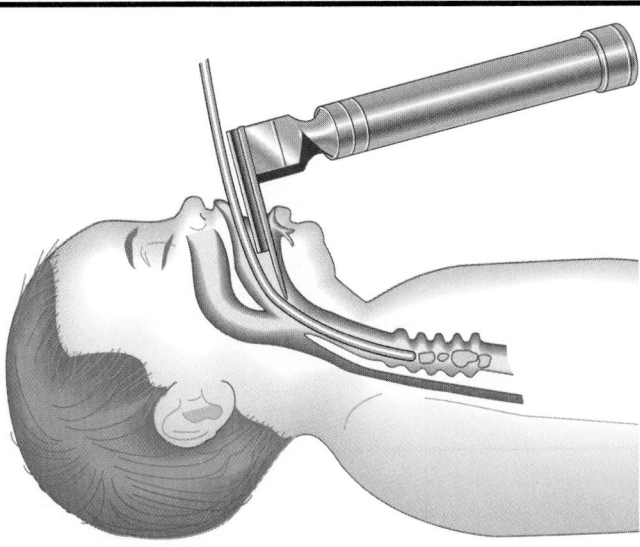

FIGURE 33-8   Tracheal suctioning is important in cases of meconium staining.

Because of this, suctioning should last no longer than 10 seconds. If meconium is present, visualize the airway with a laryngoscope and suction the meconium, preferably with a DeLee suction trap. (See Figure 33-8.) If there is a great deal of meconium, place an endotracheal tube and suction the meconium directly through the tube. (Procedure 33-2.) Next, stimulate the neonate by slapping the soles of its feet and rubbing its back.

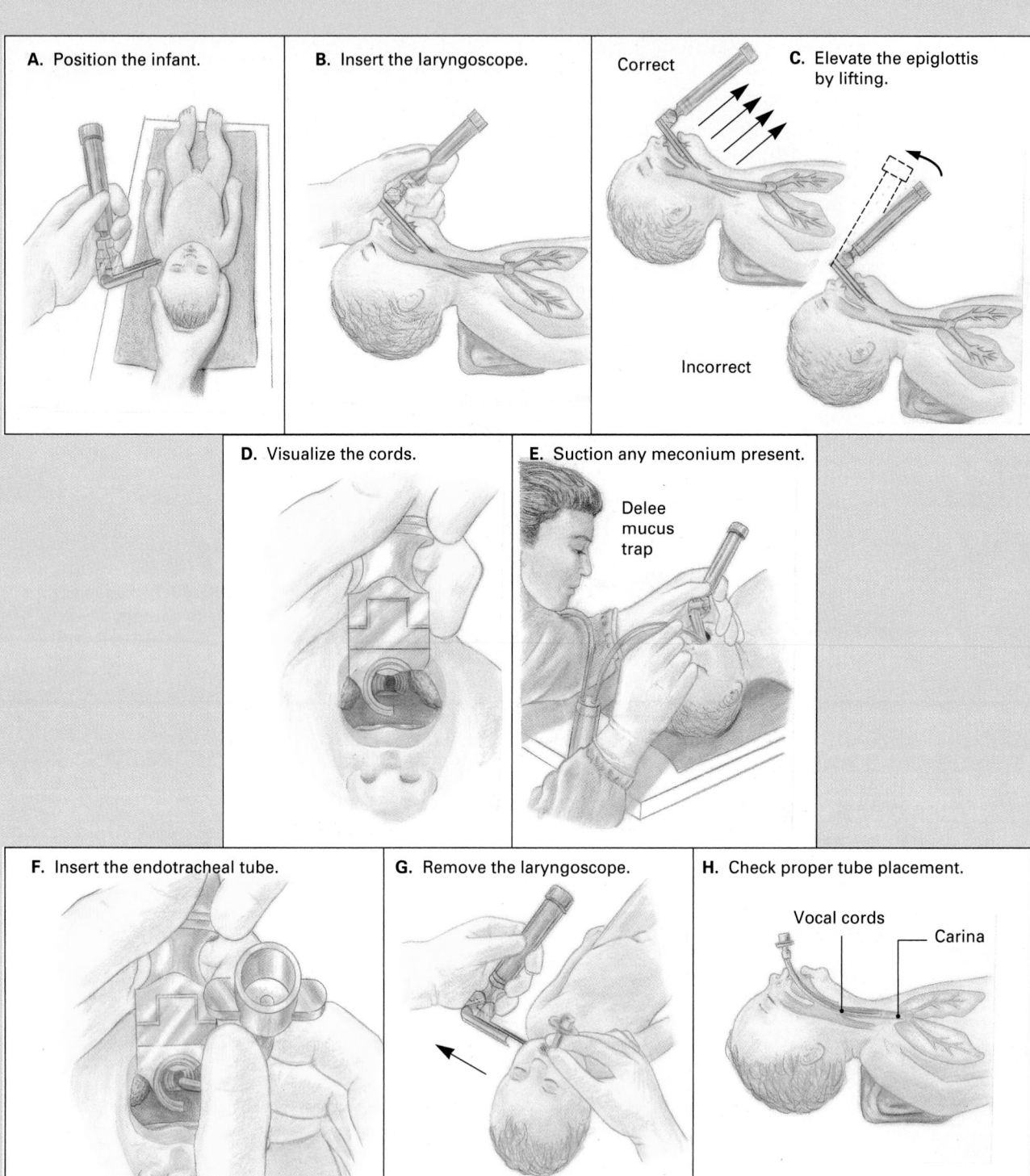

A. Position the infant.

B. Insert the laryngoscope.

Correct

C. Elevate the epiglottis by lifting.

Incorrect

D. Visualize the cords.

E. Suction any meconium present.

Delee mucus trap

F. Insert the endotracheal tube.

G. Remove the laryngoscope.

H. Check proper tube placement.

Vocal cords

Carina

After carrying out the maneuvers described above, assess the neonate. Assessment should include the following parameters:

❑ *Respiratory Effort.* The rate and depth of the neonate's breathing should increase immediately with tactile stimulation. If the respiratory response is appropriate, evaluate the heart rate next. If the respiratory rate is inappropriate, begin positive-pressure ventilation (see Step 3).

❑ *Heart Rate.* The heart rate is a critical component of neonatal resuscitation. Check the heart rate by listening to the apical area of the heart with a stethoscope, feeling the pulse by lightly grasping the umbilical cord, or feeling either the brachial or femoral pulse. If the heart rate is greater than 100 and spontaneous respirations are present, continue the assessment. If the heart rate is less than 100, begin positive-pressure ventilation immediately (see Step 3).

❑ *Color.* A neonate may be cyanotic despite a heart rate greater than 100 and spontaneous respirations. If you note *central cyanosis*, or cyanosis of the chest and abdomen, in a neonate with adequate ventilation and a pulse rate greater than 100, administer supplemental oxygen (see Step 2). Neonates with peripheral cyanosis do not usually need supplemental oxygen unless the cyanosis is prolonged.

❑ *APGAR Score.* As described previously, if resuscitation is not required, obtain 1- and 5-minute APGAR scores.

Step 2: Supplemental Oxygen. If central cyanosis is present or the adequacy of ventilation is uncertain, administer supplemental oxygen by blowing oxygen across the neonate's face. (See Figures 33-9 and 33-10.) If possible, the oxygen should be warmed. Continue oxygen administration until the neonate's color has improved throughout. Although oxygen toxicity is a concern, this condition is usually associated with prolonged usage over several days. Administration in the prehospital setting will not cause problems. NEVER DEPRIVE A NEONATE OF OXYGEN IN THE PREHOSPITAL SETTING FOR FEAR OF TOXICITY.

✱Never deprive a neonate of oxygen in the prehospital setting for fear of toxicity.

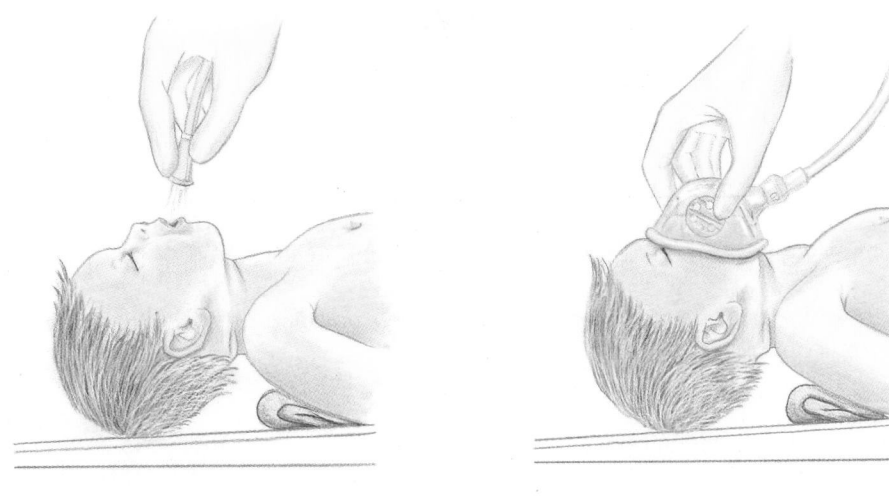

Tubing   Mask

FIGURE 33-9   Oxygen administration for the neonate.

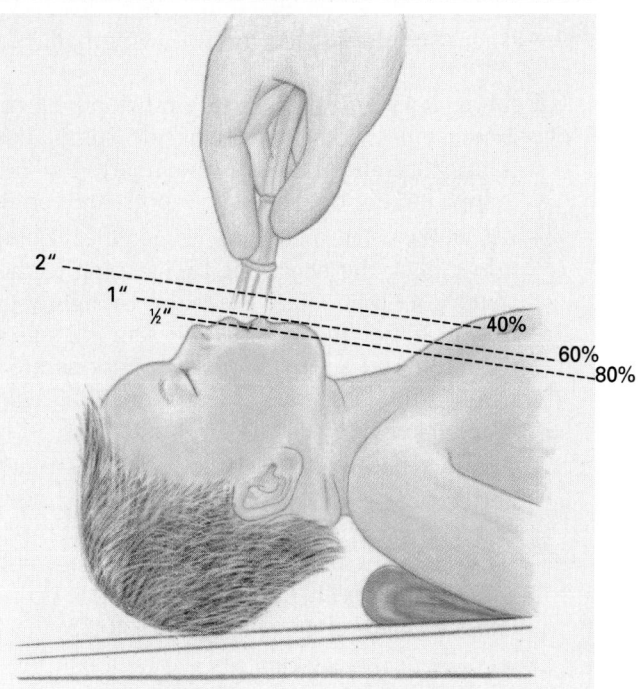

FIGURE 33-10 Guidelines for estimating oxygen concentration. Based on oxygen flow rate of 5 liters per minute.

2"
1"
½"
40%
60%
80%

Step 3: Ventilation. Begin positive-pressure ventilation if any of the following conditions are present.

❑ Heart rate less than 100 beats per minute
❑ Apnea
❑ Persistence of central cyanosis after administration of supplemental oxygen

A ventilatory rate of 40–60 breaths per minute is usually adequate. A bag-valve-mask unit is the device of choice. The initial pressures required to ventilate a neonate may be as high as 60 cm/H_2O. If the bag-valve-mask unit has a pop-off pressure valve, you may have to depress it to ensure adequate ventilation is present.

Endotracheal intubation in a neonate should be carried out under the following situations:

❑ The bag-valve-mask unit does not work.
❑ Tracheal suctioning is required (for example, for thick meconium).
❑ Prolonged ventilation will be required.

The endotracheal tube should be uncuffed. Ensure proper placement by noting symmetrical chest wall motion and equal breath sounds.

Step 4: Chest Compressions. Initiate chest compressions if either of the following conditions exists.

❑ The heart rate is less than 60 beats per minute.
❑ The heart rate is between 60 and 80, but does not increase even with 30 seconds of positive-pressure ventilation and supplemental oxygenation.

Perform chest compressions by encircling the neonate's chest and placing both of your fingers on the lower one-third of the sternum. (See Figure

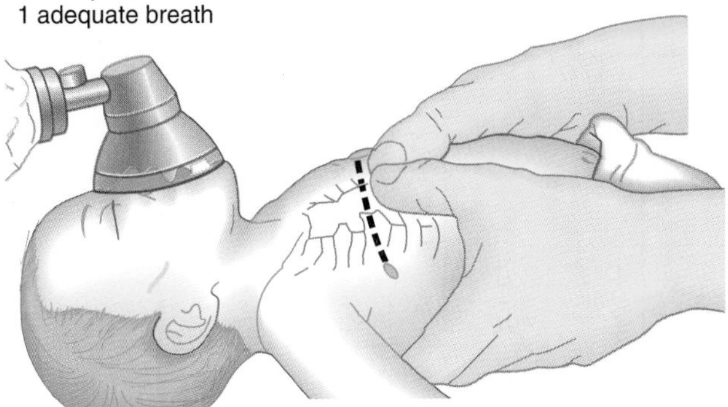

- At least 100 compressions/minute delivered midsternum with 2 or 3 finger tips, 1 fingertip below the intermammary line

- Compress ½ to 1 inch

- 5 Compressions: 1 adequate breath

FIGURE 33-11 Chest compressions in the distressed neonate.

33-11.) If the neonate is large, use two-finger compressions. Regardless of the method, the sternum should be compressed 1.5–2.0 cm at a rate of 120 times per minute. Compressions should always be accompanied by positive-pressure ventilation. Reassess the neonate periodically. Discontinue compressions if the spontaneous heart rate exceeds 80 per minute.

Step 5: Medications and Fluids. Most cardiopulmonary arrests in neonates result from hypoxia. Because of this, initial therapy consists of ventilation and oxygenation. However, when these measures fail, fluid and medications should be administered.

Fluids and drugs can be administered most readily through the umbilical vein. The umbilical cord contains three vessels—two arteries and one vein. The vein is larger than the arteries and has a thinner wall. To establish venous access, trim the umbilical cord with a scalpel blade to 1 cm above the abdomen. Insert a 5 french umbilical catheter into the umbilical vein. Connect the catheter to a three-way stopcock and fill it with saline. Insert the catheter until the tip is just below the skin and you note free flow of blood. If the catheter is inserted too far, it may become wedged against the liver, and it will not function. After it is in place, secure the catheter with umbilical tape.

If an umbilical vein catheter cannot be placed, many medications can be given via the endotracheal tube. These include atropine, epinephrine, lidocaine, and naloxone. Table 33-2 lists recommended medications and doses for the neonate. Fluid therapy should consist of 10 mL/kg of saline or lactated Ringer's solution given by syringe over a 5–10 minute period.

Continue all resuscitative measures until the neonate is resuscitated or until the emergency department staff assumes care.

NEONATAL TRANSPORT

Paramedics are frequently called upon to transport a high-risk neonate from a facility where stabilization has occurred to a neonatal intensive care unit (NICU). The trip may be across the street or across the state. Usually, a pedi-

TABLE 33-2 Neo-Natal Resuscitation Drugs

Medication	Concentration to Administer	Preparation	Dosage/Route*	Total Dose/Infant	Rate/Precautions
Epinephrine	1:10,000	1 mL	0.1–0.3 mL/kg I.V. or I.T.	*weight / total mL's* 1 kg 0.1–0.3 mL 2 kg 0.2–0.6 mL 3 kg 0.3–0.9 mL 4 kg 0.4–1.2 mL	Give rapidly
Volume Expanders	Whole Blood 5% Albumin Normal Saline Ringer's Lactate	40 mL	10 mL/kg I.V.	*weight / total mL's* 1 kg 10 mL 2 kg 20 mL 3 kg 30 mL 4 kg 40 mL	Give over 5–10 min
Sodium Bicarbonate	0.5 mEq/mL (4.2% solution)	20 mL or two 10-mL prefulled syringes	2 mEq/kg I.V.	*weight / total dose / total mL's* 1 kg 2 mEq 4 mL 2 kg 4 mEq 8 mL 3 kg 6 mEq 12 mL 4 kg 8 mEq 16 mL	Give slowly, over at least 2 min Give only if infant being effectively ventilated
Narcan Neonatal	1 mg/mL or 0.4mg/mL	2 mL	0.01 mg/kg I.V., I.M., S.Q., I.T.	*weight / total mL's* 1 kg 0.5 mL 2 kg 1.0 mL 3 kg 1.5 mL 4 kg 2.0 mL	Give rapidly
Dopamine	$$6 \times \frac{\text{weight (kg)} \times \text{desired dose (mcg/kg/min)}}{\text{desired fluid (mL/hr)}} = \text{mg of dopamine per 100 mL of solution}$$		Begin at 5 mcg/kg/min (may increase to 20 mcg/kg/min if necessary) I.V.	*weight / total mcg/min* 1 kg 5–20 mcg/min 2 kg 10–40 mcg/min 3 kg 15–60 mcg/min 4 kg 20–80 mcg/min	Give as a continuous infusion using an infusion pump Monitor HR and BP closely Seek consultation

From: *Textbook of Neonatal Resuscitation* ©1993, American Heart Association.
* I.M.–Intramuscular
I.T.–Intratracheal
I.V.–Intravenous
S.Q.–Subcutaneous

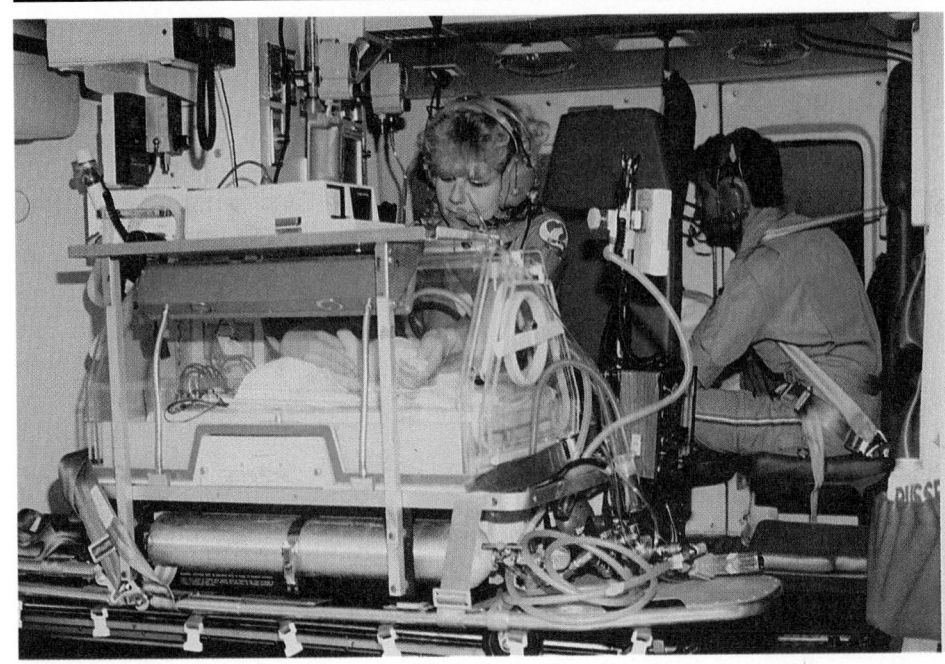

FIGURE 33-12 Neonatal transport isolette.

atric nurse, respiratory therapist, and, often, a physician accompany the neonate. During transport, it is important to maintain body temperature, control oxygen administration, and maintain ventilatory support. Often, a transport isolette with its own heat, light, and oxygen source is available. (See Figure 33-12.) In such cases, intravenous medications are usually being infused through the umbilical vein. The umbilical artery is also catheterized as well.

If a self-contained isolette is not available for transport, it is important to keep the ambulance warm. Wrap the neonate in several blankets and place hot-water bottles containing water heated to less than 40° C (104° F) near, but not touching, the neonate. Do not use chemical heat packs to keep the neonate warm.

SUMMARY

After a woman gives birth, you must care for two patients. The neonate has several special needs. The most important is protection of the airway and support of ventilation. Next, the neonate should be kept warm. If a neonate becomes distressed, you should initiate ventilatory support, stimulation, and, if required, CPR. If possible, distressed neonates should be transported to a facility with a NICU.

FURTHER READING

American Heart Association and American Academy of Pediatrics. *Textbook of Neonatal Resuscitation.* Dallas, TX: American Heart Association, 1993.

American Heart Association and American Academy of Pediatrics. *Textbook of Pediatric Advanced Life Support.* Dallas, TX: American Heart Association, 1993.

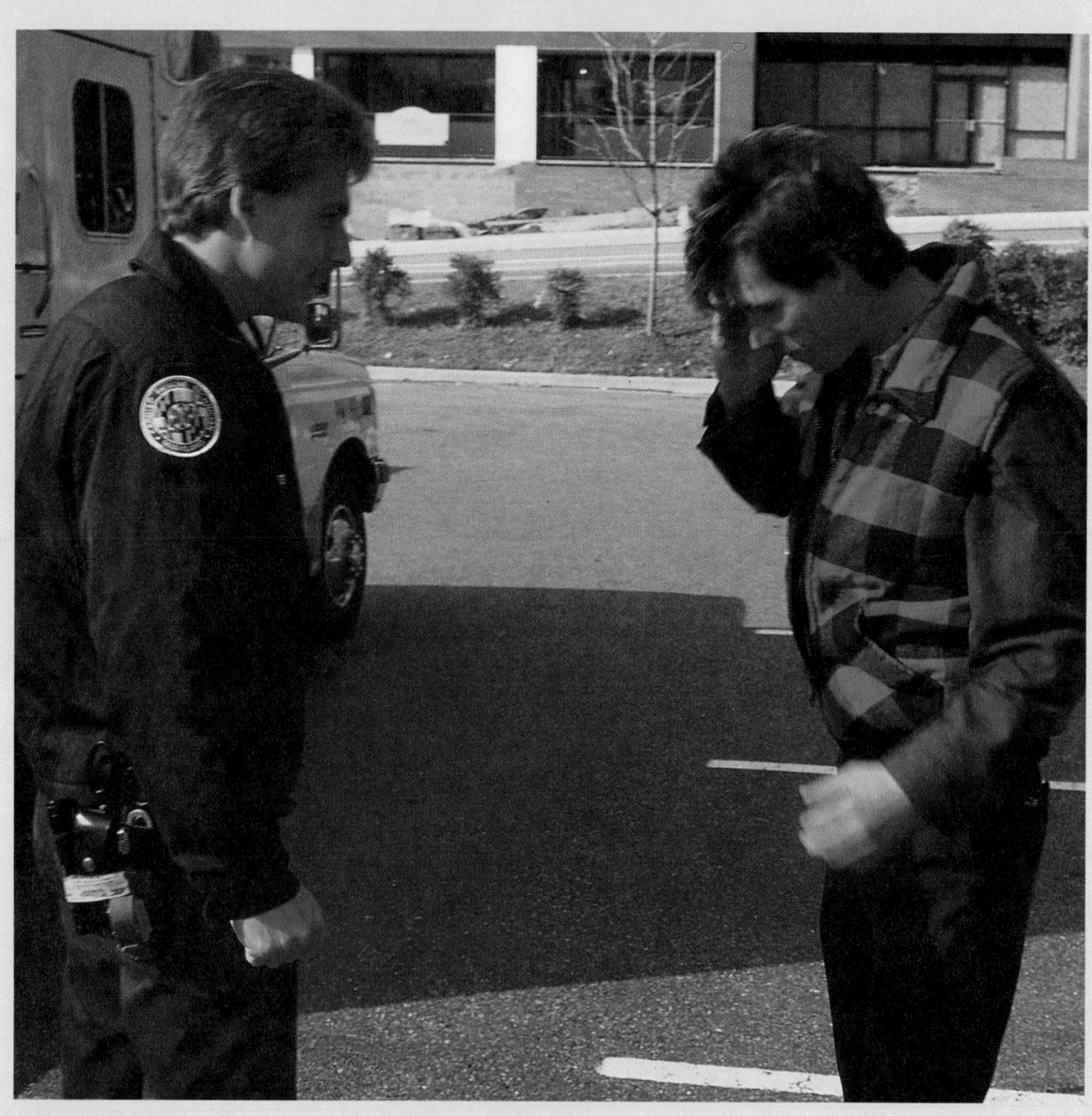

34

BEHAVIORAL AND PSYCHIATRIC EMERGENCIES

Objectives for Chapter 34

After reading this chapter, you should be able to:

1. Define the term behavioral emergency. (See p. 1014.)

2. Discuss the role of drugs and alcohol in behavioral emergencies. (See p. 1015.)

3. List physical problems that can be manifested as psychiatric problems. (See pp. 1015–1016.)

4. Describe verbal communication techniques useful in managing the emotionally disturbed patient. (See pp. 1017–1018.)

5. Describe the use of open-ended versus closed-ended questions. (See p. 1017.)

6. List factors associated with increased risk of suicide. (See p. 1020.)

7. Define and briefly describe management of the following conditions. (See below pages.)

- depression (p. 1019)
- suicide (pp. 1019–1021)
- anxiety (p. 1021)
- mania (pp. 1021–1022)
- schizophrenia (p. 1022)
- behavioral problems in the elderly (p. 1023)
- behavioral problems in children (pp. 1023–1024)
- domestic violence (p. 1029)

8. Describe the indications and procedures for restraining a violent patient. (See pp. 1024–1029.)

On Saturday night, paramedics report to an address some distance from the station. They pull up to a small frame house where a middle-aged woman meets them. "I'm sick of this," she says. "Just get him out of here." Once inside the house, the woman points to a poorly dressed young man seated in front of a television. He is wearing his socks on his hands, and his gaze is fixed on the television screen. However, the television is not turned to a station; there is only static coming from the television's speaker.

The paramedics attempt a primary and secondary survey, but the patient does not acknowledge their presence. The mother states that the young man is a patient at the mental health center but has missed his last two appointments. She shows the paramedics two empty pill bottles, one for haloperidol (Haldol) and the other unlabeled. She tells them that her son has not taken his medicine in over 3 weeks and that he has been sitting in front of the television for 2 days.

One of the paramedics turns the television off and kneels beside the patient. The patient immediately stops staring at the television and looks at the

paramedic. Finally, the patient speaks. The paramedics learn that the patient has been "receiving messages from extraterrestrial beings" through the television. These beings have given him various instructions. His most recent directive is to lead the people of Australia "out of their bondage."

The patient is oriented only to person. He denies taking any medications. He frequently stops, in mid-conversation, to listen to his hallucinations. Evidently, he is still receiving messages through the television even though it is turned off. The paramedics ask if he wants to go to the hospital. He responds, "Sure, let's go." He gets up, grabs a pack of cigarettes, and heads for the ambulance as the paramedics follow behind him. Seated in the back of the ambulance, one paramedic positions himself near the door. On the way to the hospital, he tries to learn more about the patient's television messages.

When the patient arrives at the hospital, two nurses recognize him. He has a long history of schizophrenia, and this is just one of many "breaks." The paramedics learn that the patient does well when he is taking his medications.

INTRODUCTION

The emergency department and the EMS system are now the most common points of entry by disturbed persons into the mental health system. There are several reasons for this. First, over the last 10 years there has been a trend to *deinstitutionalize* the mentally ill. These patients, formerly confined to mental hospitals, now receive care through community centers and other facilities. Second, substance abuse, a major problem in our society, is a frequent cause of behavioral and psychiatric crises. These patients are not generally enrolled in the mental health system. They enter the health care system through EMS, either seeking help or because of a drug- or alcohol-related accident or illness.

UNDERSTANDING BEHAVIORAL EMERGENCIES

A *behavioral emergency* is an intrapsychic, environmental, situational, or organic alteration that results in behavior that cannot be tolerated by the patient or other members of society. It usually requires immediate attention.

Intrapsychic Causes

Intrapsychic causes of altered behavior arise from problems within the person. Such behavior usually results from an acute stage of an underlying psychiatric condition. A wide range of behavior can be manifested. These include:

- ❏ Depression
- ❏ Withdrawal
- ❏ Catatonia
- ❏ Violence
- ❏ Suicidal acts
- ❏ Homicidal acts
- ❏ Paranoid reactions
- ❏ Phobias
- ❏ Hysterical conversion
- ❏ Disorientation and disorganization

In the field, behavioral emergencies resulting from intrapsychic causes are less common that those resulting from other causes, such as alcohol or drug abuse.

Interpersonal/Environmental Causes

Interpersonal and environmental causes of behavioral emergencies result from reactions to stimuli outside the person. They often result from overwhelming and stressful incidents, such as the death of a loved one, rape, or a disaster. The change in behavior can frequently be linked to a specific incident or series of incidents. The range of behavior manifested is broad, and a patient's specific symptoms often relate to the type of incident that precipitated them.

Organic Causes

An *organic cause* of altered behavior results from a disturbance in the patient's physical or biochemical state. Such disturbances include drugs, alcohol, trauma, illness, and dementia. The area of the brain affected by the disturbance determines the type of behavior change.

- ❏ *Alcohol Abuse. Substance abuse* is the pathological use of a substance to the point that it significantly interferes with a person's normal activities. Alcohol abuse, a common problem, often complicates an underlying medical or behavioral condition. Alcohol is a CNS depressant, and alcohol abuse should be suspected in any patient who has a breath odor of ethanol, slurred speech, or unsteady gait. Also, suspect alcohol in a person who is slow to respond to questions. Evidence of recent alcohol consumption often appears in the form of empty cans or bottles or reports from friends or bystanders.
- ❏ *Drug Abuse.* Drug abuse can result from the frequent use of either street or prescription drugs. Because of the wide variety of drugs abused today and the wide variety of clinical symptoms, the drug abuser is often much more difficult to evaluate than the alcohol abuser. Assessment of the patient suspected of drug abuse should include routine examination of the vital signs and pupillary reaction. There is often physical evidence of abuse, such as prescription bottles, drug paraphernalia, or needle tracks. The behavior of the substance-abuse patient can include withdrawal, suicidal or homicidal actions, violent behavior, or hysteria.
- ❏ *Trauma.* Trauma can also result in altered behavior. Causative factors include increased intracranial pressure, decreased circulation to the brain, or hypoxia resulting from poor perfusion.
- ❏ *Medical Illnesses.* Medical illnesses can have behavioral manifestations too. The diabetic may exhibit confusion, slurred speech, and unsteady

gait, particularly with hypoglycemia. Because of this, diabetics are occasionally thought to be drunk. In such cases, medical care may not be summoned until coma ensues. In addition to diabetes, various electrolyte imbalances can result in a behavior change such as confusion, violence, and extreme anxiety.

❏ *Dementia. Dementia* results from actual damage to brain cells. Signs of dementia often include impairment or loss of memory, impaired judgment, and confusion. These are often complicated by poor eyesight and hearing. The onset of dementia is usually slow and gradual. Because dementia occurs most frequently in the elderly, it is often associated with aging. Dementia can result from *organic brain syndrome, Alzheimer's disease,* or similar conditions. Alzheimer's disease is a progressive degenerative disease that attacks the brain and results in impaired memory, thinking, and behavior. It affects approximately 2.5 million American adults and is present in approximately 25 percent of persons age 85 and older.

It is important to consider the possibility of organic disease in *ALL* behavioral emergencies. As a result, physical assessment of patients with aberrant behavior is extremely important. It may uncover unsuspected causes of the altered behavior, such as drugs or alcohol.

ASSESSMENT OF BEHAVIORAL EMERGENCIES

A feeling of uncertainty often exists at the scene of a behavioral emergency, creating great stress for paramedics and other public safety personnel called to the incident. This uncertainty often stems from an initial inability to determine the cause of the crisis. Also, in the past, paramedic education did not cover behavioral problems thoroughly, leaving paramedics feeling unprepared. Even today, there are few protocols to guide prehospital care of behavioral emergencies, since these situations do not lend themselves to a structured approach.

Scene Survey

✱ Always evaluate the scene for danger before you leave the vehicle.

Emergency medical providers may be injured at the scene of behavioral emergencies. Therefore, before leaving the vehicle, you should evaluate the scene for possible danger. Paramedics cannot render aid if they become victims. Unless you are adequately trained, avoid the following situations.

❏ A patient armed with a weapon
❏ Riot scenes
❏ Fire scenes
❏ Hostage situations
❏ Radioactive sites

If the potential danger is minimal, then observe the scene for evidence of what may have happened. Look for evidence of violence, substance abuse, or suicide attempt.

Assessment   Perform primary and secondary assessments in addition to gathering information necessary for immediate management of life-threatening conditions. Sources of information should include observation of the patient, statements volunteered by the patient, information gained from interviewing the patient, and information obtained from family members, bystanders, and first responders. A systematic approach to assessment is critical. The information obtained should include:

- Precipitating situation or problem
- Patient's current life situation
- Patient's recent medical and psychiatric history
- Patient's past medical and psychiatric history
- Patient's mental status
- Patient's affect and physical signs
- Patient's behavior

From the assessment, you should draw conclusions about the possible cause of the behavioral change.

Interviewing Techniques

The interview is the most important part of assessing the behavioral emergency patient. The interview should be organized and logical. Use of a formal checklist is not practical, however. Only short interviews should be conducted in the field, and the situation should dictate the interview's scope. Gather only information that is critical to prehospital management and transportation of the patient, unless the patient volunteers more.

The interview should be open-ended, although both direct and indirect questions may be asked. Allow the patient to take the lead in the interview, unless you are afraid that essential information will be lost or suspect that the patient is depressed, minimally responsive, or suicidal. If the patient is reluctant to answer certain questions, do not press, as the patient may withdraw completely and provide no information. Be prepared to spend whatever time is required to obtain information. Exceptions include the patient whose physical condition requires immediate transport or the patient who may endanger himself, herself, or others. Above all, do not make judgements about the patient's behavior or answers.

The following guidelines will make your interviews more effective.

- Remove the patient from the crisis situation, and exclude the disturbing person or objects.
- Communicate self-confidence as well as honesty, firmness, and a reasonable attitude about issues important to the patient and the situation.
- It is not necessary either to agree or disagree if the patient distorts reality. Simply understand that these distortions are real for the patient.
- Encourage the patient to sit down and relax.
- Encourage the patient to speak in his or her own words, and appear interested in his or her statements.
- Interrupt the patient as little as possible, unless you must redirect a disorganized, rambling communication.
- Do not be afraid of long silent periods. Remain relaxed and attentive.
- If the patient begins to cry or laugh, do not interrupt the display of emotion by talking.
- Encourage the patient to relate his or her story. Nod your head, and say things such as: "I see, tell me more."
- If the patient views the situation as chaotic or if the patient's thoughts are disorganized, use the interview to build a sense of structure.

- Do not argue with the patient.
- If you must ask questions to keep the interview moving, avoid closed-ended questions (those that can be answered simply "yes" or "no").
- Position yourself so that you will not intimidate the patient. Look as though you are at ease.
- Do not shout at a disturbed patient.
- Do not touch a patient without the patient's permission.
- Do not judge the patient's actions or statements. Let the patient understand that you are a neutral party.
- Do not lie or be dishonest.
- Do not place the patient between yourself and the exit.

GENERAL MANAGEMENT AND INTERVENTION TECHNIQUES

The paramedic's attitude is the single most important factor in dealing with the disturbed patient. Communicate warmth, sensitivity, and compassion. (See Figure 34-1.) The patient must take you seriously. Intervene only to the extent that you feel competent, and be aware of your own professional limitations.

The following are general guidelines for managing behavioral emergencies.

1. Before intervening, assess the risk to your own safety.
2. Give first priority to life-threatening injuries.
3. Take command of the situation.
4. Assign bystanders to perform some tasks when appropriate.
5. Accept the patient's feelings. Do not tell the patient how to feel.
6. Display a calm, reassuring attitude to relax the patient.
7. Avoid severe anxiety reactions in family members, friends, and bystanders by good management. Have appropriate authorities remove unnecessary persons from the scene.

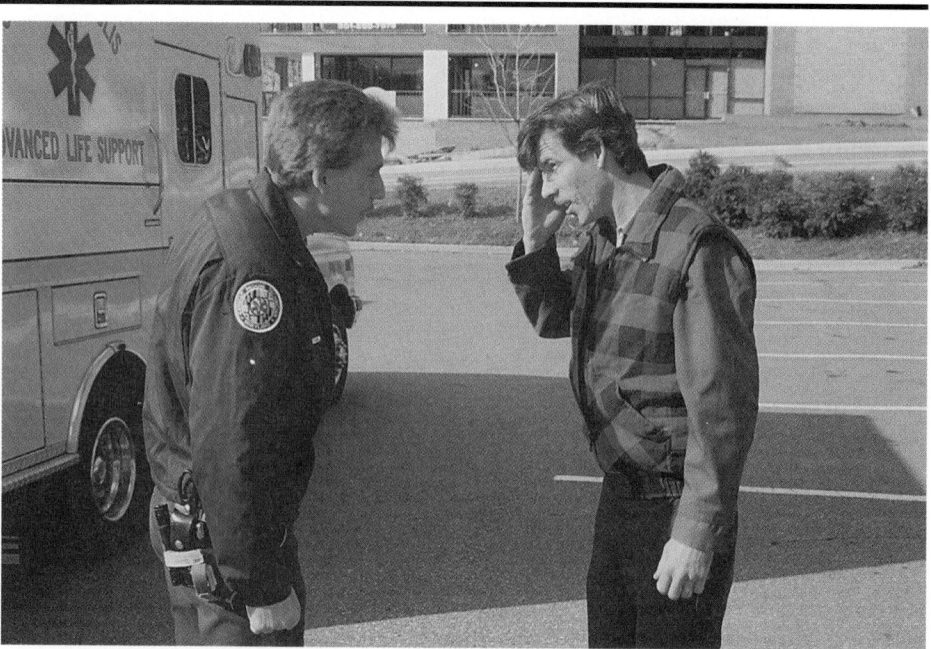

FIGURE 34-1 The psychotic patient should be dealt with in a quiet and reassuring manner.

8. Have familiar persons provide support to the patient as necessary.

9. To avoid heightening the patient's anxiety, develop some rapport with the patient before carrying out a physical examination. Maintain privacy, professionalism, and efficiency.

10. If the patient is anxious or confused, explain all procedures carefully.

Some emotionally disturbed patients are transported under police arrest. If this happens, remember that you are acting as an agent of the police. If possible, a police officer should accompany the patient in the ambulance. This is good practice for both safety and medical-legal reasons.

SPECIFIC PSYCHIATRIC DISORDERS

The psychiatric and behavioral emergencies that paramedics most often encounter fall into several categories. These include:

- ❑ Depressive disorders
- ❑ Suicide attempts
- ❑ Anxiety disorders
- ❑ Manic disorders
- ❑ Schizophrenic disorders
- ❑ Paranoid disorders
- ❑ Disorders of age (delirium and dementia)
- ❑ Substance abuse or dependence

Depression

Depression is a common psychiatric disorder. It affects over 20 percent of the population and accounts for the majority of psychiatric referrals. **Depression** is a mood disorder characterized by feelings of helplessness and hopelessness. Typically, the patient loses interest and pleasure in his or her usual activities. Depressed patients cry easily. They exhibit behavioral and physical changes, such as appetite increases or decreases, weight loss or gain, insomnia, low energy level and malaise, feelings of worthlessness or inappropriate guilt, and, in many cases, recurrent thoughts of death or suicide. The patient's home medications may give you additional insight into the patient's problem. Antidepressant medications include amitriptyline (Elavil), imipramine (Tofranil), phenelzine (Nardil), buproprion (Wellbutrin), and fluoxetine (Prozac).

■ **depression** a mood disorder characterized by hopelessness and malaise.

Management   Depressed patients should receive supportive care. Encourage them to talk, delicately raising questions about suicidal thoughts. Remember that depression often has an organic cause, such as organic brain syndrome, hypothyroidism, or chronic corticosteroid usage. The seriously depressed patient should be transported to the hospital.

Suicide

Suicide is a frequent cause of death in the United States today. It is quite prevalent in the 15–24 age group. After age 24, the incidence drops, until age 40, when it again begins to rise. Women attempt suicide more frequently than men. Yet men succeed more often, accounting for 70 percent of all suicides. Men tend to use highly lethal suicide methods, such as guns, carbon monoxide asphyxiation, or hanging. Women tend to use less violent methods, such as pills or wrist lacerations.

Assessment   Suicidal behavior is related to stress. As a paramedic you should try to evaluate the stress from the patient's point of view. If the patient's stress level is high, then the suicide potential is high. Any person who has attempted suicide, threatened suicide, revealed self-destructive thoughts, or who shows symptoms of a severe depression should be transported to the hospital for psychiatric evaluation.

When confronted by a patient who is possibly suicidal, assess the suicide potential by evaluating the risk factors. These factors include:

□ Previous attempts (80 percent of persons who successfully commit suicide have made a previous attempt).
□ Depression (suicide is 500 times more common among patients who are severely depressed than those who are not).
□ Age (incidence is high during ages 15–24 years and over age 40).
□ Alcohol or drug abuse.
□ Divorced or widowed (5 times higher rate than among other groups).
□ Giving away personal belongings, especially those the patient cherishes.
□ Living alone or increased isolation.
□ The presence of **psychosis** with depression (for example, suicidal or destructive thoughts or hallucinations about killing or death).
□ Homosexuality (especially homosexuals who are depressed, aging, alcoholic, or HIV-infected).
□ Major separation trauma (mate, loved one, job, money).
□ Major physical stresses (surgery, childbirth, sleep deprivation).
□ Loss of independence (disabling illness).
□ Lack of goals and plans for the future.
□ Suicide of same-sexed parent.
□ Expression of a plan for committing suicide.
□ Possession of the mechanism for suicide available (gun, pills, rope).

If you suspect suicide potential, do not hesitate to discuss your concerns with the patient. Ask such questions as the following.

1. How do you feel about life?
2. Do you have any thoughts about killing yourself?
3. Have you ever tried to kill yourself?

It is important to evaluate the lethality of the suicide plan (for example, a gun versus a few pills). The more lethal the plan, the higher the risk. In addition, determine whether the patient has immediate access to the suicide device (is there a gun in the house?). Also determine the specific nature of the plan. A well-organized, well-thought-out suicide plan is much more dangerous than a vague plan. Finally, determine if the patient has made a prior attempt.

Management   The first priority in the management of a suicidal patient is to protect the patient from self-harm. To do this, you must gain access to the patient. This may require breaking into a house or room, particularly if the patient is unconscious and can be readily seen. If the patient is armed, consider him or her to be homicidal as well as suicidal and do not approach.

If you can reach the patient, emergency care has the highest priority.

■ **psychosis** a personality change that prevents the patient from functioning normally. It is characterized by severe depression, excitement, illusions, delusions, or hallucinations.

Conduct a brief interview to assess the situation, and determine the need for further action. Do not leave the suicidal patient alone. Use physical restraints if necessary. Administer haloperidol (Haldol) if ordered by the medical control physician. ALL SUICIDAL PATIENTS SHOULD BE TRANSPORTED TO THE HOSPITAL.

Anxiety Disorders

Anxiety is a normal response to stress. However, it can build to such a point that it overwhelms the patient, who then feels helpless and becomes unable to function normally. Typically, these patients develop an acute onset of intense terror, accompanied by a feeling of impending doom. The patient subsequently fears loss of control. This is what is referred to as an *anxiety disorder*, or "panic attack." Typical manifestations of an anxiety disorder include:

❑ Hyperventilation
❑ Fear of going crazy, dying, or losing control
❑ Somatic complaints, such as chest discomfort, palpitations, headache, dyspnea, choking or smothering, faintness, syncope, or vertigo
❑ Feelings of unreality
❑ Trembling and sweating
❑ Urinary frequency and diarrhea

The patient's home medications can provide additional information. Examples of medications used in the treatment of anxiety disorder include: diazepam (Valium), alprazolam (Xanax), lorazepam (Ativan), and buspirone (Buspar).

Management   The management of the patient suffering an anxiety disorder is primarily supportive. Look for physical causes of the patient's symptoms before attributing them purely to anxiety. Allow the patient to talk, and provide gentle reassurance while transporting him or her to the hospital.

Manic Disorders

Mania and manic disorders can be thought of as the opposite of severe depression. Mania appears frequently in *bipolar disorder*, also called *manic-depressive disorder*. This condition causes tremendous mood swings, from near euphoria to debilitating depression.

In the manic stage, patients appear "high." Symptoms include an elevated and expansive mood. Patients have a marked increase in activity—either social, work, or sexual—and a decreased need for sleep. In addition, patients are physically restless and speak garrulously. They are unable to concentrate or complete tasks. They may have a sense of inflated self-esteem, to a point of delusion. The manic phase of bipolar disorder can last weeks or months.

Manic patients are often prescribed lithium (Lithobid, Eskolith). In addition, they may be taking antipsychotic medications such as haloperidol (Haldol) or chlorpromazine (Thorazine). Some manic states are drug-induced by the abuse of street drugs, such as cocaine ("crack"), amphetamines, or PCP ("angel dust").

Management   The management of mania depends on whether the patient is violent. If the patient is not violent, he or she should be "talked down." Sit at eye level to the patient and talk matter-of-factly. Avoid discussing the delusional symptoms. Try to determine from the patient or family members what

■ **mania** a mood characterized by great excitement and activity.

medications, if any, the patient is taking. Lithium is commonly used for the treatment of mania. If the patient takes this medication or has done so in the past, suspect bipolar disorder. If the patient has never been on medication for mania, or if the family reports that this is the first instance of manic behavior, suspect drug abuse.

Transport the patient to the emergency department for additional evaluation. The medical control physician may request the administration of haloperidol (Haldol) or another antipsychotic drug if the patient is at risk of self-harm or of harming others.

Schizophrenia

Schizophrenia is a disease characterized by deterioration from a previous level of functioning. The onset of schizophrenia commonly occurs in late adolescence and early adulthood. The onset of schizophrenia often manifests itself by a period of social withdrawal, poor hygiene, blunted emotions, and disturbed communications.

Assessment   The signs and symptoms of schizophrenia vary, but several characteristics frequently emerge. These include:

- ❑ *Hallucinations.* Most schizophrenic patients suffer **hallucinations**. These may be either auditory or visual. The patient may hear voices or see people or things that are not there. Often the hallucinations are persecutory.
- ❑ *Delusions.* Schizophrenics often cannot distinguish reality from fiction. They suffer various **delusions**. Some are persecutory, while others have religious overtones. Some patients have delusions of grandeur, in which they imagine themselves to be rich, important, or powerful.
- ❑ *Altered Thought.* Schizophrenics suffer from altered thought processes. The patients cannot reason abstractly and thought is concrete.
- ❑ *Inappropriate Affect.* The patient's **affect**, or emotional state, is generally inappropriate. For example, the patient may laugh or cry at inappropriate times.
- ❑ *Disorganization.* The schizophrenic is disorganized in thought and dress. Clothing is inappropriate or, on some occasions, absent.

Schizophrenic symptoms must be present for over 6 months before the diagnosis can be made. Patients with schizophrenic symptoms of less than 6 months duration are referred to as *schizophreniform.*

Schizophrenia takes several forms. *Catatonic schizophrenia* is a rare disorder that manifests itself by a catatonic stupor. The patient becomes detached from the environment and may maintain a rigid or bizarre posture for hours at a time. *Paranoid schizophrenia* is characterized by persecutory delusions, grandiose delusions, delusional jealousy, or hallucinations with persecutory or grandiose content. These patients often feel that someone, such as the FBI or CIA, is after them. Such paranoia often results from the patient's feeling of self-importance. Some paranoid schizophrenics become delusional and believe that they are famous figures, like Jesus Christ or Napoleon. Another form of schizophrenia, *undifferentiated schizophrenia*, includes patients who do not fit into other categories.

Schizophrenics often remain symptom-free when taking their prescribed medications. Medications commonly used in the treatment of schizophrenia include: haloperidol (Haldol), chlorpromazine (Thorazine), fluphenazine (Prolixin), thioridazine (Mellaril), and thiothixene (Navane). As an alternative,

■ **schizophrenia** a group of mental disorders characterized by disturbances in thought, mood, and overall behavior.

■ **hallucinations** sense perceptions that have no basis in reality, for example, hearing voices when no one is present.

■ **delusions** false beliefs that a patient firmly maintains despite overwhelming evidence to the contrary.

■ **affect** a patient's emotional state as perceived by the rescuer.

schizophrenic patients may receive injections of long-acting, antipsychotic medications (Haldol Deconoate and Prolixin Enanthate). The antipsychotic medications are associated with several side-effects. The most common of these are **extrapyramidal (EPS)** symptoms. They include: dystonia (impaired muscle tone), dyskinesia (a defect in voluntary movement), akathesia (inability to sit still), abnormal posture, excessive salivation, and others. To counter the undesired effects of the antipsychotics, many patients are prescribed anticholinergic drugs such as benztropine (Cogentin) and trihexyphenidyl (Artane).

■ **extrapyramidal system (EPS)** the part of the nervous system that controls movement.

Management   Management of the schizophrenic patient depends upon the situation. If the patient is nonviolent, transportation is all that is required. However, if the patient is delusional to such a degree that he or she poses a threat to others, antipsychotic medication is indicated.

Occasionally, patients taking antipsychotic medications will develop many of the extrapyramidal symptoms previously described. These most frequently occur when the dosage of medication is changed or when the patient is switched to another antipsychotic medication. Prehospital treatment of an EPS reaction should include the administration of oxygen, establishment of an IV of normal saline, and administration of 50 milligrams of diphenhydramine (Benadryl) intravenously. This usually reverses the EPS symptoms.

* Anytime you administer an antipsychotic medication, always have diphenhydramine (Benadryl) available to treat any extrapyramidal symptoms that develop.

* An extrapyramidal reaction should be treated by intravenous or intramuscular diphenhydramine.

AGE-SPECIFIC BEHAVIORAL EMERGENCIES

Chronological age is not an adequate indication of a patient's mental or physical status. Behavioral emergencies can develop at anytime, from early childhood to late adulthood. Childhood and geriatric behavioral emergencies present special challenges to the paramedic.

Behavioral Emergencies in the Aged

Common physical problems associated with the elderly include organic brain syndrome, chronic illness, and diminished eyesight and hearing. The elderly also experience depression, which is often mistaken for dementia.

When confronted with an elderly person in a crisis, you should take the following steps.

❑ Assess the patient's ability to communicate.
❑ Provide continual reassurance.
❑ Compensate for the patient's loss of sight and hearing with reassuring physical contact.
❑ Treat the patient with respect. Call the patient by name and title, such as "Mrs. Jones." Avoid such terms as "dear," "honey," and "babe."
❑ Avoid administering medication.
❑ Describe what you are going to do before you do it.
❑ Take your time. Do not convey the impression that you are in a hurry.
❑ Allow family members and friends to remain with the patient if possible.

Crisis in the Pediatric Patient

Behavioral emergencies are not limited to adults. Children also have behavioral crises. The child's developmental stage will affect his or her behavior. When confronted with an emotionally distraught or disruptive child, follow these guidelines.

- ❏ Avoid separating a young child from his or her parent.
- ❏ Attempt to prevent the child from seeing things that will increase his or her distress.
- ❏ Make all explanations brief and simple, and repeat them often.
- ❏ Be calm and speak slowly.
- ❏ Identify yourself by giving both your name and your function.
- ❏ Be truthful with the child. Telling the truth will develop trust.
- ❏ Encourage the child to help with his or her care.
- ❏ Reassure the child by carrying out all interventions gently.
- ❏ Do not discourage the child from crying or showing emotion.
- ❏ If you must be separated from the child, introduce the person who will assume responsibility for care.
- ❏ Allow the child to keep a favorite blanket or toy.
- ❏ Do not leave the child alone, even for a short period.

CONTROLLING THE VIOLENT SITUATION

You will occasionally encounter severely disturbed patients who pose a threat to themselves or others. In most jurisdictions these patients may be hospitalized against their will, at least until they have been examined by a psychiatrist. As a paramedic, you must be familiar with appropriate mental health laws in the state and city in which you work.

If, after the assessment is complete, the patient appears to be homicidal, do not attempt restraint. If the patient is armed, move everyone out of range and summon law enforcement officials. Avoid heroic efforts. If, however, the patient is not armed and you must contain his or her violent behavior, you may use "reasonable force" in restraining the patient. Before beginning this, seek police authorization. There should be at least four persons available to restrain the patient, and all must understand the plan of restraint. (See Figure 34-2.) Use only the amount of force necessary to restrain the patient. Do not be overzealous.

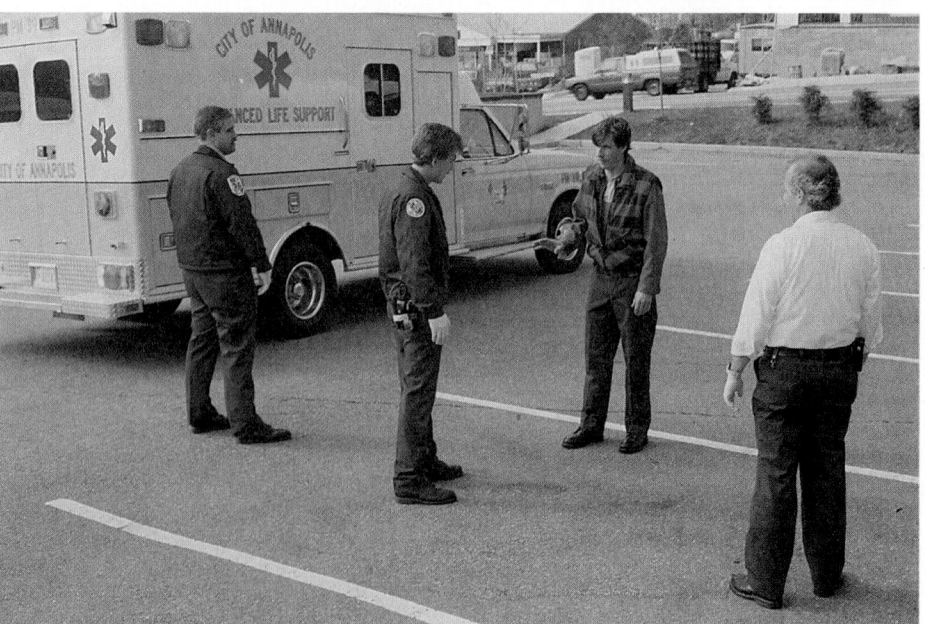

FIGURE 34-2 If it is necessary to restrain the patient, make sure you have adequate assistance.

Methods of Restraint

There are many techniques and devices for restraining the violent patient. Before restraining a person, first consider the normal range of motion for the major joints. The arms cannot flail backwards, the legs cannot kick backwards, and the spinal column cannot double over backwards. Also, consider the power of each major muscle group. For example, the flexor muscles of the arm are much stronger than the extensor muscles. Whenever possible, position the patient to limit his or her strength and range of motion.

You should become familiar with the restraint devices used in your EMS systems. Commercial leather restraints are available, but restraints can be improvised from common materials. Examples include:

❏ Small towels, cravats, or triangular bandages can be wrapped around a wrist or ankle and secured with strong tape to the cot.
❏ Webbed straps, ordinarily used with spine boards, can be used as restraints.
❏ Roll bandage (Kling) can be used to restrict movement of the extremities and thus restrain the patient.

When it becomes necessary to restrain a patient, do not attempt to hold him or her for a long period. This sets up a confrontation and aggravates the situation. It also restricts your activities, because you will be too busy holding the patient to treat him or her. Continuous restraint also requires more than one paramedic or assistant per patient.

The following sequence of actions will help you to restrain an unarmed patient.

1. Make certain you have adequate assistance, since this will reduce the likelihood of injury to both you and the patient.
2. Offer the patient one final opportunity to cooperate. (See Figure 34-3.)
3. If the patient does not respond to this request, at least two persons

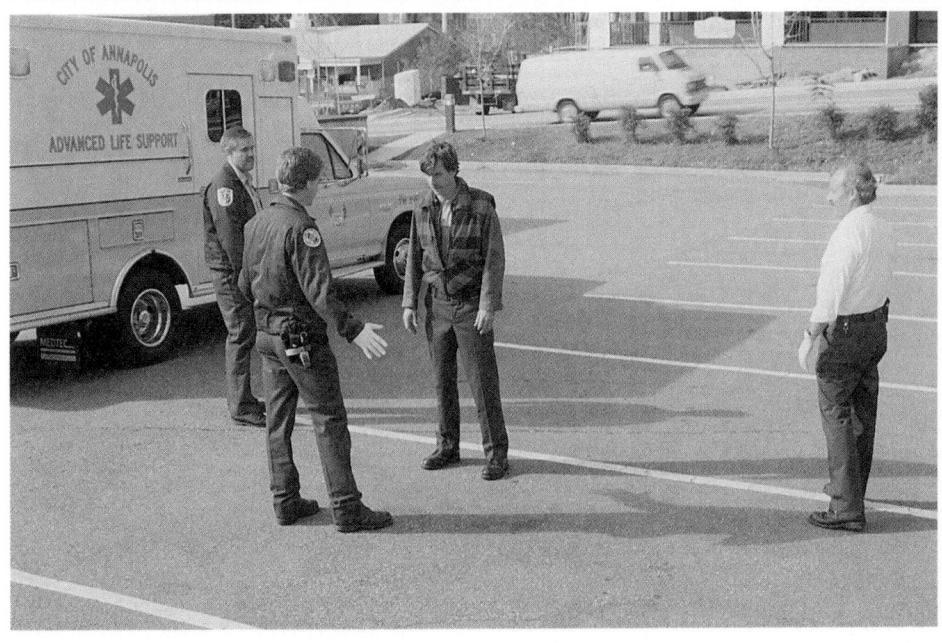

FIGURE 34-3 Offer the patient a final opportunity to cooperate, and encircle the patient.

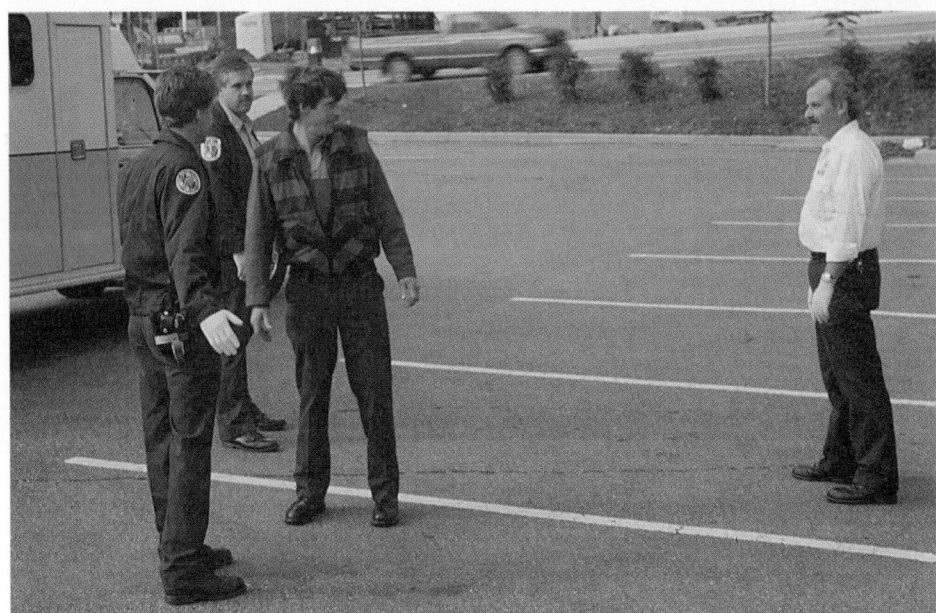

FIGURE 34-4 The patient cannot keep his eye on more than one person at a time. Two of the paramedics should rush the patient at the same time.

should move swiftly towards him or her. The patient cannot focus on both paramedics at once. (See Figure 34-4.) Also, swiftness minimizes the accuracy of a potential kick or blow. At this time, one paramedic should continue talking with the patient.

4. Both paramedics should cautiously move closer and behind the patient. They should not assume that they are in control at this point, as the patient can still kick, bend forward, bite, spit, and jerk about.

5. If the patient does calm down, you may elect to transport without restraints. In this case, continue to reassure the patient. The patient should lie down, and a paramedic should be positioned between the patient and the doors of the ambulance. However, it is likely that the

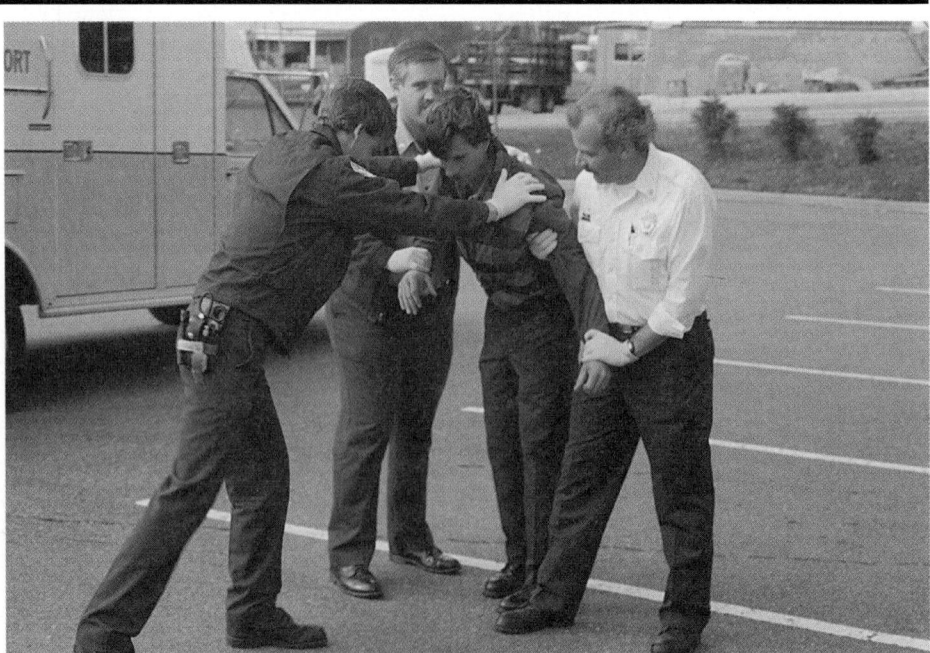

FIGURE 34-5 If necessary, "take down" the patient by placing a leg in front of the patient's leg and bringing the patient forward.

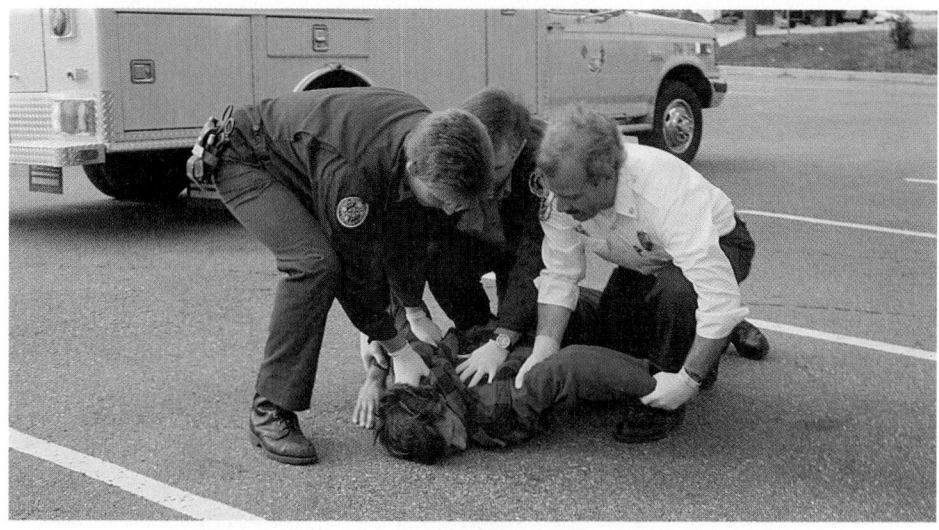

FIGURE 34-6 Maintain the patient on his stomach so that he cannot kick.

patient will again become violent. Therefore, it is best to leave the restraints in place until arrival at the hospital.

6. If the patient continues to resist, the paramedics near the patient should position their inside legs in front of the patient's leg and force the patient forward into a prone position. (See Figure 34-5.) The prone position prevents the patient from using the strong abdominal muscles to sit up. Therefore, the arms are more easily restrained and the legs can kick less effectively. (See Figure 34-6.) Also, biting and spitting are effectively controlled.

7. Continue to reassure the patient. Both paramedics should maintain a good grip on the patient's outstretched arm, while leaning their weight on the patient's back.

Positioning and Restraining Patient for Transport

Once the patient is subdued, he or she should be positioned prone or on the side. (See Figure 34-7.) This dramatically reduces resistance and allows contin-

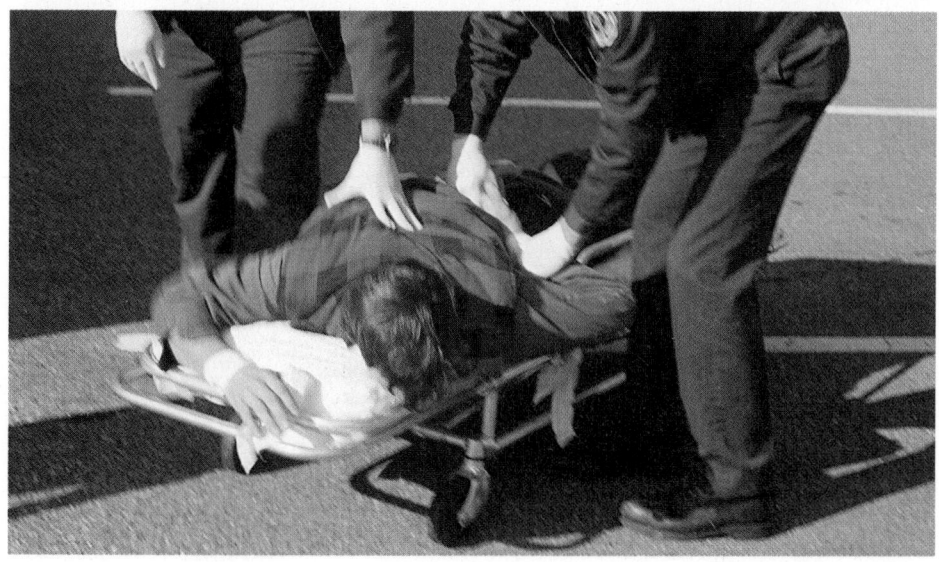

FIGURE 34-7 Place the patient on the stretcher face down and restrain as directed.

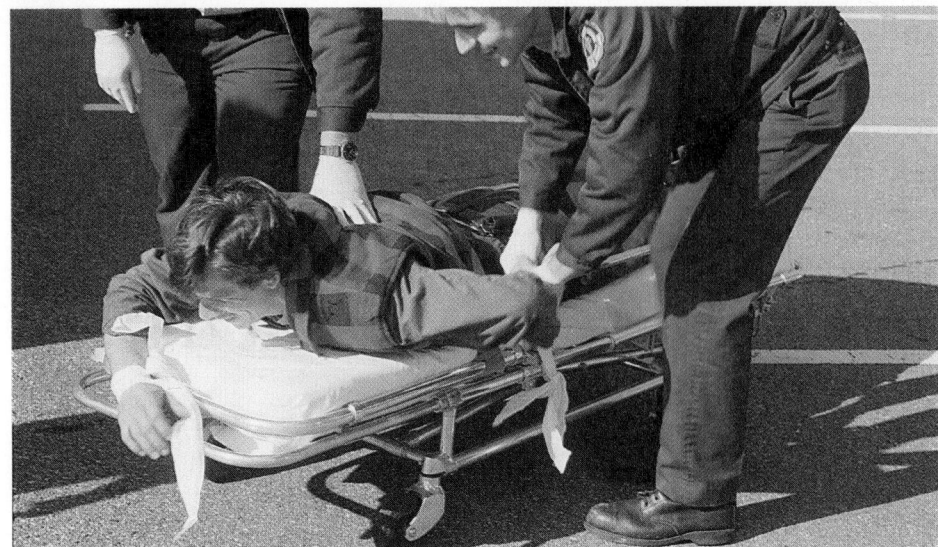

FIGURE 34-8 Secure the arms and legs.

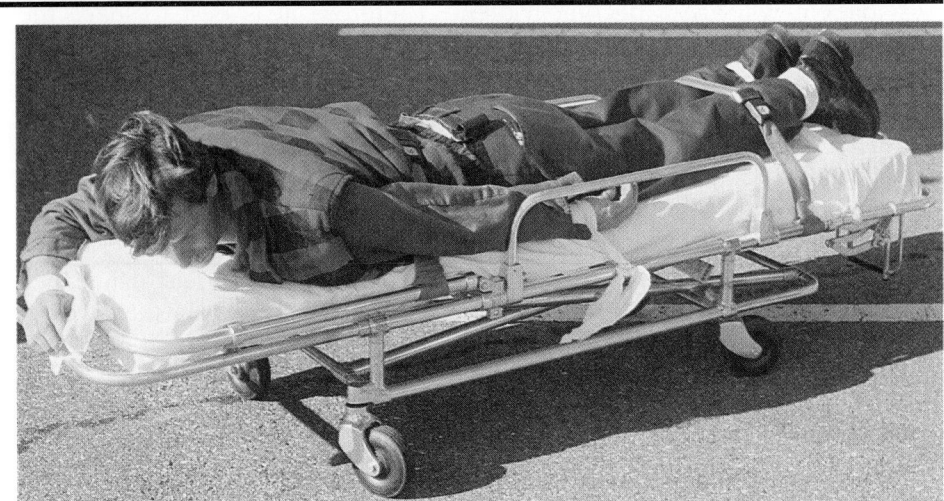

FIGURE 34-9 Patient prepared for transport.

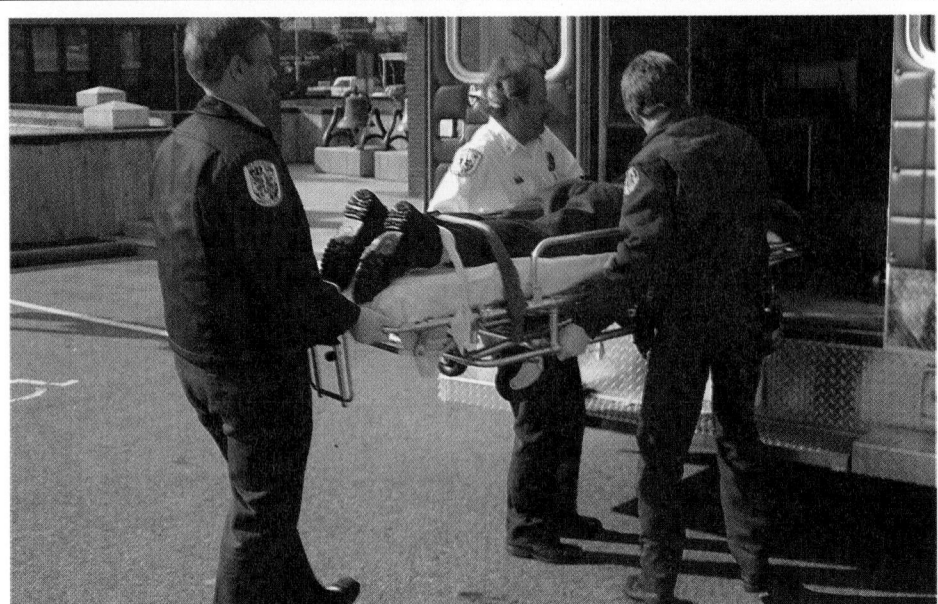

FIGURE 34-10 Transport with adequate assistance.

ued assessment and maintenance of the airway. Adjust the cot to its lowest position to improve stability, avoid lifting, and shorten the distance in case the patient falls. Do not allow the patient's large muscle groups to work together. For example, restrain one arm at the patient's side and the other above the patient's head. Place a webbed strap across the patient's lumbar region, but do not cinch it too tightly. After applying restraints to the ankles and securing the cot, tie the ankle restraints to one another. (See Figures 34-8, 34-9, and 34-10.) Do not remove the restraints until there are enough personnel present to control the patient. Always check the distal pulses after placing restraints.

Methods of Avoiding Injury to the Paramedic

The following precautions can help you to avoid injury.

In a Room With a Hostile Patient

❑ Remain at a safe distance.
❑ Do not allow the patient to block your exit.
❑ Keep furniture between you and the patient.
❑ Do not make threatening statements.
❑ If there are two paramedics, they should stand apart from each other, at equal distance from the patient.
❑ Do not allow a single paramedic to remain alone with the patient.

For Protection Against Thrown Objects

❑ Hold a folded blanket in front of your arm while holding the bottom of the blanket to the floor with your foot.
❑ Hold the blanket away from your body.
❑ Use the same blanket to wrap the violent patient.

DOMESTIC VIOLENCE

Domestic violence is the use of force by one family member with the intent to inflict emotional or physical injury, or even death, upon another family member. Its effects are both immediate and long-term. Domestic violence is a common problem in our society and poses a serious danger to emergency personnel. Emotions are high, and any family member may direct his or her anger at rescue personnel.

It is best to wait for police officers before approaching a scene where domestic violence has occurred. They have received special training in dealing with such situations and encounter them on a regular basis. If you must enter the scene, never do so alone. Also, do not take any unnecessary risks. If possible, try to separate family members into different rooms. If children are present, try to get them out of the immediate area, preferably with a non-involved adult family member. Use a calm and steady voice to gain the confidence of at least one family member. Never take sides in the conflict and try not to pay attention to any one person involved in the dispute. Concentrate on rendering emergency medical care rather than on trying to resolve the conflict. If violence again breaks out, retreat from the scene, and wait for the arrival of the police.

■ **domestic violence** the use of force by one family member against another with the intent of inflicting physical or emotional injury.

✳ It is best to await arrival of police before entering the scene of domestic violence.

SUMMARY

Paramedics do not see society at its best. Although there is a strong behavioral component to every emergency, many calls are purely behavioral in nature. Most behavioral emergencies encountered in the field require little more than reassurance of the patient. However, violent or suicidal patients require aggressive therapy. Each patient should be treated individually, based upon presenting signs and symptoms.

FURTHER READING

Dernocoeur, Kate B. *Streetsense: Communications, Safety, and Control*, 2nd ed. Englewood Cliffs, NJ: Prentice-Hall, 1990.

George, James E. *Law and Emergency Care.* Saint Louis, MO: C.V. Mosby, 1980.

Kaplan, Harold I., and Benjamin J. Sadlock. *Modern Synopsis of Comprehensive Textbook of Psychiatry/III.* 3rd ed. (revised). Baltimore, MD: Williams and Wilkins, 1987.

APPENDIX
12 LEAD ECG
MONITORING
AND INTERPRETATION

INTRODUCTION

An **electrocardiogram (ECG)** is a graphic recording of the electrical activity of the heart. For years, routine single lead monitoring has been an intrinsic part of prehospital care. Now, with the advent of portable 12 lead ECG monitors, multi-lead monitoring is available to prehospital providers.

Single lead ECG monitoring was principally designed to detect cardiac dysrhythmias. It did not allow for diagnosis of acute myocardial infarction, conduction abnormalities, and other electrophysiological problems. With the advent of thrombolytic therapy, early detection of acute myocardial infarction has become very important. There is a limited window of time following the onset of symptoms to begin thrombolytic therapy. In many instances, early diagnosis of acute myocardial infarction can be obtained in the field and thrombolytic therapy initiated either in the field or upon arrival at the emergency department.

This appendix will examine the use of 12 lead ECG monitoring in prehospital care, including relevant electrophysiology, interpretation, and techniques.

■ **electrocardiogram (ECG)** a graphic recording of the electrical activity of the heart.

THE CARDIAC CONDUCTIVE SYSTEM

The cardiac conductive system was discussed in detail in Chapter 21. The cardiac conductive system consists of specialized cardiac muscle fibers known as *conductive fibers*. These fibers are designed to transmit the depolarization potential rapidly through the heart. Transmission through these specialized conductive fibers is much faster than if the impulse were transmitted through regular myocardial cells.

The purpose of the cardiac conductive system is to stimulate the atria and the ventricles to contract in the proper direction and at the proper time. The mass of atrial tissue functions together as the *atrial syncytium*. That is, when one cell of atrial muscle becomes excited, the action potential will rapidly spread across the entire group of cells, resulting in coordinated depolarization and subsequent contraction. Likewise, the mass of ventricular tissue functions together as the *ventricular syncytium*. Once stimulated, the action potential quickly spreads across the entire group of cells, resulting in coordinated depolarization and contraction.

Knowledge of the cardiac conductive system is essential to understanding and interpreting 12 lead ECG tracings. (See Figure A-1.) The SA (sinoatrial) node, located high in the right atrium, is connected to the AV (atrioventricular) node by the internodal pathways. The internodal pathways conduct the depolarization impulse from the SA node to the atrial muscle mass and, through the atria, to the AV junction. The impulse is slowed at the AV junction, allowing time for ventricular filling. Then, as the impulse passes through the AV junction, it enters the AV node. The AV node is connected to the AV fibers, which conduct the impulse from the atria to the ventricles. The AV fibers then become the bundle of His, which transmits the impulse through the interventricular septum.

The bundle of His subsequently divides into the right and left bundle branches. The right bundle branch delivers the impulse to the apex of the right ventricle, where it is spread across the myocardium by the Purkinje system. At the same time, the impulse is carried into the left bundle branch. The left bundle branch divides into the anterior and posterior fascicles, which ultimately terminate into the Purkinje system. At the same time that the impulse is transmitted to the right ventricle, the Purkinje system spreads it across the mass of the myocardium.

Repolarization predominantly occurs in the opposite direction.

This normal series of electrophysiological events results in the normal ECG tracing. (See Figure A-2.)

ECG RECORDING

An ECG machine actually records the electrical activity of the heart as detected by the various leads attached to the body. A minimum of two electrodes are required to detect the electrical activity of the heart, so each lead is comprised of a pair of electrodes. Typically, one electrode is positive and the other negative, or one electrode is positive and the other electrode functions as a reference point. (This will be explained in more detail later.) Passage of electrical

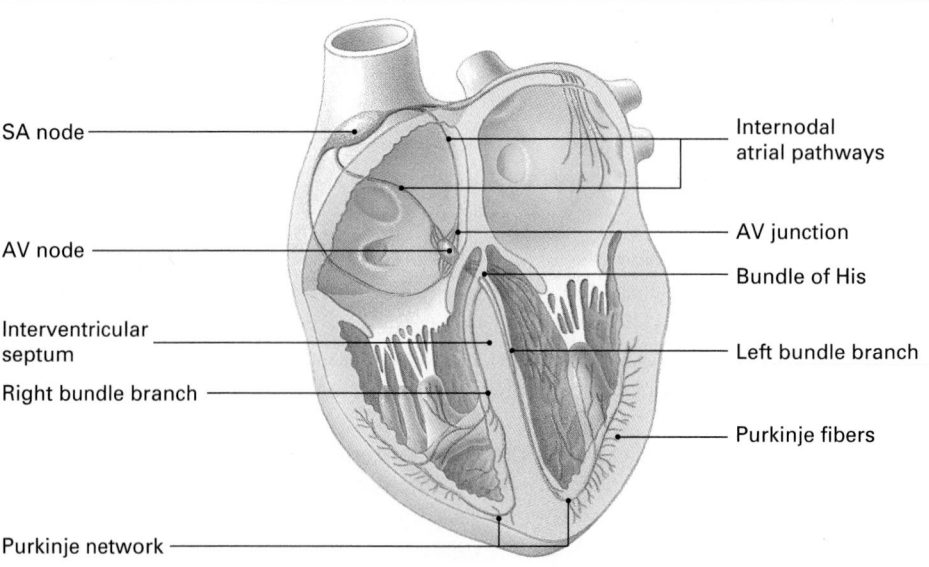

FIGURE A-1 The cardiac conductive system.

SA node

AV node

Interventricular septum

Right bundle branch

Purkinje network

Internodal atrial pathways

AV junction

Bundle of His

Left bundle branch

Purkinje fibers

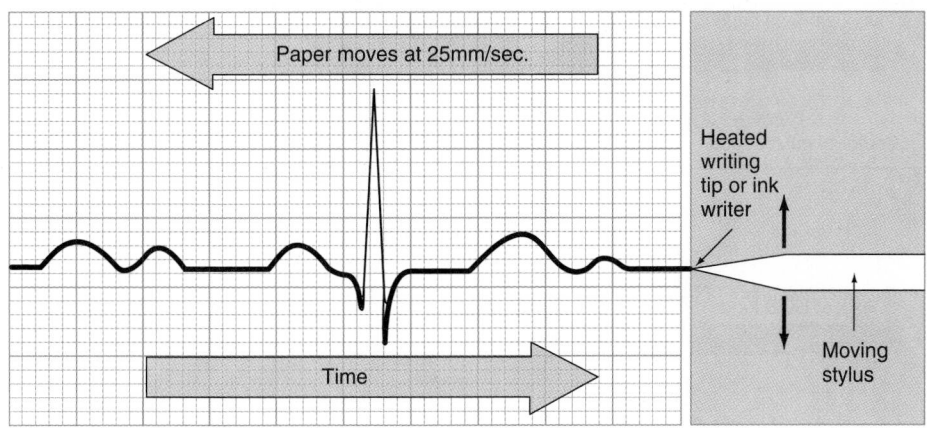

current toward the positive electrode will cause a positive deflection on the recorder. A positive deflection will cause the marker or stylus to move upward. Likewise, passage of an electrical current away from the positive electrode will cause a negative deflection on the recorder. A negative deflection will cause the marker or stylus to move downward on the recorder.

The stronger the current, the greater will be the deflection of the stylus on the ECG recorder. Electrical current that flows directly toward the positive electrode will cause a greater deflection than electrical current that flows obliquely toward the positive electrode. (See Figure A-3.) If current flow is exactly perpendicular to the axis of the ECG lead, there will be no deflection on the graph. This is due to the fact that the current is neither flowing toward nor away from the electrode. As mentioned above, current flow away from the positive electrode will result in a negative deflection of the stylus. Current flowing directly toward the negative electrode, and away from the positive electrode, produces a strong negative deflection. Current that flows obliquely toward the negative electrode, and away from the positive electrode, will produce a less negative deflection. In the absence of current flow, there will be no deflection on the ECG monitor.

In summary, the electrical activity of the heart is a complex combination of positive and negative current flows that can be graphically recorded on paper or an oscilloscope for monitoring. (See Figure A-4.)

ECG LEADS

The first ECG recording was reported by Willem Einthoven in 1903. Einthoven placed leads on the arms and legs in an effort to measure the electrical activity of the heart using a simple galvanometer. Some of the leads first utilized by Einthoven are still in use today.

An ECG lead is not a single wire, but a combination of two wires and their electrodes, which makes a complete circuit with the electrocardiograph.

There are three types of ECG leads. Leads I, II, and III are referred to as **bipolar limb leads**. Leads aVR, aVL, and aVF are referred to as **unipolar limb leads** or the **augmented limb leads**. Together, Leads I, II, III, aVR, aVL, and aVF constitute the *frontal plane leads*. That is, they record the electrical activity of the heart in the frontal plane of the body utilizing electrodes placed on the extremities. The remaining type of ECG leads is referred to as **precordial leads** or **chest leads**. The precordial leads, developed in the 1930s, are designed to look at the heart in the horizontal plane. Leads V_1, V_2, V_3, V_4,

■ **bipolar limb leads** electrocardiogram leads applied to the arms and legs that contain two electrodes of opposite (positive and negative) polarity; leads I, II, and III.

■ **unipolar limb leads** electrocardiogram leads applied to the arms and legs, consisting of one polarized (positive) electrode and a nonpolarized reference point that is created by the ECG machine combining two additional electrodes; also called *augmented limb leads*; leads aVR, aVL, and aVF.

■ **augmented limb leads** another term for unipolar limb leads (see definition), reflecting the fact that the ground lead is disconnected, which increases the amplitude of deflection on the ECG tracing.

■ **precordial (chest) leads** electrocardiogram leads applied to the chest in a pattern that permits a view of the horizontal plane of the heart; leads V_1, V_2, V_3, V_4, V_5, and V_6.

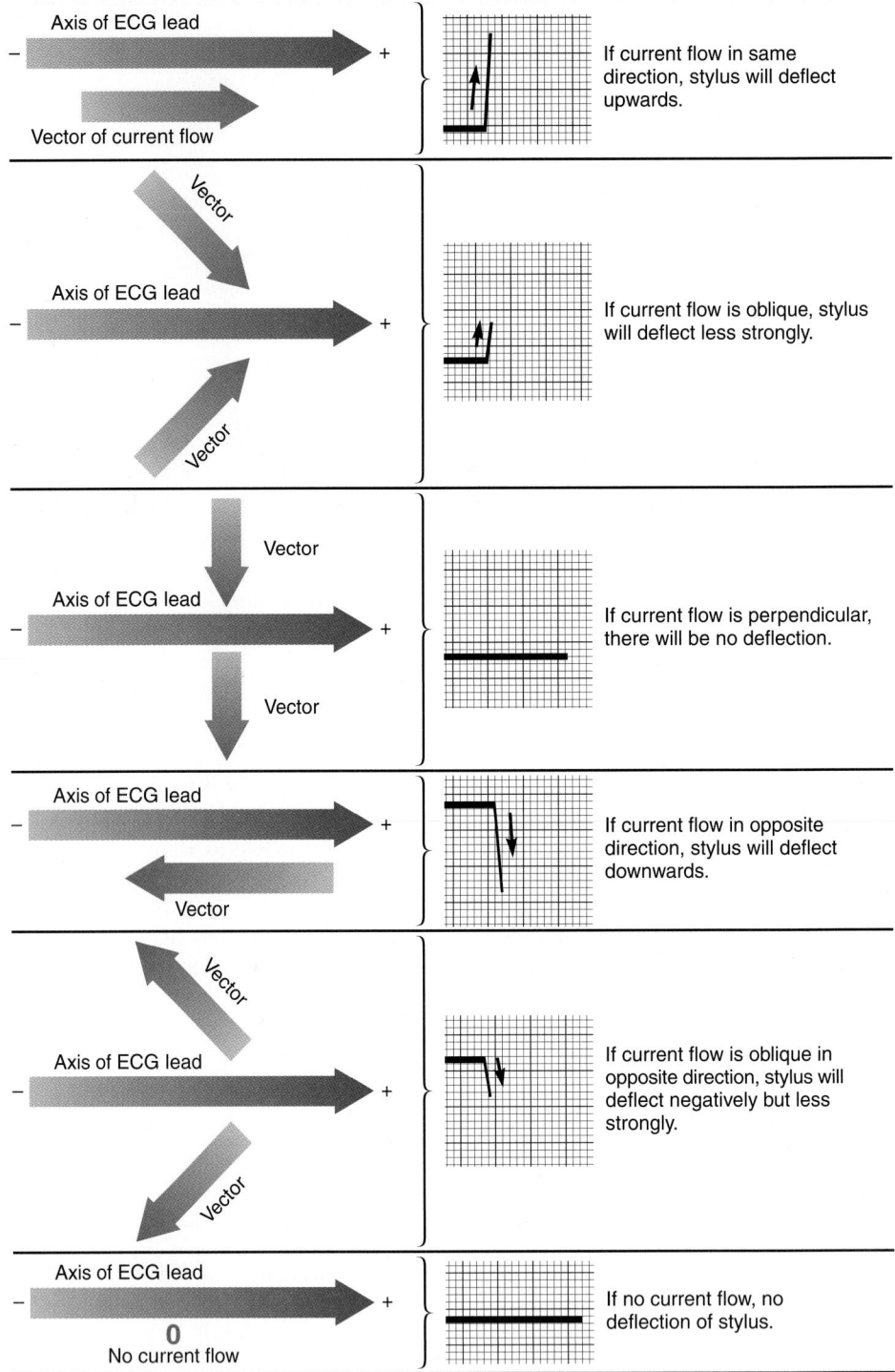

FIGURE A-3 Results of relationships between current flow direction and ECG lead axis.

V₅, and V₆ are called precordial leads. (See Figure A-5.) Additional information pertaining to the ECG leads is detailed below.

Bipolar Limb Leads

Leads I, II, and III are referred to as bipolar limb leads because two electrodes of opposite polarity (positive and negative) are utilized. These leads record the difference in electrical potential between two limbs.

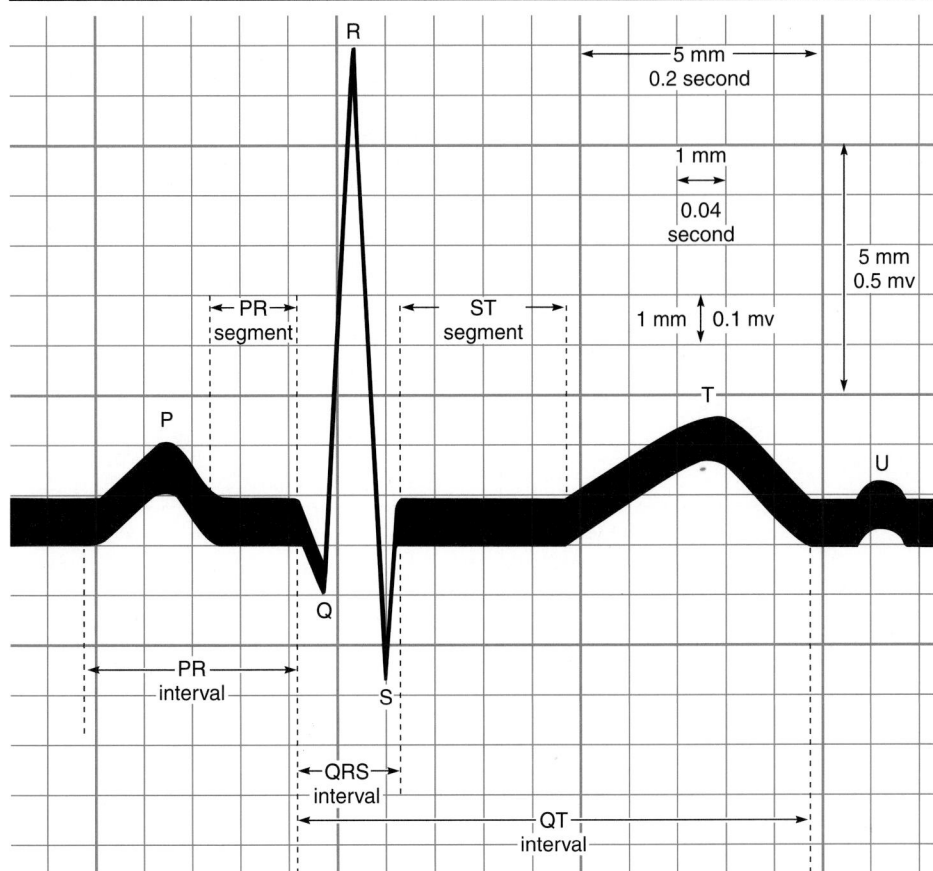

FIGURE A-4 Electrocardiograph waves.

❑ **Lead I.** In Lead I, the negative electrode is placed on the right arm and the positive electrode is placed on the left arm. Thus, when the electrical current moves through the heart from the right arm toward the left arm, a positive deflection will be recorded in Lead I.

❑ **Lead II.** In Lead II, the negative electrode is placed on the right arm and the positive electrode is placed on the left leg. Thus, when the electrical current moves through the heart from the right arm toward the left leg, a positive deflection will be recorded in Lead II.

❑ **Lead III.** In Lead III, the negative electrode is placed on the left arm and the positive electrode is placed on the left leg. Thus, when the electrical current moves through the heart from the left arm toward the left leg, a positive deflection will occur in Lead III.

The triangle around the heart that is formed by these leads is referred to as **Einthoven's Triangle**. (See Figure A-6.) The two arms and the left leg form the corners of the triangle. It is important to point out that electrodes are typically attached to both legs. The right leg is typically used as a ground or a spare as recordings obtained from either leg are virtually identical.

■ **Einthoven's triangle** the triangle around the heart formed by the bipolar limb leads.

Unipolar or Augmented Limb Leads

The unipolar or augmented limb leads utilize the same electrodes as used for the bipolar limb leads. These leads allow a different "look" at the heart by using two of the electrodes as a single electrode. To achieve this, two selected leads are combined in the ECG machine after each has been run through a

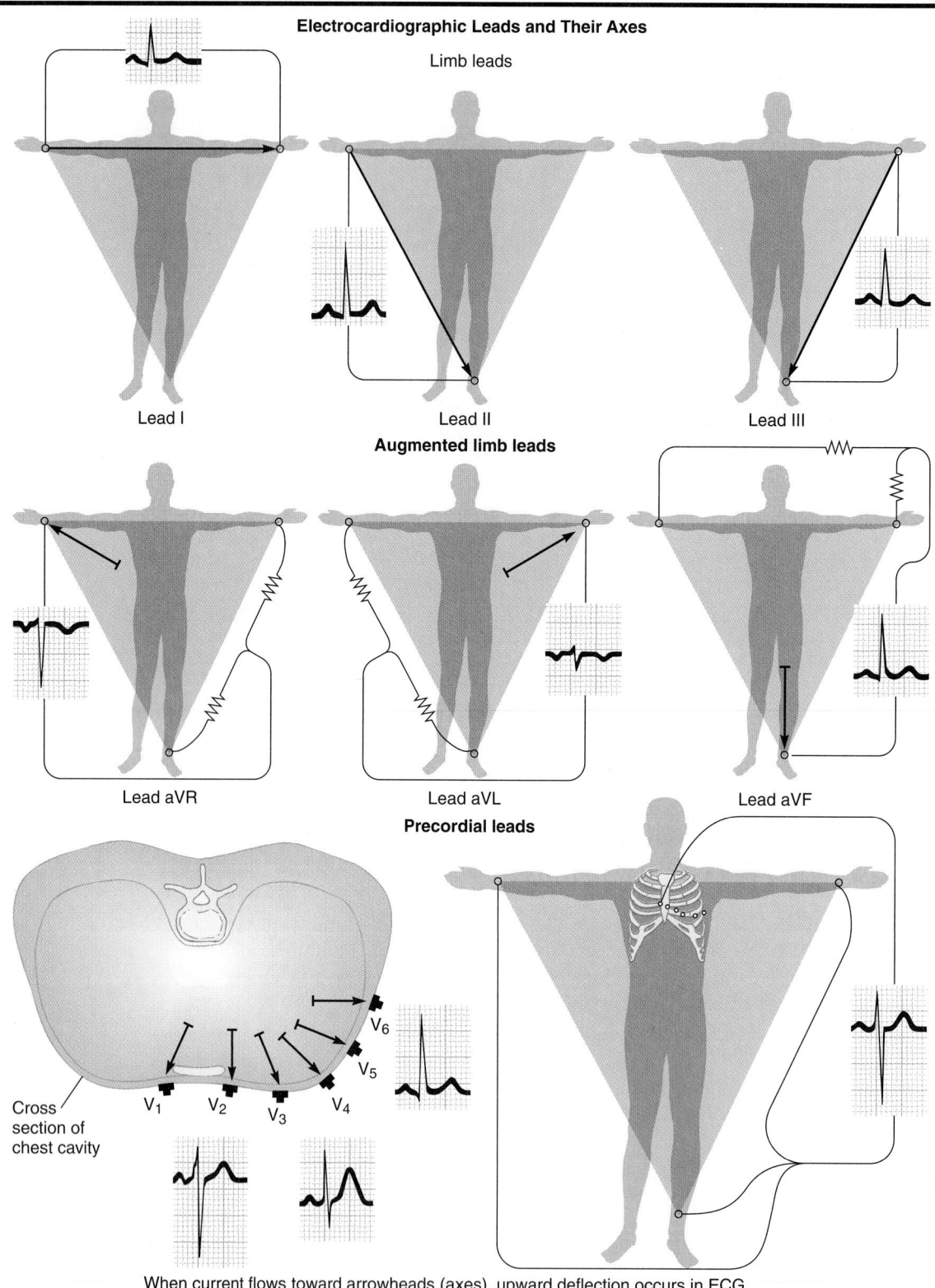

Electrocardiographic Leads and Their Axes

Limb leads

Lead I

Lead II

Lead III

Augmented limb leads

Lead aVR

Lead aVL

Lead aVF

Precordial leads

Cross section of chest cavity

V₁ V₂ V₃ V₄ V₅ V₆

When current flows toward arrowheads (axes), upward deflection occurs in ECG
When current flows away from arrowheads (axes), downward deflection occurs in ECG
When current flows perpendicular to arrows (axes), no deflection occurs

FIGURE A-5   ECG leads and their axes.

resistor to reduce the current flow. This effectively provides a functional electrode halfway between the combined leads. The term *unipolar* refers to the resulting arrangement of one polarized (positive) electrode and the combined

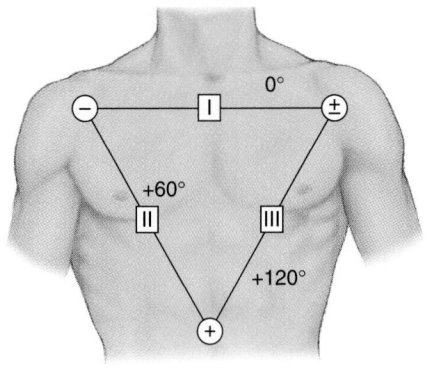

FIGURE A-6 Einthoven's Triangle as formed by the bipolar leads.

leads, which serve as a non-polarized reference point. To increase the amplitude of the deflection, the ground lead is disconnected, thus giving rise to the term *augmented lead*. (See Figure A-7.)

- ❏ **Lead aVR.** In Lead aVR, the positive electrode is placed on the right arm. The negative electrode is a combination of the left arm and left leg electrode.
- ❏ **Lead aVL.** In Lead aVL, the positive electrode is placed on the left arm. The negative electrode is a combination of the right arm and left leg.
- ❏ **Lead aVF.** In Lead aVF, the positive electrode is placed on the left foot. The negative electrode is a combination of the right arm and the left arm.

All of the limb leads are in the frontal plane. If you superimpose the direction of each of these leads on a single diagram, you will notice that these six leads constitute a complete 360 degree circle. (See Figure A-8.) By established convention, the direction toward the left arm is considered to be 0 degrees. Starting clockwise, the radials increase in a positive fashion. Some systems will use the full 360 degree circle to describe the axis of the lead in question. Others will divide the circle into positive and negative halves (semicircles). Using this system, moving clockwise, the radial coordinates are positive up to 180 degrees. Moving counterclockwise from 0 degrees, the radial coordinates are negative up to −180 degrees. Each lead can be measured on this coordinate system.

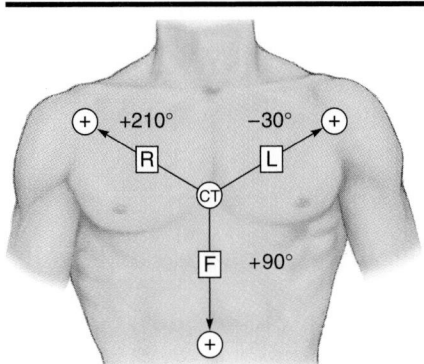

FIGURE A-7 The pattern formed by the unipolar/augmented leads.

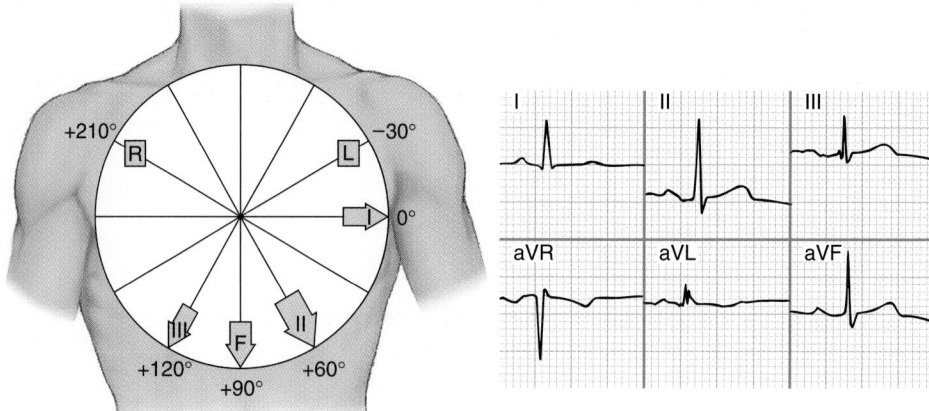

FIGURE A-8 The hexaxial (six axes) reference system.

The following is a listing of the limb leads and the direction in which they point:

Lead	Full Circle	Semi-Circle
Lead I	0 degrees	0 degrees
Lead II	60 degrees	+60 degrees
Lead III	120 degrees	+120 degrees
aVR	210 degrees	−150 degrees
aVL	330 degrees	−30 degrees
aVF	90 degrees	+90 degrees

The semi-circle system is more commonly used and is the system we have chosen to utilize in this discussion. Please remember that both systems describe the same radials, but each uses a different frame of reference.

Precordial Leads

The precordial leads provide a look at the horizontal plane of the heart. The horizontal plane is the plane that results from a section taken from front to back, from the sternum to the spine. The negative pole for the precordial leads is a common ground arranged electronically within the ECG machine by connecting all limb leads together. The positive electrode is placed on the anterior surface of the chest in positions ranging from V_1 to V_6.

- ❑ **Lead V_1.** Lead V_1 is obtained by placing the positive electrode to the right of the sternum at the fourth intercostal space.
- ❑ **Lead V_2.** Lead V_2 is obtained by placing the positive electrode to the left of the sternum at the fourth intercostal space.
- ❑ **Lead V_3.** Lead V_3 is obtained by placing the positive electrode in a line midway between Lead V_2 and Lead V_4.
- ❑ **Lead V_4.** Lead V_4 is obtained by placing the positive electrode at the mid-clavicular line at the fifth intercostal space.
- ❑ **Lead V_5.** Lead V_5 is obtained by placing the positive electrode at the anterior axillary line at the same level as V_4.

❑ **Lead V$_6$.** Lead V$_6$ is obtained by placing the positive electrode to the mid-axillary line at the same level as V$_4$.

It is important to point out that all 12 leads described record exactly the same electrical events occurring within the heart. Each lead, however, allows us to look at these events from a different perspective.

MEAN QRS AXIS DETERMINATION

The electrical energy of the heart is the sum total of the electricity generated by each individual cardiac muscle cell. The electrical energy of the heart exhibits both *magnitude* and *direction*. Any force that has both magnitude and direction is referred to as a **vector**. In actuality, the electrical forces of the heart move in three dimensions simultaneously during the course of each cardiac cycle. However, these forces can be averaged together at any given point in time. This averaged vector is referred to as the **instantaneous vector**. Ultimately, we can combine all of the instantaneous vectors occurring during the cardiac cycle into a single, averaged vector referred to as the **resultant cardiac vector** or **mean cardiac vector.** In this case, all of the electrical forces generated by the millions of cardiac cells of the heart can be reduced to a single vector represented by an arrow moving in a single plane (the QRS axis).

AXIS DEVIATION

The normal electrical axis of the heart is 59 degrees (−29 to +105 degrees). In the normal tracing, Lead II should have the most positive deflection as the axis of Lead II is +60 degrees. If the calculated axis of the heart falls outside of normal, an **axis deviation** is said to exist. Any time the axis equals or exceeds +105 degrees the patient is said to have a **right axis deviation**. Right axis deviation is abnormal and often associated with chronic obstructive pulmonary disease, and pulmonary hypertension. Any time the axis of the heart is greater than or equal to −30 degrees, a **left axis deviation** is said to exist. Left axis deviation can be associated with high blood pressure, valvular heart disease, and other disease processes.

To simplify matters, the frontal plane can be divided into quadrants. (See Figure A-9.) The quadrant from 0 to +90 degrees is considered *normal.* The

■ **vector** a force that has both magnitude and direction.

■ **instantaneous vector** the vectors of electrical energy of the heart, from all three dimensions, that are averaged together at a point in time.

■ **resultant cardiac vector (mean cardiac vector)** all of the instantaneous vectors occurring during a cardiac cycle, averaged together.

■ **axis deviation** a calculated axis of the heart's electrical energy that is outside the normal quadrant of −29 to +105 degrees.

■ **right axis deviation** a calculated axis of the heart's electrical energy that equals or exceeds +105 degrees (or, in a simplified formula, from +90 to +180 degrees).

■ **left axis deviation** a calculated axis of the heart's electrical energy that equals or exceeds −30 degrees (or, in a simplified formula, from 0 to −90 degrees).

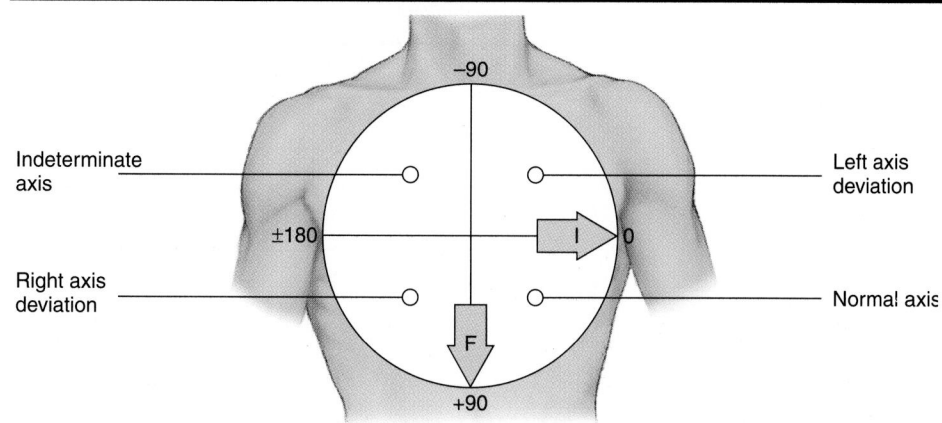

FIGURE A-9 Axis determination.

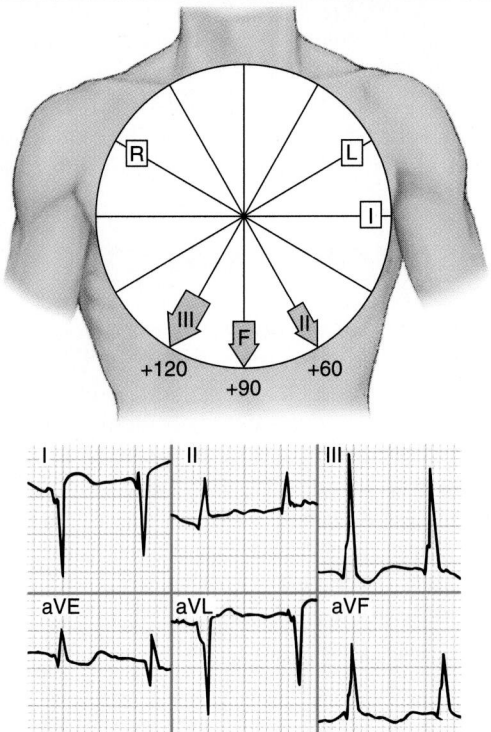

FIGURE A-10 Right axis deviation.

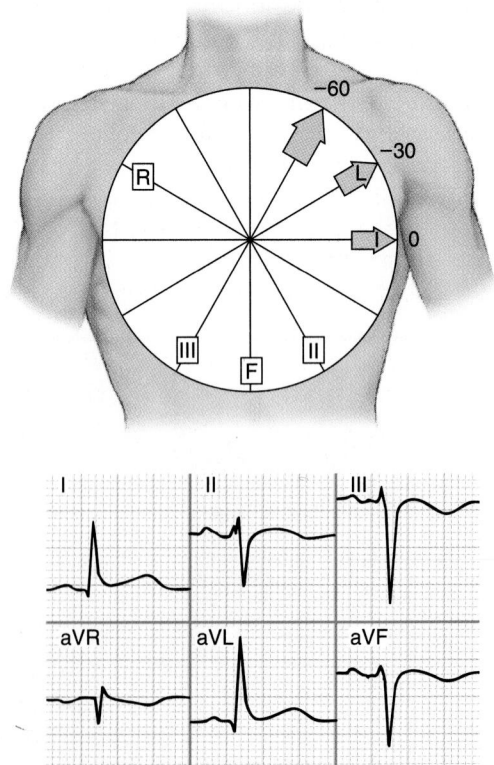

FIGURE A-11 Left axis deviation.

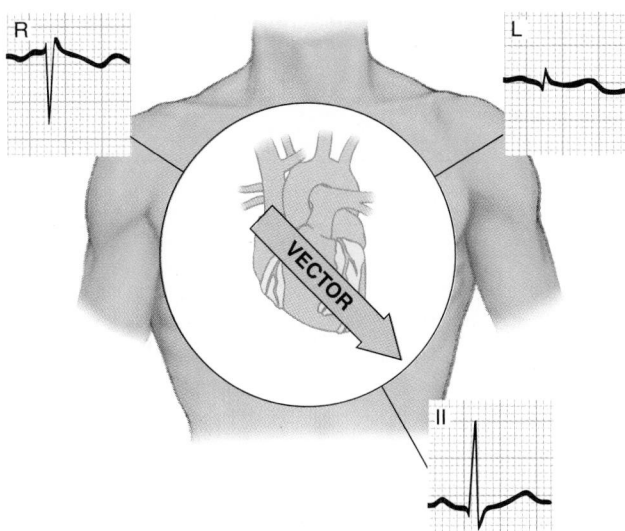

FIGURE A-12 Resultant cardiac vector (QRS axis) calculated from leads I, II, and III.

quadrant from +90 to +180 degrees is considered *right axis deviation*. (See Figure A-10.) The quadrant from 0 to −90 degrees is considered *left axis deviation*. (See Figure A-11.) Finally, the quadrant from −90 to −180 degrees is considered **indeterminate axis**. Indeterminate axis is often considered extreme right axis deviation. While not quite as accurate, this system is effective in detection of abnormal ECG axis.

Most modern 12 lead ECG machines will electronically calculate the axis of the various waves of the ECG (P, QRS, T). These can be used to determine whether an axis deviation exists. In our discussion of cardiac axis, we have been referring to the QRS axis as it represents ventricular depolarization.

In situations where the machine does not calculate the QRS axis, it can be calculated based on Leads I, II, and III. (See Figure A-12.) The heights of the QRS complexes can be measured and plotted on a triaxial reference system. Then, the cardiac axis can be calculated and determined. This system is of little use in the prehospital setting as it is time-consuming and requires calipers and graph paper. Alternatively, a practical system is available for rapid estimation of the electrical axis of the heart.

To rapidly determine the electrical axis of the heart, you must look at Leads I, II, and III. The system is as follows (see Figure A-13):

1. Look at the QRS in Leads I, II, and III. If the QRS is NOT negative in any of these leads, the axis is within *normal range*.
2. Examine Lead I. If the QRS is negative in Lead I, look at Leads II and III. If the QRS is negative in all three leads, the axis is *indeterminate*. If the QRS is variable in Lead II (positive, intermediate, negative), and positive in Lead III, a *right axis deviation* is present.
3. Examine Lead III. If the QRS is negative in Lead III, look at Lead II. If both Lead II and III are negative, a *left axis deviation* is present.

Axis determination is important in interpretation of the 12 lead ECG. Bundle branch blocks, chamber enlargement, and other factors can affect the QRS axis. The role of axis determination will be discussed in greater detail later in this appendix.

■ **indeterminate axis** a calculated axis of the heart's electrical energy from −90 to −180 degrees. (Indeterminate axis is often considered to be extreme right axis deviation.)

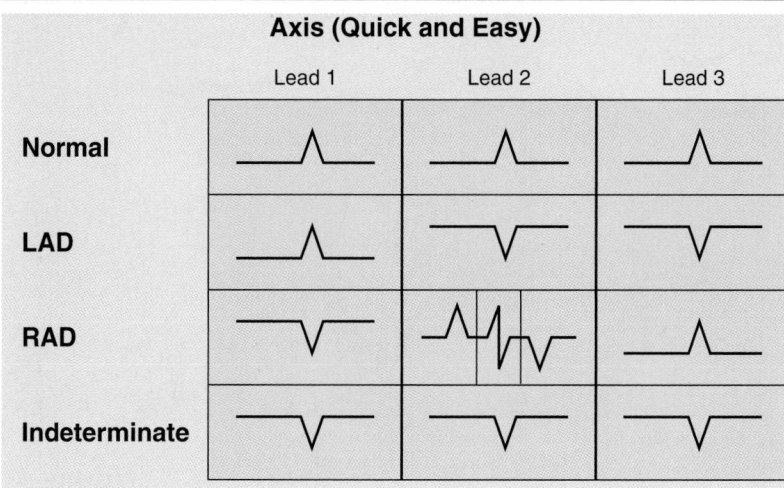

Axis (Quick and Easy)

	Lead 1	Lead 2	Lead 3
Normal			
LAD			
RAD			
Indeterminate			

FIGURE A-13 Rapid axis determination.

THE NORMAL 12 LEAD ECG

Each lead of the normal 12 lead ECG records exactly the same series of electrical events occurring within the heart, but from 12 different perspectives. (See Figure A-14.) This allows for examination of the heart in two planes. Many abnormalities can be detected with the 12 lead ECG. It is important to point out that the ECG records only the electrical events that occur. It does not provide any information about the efficiency of the heart as a pump. The ECG, like other pieces of medical information, must be used in association with a good history and physical examination, vital sign determination, and use of other ancillary testing and diagnostic equipment available for advanced prehospital care.

The 12 lead ECG can be presented in several fashions depending on the machine being used. The most common 12 lead presentation is a 3-channel machine that provides short strips of each lead. (See Figure A-15.) The most common format is to place the bipolar limb leads on the left with Lead I at the top, Lead II in the middle, and Lead III at the bottom. To the right of this, in the second column, are placed the augmented limb leads with aVR at the top, aVL in the middle, and aVF at the bottom. To the right of the augmented limb

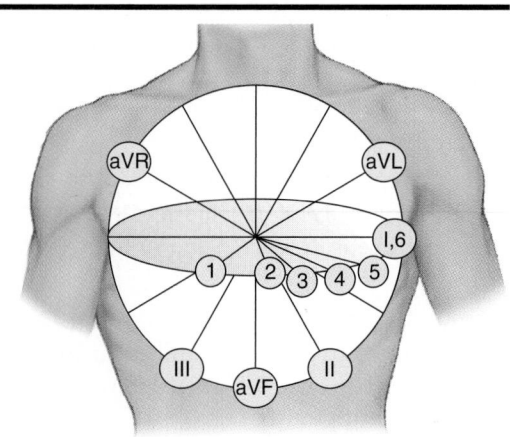

FIGURE A-14 12 lead ECG perspectives.

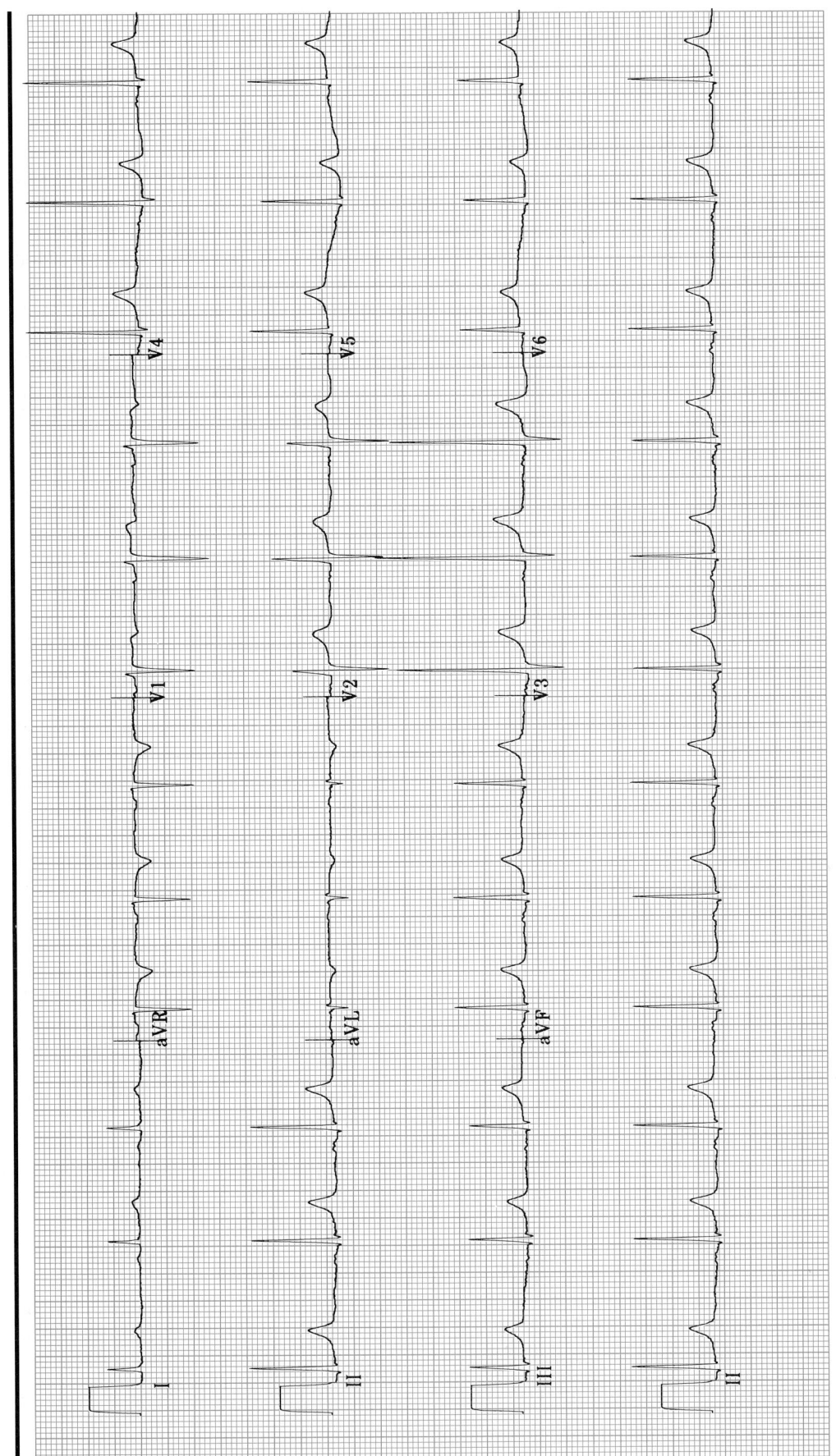

FIGURE A-15 Normal 12 lead ECG.

leads are the precordial leads. Leads V_1 through V_3 are placed in the third column with Leads V_4 through V_6 in the fourth column. This system functionally groups the leads based upon their view of the heart.

DISEASE FINDINGS

Many disease processes can affect the ECG. Among the most important of these is myocardial ischemia, injury, and infarction. A myocardial infarction is the death of a portion of the myocardium due to a loss of blood flow. Most commonly, a blood clot will form in a diseased coronary artery. This clot results in complete occlusion of the artery and stoppage of blood flow through that artery to the part of the myocardium it serves.

Initially, this will result in myocardial ischemia. **Myocardial ischemia** occurs almost immediately following loss of blood supply. The ischemic tissue is deprived of oxygen and other nutrients. Ischemic tissue can still depolarize. However, ischemia tends to affect repolarization. Myocardial ischemia can cause depression of the ST segment and inversion of the T wave on the ECG. Both of these findings are due to abnormalities of repolarization. If blood supply is restored promptly to ischemic tissue, then permanent myocardial injury can often be avoided.

If myocardial ischemia is allowed to progress untreated, myocardial injury will occur. **Myocardial injury** reflects actual injury to the myocardium. The degree of injury is dependent upon how quickly blood supply is restored. Injured myocardium tends to be partially or completely depolarized. This tissue, often called "stunned myocardium," does not contract and does not contribute to the pumping ability of the heart. In addition, injured myocardium can be very irritable and can be a source of serious, and potentially life-threatening, dysrhythmias. With myocardial injury, current flows between the pathologically depolarized area and the normally depolarized areas. This current flow is referred to as a **current of injury** or **injury current**. Thus, with myocardial injury, the injured tissue remains depolarized. It effectively emits a negative electrical charge into the surrounding fluids when the surrounding normal myocardium is positively charged. This current of injury can sometimes be seen on the ECG as elevation of the ST segment.

If the coronary occlusion persists, the myocardial tissue will subsequently die. Death of the myocardial tissue is called **myocardial infarction**. Eventually, the infarcted myocardium will be replaced by fibrous scar tissue. The scar tissue does not contract and does not depolarize in the course of cardiac depolarization. In major infarctions, the scar tissue will result in the formation of significant Q waves in the affected leads. Large areas of scar tissue can result in a ventricular aneurysm. Large aneurysms can cause chronic elevation in the ST segment, often mimicking acute myocardial injury.

All three areas (areas of ischemia, injury, and infarction) can typically be found following coronary occlusion. The outermost tissue will be *ischemic* (zone of ischemia). Because of collateral blood supply, oxygen and nutrients are often re-supplied to this tissue before permanent injury occurs. The intermediate area will be *injured* (zone of injury). This area has sustained some permanent injury but still maintains some capacity for recovery. At the center of the lesion will be the most compromised tissue, or *infarcted* tissue (zone of infarction). This part of the myocardium will die and eventually be replaced by scar tissue. Figure A-16 illustrates the effects of myocardial ischemia, injury, and infarction. It also illustrates the ECG changes commonly associated with each.

Myocardial infarctions may involve the whole thickness of the myocardium or only a partial thickness. The coronary arteries lie on the surface of the

■ **myocardial ischemia** deprivation of oxygen and other nutrients to the myocardium (heart muscle), typically causing abnormalities in repolarization.

■ **myocardial injury** injury to the myocardium (heart muscle), typically following myocardial ischemia that results from loss of blood and oxygen supply to the tissue. The injured myocardium tends to be partially or completely depolarized.

■ **current of injury (injury current)** the flow of current between the pathologically depolarized area of myocardial injury and the normally depolarized areas of the myocardium.

■ **myocardial infarction** death of myocardial tissue. A major infarction will result in significant Q waves in the affected leads.

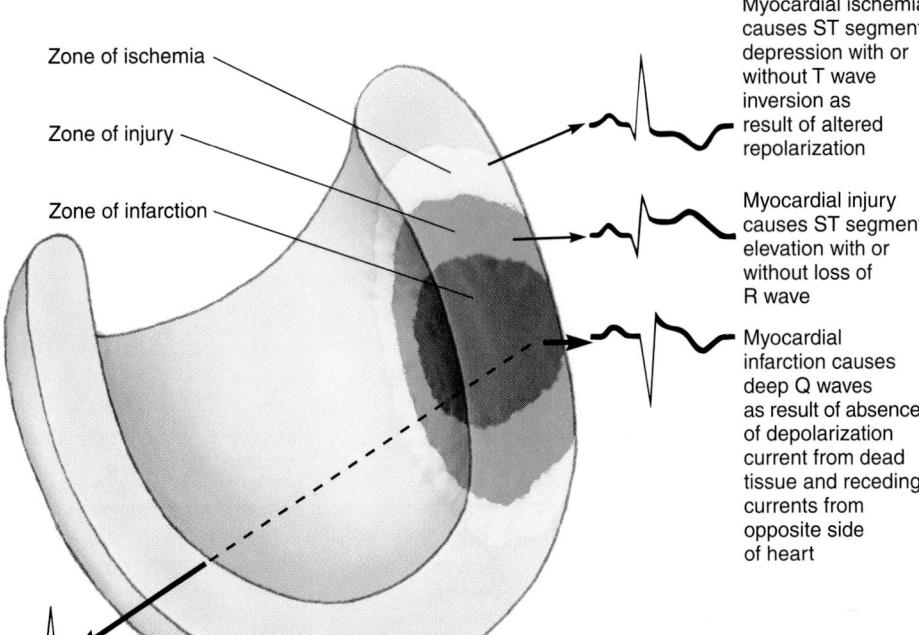

Myocardial ischemia causes ST segment depression with or without T wave inversion as result of altered repolarization

Myocardial injury causes ST segment elevation with or without loss of R wave

Myocardial infarction causes deep Q waves as result of absence of depolarization current from dead tissue and receding currents from opposite side of heart

Zone of ischemia

Zone of injury

Zone of infarction

FIGURE A-16 The effects of myocardial ischemia, injury, and infarction.

heart (at the epicardial level). Interruption of blood supply threatens the deeper layers (subendocardium) of the myocardium more than the superficial layers. A myocardial infarction that affects only the deeper part of the myocardium is called a **subendocardial infarction**. The amount of tissue affected in a subendocardial infarction is typically less than in full-thickness infarctions. Subendocardial infarctions typically do not result in the development of a significant Q-wave in the affected lead. Because of this, subendocardial infarctions are often called *non-Q-wave infarctions.*

Infarctions that affect the full thickness of the myocardium are called **transmural infarctions**. Both types of infarction can result in permanent myocardial death if appropriate intervention, such as thrombolytic therapy or percutaneous transluminal coronary angioplasty (PTCA), is not completed early in the course of the event. Transmural infarctions almost always result in the formation of a significant Q wave in the affected leads.

The goal of emergency care is to identify myocardial ischemia long before it becomes myocardial injury and infarction.

Evolution of Acute Myocardial Infarction

The precipitating event in acute myocardial infarction is occlusion of a coronary artery and interruption of blood flow to a portion of the myocardium it supplies. It is at this precise moment that the clock starts running. In the field of emergency care, *time is myocardium!*

The evolution of myocardial infarction has been extensively studied. Figures A-17 and A-18 illustrate the events that occur in transmural and subendocardial myocardial infarctions. The following description details the evolution of a transmural myocardial infarction.

Initially, following coronary occlusion, the affected tissue will become deprived of oxygen and other nutrients and will become ischemic. Myocardial ischemia can often be demonstrated on the ECG as ST segment depression

■ **subendocardial infarction** myocardial infarction that affects only the deeper levels of the myocardium; also called *non-Q-wave infarction* because it typically does not result in a significant Q wave in the affected lead.

■ **transmural infarction** myocardial infarction that affects the full thickness of the myocardium and almost always results in a significant Q wave in the affected leads.

* Time is myocardium!

Transmural Infarction

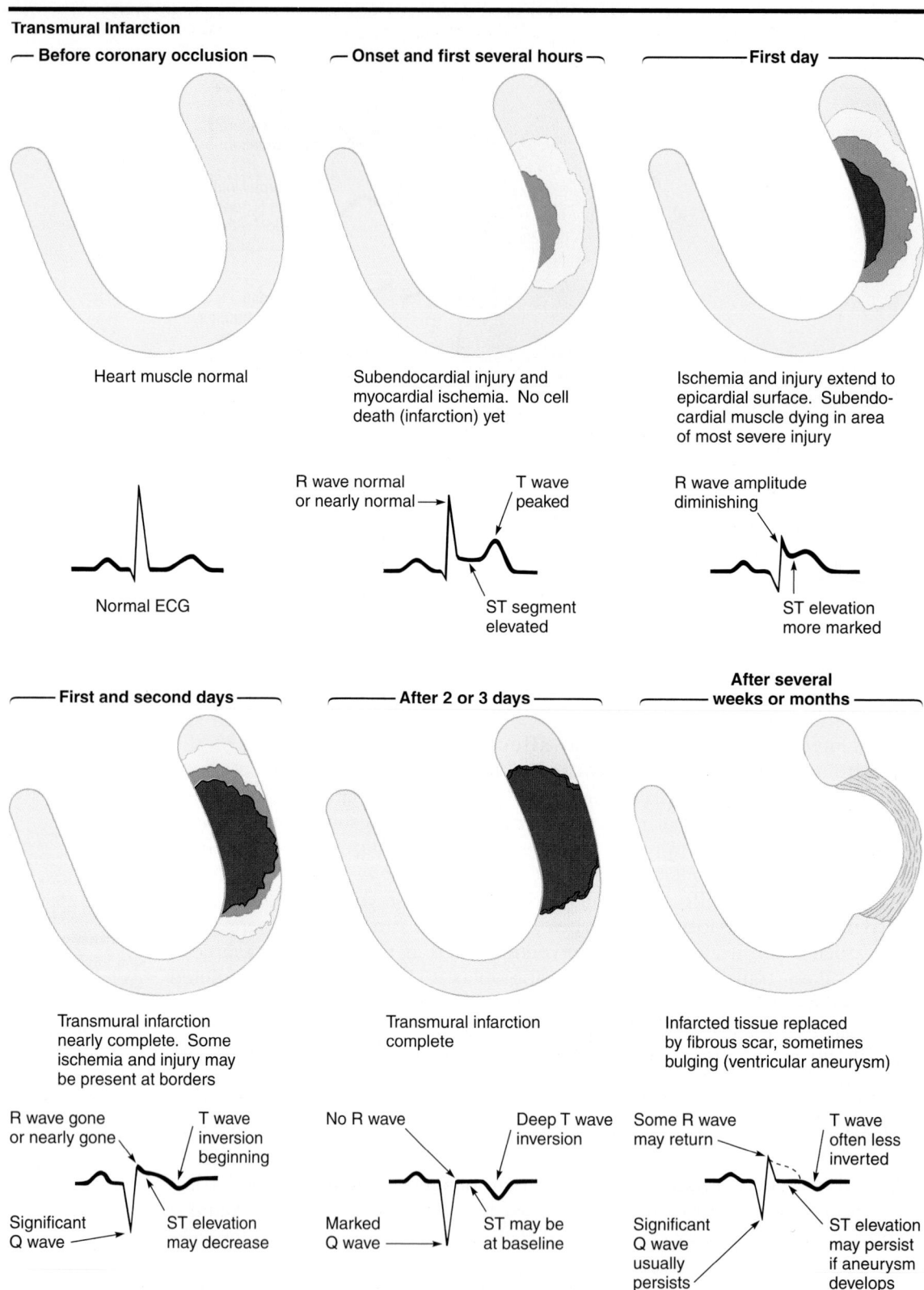

Before coronary occlusion

Heart muscle normal

Normal ECG

Onset and first several hours

Subendocardial injury and myocardial ischemia. No cell death (infarction) yet

R wave normal or nearly normal →

T wave peaked

ST segment elevated

First day

Ischemia and injury extend to epicardial surface. Subendo-cardial muscle dying in area of most severe injury

R wave amplitude diminishing

ST elevation more marked

First and second days

Transmural infarction nearly complete. Some ischemia and injury may be present at borders

R wave gone or nearly gone

T wave inversion beginning

Significant Q wave

ST elevation may decrease

After 2 or 3 days

Transmural infarction complete

No R wave

Deep T wave inversion

Marked Q wave

ST may be at baseline

After several weeks or months

Infarcted tissue replaced by fibrous scar, sometimes bulging (ventricular aneurysm)

Some R wave may return

T wave often less inverted

Significant Q wave usually persists

ST elevation may persist if aneurysm develops

FIGURE A-17 Transmural infarction.

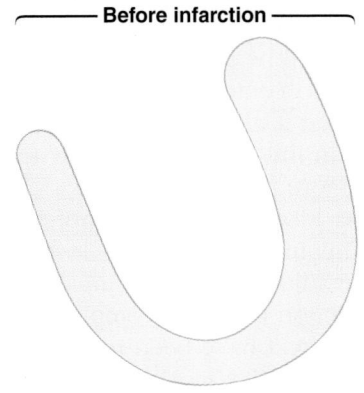

── Before infarction ──

Heart muscle normal

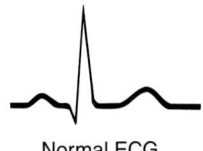

Normal ECG

── First few hours ──

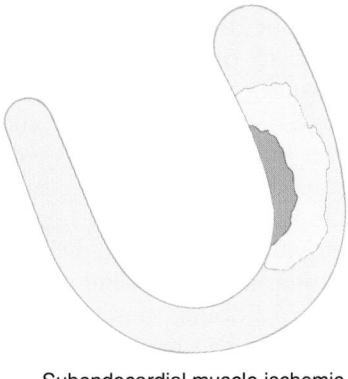

Subendocardial muscle ischemic
and injured but not dead

ST depressed
or
elevated

── First several days ──

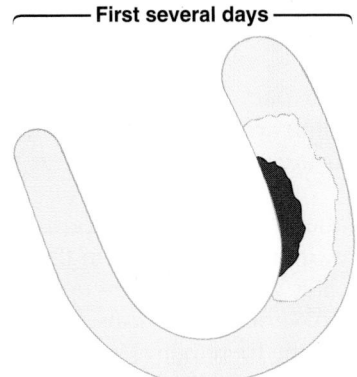

Some subendocardial muscle dies,
but lesion does not extend through
entire heart wall

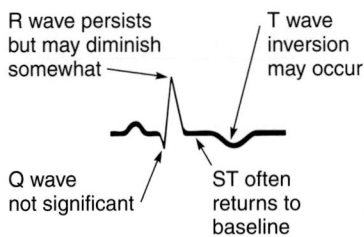

R wave persists
but may diminish
somewhat

T wave
inversion
may occur

Q wave
not significant

ST often
returns to
baseline

After several
── weeks or months ──

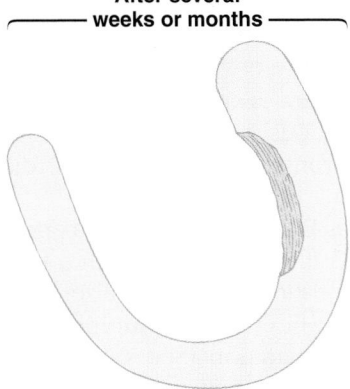

Lesion heals. Some subendocardial
fibrosis may occur but does not
involve entire thickness of heart wall

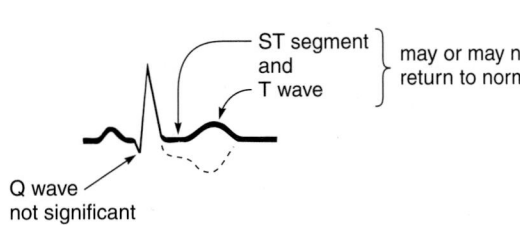

ST segment
and
T wave

may or may n
return to norm

Q wave
not significant

FIGURE A-18 Subendocardial infarction.

and T wave inversion in the affected leads. ST segment depression and T wave inversion may not be present at the same time. The larger the quantity of ischemic tissue, the more significant, as a rule, will be the ECG findings.

If allowed to progress untreated, tissue at the center of the myocardial injury will transition from ischemia to injury. When a critical mass of tissue is affected, the ST segments will become elevated in the affected leads. In addition, T waves in the affected leads will become more peaked.

After approximately 6 hours, and provided blood supply has not been restored, the injured tissue will begin to die. This infarcted tissue is lost. The ST segment will remain elevated (because of the adjoining zone of injury) and the R wave amplitude will diminish. As the infarction becomes complete over the next 48 to 72 hours, most ischemia and injury will have been replaced by infarcted tissue or will have been reperfused. This results in a decrease in ST segment elevation. Also, however, a significant Q wave will develop. A significant Q wave is one with a width greater than or equal to 0.04 second (one small box) or amplitude (depth) greater than or equal to one-fourth of the R wave in the same lead. T wave inversion will continue. After several months, the infarcted tissue will be replaced with a fibrous scar. By this time, the ST segment will usually return to normal and some R wave may return. T wave inversion often persists. A significant Q wave usually persists and is an indicator of an old transmural infarction.

The evolution of a subendocardial infarction is similar to that described above for a transmural infarction. However, significant Q waves typically do not occur. In addition, as the lesion heals, the ECG may return to normal, leaving no indication of a prior infarct.

Localization of Acute Myocardial Infarction

Each ECG lead is designed to visualize a particular part of the heart. As mentioned previously, the bipolar and augmented limb leads evaluate the heart from the frontal plane. The precordial leads, on the other hand, look at the heart from a horizontal plane.

Various ECG leads "look" at a specific part of the myocardium. Abnormalities of the ECG in certain leads, with a few exceptions, indicate problems in the part of the heart those leads visualize. The following is a generalized description of the various ECG lead groupings associated with various locations of acute myocardial infarction (See Table A-1). It is important to remember that these descriptions are generalized and some overlapping may occur.

❑ **Anterior.** Leads I, V_2, V_3, and V_4 are immediately over the anterior surface of the heart. ST segment elevation, T wave inversion, and the devel-

TABLE A-1	Localization of Myocardial Ischemia/Infarction
Location	**Indicative Changes** **(Q Waves, S-T Elevation, T-Wave Inversion)**
Anterior	I, V_2, V_3, and V_4
Anteriolateral	I, aVL, V_5, and V_6
Lateral	V_5 and V_6
High lateral	I and aVL (often with V_5 and V_6)
Inferior	II, III, and aVF
Inferolateral	II, III, aVF, and V_6
True posterior	Reciprocal changes in V_1 and V_2

opment of significant Q waves in these leads indicate myocardial infarction involving the anterior surface of the heart. (See Figure A-19.) Leads V_2 and V_3 overlie the ventricular septum. Ischemic changes in these leads, and possibly in the adjoining precordial leads, are often referred to as *septal infarctions.*

❑ **Anterolateral**. Leads I, aVL, V_5 and V_6 examine the anterior and lateral surface of the heart. ST segment elevation, T wave inversion, and the development of significant Q waves in these leads indicate myocardial infarction involving the anterolateral surface of the heart (See Figure A-20).

❑ **Lateral.** Leads V_5 and V_6 visualize the lateral surface of the heart. ST segment elevation, T wave inversion, and the development of significant Q waves in these leads indicate myocardial infarction involving the lateral surface of the heart.

❑ **High lateral**. Leads I and aVL visualize the high lateral surface of the heart. Changes in these leads can often be seen in the other lateral leads (Leads V_5 and V_6). ST segment elevation, T wave inversion, and the development of significant Q waves in these leads indicate myocardial infarction involving the high lateral surface of the heart.

❑ **Inferior.** Leads II, III, and aVF visualize the inferior (diaphragmatic) surface of the heart. ST segment elevation, T wave inversion, and the development of significant Q waves in these leads indicate myocardial infarction involving the inferior surface of the heart. (See Figure A-21.)

❑ **Inferolateral**. Leads II, III, aVF, and V_6 visualize the inferolateral portion of the heart. ST segment elevation, T wave inversion, and the development of significant Q waves in these leads indicate myocardial infarction involving the inferolateral surface of the heart.

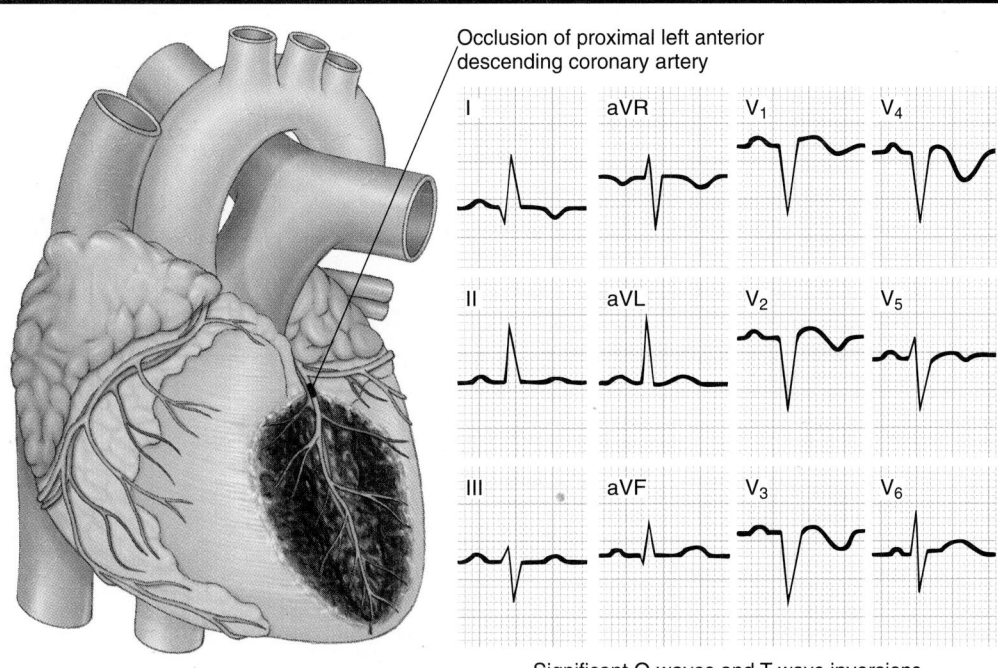

Occlusion of proximal left anterior descending coronary artery

Significant Q waves and T wave inversions in leads I, V_2, V_3 and V_4

FIGURE A-19   Anterior infarct.

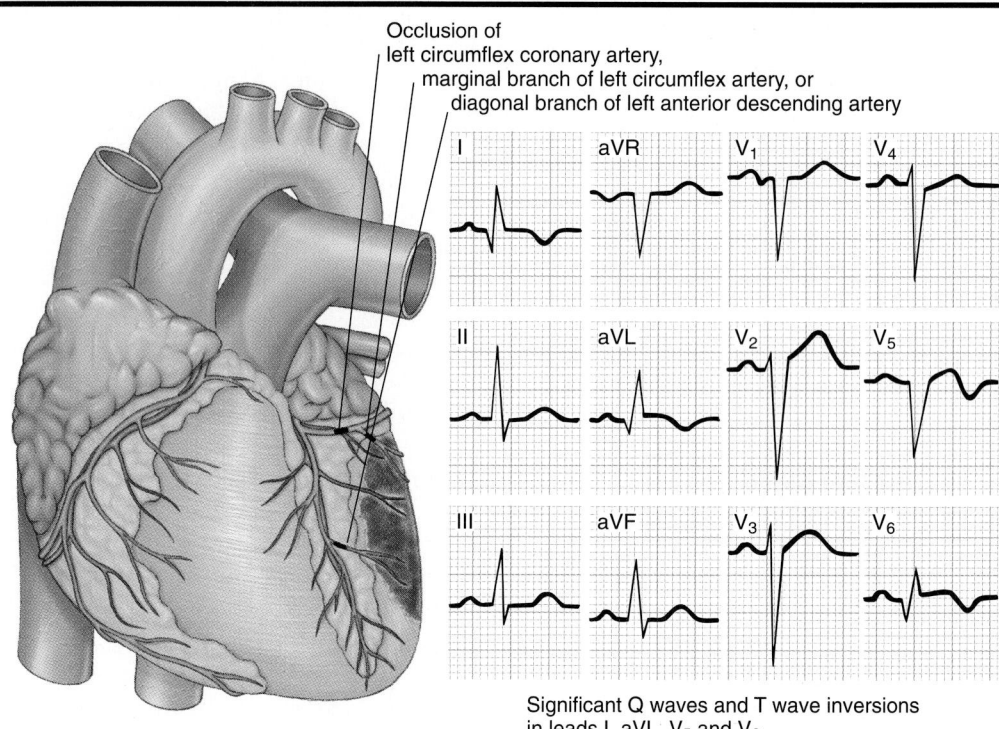

Occlusion of
left circumflex coronary artery,
marginal branch of left circumflex artery, or
diagonal branch of left anterior descending artery

Significant Q waves and T wave inversions
in leads I, aVL, V$_5$ and V$_6$

FIGURE A-20   Anterolateral infarct.

❑ **True posterior**. There are no ECG leads over the posterior surface of the heart. True posterior infarctions, although rare, can be diagnosed by looking for reciprocal changes in the anterior leads (V$_1$ and V$_2$). Normally, the R wave in Leads V$_1$ and V$_2$ is principally negative. An

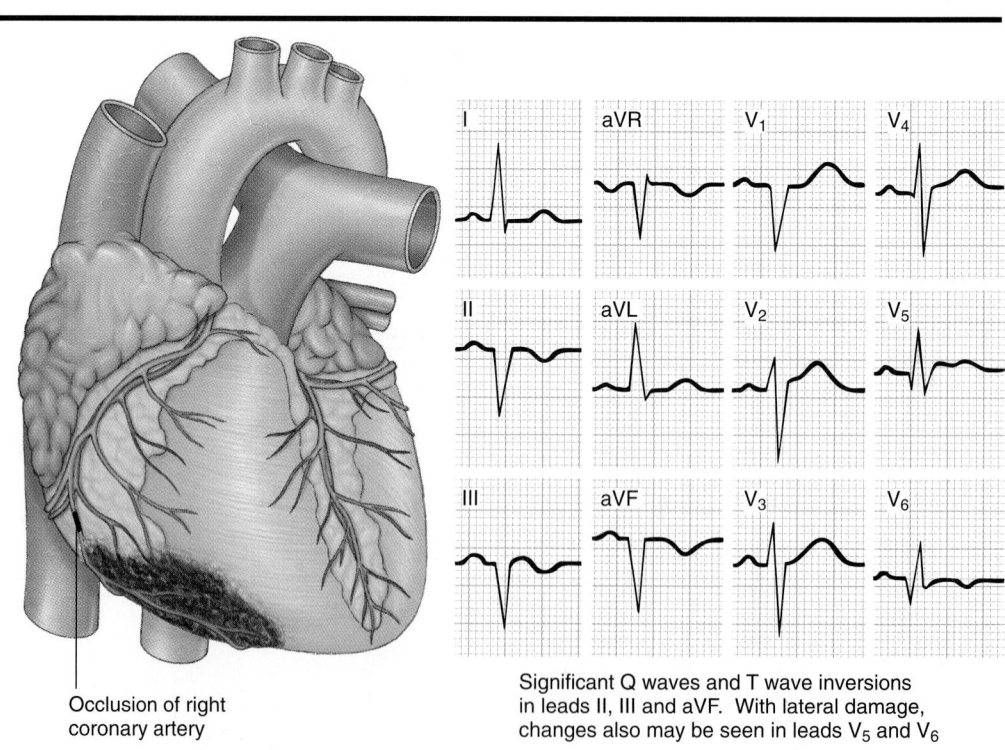

Occlusion of right
coronary artery

Significant Q waves and T wave inversions
in leads II, III and aVF. With lateral damage,
changes also may be seen in leads V$_5$ and V$_6$

FIGURE A-21   Inferior infarct.

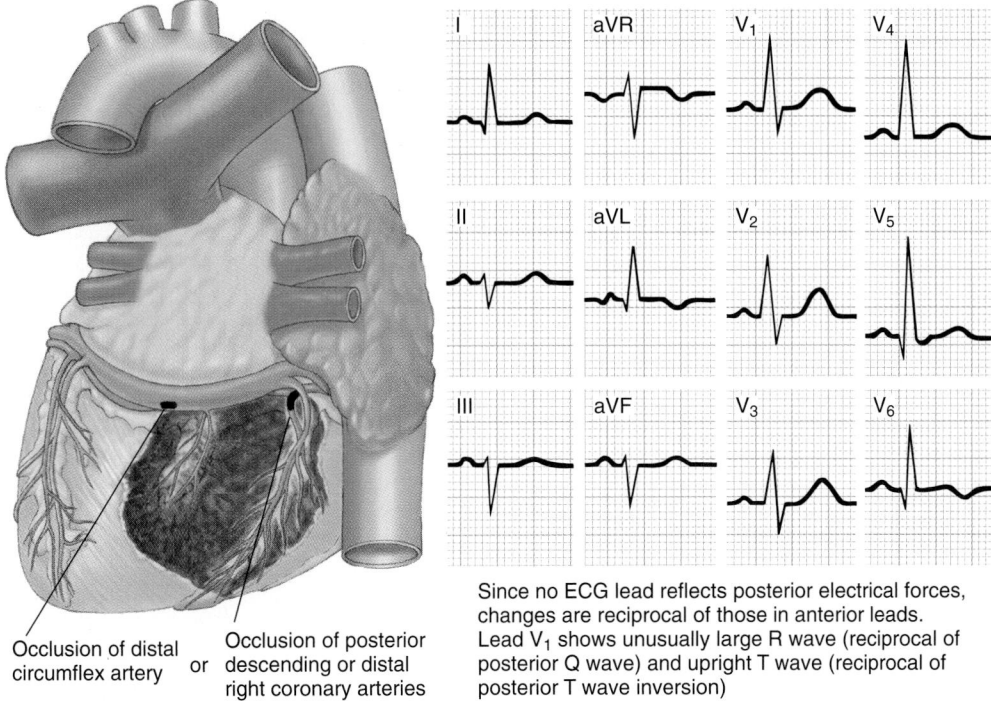

Since no ECG lead reflects posterior electrical forces, changes are reciprocal of those in anterior leads. Lead V_1 shows unusually large R wave (reciprocal of posterior Q wave) and upright T wave (reciprocal of posterior T wave inversion)

Occlusion of distal circumflex artery   or   Occlusion of posterior descending or distal right coronary arteries

FIGURE A-22   True posterior infarct.

unusually large R wave in Lead V_1 and V_2 can actually be a reciprocal of a posterior Q wave. Likewise, an upright T wave in these leads would be a reciprocal of posterior T wave inversion. (See Figure A-22.) These findings are subtle and require practice to learn. Alternatively, posterior leads (V_7 through V_{12}) can be applied to the back to confirm the presence of a true posterior myocardial infarction.

It is important to point out that the guidelines presented above are generalized. Individual ECG tracings will vary due to variances in body structure, underlying heart and lung disease, and other factors which can affect the ECG tracing. Thus there may be some overlapping of abnormal findings in various leads. Figure A-23 is an actual 12 lead tracing from a patient suffering an acute anterior wall myocardial infarction. Figure A-24 is an actual 12 lead ECG from a patient with an acute anterior wall myocardial infarction with lateral extension of the infarction (anterolateral MI). Finally, Figure A-25 is an actual 12 lead tracing taken from a patient suffering an acute inferior wall (diaphragmatic) myocardial infarction. It is important to study and periodically review actual patient ECG tracings in order to learn the various pathological changes described in this text.

CONDUCTION ABNORMALITIES

Conduction abnormalities occur when there is a delay or blockage of a part or parts of the cardiac conductive system. Conduction abnormalities can be caused by disease, drugs, and various electrolyte abnormalities.

AV Blocks

AV heart blocks (which were discussed in Chapter 21) are some of the more common types of conduction abnormalities. AV blocks result from a delay in impulse transmission through the AV node from the atria to the ventricles.

✱ AV blocks are among the more common types of conduction abnormalities.

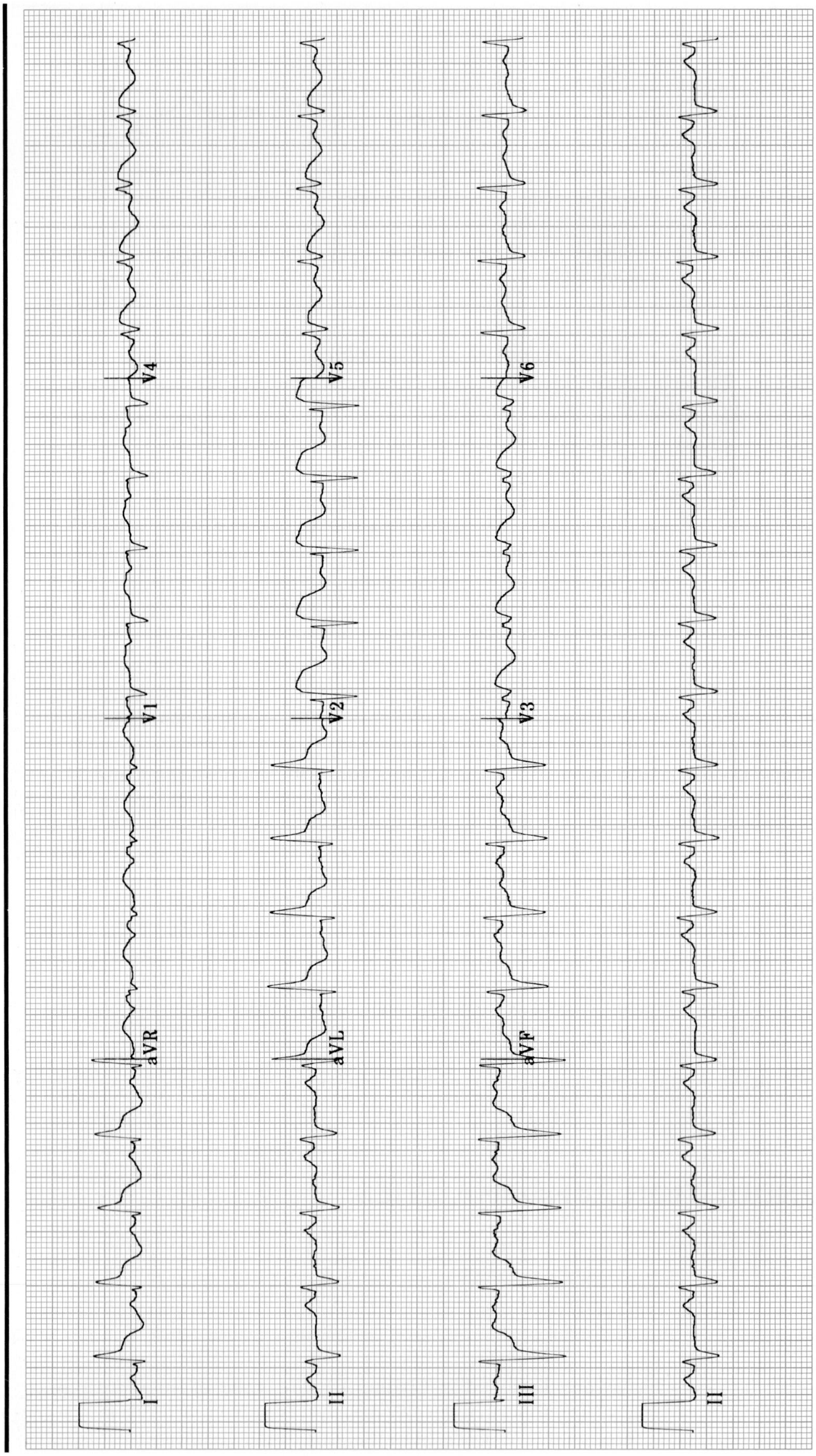

FIGURE A-23 Tracing from patient with acute anterior wall infarct.

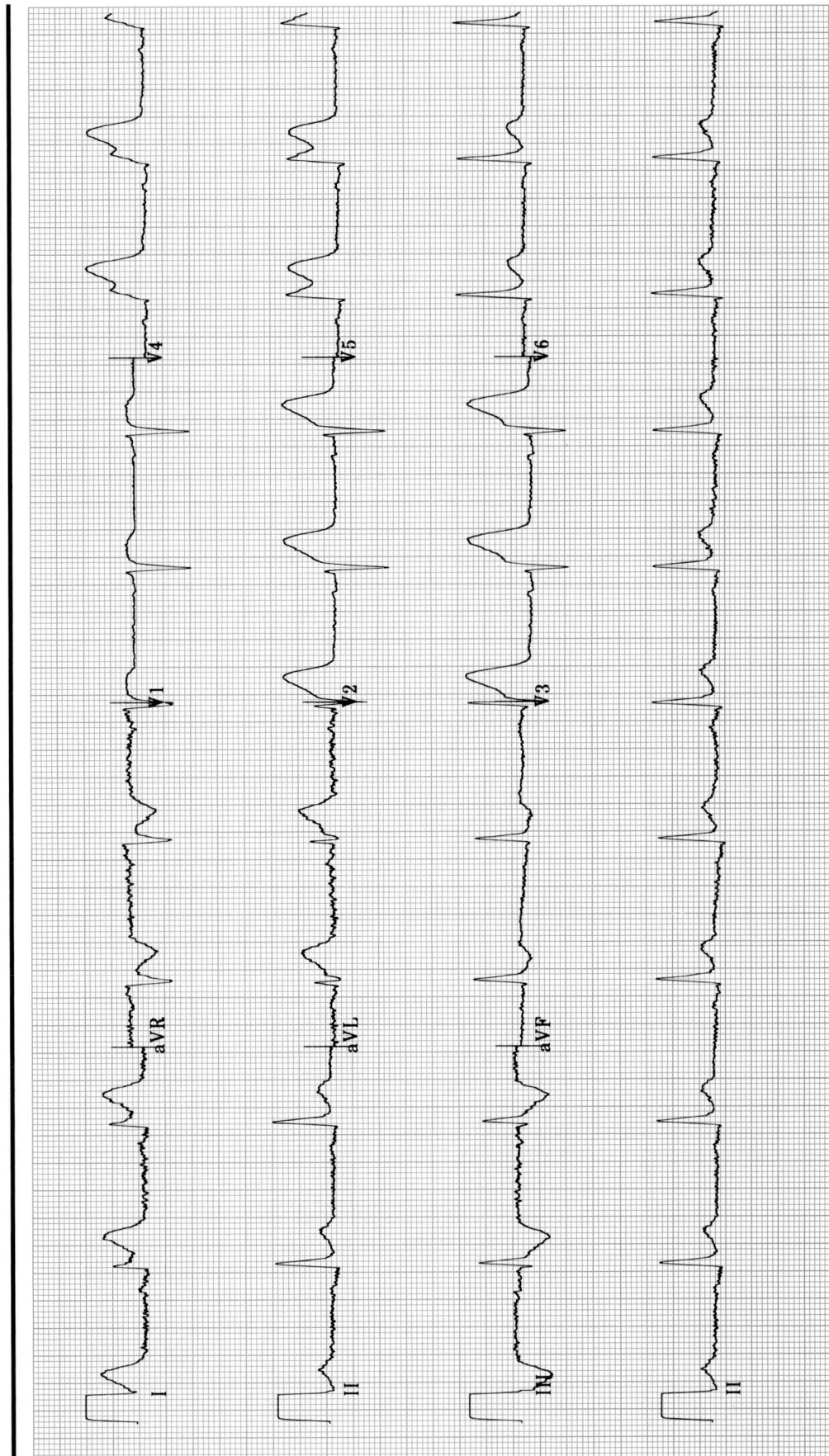

FIGURE A-24 Tracing from patient with acute anterior wall infarct with lateral extension of the infarction (anterolateral infarct).

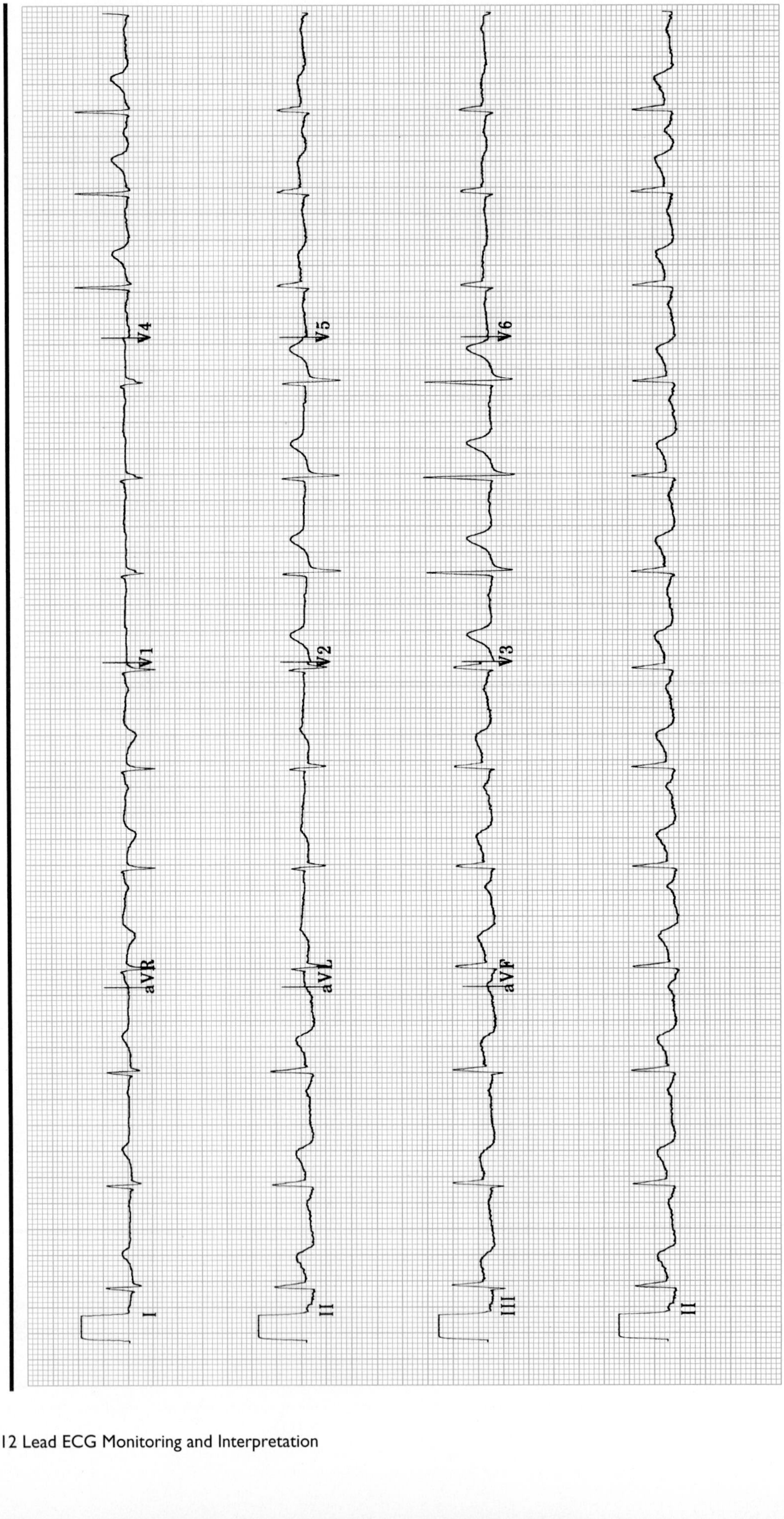

FIGURE A-25 Tracing from a patient with acute inferior wall (diaphragmatic) infarct.

- **First-Degree AV Block** The simplest type of AV heart block is a First-Degree AV Block. In a First-Degree AV Block, there is a delay in transmission of the electrical impulse from the atria to the ventricles. This can be detected on the ECG by noting a PR interval of greater than 0.21 second. In a First-Degree Block, there is not a complete blockage of AV transmission, only a slowing of the impulse in the AV node.
- **Second-Degree AV Block (Mobitz I)** The next type of heart block is a Second-Degree AV Block (Mobitz I). This unique type of block, also referred to as a Wenckebach phenomenon, involves a delay of impulse conduction at the AV node. Each impulse arriving at the AV junction is progressively delayed until, eventually, AV conduction is completely blocked. This results in failure of the impulse to be transmitted through to the ventricles. Typically, following the dropped beat, the cycle will repeat itself.
- **Second-Degree AV Block (Mobitz II)** A more severe form of AV heart block is a Second-Degree AV Block (Mobitz II). In this block, certain of the impulses are conducted through the AV node while others are blocked. There is usually a recognized pattern in that one, two, or three impulses are conducted, and then one is blocked.
- **Third-Degree AV Block** The most serious type of AV heart block is a Third-Degree AV Block, also called a Complete Heart Block. In a Third-Degree Heart Block, none of the impulses originating in the atria are conducted into the ventricles. This results in the atria and ventricles each having their own intrinsic rate. This can lead to severe bradycardia, heart failure, and, in certain situations, cardiac arrest.

Bundle Branch Blocks

Conduction abnormalities are not limited to the AV node. Conduction defects can also occur in the right bundle branch, the left bundle branch, or even in one of the fascicles of the left bundle branch. AV blocks can be detected by single lead monitoring. Bundle branch blocks, on the other hand, can only be diagnosed with a 12 lead tracing.

✱ AV blocks can be detected by single lead monitoring. Bundle branch blocks can only be diagnosed with a 12 lead tracing.

In a bundle branch block, ventricular depolarization is abnormal. The impulse will originate in the SA node, be transmitted through the internodal pathways, through the AV node, and into the bundle of His. After entering the bundle of His, the impulse is transmitted into the left and right bundle branches, and into the Purkinje system. If the right bundle branch is blocked, the impulse will proceed down the left bundle branch. The block will prevent transmission of the impulse through the right bundle branch. The impulse must then spread from the left bundle branch, through the myocardial cells of the interventricular septum, and into the right ventricle. Likewise, blockage of the left bundle branch will cause the impulse to be spread from the right bundle branch, through the interventricular septum, and into the left ventricle.

In the case of a bundle branch block, the electrical forces traveling across the interventricular septum are unable to utilize the rapid fibers of the ventricular conductive system. Because the impulse must be transmitted through the interventricular septum itself, from the functioning bundle branch to the side with the non-functioning bundle branch, there will be a delay in depolarization of the affected ventricle. This can be detected on the ECG as prolongation of the QRS complex of greater than or equal to 0.12 second. In addition, the delay in depolarization of the ventricle on the affected side can result in abnormal formation of the QRS complex.

The following discussion will address the common bundle branch blocks and hemiblocks.

□ **Right Bundle Branch Block** A right bundle branch bloc results from blockage of some portion of the right bundle branch. In this case, the impulse must continue down the left bundle branch and spread through the interventricular septum until the right ventricle is depolarized. This results in a delay of impulse transmission into the right ventricle causing a prolongation of the QRS complex (greater than or equal to 0.12 second). The right ventricle is a low pressure pump. Because of this, the right ventricular muscle mass is considerably smaller than the left. In the normal ECG, the electrical forces of the right ventricle are overshadowed by the more massive forces of the left ventricle. In the case of a right bundle branch block, right ventricular depolarization occurs after left ventricular depolarization. The vector of the right ventricular depolarization is rightward and anterior as compared to the left. This is due to the fact that the impulse is spreading from the left ventricle to the right ventricle instead of the normal scenario where the right ventricle is stimulated by the right bundle branch.

A complete right bundle branch is typically characterized by a prolonged QRS complex of greater than or equal to 0.12 second. In addition, there is an abnormal late portion of the QRS directed toward the right ventricle and away from the left ventricle. This is typically seen as a broad S wave in Lead I. Also, a characteristic RSR′ (R-S-R prime) complex will be seen in Lead V_1. (See Figure A-26.) The RSR′ (also called a "rabbit ear") reflects the abnormal septal depolarization and subsequent right ventricular depolarization. Lead V_1 lies immediately over the right ventricle and is a good lead for detecting right ventricular abnormalities.

Right bundle branch block is a rather common finding. It is a relatively thin bundle of fibers compared to the left bundle branch and is thus more susceptible to injury. Right bundle branch block can result

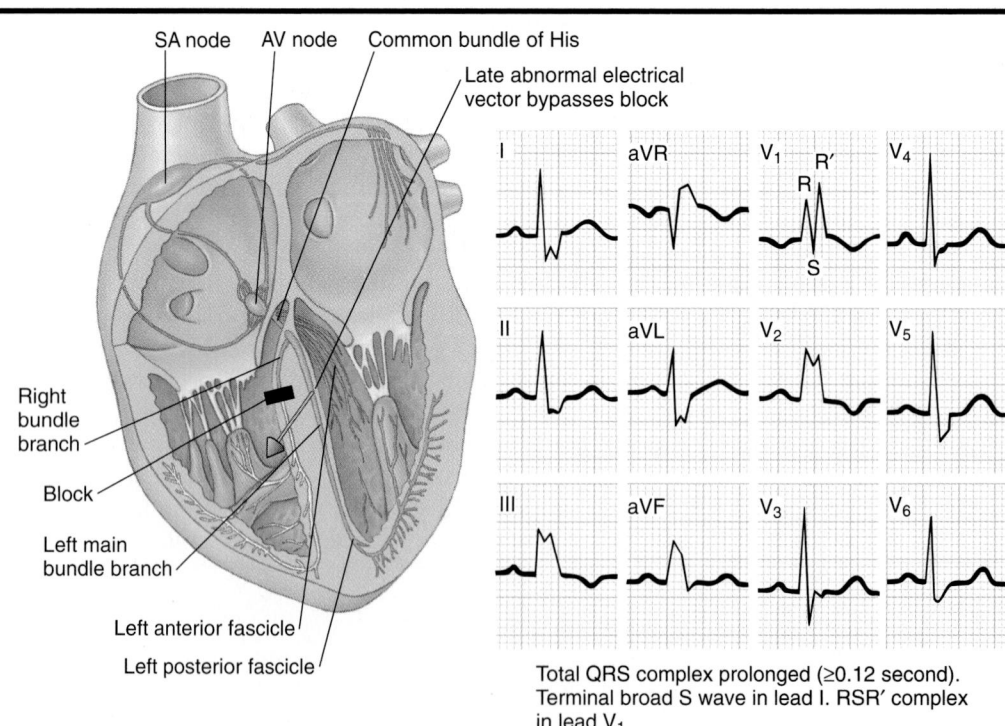

Total QRS complex prolonged (≥0.12 second). Terminal broad S wave in lead I. RSR′ complex in lead V_1

FIGURE A-26 Right bundle branch block.

from acute MI, drugs, electrolyte abnormalities, or general age-related deterioration of the cardiac conductive system.

❑ **Left Bundle Branch Block** The left bundle branch is derived from the bundle of His. It subsequently divides into the anterior and posterior fascicles before it terminates in the Purkinje system of the left ventricle. When a left bundle branch block occurs, the left ventricle cannot be depolarized normally. Thus, the electrical impulse must be transmitted from the right ventricle, through the interventricular septum, and then into the left ventricle. As with a right bundle branch block, the depolarization impulse must spread through the interventricular septum without the aid of specialized conductive fibers. This causes a delay in impulse transmission through the interventricular septum and results in a prolongation of the QRS complex. Unlike a right bundle branch block, the forces in a left bundle branch block are from right to left which is nearly the same direction as occurs in the normal heart.

The QRS complexes in left bundle branch block are prolonged (greater than or equal to 0.12 second) and bizarre in appearance. Typically, wide, notched QRS complexes are seen in leads I, aVL, V_5 and V_6. (See Figure A-27.) The changes are more pronounced in these leads, as they visualize the lateral aspect of the heart which is principally the left ventricle. Deep S waves can be seen in lead V_1, V_2, or V_3 or tall R waves seen in lead I, aVL, V_5 and V_6 (as described previously).

A left bundle branch block usually indicates significant and widespread myocardial disease. Like the right bundle branch block, it too results from MI, drugs, electrolyte abnormalities, and degenerative disease of the conductive system. Most myocardial infarctions primarily affect the left ventricle. The presence of a left bundle branch block will mask ischemic changes associated with MI. Thus, a patient can suffer a

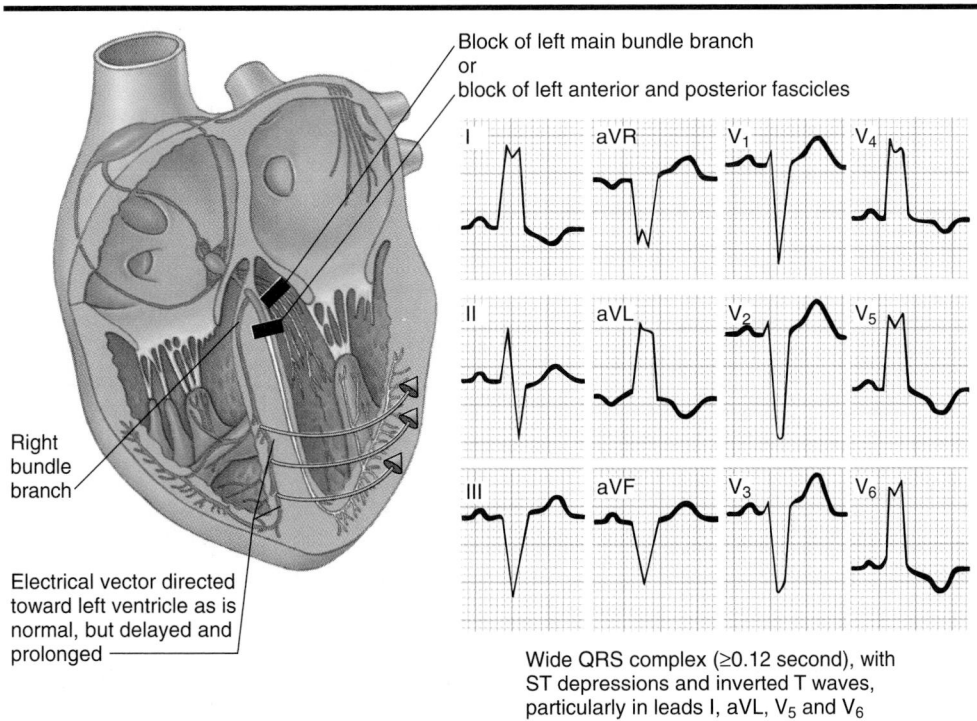

FIGURE A-27 Left bundle branch block.

significant MI, and ECG changes will not be seen because of the left bundle branch block. In fact, the presence of a left bundle branch block negates any chance of localizing an MI with a 12 lead ECG.

❑ **Hemiblocks** The left bundle branch divides into the left anterior and left posterior fascicles. Blocks can occur in either of these fascicles and are a fairly common finding.

Left Posterior Hemiblock A left posterior hemiblock, also called a left posterior fascicular block, results from blockage of the left posterior fascicle. Blockage of the left posterior fascicle results in a delay in depolarizing the portion of the left ventricle it innervates. A left posterior hemiblock does not, typically, result in prolongation of the QRS interval. In addition, the shape of the QRS complex remains relatively normal. The principal finding in a left posterior hemiblock is a rightward shift in the QRS axis. This is often difficult to diagnose, particularly if there is underlying right ventricular or pulmonary disease. Generally, the QRS axis must be greater than or equal to +120 degrees to consider a left posterior hemiblock. (See Figure A-28.) Left posterior hemiblock is usually due to degenerative disease of the conductive system or ischemic heart disease.

Left Anterior Hemiblock A left anterior hemiblock, also called a left anterior fascicular block, results from blockage of the left anterior fascicle. This block is similar to what occurs with a bundle branch block but does NOT result in a delay in ventricular depolarization. Thus, the QRS complex is of normal duration and is generally of normal shape, without the unusual notching seen in the bundle branch blocks. The principal abnormality in a left anterior hemiblock is a shift in the QRS axis far to the left (typically more negative than −30 degrees). This results in a negative QRS complex in Leads II, III, and aVF. (See Figure A-29.) A left anterior

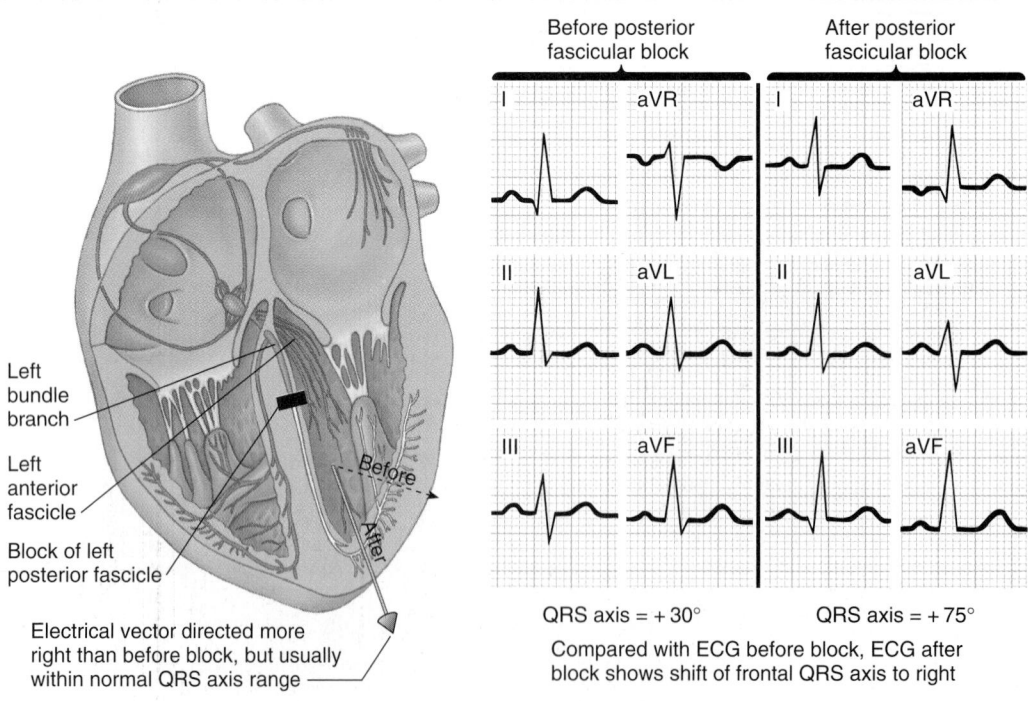

FIGURE A-28 Left posterior hemiblock (left posterior fascicular block).

hemiblock is usually caused by degeneration of the cardiac conductive system or ischemic heart disease. It is usually a benign finding.

Figure A-30 is an actual tracing from a patient with a left bundle branch block. Figure A-31 is an actual tracing from a patient with a complete right bundle branch block. Both are common findings in 12 lead ECG interpretation. Remember, a left bundle branch block renders the ECG relatively useless for detecting injury or ischemia.

✱ A left bundle branch block renders the ECG relatively useless for detecting injury or ischemia.

PREHOSPITAL ECG MONITORING

Prehospital technology has evolved to a point where portable 12 lead ECG monitoring is readily available. Many manufacturers now have 12 lead machines available for prehospital care. Most machines have sophisticated electronics, many with ECG diagnostic packages. Some machines now have a defibrillator/pacer unit available. (See Figure A-32.). The principles of 12 lead monitoring are similar to those described in Chapter 21 for routine ECG monitoring.

Prehospital 12 Lead ECG Monitoring

The following skill sequence details application of 12 lead prehospital ECG monitoring.

1. Explain what you are going to do to the patient. Reassure him or her that the machine will not "shock you."

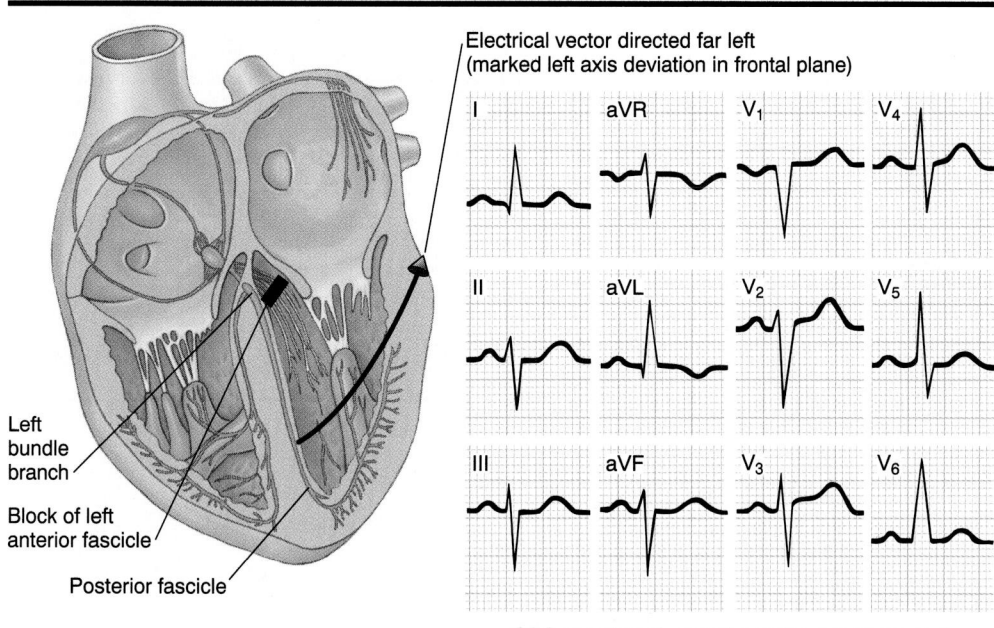

Electrical vector directed far left (marked left axis deviation in frontal plane)

Left bundle branch

Block of left anterior fascicle

Posterior fascicle

QRS complex of normal duration (<0.11 second) in all leads. S wave > R wave in leads II, III and aVF (marked left axis deviation)

FIGURE A-29 Left anterior hemiblock (left anterior fascicular block).

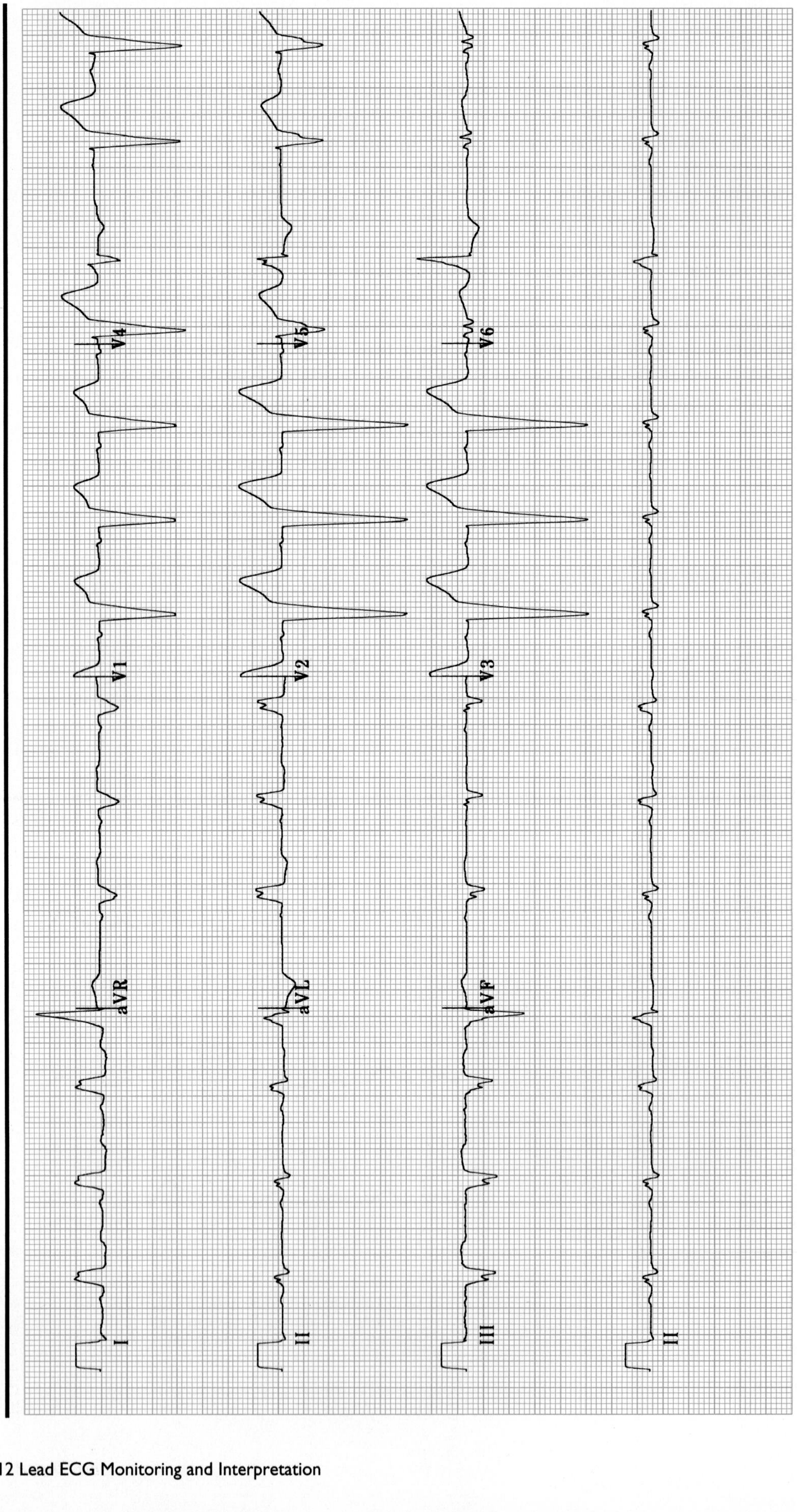

FIGURE A-30 Tracing from patient with left bundle branch block.

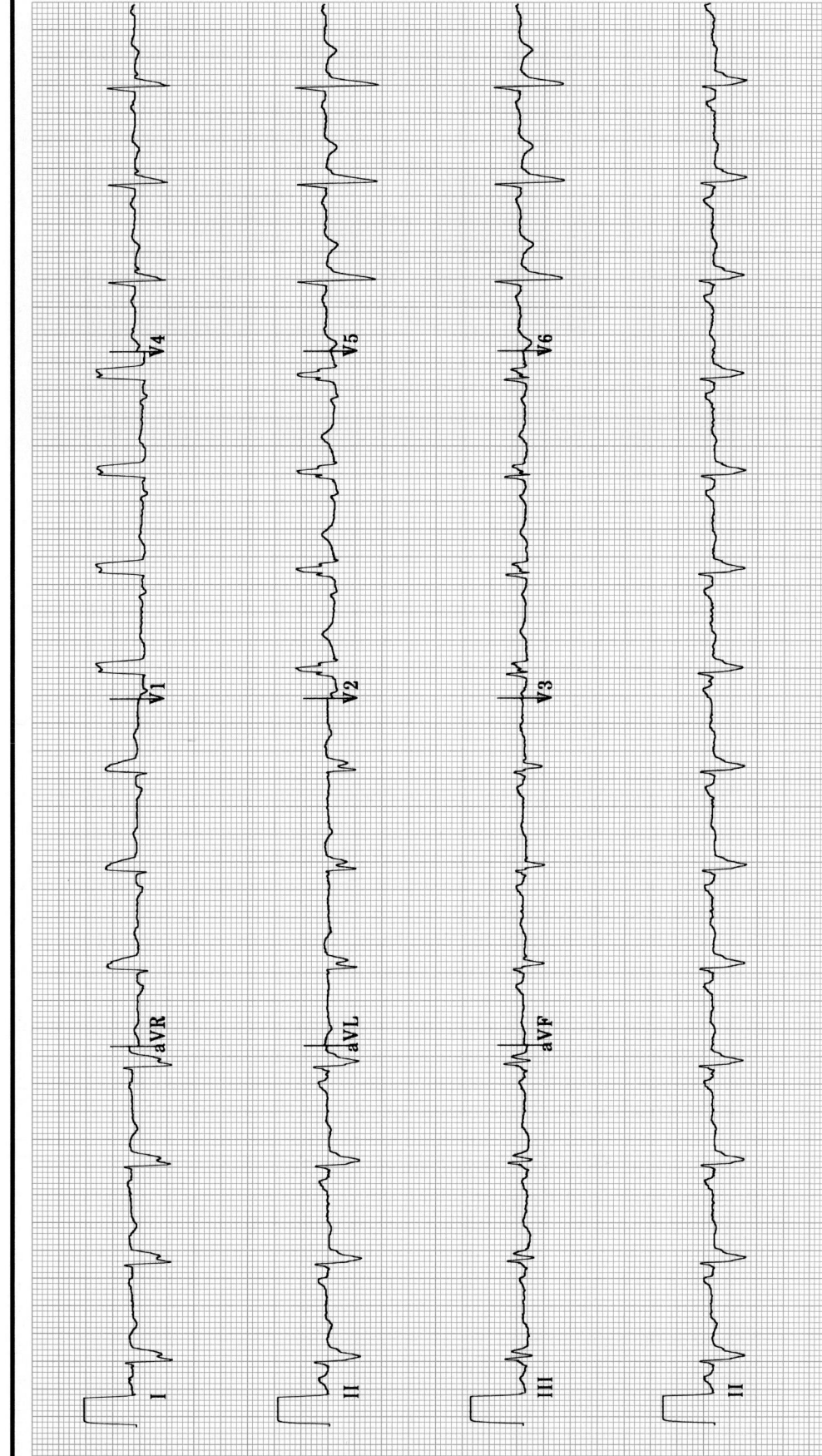

FIGURE A-31 Tracing from patient with complete right bundle branch block.

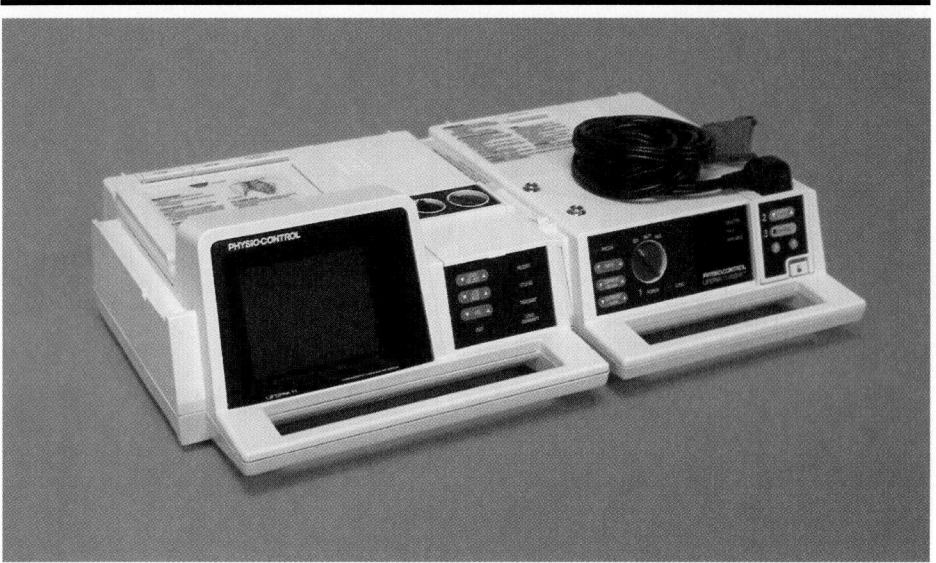

FIGURE A-32 Prehospital 12 lead monitor.

2. Prepare all of the equipment and assure the cable is in good repair. Check to make sure there are adequate leads and materials for prepping the skin.

3. Prep the skin. (See Procedure A-1A.) Dirt, oil, sweat, and other materials on the skin can interfere with obtaining a quality tracing. The skin should be cleansed with an appropriate substance. If the patient is diaphoretic, dry the skin with a towel. On very hot days, or in situations where the patient is very diaphoretic, tincture of Benzoin can be applied to the skin before attaching the electrode. Occasionally, it may be necessary to slightly abrade the skin to obtain a good interface. Patients with a lot of body hair may need to have the area immediately over the electrode site shaved to assure good skin/electrode interface.

4. Place the four limb leads according to the manufacturer's recommendations. (See Procedure A-1B.)

5. Following placement of the limb leads, prepare for placement of the precordial leads. Procedure A-1C illustrates proper placement of the precordial leads.

6. First, place Lead V_1 by attaching the positive electrode to the right of the sternum at the fourth intercostal space. (See Procedure A-1D.)

7. Next, place Lead V_2 by attaching the positive electrode to the left of the sternum at the fourth intercostal space. (See Procedure A-1E.)

8. Next, place Lead V_4 by attaching the positive electrode at the mid-clavicular line at the fifth intercostal space. (See Procedure A-1F.)

9. Next, place Lead V_3 by attaching the positive electrode in a line midway between Lead V_2 and Lead V_4. (See Procedure A-1G.)

10. Next, place Lead V_5 by attaching the positive electrode at the anterior axillary line at the same level as V_4. (See Procedure A-1H.)

11. Finally, place V_6 by attaching the positive electrode to the mid-axillary line at the same level as V_4. (See Procedure A-1I.)

12. Assure that all leads are attached. (See Procedure A-1J.)

13. Turn on the machine. (See Procedure A-1K.)

14. Check to assure all leads are properly attached and a good tracing is being received from each channel.(See Procedure A-1L.)

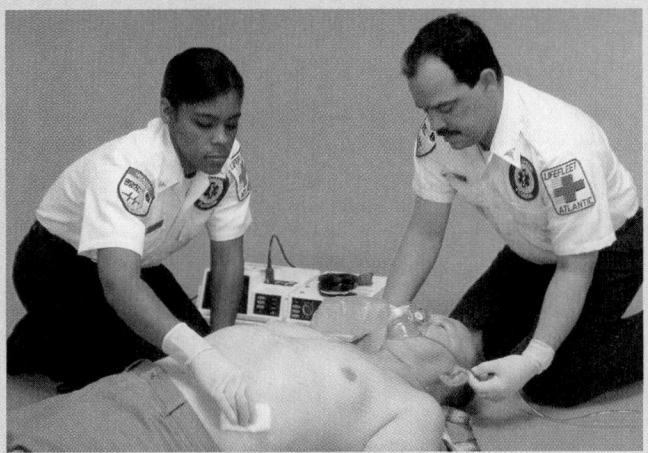

A-1A. Prep the skin.

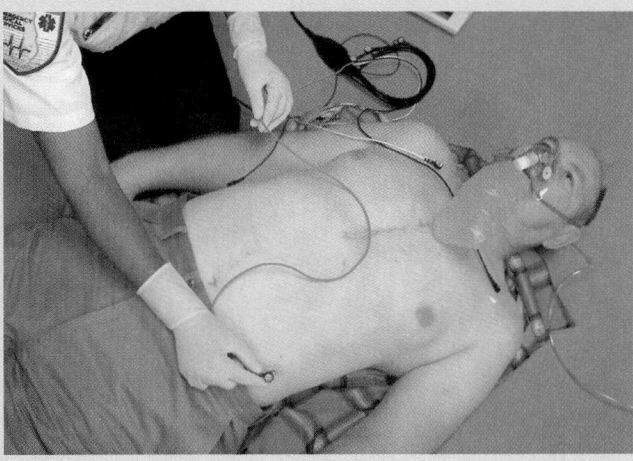

A-1B. Place the four limb leads according to the manufacturer's recommendations.

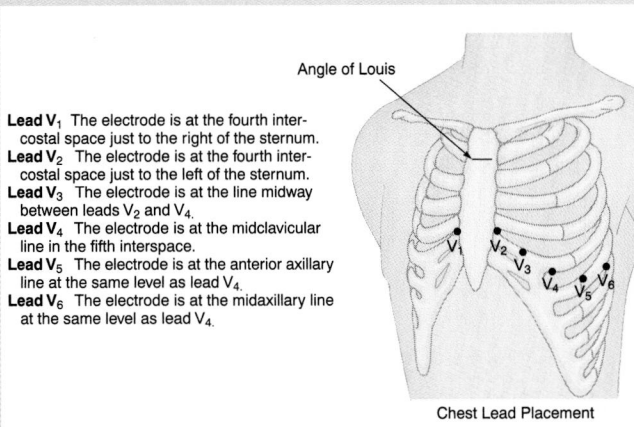

Angle of Louis

Lead V₁ The electrode is at the fourth intercostal space just to the right of the sternum.
Lead V₂ The electrode is at the fourth intercostal space just to the left of the sternum.
Lead V₃ The electrode is at the line midway between leads V₂ and V₄.
Lead V₄ The electrode is at the midclavicular line in the fifth interspace.
Lead V₅ The electrode is at the anterior axillary line at the same level as lead V₄.
Lead V₆ The electrode is at the midaxillary line at the same level as lead V₄.

Chest Lead Placement

A-1C. Proper placement of the precordial leads.

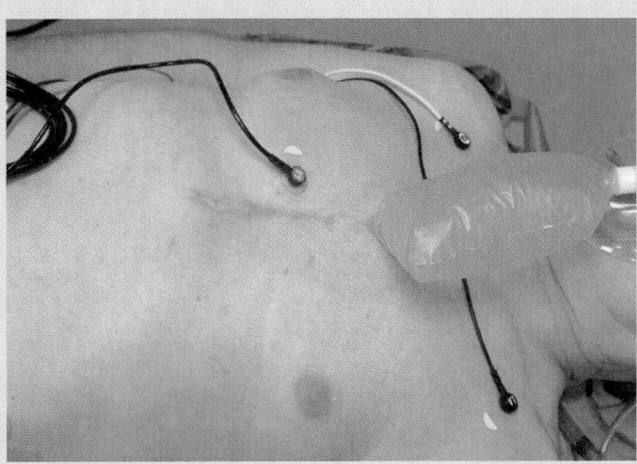

A-1D. Place lead V_1.

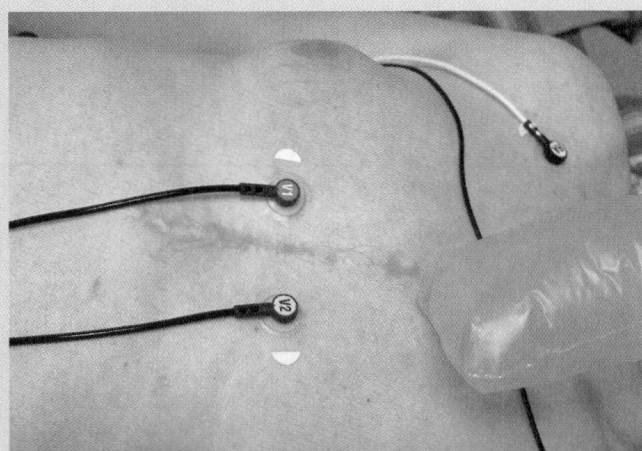

A-1E. Place lead V_2.

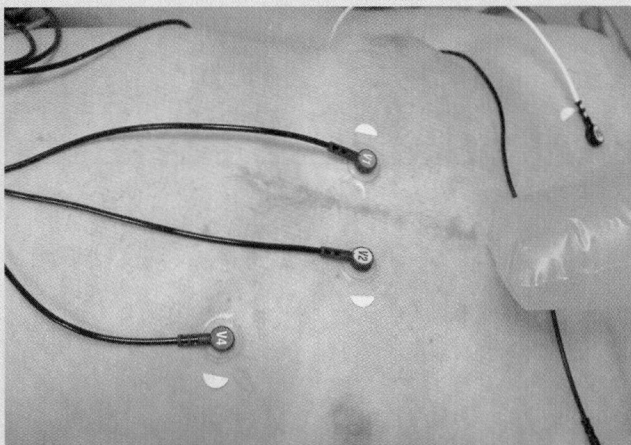

A-1F. Place lead V_4.

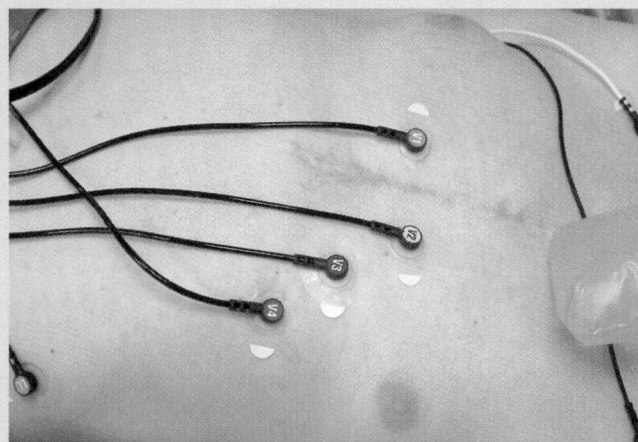

A-1G. Place lead V₃.

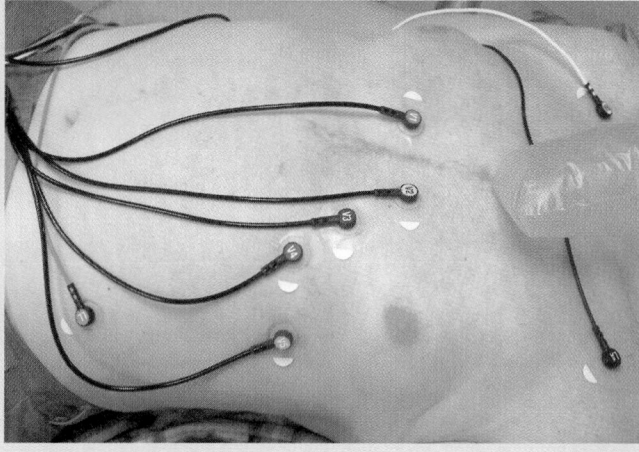

A-1H. Place lead V₅.

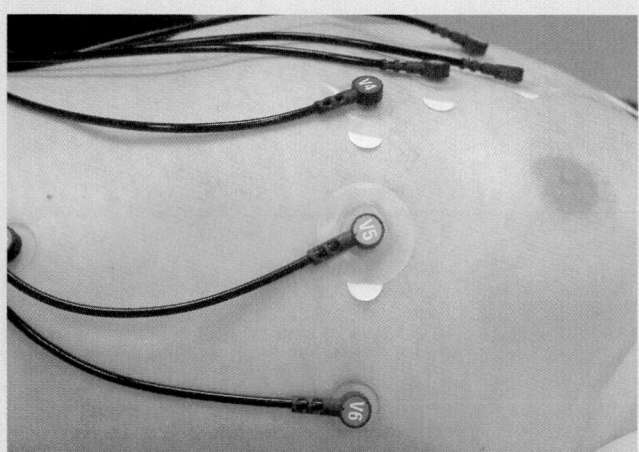

A-1I. Place lead V₆.

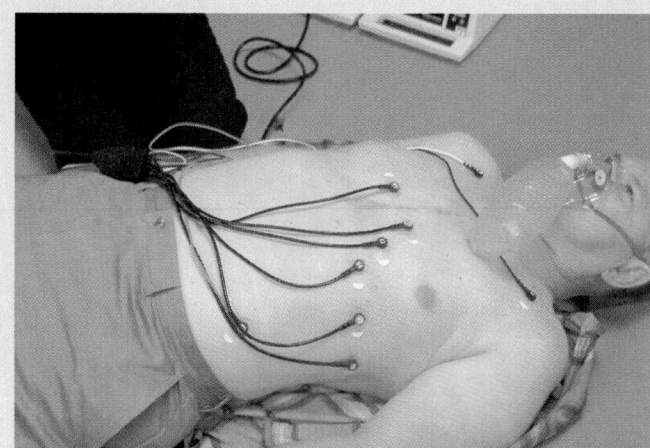

A-1J. Assure that all leads are attached.

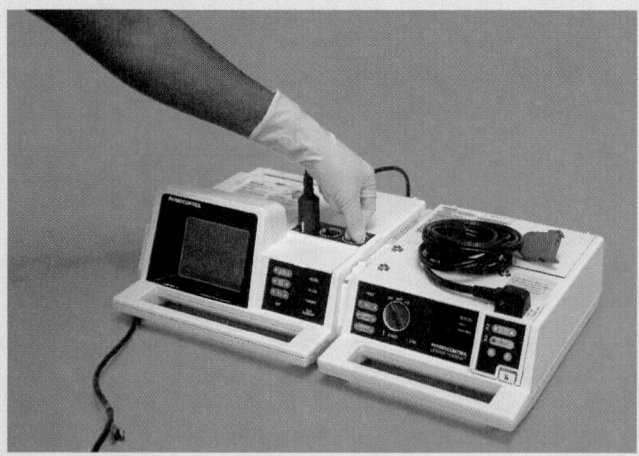

A-1K. Turn on the machine.

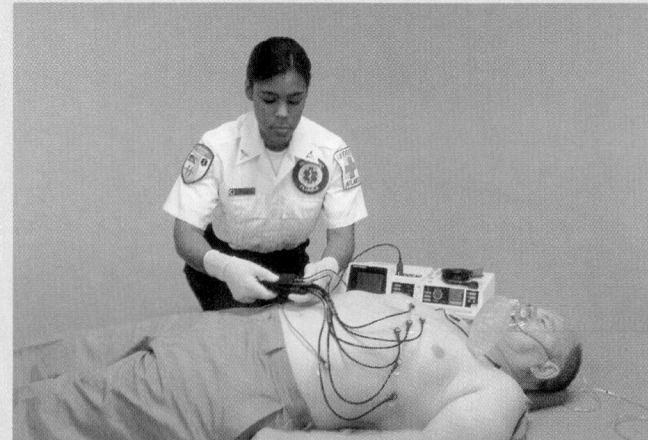

A-1L. Check the quality of the tracing being received from each channel.

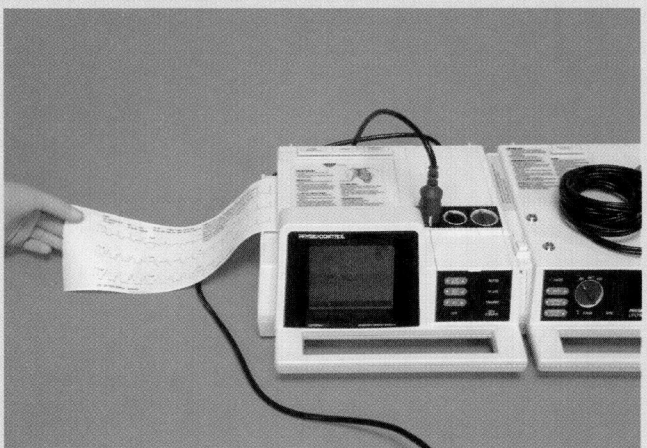

A-1M.   Record the tracing.

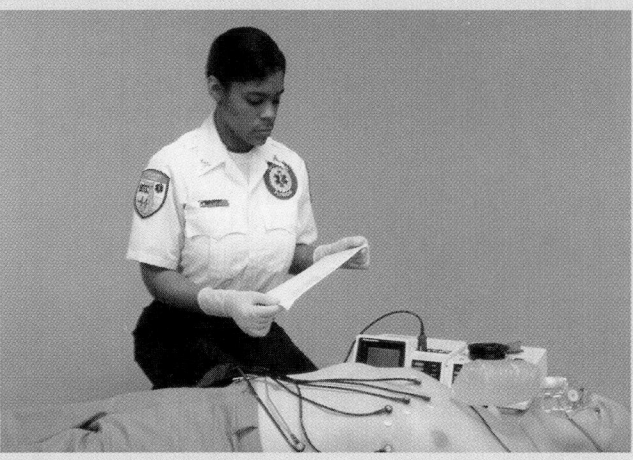

A-1N.   Examine the tracing.

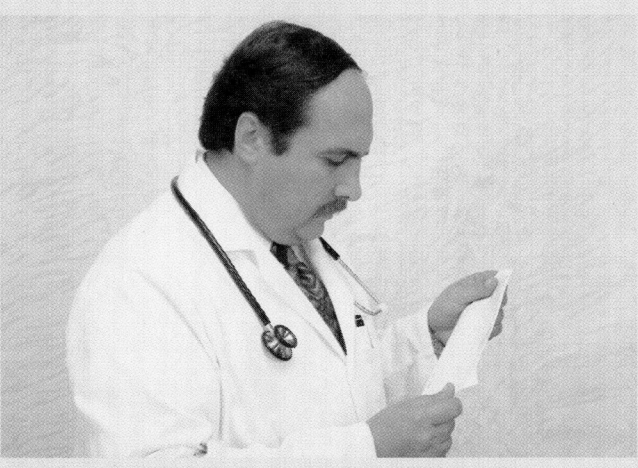

A-1O.   Transmit the tracing to the receiving hospital.

15. Record the tracing. (See Procedure A-1M.)
16. Examine the tracing. Do not completely rely on the machine interpretation of the tracing. If necessary, confirm with medical control. (See Procedure A-1N.)
17. Provide the tracing to the receiving hospital. (See Procedure A-1O.) If thrombolytic therapy is not started in the field, the door to needle time can be reduced by providing a quality 12 lead tracing to the emergency department staff as soon as the patient arrives.
18. Perform patient pass-off to the hospital personnel.
19. Restock equipment for next call.
20. Compare field interpretation with emergency department and cardiology interpretation.

SUMMARY

With the advent of thrombolytic therapy for acute myocardial infarction, 12 lead ECG monitoring and interpretation may become an important part of advanced prehospital care. Even if thrombolytic therapy is not initiated in the field, prehospital 12 lead ECG therapy can be used to screen patients for delivery to hospitals with thrombolytic capabilities as well as to make early identification of patients who may benefit from thrombolytic therapy.

FURTHER READING

Abedin, Zainul and Robert Conner. *12 Lead ECG Interpretation: The Self-Assessment Approach*. Philadelphia: W.B. Saunders Company, 1989.

Dernocer, Kate, Charley Miller, and Mike Taigman. *Taigman's Advanced Cardiology (In Plain English)*. Upper Saddle River, NJ: Brady/Prentice Hall, 1995.

Guyton, Arthur. *Textbook of Medical Physiology*, 8th ed. Philadelphia: W.B. Saunders Company, 1991.

Scheidt, Stephen and Frank Netter. *Basic Electrocardiography*. West Caldwell, NJ: Ciba-Geigy, 1986.

GLOSSARY

abandonment   the termination of a health care provider-patient relationship, without assurance that an equal or greater level of care will continue.

abdomen   portion of the body located between the thorax and the pelvis; the superior portion of the abdominopelvic cavity.

abduction   movement of a body part or extremity away from the midline.

aberrant conduction   conduction of the electrical impulse through the heart's conductive system in an abnormal fashion.

abortion   the termination of pregnancy before the twentieth week of gestation. The term "abortion" refers to both miscarriages and induced abortions. Generally, however, "abortion" is used for elective termination of pregnancy and *miscarriage* for the loss of a fetus, before 20 weeks, by natural means.

ABO system   system of blood typing based on the presence of proteins on the surface of the red blood cells.

abrasion   scraping or abrading away of the superficial layers of the skin. An open soft-tissue injury.

absolute refractory period   the period of the cardiac cycle when stimulation will not produce any depolarization whatever.

acceleration   the rate at which speed or velocity increases.

acid   a chemical substance that liberates hydrogen ions (H_+) when in solution.

acidosis   a state where the pH is lower than normal due to an increased hydrogen ion concentration.

acquired immune deficiency syndrome (AIDS)   fatal illness caused by infection with the Human Immunodeficiency Virus (HIV). Because AIDS destroys the ability of the immune system to fight infection, patients die from overwhelming infection. Also called HIV infection.

action potential   the stimulation of myocardial cells, as evidenced by a change in the membrane electri-cal charge, that subsequently spreads across the myocardium.

active transport   biochemical process where a substance is moved across a cell membrane, often against a gradient, using energy.

acute   having a rapid onset and a short course.

acute abdomen   a rapid onset of severe abdominal pain.

acute myocardial infarction   death and subsequent necrosis of the heart muscle caused by inadequate blood supply.

acute stress reaction   reaction that occurs soon after a catastrophic event that has a powerful emotional impact on the rescuer.

adduction   movement of a body part or extremity toward the midline.

adrenergic   pertaining to synapses that use the neurotransmitter norepinephrine.

adrenergic receptors   receptors specific to norepinephrine and epinephrine-like substances.

affect   a patient's appearance as perceived by the rescuer.

afferent fibers   carrying impulses toward the center of the body. Sensory nerves send messages toward the brain and are thus afferent.

afterload   the pressure or resistance against which the heart must pump.

aggravate   to worsen or increase in severity.

agonist   a drug or other substance that causes a physiological response.

air embolism   presence of an air bubble in the circulatory system.

alarms   term used by the fire service to identify groups of fire apparatus and personnel called to assist on-scene personnel at major events. Each alarm brings a given amount of personnel and apparatus to the scene.

albumin protein found in almost all animal tissues that constitutes one of the major proteins in human blood.

alkali a strong base; a substance that liberates hydroxyl ions (OH⁻) when in solution.

alkalosis a state where the pH is higher than normal due to a decreased hydrogen ion concentration.

allergic reaction hypersensitivity to a given antigen. A reaction more pronounced than would occur in the general population.

alleviate to reduce or eliminate. It usually refers to a problem or discomforting feeling.

allied health term used to describe ancillary health care professionals, apart from physicians and nurses, such as paramedics, respiratory therapists, and physical therapists.

alpha radiation lowest level of nuclear radiation. A weak source of energy, it is stopped by clothing or the first layers of skin.

ALS Advanced Life Support. EMS personnel trained to use intravenous therapy, drug therapy, intubation, and defibrillation.

alveoli the microscopic air sacs where the oxygen–carbon dioxide exchange takes place.

alveolus one of the millions of microscopic chambers within the lung. It is the location where the gasses of respiration are exchanged. (pl. alveoli)

Alzheimer's Disease a progressive, degenerative disease that attacks the brain and results in impaired memory, thinking, and behavior. It affects an estimated 2.5 million American adults.

ambient surrounding on all sides.

amniotic fluid clear, watery fluid that surrounds and protects the developing fetus.

amniotic sac the membranes that surround and protect the developing fetus throughout intrauterine development.

amputation severance, removal, or detachment, either partial or complete, of a body part.

anaphylaxis an acute, generalized, and violent antigen-antibody reaction that can be rapidly fatal.

anastomosis a communication between two or more vessels.

anatomy the study of body structure.

aneurysm the ballooning of an arterial wall, resulting from a defect or weakness in the wall.

anion a negatively charged ion. It is attracted to the positive pole of an electrode (anode), hence the name.

anisocoria pupils of unequal size.

anorexia lack of or loss of appetite.

antagonist a drug or other substance that blocks a physiological response or the action of another drug or substance.

antibiotics medications effective in inhibiting the growth of or killing bacteria. They have no impact on viruses.

antibodies proteins, produced by plasma cells, released in response to an antigen. Antibodies bind to antigens to facilitate their removal by scavenger cells such as macrophages and neutrophils.

antidote a substance that neutralizes a poison or the effects of a poison.

antigen any substance capable of inducing an immune response.

anxiety an emotional state caused by stress. It is characterized by increase in sympathetic nervous system tone.

aortic dissection a degeneration of the wall of the aorta.

APGAR scoring a numerical system of rating the condition of a newborn. It evaluates the neonate's heart rate, respiratory rate, muscle tone, reflex irritability, and color.

apnea the absence of breathing.

apothecary's system an antiquated system of weights and measures used widely in early medicine.

arachnoid membrane middle layer of the meninges.

arachnoid weblike in appearance.

arrhythmia the absence of cardiac electrical activity; often used interchangeably with dysrhythmia.

arteriosclerosis a thickening, loss of elasticity, and hardening of the walls of the arteries from calcium deposits.

articulate to join together and permit motion.

arytenoid folds cupped- or ladle-shaped tissues found posterior to the vocal cords.

ascites the presence of fluid within the abdominal cavity, often associated with congestive heart failure and alcoholism, among other causes.

ascites accumulation of fluid within the peritoneal cavity.

asphyxia a decrease in the amount of oxygen and an increase in the amount of carbon dioxide as a result of some interference with respiration.

aspiration the act of taking foreign material into the lungs during inhalation.

assault an action that places a person in immediate fear of bodily harm.

atelectasis a collapse of the alveoli, which in turn decreases ventilatory effectiveness.

atherosclerosis a progressive, degenerative disease of the medium-sized and large arteries.

atopy   patients with a group of diseases of an allergic nature. Included in these diseases are asthma, eczema, and allergic rhinitis. Such diseases have a strong hereditary component.

attenuated   diluted or weakened. Applied to organisms that are weakened so as not to be infectious, in order that they may be administered to provoke an immune response.

audiovestibular system   the organs and structure of the inner ear associated with hearing and balance.

auscultation   the process of listening to sounds made by the internal organs; usually associated with the use of the stethoscope.

automaticity   the capability of self-depolarization. Refers to the pacemaker cells of the heart.

autonomic dysfunction   an abnormality of the involuntary aspect of the nervous system.

autonomic ganglion   a group of autonomic nerve cells located outside the central nervous system.

autonomic nervous system   part of the nervous system controlling involuntary bodily functions. It is divided into the sympathetic and the parasympathetic systems.

autotransfusion   a process that causes the displacement of the patient's blood from one region to another.

avulsion   forceful tearing away or separation of body tissue. The avulsion may be partial or complete.

axial loading   extreme compressional forces applied to the axis of the vertebral spine.

bacteria   small, unicellular organisms present throughout the environment. They are capable of life independent of other organisms.

ballistics   the study of projectile motion and its effects upon any object it impacts.

band   a group of radio frequencies close together on the electromagnetic spectrum.

battery   the unlawful touching of a person without his or her consent.

Battle's sign   black-and-blue discoloration over the mastoid process (just behind the ear) that is characteristic of a basilar skull fracture.

bend fracture   fracture seen in children characterized by angulation and deformity in the bone without obvious break.

benzodiazepines   general term to describe a group of tranquilizing drugs with similar chemical structures.

beta radiation   medium-strength radiation stopped with light clothing or the uppermost layers of skin.

bilateral periorbital ecchymosis   black-and-blue discoloration of the area surrounding the eyes. It is usually associated with basilar skull fracture. (Also called raccoon eyes.)

bile   a yellow to green viscous fluid secreted by the liver and stored in the gall bladder. It is secreted into the small bowel, aids in digestion of fats, and gives the stool its normal coloration.

biochemistry   the study of chemical events occurring within a living organism.

biophysics   the application of the principles of physics to body mechanics.

biotelemetry   the process of transmitting physiological data, such as an electrocardiogram, over distance, usually by radio.

Biot's respirations   breathing pattern characterized by irregular periods of apnea and hyperpnea, generally associated with increased intracranial pressure.

blood brain barrier   a protective mechanism that selectively allows the entry of only a limited number of compounds into the brain.

bradycardia   a heart rate less than 60.

brainstem   that part of the brain connecting the cerebral hemispheres with the spinal cord. It is comprised of the medulla oblongata, the pons, and the midbrain.

bronchiolitis   viral infection of the medium-sized airways, occurring most frequently during the first year of life.

bruit   the sound of turbulent blood flow through a vessel; usually associated with atherosclerotic disease.

buckle fracture   fracture seen in children characterized by a raised or bulging projection at the fracture site.

buffer   substance that neutralizes or weakens a strong acid or base.

bundle branch block   a kind of interventricular heart block where conduction through either the right of left bundle branches is blocked or delayed.

bundle of Kent   an accessory AV conduction pathway that is thought to be responsible for the ECG findings of pre-excitation syndrome.

burnout   burnout occurs when coping mechanisms no longer buffer the job stressors. It can compromise personal health and well-being.

cancellous   having a lattice-work structure, as in the spongy tissue of the bone.

cancellous bone   spongy bone tissue found at the distal and proximal ends of the long bones.

capillary refill   diagnostic sign for evaluating peripheral circulation. A capillary bed, such as a fingernail, is compressed. The time taken for color to return to the bed is the capillary refill time, usually 2 seconds or less.

carcinoma malignant (cancerous) growth arising from epithelial cells.

cardiac contractile force the force generated by the heart during each contraction.

cardiac cycle the period of time from the end of one cardiac contraction to the end of the next.

cardiac output the amount of blood pumped by the heart in one minute.

cardiogenic shock the inability of the heart to meet the metabolic needs of the body, resulting in inadequate tissue perfusion.

cardiovascular disease diseases affecting the heart, peripheral blood vessels, or both.

cardioversion the passage of an electric current through the heart during a specific part of the cardiac cycle to terminate certain kinds of dysrhythmias.

carina the point at which the trachea bifurcates into the right and left mainstem bronchi.

cartilage connective tissue providing the articular surfaces of the skeletal system.

cataracts medical condition in which the lens of the eye loses its clearness.

catecholamine class of hormones that act upon the autonomic nervous system. They include epinephrine, norepinephrine, and similar compounds.

cathartic an agent or substance that causes evacuation of the bowels.

cation a positively charged ion. It is attracted to the negative pole of an electrode (cathode), hence the name.

cauda equina terminal portion of the spinal cord shaped much like the tail of a horse (Cauda Equina is Latin for tail of a horse).

caudally of, at, or near the foot end of the body.

cavitation formation of a partial vacuum, and subsequent cavity, within a liquid. This describes the action of a high-velocity projectile on the human body, which is 60 percent water.

cavity a hollow space in a larger structure, a space which holds the organs of the body.

cell the basic unit of life and the fundamental element of which an organism, such as the human body, is composed.

cell membrane structure which surrounds the cell. It plays a major role in maintaining the internal environment of the cell.

cerebellum portion of the brain located dorsally to the pons and medulla oblongata. It plays an important role in the fine control of voluntary muscular movements.

cerebrospinal fluid watery, clear fluid that acts as a cushion, protecting the brain and spinal cord from physical impact. The cerebrospinal fluid also serves as an accessory circulatory system for the central nervous system.

cerebrum largest part of the brain. It consists of two hemispheres separated by a deep longitudinal fissure. The cerebrum is the seat of consciousness and the center of the higher mental functions such as memory, learning, reasoning, judgement, intelligence, and the emotions.

certification the process by which an organization or governmental agency grants permission to engage in a given occupation to an applicant who has attained the degree of competency required to ensure the public's protection.

Cheyne-Stokes respirations breathing pattern characterized by progressive increase in the rate and volume of respirations that later gradually subsides. It is usually associated with a disturbance in the respiratory center of the brain.

cholinergic pertaining to synapses that use the neurotransmitter acetylcholine.

chronic obstructive pulmonary disease (COPD) characterized by a decreased ability of the lungs to perform the function of ventilation.

chronic of long duration.

chronotrope a drug or other substance that affects the heart rate.

chronotropy pertaining to heart rate.

ciliated having hairlike processes projecting from the cells that propel mucus.

circumferential encircling or going around the complete exterior.

civil law the division of the legal system that deals with non-criminal issues and conflicts between two parties.

clonic alternating contraction and relaxation of muscles.

clubbing the enlargement of the distal fingers and toes, often due to chronic respiratory or cardiovascular disease.

cochlea snail-shaped structure within the inner ear containing the receptors for hearing.

colloid osmotic pressure pressure generated by the presence of colloids in the vascular system or interstitial space.

coma a state of unconsciousness from which the patient cannot be aroused.

command post a fixed location where the incident commander is located. Typically a vehicle with radio communications, it is often staffed by a number of other agency representatives, who will provide support and coordination in the rescue effort.

compensated shock a hemodynamic insult to the body in which the body responds effectively. Signs and symptoms are limited, and the human system functions normally.

compensatory pause the pause following an ectopic beat where the SA node is unaffected and the cadence of the heart is uninterrupted.

computer-aided-dispatch enhanced dispatch system in which computerized data is used to assist dispatchers in selection and routing of emergency equipment and resources.

concussion a transient period of unconsciousness. In most cases, the unconsciousness will be followed by a complete return of function.

conduction moving electrons, ions, heat, or sound waves through a conductor or conducting medium.

congenital present at birth.

consent the granting of permission to treat, by a patient to a health care provider.

contiguous in contact or closely related.

contralateral relating to the opposite side of the body.

contrecoup occuring on the opposite side; an injury to the brain opposite the site of impact.

contusion closed wound in which the skin is unbroken, although damage has occurred to the immediate tissue beneath.

convection transferring of heat via currents in liquids or gases.

cor pulmonale hypertrophy of the right ventricle resulting from disorders of the lung.

cranium vault-like portion of the skull encasing the brain.

crepitation a grating or crackling sensation, felt or heard in such conditions as subcutaneous emphysema, or bone fracture.

cribriform plate thin, sharp plate in the central cranium.

cricothyroid membrane the membrane located between the cricoid and thyroid cartilages of the larynx.

criminal law the division of the legal system that deals with wrongs against society or its members.

critical/immediate category a triage term used to describe critically injured patients requiring immediate transportation.

Critical Incident Stress Debriefing (CISD) form of group support developed by Jeff Mitchell, Ph.D., to assist rescuers in coping with highly stressful events.

critical incidents an event that has a powerful emotional impact on a rescuer that causes an acute stress reaction.

critical incident stress reaction that occurs soon after a catastrophic event that has a powerful emotional impact on the rescuer. It is synonymous with acute stress reaction.

croup laryngotracheobronchitis, a common viral infection of young children, resulting in edema of the sub-glottic tissues. Characterized by barking cough and inspiratory stridor.

crowning the bulging of the fetal head past the opening of the vagina during a contraction. Crowning is an indication of impending delivery.

Cullen's sign a bluish discoloration of the area around the umbilicus, caused by intra-abdominal hemorrhage.

cumulative stress reaction stress reaction that results from continuous exposure to work and non-work stressors. This reaction, also called "burnout," usually is not associated with a critical incident.

CVA (cerebrovascular accident) caused by either ischemic or hemorrhagic lesions to a portion of the brain, resulting in damage or destruction of brain tissue. CVA is commonly referred to as "stroke."

cyanosis bluish discoloration of the skin due to an increase in reduced hemoglobin in the blood. The condition is directly related to poor ventilation.

cystic medial necrosis a death or degeneration of a part of the wall of an artery.

cytoplasm material within the cell that provides for structure, support, and certain biochemical functions.

dead/nonsalvageable category a triage term used to describe patients who are obviously dead or who have mortal wounds.

deceleration the rate at which speed or velocity decreases.

decerebrate posture sustained contraction of extensor muscles of the extremities resulting from a lesion in the brain stem. The patient presents with stiff and extended extremities and retracted head.

decoder a device that receives and recognizes unique codes or tones sent over the air.

decompensated shock a continuing hemodynamic insult to the body in which the compensatory mechanisms break down. The signs and symptoms become very pronounced, and the patient moves rapidly toward death.

decompression sickness condition, commonly known as "the bends," in which nitrogen bubbles develop within the tissues due to a rapid reduction of air pressure after a diver returns to the surface following exposure to compressed air.

decorticate posture characteristic posture of a patient with a lesion at or above the upper brainstem. He or she presents with the arms flexed, fists clenched, and legs extended.

defense mechanisms adaptive functions of the personality that help an individual adjust to stressful situations.

defibrillation the process of passing a DC electrical current through a fibrillating heart to depolarize a "critical mass" of mycardial cells, allowing them to depolarize uniformly, resulting in an organized rhythm.

dehydration an abnormal decrease in total body water.

delay category a triage term used to describe injured patients who do not have immediate life-threatening injuries and who can wait a period of time for definitive treatment and transportation.

delayed stress reactions a stress reaction that occurs days, weeks, or months after a critical incident, also called post-traumatic stress syndrome.

DeLee trap suction a suction device that contains a suction trap connected to a suction catheter. The negative pressure that powers it can come either from the mouth of the operator or, preferably, from an external vacuum source.

delegation of authority the granting of privileges by a physician to a non-physician to perform well-delineated skills and procedures.

delirium tremens (DTs) disorder found in habitual and excessive users of alcoholic beverages after cessation of drinking for 48-72 hours. Patients experience visual, tactile, and auditory hallucinations.

delirium an acute alteration in mental functioning that is often reversible.

delusion a false belief that a patient firmly maintains despite overwhelming evidence to the contrary.

dementia a deterioration of mental status that is usually associated with structural neurological disease. It is often progressive and irreversible.

depression a mood disorder characterized by hopelessness and malaise.

dermatome topographical region of the body surface innervated by one specific nerve root.

dermis true skin, also called the corium. It is the layer of tissue producing the epidermis and housing the structures, blood vessels, and nerves normally associated with the skin.

diabetes mellitus endocrine disorder characterized by inadequate insulin production by the beta cells of the islets of Langerhans in the pancreas.

dialysate physiologic solution used in renal dialysis.

dialysis process of exchanging various biochemical substances across a semipermeable membrane to remove toxic substances.

diaphysis hollow shaft of the long bones.

diastole the period of time when the myocardium is relaxed and cardiac filling and coronary perfusion occur.

diffusion the movement of solutes (substances dissolved in a solution) from an area of greater concentration to an area of lesser concentration.

direct medical control communications between field personnel and a medical control physician during an emergency run.

disentanglement the processes of freeing a patient from wreckage, to allow for proper care, removal, and transfer.

dislocation displacement of a long bone or other structure from its normal anatomical location.

dispatch term used to describe the dispatch center for emergency medical services. Also called alarm headquarters.

diuretic a medication that stimulates the kidneys to excrete water.

diverticula small finger-like pouches on the colon associated with degeneration of the muscular layer of the organ.

diverticulitis an inflammation or infection of a diverticulum.

diverticulosis the presence of diverticula on the colon.

division used by some agencies in place of the term "sector" to describe a group of rescuers working for a supervisor. The supervisor is commonly called a divisional officer.

doll's eye reflex the eyes turning as the head is turned. An unnatural response, indicative of head injury.

domestic violence the use of force by one family member against another with the intent of inflicting physical or emotional injury.

drug a chemical agent used in diagnosis, treatment, and prevention of disease.

duodenum first part of the small bowel. About 10 inches in length, it receives the secretions of the liver and the pancreas.

duplex transmissions method of radio transmission in which simultaneous transmission and reception occur using two frequencies.

dura mater tough layer of the meninges firmly attached to the interior of the skull.

Durable Power of Attorney for Health Care a legal document whereby a patient designates another person to make health care decisions for them.

dysconjugate gaze failure of the eyes to rotate simultaneously in the same direction.

dyspnea difficult or labored breathing.

dysrhythmia any deviation from the normal electrical rhythm of the heart.

ecchymosis blue-black discoloration of the skin due to leakage of blood into the tissues.

ectopic beats cardiac depolarization resulting from depolarization of cells in the heart that are not a part of the heart's normal pacemaker.

ectopic pregnancy the implantation of a developing fetus outside of the uterus, often in a fallopian tube.

effacement the thinning of the cervix during labor.

efferent fibers carrying conducted impulses away from the brain or spinal cord to the periphery.

effusion the escape of fluid, normally from the vascular space, into a cavity (e.g., pleural effusion).

elderly a person age 65 years or older.

electrocardiogram (ECG) the graphic recording of the heart's electrical activity. It may be displayed either on paper or on an oscilloscope.

electrolytes chemical substances that dissociate into charged particles when placed in water.

emboli a clot or other particle brought by the blood from another vessel and forced into a smaller one.

emergency medical dispatcher person responsible for assignment of emergency medical resources to a medical emergency.

emergency medical services a complex health care system that provides immediate, on-scene patient care to those suffering sudden illness or injury.

EMS System a comprehensive approach to providing emergency medical services.

EMT-Basic a person, currently certified, who has successfully completed the U.S. Department of Transportation (USDOT) National Standard Curriculum for EMT-Basic.

EMT-Intermediate a person, currently certified, who has successfully completed the USDOT National Standard Curriculum for EMT-I.

EMT-Paramedic a person, currently certified, who has successfully completed the USDOT National Standard Curriculum for EMT-P.

encoder a device for generating unique codes or tones that are recognized by another radio's decoder.

endocrine glands glands that secrete hormones directly into the blood.

endometrium the inner lining of the uterus where the fertilized egg implants.

energy the capacity to do work in the strict physical sense.

enzyme biochemical catalyst that speeds chemical reactions. The enzyme itself does not normally change during the process.

epidermis outermost layer of the skin comprised of dead or dying cells.

epidural hematoma accumulation of blood between the dura mater and the cranium.

epigastrium portion of the abdomen immediately below the xiphoid process.

epiglottitis bacterial infection of the epiglottis, usually occurring in children older than age 4. A serious medical emergency.

epinephrine major hormone secreted by the adrenal medulla in response to sympathetic stimulation; a major mediator of the sympathetic response.

epiphysis ends of the long bone, including the epiphyseal, or growth plate, and support structures underlying the joint.

erythema general reddening of the skin due to dilation of the superficial capillaries.

eschar hard, leathery product of deep third-degree burn. It consists of dead and denatured skin.

estimated date of confinement (EDC) the approximate day the child will be born. This date is usually based on the date of the mother's last menstrual period (LMP).

ethics the rules, standards, and morals governing the activities of a group or profession.

eustachian tube a tube connecting the pharynx and the middle ear.

evaporation change from liquid to a gaseous state.

excursion extent of movement of a body part such as the chest during respiration.

expressed consent verbal, non-verbal, or written communication by a patient that he or she wishes to receive medical care.

extracellular fluid   portion of the body fluid outside the body's cells.

extrapyramidal system (EPS)   the part of the nervous system that controls movement.

extravasation   the leakage of fluid or medication outside a blood vessel.

extrication   the use of force to free a patient from entrapment.

extrication officer   title of an individual who supervises all personnel and activities related to an extrication process.

extrication sector   the component of the incident command system that is responsible for freeing victims from wreckage and managing them at an accident site.

facilitated diffusion   biochemical process where a substance is selectively transported across a membrane, using "helper proteins" and energy.

fibrosis   the formation of fiber-like connective tissue, also called scar tissue, in an organ.

FiO$_2$ the concentration of oxygen in inspired air.

flaccid   relaxed, flabby, or without muscle tone.

flail chest   a defect in the chest wall that allows for free movement of a segment. Breathing will cause paradoxical chest wall motion.

fontanelles   areas in the infant skull where bones have not yet fused. Posterior and anterior fontanelles are present at birth.

fracture   disruption of the bone tissue. Types of fractures include: comminuted, greenstick, impacted, linear, oblique, spiral, and reverse.

fungi   class of organisms containing yeast and molds.

gag reflex   the act of retching or striving to vomit; a normal reflex triggered by touching the soft palate or the throat.

gamma radiation   powerful electromagnetic radiation emitted by radioactive substances. It is stronger than alpha and beta radiation.

genitalia   reproductive organs of either the male or the female.

geriatric abuse   a syndrome in which an elderly person is physically or psychologically injured by another person.

geriatrics   the study and treatment of diseases of the aged.

Glasgow Coma Scale   scoring system for monitoring the neurological status of patients with head injuries.

glaucoma   medical condition where the pressure within the eye increases.

glottis   the slit-like opening between the vocal cords.

Golden Hour   the one-hour period following a severe injury. Based on research, it has been demonstrated that severe trauma patients who reach surgery within this period have a higher survival rate.

Good Samaritan Laws   laws designed to protect from liability persons who assist at the scene of a medical emergency.

grand mal seizure   form of seizure characterized by tonic-clonic muscle contractions. It may occur with or without coma.

grand multipara   a woman who has delivered at least seven babies.

greenstick fracture   fracture seen in children characterized by an incomplete break in the bone.

Grey Turner's sign   the ecchymotic discoloration of the flanks and umbilical region, associated with intra-abdominal hemorrhage, often of pancreatic origin.

guarding   voluntary or involuntary contraction of the abdominal muscles in response to severe abdominal pain.

gynecology   the branch of medicine that treats disorders of the female reproductive system.

half-life   time required for half of the nuclei of a radioactive substance to lose activity by undergoing radioactive decay.

hallucination   a sense perception that has no basis in reality, for example, hearing voices when no one is present.

haversian canals   small perforations of the long bones through which the blood vessels and nerves travel into the bone itself.

hazard zone   an area of rescue operations that poses a significant physical threat to rescuers.

heat cramps   acute painful spasms of the voluntary muscles following strenuous activity in hot environment without adequate fluid or salt intake.

heat exhaustion   acute reaction to heat exposure. Blood pools in the vessels as the body attempts to give off excessive heat. It can lead to collapse due to inadequate blood return to the heart.

heat stroke   acute, dangerous reaction to heat exposure, characterized by a body temperature usually above 106° F (41.1° C). The body ceases to perspire.

hematemesis   the vomiting of blood.

hematocrit   the percentage of the blood consisting of the red blood cells, or erythrocytes (usually 35–45 percent).

hematoma   collection of blood beneath the skin or trapped within a body compartment.

hematuria   presence of blood in the urine.

hemodialysis   a medical procedure whereby waste products and fluid, normally excreted by the kidneys, are removed by a machine.

hemoglobin   an iron-containing compound, found within the red blood cell, that is responsible for the transport and delivery of oxygen to the body cells.

hemoptysis   expectoration of blood from the respiratory tree.

hemothorax   blood within the pleural cavity.

Hertz   a measurement of radio frequency, one cycle per second.

histamine   a chemical released by mast cells and basophils upon stimulation. It is one of the most powerful vasodilators known and a major mediator of anaphylaxis.

homeostasis   the natural tendency of the body to maintain the internal environment relatively constant.

hormones   chemical substances released by a gland that control or affect other glands or body systems.

hypercarbia   an increased level of carbon dioxide in the body.

hyperpyrexia   elevation of body temperature, due to fever, above 106° F (41.1° C).

hypertension   a common disorder characterized by a persistent elevation of the blood pressure above 140/90 mmHg.

hypertensive emergency   an acute elevation of blood pressure that requires the blood pressure be lowered within one hour; characterized by end-organ changes such as hypertensive encephalopathy, renal failure, or blindness.

hypertensive encephalopathy   a cerebral disorder of hypertension indicated by severe headache, nausea, vomiting and altered mental status. Neurological symptoms may include blindness, muscle twitches, inability to speak, weakness, and paralysis.

hyperthermia   unusually high body temperature.

hypertonic   a state in which a solution has a higher solute concentration on one side of a semi-permeable membrane compared to the other side.

hypertonic phase   phase of a seizure when muscles are in a state of greater than normal tension or of incomplete relaxation.

hypertrophy   an increase in the size or bulk of an organ.

hypoglycemia   complication of diabetes characterized by low levels of blood glucose. This often occurs from too high a dose of insulin or from inadequate food intake following a normal insulin dose. Sometimes called *insulin shock*, hypoglycemia is a true medical emergency.

hypoglycemic seizure   seizure that can occur when blood glucose levels fall dangerously low, seriously altering the brain's energy supply.

hypothalamus   portion of the diencephalon producing neurosecretions important in the control of certain metabolic activities, including body temperature regulation.

hypothermia   having a body temperature below normal.

hypotonic   a state in which a solution has a lower solute concentration on one side of a semi-permeable membrane compared to the other side.

hypoxemia   a condition of reduced partial pressure of oxygen in the blood.

hypoxia   state in which insufficient oxygen is available to meet the oxygen requirements of the cells.

ileum   third and longest portion of the small bowel. It is approximately 12 feet in length and extends from the jejunum to the ileo-cecal valve.

immune response   the sequence of events that occurs following entry of an antigenic substance into the body.

immunity   a heightened responsiveness to an antigenic stimulus resulting in more rapid binding and elimination of the antigen as compared to the non-immune state.

immunoglobulin E (IgE)   antibody responsible for mediating allergic and anaphylactic reactions in a patient.

impact   the forceful contact or collision. It is the forceful exchange of energy that frequently results in trauma.

implied consent   situation involving an unconscious patient where care is initiated under the premise that the patient would desire such care if they were conscious and able to make the decision.

incident command system   a management program designed for controlling, directing, and coordinating emergency response resources. It applies in managing fires, hazardous materials, and mass-casualty incidents, as well as during other rescue operations. Major components of the system include the incident commander and a subdivided, subordinate management team in charge of sectors or divisions.

incident commander   the individual in charge of and responsible for all activities at an incident when the incident command system is in effect.

incision very smooth or surgical laceration, frequently caused by a knife, scalpel, razor blade, or piece of glass.

index of suspicions the anticipation of injuries based on analysis of the mechanism of injury.

indirect medical control the establishment of system policies and procedures, such as treatment protocols and case reviews.

inertia the tendency of an object to remain at rest or remain in motion unless acted on by an external force.

informed consent consent obtained only after the patient has had the risks and benefits of treatment explained in a manner which the patient understands.

ingestion the entrance of a substance into the body through the gastrointestinal tract.

inhalation the entrance of a substance into the body through the respiratory tract.

injection the entrance of a substance into the body through a break in the skin.

inotrope a drug or other substance that affects the contractile force of the heart.

inotropy pertaining to cardiac contractile force.

insertion attachment of a muscle to the bone that moves when the muscle contracts.

inspection the physical assessment skill of visually examining a patient.

insulin pancreatic hormone needed to transport simple sugars from the interstitial spaces into the cells.

integumentary system skin, consisting of the epidermis and dermis.

intercalated discs specialized band of tissue inserted between myocardial cells that increase the rate in which the action potential is spread from cell to cell.

intercostal muscles muscles between the ribs that serve to expand the chest.

interpolated beat a PVC that falls between two sinus beats without effectively interrupting this rhythm.

interstitial fluid portion of the body fluid found outside the body's cells, yet not within the circulatory system. Interstitial fluid is that fluid found within the interstitial space between the cells.

intervener physician a licensed physician, professionally unrelated to patients on the scene, who attempts to assist paramedic field crews.

intracellular fluid portion of the body fluid inside the body's cells.

intracerebral hemorrhage bleeding directly into the tissue of the brain.

intracranial pressure pressure exerted on the brain by the blood and cerebrospinal fluid.

intractable resistant to cure, relief, or control.

intrathoracic within the thoracic cage.

intravascular fluid portion of the body's fluid outside the body's cells and within the circulatory system.

intubation to pass a tube into an opening of the body.

involuntary consent consent to treat based upon a court order or magistrate's order which is against the desires expressed by the patient.

ion a charged particle.

ionization the process of changing a substance into separate charged particles (ions).

ionizing radiation electromagnetic radiation (e.g., X-ray) or particulate radiation (e.g., alpha particles, beta particles, and neurons) capable of producing ions by direct or secondary processes.

ipsilateral on, or referring to, the same side.

iris pigmented portion of the eye. It is the muscular area that constricts or dilates to change the size of the pupil.

Irreversible shock the final stage of shock where organs and cells are so damaged that recovery is impossible.

isotonic a state in which solutions on opposite sides of a semi-permeable membrane are in equal concentration.

J wave ECG deflection found at the junction of the QRS complex and the ST segment. It is associated with hypothermia and seen at core temperatures below 32° C, most commonly in leads II and V$_6$. Also called the Osborn wave.

jejunum second portion of the small bowel. It is approximately 8 feet in length and is located between the duodenum and ileum.

ketoacidosis complication of diabetes due to decreased insulin secretion or intake. It is characterized by high levels of glucose in the blood, metabolic acidosis, and, in advanced stages, coma. Ketoacidosis is often called *diabetic coma*.

kinetic energy the energy an object has while it is in motion. It is related to the object's velocity and mass.

kinetics the branch of dynamics that deals with motion, taking into consideration mass and force.

Korsakoff's syndrome psychosis characterized by disorientation, muttering delirium, insomnia, delusions, and hallucinations. Symptoms include painful extremities, bilateral wrist drop (rarely), bilateral foot drop (frequently), and pain on pressure over the long nerves.

Kussmaul respirations   a very deep gasping respiratory pattern, found in diabetic coma.

kyphosis   exaggeration of the normal posterior curvature of the spine.

labor   the time and processes that occur during childbirth.

laceration   open wound, normally a tear with jagged borders.

lacrimal ducts   passageways carrying the lacrimal fluid (tears) from the lacrimal glands to the eye.

landing zone   an area or sector designated as a landing point for helicopters.

laryngospasm   a spasm of the vocal folds that may occlude the airway. It is a protective mechanism to prevent the aspiration of foreign bodies into the airway.

libel   the act of injuring a person's character, name, or reputation by false or malicious writings.

licensure   the process by which a governmental agency grants permission to engage in a given occupation to an applicant who has attained the degree of competency required to ensure the public's protection.

ligament   connective tissue connecting bone to bone and holding the joints together. The ligaments will stretch to allow joint movement.

litigation   the act or process of carrying on a lawsuit.

living will   a written request to withhold heroic life support measures from a patient with a terminal condition. A living will is usually executed before the person becomes ill or injured and is used to express that person's wishes.

logarithm   mathematical concept that eases calculation of large numbers. The log of a number is the exponent of the power to which a given base must be raised to equal that number. For example, the log of 100 is 2 ($100 = 10^2$), and the log of 1,000 is 3 ($1,000 = 10^3$).

lumen   opening, or space, within a needle, artery, vein, or other hollow vessel.

lymphatic system   a complex network of small thin vessels, valves, ducts, lymph nodes, and organs that helps to protect and maintain the fluid environment of the body. The lymphatic system plays a major role in fighting disease. The lymph is restored to the regular circulation by the thoracic duct and the lymphatic duct.

Magill forceps   instrument used in airway management for reaching into the oropharynx to manipulate a foreign body, endotracheal tube, or similar item.

malaise   discomfort or uneasiness often associated with disease.

mammalian diving reflex   a complex cardiovascular reflex, resulting from submersion of the face and nose in water, that constricts blood flow everywhere except to the brain. It decreases cardiac output and rate, and produces stable or slightly increased arterial blood pressure.

mania   a mood characterized by great excitement and activity.

maxillary   having to do with, or related to, the maxilla, on the bone of the upper jaw.

mechanism of injury   the strength, direction, and nature of forces that cause injury to a patient.

meconium   dark-green material found in the intestine of the full-term neonate. It can be expelled from the intestine into the amniotic fluid during periods of fetal distress.

mediastinum   central cavity within the thorax containing the heart, great vessels, trachea, and esophagus.

medical director   a physician, who by experience or training, handles the clinical and patient care aspects of the EMS system.

medical terminology   the language and terms of medicine, based mostly on Latin and Greek.

medulla oblongata   lower portion of the brainstem.

melena   black, tar-like feces due to gastrointestinal bleeding.

menarche   the onset of menses, usually occurring between ages 12 and 14.

Meniere's disease   a disease of the inner ear characterized by vertigo, nerve deafness, and a roaring or buzzing in the ear.

meninges   membranes covering and protecting the brain and spinal cord. They consist of the pia mater, arachnoid membrane, and dura mater.

meningitis   infection and inflammation of the meninges, the covering of the brain and spinal cord.

menopause   the cessation of menses and the end of a woman's reproductive life.

mesentery   double fold of peritoneum that supports the major portion of the small bowel, suspending it from the posterior abdominal wall.

metaphysis   growth zone of the bone, active during the development stages of youth. It is located between the epiphysis and the diaphysis.

metric system   a system of weights and measures widely used in science and medicine. It is based on a unit of 10.

midbrain   portion of the brain connecting the pons and cerebellum with the cerebral hemispheres.

milliequivalent weight of a substance contained in one milliliter of a normal solution.

minute volume (V_{min}) the amount of air inhaled and exhaled in one minute; it equals the respiratory rate times the tidal volume.

mitochondria organelle responsible for provision of cellular energy.

modulator a device that transforms electrical energy into sound waves.

morality the principles of right and wrong as governed by individual conscience.

motion the process of changing place; movement.

mucous membrane a membrane lining many of the body cavities that handle air transport; it usually contains small, mucous-secreting glands.

mucus a thick, slippery secretion that functions as a lubricant and protects various surfaces.

multiparity a woman who has delivered more than one baby.

multiplex transmissions method of radio transmission in which voice and other data can be transmitted simultaneously by use of multiple frequencies.

nares the openings of the nose that lead into the nasal cavity.

nasal flaring excessive widening of the nares with respiration.

National Standard Curriculum paramedic training curriculum published by the United States Department of Transportation, widely used as the standard guidelines for paramedic education.

negligence a deviation from an accepted standard of care. It is synonymous with malpractice in the context of medical care.

neonate an infant from the time of birth to one month of age.

nephron the functional unit of the kidney.

nerve conduction velocity the rate at which a nervous impulse is transmitted along a nerve.

neurilemma thin, fibrous sheath surrounding the peripheral nerve fiber.

neuroeffector junction a specialized synapse between a nerve cell and the organ or tissue that it innervates.

neuron the nerve cell, the fundamental component of the nervous system.

neurotransmitter a substance that is released from the axon terminal of a presynaptic neuron upon excitation and that travels across the synaptic cleft to either excite or inhibit the target cell. Examples include acetylcholine, norepinephrine, and dopamine.

noncompensatory pause the pause following an ectopic beat where the SA node is depolarized and the underlying cadence of the heart is interrupted.

norepinephrine neurotransmitter of the postganglionic sympathetic nerves and a hormone secreted by the adrenal medulla.

nucleus cellular organelle which contains the genetic material (DNA).

nullipara a woman who has never delivered a baby.

oblique having a slanted position or direction.

odontoid process fingerlike projection of the second cervical vertebra, around which the first cervical vertebra rotates.

"old-old" an elderly person age 75 years or older.

omentum sheet of peritoneum and fat tissue, covering and protecting the anterior surface of the interior abdomen.

organ a group of tissues with a common function.

organelles specialized structures within the cell which provide for cellular needs.

organism a group of organ systems; the functional unit of life.

origin attachment of a muscle to the bone that does not move (or experiences the least movement) when the muscle contracts.

osmosis the movement of a solvent (water) across a semi-permeable membrane from an area of lesser (solute) concentration to an area of greater (solute) concentration. Osmosis is a form of diffusion.

osteoporosis softening of bone tissue due to the loss of essential minerals, principally calcium.

overdose a dose of a drug in excess of that usually prescribed. An overdose can adversely affect the patient's health.

overhydration an excess of total body water.

ovulation the growth and discharge of an egg from the ovary.

packaging the completion of emergency care procedures needed for transferring a patient from the scene to an ambulance.

palpation the physical assessment skill of examining a patient by touch.

palpitation a sensation that the heart is pounding, racing, or skipping a beat.

paradoxical breathing an asymmetrical chest wall movement caused by a defect (flail chest) that lessens respiratory efficiency.

paradoxical movement moving in a fashion opposite to that expected. It is often seen in flail chest injuries, where the flail segment moves in an opposite direction compared to the rest of the chest.

parasympathetic nervous system division of the autonomic nervous system that is responsible for controlling vegetative functions.

parasympatholytic a drug or other substance that blocks or inhibits the actions of the parasympathetic nervous system (also called anticholinergic).

parasympathomimetic a drug or other substance that causes effects like those of the parasympathetic nervous system (also called cholinergic).

parenchyma the principle or essential parts of an organ.

parenteral drugs drugs administered into the body without going through the digestive tract.

parietal pleura fine fibrous sheath covering the interior of the thorax.

paroxysmal nocturnal dyspnea (PND) a sudden episode of difficult breathing that occurs after lying down; most commonly caused by left heart failure.

patent open.

patient assessment that act of examining a patient in order to detect a medical problem.

percussion the act of striking an object or area to elicit a sound or vibration.

perfusion fluid passing through an organ or a part of the body.

pericardial tamponade filling of the pericardial sac with fluid, which in turn limits the filling of the heart.

pericardium two-layered sac surrounding the heart.

periosteum the exterior covering of a bone.

periosteum tough, hard covering of bone.

peripheral vascular resistance the resistance to blood flow due to the peripheral blood vessels. This pressure must be overcome for the heart to pump blood effectively.

peristalsis wavelike muscular motion of the esophagus and bowel that moves food through them.

peristalsis wavelike muscular motion of the esophagus and bowel that moves food through the digestive system.

peritoneum fine fibrous tissue surrounding the interior of most of the abdominal cavity and covering most of the small bowel and some of the abdominal organs.

petit mal seizure form of seizure where consciousness may or may not be lost.

pH scientific method of expressing the acidity or alkalinity of a solution. It is the logarithm of the hydrogen ion concentration divided by one. The higher the pH, the more alkaline the solution. The lower the pH, the more acidic the solution.

pharmacodynamics the study of a drug's action upon the body.

pharmacokinetics the study of how drugs enter the body, reach their site of action, and eventually are eliminated.

pharmacology the study of drugs and how they affect the body.

phonation the process of generating speech and other sounds.

physiology the study of body function.

pia mater inner and most delicate layer of the meninges. It covers the convolutions of the brain and spinal cord.

placenta the organ that supports the fetus during intrauterine development. The placenta is attached to the wall of the uterus and the umbilical cord.

plasma the fluid portion of the blood consisting of serum and protein substances in solution.

pleura a membrane covering the lungs and the interior of the thoracic cage.

pneumomediastinum the presence of air in the mediastinum.

Poiseuille's Law a law of physiology stating that blood flow through a vessel is directly proportional to the radius of the vessel to the fourth power.

poison control center information center staffed by trained personnel that provides up-to-date toxicologic information.

poisoning taking a substance into the body that interferes with normal physiological functions.

polycythemia an excess of red blood cells.

pons process of tissue connecting two or more parts of an organ.

portal system circulatory system that collects blood from parts of the abdominal viscera and transports it to the liver.

portal system part of the circulatory system consisting of the veins that drain some of the digestive organs. The portal system delivers blood to the liver.

post-ganglionic nerves nerve fibers that extend from the autonomic ganglia to the target tissues.

postpartum the time period after delivery of the fetus.

pre-ganglionic nerves nerve fibers that extend from the central nervous system to the autonomic ganglia.

prefix one or more syllables affixed to the beginning of a word to modify its meaning.

preload the pressure within the ventricles at the end of the diastole.

preload the volume of blood delivered to the atria prior to ventricular diastole.

preload the pressure within the ventricles at the end of diastole; commonly called the end-diastolic volume.

prenatal means essentially the same thing as "antepartum" and refers to the time period before birth. Health care visits during pregnancy are referred to as "prenatal visits" or "prenatal care."

presacral edema an accumulation of fluid in the sacral area in the recumbent patient, usually related to congestive heart failure.

priapism a painful, prolonged erection of the male penis, due to spinal injury or disease process. (It may occur in sickle cell anemia).

primary assessment first aspect of the patient assessment designed to determine any immediate threats to the patient's life. It assesses airway, breathing, and circulation, and looks for significant hemorrhage.

primary treatment patient treatment that targets three life-threatening medical problems: breathing trouble, hemorrhaging, and circulation trouble.

primary ventricular fibrillation ventricular fibrillation due to a problem occurring within the heart itself, such as acute myocardial infarction.

Prinzmetal's angina variant of angina pectoris caused by vasospasm of the coronary arteries; not blockage *per se.*

professional a person who exhibits the conduct or qualities that characterize a practitioner in a particular field or occupation.

profile the size and shape of a projectile as it contacts a target.

pronation turning of the palm or foot downward.

protocols a set of policies and procedures for all components of an EMS system.

proximate cause a legal concept describing a person, who, through his or her actions, does something that produces an effect. In current usage, it usually means that a person was the immediate causative factor in a civil or criminal wrong.

psychomotor mental processes causing or associated with physical activity.

psychomotor seizure type of seizure usually originating in the temporal lobe characterized by an aura and focal findings such as alterations in mental status or mood.

psychosis a personality change that prevents the patient from functioning normally. It is characterized by severe depression, excitement, illusions, delusions, or hallucinations.

pulmonary embolism blood clot or other thrombus in the pulmonary circulation that adversely affects oxygenation of the blood.

pulse oximetry assessment modality that measures the oxygen saturation level of the blood through a noninvasive sensor placed on a finger or ear lobe.

puncture specific soft-tissue injury involving a deep, narrow wound to the skin and underlying organs. It carries an increased danger of infection.

pyrexia fever, or above normal body temperature, fever.

pyrogen any substance capable of causing fever.

Quality Assurance (QA) quality evaluation program that is designed to objectively identify problems within the system. A QA program deals primarily with clinical issues.

Quality Improvement (QI) quality evaluation program that emphasizes service and uses customer satisfaction as the ultimate indicator of system performance.

radio an electronic device that transmits sound waves and telemetry over distances using electromagnetic waves.

rales abnormal breath sound due to the presence of fluid in the smaller airways.

rebound tenderness tenderness on release of the examiner's hands, allowing the patient's abdominal wall to return to its normal position. Rebound tenderness is associated with peritoneal irritation.

reciprocity the process by which an agency grants certification or licensure to an individual who has comparable certification or licensure from another agency.

recompression the restoration of pressure, often used in the treatment of diving emergencies so that a patient can be slowly decompressed.

refractory a disorder or condition that resists treatment.

refractory period the period of time when myocardial cells have not yet completely repolarized and cannot be stimulated again.

relative refractory period the period of the cardiac cycle when a sufficiently strong stimulus may produce depolarization.

repeater a radio base station modified to retransmit a radio broadcast so the range of the broadcast can increase.

repolarization   the return of a muscle cell to its pre-excitation resting state.

rescue   to free from confinement or danger.

research   diligent and scientific study, investigation, and experimentation in order to establish facts and determine their significance.

res ipsa loquitur   a Latin phrase meaning "the thing speaks for itself," used in negligence proceedings.

resource   term applied to all personnel, vehicles, apparatus, equipment, and medical supplies that respond to an emergency incident.

respiration   the exchange of gases between a living organism and its environment.

resting potential   the normal electrical state of cardiac cells.

reticular activating system   the system responsible for consciousness. A series of nervous tissues keeping the human system in a state of consciousness.

retraction   the act of drawing back or inward (e.g., acute airway obstruction when the intercostal spaces and sternal notch retract).

retroperitoneal   behind the layers of the peritoneum. The organs within this space include the kidneys, spleen, and part of the pancreas.

Reye's syndrome   illness of uncertain etiology that results in alteration of mental function in children. Often associated with viral infections and the use of aspirin.

rhonchi   abnormal breath sound due to the presence of fluid or mucous in the larger airways.

root word   a word to which a suffix, prefix, or both is affixed.

safety officer   a person with the knowledge and authority to intervene in unsafe rescue situations. The person who makes the "go/no go" decision for the rescue operation.

scapula   large, flat, and irregular bone located in the posterior shoulder that articulates with the humerus.

schizophrenia   a group of mental disorders characterized by disturbances in thought, mood, and behavior.

SCUBA   abbreviation for Self-Contained Underwater Breathing Apparatus.

sebaceous glands   glands within the dermis secreting sebum.

sebum   fatty secretion of the sebaceous gland. It helps keep the skin pliable and waterproof.

secondary assessment   part of the physical assessment process where detailed historical and physical findings are evaluated in order to determine the patient's medical or traumatic problem.

secondary ventricular fibrillation   ventricular fibrillation due to a problem elsewhere in the body that secondarily affects the heart (e.g., electrolyte abnormalities, hypoxia, and hypovolemia).

sector   a component of the incident command system consisting of a group of rescuers working for a supervisor within the sector. The supervisor is commonly referred to as the sector officer.

sector officer   the person supervising a group of rescuers. The sector officer is subordinate to the incident commander and receives direction from incident command.

sector vest   a vest worn by sector or divisional officers and their aides to identify them as having incident management responsibilities. They are typically brightly colored and bear titles.

seizure   a disorder of the nervous system due to a sudden, excessive, disorderly discharge of the brain neurons.

Seldinger technique   a technique for guiding a larger catheter into a vein previously entered with a small catheter, using a wire dilator.

semicircular canals   the three rings of the inner ear. They sense the motion of the head and provide positional sense for the body.

semi-permeable membrane   specialized biological membrane, such as that which encloses the body's cells, that allows the passage of certain substances and restricts the passage of others.

senescence   the process of growing old.

senile dementia   general term used to describe an abnormal decline in mental functioning seen in the elderly.

sepsis   the presence of an infectious agent, usually bacteria, in the blood stream.

septic shock   type of shock which accompanies a bacterial infection, often due to release of endotoxins by the bacteria.

septum   a wall that divides a chamber into two cavities.

shock   a state of inadequate tissue perfusion.

sick sinus syndrome   a group of disorders characterized by dysfunction of the sinoatrial node in the heart.

silent myocardial infarction   a myocardial infarction that occurs without exhibiting obvious signs or symptoms.

simplex transmissions   method of radio transmission in which both transmission and reception occur on the same frequency.

size up a quick assessment of a situation to determine the nature and extent of the emergency scene and to decide what resources will be needed to resolve the emergency.

slander the act of injuring a person's character, name, or reputation by false or malicious spoken words.

snoring upper airway noise caused by the partial obstruction of the airway by the tongue or some similar materials.

somatic nervous system portion of the nervous system responsible for control of the skeletal muscles and dermatomes.

spinal foramen the opening in the vertebrae through which the spinal cord passes.

spondylolysis a degeneration of the vertebral body.

staging the collection of vehicles at a central location for distribution as needed at a major incident scene.

staging sector the component of the incident command system that is responsible for managing a staging area.

standing orders paramedic field interventions that are completed before contacting the direct medical control physician.

Starling's Law of the Heart law of physiology stating that the more the myocardium is stretched, up to a certain amount, the more forceful the subsequent contraction will be.

START the acronym for Simple Triage and Rapid Treatment. The START program describes a rapid method of triaging large numbers of patients at an emergency incident.

status epilepticus act of having two or more successive seizures without any intervening periods of consciousness.

sternocleidomastoid muscle of the lateral neck and anterior thorax attaching at the mastoid, clavicle and sternum. It serves as an accessory muscle of respiration and lifts the sternum and anterior chest during deep respiration.

stimulus (pl. stimuli) any factor or input into the sensory system that causes an action or response.

Stokes-Adams syndrome a series of symptoms resulting from heart block, most commonly syncope. The symptoms result from decreased blood flow to the brain caused by the sudden decrease in cardiac output.

stress a state of physical or psychological arousal.

stressor any agent or situation that causes stress.

stress reaction complex response of the body to stress that prepares the body to deal with any perceived threats.

stridor a high-pitched "crowing" sound, caused by restriction of the upper airway.

stroke an interruption of blood flow—from emboli, thrombus, or hemorrhage—to an area of the brain.

stroke volume the amount of blood ejected by the heart in one cardiac contraction.

subcutaneous emphysema the presence of air within the subcutaneous tissues, often associated with pneumothorax.

subdural hematoma collection of blood directly beneath the dura mater.

subluxation incomplete dislocation of a joint. The surfaces remain in contact, while the joint is somewhat deformed.

sudden death death within one hour after the onset of symptoms.

sudden infant death syndrome (SIDS) illness of unknown etiology that occurs during the first year of life.

suffix one or more syllables affixed to the end of a word to modify its meaning.

supination turning of the palm or foot upward.

supply sector the title for a sector within the incident command system that is responsible for obtaining and distributing additional supplies at a major incident. A sector officer is assigned as the supervisor.

surface absorption the entrance of a substance into the body directly through the skin.

surfactant a compound secreted by cells in the lungs that contributes to the elastic properties of the pulmonary tissue.

sutures pseudo-joints that join the various bones of the skull to form the cranium.

sympathetic nervous system division of the autonomic nervous system that prepares the body for stressful situations.

sympathetic stimulation a stimulus that triggers the sympathetic nervous system, increasing heart rate and blood pressure, as well as other actions of the sympathetic nervous system.

sympatholytic a drug or other substance that blocks the actions of the sympathetic nervous system (also called antiadrenergic).

sympathomimetic a drug or other substance that causes effects like those of the sympathetic nervous system (also called adrenergic).

synapse a connection between nerve cells. Electrical impulses are transmitted across the synaptic cleft by special messenger chemicals called neurotransmitters.

syncope transient loss of consciousness due to inadequate flow of blood to the brain; fainting.

syncytium group of cardiac muscle cells that physiologically function as a unit.

synovial having to do with, or relating to, the lubrication of the joint.

systole the period of the cardiac cycle when the myocardium is contracting.

tachycardia a heart rate greater than 100.

tachypnea rapid respiration.

tactile fremitus vibratory tremors felt through the chest by palpation.

ten-code system radio code system published by the Association of Public Safety Communications Officers that uses the number "10" followed by another code number.

tendon band of connective tissue that attaches muscle to bone.

tension pneumothorax buildup of air under pressure within the thorax. By compressing the lung, it severely reduces the effectiveness of respiration.

tentorium extension of the dura mater separating the cerebrum from the cerebellum.

thermal gradient the difference in temperature between the environment and the body.

thermogenesis the production of heat, especially within the body.

thyrotoxicosis toxic condition characterized by tachycardia, nervous symptoms, and rapid metabolism due to hyperactivity of the thyroid gland.

TIA (transient ischemic attack) temporary interruption of blood supply to the brain.

tiered response a type of EMS system where BLS-level vehicles are initially dispatched to all calls unless ALS-level care is needed.

tilt test drop in the systolic blood pressure of 15 mmHg or an increase in the pulse rate of 15 beats per minute when a patient is moved from a supine to a seated position. Such a condition is considered positive and suggestive of a relative hypovolemia. Also called orthostatic vital signs.

tissue a group of cells, which, together, have a common function or purpose.

titration estimation of the appropriate dosage by slowly changing the rate of administration.

tonicity the number of particles present per unit volume.

tonic phase phase of a seizure characterized by tension or contraction of muscles.

tort law a branch of civil law concerning civil wrongs between two parties.

toxicology medical and biological science that studies the detection, chemistry, pharmacological actions, and antidotes of toxic substances.

toxins poisonous chemicals secreted by bacteria or released following destruction of the bacteria.

tracheal tugging retraction of the tissues of the neck due to airway obstruction or dyspnea.

trajectory the path a projectile follows. It is typically curved because of the effect of gravity.

transfer of command a process of transferring command responsibilities from one individual to another. Commonly a formal procedure of face-to-face communication, followed by a briefing on the situation, and then a radio announcement to a dispatch center that a certain individual has now assumed command of the incident. This process also applies to the transfer of sector or division responsibilities.

transient ischemic attack reversible interruption of blood flow to the brain. Often seen as a precursor to major stroke.

transportation the act of moving a patient from the scene into the ambulance or from the ambulance into the emergency department.

transportation sector the title for a sector within the incident command system that is responsible for obtaining and coordinating all patient transportation. A sector officer is assigned as the supervisor.

trauma a physical injury or wound caused by external force or violence.

trauma center hospital that has the capability of caring for the acutely injured patient. Trauma centers must meet strict criteria to use this designation.

trauma triage protocols guidelines to aid prehospital personnel in determining which patients require urgent transportation to a trauma center.

traumatic asphyxia compression of the chest due to a crush injury. It limits chest excursion yet tamponades hemorrhage.

treatment sector the title for a sector within the incident command system that is responsible for collecting and treating patients in a centralized treatment area. A sector officer is assigned as the supervisor.

triage the act of sorting patients by the severity of their injuries.

triage sector the title for a sector within the incident command system that is responsible for triaging all patients. A sector officer is assigned as the supervisor.

trunking a system to expedite radio transmissions by automatically routing, usually by computer, the transmissions to the next available frequency in the order they are received.

tunica adventitia   outer fibrous layer of the blood vessels. It maintains their maximum size.

tunica intima   interior layer of the blood vessels. It is smooth and provides for the free flow of blood.

tunica media   the middle, muscular layer of the blood vessels. It controls the vessel lumen size.

umbilical cord   structure containing 2 arteries and 1 vein that connects the placenta and the fetus.

umbilicus   the navel, the remnant of the umbilical cord.

universal precautions   set of procedures and precautions published by the Centers for Disease Control to assist health care personnel in protecting themselves from infectious disease.

untoward   an unexpected reaction, usually associated with the administration of a drug.

uremia   toxic condition caused by the retention of nitrogen-based substances (urea) in the blood, normally excreted by the kidneys.

urticaria   name given to the raised areas that occur on the skin associated with vasodilation due to histamine release. Commonly referred to as "hives."

vallecula   the depression between the epiglottis and the base of the tongue.

Valsalva's maneuver   forced exhalation against a closed glottis. This maneuver increases intra-abdominal and intra-thoracic pressure, which in turn slows the pulse.

varices   an enlarged and tortuous vein, artery, or lymphatic vessel.

varicosities   an abnormal dilation of a vein or group of veins.

velocity   the rate of motion in a particular direction in relation to time.

vertigo   loss of positional sensation and the perception that the horizon and all points of reference are moving.

vesicular breath   sound heard in the normal lung.

virus   microscopic organism, smaller than bacteria, that requires the assistance of another organism for its survival. Viruses are a common cause of human disease.

visceral pleura   fine lining covering the lungs. With the parietal pleura, it forms the seal holding the lungs to the interior of the thoracic cage.

vitreous humor   clear watery fluid filling the posterior chamber of the eye. It is responsible for giving the eye its spherical shape.

voting   a process by which the repeater station receiving the strongest incoming signal is chosen to rebroadcast that signal.

water   the universal solvent. Approximately 60 percent of the weight of the human body is due to water.

watt   a fundamental unit of electrical power.

Wernicke's syndrome   condition characterized by loss of memory and disorientation; associated with chronic alcohol intake and a diet deficient in thiamine.

wheezing   whistling type breath sound associated with narrowing or spasm of the smaller airways.

Wolf-Parkinson-White   a disorder of the heart characterized by early contraction of the heart muscle.

INDEX

Abandonment, 46
Abbreviations, medical, 134-39
ABCDE of primary assessment,
    170-74, 555. *See also*
    Airway assessment;
    Breathing; Circulation;
    Disability assessment;
    Exposure of injury
Abdomen. *See also* Abdominal
    emergencies; Body cavity
    trauma
  anatomy and physiology of,
    771-76
    topographical anatomy, 161-
    62
  assessment of, 187, 484-85, 487-
    88
  quadrants of, 161
Abdominal aorta, 475
Abdominal aortic aneurysm, 705-6
Abdominal cavity, 162, 471, 474
Abdominal emergencies, 481-82,
    769-91
  acute abdomen, 770, 776
    assessment of, 783-86
    management of, 786-87
  dialysis, 787-90
    complications of, 788-90
    management of patient on,
    790
    types of, 787-88
  gastrointestinal system emergen-
    cies, 776-79
  genitourinary system emergen-
    cies, 779-81
  pediatric, 922-23
  reproductive system emergen-
    cies, 781-82
  trauma
    management of, 495-96
    penetrating, 431
  vital signs and, 488
Abdominal pain
  gynecological, 959-60
  in poisoned patient, 812
Abdominal space, 474
Abdominal symptoms, history of,
    489
Abdominopelvic cavity, 162
Abduction, 506
Aberrant conduction, 682
Abortion, 974-75
ABO system, 295-96
Abrasion, 526
Abruptio placentae, 973, 975-77
Absolute refractory period, 625
Absorbed poisons, 807, 808-9,
    829-30

Absorbents, 396-97
Absorption
  of drug, 337
  poisoning through, 807, 808-9
Abuse
  of children, 923-27
  of elderly, 909
Accelerated junctional rhythm,
    656-57
Acceleration, 407
Acceptance stage of grief, 121
Access, gaining, 76-78
Accessory organs, 474-75
Accessory respiratory muscles, 212
Accident(s)
  automobile, 402, 408-19
    evaluation of, 419
    events of impact, 408-10
    intoxication and, 418
    mortality from, 418-19
    pneumothorax from, 478
    restraints and, 410-11
    types of impact, 411-18
  motorcycle, 419-20
  pedestrian, 420-21
"Accidental Death and Disability:
    The Neglected Disease of
    Modern Society" ("The
    White Paper"), 5
Acetabulum, 504
Acetaminophen, 833
Acetic acid, 347
Acetylcholine, 341, 347, 348, 375-
    76, 612, 741, 747, 829
Acetylcholinesterase, 347, 376
Achilles tendon, 505
Acid-base balance, 299-303
  bodily regulation of, 299-302
  derangements of, 302-3
Acid burns, 549
Acidosis, 299, 302, 377
Acids, 812
  organic, 731
Acquired immune deficiency syn-
    drome (AIDS), 841, 858-61
ACTH (adrenocorticotropin hor-
    mone), 727, 728
Action potential, 613, 741
Activated charcoal, 396-97, 810, 813
Active transport, 293
Acute, defined, 770
Acute abdomen, 770, 776
  assessment of, 783-86
  management of, 786-87
Acute arterial occlusion, 707
Acute pulmonary embolism, 707-8
Acute retinal artery occlusion, 452-
    53

Acute stress reaction, 113-14
Adalat (nifedipine), 381, 382-83,
    690, 709
Adduction, 506
Adenosine (Adenocard), 374-75,
    645, 659, 693, 710, 950
Adenosine triphosphate (ATP), 144
ADH, 289, 727, 728, 980
Adhesions, 959
Adrenal glands, 727, 729-30
Adrenaline. *See* Epinephrine
Adrenal medulla, 343
Adrenergic receptors, 339, 344-45
Adrenergic synapses, 341, 345
Adrenocorticotropin hormone
    (ACTH), 727, 728
Advanced life support, 29
Advanced Trauma Life Support
    (ATLS), 554
Aerobic metabolism, 309
Aeromedical transport, 31-32
Aeromedical transportation, 31-32
Affect, inappropriate, 1022
Afferent fibers, 746-47
Afferent receptors, 866
Afterload, 304, 557, 610
Aggravate, defined, 197
Aging, anatomy and physiology of,
    895-96. *See also* Elderly
Agonists, 339, 345. *See also specific*
    drugs
AHA, 24
AIDS, 841, 858-61
Air, transport by, 31-32
Air bags, 410, 411
Airborne diseases, 843
Air embolism, 327, 886, 890
  from dialysis, 789-90
Air Force Rescue Coordination
    Center, 84
Air medical transport, 567-69
Air splint, 518-19
Airway
  anatomy of, 207-10
    in children, 256
  head injury and, 461
  obstruction of, 185, 218-20
  shock assessment and, 312
  thermal burns of, 532-33
Airway adjunct, placement of, 222
Airway assessment, 170-72, 555
  in body cavity trauma, 483
  in critical life threatening situa-
    tions, 564
  primary, 454
  shock and, 560
  of thermal burn patient, 540
Airway management, 225-79

  in elderly patient, 900
  laryngopharynx and, 208
  manual airway maneuvers, 226-
    28
  mechanical airways, 228-74
    endotracheal intubation, 232,
    236-64
    esophageal gastric tube air-
    way (EGTA), 236
    esophageal obturator airways
    (EOA), 232-36, 247-48
    Esophageal Tracheal
    CombiTube (ETC) airway,
    267-69
    nasopharyngeal airways, 230-
    32
    oropharyngeal airways, 228-
    30, 240
    Pharyngeo-tracheal Lumen
    (PtL) airway, 264, 265-66
    surgical airways, 269-74
  neonatal, 998
  oxygenation, 223, 242, 276-79,
    317
  pediatric, 945-46
  shock and, 315-17
  suctioning, 275-76
  ventilation, 279-82
"Alarm reaction," 113
Albumin, 298
Albuterol (Proventil, Ventolin),
    387-88, 590, 802-3, 934
Alcohol abuse (alcoholism), 830-36
  alcoholic profile, 834-35
  altered behavior and, 1015
  chronic alcoholism, 758-59
  consequences of, 835
  defined, 832
  in-field treatment of, 836
  pancreatitis and, 779
  physiological effects of, 833-34
  withdrawal syndrome, 835-36
Alimentary canal, 474
Alkali, 299, 812
Alkali burns, 549
Alkalinizing drugs, 377-78
Alkalosis, 299, 302-3
  metabolic, 377
Allergen, 797
Allergic reactions, 395
Allergies, 198-99, 796-97. *See also*
    Anaphylaxis
  questioning patients about, 199
Alleviate, defined, 197
Allied health profession, 7
All-terrain vehicles (ATV), 422
Alpha (α) cells, 729
Alpha radiation, 531, 880

alpha receptors, 339
Altered mental status, 754-55
  in elderly patient, 903-4
  respiratory system assessment, 220
Alupent (metaproterenol), 591, 803
Alveolar/capillary membranes, 213
Alveolar ducts, 211, 573
Alveolar sacs, 155, 211, 573
Alveolar ventilation, 214
Alveolar volume, 217
Alveoli, 155, 210, 211, 307, 473, 574
  gas exchange in, 218
Alzheimer's Disease, 905, 1016
AMA Drug Evaluations, 334
Amanita, 816
Ambient temperature, 865, 998
Ambulance report form, 201-2
Ambulances, 29-31
  in mass-casualty events, 108
  types of, 29-31
American Heart Association
  (AHA), 24
American Red Cross, 83
Americans with Disabilities Act,
  xxx
Aminophylline (Somophyllin), 384,
  385-86, 589, 594, 711, 803
Ammonia poisoning, 820
Amnesia, 459
Amniotic fluid, 968
Amniotic sac, 968
Amperage, 529
Amphetamines, 831
AMPLE, 198-99
  allergies, 198-99
  events preceding the emer-
    gency, 198-99
  last oral intake, 198-99
  medications, 198-99
  past medical problems, 198-99
Amplitude modulation (AM), 58
Ampules, 335
Amputated parts, management of,
  546
Amputations, 528, 565
Amyl nitrite, 819
Anaerobic metabolism, 309
Analgesics, 378-80, 399
Anaphylaxis, 384, 392-93, 395, 793-
  803
  assessment of, 798-99
  causes of, 795, 796
  clinical features of, 798
  defined, 794
  epinephrine for, 363
  from *hymenoptera* stings, 822
  immune system and, 794-96
  management of, 799-803
Anastomoses, 607
Anatomy and physiology, 140-63
  of abdomen, 771-76
    circulatory system, 773
    gastrointestinal system, 772-73
    genitourinary system, 774
    reproductive system, 774-76
  of aging, 895-96
  of airway, 207-10
    in children, 256
  of autonomic nervous system,
    340-41
  of body cavities, 162-63
  of cardiovascular system, 145,
    146, 151, 602-16
    electrolytes' role, 612
    electrophysiology, 612-16
    heart, 603-7
    peripheral circulation, 607-9

of cell, 143-44
of central nervous system, 435-
  44
  brain, 439-40
  circulation in, 442
  neck, 443-44
  protective mechanisms, 435-
    39
  sense organs, 442-43
  spinal cord, 440-42
of circulatory system, 152
defined, 142
of digestive system, 156
of endocrine system, 146, 726-
  30
of external jugular vein, 325
of eye and ear, 147
of gastrointestinal system, 145
of genitourinary system, 146
of heart, 472-73
of lower extremity, 504-5
of lymphatic system, 146
of membranes, 148
of muscular system, 146, 150
of neonate, 997-98
of nervous system, 146, 153-54,
  740-48
of obstetric patient, 966-69
of organisms, 146
of organs, 144-45
of organ systems, 145-46
of reproductive system, 146,
  158, 774-76, 954-57
of respiratory system, 145, 155,
  206-17
  lower airway, 210-11
  upper airway, 207-10
of skeletal system, 146, 149
of tissues, 144
topographical anatomy, 159-62
  of abdomen, 161-62
  of chest, 160-61
  terminology, 159
of upper extremity, 504
of urinary system, 157
Androgenic hormones, 729
Anectine (succinylcholine), 260
Anemia, pulse oximeter and, 195
Aneurysms, 187, 480, 705-7, 765
  aortic, 494, 779, 785
  ventricular, 691
Anger stage of grief, 120
Angina
  preinfarction, 690
  Prinzmetal's, 689
Angina pectoris, 381-83, 689-90
Angular impact, 420
Animals, drugs from, 332
Anions, 290, 291, 292
Anisocoria, 182, 457
Ankle, 505
  fractures of, 511-12
Anorexia, 777
Antacids, 777
Antagonism, defined, 336
Antagonists, 339, 345
  narcotic, 397-98
Antegrade amnesia, 459
Antegrade conduction, 628
Anterior spinal artery, 442
Antianginal agents, 381-83
Antibiotics, 841
Antibodies, 796, 797, 842
  as indicators of exposure, 844
Anticholinergics (parasympatholyt-
  ics), 347, 375-77, 388-89
Anticonvulsant medications, 391-
  92, 762
Anti-diuretic hormone (ADH), 289,

727, 728, 980
Antidote, 809
Antidysrhythmic medications, 369-
  76, 710
  adenosine, 374-75, 645, 659,
    693, 710, 950
  bretylium tosylate, 372-74
    lidocaine, 353, 369-71, 663,
      667, 693, 710, 950, 951
    procainamide, 371-72, 667,
      693, 710
    verapamil, 375-76, 645, 659,
      693, 710
Antiemetics, 398-99, 814-15
Antigen-antibody complex, 796,
  842
Antigens, 295, 796, 842
Antihistamines, 395, 398-99, 801-2
Antihypoglycemic agents, 390-91
Anti-inflammatory agents, 392-93,
  777
Anus, 474
Anxiety, 116-17, 217
Anxiety disorders, 1021
Aorta, 472
  abdominal, 475
  descending, 773
Aortic aneurysm, 494, 779, 785
Aortic dissection, 902
Aortic valve, 606
Apex of heart, 603
APGAR score, 999-1000, 1007
Apnea, 172
Apneustic center, 215
Apneustic respirations, 750, 751
Apothecary's system, 348, 349
Appendicitis, 777, 960
Appendicular skeleton, 501
Appendix, 773
Aqueous humor, 442
Arachnoid membrane, 438, 744
Areterial puncture, inadvertent,
  327
Aretrio-venous malformations, 907
Arrest. *See* Cardiac arrest
Arrhythmias, 627
  from digitalis toxicity, 373
  drug therapy for, 369-75
    adenosine (Adenocard), 374-
      75
    bretylium tosylate (Bretylol),
      372-74
    lidocaine (Xylocaine), 369-71
    procainamide (Pronestyl),
      371-72
Arterial occlusion, acute, 707
Arterial system, 608
Arteries, 152, 306, 608
  bronchial, 213, 575
  carotid, 444, 453
  circumflex, 607
  coronary, 151, 607
  iliac, 773
  marginal, 607
  mesenteric, 773
  peripheral, 608
  pulmonary, 212, 575, 605, 606
  spinal, 442
  vertebral, 442
Arterioles, 306, 556, 608
Arteriosclerosis, 689
Arteriovenous malformations, 765
Articulation, 501
Artifacts, 625
Arytenoid cartilages, 209
Arytenoid folds, 209
Ascites, 187, 781
Asendin, 833
Aseptic meningitis, 928

ASHD, 690
Asphyxia, 576
  traumatic, 476-77
    management of, 492-93
Asphyxiant, cellular, 818
Aspiration, 220
Aspiration pneumonia, 812
Aspirin, 777, 833
  poisoning by, 808
Assault, sexual, 961-62
Assessment, 165-203. *See also specific emergencies and body
  systems*
  communication and documenta-
    tion of, 200-202
  defined, 166
  head-to-toe evaluation, 178-91
    abdomen, 180, 187
    analysis of, 189
    chest, 180, 185-87
    facial region, 179, 182-83
    genitalia, 188
    head, 178-82
    lower extremities, 181, 188-89
    neck, 180, 184
    neurological assessment, 189-
      91, 750-52
    pelvis, 181, 187-88
    posterior body, 181, 189
    upper extremities, 181, 189
  ongoing, 200
  patient history. *See* History of
    patient
  phases of, 166-67
  primary, 170-78
    ABCDE of, 170-74
    critical management priorities,
      174-75
    defined, 170
  scene size-up, 167-69
  secondary, 175-78
  of terrain, 81
  for trauma vs. medical illness,
    167
  vital signs. *See* Vital signs
Asthma, 392-93, 586-94
  assessment of, 587-88
  bronchial, 384, 385, 387-89
  epinephrine for, 363
  management of, 588-93
  pathophysiology of, 586-87
  pediatric, 934-35
  special cases, 594-95
Asystole, 376-77, 670-71
  cardiac arrest secondary to,
    702-3
  pediatric, 937, 939
Atarax (hydroxyzine), 802
Ataxis respirations, 750, 751
Atelectasis, 215, 476
Atherosclerosis, 688-94
  acute myocardial infarction (MI)
    and, 690-94
  angina pectoris and, 689-90
Atherosclerotic disease, peripheral
  arterial, 708
Atherosclerotic heart disease
  (ASHD), 690
Ativan, 832
Atlas, 436
ATLS, 554
Atom, 290
Atopy, 797
ATP, 144
Atria, 604, 605
  dysrhythmias originating in, 628,
    638-51
    atrial fibrillation, 648-51
    atrial flutter, 646-47

paroxysmal supraventricular tachycardia (PSVT), 642-45, 658
premature atrial contractions (PAC), 640-41
wandering pacemaker, 638-39
Atrial excitation, 621, 622
Atrial fibrillation, 648-51, 901
Atrial flutter, 646-47
"Atrial kick," 649
Atrial syncytium, 612, 1031-32
Atrioventricular (AV) blocks, 675-81, 1051-54
first-degree, 675
second-degree, 676-79
third-degree, 680-81
Atrioventricular (AV) bundle, 612
Atrioventricular (AV) junction, 1032
dysrhythmias originating in, 629, 652-59
junctional rhythm, 654-57
paroxysmal junctional tachycardia (PJT), 658-59
premature junctional contractions (PJCs), 652, 653
impulse delay at, 623
Atrioventricular (AV) node, 1032
Atrioventricular (AV) sequential pacemakers, 672
Atrioventricular (AV) valves, 604
Atropine, 347, 353, 376, 677, 679, 681, 830
Atropine sulfate, 376-77, 631, 637, 655, 661, 693, 710, 950
Atrovent (ipratropium), 388-89
ATVs, 422
Atypical bacteria, 852
Audiovestibular system, 888
Augmented limb leads, 618, 1033, 1035-38
Aura, 760
Auscultation, 177-78
Authority, delegation of, 41
Automaticity, 615
enhanced, 628
Automatic ventilators, 281-82
Automobile accidents, 402, 408-19
evaluation of, 419
events of impact, 408-10
intoxication and, 418
mortality, 418-19
pneumothorax from, 478
restraints and, 410-11
types of impact, 411-18
frontal, 412-14
lateral, 414-16
rear-end, 416-17
rollover, 417-18
rotational, 416
Autonomic dysfunction, 903
Autonomic ganglia, 340-41
Autonomic nervous system, 340-48, 440, 747
adrenergic receptors, 344-45
anatomy and physiology of, 340-41
parasympathetic nervous system, 154, 340, 345-48
sympathetic nervous system, 340, 341-44
Autotransfusion, 565
AV. See Atrioventricular (AV) blocks; Atrioventricular (AV) bundle; Atrioventricular (AV) junction; Atrioventricular (AV) node; Atrioventricular (AV) sequential pacemakers; Atrioventricular (AV) valves

AVPU method, 173, 752-53
Avulsions, 527-28
Axial loading, 414, 447
Axial skeleton, 501
Axis, 436
Axis deviation, 1039-42
Axon, 439

Bacteria
atypical, 852
infectious diseases from, 841
Bacterial food poisonings, 815
Bag-valve-mask (BVM) device, 221, 222-23, 280, 946
Ballistics, 426-28
Band, 58
Bandaging, 544-45
Bargaining stage of grief, 121
Bark scorpion, 824
Baroreceptors, 305-6
Barotrauma ("squeeze"), 88-90, 885-86, 887-90
Base, 299
Base of heart, 603
Base station, 54-55
Basic life support (BLS)
in cardiovascular emergencies, 712
pediatric, 945-46
procedures, 25
Basic Trauma Life Support (BTLS), 554
Basilar skull fractures, 445-46
Basophiles, 797
Battle's sign, 182, 445, 446, 456
Bayer, 833
Beat, interpolated, 662
Beer, 831
Behavioral emergencies, 1013-19. See also Psychiatric disorders
age-specific, 1023-24
assessment of, 1016-18
defined, 1014
domestic violence, 1029
drugs for, 398
interpersonal and environmental causes of, 1015
intrapsychic causes of, 1014-15
management and intervention techniques, 1018-19
organic causes of, 1015-16
violent situations, 1024-29
Bellows system, 473, 477
"Belly breathing," 456
Benadryl (diphenhydramine), 297, 395, 801-2, 814
Bend fractures, 923
"Bends" (Caisson disease), 886, 887-89
Benzedrine, 831
Benzodiazepines, 832
Beta agonists, 589, 802-3
Beta blockers, 339, 368-69, 712
Beta (ß) cells, 729
Beta radiation, 531, 880, 881
beta receptors, 339
Bicarbonate, 215, 292
Bicarbonate buffer system, 300-301
Bicarbonate ion, 300
Bigeminy, 662
Bilateral periorbital ecchymosis (Raccoon eyes), 182, 445-46
Bile, 475
Biochemistry, 142
Biophysics, 142
Biotelemetry, 59-60, 66
Biotransformation, 338
Biot's respirations, 187

Bipolar disorder, 1021
Bipolar limb leads, 616-18, 1033, 1034-35
Bites
black widow spider, 824
brown recluse spider, 822-24
snake, 825-28
Bladder, urinary, 774
infection of (cystitis), 780, 960
ruptured, 482
Blades, laryngoscope, 237-38
Blankets, protective, 72-73
Blast injuries, 424-25
Bleeding, 172. See also Hemorrhage
compartment syndrome and, 514
control of, with PASG, 317, 319
from scalp and facial areas, 444
in shock patient, 317
soft-tissue, 526
vaginal, 960-61
during pregnancy, 970, 973, 974, 977
third-trimester, 973, 975-77
Blind nasotracheal intubation, 261, 262-63
Blindness, 898
Blood, 294-96, 556
carbon dioxide concentrations in, 215
components of, 294-96
oxygen concentrations in, 214-15
perfusion and, 306
spilling into peritoneal space, 482
vomiting of, 778
whole, 296
Bloodborne diseases, 843
Bloodborne pathogens, precautions on, xxx-xxxi
Blood brain barrier, 338
Blood cells
red, 294-95, 296, 310, 530, 556
white, 294, 295, 842
Blood glucose, test for, 733, 734
Blood pressure, 191-92, 193, 305-6, 556, 610. See also Hypotension
body cavity trauma and, 488
CNS injury and, 458
PASG to elevate, 319, 320
pediatric, 943
Blood types, 295-96
Blood vessels, 306, 524-25, 556
Blowout fracture, 453
BLS. See Basic life support (BLS)
"Blue bloaters," 586
Blunt trauma, 407-25
to abdomen, 481-82
care of, 496
of children, 923
automobile accidents, 402, 408-19
evaluation of, 419
events of impact, 408-10
intoxication and, 418
mortality, 418-19
restraints, 410-11
types of impact, 411-18
blast injuries, 424-25
contusion from, 506-7, 525-26
to eye, 452
falls, 422-23
motorcycle accidents, 419-20
pedestrian accidents, 420-21
recreational vehicle accidents, 421-22

sports injuries, 423-24
B lymphocytes, 794, 796, 842
Board, padded, 518-19
Body, vertebral, 437, 438
Body cavities, anatomy and physiology of, 162-63
Body cavity trauma, 469-97
abdominal injuries. See Abdominal emergencies
assessment of, 471, 482-89
mechanism of injury, 482-83
primary, 483-85
secondary, 485-89
chest injuries, 430, 476-81, 488, 490, 491, 922-23
genitalia injury, 482
management of, 489-96
Body collision, 409
Body substance isolation (BSI), xxxi, 168
Body temperature, 192-94
shock patient and, 328
Bolus
defined, 336
intravenous, 352, 356
Bone(s)
cancellous, 435-36, 503
carpal, 504
extremity long, 501-3
facial, 435, 442
nasal, 435
of skull, 742-44
Bone marrow, 501, 503
Boots, 71
Botulism, 815
Bowel, protrusion of, 481
Bowel obstruction, 778, 907
Boyle's Law, 885
Brachial plexus, 747
Bradycardia, 376-77
defined, 626
pediatric, 937-38, 950
sinus, 630, 631
Brain, 153, 744-46
anatomy and physiology of, 439-40
areas of specialization, 745-46
divisions of, 744-45
injury to, 447-50
concussion/contusion, 448-49
hemorrhage inside, 764-65
intracranial hemorrhage, 449-50
intracranial pressure, 450
posturing and, 191
vascular supply to, 746
Brainstem, 448, 744
Braxton-Hicks contractions, 980
Breast, 157
Breathing
assessment of, 170-72, 555
in body cavity trauma, 483
in critical life threatening situations, 564-65
in poisoned patient, 811
primary, 454-55
shock and, 312, 560
"belly breathing," 456
diaphragmatic, 750
paradoxical, 220
Breath sounds
abnormal, 186
absence of, 222
auscultation, 245
in cardiac patient, 687
Breech presentations, 988, 989
Brethine (terbutaline), 387, 591
Bretylium tosylate (Bretylol), 372-74, 667, 694, 710, 950

Index **1087**

Bricanyl (terbutaline), 387, 591
Bronchi, 210, 211, 573
Bronchial arteries, 213, 575
Bronchial asthma, 384, 385, 387-89
Bronchial veins, 213, 575
Bronchioles, 211, 573
Bronchiolitis, pediatric, 933-34
Bronchitis, chronic, 585-86
Bronchospasm, 385
 reversible, 387-89
Bronkosol (isoetharine), 590, 803
Brown recluse spider bites, 822-24
Bruits, carotid, 645, 687-88
BSI, xxxi, 168
BTLS, 554
Buckle fractures, 923
Buffer, 292
Bufferin, 833
Buffer system, 300-301
Bundle branch blocks, 682, 1055-59, 1060-61
Bundle of Kent, 682
Burnout (cumulative stress reaction), 112, 116
Burns, 523, 528-38
 assessment of, 539-42
 burn surface area, 535-36, 541
 chemical, 523, 530, 542-43, 548-50
 degree of, 533-34, 541
 electrical, 529-30, 543, 548
 inhalation injury accompanying, 523, 532-33
 local, 548
 management of, 548-51
 minor, 548
 moderate, 548
 pediatric, 923
 radiation injury, 530-32, 543, 550-51
 severe, 548
 shock due to, 297
 special field considerations, 537
 systematic complications of, 536-37
 thermal, 529, 532-33, 539-42, 548
BVM device, 221, 222-23, 280, 946
Bystander, role of, 25

CAD, 62
Cafe coronary, 219, 582
Caffeine, 384
Caisson disease ("bends"), 886, 887-88
Calan (verapamil), 375-76, 645, 659, 693, 710
Calcitonin, 728
Calcium, 292
Calcium channel blockers, 375, 382-83, 712
 toxicity to, 383
Calcium chloride, 383-84, 950
Cancellous bone, 435-36, 503
Cancer, 402
 in elderly, 901
Cannula
 intravenous, 322-23
 nasal, 277-78
Capillaries, 306, 525, 608
 pulmonary, 212-13, 574
Capillary refill, 173
 of cardiac patient, 686
 testing, 313-14
 time for, 104
Capnography, 225
Capsules, 335
Carbohydrates, 389-90, 730-31
Carbon dioxide, 206-7

levels of, 213, 215, 751
 measurement of, 213-14
Carbon dioxide detectors, end-tidal, 225, 245
Carbonic acid, 300-301
Carbonic anhydrase, 301
Carbon monoxide poisoning, 523, 533, 596-97, 819
Carcinoma of colon, 777
Cardiac arrest, 701-4
 epinephrine for, 363
 incidence of, 24-25
 pediatric, 950
 sinus arrest, 636-37
 sodium bicarbonate for, 377
Cardiac conductive system, 1031-32
Cardiac contractile force, 304
Cardiac contusion, 494
Cardiac cycle, 609
Cardiac dysrhythmias. See Dysrhythmias
Cardiac enzymes, 694
Cardiac injury, 480
Cardiac monitoring, 194
Cardiac muscle, 144, 145, 473, 612
Cardiac output, 304-5, 610
 elimination of heat through, 867
 shock and, 308
Cardiac plexus, 610-11
Cardiac resuscitation, 44
Cardiac standstill. See Asystole
Cardiac syncope, 903
Cardinal Positions of Gaze, 750
Cardiogenic shock, 311, 328, 691, 699-701
 dopamine for, 365
Cardiopulmonary arrest, pediatric, 941-51
 airway management, 945-46
 anticipating, 941
 electrical therapy, 951
 medications, 949-51
 rapid assessment, 941-45
 vascular access and fluid therapy, 946-49
 ventilation, 946
Cardiopulmonary resuscitation (CPR), 25
Cardiovascular disease, 184, 402
 defined, 602
 among elderly, 902-3
Cardiovascular emergencies, 601-723
 acute arterial occlusion, 707
 acute pulmonary embolism, 707-8
 aneurysm, 705-7
 assessment of cardiac patient, 683-88
 chief complaints and symptoms, 683-85
 past medical history, 685
 physical examination, 685-87
 atherosclerosis, 688-94
 acute myocardial infarction (MI) and, 690-94
 angina pectoris and, 689-90
 cardiac arrest, 24-25, 363, 377, 636-37, 691, 701-4, 950
 cardiogenic shock, 311, 328, 365, 691, 699-701
 drugs for, 361-84
 adenosine (Adenocard), 374-75
 atropine sulfate, 376-77
 bretylium tosylate (Bretylol), 372-74
 calcium chloride, 383-84
 dobutamine (Dobutrex), 366-67

dopamine (Intropin), 365-66
 epinephrine, 362-63
 furosemide (Lasix), 380-81
 labetalol (Trendate, Normodyne), 368-69
 lidocaine (Xylocaine), 369-71
 morphine sulfate, 378-79
 nifedipine (Procardia, Adalat), 381, 382-83
 nitroglycerin (Nitrostate), 381-82
 nitrous oxide (Nitronox), 379-80
 norepinephrine (Levophed), 363-65
 oxygen, 361-62
 procainamide (Pronestyl), 371-72
 sodium bicarbonate, 377-78
 verapamil (Isoptin, Calan), 375-76
 dysrhythmias. See Dysrhythmias
 hypertensive emergency, 709
 left ventricular failure with pulmonary edema, 694-97
 management of, 709-21
 basic life support, 712
 carotid sinus massage, 717-21
 defibrillation, 715-17, 718
 drug therapy, 710-12
 ECG monitoring, 712-15
 emergency synchronized cardioversion, 717, 719
 precordial thump, 715
 transcutaneous cardiac pacing (TCP), 721, 722
 pediatric, 936-39
 peripheral vascular conditions, noncritical, 708
 right ventricular failure, 697-99
 sudden death, 27-28, 691, 701-4
Cardiovascular system
 aging and, 896
 anaphylaxis and, 798
 anatomy and physiology of, 145, 146, 151, 602-16
 electrolytes' role, 612
 electrophysiology, 612-16
 heart, 603-7
 peripheral circulation, 607-9
Cardioversion, 647, 667
 emergency synchronized, 717, 719
Cardizem (diltiazem), 381, 647, 651
Care
 patient, 79-80
 prolonged, 79-80
 standard of, 44-45
Career mobility, 118
Carina, 211, 573
Carotid arteries, 444, 453
Carotid bruit, 645, 687-88
Carotid sinus massage, 717-21
Carotid system, 746
Carpal bones, 504
Carrier state, 856
Cartilage, 503-4
Cataracts, 898
Catatonic schizophrenia, 1022
Catecholamines, 304, 362, 558, 729
Cathartic, 778
Catheters
 shock/trauma resuscitation and, 566
 suction, 275-76
Catheter shear, 327
Cation, 290, 291-92
Cauda equina, 440
Caudally, defined, 254

Cause, proximate, 44
Cavitation, 426-28
C-cells, 728
Cecum, 772, 773
Cell-mediated immunity, 842
Cell membrane, 143, 144
Cells, anatomy and physiology of, 143-44. See also specific types of cells
Cellular asphyxiant, 818
Cellular immunity, 794
Cellular-level shock, 308-9
Cellular respiration, 212, 575
Cellular telephones, 57-58
Centers for Disease Control (CDC), infection control guidelines, xxx
Central cyanosis, 189, 1007
Central nervous system, 741-47
 anatomy and physiology of, 435-44, 741-47
 brain, 439-40
 circulation in, 442
 neck, 443-44
 protective mechanisms, 435-39
 sense organs, 442-43
 spinal cord, 440-42
 brain, 153, 744-46
 areas of specialization, 745-46
 divisions of, 744-45
 vascular supply, 746
 dysfunctional, 598
 injury to, 447-52
 assessment of, 455, 458-60
 brain injury, 191, 447-50, 764-65
 pathway of deterioration following, 451
 spinal cord injury, 189, 392-93, 430, 450-52, 922
 neuron, 341, 741-42
 protective structures, 435-39, 742-44
 spinal cord, 153, 746-47
Central neurogenic hyperventilation, 186, 750, 751
Centrax, 832
Centruroides exilicauda, 824
Cerebellum, 440, 745
Cerebral cortex, 113, 744
Cerebrospinal fluid (CSF), 435, 439, 744
Cerebrovascular accident (CVA). See Stroke
Cerebrovascular disease in elderly, 904
Cerebrum, 439-40, 744, 745
Certification, 12, 28-29
Cervical collar, 184, 462, 463, 465
Cervical immobilization device (CID), 463-64
Cervical spine, 436, 447
 of elderly, 900
 immobilization of, 460
 injury to, 452
 stabilization of, 560
Cervix, 775, 955, 956
 dilation of, 982
 effacement of, 977, 982
Chancre, 857
Charcoal, activated, 396-97, 810, 813
Cheek, impaled object in, 465
Chemical burns, 523, 530
 assessment of, 542-43
 management of, 548-50
"Chemical code only," 44

Chemical emergencies or spills, 809
Chemical name of drugs, 334
Chemical notation, 290-91
Chemical phlebotomy, 378
Chemoreceptors, 216
Chest
  assessment of, 484, 485-87
  auscultation of, 222, 223, 486-87
  evaluation of, 180, 185-87
  flail, 220, 476, 477, 491-92
  hyperinflated, 478
  palpation of, 486, 487
  percussion of, 487
  topographical anatomy of, 160-61
Chest injuries, 476-81
  pediatric, 922-23
  respirations and, 488
  wounds
    open, 490
    sucking, 430, 490, 491
Chest pain
  cardiac disease and, 683-84
  from dialysis, 789
  left ventricular failure and, 696
Chest (precordial) leads, 618, 1033, 1038-39
Cheyne-Stokes respiration, 750, 751
Chicken pox (varicella), 854
"Chicken with its head cut off" syndrome, 91
Chief complaint, 196-98
Child abuser, 924
Childbirth. See Labor; Neonate(s); Pregnancy
Childhood diseases, 854-55
Children. See also Pediatric emergencies; Pediatric patient(s)
  asthma in, 594
  fears of, 912-13
  mechanisms of injury in, 169
  rule of nines for, 535
  sexual abuse of, 961
  as vehicular accident victims, 420
Chin-lift/head tilt method, 942
Chlamydia, 857-58
Chlamydia trachomatous, 858
Chloride, 292
Chlorpromazine (Thorazine), 1021
"Chokes, the," 888
Cholecystitis, 779, 972
Choline, 347
Cholinergics (parasympathomimetics), 347
Cholinergic synapses, 341, 348
Cholinesterase, 829
Chordae tendonae, 604, 605
Chronic, defined, 780
Chronic hepatitis, 856
Chronic obstructive pulmonary disease (COPD), 384, 392-93, 577, 698
  in elderly, 900, 901
  oxygen therapy for, 581
Chronotropy, 363, 612
Chyme, 474
Cheyne-Stokes pattern, 186-87
CID, 463-64
Ciguatera poisoning, 815
Cilia, 143, 208
Cimetadine (Tagamet), 802
Circle of Willis, 442, 746
Circulation
  assessment of, 171, 555
    in body cavity trauma, 484
    in critical life threatening situ-

ations, 565
  of poisoned patient, 811
  shock and, 561
fetal, 968-69
peripheral, 607-9
physiology of, 609-10
primary assessment of, 455
pulmonary, 212-13
shock assessment and, 312-14
Circulatory overload, 327
Circulatory system
  anatomy and physiology of, 152, 773
  components of, 305
  perfusion and, 304-6
Circumferential burns, 536-37
Circumflex artery, 607
Citizens, stress from angry or confused, 117
Citric acid (Krebs) cycle, 309
Civil law, 41
Claudication, 689
  intermittent, 708
Clavicle, 504
  evaluation of, 180, 185
Clean radiation accident, 882
Clonic movements, 760
Closed fracture, 508
Closed pneumothorax, 478
Clostridium botulinum, 815
Clostridium tetani, 841
Clotting, dialysis and, 790
Clubbing, 189
CO2 detectors, end-tidal, 225, 245
Coats, turnout, 72
COBRA, 21
Cocaine, 831
Coccygeal vertebra, 744
Coccyx, 437
Cochlea, 443
Codeine, 831
Code of Ethics, 7, 8
Codes, radio, 63, 106
Cold, extremes of, 194
Colitis, ischemic, 907
Collar, cervical, 184, 462, 463, 465
Collateral circulation, 607
Collateral ganglia, 341, 343
Colle's fracture, 512
Collisions, types of, 408-10. See also Blunt trauma
Colloid osmotic pressure, 297
Colloids, 297-98, 320-22, 728
Colon, 772, 773
  carcinoma of, 777
  tumors of, 906
Color
  neonatal, 1007
  of skin, 172, 176, 686
Coma, 190, 755
  diabetic (diabetic ketoacidosis), 732-33, 735, 736
  drugs for managing, 389-90
  naloxone for, 397
  nonketotic hyperosmolar, 732
"Coma cocktail," 814
Command, transfer of, 91, 96
Comminuted fractures, 445
Communication(s), 25-26, 27, 32, 51-67
  of assessment, 200-202
  base station, 54-55
  encoders and decoders, 56-57
  equipment maintenance, 61
  hardware, 26
  in ICS, 105-6
  links, 52-54
  medical control, 23
  of medical information, 64-66

mobile telephones, 57-58
  order of events and, 53
  radios, 55, 58-61
  remote consoles, 56, 57
  repeater systems, 55-56
  rules and operating procedures, 61-64
  satellite receivers, 56, 57
  software, 26
Compartment syndrome, 514
Compensated shock, 309-10, 557-58
Compensatory mechanisms, 308, 309
Compensatory pause, 653
Complaint, chief, 196-98
Compliance, 222-23
Computer-aided dispatch (CAD), 62
Concentration
  of drug, 350
  minimum effective, 339
Conception, 968
Conchae, 207, 208
Concussion, 448
Condensation in endotracheal tube, 246
Conduction, heat loss through, 865, 866, 998
Conduction disorders, 629, 674-83, 1051-59
  atrioventricular (AV) blocks, 675-81, 1051-55
    first-degree, 675
    second-degree, 676-79
    third-degree, 680-81
  bundle branch blocks, 682, 1055-59, 1060-61
  disturbances of ventricular conduction, 682
  pre-excitation syndromes, 682-83
Conductive fibers, 614, 1031
Confined-space rescues, 78
Congenital heart disease, pediatric, 938-39
Congestion, pulmonary, 695
Congestive heart failure, 380-81, 385, 691
  dobutamine for, 367
  in elderly, 902
Conjunctiva, 442
Conjunctival hemorrhage, 452
Connective tissue, 144
Consciousness
  continuum of, 190
  left ventricular failure and, 696
  loss of, 760
  shock assessment and, 314
Consent, 45-46
Conservation of Energy, Law of, 406, 425
Consoles, remote, 56, 57
Consolidated Omnibus Budget Reconciliation Act (COBRA) of 1981, 21
Constrict, defined, 182
Continuing education, 13, 28
Contraceptives, 958
Contractions, Braxton-Hicks, 980
Contraindications, defined, 336
Contralateral, defined, 184
Contrecoup injury, 448
Controlled Substances Act of 1970, 333-34
Contusion(s), 174, 448-49, 506-7, 525-26
  bandaging of, 545
  cardiac, 494

myocardial, 414, 480
  pulmonary, 476
Convection, heat loss through, 865, 866, 998
COPD. See Chronic obstructive pulmonary disease (COPD)
Coral snake, 826, 827-28
Core temperature, 864
Cornea, 442-43
Coronary arteries, 151, 607
Coronary sinus, 607
Coronary veins, 607
Cor pulmonale, 583
Corpus callosum, 744
Corticosteroids, 392-93, 802
Costovertebral angle (CVA), 161
Coughing, 216
Coup injury, 448
Coveralls, 71-72
Crack, 831
Cramps, heat (muscle), 507, 867-69, 872
Cranial cavity, 741
Cranial nerves, 443, 747, 748
Cranial vault, 162
Cranium, 162, 435-36
  evaluation of, 178-82
  penetrating injuries to, 430
Crepitation, 176
Cribriform plate, 440
Cricoid cartilage, 207, 209
Cricothyroid membrane, 209, 270, 271, 272
Cricothyrotomy, 270-71, 274
Criminal abortion, 974
Criminal law, 41
Critical/immediate patients, 103
Critical incidents, 113
Critical-incident stress, 12, 113, 119-20
Cromolyn sodium (Intal), 803
Croup (laryngotracheobronchitis), 386, 931-32
  endotracheal intubation for, 257
Crowing (stridor), 172, 186, 222, 578
Crowning, 971
Crushing wound, 528
Crush injury, hemorrhage control in, 544-45
Crystalloids, 298-99, 320
CSF, 435, 439, 744
Cullen's sign, 187
Cumulative action, defined, 336
Cumulative stress reaction (burnout), 112, 116
Current of injury (injury current), 1044
Curved (MacIntosh) blade, 237-38, 239
Cushing's disease, 730
Cushing's Reflex, 450, 451, 752
Customer satisfaction, 33
CVA. See Stroke
Cyanide poisoning, 818-19, 829
Cyanosis, 176, 222, 577
  central, 189, 1007
  left ventricular failure and, 695
  pediatric, 938-39
Cyanotic spells, 938-39
Cyclopeptide group, 816
Cyst, ovarian, 781-82
Cystic duct, 773
Cystic medial necrosis, 706
Cystitis (bladder infection), 780, 960
Cysts, ovarian, 960
Cytoplasm, 144
Cytosol, 143

D50W (50% dextrose in water), 299, 389-90

Dalmane, 832
Dane particle, 855
Darvocet, 831
Darvon, 831
Dead/non-salvageable patients, 103
Dead space volume, 217
Death
   stress management and, 120-21
   sudden, 27-28, 691, 701-4
Debriefing, 119, 120
Decadron (dexamethasone), 759, 802
Deceleration, 407
Decerebrate posturing, 191, 753
Decoders, 56-57
Decompensated shock, 310, 557, 558-59
Decompression sickness, 887-89
Decontamination, 810, 849-50
Decorticate posturing, 191, 753
Deep frostbite, 876
Deep venous thrombosis, 708
Defective virus, 856
Defense mechanisms, 116, 121
Defense wounds, 428
Defibrillation, 715-17, 718
   by bystander, 25
   negligence in, 45
Defibrillator paddles, 712-14
Definitive patient care rescue operations, 79
Degloving injury, 527-28
Degranulation, 797
Dehydration, 289, 297
   pediatric, 935, 936
Deinstitutionalization, 1014
Delayed hypersensitivity, 796
Delayed stress reactions, 114-15
DeLee suction trap, 998
Delegation of authority, 41
Delirium, 905
Delirium tremens (DTs), 390, 836
Deliveries, 981-82
   abnormal presentations, 988-89
   cephalopelvic disproportion, 987
   maternal complications of, 991-92
   multiple births, 989-91
   normal, 984-86
   precipitous, 991
   prolapsed cord, 971, 989, 990
   shoulder dystocia, 991
   unscheduled field delivery, 983-87
Delta (∂) cells, 729
Delta hepatitis, 856
Delta wave, 682, 683
Delusions, 1022
Demand pacemakers, 672
Demand valve resuscitator (manually triggered oxygen-powered breathing device), 280-81
Dementia, 905, 909, 1016
Denial stage of grief, 120
Depolarization, 613-14
Depolarization impulse, 628
Depolarizing drugs, 260
Depressant, defined, 336
   depressant drugs, 217
Depressed fractures, 445, 462
Depression, 1019, 1020
   from narcotics, 397
   as stage of grief, 121
Dermatomes, 440-42, 747
Dermis, 524

Detrimental anxiety levels, 116-17
Development
   child, 913-17
   fetal, 968
Dexamethasone (Decadron, Hexadrol), 759, 802
Dexedrine, 831
Dextran, 298
Dextrose, 730-31, 757, 758
Dextrose in water (D50W), 299, 389-90
Dextrostix, 195
Diabetes, gestational, 972
Diabetes mellitus, 730-32, 978
Diabetic ketoacidosis (diabetic coma), 732-33, 735, 736
Dialysate, 787-88
Dialysis, 787-90
   complications of, 788-90
   management of patient on, 790
   types of, 787-88
Diaphoresis, 289, 695
Diaphragm, 471
   rupture of, 481
Diaphragmatic breathing, 750
Diaphysis, 501
Diarrhea
   melanotic, 778
   pediatric, 935
Diastole, 609, 610
Diazepam (Valium), 338, 353, 391-92, 466-67, 693, 711, 764, 832, 928
Dictation, 48
Dictionary, medical, 125
Diencephalon, 744
Diffusion, 214, 292-94
   facilitated, 731
Digestive system, anatomy and physiology of, 156
Digital intubation, 248-51, 461
Digitalis (Digoxin, Lanoxin), 649, 712
Digitalis toxicity, 373
Dilate, defined, 182
Dilation of cervix, 982
Dilemma, moral, 8-9
Diltiazem (Cardizem), 381, 647, 651
Dinoflagellate, 815
Diphenhydramine (Benadryl), 297, 395, 801-2, 814
Director, medical, 22
Direct pressure to control hemorrhage, 544
Dirty radiation accident, 882-83
Disability assessment, 173, 455-56, 555
   in body cavity trauma, 484
   shock and, 562
Disaster/catastrophic incident, 90
Discolorations, ecchymotic, 187
Discs, 437-38
   intercalated, 612, 613
Diseases, infectious. See Infectious diseases
Disentanglement, 80-81
Disequilibrium syndrome, from dialysis, 789
Dislocation(s), 507-8, 512-13
   of hip, 510, 518
   of knee, 511, 518
   near joint, 510
   on-scene care of, 516-19
   partial, 507
   shoulder, 512
Disorganization, 1022
Dispatch, computer-aided (CAD), 62

Dispatch information, 167
Dispatching, 26-28, 61-62, 167
   rules and operating procedures for, 61-63
   training for, 27
Dissecting aortic aneurysm, 706
Dissociative reactions, 291
Distress signals, 114, 115
Distribution of drug, 337-38
Diuresis, osmotic, 732
Diuretics, 303, 380-81
Diverticula, 777
Diverticulitis, 777
Diverticulosis, 777, 906
Diving emergencies, 423, 884-90
   assessment of, 886-87
   common injuries, 885-86
   pressure disorders (barotrauma), 88-90, 885-86, 887-90
Diving reflex, mammalian, 879
Dizziness among elderly, 904
DNA, 144
Dobutamine (dobutrex), 328, 366-67, 697, 711
Dobutamine hydrochloride, 950, 951
Documentation, 11-12, 48
   of assessment, 200-202
   post-call, 66
Doll's eye response, 183
Domestic violence, 1029
Donor, universal, 296
"Do not resuscitate" (DNR) orders, 42-44
Dopamine hydrochloride, 328, 365-66, 699, 711, 950, 951, 1010
Dopamine (Intropin), 328, 365-66, 699, 711, 1010
Dopaminergic receptors, 345
Doppler, ultrasonic, 192, 193
Dorsalis pedis pulse, 181, 188
Down-and-under pathway of injury, 412, 413
Doxepin, 833
Drowning and near-drowning, 877-80
Drug(s), 332-99. See also Medication(s); Pharmacology; *specific drugs*
   actions of, 337-40
   administration of, 348-60
     enteral routes for, 335, 360
     parenteral routes for, 335, 352-59
     precautions, 360
     weights and measures, 348-52
   anti-inflammatory, 392-93, 777
   for behavioral emergencies, 398
   for cardiovascular emergencies, 361-84, 710-12
     adenosine (Adenocard), 374-75
     atropine sulfate, 376-77
     bretylium tosylate (Bretylol), 372-74
     calcium chloride, 383-84
     dobutamine (Dobutrex), 366-67
     dopamine (Intropin), 365-66
     epinephrine, 362-63
     furosemide (Lasix), 380-81
     labetalol (Trendate, Normodyne), 368-69
     lidocaine (Xylocaine), 369-71
     morphine sulfate, 378-79
     nifedipine (Procardia, Adalat), 381, 382-83

     nitroglycerin (Nitrostate), 381-82
     nitrous oxide (Nitronox), 379-80
     norepinephrine (Levophed), 363-65
     oxygen, 361-62
     procainamide (Pronestyl), 371-72
     sodium bicarbonate, 377-78
     verapamil (Isoptin, Calan), 375-76
   chronotropic agents, 612
   defined, 332
   depolarizing, 260
   for elderly, 908
   for endocrine and metabolic emergencies, 389-91
     D50W (50% dextrose in water), 389-90
     glucagon, 390-91
     thiamine, 390
   forms of, 334-35
   for head, neck, and spinal trauma, 466-67
   for hypertensive emergencies, 709
   for ingested poisons, 813-14
   inotropic agents, 612
   laws on, 333-34
   for myocardial infarction, 693-94
   names of, 334
   for neurological emergencies, 391-93
     diazepam (Vallium), 391-92
     methylprednisolone (Solu-Medrol), 392-93
   neuromuscular blocking, 259-61
   non-depolarizing, 260
   for obstetrical and gynecological emergencies, 393-94
     magnesium sulfate, 394
     oxytocin (Pitocin), 393-94
   references, 334
   for respiratory emergencies, 384-89
     albuterol (Proventil, Ventolin), 387-88
     aminophylline (Somophyllin), 384, 385-86
     epinephrine, 384-85
     ipratropium (Atrovent), 388-89
     racemic epinephrine (microNEFRIN, Vaponefrin), 386-87
     terbutaline (Brethine, Bricanyl), 387
   sources of, 322
   terminology, 335-36
   for toxicological emergencies, 394-98
     activated charcoal, 396-97
     diphenhydramine (Benadryl), 395
     naloxone (Narcan), 397-98
     syrup of ipecac, 395-96
Drug abuse
   altered behavior and, 1015
   overdose, 830, 831-33
     esophageal obturator airways and, 234
Drug Inserts, 334
Drug receptors, 339
Dry drowning, 878
"Dry mouth" syndrome, 834
DTs, 390, 836
Ductus arteriosus, 969, 997
Ductus venosus, 969

Due date, 968
Duodenum, 474, 773
Duplex transmissions, 60-61
Durable power of attorney for
health care, 42
Dural sinuses, 442
Dura mater, 438, 744
Duties of paramedic, 107-9
Duty to act, 44
Dysconjugate gaze, 183, 756
Dyspnea, 575
cardiac disease and, 684
paroxysmal nocturnal (PND),
197, 695
Dysrhythmias, 314, 328, 480, 627-83
cardiac arrest and, 701
causes of, 627
classification of, 628-29
conduction disorders, 629, 674-
83, 1051-59
atrioventricular (AV) blocks,
675-81, 1051-55
bundle branch blocks, 682,
1055-59, 1060-61
disturbances of ventricular
conduction, 682
pre-excitation syndromes,
682-83
defined, 627
from dialysis, 789
in elderly, 902
as MI complication, 691, 692
originating in atria, 628, 638-51
atrial fibrillation, 648-51
atrial flutter, 646-47
paroxysmal supraventricular
tachycardia (PSVT), 642-45,
658
premature atrial contractions
(PAC), 640-41
wandering pacemaker, 638-39
originating in AV junction, 629,
652-59
junctional rhythm, 654-57
paroxysmal junctional tachycardia (PJT), 658-59
premature junctional contractions (PJCs), 652, 653
originating in SA node, 628,
630-37
sinus arrest, 636-37
sinus bradycardia, 630, 631
sinus dysrhythmia, 634-35
sinus tachycardia, 632-33
originating in ventricles, 629,
660-73
artificial pacemaker rhythm,
672-73
asystole (cardiac standstill),
670-71
premature ventricular contraction (PVC), 662-63
ventricular escape complexes
and rhythms (idioventricular rhythm), 660, 661
ventricular fibrillation, 668-69
ventricular tachycardia, 664-67
pediatric, 937-38, 939
syncope caused by, 903
Dystocia, shoulder, 991
Dystonic (extrapyramidal) reactions, 395, 814

Ears, 443
anatomy and physiology of, 147
evaluation of, 182
injury to, 453
Ecchymosis, 176, 526
bilateral periorbital, 182, 445-46

Ecchymotic discolorations, 187
ECF, 288
ECG monitoring, 54, 616-27, 1031
cardiac conductive system
anatomy and, 615
cardiac depolarization and, 613
in cardiovascular emergencies,
712-15
of dysrhythmias
accelerated junctional rhythm,
656, 658
artificial pacemaker rhythm,
672, 673
asystole, 670, 671
atrial fibrillation, 648, 649
atrial flutter, 646, 647
AV blocks, 674-81
idioventricular rhythm, 660,
661
junctional escape complex
and rhythm, 654, 655
originating in atria, 639
originating in AV junction,
653
originating in SA node, 631
originating in ventricles, 661
paroxysmal junctional tachycardia, 658, 659
paroxysmal supraventricular
tachycardia, 642, 643
premature atrial contractions,
640, 641
premature junctional contractions, 652, 653
premature ventricular contractions, 662, 663
sinus arrest, 636, 677
sinus bradycardia, 630, 632
sinus dysrhythmia, 634, 635
sinus tachycardia, 632, 633
ventricular conduction disturbances, 682
ventricular fibrillation, 668,
669
ventricular tachycardia, 664,
665
wandering pacemaker, 638,
639
ECG graph paper, 619
electrical events in heart, 619-25
electrode leads, 616-18, 712,
1033-39
normal sinus rhythm, 627
rhythm strips interpretation,
625-27
routine, 618
12 lead, 1031-66
axis deviation, 1039-42
conduction abnormalities,
1051-59
disease findings, 1044-51
leads, 1033-39
mean QRS axis determination,
1039
normal, 1042-44
prehospital, 1059-65
recording, 1032-33
"Echo" procedure, 64
Eclampsia, 394, 978, 979
Ectopic beats, 628
Ectopic pregnancy, 782, 960, 975
EDC, 968
Edema, 174
laryngeal, 532-3, 596
overhydration and, 289
peripheral, 687
right heart failure and, 698
pitting, 189
presacral, 187, 687

pulmonary, 378, 381, 385, 696-
97
in elderly, 901
left ventricular failure with,
694-97
PASG and, 565
Education
continuing, 13, 28
in EMS, 28-29
original, 28
of public, 24-25
Effacement of cervix, 977, 982
Efferent fibers, 746-47
Effusion, 186
EGTA, 236
Einthoven's Triangle, 617, 1035,
1037
Ejection, injury from, 414, 420
Elapidae, 826, 827-28
Elavil, 833
Elbow injury, 516
fracture, 512
splinting, 518
Elderly, 893-909
abuse/neglect of, 909
assessment of, 897-99
behavioral emergencies in, 1023
burns on, 537, 542
cardiovascular disease in, 902-3
defined, 894
drug therapy for, 908
environmental emergencies
among, 907-8
fractures in, 509-10
gastrointestinal emergencies
among, 906-7
musculoskeletal injuries in, 515
neurological emergencies in,
903-5
psychiatric disorders in, 905-6
respiratory emergencies in, 900-
901
trauma in, 899-900
Elective abortion, 974
Electrical burns, 529-30
assessment of, 543
management of, 548
Electrical therapy
for atrial fibrillation, 651
for atrial flutter, 646
for paroxysmal junctional tachycardia, 659
for pediatric cardiopulmonary
arrest, 951
for PSVT, 645
Electrocardiogram. See ECG monitoring
Electrolyte abnormalities, pediatric,
935
Electrolytes, 287, 289-92, 394, 612
Electrons, 290, 291, 880
Electrophysiology, 612-16
cardiac conductive system, 614-
16
cardiac depolarization, 613-14
Elevation to control hemorrhage,
544
Elimination of drugs, 338
Elixirs, 335
Emboli, 184, 763-64
mural, 707
transient ischemic attacks and,
765-66
Embolism
air, 327, 886, 890
from dialysis, 789-90
pulmonary, 215, 597, 698
acute, 707-8
in elderly, 901

after pregnancy, 992
Emergency department, arrival at,
201
Emergency medical dispatch
(EMD) systems, 167. See
also Dispatching
Emergency Medical Services (EMS)
systems, 4, 17-37
communications network, 25-26,
27, 32
components of, 18-20
defined, 18
demonstration projects, 20
design of, 36
dispatching, 26-28
education and certification, 28-
29
financing of, 21, 36
history of, 20-21
medical control, 21, 22-24
direct, 22-23
indirect, 22, 23-24
mutual aid/mass casualty preparation, 36
patient transportation, 29-32
aeromedical, 31-32
ambulances, 29-31
public information and education, 24-25
Quality Assurance (QA) and
Quality Improvement (QI)
programs, 32-33
receiving facilities, 34-35
research, 34
system administration, 21-22
tiered response of, 19
Emergency Medical Services
Systems Act (1973), 20-21
Emergency medical technician
(EMT), 5, 6, 19
levels of, 28-29
Emergency operations center
(EOC), 90
Emergency (TV series), 6
Emesis, 183
Emetic agents, 395-96
Emphysema, 583-85, 586
subcutaneous, 184, 185
EMT Oath, 7
Emulsions, 335
Encephalopathy, AIDS, 859
Encoders, 56-57
End-diastolic volume (preload),
304, 557, 609
Endobronchial intubation, 246-47
Endocardium, 473, 603, 604
Endocrine emergencies, 730-36
diabetes mellitus, 730-32, 978
iabetic ketoacidosis (diabetic
coma), 732-33, 735, 736
drugs for, 389-91
D50W (50% dextrose in
water), 389-90
glucagon, 390-91
thiamine, 390
hypoglycemia (insulin shock),
234, 391, 733-36
Endocrine glands, 389, 726
Endocrine system, 113
anatomy and physiology of,
146, 726-30
Endometritis, 960
Endometrium, 956
End-organ perfusion, 944
Endotoxins, 841
Endotracheal drug administration,
352-53, 358
Endotracheal intubation, 232, 236-
64

Endotracheal intubation *(con't)*
  in children, 256-59
  digital intubation, 248-51
  with EOA in place, 247-48
  equipment, 236-40
  for head, neck, and spinal trauma, 461
  indications, advantages, and disadvantages, 240-41
  insertion
    nasotracheal route, 254, 261-64
    orotracheal route, 242-45, 254
  in neonate, 1006
  precautions, 241-42
  rapid sequence intubation with neuromuscular blockade, 259-61
  of shock patient, 316
  of thermal burn patient, 540
  transillumination (lighted stylet) intubation, 251-54
  in trauma patient, 254-55
  verification of tube placement, 245-47
End-tidal carbon dioxide (ETCO2) detectors, 225, 245
Energy, 406
  dissipation of, 426
Enhanced 9-1-1 (E-911), 25-26
Environment, defined, 864
Environmental emergencies, 863-91
  diving emergencies, 423, 884-90
    assessment of, 886-87
    common injuries, 885-86
    pressure disorders (barotrauma), 88-90, 885-86, 887-90
  among elderly, 907-8
  near-drowning and drowning, 877-80
  nuclear radiation, 880-84
    dose-effect relationship to, 881, 882
    prehospital management of, 883-84
    safety principles in, 881
  thermal disorders, 867-77
    fever (pyrexia), 217, 871, 914
    frostbite, 876-77
    hyperpyrexia, 871
    hyperthermia, 867-71
    hypothermia, 867, 871-76
Environmental extremes, body temperature, 193-94
Environmental Protection Agency (EPA), 83
Enzymes, 474
  cardiac, 694
EOA, 232-36, 247-48
EOC, 90
Epicardium, 603, 604
Epidermis, 523
Epididymis, 775, 776
Epididymitis, 782
Epidural hematoma, 449-50
Epidural space, 744
Epigastrium, 771
Epiglottis, 207, 208
Epiglottitis
  endotracheal intubation for, 241, 257
  pediatric, 931, 932-33
Epilepsy, idiopathic, 760
Epinephrine
  administration of, 353
  from adrenal glands, 729
  for anaphylaxis, 800-801
  biotransformation of, 338

cardiac contractile strength and, 304
  for cardiovascular disease, 693
  for cardiovascular emergencies, 362-63, 710
  heat generation and, 867
  for pediatric asystolic or pulseless arrest, 950
  for pediatric bradycardia, 950
  pharmacodynamics of, 339
  preparation of infusions, 951
  release of, 343-44, 558
  for respiratory emergencies, 384-85, 589
  to resuscitate neonates, 1010
  stress and, 113
  for toxicological emergencies, 395
  for ventricular fibrillation, 669
Epiphysis, 501, 503
Epithelial tissue, 144
EPS, 1023
Equipment
  for patient safety, 72-73
  for personal safety, 70-72
  for removal, 81
  standard set of, 29
  for suctioning, 275-76
Erythema, 176, 526
Erythrocytes (red blood cells), 294-95, 296, 310, 530, 556
Eschar, 536-37, 542
Eskolith (lithium), 1021, 1022
Esophageal detectors, 245-46
Esophageal gastric tube airway (EGTA), 236
Esophageal injury, 481
Esophageal intubation, 246
Esophageal obturator airways (EOA), 232-36
  endotracheal intubation with, 247-48
Esophageal Tracheal CombiTube (ETC) airway, 267-69
Esophageal varices, 776-77, 906
Esophagus, 207, 209, 444, 472, 772, 773
Estimated date of confinement (EDC), 968
Estrogen, 730, 957, 966
Ethics, 6-9
Ethmoid bone, 742, 743
Ethylene glycol poisoning, 816-17, 836
Eustachian tube, 208
Evaporation, heat loss through, 865, 866, 998
Events, order of, 52-53
Evidence, rules of, 33
Evisceration, 481
Excedrin, 833
Excursion, 185, 476
Exhaustion, heat, 867-68, 869, 872
Exhaustion, stage of stress response, 113
Exotoxins, 841
Expiration, 212, 215, 472
Exposure control plan, xxxi
Exposure of injury, 173-74, 456, 555
  shock and, 562
Expressed consent, 45
Extension, 506
Extracellular compartment, 288
Extracellular fluid (ECF), 288
Extraocular movements, 756
Extrapyramidal (dystonic) reactions, 395, 814
Extrapyramidal system (EPS), 1023

Extravasation, 325, 327
Extremity injuries
  pediatric, 923
    penetrating injury, 430
    splinting of, 516-19
Extremity long bones, 501-3
Extrication, 81
  of potential spinal injury patient, 462
Extrication sector, 97-98
Eye injuries, 452-53
  management of, 465-66
Eyes, 442-43
  anatomy and physiology of, 147
  assessment of, 457
  evaluation of, 179, 182
  of poisoned patient, 811
  protection for, xxxi, 71, 72
  raccoon, 446
  shock symptoms manifested in, 558

Face mask for oxygenation, 278
Facial bones, 435, 442
Facial region, evaluation of, 179, 182-83
Facial trauma, 447
  airway and, 454
  nosebleeds and, 465
  pediatric, 922
  penetrating, 429-30
Facilitated diffusion, 293, 294, 731
Failsafe franchise, 36
Fallopian tubes (uterine tubes), 775, 954, 955
Falls, 422-23
  as mechanisms of injury, 169
False imprisonment, 46
False labor, 980
False vocal cords, 209
Falx cerebri, 439
Family of dead patient, 121
Fascicles, anterior and posterior, 615-16
Fasciculations, 260
Fears of children, 912-13
Febrile seizures, 927-28
Fecal-oral route of disease transmission, 843
Federal Communications Commission (FCC), 58, 59, 60
Federal Emergency Management Agency (FEMA), 84
Federal Food, Drug, and Cosmetic Act of 1938, 333
"Feed-or-breed" ("rest-and-repose") system, 340, 747
Feet. *See* Foot/feet
Femur, 504-5
  fractures of, 511, 518
Fertilization, 966, 967
Fetal circulation, 968-69
Fetal development, 968
Fetal heart tones (FHTs), 968
Fever (pyrexia), 217, 871, 914
Fibrillation
  atrial, 648-51, 901
  ventricular, 373, 701-2
    duration of, 716
    primary and secondary, 701
    refractory, 370-71
Fibrosis, 896
Fibula, 505
Fick Principle, 307
Fiddleback spider, 822-24
"Fight-or-flight" system, 113, 340, 747
Financing of EMS, 21, 36

Fire departments, 5
First-degree burns, 533-34, 541
First responder, 19
Fixed-rate pacemakers, 672
Flaccidity, 458
Flagg blade, 237-38, 239
Flail chest, 220, 476, 477, 491-92
Flank, 161, 771
Flexion, 506
Fluids, body, 287-99
  hydration, 288-89
  osmosis and diffusion, 292-94
  water, 287-89
Fluid therapy. *See also* Intravenous (IV) therapy
  for anaphylaxis, 799-800
  for distressed neonate, 1009
  for ingested poisons, 813-14
  for pediatric cardiopulmonary arrest, 946-49
  for shock/trauma, 566-67
Flumazenil (Romazicon), 392
FM, 58
Focal motor seizures, 761
Follicle-stimulating hormone (FSH), 727, 728, 954, 957
Fontanelles, 919
Foodborne diseases, 843
Food poisoning, 815, 855
Foot/feet, 148
  burns involving, 541
  fractures of, 511-12
Foramen magnum, 440, 746
Foramen ovale, 969
Foramina, 445
Force, 407
Forceps, Magill, 183, 240, 263
Forearm fracture, 512
Foreign body
  airway obstruction from, 219
  aspirated, 930-31
  removal under direct laryngoscopy, 264
Formed elements of blood, 294-95
Fossa, 504
Fractionation, 296
Fracture(s), 508-10
  aligning, 517
  bend, 923
  blowout, 453
  buckle, 923
  closed, 508
  depressed, 445, 462
  effects of, 512-13
  of elbow, 512
  of facial bones, 447
  of femur, 511, 518
  of foot/ankle, 511-12
  of forearm, 512
  in geriatric patient, 509-10
  greenstick, 508, 509, 923
  hairline, 509
  of hand, 512
  in head and neck areas, 445-47
  of hip, 518
  of humerus, 512, 518
  impacted, 508, 509
  of knee, 511, 518
  long bone, 510
  lower-leg, 511
  near joint, 510
  on-scene care of, 516-19
  open, 508
  pelvic, 510-11, 517
  prioritizing care of, 516
  of rib, 430, 476
  skull, 462
  spinal, 447, 450
  stabilization of, 319

wrist, 512
Frank-Starling mechanism, 304
"Freelancing," 91
Freon poisoning, 819-20
Frequencies, radio, 58-59
Frequency modulation (FM), 58
Fresh frozen plasma, 296
Fresh-water drowning, 878
Friction rub, 579
Frontal bone, 742, 743
Frontal (head-on) impact, 412-14, 420
Frostbite, 876-77
FSH, 727, 728, 954, 957
Full-thickness burns (third-degree burns), 534, 541
Functional reserve capacity (FRC), 217
Fundal height, 971
Fundus, 775, 956
Funeral homes, 5
Fungi, infection from, 842
Furosemide (Lasix), 297, 380-81, 466, 697, 711

Gag reflex, 208, 229, 232
Galerina, 816
Gall bladder, 474-75, 773, 779
Gamma radiation, 531, 881
Ganglia
    autonomic, 340-41
    collateral, 343
    parasympathetic, 345-46
    sympathetic, 341-43
Gas exchange in lungs, 213-15, 218
Gastric distention, 281
Gastritis, 777, 906
Gastroenteritis, 855, 935
Gastrointestinal emergencies, 776-79
    in children, 919
    in elderly, 906-7
    hemorrhage, 778-79, 906-7
    pediatric, 935
    water loss, 289
Gastrointestinal system
    aging and, 896
    anaphylaxis and, 798
    anatomy and physiology of, 145, 772-73
    infections of, 855-57
    shock and, 308
Gaze
    Cardinal Positions of, 750
    dysconjugate, 183, 756
Geiger counter, 881
Generalized seizures, 760
Generic name of drugs, 334
Genitalia, 474
    evaluation of, 188
    injury to, 482
Genitourinary system
    anatomy and physiology of, 146, 774
    emergencies of, 779-81
Geriatric patient. *See* Elderly
Geriatrics, 894
Gestational diabetes, 972
GH, 727, 728
Gin, 831
Gland(s)
    adrenal, 727, 729-30
    endocrine, 389, 726
    parathyroid, 727, 728
    pituitary, 726-28, 745
    sebaceous, 524
    thyroid, 727, 728
Glasgow Coma Scale, 174, 175,

191, 458, 459, 753-54
Glaucoma, 898
Glenoid depression, 504
Glossary, 1067-84
Glottic opening, 209
Glottis, 269
Gloves, protective, xxxi, 71
Glucagon, 390-91, 729
Glucocorticoids, 729-30
Glucometer, 195
Gluconeogenesis, 729
Glucose
    in blood, 733, 734
    metabolism of, 730-32
Glycolysis, 309
Golden Hour, 174, 404, 559
Gonads, 727, 730
Gonorrhea, 857-58
Good Samaritan laws, 41
Gowns, protective, xxxi
Grains, 349
Gram (G), 348
Gram stain, 841
Grand mal seizure, 760
Grand multipara, 991
Granules, 797
Granulocytes, 797
Graves' disease, 728
Gravidity, 958
"Great Imitator," 888
Great vessels, 606
Greenstick fractures, 508, 509, 923
Grey Turner's sign, 187
Grief process, 120-21
Group discussions, 119, 120
    critical incident stresses and, 119-20
    daily routines for, 119
    death and dying, 120-21
Growth hormone (GH), 727, 728
Grunting, 217
Guarding, 770
Gums, 208
Gunshot wound, 407
Gurgling, airflow compromise and, 222
Gynecological emergencies, 959-63
    assessment of, 957-58
    drugs for, 393-94
    medical, 959-60
    traumatic, 960-62
Gynecology, 954

Habituation, defined, 336
Haemophilus influenza, 851, 854, 929, 932
Hairline fracture, 509
Halcion, 832
Half-life, 880
Hallucinations, 1022
Hallucinogens, 832
Haloperidol (Haldol), 398, 1021
Hand, 148
Hands, 148
    burns involving, 541
    fractures of, 512
    splinting, 516-17
Hand-washing, 848
Harrison Narcotic Act of 1914, 333
Haversian canals, 503
Hazardous materials, 82
Hazardous-materials suits, 72
Hazards
    identifying potential, 168
    scene, 75-76
Hazard zone, 97
Head, neck, and spinal trauma, 444-67
    assessment of, 453-60

primary, 454-56
secondary, 456-60
internal CNS injury, 447-52
    brain injury, 447-50
    pathway of deterioration following, 451
    spinal cord injury, 450-52
management of, 460-67
    drug therapy, 466-67
    endotracheal intubation, 461
    hemorrhage control/shock care, 461
    oxygen and hyperventilation, 460-61
    spinal immobilization, 460, 461-64
    wound care, 464-66
neck injury, 453
pediatric, 922
penetrating, 429-30
respiratory evaluation and, 454
sense organ injury, 452-53
superficial injury, 444-47
Head-on (frontal) impact, 412-14, 420
Head region, sense organs in, 442-43
Head-tilt/chin-lift maneuver, 226, 227
Head-to-toe evaluation, 178-91.
    See also specific injuries and disorders
    abdomen, 180, 187
    analysis of, 189
    chest, 180, 185-87
    facial region, 179, 182-83
    genitalia, 188
    head, 178-82
    lower extremities, 181, 188-89
    neck, 180, 184
    neurological assessment, 189-91, 750-52
    pelvis, 181, 187-88
    posterior body, 181, 189
    upper extremities, 181, 189
Hearing, 443
    diminished, 898
    protection of, 71, 72
Heart, 151, 556, 557, 603-7
    anatomy and physiology of, 472-73
    blood flow through, 605
    chambers of, 604, 605
    electrical energy of, 1039
    location within chest, 603
    nervous control of, 610-12
    perfusion and, 304-6
    tissue layers of, 603-4
    valves of, 604-6
    vessels of, 606-7
Heart disease
    atherosclerotic (ASHD), 690
    pediatric, 938-39
    pregnancy and, 972
Heart failure, congestive, 380-81, 385, 691, 902
    dobutamine for, 367
Heart rate, 612
    analysis of, 626
    neonatal, 1007
    pediatric, 943
Heart rate calculator rulers, 626
Heart sounds in cardiac patient, 687
Heat. *See also* Thermal disorders
    extremes of, 193-94
    generation and loss of, 864-65
    in neonate, 998-99
Heat-controlling mechanisms, 865-67

Heat exhaustion, 867-68, 869, 872
Heat (muscle) cramps, 507, 867-69, 872
Heat stroke, 867-68, 870-71, 872
Helicopter transport, 31, 567-69
Helmets, 71, 72
Helper proteins, 294
Hematemesis, 778
Hematocrit, 195, 295
Hematoma, 526
    epidural, 449-50
    from intravenous therapy, 325
    subdural, 449
Hematuria, 780
Hemodialysis, 787
Hemodilution, 878
Hemoglobin, 195, 214, 294, 307
Hemoptysis, 575
Hemorrhage, 764-65. *See also* Bleeding
    assessment of, 538
    bandaging to control, 544-45
    conjunctival, 452
    control of, 461
    in critical life threatening situations, 565
    dialysis and, 790
    gastrointestinal, 778-79, 906-7
    intracerebral, 764-65
    intracranial, 449-50
    postpartum, 393-94, 991-92
    from soft-tissue injuries, 528
    subarachnoid, 765
Hemorrhagic shock, 297, 310
Hemorrhoids, 776-77
Hemothorax, 185, 186, 484
    pediatric, 922-29
    pneumothorax and, 478-79
Henry's Law, 885
Hepatitis, 779, 855-56
Hepatitis B virus (HBV), 847
    vaccine for, xxxi
Hering-Breuer reflex, 216
Heroin, 831
Herpes, 858
Hertz (Hz), 58
Hetastarch (Hespan), 298
Hexadrol (dexamethasone), 759, 802
Hiccoughing, 216
High-angle rescue, 83
High-impact incident, 88-90
High-velocity injuries, 429
Hip
    dislocations of, 510, 518
    fractures of, 518
His, bundle of, 615-16, 1032
Histamine, 587, 797
Histamine (scombroid) poisoning, 815
History of patient, 196-99
    with acute abdomen, 786
    with body cavity trauma, 489
    with cardiac emergency, 685
    chief complaint, 196-98
    circumstances of present illness or injury, 197-98
    in diving-related emergency, 886-87
    elderly, 898
    gynecological patient, 957
    with head or spinal injury, 458-60
    menstrual activity, 786
    with musculoskeletal injuries, 515
    with neurological disorder, 749-50
    obstetrical patient, 970-71

History of patient *(con't)*
past medical history, 198-99
pediatric patient, 917-18
poisoned patient, 811
questioning techniques, 196
respiratory system assessment
and, 221
with right heart failure, 698-99
HIV (human immunodeficiency
virus), 594, 844, 847, 858-61
"Hold-up" position, 452
Hollow-organ injury, 481
Hollow organs, 772
Homan's sign, 708
Homeostasis, 146, 288, 293, 557
Hormone(s), 390-91, 393-94, 728,
966
from adrenal glands, 729-30
from gonads, 730, 954, 957
from pancreas, 729
parathyroid, 728
from pituitary gland, 726-28
from thyroid gland, 727, 728
Hospital component of EMS, 18
Hospitals
categorization of, 34, 35
direct communication with, 54
Host resistance, 844
Human Immunodeficiency Virus.
See HIV (human immunod-
eficiency virus)
Humerus, 504
fracture of, 512, 518
Humoral immunity, 794, 796, 842
Hydration, 288-89
Hydrocortisone (Solu-Cortef), 802
Hydrogen ion concentration. *See*
Acid-base balance
Hydromorphone, 831
Hydroxyzine (Atarax, Vistaril), 802
Hymenoptera, 808, 821-22
Hyoid bone, 208
Hyperbilirubinemia, 999
Hypercalcemia, 292, 612
Hypercarbia, 182, 215, 220, 450
Hyperkalemia, 292, 377, 383, 612
Hypernatremia, 292, 730
Hyperpyrexia, 871
Hypersensitivity, 336, 796
Hypertension, 191, 709
defined, 709
labetalol for, 368
portal, 776-77
pregnancy and, 972
right ventricular failure and, 698
Hypertensive disorders of preg-
nancy, 977-79
Hyperthermia, 867-71
malignant, 871
Hyperthyroidism, 728
Hypertonic phase, 760
Hypertonic solutions, 298-99
Hypertonic state, 292
Hypertrophy, 896
Hyperventilation, 460-61, 466
central neurogenic, 186, 750,
751
endotracheal intubation, 242
before suctioning, 276
Hyperventilative syndrome, 597-98
Hyphema, 452
Hypocalcemia, 292, 383, 612
Hypoglycemia (insulin shock),
733-36
drugs for managing, 389-90
EOA and, 234
glucagon for, 391
Hypoglycemic seizure, 735
Hypokalemia, 292, 733

Hyponatremia, 292
Hypoperfusion, 314
Hypopharynx, 208
Hypotension, 191
from dialysis, 789
dopamine for, 365
management of, 317-27
intravenous fluid therapy,
320-27
patient positioning, 317-18
pneumatic anti-shock garment
(PASG), 318-20
norepinephrine for, 364
orthostatic, 289
Hypothalamic thermostat, 866
Hypothalamus, 113, 727, 744, 745,
866
Hypothermia, 867, 871-76
from burns, 536
management of, 874-76
metabolic factors in, 874
presentation, 873-74
spine injury and, 464
Hypothyroidism, 728
Hypotonic solutions, 298-99
Hypotonic state, 292
Hypovolemia, 173, 192
from burns, 536
pulse oximeter and, 195
Hypovolemic shock, 174, 310-11
medications for, 328
Hypoxemia, 216, 220
from carbon monoxide poisoning, 533
Hypoxia, 182, 314, 576, 585
intubation and, 242
irreversible shock and, 559
myocardial, 381
oxygen for, 361
respiratory rate and, 217
suctioning and, 276
Hypoxic drive, 216, 277
Hysterical seizures, 761

ICF, 288
ICS. *See* Incident Command System
(ICS)
Idiopathic epilepsy, 760
Idiosyncrasy, defined, 336
Idioventricular rhythm (ventricular
escape complexes and
rhythms), 660, 661
Ileocecal valve, 474, 773
Ileum, 474, 773
Iliac arteries, 773
Illness, nature of, 167, 168-69
Ill patients, burns on, 537-38, 542
Immediate hypersensitivity, 797
Immobilization, bandaging to
ensure, 545
Immune response, 794, 842-43
Immune system, anaphylaxis and,
794-96
Immunity, 842-43
Immunoglobulins, 796, 797
Impact, 406
Impacted fracture, 508, 509
Impaled objects, 464-65
care of, 494-95
PASG and, 565
Implantation, 966, 967
Implied consent, 45
Imprisonment, false, 46
Incident Command System (ICS),
90-106
benefits of, 90-92
communications in, 105-6
extrication sector, 97-98
Incident Commander, 91, 92,

93-96
staging sector, 101-2
supply sector, 102
transfer of command, 96
transportation sector, 99-101, 108
treatment sector, 98-99
triage sector, 102-5, 106
Incisions, 526
Incomplete abortion, 974
Incubation period, 845
Inderal (propranolol), 339
Indeterminate axis, 1041
Index, therapeutic, 339-40
Index of suspicion, 404
Indication, defined, 336
Inertia, 406
Law of, 407
Inevitable abortion, 974
Infant(s). *See also* Neonate(s)
mechanisms of injury in, 169
premature, 277, 1000-1001
rule of nines for, 535
Infarction, 763-64, 765. *See also*
Myocardial infarction (MI)
zone of, 1044
Infection(s)
of bladder (cystitis), 780, 960
control of, xxx-xxxi, 845-50
from intravenous therapy, 327
of kidney (pyelonephritis), 780
of liver, 779
urinary tract (UTI), 780
Infectious diseases, 839-61
of childhood, 854-55
defined, 840
of gastrointestinal system, 855-
57
HIV infection, 858-61
immune response to, 842-43
of nervous system, 850-51
pathogenesis of, 841-42
precautions on, xxx-xxxi
of respiratory system, 851-53
sexually transmitted, 857-58
of skin, 853-54
transmission of, 843-45
Inferior conchae, 207, 208
Inferior vena cava, 606
Infiltration from intravenous therapy, 325
Information from dispatch, 167
Informed consent, 45
Infusion, intraosseous, 947, 949
Infusion rate, 351
Ingested poisons, 807-8, 810-17
antiemetics, 814-15
assessment of, 810-12
contaminated foods, 815, 855
ethylene glycol and methanol,
816-17
management of, 812-14
niacin (nicotinic acid), 816
poisonous plants, 815-16
Inhalation
injury due to, 523, 532-33
of therapeutic drugs, 353
toxic, 595-96, 807, 808, 817-21
ammonia, 820
carbon monoxide, 596-97,
819
cyanide, 818-19, 829
freon, 819-20
management of, 818
methylene chloride, 820-21
presentation of, 817-18
Injection(s)
intracardiac, 353
intramuscular, 352, 353, 355
intraosseous, 353, 359

poisoning through, 807, 808,
821-28
black widow spider bites, 824
brown recluse spider bites,
822-24
insect stings, 821-22
management of, 821
marine animal injection, 828
scorpion stings, 824-25
snake bites, 825-28
Injury, zone of, 1044
Injury current (current of injury),
1044
Injury mechanisms. *See*
Mechanism(s) of injury
Innominates, 504
Inotropy, 363, 612
Insect stings, 821-22
Insensible loss of water, 289
Insertion, 505
Inspection, 177
Inspiration, 212, 472
Instantaneous vector, 1039
Insulin, 475, 729, 731
Insulin shock. *See* Hypoglycemia
(insulin shock)
Insurance, malpractice, 48
Intal (cromolyn sodium), 803
Integumentary system, 522-23. *See
also* Burns; Wound(s)
Interatrial septum, 604, 605
Intercalated discs, 612, 613
Intercostal muscles, 472
Intermittent claudication, 708
Intermittent positive pressure ven-
tilation (IPPV), 478
Internal ("third space") losses of
water, 289
International Fire Service Training
Association, 82
Internodal pathways, 615
Interpolated beat, 662
Interstitial fluid, 288
Intervener physician, 23
Interventricular septum, 604, 605
Interviews, during behavioral
emergencies, 1017-18
Intestines, 156, 772, 773
Intoxication, 47
automobile accidents and, 418
water, 867-68, 869-70
Intracardiac injections, 353
Intracellular compartment, 288
Intracellular fluid (ICF), 288
Intracellular parasites, 841
Intracerebral hemorrhage, 449,
764-65
Intracranial hemorrhage, 449-50
Intracranial pressure, 440, 450,
759-60
Intractable vertigo, 904
Intradermal drug administration,
352
Intramuscular injection, 352, 353,
355
Intraosseous infusion, 947, 949
Intraosseous injection, 353, 359
Intrathoracic pressure, 473
Intrauterine devices (IUD), 958
Intravascular fluid, 288
Intravenous (IV) therapy, 294-99,
329. *See also* Fluid therapy
for hypotension, 320-27
kit for, 566
Introitus, 775
Intropin (dopamine), 328, 365-66,
699, 711, 1010
Intubation, 232. *See also*
Endotracheal intubation

in critical life threatening situations, 564
endobronchial, 246-47
esophageal, 246
Inversion, uterine, 992
Involuntary consent, 45
Ionization, 530-31
Ionizing radiation. *See* Nuclear radiation
Ions, 290, 291
Ipecac, syrup of, 395-96, 810, 813
IPPV, 478
Ipratropium (Atrovent), 388-89
Ipsilateral, defined, 184
Iris, 442
Irreversible shock, 310, 557, 559
Ischemia, 682
myocardial, 1044, 1045
zone of, 1044
Ischemic colitis, 907
Islets of Langerhans, 729
Isoelectric line, 616
Isoetharine (Bronkosol), 590, 803
Isolation stage of grief, 120
Isolette, neonatal transport, 1011
Isomers, 386
Isoproterenol, 710-11
Isoptin (verapamil), 375-76, 645, 659, 693, 710
Isotonic solutions, 298-99
Isotonic state, 292
Isotopes (radioisotope), 880
Isthmus, 728
IUD, 958

Jaundice, 176, 855
Jawbone (mandible), 435, 447
Jaw-thrust maneuver, 226, 315
modified, 226-27, 228
Jejunum, 474, 773
Job stress, 117-20
Joints, 504
burns involving, 541
injury to, 507-8, 510
splinting, 517
Journals, professional, 14
Jugular vein, 444, 453
anatomy of, 325
Jugular vein distention (JVD), 184, 484
of cardiac patient, 686
left ventricular failure and, 696
right heart failure and, 698
Junctional rhythm, 654-57
J waves, 873

Kaposi's sarcoma, 859
Ketoacidosis, 731
diabetic, 732-33, 735, 736
Ketones, 731
Kidney(s), 157, 475, 774
acid-base balance and, 301
failure of, 780-81, 787-88
infection of (pyelonephritis), 780
Kidney stone, 779-80
Kinetic energy, 406-7
Kinetics of trauma, 406-7
KKK-A-1822 Federal Specifications for Ambulances, 29, 31
Knee dislocation/fracture, 511, 518
Korsakoff's psychosis, 390, 758, 759
Krebs (citric acid) cycle, 309
Kubler-Ross, Elizabeth, 120
Kussmaul respirations, 186, 733
Kyphosis, 896

Labetolol (Trendate, Normodyne), 368-69, 709
Labia, 775, 955, 956

Labor
defined, 981
false, 980
management of patient in, 982-83
maternal complications of, 991-92
preterm, 394, 727-28, 980
stages of, 981-82
Lacerations, 526-27
Lacrimal ducts, 442
Lactated Ringer's solution, 298, 299, 567
Lactic acid, 309
Lanoxin (digitalis), 649, 712
Lap belts, 410-11
Large intestine, 156
Laryngeal edema, 532-3, 596
Laryngeal spasm, 219-20
Laryngopharynx, 207, 208
Laryngoscope, 236-38
placement in pediatric patient, 257
Laryngospasm, 186, 269
Laryngotracheobronchitis (croup), 386, 931-32
endotracheal intubation for, 257
Larynx, 208-10, 444
injury to, 453
Lasix (furosemide), 297, 380-81, 466, 697, 711
Last menstrual period (LMP), 786, 958
Last oral intake, questioning patients about, 198-99
Lateral impact, 414-16
Lateral malleolus, 505
Law(s). *See also* Medical-legal considerations
on drugs, 333-34
infection-control, xxx-xxxi
of motion, 407, 422
Leadership by EMT, 10, 11
Leads, ECG, 616-18, 712, 1033-39
augmented, 1033, 1035-38
bipolar, 616-18, 1033, 1034-35
precordial (chest), 618, 1033, 1038-39
unipolar, 1033, 1035-38
Left axis deviation, 1039, 1040, 1041
Left ventricular failure with pulmonary edema, 694-97
Legal considerations. *See* Law(s); Medical-legal considerations
Length, 348
Lens, 442
Leukocytes (white blood cells), 294, 295, 842
Levophed. *See* Norepinephrine (noradrenalin)
LH, 727, 728, 954, 957
Liability, medical, 45-48
Libel, 47
Librium, 832
Lice, 853
Licensure, 13
Lidocaine (Xylocaine), 353, 369-71, 663, 667, 693, 710, 950, 951
Ligaments, 504
Ligamentum arteriosum, 473
Ligamentum teres, 482
Limbic system, 113, 744
Limb leads, 617
Lime, dry, 549-50
Linear fractures, 445
Lips, 208
Liquid drugs, 334
Liter (L), 348

Lithium (Lithobid, Eskolith), 1021, 1022
Litigation, 41
Liver, 156, 474, 773
blunt trauma to, 407-8
deceleration injury to, 482
inflammation/infection of, 779
right heart failure and engorgement of, 698
Living wills, 42, 43
LMP, 786, 958
Loading, axial, 414, 447
Lobes of lungs, 473
Logarithm, 299
Long bones
extremity, 501-3
fracture of, 510
Lower airway, 572, 574
Lower extremities
anatomy and physiology of, 504-5
assessment of, 181, 188-89, 513-14, 515
injuries to, 510-12
management of, 517-18
Lower-leg fractures, 511
Low-impact incident, 88
Low-velocity injury, 428
LSD, 832
Lubricants, water-soluble, 240
Lucid interval, 450
Lumbar spine, 436
Lumen, 525, 608, 777
Lung disease, obstructive, 583-94
asthma, 586-94
assessment of, 587-88
management of, 588-93
pathophysiology, 586-87
special cases, 594-95
chronic bronchitis, 585-86
emphysema, 583-85, 586
Lung parenchyma, 211
Lungs, 212, 471, 473
gas exchange in, 213-15
injuries to
from overinflation, 889-90
SCUBA diving and, 886
penetrating injuries to, 430
Lung sounds, adventitious, 695
Luteinizing hormone (LH), 727, 728, 954, 957
Lymph, 843
Lymphatic system, 146, 843
Lymphocytes, 794, 796, 842
Lysosome, 143

MacIntosh (curved) blade, 237-38, 239
Macrodrip, 322, 323
Macrophages, 796, 842
Magill forceps, 183, 240, 263
Magnesium, 292
Magnesium sulfate, 394
Major incident response, 87-109
Incident Command System (ICS), 90-106
benefits of, 90-92
communications in, 105-6
extrication sector, 97-98
Incident Commander, 91, 92, 93-96
staging sector, 101-2
supply sector, 102
transfer of command, 96
transportation sector, 99-101, 108
treatment sector, 98-99
triage sector, 102-5, 106
plans, procedures, and equip-

ment, 107-9
prehospital emergency response, 88-90
Malaise, 595
Malignant hyperthermia, 871
Mallory-Weiss tear, 906
Malpractice insurance, 48
Mammalian diving reflex, 879
Management. *See specific emergencies and body systems*
Mandible (jawbone), 435, 447
Manic disorders, 1021-22
Mannitol (Osmotrol), 297, 759-60
Manually triggered oxygen-powered breathing device (demand valve resuscitator), 280-81
Marfan's syndrome, 705
Marginal artery, 607
Marijuana, 831
Marine animal injection, 828
Marrow, bone, 501, 503
Maryland Institute for emergency medical services (MIEMSS), 32, 404
Masks
protective, xxxi
ventilating, 278-79
Mass, 348, 406
Massage, carotid sinus, 717-21
Mass-casualty incident (MCI), 88. *See also* Major incident response
categories of, 88-90
defined, 88
preparation for, 36
Mast cells, 797
MAST program, 31
Maxilla, 435
Maxillary fractures, 447
Mean cardiac vector (resultant cardiac vector), 1039
Measles, 854
Mechanical ventilators, 281-82
Mechanism of action, 337. *See also specific drugs*
Mechanism(s) of injury, 167, 168-69, 403
of body cavity trauma, 482-83
decision to transport and, 405
falls, 169
for frontal impacts, 412-14
of genitalia, 482
from lateral impact, 414-16
motorcycle, 169
motor vehicle collisions, 169
musculoskeletal injuries, 515
penetrating injuries, 169
rapid transport and, 563
from rear-end impact, 416-17
from rollover, 417-18
from rotational impact, 416
Meconium staining, 983, 1001, 1002, 1005
Medial malleolus, 505
Mediastinum, 471, 472-73
injuries to structures in, 480-81
Medical control, 21, 22-24
communications between paramedic and, 54
Medical control *(con't)*
direct, 22-23
indirect, 22, 23-24
Medical dictionary, 125
Medical director, 22
Medic alert identification, 189
Medical illnesses, altered behavior and, 1015-16
Medical-legal considerations, 39-49

Medical-legal considerations *(con't)*
  laws affecting EMS, 41-44
  legal principles, 41
  medical liability, 45-48
  standard of care, 44-45
Medical patient. *See also* Patient(s);
    *specific disorders and
    emergencies*
  assessment of, 176, 203
  critical management priorities
    for, 174-75
  secondary, 176
Medical practice act, 41
Medical record, 48
Medical terminology, 123-39
  abbreviations, 134-39
  defined, 124
  prefixes, 125, 130-32
  root words, 125-29
  suffixes, 125, 130, 133
Medication(s), 198-99. *See also*
    Drug(s); *specific drugs*
  for anaphylaxis, 799-803
  anticonvulsant, 391-92, 762
  antidysrhythmic, 369-76, 710
  for anxiety disorders, 1021
  for cardiogenic shock, 699-700
  for distressed neonate, 1009,
    1010
  for left ventricular failure, 696-97
  for musculoskeletal injuries, 519
  for pediatric cardiac arrest, 949-
    51
  for pediatric cardiopulmonary
    arrest, 949-51
  for pulmonary edema, 696-97
  questioning patients about, 199
  for schizophrenics, 1022-23
  shock signs and symptoms hid-
    den by, 310
  in shock treatment, 328
  for thoracic trauma, 490-91
Medulla, 215
Medulla oblongata, 440, 450, 745
Melena, 778, 907
Membranes, anatomy and physiol-
    ogy of, 148
Menarche, 957
Meniere's disease, 904
Meninges, 435, 438-39, 744
Meningitis, 850-51, 854
  pediatric, 928-29
  sepsis and, 936
Menopause, 957
Menstrual activity, history of, 786
Menstrual cycles, 957
Menstrual period, 956
Menstrual phase, 957
Mental status
  altered, 754-55
    in elderly patient, 903-4
    respiratory system assessment
      and, 220
  assessment of, 173
  of elderly patient, 898
Meperidene, 831
Mescaline, 832
Mesencephalon, 745
Mesenteric arteries, 773
Mesentery, 475
Metabolic acidosis, 302, 303
Metabolic alkalosis, 302, 303
Metabolic emergencies, drugs for,
    389-91
  D50W (50% dextrose in water),
    389-90
  glucagon, 390-91
  thiamine, 390
Metabolism, 308-9

defined, 286
  of glucose, 730-32
  hypothermia and, 874
  steady-state, 864
Metabolites, 338
Metacarpals, 504
Metaphysis, 501, 503
Metaproterenol (Alupent), 591, 803
Metatarsals, 505
Meter (M), 348
Methadone, 831
Methanol poisoning, 816-17, 836
Methylene chloride poisoning,
    820-21
Methylprednisolone (Solu-Medrol),
    392-93, 466, 593, 802
Methylxanthines, 374
Metric system, 348
METTAG system, 105, 106
MI. *See* Myocardial infarction (MI)
Microdrip, 322, 323
Microfilament, 143
MicroNEFRIN (racemic epineph-
    rine), 386-87
Microtubule, 143
Mid-axillary line, 160
Midbrain, 745
Middle conchae, 207, 208
Mid-spinal line, 160
Mid-sternal line, 160
MIEMSS, 32, 404
Military assistance to safety and
    traffic (MAST) program, 31
Miller blade, 237-38, 239
Milliequivalent, 292
Mineralocorticoids, 729, 730
Minerals, drugs from, 332
Minimum effective concentration,
    339
Mini-neuro examination, 685
Minute volume, 217
Miscarriage, 974
Mitochondria, 143, 144
Mitral valve, 604, 605
Mittelschmerz, 782, 960
Mobile telephones, 57-58
Mobile two-way radios, 55
Modified chest lead 1 (MCL$_1$), 618
Modified jaw-thrust maneuver,
    226-27, 228
Modulator, 59
Molecule, 290
Monitoring, non-invasive, 920-21
Moral dilemma, 8-9
Morbidity, 402
Morphine, 831
Morphine sulfate, 378-79, 491, 693,
    696, 709, 711
Mortality, 402
  from automobile accidents, 418
Motion, 406
  laws of, 407, 422
  paradoxical, 170, 476, 477
Motion sense, 443
Motion sickness, 399
Motorcycle, as mechanisms of
    injury, 169
Motorcycle accidents, 419-20
Motor vehicle accidents. *See* Blunt
    trauma
Motor vehicle collisions, as mecha-
    nisms of injury, 169
Motor vehicle laws, 41-42
Mountain Rescue Association, 84
Mouth, 208, 772
  evaluation of, 179, 183
  fluids in, 183
  odor from, 183
  of poisoned patient, 811

Mouth-to-mouth breathing, 279
Mouth-to-nose breathing, 279
Mucous membrane, 208
Mucous production, chronic, 585
Mucus, 208
Multiparity, 976
Multiple casualty incidents. *See*
    Mass-casualty incident (MCI)
Multiplex communications, 60, 61
Mumps, 854
Mural emboli, 707
Muscle(s)
  accessory respiratory, 212
  cardiac, 473, 612
  electrocution and, 530
  intercostal, 472
  papillary, 604, 605
  respiratory, 598-99
  skeletal, 505
  smooth, 505
  sternocleidomastoid, 472
Muscle (heat) cramps, 507, 867-69,
    872
Muscle tissue, 144, 145, 150
Muscle tone, neurologic assess-
    ment of, 191
Muscular control, pediatric, 914
Muscular system, anatomy and
    physiology of, 146, 150
Musculoskeletal injuries, 499-519
  assessment of, 500, 513-15
  dislocations, 507-8, 512-13
  fractures. *See* Fracture(s)
  joint injury, 507-8, 510, 517
  to lower extremities, 510-12
  management of, 500, 515-19
  muscular injury, 506-7
  to upper extremities, 512
Musculoskeletal system, aging and,
    896
Mushroom poisonings, 816
Mutual-aid agreements, 36
Mycobacterium tuberculosis, 849,
    851
Mycoses, 842
Myocardial contusion, 414, 480
Myocardial hypoxia, 381
Myocardial infarction (MI), 684,
    690-94, 1044-45
  acute, 690-94
    evolution of, 1045-48
    localization of, 1048-51, 1052-
      54
  cardiogenic shock and, 699
  defined, 1044
  in elderly, 902
  in-hospital management of, 694
  prehospital management of,
    692-94
  signs and symptoms of, 691-92
  silent, 902
  subendocardial, 1045, 1047
  transmural, 1045, 1046
Myocardial injury, 1044, 1045
Myocardial ischemia, 1044, 1045
  drugs for, 711
Myocardium, 505, 603, 604
  condition of, 716
Myxedema, 728

Nagel, Eugene, 6
Nalbuphine (Nubain), 693
Naloxone (Narcan), 195, 339-40,
    353, 397-98, 519, 757-58
Narcan Neonatal, 1010
Narcotic antagonists, 397-98
Narcotics, abuse and overdose of,
    831
Nares, 183, 207-8

Nasal bones, 435
Nasal cannula, 277-78
Nasal cavity, anatomy of, 207-8
Nasal flaring, 577
Nasal intubation, for spinal injury
    patients, 461
Nasopharyngeal airways, 230-32
Nasopharynx, 207, 208
Nasotracheal intubation, 254, 261-
    64
  blind, 261, 262-63
  under direct visualization, 263-
    64
  of thermal burn patient, 540
National Association for Research
    and Rescue (NASAR), 84
National Association of
    Underwater Instructors, 84
National Cave Rescue Commission
    (NCRC), 84
National Fire Academy (NFA), 83,
    107
National Fire Protection
    Association, xxxi, 84
National Highway Safety Act
    (1966), 20
National Institute of Occupational
    Safety and Health (NIOSH),
    83
National Registry of EMTs, 14
National Standard Curriculum for
    EMT-P, 12
Nausea
  drugs to manage, 399
  pediatric, 935
Neck. *See also* Head, neck, and
    spinal trauma
  anatomy and physiology of,
    443-44
  evaluation of, 180, 184
    for body cavity trauma, 484
  injuries to
    pediatric, 922
    penetrating, 430
Necrosis, cystic medial, 706
Needle cricothyrotomy, 270-71
Needles, disposal of, 848
Negatives, pertinent, 198
Neglect
  of children, 923-27
  of elderly, 909
Negligence, 44-45
Neisseria gonorrhea, 858
Neisseria meningitides, 929
Neisseria meningitis, 851
Neonate(s), 913-14, 991-1011
  anatomic and physiologic
    changes at birth, 997-98
  defined, 996
  distressed, 1001-9
    chest compressions in, 1008-9
    drying, warming, positioning,
      suctioning, and tactile stim-
      ulation of, 1003-7
    fetal heart rate of, 1001
    meconium staining, 983,
      1001, 1002, 1005
    medications and fluids for,
      1009, 1010
    supplemental oxygen for,
      1007-8
    ventilation of, 1008
  heat loss in, 998-99
  premature, 277, 1000-1001
  routine care of, 998-1000
  transport of, 1009-11
Nephrons, 157, 896
Nerve(s)
  cranial, 443, 747, 748

dysfunction of, 598-99
parasympathetic, 347
peripheral, 440, 747
post-ganglionic, 340, 342-43, 344
post-synaptic, 344, 346
pre-ganglionic, 340, 341-42
pre-synaptic, 344
spinal, 746-47
vagus, 375, 611-12, 625
Nerve conduction velocity, 896
Nerve roots, 440
Nerve tissue, 144
Nervous impulses from respiratory center, 215
Nervous system, 740-48
aging and, 896
anaphylaxis and, 798
anatomy and physiology of, 146, 153-54, 740-48
assessment of, 749-54
Glasgow Coma Scale, 174, 175, 191, 458, 459, 753-54
neurological, 752-53
primary, 749
secondary, 749-54
central. *See* Central nervous system
infections of, 850-51
peripheral, 747-48
Nervous system emergencies, 754-67
altered mental status, 754-55
management of, 757-60
primary assessment, 756
secondary assessment, 756-57
seizures. *See* Seizures
status epilepticus, 763, 927
stroke, 763-67
categories of, 763-65
clinical presentation of, 765
in elderly, 904
management of, 766-67
transient ischemic attack and, 765-66
Neurilemma, 439
Neuroeffector junction, 341
Neurogenic shock, 311, 328
norepinephrine for, 364
Neurological assessment, 189-91, 752-53
Neurological emergencies
drugs for, 391-93
diazepam (Vallium), 391-92
methylprednisolone (Solu-Medrol), 392-93
among elderly, 903-5
pediatric, 927-29
Neuromuscular blockade, rapid sequence intubation with, 259-61
Neuron, 341, 741-42
CNS, 435, 439
Neurotransmitter, 341, 742
Neutralizing agents on chemical burns, 549
Neutrons, 290, 291, 880, 881
Newborn. *See* Neonate(s)
Newton, Isaac, 406
NFA, 83, 107
Niacin (nicotonic acid), 816
Nifedipine (Procardia, Adalat), 381, 382-83, 690, 709
9-1-1 Telephone service, 25-26
NIOSH, 83
Nipride (sodium nitroprusside), 709
Nitrates, 381-82
Nitrogen narcosis, 886

Nitroglycerin (Nitrostate), 381-82, 690, 693, 697, 711
Nitrous oxide (Nitronox), 379-80, 490-91, 519, 693, 711
Noncompensatory pause, 641
Nonketotic hyperosmolar coma, 732
Non-Q-wave infarctions, 690, 1045
Nonrebreather mask, 278
Norcuron (vecuronium), 260
Norepinephrine (noradrenalin), 363-65
cardiac contractile strength and, 304
for cardiovascular emergencies, 710
heat generation and, 867
as neurotransmitter, 341, 611, 742
release of, 343-44, 345, 558, 729
for shock, 328, 700
stress and, 113
Normal anxiety levels, 116
Normal saline, 299
Normodyne (labetolol), 368-69, 709
Norpramin, 833
Nose, evaluation of, 179, 183
Nosebleeds
facial trauma and, 465
nasopharyngeal airway, 231
Notification of EMS personnel, 53
Nubain (nalbuphine), 693
Nuclear radiation, 880-84
dose-effect relationship to, 881, 882
prehospital management of, 883-84
safety principles in, 881
Nucleolus, 143
Nucleus, 144
Nullipara, 982

Oath of Geneva, 7
Oblique angle, 416
Obstetrical emergencies, 965-93
deliveries, 981-82
abnormal presentations, 988-89
cephalopelvic disproportion, 987
maternal complications of, 991-92
multiple births, 989-91
precipitous, 991
prolapsed cord, 971, 989, 990
shoulder dystocia, 991
unscheduled field delivery, 983-87
drugs for, 393-94
labor
false, 980
management of patient in, 982-83
maternal complications of, 991-92
preterm, 394, 727-28, 980
pregnancy, 971-80
abortion, 974-75
abruptio placentae, 973, 975-77
Braxton-Hicks contractions, 980
ectopic, 782, 960, 975
hypertensive disorders of, 977-79
placenta previa, 973, 977
pre-existing or aggravated medical conditions and,

972
supine-hypotensive syndrome, 979
trauma during, 971-72
vaginal bleeding during, 970, 973, 974, 977
puerperium, 981
Obstetrical patient
anatomy and physiology of, 966-69
assessment of, 970-71
Obstructive lung disease. *See* Lung disease, obstructive
Occipital bone, 742, 743
Occiput posterior position, 988
Occupational exposure to blood-borne pathogens, xxx-xxxi
Occupational Safety and Health Administration (OSHA), xxx-xxxi, 83
Ocean Corporation, 84
Odontoid process, 436
Official names of drugs, 334
Ohio Department of Natural Resources, 83
Oil of Wintergreen, 833
Oklahoma City federal building bombing (1995), 89
"Old-old," defined, 894
Omentum, 475
Ongoing assessment, 200
On-line physician, 23, 24
Onset of chief complaint, 197
Open chest wound, 490
Open fracture, 508
Open pneumothorax, 174, 430, 478
Opium, 333
OPQRST method, 197
Oral administration of medication, 360
Oral cavity. *See* Mouth
Oral intubation, 461, 540
Orbit, 452-53
Organ collision, 409, 410
Organelles, 143
Organic acids, 731
Organic brain syndrome, 905, 1016
Organisms, anatomy and physiology of, 146
Organizations, professional, 13
Organophosphates, 376, 829-30
Organs
anatomy and physiology of, 144-45
hollow, 772
solid, 772
Organ systems, anatomy and physiology of, 145-46
Origin, 505
Original education, 28
Ornato, Joseph P., 33
Oropharyngeal airways, 228-30, 240
Oropharynx, 207, 208
Orotracheal intubation, 242-45, 254
Orthostatic hypotension, 289
Orthostatic syncope, 903
Osborn waves, 873
OSHA, xxx-xxxi, 83
Osmosis, 292-94
Osmotic diuresis, 732
Osmotic gradient, 292
Osmotrol (mannitol), 297
Ossicles, 443
Osteoporosis, 896, 900
Ovarian cysts, 781-82, 960
Ovaries, 157, 727, 730, 774-75, 954, 955
Overdose, 47, 806. *See also*

Poisoning; Substance abuse
drug, 234, 830, 831-33
emetics to manage, 395-96
Overhydration, 289
Ovulation, 957, 966
Ovum, 966, 967
Oximetry, pulse, 194-95, 223, 486, 580-81, 920
Oxmotrol (mannitol), 759-60
Oxygen, 206
blood concentrations of, 214-15
for cardiac emergencies, 711
for cardiovascular emergencies, 361-62
for chronic obstructive pulmonary disease, 581
for distressed neonate, 1007-8
for head, neck, and spinal trauma, 460-61, 466
hyperbaric, 596-97
levels of, 213
measurement of, 213-14
for myocardial infarction, 692-93
for respiratory emergencies, 384
Oxygenation, 276-79
delays in, 242
monitoring, 223
of shock patient, 317
Oxygen saturation percentage (SpO$_2$), 224
Oxygen transport, 307
Oxytocin (Pitocin), 393-94, 727, 728, 980

PAC, 640-41
Pacemaker, 672-73
artificial rhythm, 672-73
insertion of, 679, 681
wandering, 638-39
Packaging of patients, 79, 329
Packed red blood cells, 296
Padded board, 518-19
Palates, 208
Pallor, 176
Palmar surface, 535
Palpation, 177
Palpitations, 685
Pamelor, 833
Pancreas, 156, 475, 727, 729, 773
Pancreatitis, 779
Pancuronium (Pavulon), 260
Panic attack, 1021
Pantridge, J. Frank, 6
Pants, turnout, 72
Paper bag syndrome, 415, 478
Papillary muscles, 604, 605
Paradoxical breathing, 220
Paradoxical motion, 170, 476, 477
Paramedic roles and responsibilities, 10-12
after patient delivery, 11-12
post-graduate, 12-14
primary, 4, 12
during removal, 81
Paranoid schizophrenia, 1022
Parasites, 841, 842
Parasympathetic control of heart, 611-12
Parasympathetic ganglia, 345-46
Parasympathetic nerves, 347
Parasympathetic nervous system, 154, 340, 345-48
Parasympatholytics (anticholinergics), 347, 375-77, 388-89
Parasympathomimetics (cholinergics), 347
Parathyroid glands, 727, 728
Parathyroid hormone, 728
Parenchyma, lung, 211

Parenteral drugs, 335
Parietal bone, 742, 743
Parietal pericardium, 603
Parietal pleura, 211, 473, 574
Parity, 958
Parkland formula, 548
Paroxysmal junctional tachycardia (PJT), 658-59
Paroxysmal nocturnal dyspnea (PND), 197, 695
Paroxysmal supraventricular tachycardia (PSVT), 374, 375, 642-45, 658
Partial pressure, 213-14
    of oxygen in the blood (PaO2), 224
Partial seizures, 760
Partial-thickness burns, 541
PASG. See Pneumatic anti-shock garment (PASG)
Patellar dislocations, 511
Patent, defined, 220
Pathogens, bloodborne, xxx-xxxi
Pathway expansion, 426
Patient(s). See also Assessment; Elderly; History of patient; Pediatric patient(s); Transport of patient
    abusive, 118
    assessment in rescue operations, 78-79
    communication of information on, 65-66
    critical/immediate, 103
    critically ill or dying, 118
    dead/non-salvageable, 103
    dying, 120-21
    gaining access to, 76-78
    level of orientation, 189-90
    location of, 76, 169
    obstetrical, 966-69, 970-71
    packaging of, 79, 329
    problem, 47
    psychological support for, 80, 519
    safety of, 72, 81
    specific, 76
    suicidal, 809, 811
    unresponsive, 190
Patient report, 64, 65, 66
    written, 66
Pause, compensatory, 653
Pavulon (pancuronium), 260
PCP, 832
PEA, 661, 703-4
Peak Expiratory Flow Rate (PEFR), 588
Pedestrian accidents, 420-21
Pediatric emergencies, 911-51
    assessment of, 917-21
        development stages and, 913-17
    cardiopulmonary arrest, 941-51
        airway management, 945-46
        anticipating, 941
        electrical therapy, 951
        medications, 949-51
        rapid assessment, 941-45
        vascular access and fluid therapy, 946-49
        ventilation, 946
    cardiovascular emergencies, 936-39
    child's response to, 912-13
    gastrointestinal emergencies, 935
    neurological emergencies, 927-29
    parents' response to, 917

pediatric advanced life support (PALS) for, 941-51
    respiratory emergencies, 930-35
        aspirated foreign body, 930-31
        asthma, 934-35
        bronchiolitis, 933-34
        croup, 931-32
        epiglottitis, 931, 932-33
        status asthmaticus, 935
    sudden infant death syndrome (SIDS), 940
    trauma, 921-27
        burns, 923
        chest and abdomen injuries, 922-23
        child abuse/neglect, 923-27
        extremity injuries, 923
        head, face, and neck injuries, 922
Pediatric immobilization devices, 464
Pediatric patient(s)
    behavioral emergencies in, 1023-24
    burns on, 537, 542
    endotracheal intubation in, 256-59
    endotracheal intubation of, 256-59
PEFR, 588
Pelonephritis (kidney infection), 780
Pelvic cavity, 162, 474. See also Body cavity trauma
Pelvic inflammatory disease (PID), 781, 959
Pelvic ring, 504
Pelvis, 504
    evaluation of, 181, 187-88
    fractures of, 510-11
        management of, 517
Penetrating trauma, 408, 425-31
    to abdomen, 481, 496
    blast injuries, 424-25
        ballistics, 426-28
        high velocity, 429
        low velocity, 428
        pathologies of, 429-31
    to chest, 565
    as mechanisms of injury, 169
    to muscles, 507
    punctures, 527
Penis, 775, 776
Pentazocine, 831
Peptic ulcer disease, 777, 906
Percussion, 177, 178
Perforated abdominal viscus, 778
Perfusion, 104
    defined, 304
    evaluation of, 173
    physiology of, 304-6
    tissue, 307-8
Pericardial fluid, 603
Pericardial tamponade, 430, 480, 494
Pericardiocentesis, 494, 495
Pericardium, 473, 603, 604
Perineum, 956
Periosteum, 438, 503
Peripheral arterial atherosclerotic disease, 708
Peripheral arteries, 608
Peripheral circulation, 607-9
    pediatric, 943
Peripheral edema, right heart failure and, 698
Peripheral nerves, 440
Peripheral nervous system, 747-48

Peripheral resistance, 306, 318
Peripheral vascular conditions, noncritical, 708
Peripheral vascular resistance, 305
Peristalsis, 474, 773
Peritoneal dialysis, 788, 789
Peritoneal space, spilling of abdominal contents or blood into, 482
Peritoneum, 148, 187, 475, 771
Peritonitis, 772
Personal protective equipment (PPE), xxxi, 845
Personal safety, 70-72
Personnel
    direct communication with, 54
    for removal operations, 81
    screening of, 73
    support, 18
Perspiration, 289, 867
Pertinent negatives, 198
Petit mal seizures, 761
Phalanges, 504, 505
Pharmacodynamics, 337, 339-40
Pharmacokinetics, 337
Pharmacology. See also Drug(s); Medication(s)
    autonomic nervous system and, 340-48
        adrenergic receptors, 344-45
        anatomy and physiology of, 340-41
        parasympathetic nervous system, 340, 345-48
        sympathetic nervous system, 340, 341-44
    defined, 332
    in geriatrics, 905
Pharyngeo-tracheal Lumen (PtL) airway, 264, 265-66
Pharynx (throat), 208
Phenergan (promethazine), 398-99, 802
Phenobarbital, 377, 832
Phenol, 549
Phenothiazines, 814
Phentolamine (Regitine), 364
Phlebotomy, chemical, 378
Phonation, 246
Phosphate, 292
pH scale, 299, 300
PHTLS, 554-55
Physical examination
    of cardiac patient, 685-87
    of elderly patient, 899
    of gynecological patient, 958
    of obstetric patient, 971
    of pediatric patient, 918-19
    of poisoned patient, 811-12
    of respiratory distress, 221-23
    techniques for conducting, 177-78
Physician
    intervener, 23
    on-line, 23, 24
Physicians' Desk Reference (PDR), 334
Physiology. See also Anatomy and physiology
    of adrenergic synapse, 345
    of cholinergic synapse, 348
    of perfusion, 304-6
Pia mater, 438, 744
PID, 781, 959
"Piggyback" infusion, 352, 357
PIH, 978
Pills, 335. See also Drug(s)
Piloerection, 867
"Pink puffer," 586

Pitocin (oxytocin), 393-94, 727, 728, 980
Pitting edema, 189
Pituitary gland, 726-28, 745
Pit vipers, 825-27
PJCs, 652, 653
PJT, 658-59
Placenta, 966-67, 987
Placenta previa, 973, 977
Plans
    multiple casualty incident (MCI), 88
    rescue, 77
Plants
    drugs from, 332
    poisonous, 815-16
Plasma, 294, 295, 528, 556
    fresh frozen, 296
Plasma losses, 289
    shock due to, 297
Plasma protein fraction (Plasmanate), 298
Platelets (thrombocytes), 294, 295, 528
Pleura, 148, 185, 211, 473, 573-74
    decompression of, 493
Pleural fluid, 211
PND, 197, 695
Pneumatic anti-shock garment (PASG), 33, 316, 329
    application of, 321
    control of bleeding with, 317, 319
    elevation of blood pressure with, 319, 320
    for hypotension, 318-20
    shock/trauma resuscitation and, 565-65
Pneumocystis carinii, 859
Pneumomediastinum, 890
Pneumonia, 594-95
    in AIDS patients, 859
    aspiration, 812
    in elderly, 901
Pneumotaxic center, 215
Pneumothorax, 185, 477-78, 484
    closed, 478
    open, 174, 430, 478
    pediatric, 922-29
    tension, 175, 185, 186, 478-79
        management of, 493-94
Pocket mask, 279-80
Poiseuille's Law, 566, 608
Poison control center, 806
Poison information centers, 809
Poisoning, 805-30
    by absorption, 807, 808-9, 829-30
    carbon monoxide, 523, 533
    defined, 807
    emetics to manage, 395-96
    by ingestion, 807-8, 810-17
        antiemetics, 814-15
        assessment of, 810-12
        contaminated foods, 815, 855
        ethylene glycol and methanol, 816-17
        management of, 812-14
        niacin (nicotinic acid), 816
        poisonous plants, 815-16
    by inhalation, 807, 808, 817-21
        ammonia, 820
        carbon monoxide, 819
        cyanide, 818-19, 829
        freon, 819-20
        management of, 818
        methylene chloride, 820-21
        presentation of, 817-18
    by injection, 807, 808, 821-28

black widow spider bites, 824
brown recluse spider bites, 822-24
insect stings, 821-22
management of, 821
marine animal injection, 828
scorpion stings, 824-25
snake bites, 825-28
routes of exposure, 807
Polycythemia, 585, 999
Pons, 440, 745
Portable radios, 55
Portal hypertension, 776-77
Portal system, 187, 773
Positional sense, 443
Post-call documentation, 66
Post-capillary sphincter, 306
Posterior body, evaluation of, 181, 189
Posterior spinal artery, 442
Posterior tibial pulse, 188
Post-ganglionic nerves, 340, 342-43, 344
Postictal phase, 760
Postpartum hemorrhage, 393-94, 991-92
Post-seizure, 760
Post-synaptic nerves, 344, 346
Post-traumatic stress disorder, 114-15
Posturing
brain injury and, 191
decerebrate, 191, 753
decorticate, 191, 753
Potassium, 292, 612
Potentiation, defined, 336
Powders, 335
PPD skin test, 852
PPE, xxxi, 845
PQRST method, 786
Practice, restrictions on, 118
Pralidoxime (2-PAM), 376
Pre-arrival instruction program, 27
Pre-capillary sphincter, 306
Precautions, universal, 860-61
Precipitous delivery, 991
Precordial (chest) leads, 618, 1033, 1038-39
Precordial thump, 715
Preeclampsia, 978-79
Pre-excitation syndromes, 682-83
Prefixes, metric system, 348-49
Pre-ganglionic nerves, 340, 341-42
Pregnancy, 971-80
abortion, 974-75
abruptio placentae, 973, 975-77
Braxton-Hicks contractions, 980
ectopic, 782, 960, 975
fetal circulation, 968-69
fetal development, 968
hemodynamic changes of, 973
hypertensive disorders of, 977-79
PASG and, 565
placenta previa, 973, 977
pre-existing or aggravated medical conditions and, 972
supine-hypotensive syndrome, 979
trauma during, 971-72
vaginal bleeding during, 970, 973, 974, 977
Pregnancy-induced hypertension (PIH), 978
Prehospital component of EMS, 18
Prehospital Trauma Life Support (PHTLS), 554-55
Preinfarction angina, 690
Preload (end-diastolic volume),

304, 557, 609
Premature atrial contractions (PAC), 640-41
Premature junctional contractions (PJCs), 652, 653
Premature neonates, 1000-1001
Premature ventricular contraction (PVC), 662-63
Prenatal care, 970
Prenatal period. See Pregnancy
"Prepatory depression," 121
Preplanning of rescue operations, 73
Presacral edema, 187
Presenting part, 982
Pressure
intracranial, 440, 450, 759-60
intrathoracic, 473
partial, 213-14
physical principles of, 884-85
Pressure disorders (barotrauma), 88-90, 885-86, 887-90
Pre-synaptic nerves, 344
Priapism, 188, 452
Primary assessment, 170-78. See also Assessment; specific emergencies and body systems
ABCDE of, 170-74, 555
critical management priorities, 174-75
defined, 170
Primary motor center, 867
Primary pulmonary lobules, 211
Primary response, 796
Primary triage and treatment, 97
P-R interval, 620, 623, 627
Prinzmetal's angina, 689
Priority dispatching, 27
Problem patients, 47
Procainamide (Pronestyl), 371-72, 667, 693, 710
Procardia (nifedipine), 381, 382-83, 690, 709
Professionalism, 9
Professional organizations, 13
Profile of bullet, 426, 427
Progesterone, 730, 957, 966
Projectile injury, 425-29
Prolactin, 727
Prolapsed cord, 971, 989, 990
Proliferative phase, 957
Promethazine (Phenergan), 398-99, 802
Pronation, 504
Propranolol (Inderal), 339
Prostate, 775, 776
Prostatitis, 782
Protective gear, xxxi, 72-73
Protein(s)
antigens, 295
helper, 294
pyrogens, 327
Protocols, 24
for priority dispatching, 27
for prolonged patient care, 79-80
Protons, 290, 291, 880
Proventil (albuterol), 387-88, 590, 802-3, 934
Provocation of chief complaint, 197
Proximate cause, 44
Pruritus, 798
Psilocybin, 832
PSVT, 374, 375, 642-45, 658
Psychiatric disorders, 1019-23. See also Behavioral emergencies
anxiety disorders, 1021

depression, 397, 1019, 1020
in elderly, 905-6
manic disorders, 1021-22
schizophrenia, 1022-23
suicide, 906, 1019-21
Psychological stability of EMT, 10
Psychological support for patients, 80, 519
Psychomotor processes, 760
Psychomotor seizures, 761
Psychosis, 1020
acute episodes of, 398
Korsakoff's, 390, 758, 759
PtL airway, 264, 265-66
Public information and education, 24-25
Public utility model, 36
Puerperium, 981
Pulmonary arteries, 212, 575, 605, 606
Pulmonary capillaries, 212-13, 574
Pulmonary circulation, 212-13
Pulmonary congestion, 695
Pulmonary contusion, 476
Pulmonary disease, 184
Pulmonary edema, 378, 381, 385, 696-97
in elderly, 901
left ventricular failure with, 694-97
PASG and, 565
Pulmonary embolism, 215, 597, 698
acute, 707-8
in elderly, 901
after pregnancy, 992
Pulmonary lobules, primary, 211
Pulmonary membrane, diffusion across, 214
Pulmonary overpressure accidents, 889-90
Pulmonary respiration, 212, 575
Pulmonary veins, 213, 575, 604, 605, 606
Pulmonic valve, 606
Pulse, 172, 192, 193
abdominal injury and, 488
of cardiac patient, 688
CNS injury and, 458
distal, 181, 188
radial, 181, 189
shock assessment and, 312-14
Pulse deficit, 649
Pulseless electrical activity (PEA), 661, 703-4
Pulse oximetry, 194-95, 223, 486, 580-81, 920
Pulse pressure, 192
Pulse rate, respiratory compromise and, 223
Pulsus paradoxus, 577
Pump failure, 691
Punctures, 527
Pupillary reflexes, 756
Pupils, 442
assessment of, 179, 182, 457
Purkinje system, 615-16, 1032
Purposeful responses, 190
Purposeless responses, 190
PVC, 662-63
P waves, 619, 621, 627
Pyrexia (fever), 217, 871, 914
Pyriform fossa, 208
Pyrogenic reaction to intravenous therapy, 327
Pyrogens, 871

QRS complex, 619, 623, 627
QRS duration, 620
Quadrants, abdominal, 474, 771

Quadrigeminy, 663
Quality Assurance (QA) and Quality Improvement (QI) programs, 32-33
Quality factor (QF), 881
Quality of chief complaint, 198
Questioning techniques, 196
"Quick-look" paddle electrodes, 712-14
Q wave, 619
Q wave infarction, 690

R. Adams Cowley "Shock Trauma Center," 35
Raccoon eyes (bilateral periorbital ecchymosis), 182, 445-46
Racemic epinephrine (microNEFRIN, Vaponefrin), 386-87
Radial pulse, 172
Radiation
of chief complaint, 198
defined, 880
heat loss through, 865, 866, 998
types of, 531, 880, 881
Radiation absorbed dose (RAD), 881
Radiation exposure, 530-32. See also Nuclear radiation
assessment of, 543
management of, 550-51
Radio codes, 63, 106
Radionuclide (radioisotope), 880
Radios, 55, 58-61
biotelemetry, 59-60, 66
to communicate patient assessment, 200-201
communications techniques, 63-64
defined, 54
frequencies, 58-59
maintenance of, 61
transmission types, 60-61
Radius, 504
Rales, 186, 579, 695
Ranitidine (Zantac), 802
Rape, 961
trauma to genitalia from, 180
Rapid Cardiopulmonary Assessment, 941-45
"Raptures of the deep," 886
Rattlesnake bite, 826, 827
Reactions, chemical, 291
"Reactive depression," 121
Rear-end impact, 416-17
Reassessment during removal, 81
Rebound tenderness, 187, 482, 772, 784-85
Receivers, satellite, 56, 57
Receiving facilities, 34-35
Receptors
adrenergic, 339, 344-45
deep body temperature (afferent), 866
dopaminergic, 345
drug, 339
Recipients, universal, 295
Reciprocity, 13
Recognition, lack of, 118
Recompression, 888
Record, medical, 48
Recreational vehicle accidents, 421-22
Rectal administration of medication, 360
Rectum, 474, 772, 773
Red blood cells (erythrocytes), 294-95, 296, 310, 530, 556
Red bone marrow, 503

Reentry, phenomenon of, 628
Reflex(es), 746
  Cushing's, 450, 451, 752
  diving, 879
  Hering-Breuer, 216
  pupillary, 756
Refractory, defined, 336
Refractory period, 625
Refusal of service, 46
"Refusal of transport" form, 46
Regionalizing services, 34
Regitine (phentolamine), 364
Regulations, infection-control, xxx-xxxi
Regurgitation, Sellick's maneuver to prevent, 227-28. See also Vomiting
Relationship quality, 33
Relative refractory period, 625
"Release from liability" form, 46
REM, 881
Remote consoles, 56, 57
Removal of patient, 80-81
Renal failure, 780-81, 787-88
Renal system, aging and, 896
Repeater systems, 55-56, 60
Repolarization, 614, 624
Reports
  patient, 64, 65, 66
  radio/phone, 200-201
Reproductive system, anatomy and physiology of, 146, 158, 774-76, 954-57
Reproductive system emergencies, 781-82
Rescue operations, 3, 69-85
  defined, 70
  high-angle, 83
  phases of, 74-82
    assessment, 74-76
    disentanglement and removal, 80-81
    gaining access, 76-78
    on-scene emergency care, 78-80
    transportation, 82
  resources for, 82-84
  safety and, 70-74
  special, 77-78
  training for, 79-80
  vertical, 76
  water, 83
Rescue plan, 77
Research, EMS, 34
Res ipsa loquitur, 44-45
Resistance, 529
  host, 844
  as stage of stress response, 113
Respiration(s), 192, 193
  acid-base balance and, 301-2
  cellular, 212, 575
  chest trauma and, 488
  CNS injury and, 458
  defined, 212
  heat loss through, 866, 867
  Kussmaul's, 186, 733
  modified forms of, 216-17
  pulmonary, 212, 575
  regulation of, 215-16
  rib fracture and, 476
Respiratory acidosis, 302
Respiratory alkalosis, 302-3
Respiratory bronchioles, 211, 573
Respiratory cycle, 212
Respiratory depression, narcotic overdosage and, 814
Respiratory disorders, from inhaled poisons, 817-18
Respiratory distress, left ventricular

failure and, 695
Respiratory effort, neonatal, 1007
Respiratory emergencies, 581-99
  carbon monoxide inhalation, 523, 533, 596-97, 819
  central nervous system dysfunction, 598
  drugs for, 384-89
    albuterol (Proventil, Ventolin), 387-88
    aminophylline (Somophyllin), 384, 385-86
    epinephrine, 384-85
    ipratropium (Atrovent), 388-89
    racemic epinephrine (microNEFRIN, Vaponefrin), 386-87
    terbutaline (Brethine, Bricanyl), 387
  dysfunction of spinal cord, nerves, or respiratory muscles, 598-99
  among elderly, 900-901
  hyperventilative syndrome, 597-98
  management principles, 581
  obstructive lung disease, 583-94
    asthma, 586-94
    chronic bronchitis, 585-86
    emphysema, 583-85, 586
  pediatric, 930-35
    aspirated foreign body, 930-31
    asthma, 934-35
    bronchiolitis, 933-34
    croup, 931-32
    epiglottitis, 931, 932-33
    status asthmaticus, 935
  pneumonia, 594-95
  pulmonary embolism, 215, 597, 698, 707-8, 901, 992
  toxic inhalation, 532, 595-96
  upper-airway obstruction, 218, 581-83
Respiratory function of shock patient, 316
Respiratory patterns
  abnormal, 186-87
  nervous system emergencies and, 757
Respiratory protection, 71, 72
Respiratory rate, 217, 222
Respiratory syncytial virus (RSV), 933
Respiratory system. See also Airway management
  aging and, 896
  anaphylaxis and, 798
  anatomy and physiology of, 145, 155, 206-17
    lower airway, 210-11
    upper airway, 207-10
  assessment of, 220-25, 575-81
    history, 575
    physical examination, 575-79
    primary, 220-21
    pulse oximetry, 580-81
    secondary, 221-25
  infections of, 851-53
  problems with, 217-20
  shock and, 308
Responsibilities
  of incident commander, 94
  of paramedic, 10-12
    after patient delivery, 11-12
    post-graduate, 12-14
    primary, 4, 12
    during removal, 81
  stress from, 117

Responsiveness, continuum of, 190
"Rest-and-repose" ("feed-or-breed") system, 340, 747
Resting potential, 613
Restoril, 832
Restraint, methods of, 1025-27
Resultant cardiac vector (mean cardiac vector), 1039
Resuscitation, cardiac, 44
Resuscitation equipment, disposable, xxxi
Reticular activating system, 450
Retinal artery occlusion, acute, 452-53
Retinal detachment, 453
Retraction, 172
Retrograde amnesia, 459
Retrograde conduction, 628
Retroperitoneal organs, 771-72
Retroperitoneal space, 474
Return to service, notification of, 54
Reversible bronchospasm, 387-89
Reversible reactions, 291
Revised trauma score, 174, 175
Reye's syndrome, 929
Rh factor, 296
Rhonchi, 186, 578, 695
Rib fractures, 430, 476
Ribosomes, 143
Right axis deviation, 1039-41
Right to die, 42-44
Right ventricular failure, 697-99
Ring injury, 528
Ritalin, 831
Robert Wood Johnson Foundation, 20
Rock, 831
Roentgen equivalent in man (REM), 881
Role of paramedic, 10-12
Rollover impact, 417-18
Romazicon (flumazenil), 392
Rotational impact, 416
Rotohalers, 353
Rough endoplasmic reticulum, 143
Rouleaux formation, 310
R-R interval, 626
R-R rhythm, 626
RSV, 933
Rule of nines, 535, 541
Rules of evidence, 33
Rum fits, 835
Run report, 48
Rupture, uterine, 992
R wave, 619
Ryan White Act (1990), xxx

Sacral vertebra, 744
Sacrum, 437
Sacs
  alveolar, 155, 211, 573
  amniotic, 968
Safety, 70-74
  paramedic/personal, 70-72. See also Infectious diseases
  in nuclear radiation emergencies, 881
  patient, 72, 81
  procedures, 73-74
  during rescue operations, 70-74
Safety Officer, 73
Salicylates, 833
Saline, normal, 299
Salivary glands, 773
Salt-poor albumin, 298
SA node. See Sinoatrial (SA) node
Sarcoma, Kaposi's, 859
Satellite receivers, 56, 57

Scabies, 853
Scalp, 435, 444
Scanners, 47
Scapula, 447, 504
Scene hazards, 75-76
Scene survey, 167-69
  during behavioral emergencies, 1016-17
  of major incident, 94-95
  thermal burn assessment and, 539-40
  in toxicological emergencies, 809
Schizophrenia, 1022-23
Schizophreniform, 1022
Sclera, 442
Scombroid (histamine) poisoning, 815
Scorpion stings, 824-25
Screening, personnel, 73
SCUBA, 72
SCUBA diving, 884, 885
Seafood poisonings, 815
Seatbelts, 410-11
Sea-water drowning, 879
Sebaceous glands, 524
Sebum, 523, 524
Seconal, 832
Secondary assessment, 175-78. See also Assessment; specific emergencies and body systems
Secondary collisions, 409, 410
Secondary response, 796
Second-degree burns, 533-34, 541
Secretory phase, 957
Sector officers, 92
  duties of, 108
  responsibilities, 96
    of Extrication Officer, 96, 98
    of Staging Officer, 100, 101
    of Supply Officer, 102
    of Transportation Officer, 99-101
    of Treatment Officer, 98-99
    of Triage Officer, 102-3
Sectors in ICS, 91-92, 97-106, 107
Sector vests, 108
Sedation, 399
Sedatives, 391-92, 832
Seizures, 760-63, 903
  from alcohol withdrawal syndrome, 835
  assessment of, 761-62
  among elderly, 904
  febrile, 927-28
  hypoglycemic, 735
  management of, 762-63
  pediatric, 927
  syncope vs., 762
  types of, 760-61
Seldinger technique, 566
Self-contained breathing apparatus (SCUBA), 72
Sellick's maneuver, 227-28
Semicircular canals, 443
Semilunar valves, 605, 606
Semi-permeable membrane, 292
Senescence, 909
Sengstaken-Blakemore tube, 776-77
Senile dementia, 905, 909
Sense organ injury, 452-53
Sense organs in head region, 442-43
Sensitization, 796
Sepsis, 936-37
Septa, cardiac, 604, 605
Septic shock, 841, 937

Septum, nasal, 207
Serax, 832
Seroconversion, 845
Serous cavities, fluid accumulation in, 698
Serum hepatitis, 855-56
Service, refusal of, 46
Service quality, 33
"Seven year itch," 853
Severity of chief complaint, 198
Sexual abuse
    of children, 924
    trauma to genitalia from, 180
Sexual assault, 961-62
Sexually transmitted diseases, 857-58
Shielding, protective, 73
Shingles, 854
Shivering (thermogenesis), 865, 867
Shock, 192, 303-29, 553-69
    air medical transport, 567-69
    assessment of, 559-64
        decision to transport, 563-64
        primary assessment, 560-62
        review of dispatch informa-
            tion, 560
        scene survey, 560
        Trauma Score, 564
    cardiogenic, 311, 328, 691, 699-701
        dopamine for, 365
    care of, 461
    causes and manifestations of, 555-56
    at cellular level, 308-9
    compensated, 309-10, 557-58
    decompensated, 310, 557, 558-59
    defined, 303, 557
    evaluation of, 311-14
    hemorrhagic, 297, 310
    hypovolemic, 174, 310-11, 328
    insulin (hypoglycemia), 733-36
    irreversible, 310, 557, 559
    management of, 315-28
        airway management, 315-17
        bleeding, 317
        body temperature, 328
        hypotension, 317-27
        medications, 328
    neurogenic, 311, 328
        norepinephrine for, 364
    physiological background to, 303-8
    due to plasma loss (burns), 297
    rapid packaging and transport, 329
    resuscitation from, 564-67
        critical life threats, 564-65
        fluid therapy, 566-67
        PASG application, 565-66
    septic, 841, 937
    signs and symptoms of, 308, 310
    stages of, 309-10
    systemic response to, 308
    trauma-related, 314-15
    from uterine inversion, 992
    from uterine rupture, 992
Shoulder, 504
    dislocation of, 512
    management of injuries to, 518
    muscles of, 506
    nerves of, 154
Shoulder dystocia, 991
Shoulder straps, 410
Sick sinus syndrome, 903
Side effects, defined, 336
SIDS, 940

Sighing, 216
Silent myocardial infarction, 902
Simple triage and rapid treatment
    (START) method, 103-5
Simplex transmissions, 60
Sinequan, 833
Single system communications
    center (SYSCOM), 32
Sinoatrial (SA) node, 615, 1032
    dysrhythmias originating from,
        628, 630-37
        sinus arrest, 636-37
        sinus bradycardia, 630, 631
        sinus dysrhythmia, 634-35
        sinus tachycardia, 632-33
    impulse initiation in, 621
Sinus(es)
    coronary, 607
    dural, 442
Sinus arrest, 636-37
Sinus bradycardia, 630, 631
Sinus dysrhythmia, 634-35
Sinus tachycardia, 632-33
Site Safety Officer, 98
Six-second method, 626
Skeletal muscle, 144, 145, 150, 505
Skeletal system, anatomy and
    physiology of, 146, 149
Skin, 148, 522-23. See also Burns;
    Wound(s)
    anaphylaxis and, 798
    assessment of, 172, 173, 538
    of cardiac patient, 688
    color of, 172, 176, 686
    infections of, 853-54
    of poisoned patient, 811
    shock assessment and, 313
    temperature of, 172
Skull, 148, 435-36, 439
    bones of, 742-44
Skull fracture, 445-46
    depressed, 462
    raccoon eyes and, 182
Slander, 47
Sleep, respiratory rate and, 217
Sliding impact, 420
"Slow code," 44
Slow-reacting substance of ana-
    phylaxis (SRA), 798
SLUDGE, 829
Small bowel obstruction, 778
Small intestine, 156, 772, 773
Smooth endoplasmic reticulum,
    143
Smooth muscle, 144, 145, 505
Snake bites, 825-28
Sneezing, 216
Snoring, 172, 578
    airflow compromise, 222
Snowmobile accidents, 421
Sodium, 291-92, 293, 550
Sodium bicarbonate, 291, 377-78,
    492-93, 950, 1010
Sodium nitrite, 819
Sodium nitroprusside (Nipride),
    709
Sodium-potassium pump, 293
Sodium thiosulfate, 819
Soft-tissue trauma. See Burns;
    Wound(s)
Solid drugs, 335
Solid organs, 481, 772
Solu-Cortef (hydrocortisone), 802
Solu-Medrol (methylprednisolone),
    392-93, 466, 593, 802
Solute, 288, 334
Solution, 288, 334
Solvent, 288, 334
Somatic nervous system, 440

Somatostatin, 729
Somophyllin (aminophylline), 384,
    385-86, 589, 594, 711, 803
Spasm
    laryngeal, 219-20
    muscle, 507, 510
Speed, 406-7, 831
"Speedball," 812
Sphenoid bone, 742, 743
Sphincters, capillary, 306
Spider bites, 822-24
Spinal arteries, 442
Spinal cavity, 741
Spinal column injury, 447
Spinal cord, 153, 746-47. See also
    Head, neck, and spinal
    trauma
    anatomy and physiology of,
        440-42
    dysfunction of, 598-99
    injury to, 392-93, 450-52
        male genitalia and, 188
        pediatric, 922
        penetrating neck injuries and,
            430
        posterior body evaluation
            and, 189
Spinal foramen, 438
Spinal nerves, 746-47
Spineboard, 464, 465, 516
Spine (vertebral column), 148, 436-
    38, 742-44
    immobilization of, 460, 461-64
Spinous process, 438
Spirits, 335
Spleen, 475, 843
Splinting of extremity, 516-19
Splints, air, 518-19
Spondylolysis, 900
Spontaneous abortion, 974
Sports injuries, 423-24
Spotting, 970
Sprains, 507
"Squeeze" (barotrauma), 88-90,
    885-86
SRA, 798
Stable angina, 689
Staging sector, 101-2
Standard of care, 44-45
Standards, infection-control, xxx-
    xxxi
Standing orders, 24
Starling's Law of the Heart, 609
"Star of Life" symbol, 31
START method, 103-5
Status asthmaticus, 593, 935
Status epilepticus, 763, 927
Steady-state metabolism, 864
Sterility, bandaging to ensure, 545
Sterilization, 850
Sternocleidomastoid muscles, 472
Steroids, 729-30
Stethoscope, 177-78
Stimulant, defined, 336
Stimulation, sympathetic, 192, 867
Stimuli, 189
Sting-ray, 828
Stings
    insect, 821-22
    scorpion, 824-25
Stokes-Adams syndrome, 903
Stomach, 156, 772, 773
STP, 832
Straight blade, 237-38, 239
Strains, 507
Streptococcus pneumoniae, 851,
    929
Streptokinase, 694
Stress, 112-16

body's response to, 113
critical-incident, 12, 113, 119-20
defined, 112
job, 117-20
management of, 111-21
physiology of, 113
reactions to, 113-16
suicidal behavior and, 1020
types of, 113-16
Stressor, 112
Stretch receptors, 216
Stridor (crowing), 172, 186, 222,
    578
Stroke, 763-67
    categories of, 763-65
    clinical presentation of, 765
    in elderly, 904
    heat, 867-68, 870-71, 872
    management of, 766-67
    transient ischemic attack and,
        765-66
Stroke volume, 304, 609, 610
S-T segment, 620
Stylet, malleable, 240
Subarachnoid hemorrhages, 765
Subarachnoid space, 744
Subcutaneous drug administration,
    352, 354
Subcutaneous emphysema, 184,
    185
Subcutaneous tissue, 524
Subdural hematoma, 449
Subdural space, 744
Subendocardial infarction, 690,
    1045, 1047
Sublingual administration of med-
    ication, 360
Subluxation, 507
Substance abuse, 830, 831-33. See
    also Alcohol abuse (alco-
    holism)
    altered behavior and, 1015
Succinylcholine (Anectine), 260
Sucking chest wound, 430, 490,
    491
Suctioning, 275-76
Suction units, 240
Sudden death, 691, 701-4
    defibrillation in, 27-28
Sudden infant death syndrome
    (SIDS), 940
Sugars, 730-31
Suicidal patients, 809, 811
Suicide, 1019-21
    by elderly, 906
Sunburn, 534
Superficial frostbite, 876
Superior conchae, 207, 208
Superior vena cava, 606
Supination, 504
Supine-hypotensive syndrome, 979
Supplemental restraint systems (air
    bags), 410, 411
Supply sector, 102
Support personnel, 18
Suppositories, 335
Supraventricular tachycardia, 682,
    937
Surface absorption poisons, 807,
    808-9, 829-30
Surfactant, 211, 573, 878
Surgical airways, 269-74
    needle cricothyrotomy, 270-71
    transtracheal jet ventilation, 272-74
Suspensions, 335
Suspicion, index of, 404
Sutures, 435
S wave, 619

, 289, 869
ater rescues, 77-78
thetic blockers, 367-69
pathetic ganglia, 341-43
npathetic nervous system, 154, 340, 341-44
innervation of heart, 610-11, 612
Sympathetic stimulation, 192, 867
Sympatholytics, 345
Sympathomimetics, 345, 362-67, 710-11
albuterol, 387-88, 590, 802-3, 934
dobutamine, 328, 366-67, 697, 711
dopamine, 328, 365-66, 699, 711, 1010
epinephrine. See Epinephrine
norepinephrine. See Norepinephrine (noradrenalin)
Synapses, 341, 345, 348, 741-42
Syncope
cardiac disease and, 684
in elderly, 902-3
seizures vs., 762
Syncytium, 612, 1031-32
Synergism, defined, 336
Synovial capsule, 504
Synovial joint, 148
Synthetic medications, 332
Synthetic reactions, 291
Syphilis, 857
Syringes, prefilled, 335
Syrups, 335
SYSCOM, 32
Systole, 609, 610

Tabes dorsalis, 857
Tablets, 335
Tachycardia
defined, 626
paroxysmal junctional (PJT), 658-59
paroxysmal supraventricular (PSVT), 374, 375, 642-45, 658
right heart failure and, 698
sinus, 632-33
supraventricular, 682, 937
ventricular, 373, 664-67, 702
with pulse and malignant PVCs, 371
pulseless, 370-71
Tachydysrhythmias, 628
Tachypnea, 587
Tactile fremitus, 578
Tagamet (cimetidine), 802
"Take-it-for-granted" quality, 32-33
Talus, 505
Tape, umbilical, 240
Tarsals, 505
TBW, 287
TCP, 637, 655, 661, 677, 679, 681, 721, 722
Teeth, 208, 773
Telemetry, 66
Telephones, 57-58
Temperature, 529
ambient, 865, 998
body, 192-94
shock patient and, 328
core, 864
skin, 172
Temporal bone, 742, 743
Tempra, 833
Ten-code system, 63
Tenderness, rebound, 187, 482, 772, 784-85
Tendons, 505

Tension pneumothorax, 175, 185, 186, 478-79
management of, 493-94
pediatric, 923
Tentorium, 440
Tequila, 831
Terbutaline (Brethine, Bricanyl), 387, 591
Term, 968
Terminology. See also Medical terminology
of drugs, 335-36
obstetric, 969-70
in topographical anatomy, 159
Terrain, assessment of, 81
Testes, 730, 775, 776
Testicular torsion, 782
Testing, standardized, 14
Tetanospasmin, 841
Tetanus, 841
Thalamus, 744, 745
Therapeutic abortion, 974
Therapeutic action, defined, 336
Therapeutic index, 339-40
Therapeutic threshold, 339
Thermal burns, 529
of airway, 532-33
assessment of, 539-42
management of, 548
Thermal disorders, 867-77
fever (pyrexia), 217, 871, 914
frostbite, 876-77
hyperpyrexia, 871
hyperthermia, 867-71
hypothermia, 867, 871-76
Thermal gradient, 865
Thermogenesis (shivering), 865, 867
Thermometers, 193
Thermoregulation, 864-67
Thermostat, hypothalamic, 866
Thiamine, 390
Thiamine deficiency, 758
Third-degree burns (full-thickness burns), 534, 541
"Third space" (internal) losses of water, 289
Thirst, 289
Thoracic cage, 472
Thoracic cavity, 162, 212
Thoracic spine, 436
Thoracic symptoms, history of, 489
Thoracic trauma
management of, 490-95
penetrating, 430
Thorax. See Body cavity trauma
Thorazine (chlorpromazine), 1021
Thought, altered, 1022
Threatened abortion, 974
Throat (pharynx), 208
Thrombocytes (platelets), 294, 295, 528
Thrombolytic therapy, 694
Thrombophlebitis, 327
Thrombosis, deep venous, 708
Thrombus, 690, 763
Thymus, 794
Thyrohyoid membrane, 209
Thyroid cartilage (Adam's apple), 207, 209
Thyroid gland, 727, 728
Thyroid-stimulating hormone (TSH), 727, 728
Thyroid storm, 389
Thyrotoxicosis, 726, 728
Thyroxine, 728
TIAs, 765-66, 903, 904
Tibia, 505
Tidal volume, 217

Tie-down, 240
Tiered response, 19
Tilt test, 778-79, 785
Time constraints, stress from, 118
Time of chief complaint, 198
Tinctures, 335
Tissue perfusion, 307-8
Tissue plasminogen activator (tPA), 694
Tissues, anatomy and physiology of, 144
Titration, 394
T lymphocytes, 794, 842
Tocolysis, 980
Tofranil, 833
Tolerance, defined, 336
Tongue, 208
airway obstruction by, 219
Tonicity, 298-99
Tonic phase of seizure, 760
Tonsil tip suction devices, 275
Topographical anatomy, 159-62
of abdomen, 161-62
of chest, 160-61
terminology, 159
Tort law, 41
Total body water (TBW), 287
Total lung capacity (TLC), 217
Tourniquet, 544-45
Toxemia of pregnancy, 977
Toxic inhalation, 532, 595-96
Toxicological emergencies, drugs for, 394-98. See also Poisoning; Substance abuse
activated charcoal, 396-97, 810, 813
diphenhydramine (Benadryl), 395
naloxone (Narcan), 397-98
syrup of ipecac, 395-96
Toxicology, 806
Toxins, 841
tPA, 694
Trachea, 207, 210, 444, 453, 472
deviation of, 184
displacement of, 484
tear of, 480-81
Tracheal tugging, 577
Traction
axial, 516
distal, 518
Trade name of drugs, 334
Training
emergency medical dispatch (EMD), 27
physical, 10
for rescue operations, 79-80
Trajectory of bullets, 426
Trandate (labetalol), 709
Tranquilizers, 398
Transcutaneous cardiac pacing (TCP), 637, 655, 661, 677, 679, 681, 721, 722
Transdermal drug administration, 352
Transfer of command, 91, 96
Transfer protocols, 24
Transfusion reaction, 297
Transient ischemic attacks (TIAs), 765-66, 903, 904
Transillumination (lighted stylet) intubation, 251-54
Transmural infarctions, 690, 1045, 1046
Transportation, Department of (DOT), 83
Transportation sector, 99-101, 108
Transport of patient, 29-32, 82
by air, 567-69

by air (aeromedical), 31-32
by ambulances, 29-31
decision to, 404-5
with musculoskeletal injuries, 515-16
of neonatal patient, 1009-11
of non-stabilized patient, 79
positioning and restraining patient for, 1027-29
protocols, 24
in shock, 329, 563-64
Trauma, 401-31. See also Blunt trauma; Body cavity trauma; Head, neck, and spinal trauma; Penetrating trauma
airway obstruction from, 219
altered behavior and, 1015
assessment of, 167
defined, 402, 407
in elderly, 899-900
kinetics of, 406-7
management of, 554-56
mortality from, 554
pediatric, 921-27
burns, 923
chest and abdomen injuries, 922-23
child abuse/neglect, 923-27
extremity injuries, 923
head, face, and neck injuries, 922
during pregnancy, 971-72
resuscitation from, 564-67
critical life threats, 564-65
fluid therapy, 566-67
PASG application, 565-66
triage protocols, 403-5
Trauma center, 174
Trauma patient
assessment of, 176, 203
critical management priorities for, 174
digital intubation of, 249
endotracheal intubation of, 254-55
modified jaw-thrust maneuver for, 226-27
Trauma score, 174, 175, 564
Traumatic aortic aneurysm (rupture), 706-7
Traumatic asphyxia, 476-77, 492-93
Treatment protocols, 24
Treatment sector, 98-99
Trendate (labetalol), 368-69
Treponema palladium, 857
Triage, 24, 91, 97
Triage Officer, 97
Triage protocols, 403-5
Triage sector, 102-5, 106
Triavil, 833
Tricuspid valve, 604
Tricyclic antidepressants, 377, 833
Trigeminy, 662
Triggers of asthma, 934
Triiodothyronine, 728
Trimesters, 968
Triplicate method, 626
Trouser, pneumatic anti-shock. See Pneumatic anti-shock garment (PASG)
True vocal cords, 207, 209
Trunking, 58
TSH, 727, 728
Tubal pregnancy, 782
Tuberculosis, 851-52
Tumors of colon, 906
Tungsten, 529
Tunica adventitia, 524-25, 608
Tunica intima, 524-25, 608

Tunica media, 524-25, 608
Turbinates, 208
Turgor, 289-92
T wave, 620, 624
Two-way radios, mobile, 55
Tylenol, 833
Type I diabetes mellitus, 731-32
Type II diabetes mellitus, 732

Ulcer, peptic, 777, 906
Ulna, 504
Ultrasonic Doppler, 192, 193
Umbilical cord, 967
cutting, 999
prolapsed, 971, 989, 990
Umbilical tape, 240
Umbilical vein, 969, 1009
Umbilicus, 187
Undifferentiated schizophrenia, 1022
Unipolar limb leads, 618, 1033, 1035-38
Universal donor, 296
Universal precautions, 860-61
Universal recipients, 295
Unstable angina, 689-90
Untoward effect, defined, 336
Up-and-over pathway of injury, 412, 413
Upper airway, 572
anatomy of, 573
obstruction of, 218, 581-83
Upper extremities
anatomy and physiology of, 504
assessment of, 514-15
evaluation of, 181, 189
injuries to, 512
management of, 518-19
Urea, 781
Uremia, 781
Ureters, 774
Urethra, 774, 775, 776, 956-57
Urinary bladder, 774
infection of (cystitis), 780, 960
ruptured, 482
Urinary system
anatomy and physiology of, 157
shock and, 308
Urinary tract infections (UTI), 780
Urine, bloody (hematuria), 780
Urokinase, 694
Urticaria, 798
Uterine atony, 991
Uterine inversion, 992
Uterine rupture, 992
Uterine stimulants, 393-94
Uterine tubes (fallopian tubes), 775, 954, 955
Uterus, 775, 954-56
U wave, 620

Vaccine, Hepatitis B, xxxi, 857
Vagina, 775, 955, 956
discharge from, 188
Vaginal bleeding, 960-61
during pregnancy, 970, 973, 974, 977
third-trimester, 973, 975-77
Vagus nerve, 375, 611-12, 625
Valium (diazepam), 338, 353, 391-92, 466-67, 693, 711, 764, 832, 928

Vallecula, 208
Valsalva maneuver, 612, 645, 659, 903
Vaponefrin (racemic epinephrine), 386-87
Varicella (chicken pox), 854
Varices, esophageal, 776-77, 906
Varicose veins, 708
Varicosities, 903
Vas deferens, 775, 776
Vasectomy, 776
Vasoconstriction, 867
shock and, 308
Vasodepressor syncope, 902
Vasodilation, 866-67
Vasopressin, 727, 834
Vasospastic angina (Prinzmetal's angina), 689
Vasovagal syncope, 903
Vector, 1039
Vecuronium (Norcuron), 260
Vehicle collision, 408-9
Vein(s), 152, 306
bronchial, 213, 575
coronary, 607
for intravenous cannulation, 323-24
jugular, 325, 444, 453
pulmonary, 213, 575, 604, 605, 606
umbilical, 969, 1009
varicose, 708
Velocity, 406
Vena cavae, 472, 475, 481, 604, 605, 606, 773
Venipuncture, 195-96
Venous congestion, right heart failure and, 698
Venous system, 608-9
Ventilation, 279-82
alveolar, 214
defined, 212
of distressed neonate, 1008
inadequate, 220
monitoring, 223
of pediatric patient, 944, 946
Ventilation/perfusion mismatch, 215
Ventolin (albuterol), 387-88, 590, 802-3, 934
Ventricles, 603, 604, 746
dysrhythmias originating in, 629, 660-73
artificial pacemaker rhythm, 672-73
asystole (cardiac standstill), 670-71
premature ventricular contraction (PVC), 662-63
ventricular escape complexes and rhythms (idioventricular rhythm), 660, 661
ventricular fibrillation, 668-69
ventricular tachycardia, 664-67
electrical excitation of, 623
failure of, 694-99
left ventricle, 694-97
right, 697-99
Ventricular aneurysm, 691
Ventricular contraction (systole), 609, 610

Ventricular fibrillation, 373, 701-2
duration of, 716
primary and secondary, 701
refractory, 370-71
Ventricular repolarization, 624
Ventricular syncytium, 612, 1032
Ventricular tachycardia, 373, 664-67, 702
with pulse and malignant PVCs, 371
pulseless, 370-71
Venturi mask, 278-79
Venules, 556, 609
Verapamil (Isoptin, Calan), 375-76, 645, 659, 693, 710
Vermiform appendix, 777
Vertebrae, 744
Vertebral arteries, 442
Vertebral column (spine), 148, 436-38, 742-44
immobilization of, 460, 461-64
Vertebrobasilar system, 746
Vertical rescue, 76, 77
Vertigo, 443, 904
Vesicular sounds, 186
Vests, sector, 108
Vials, 335
Victims, number of, 76
Violence, domestic, 1029
Violent situations, controlling, 1024-29
Virulence, 843
Virus(es)
defective, 856
herpes class of, 858
HIV, 594, 844, 847, 858-61
infectious diseases from, 841
Visceral pericardium, 603
Visceral pleura, 211, 473, 574
Viscosity, 295
Vistaril (hydroxyzine), 802
Vital signs, 191-96
abdominal injury and, 488
acute abdomen and, 785
anaphylaxis and, 799
blood pressure, 191-92, 193
body temperature, 192-94
CNS injury and, 458
hypothermia and, 874-76
left ventricular failure and, 696
nervous system emergencies and, 757
normal adults, 192
other assessment techniques, 194-96
pediatric, 919-20
in pregnant patient, 971
pulse, 192, 193
respiration, 192, 193
Vitamins, 390
Vitreous humor, 442
Vocal cords, 207, 209
Vodka, 831
Voltage, 529
Volume, 348
of drug, 350-51
Volume expanders, 1010
Vomiting
of blood, 778
drugs to manage, 399
inducement of, 812-13
pediatric, 935

rapid sequence intubation and, 260
Vomitus
airway obstruction by, 220
through endotracheal tube, 246
Voting, 55-56
Vulva, 775

Wandering pacemaker, 638-39
Water, 287-89
diffusion of, 293-94
irrigation of burns with, 548-49, 550
Water intoxication, 867-68, 869-70
Water-related emergencies. *See* under Environmental emergencies
Water rescue, 83
Watt, 54
Weight, 406
Wernicke's syndrome, 390, 758-59
Wet drowning, 878
Wheezing, 172, 186, 578, 587
left ventricular failure and, 696
Whiskey, 831
"Whistle-tip" suction device, 275
White blood cells (leukocytes), 294, 295, 842
"White Paper, The" ("Accidental Death and Disability: The Neglected Disease of Modern Society"), 5
Whole blood, 296
Wilderness EMT course, 79
Wilderness Medical Society, 79, 84
Wills, living, 42, 43
Window phase, 845
Wine, 831
Wisconsin blade, 237-38, 239
Withdrawal syndrome, 835-36
Wolff-Parkinson-White (WPW) syndrome, 374, 682-83
Workplace, stress from changes in, 118
World Trade Center bombing (1993), 89
Wound(s)
care of, 464-66
chest
open, 490
sucking, 490, 491
crushing, 528
defense, 428
gunshot, 407
sucking chest, 430
Wright meter, 588
Wrist fractures, 512

Xanax, 832
Xanthines, 384, 385-86
X-rays, 531, 881
Xylocaine (lidocaine), 353, 369-71, 663, 667, 693, 710, 950, 951

Yankauer "tonsil tip" suction device, 275
Yellow bone marrow, 501

Zantac (ranitidine), 802
Zygoma, 435
Zygomatic fractures, 447